PHARMACOLOGY
for the
PRIMARY CARE PROVIDER

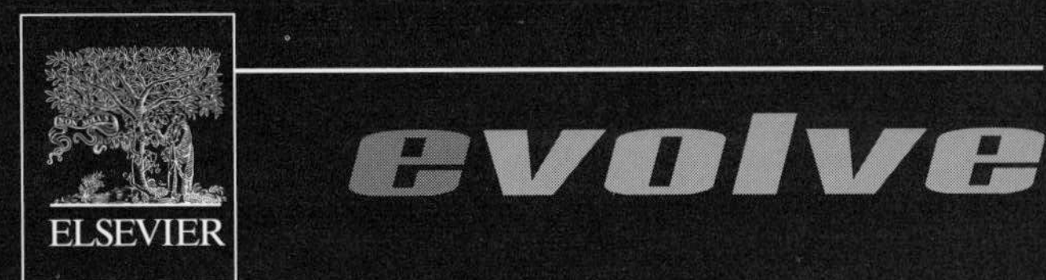

To access your Student Resources, visit the web address below:

http://evolve.elsevier.com/Edmunds/NP/

- **WebLinks**
  Organized by chapter, WebLinks are provided for all of the "Resources for Patients and Providers" in the textbook. Additional websites have been carefully chosen to supplement the content of the textbook, and all websites are updated regularly.

- **Bonus Reference Tables**
  More than 30 additional tables, organized by chapter and offering valuable information and enrichment.

- ***Mosby's Drug Consult* Internet Edition**
  Basic-level access to this comprehensive database of the most current, unbiased, accurate, and reliable drug information available. Includes Drug Updates, free information on the top 200 drugs by prescription, and Online Extras, including new drug approvals, safety notices, new drug indications, and links to pharmaceutical manufacturers for more information.

- **Sign-up page for the Mosby/Saunders ePharmacology Update newsletter**
  An informative, full-color, quarterly newsletter written by Evelyn Salerno, PharmD, the ePharmacology Update provides current and well-documented information on new drugs, drug warnings, medication errors, and more.

- **Link to the FDA's "Catalog of FDA Approved Drug Products"**
  A comprehensive and up-to-date database of FDA drug approvals and withdrawals.

PHARMACOLOGY
for the
PRIMARY CARE PROVIDER

Marilyn Winterton Edmunds PhD, ANP/GNP

Adjunct Faculty
Johns Hopkins University, School of Nursing
Baltimore, Maryland

Maren Stewart Mayhew MS, ANP/GNP

Nurse Practitioner
Private Practice
Bethesda, Maryland

SECOND EDITION

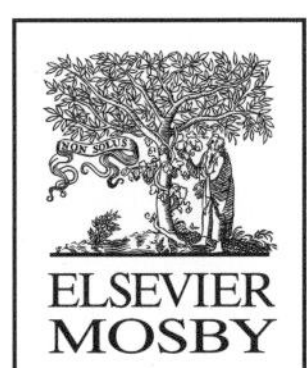

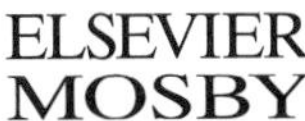

ELSEVIER
MOSBY

11830 Westline Industrial Drive
St. Louis, Missouri 63146

PHARMACOLOGY FOR THE PRIMARY CARE PROVIDER

NOTICE

Pharmacology is an ever-changing field. Standard safety precautions must be followed, but as new research and clinical experience broaden our knowledge, changes in treatment and drug therapy may become necessary or appropriate. Readers are advised to check the most current product information provided by the manufacturer of each drug to be administered to verify the recommended dose, the method and duration of administration, and contraindications. It is the responsibility of the licensed prescriber, relying on experience and knowledge of the patient, to determine dosages and the best treatment for each individual patient. Neither the publisher nor the author assumes any liability for any injury and/or damage to persons or property arising from this publication.

The Publisher

First edition 2000.

ISBN-13: 978-0-323-02403-7
ISBN-10: 0-323-02403-3

Acquisitions Editor: Barbara Cullen
Managing Editor: Lee Henderson
Developmental Editor: Maureen Iannuzzi
Publishing Services Manager: Catherine Albright Jackson
Senior Project Manager: Mary G. Stueck
Design Manager: Gail Morey Hudson

Printed in the United States of America

Last digit is the print number: 9 8 7 6 5 4 3

Contributors to the First Edition

The authors wish to express their deep appreciation for the generosity of these contributors to the first edition who shared with us their time and expertise. Their efforts created the foundation on which the current edition is built.

Susan E. Appling, RN, MS, CRNP
Assistant Professor
Johns Hopkins University School of Nursing
Baltimore, Maryland

JoAnne T. Baker, RN, MSN, FNP
Family Nurse Practitioner
Family Health Services
Cranston, Rhode Island

Elizabeth Blair, MSN, CS-ANP, CDE
Adult Nurse Practitioner
Manager of Clinical Services for Affiliated Center's Program
Joslin Diabetes Center
Boston, Massachusetts

Bonnie R. Bock, RN, BSN, MS, CRNP
Adult Nurse Practitioner
Ellicott City, Maryland

Alice M. Brazier, MS, CRNP, GNP
Clinical Systems Manager
Evercare of Maryland
Baltimore, Maryland

James Cawley, MPH, PA-C
Associate Professor
School of Medicine and Health Sciences
The George Washington University
Washington, DC

Susan E. Childs, RN, MS, CRNP
Adult Nurse Practitioner
Private Practice
Columbia, Maryland

Sandra L. Cotton, MS, C-ANP
Assistant Professor
Department of Health Promotion/Risk Reduction
West Virginia University
School of Nursing
Morgantown, West Virginia

Christy L. Crowther, RN, MS, CRNP
Clinical Instructor
Department of Family Medicine
Univesity of Maryland
School of Medicine
Baltimore, Maryland
Private Orthopaedic Surgery Practice
Glen Burnie, Maryland

Charles E. Daniels, RPh, PhD, FASHP
Chief, Clinical Center Pharmacy Department
National Institutes of Health
Bethesda, Maryland

George DeMaagd, PharmD, BCPS
Assistant Professor
College of Pharmacy
Ferris State University
Big Rapids, Michigan

Gloria A. Deniz, RN, MS, ARNP
Pediatric Nurse Practitioner
Pediatric Care Clinic
Sacred Heart Children's Hospital
Pensacola, Florida

Jan DiSantostefano, MS, CRNP
Nurse Practitioner
Airpark Primary Care
Westminster, Maryland

Susan Waldrop Donckers, RN, EdD, CS, FNP
Nurse Practitioner
Fort Lewis Family Practice
Salem, Virginia

Michael Dreis, PharmD, MPH
Deputy Chief, Operations and Analysis Branch
Division of Transplantation
Office of Special Programs
Health Resources and Services Administration
Rockville, Maryland

Diane Fatica, RN, MSN, FNP
Monterey Family Practice
Monterey, California

Kathleen Ryan Fletcher, RN, CS, MSN, GNP
Director, Senior Services
University of Virginia Health System
Charlottesville, Virginia

Annette Galassi, RN, MA, CANP, AOCN
Georgetown University Medical Center
Lombardi Cancer Center
Washington, DC

Susanne Scharnhorst Gibbons, ANP, GNP, MS
Assistant Professor
Family Nurse Practitioner Program
Uniformed Services University of the Health Sciences
Graduate School of Nursing
Bethesda, Maryland

Cynthia Knoll Grandjean, RN, MGA, MSN, NP
Adult and Geriatric Nurse Practitioner
Calvert Internal Medicine
Prince Frederick, Maryland
Assistant Professor
Uniformed Services University of the Health Sciences
Bethesda, Maryland

Catherine Hagan, MSN, RN, CNS
Director, Breast Health Services
Presbyterian Cancer Center
Charlotte, North Carolina

Nancy (Jo) Heisterman, BS, FNP
Major, United States Air Force
Tinker Air Force Base
Norman, Oklahoma

Linda C. Hersey, MS, CRNP
OB-GYN and Adult Nurse Practitioner
Nurse Practitioner Option
Waldorf, Maryland

James D. Hoehns, PharmD, BCPS
Clinical Assistant Professor
University of Iowa
College of Pharmacy
Iowa City, Iowa

Karen Huss, RN, DNSc, CANP, FAAN
Associate Professor
The Johns Hopkins University
School of Nursing
Joint Appointment, Department of Medicine
Baltimore, Maryland

Pamela Lynn Jamieson, RNC, MS, NP
Geriatric Nurse Practitioner
Primary Care/Sub-Acute Unit
University of Massachusetts Medical Center
Worcester, Massachusetts

†Bonnie Kohl, RN, MS, CRNP
Geriatric Adult Nurse Practitioner
Private Group Practice—Asher, Rosenbaum, Shargel, MD, PA
Kensington, Maryland

M. Lauren Lemieux, MS
Adjunct Assistant Professor of Nursing
Uniformed Services University of the Health Sciences
Graduate School of Nursing
Bethesda, Maryland
Women's Health Nurse Practitioner
Private Practice
Washington, DC

Marilyn Little, BS, MS, CS
Associate Professor
Director of Nursing Program
Department of Health Science
Salt Lake Community College
Salt Lake City, Utah

Jennifer Loud, MSN, CRNP
Nurse Practitioner
Medical Oncology Branch, Division of Clinical Sciences
National Cancer Institute
Bethesda, Maryland

Karen MacKay, MD
Associate Professor of Medicine
Section of Nephrology
West Virginia University
Morgantown, West Virginia

Douglas Matthews, MS, CRNP
Nurse Practitioner
Medicine Branch
National Cancer Institute
Bethesda, Maryland

Elaine McIntosh, RN, CS, FNP
Director, Nurse Managed Centers
University of Michigan
School of Nursing
Ann Arbor, Michigan

Patricia C. McMullen, CRNP, MS, JD
Associate Professor
Department of Nurse Practitioners
Uniformed Services University of the Health Sciences
Bethesda, Maryland

Carolyn S. Melby, DNSc, CRNP
Assistant Professor
Department of Nursing, Faculty of Medicine
University of Hong Kong
Hong Kong

Karen L. Minor, RN, MS, CRNP
Adult and Geriatric Nurse Practitioner
Maryland Personal Physicians, Inc.
Reisterstown, Maryland

† Deceased.

Maureen Moriarty-Sheehan, RN, MS, CRNP
Adult Nurse Practitioner
Speed Headache Associates PA
Towson, Maryland

Candis Morrison, PhD, ACNP
Associate Professor
Johns Hopkins University
School of Nursing
Baltimore, Maryland

Kathleen Murphy, RN, MS, CRNP
Pediatric Nurse Practitioner
Assistant Professor
Uniformed Services University of the Health Sciences
Bethesda, Maryland

Julie C. Novak, DNSc, RN, CPNP
Theresa A. Thomas Professor of Primary Care
Director, Primary Care Nurse Practitioner Program
Chair, Family Health Care Division
University of Virginia
Charlottesville, Virginia

Katherine M. O'Rourke, MSN, FNP
Flight Commander
Family Practice Clinic
Patrick Air Force Base, Florida

Katherine M. Pabst, CRNP, MPH
Research Nurse Practitioner
Gerontology Research Center, NIA
Johns Hopkins Bayview Medical Center
Baltimore, Maryland

Julianne B. Pinson, PharmD
Assistant Professor of Primary Practice
School of Pharmacy
Campbell University
Buies Creek, North Carolina

Stevelynn J. Pogue, MSN, RN, CS, A/GNP, ET
Geriatric Nurse Practitioner
Department of Geriatrics
Parkland Health and Hospital System
Dallas, Texas

Barbara E. Pokorny, MSN, RN, CS
Family Nurse Practitioner
Community Health Center of New London
New London, Connecticut

Jacqueline Rhoads, PhD, RN, CCRN, ACNP, CS
Professor
Louisiana State University
School of Nursing
New Orleans, Louisiana

Laurie Scudder, MS, PNP
Private Practice
Vice-President, Nurse Practitioner Alternatives in Education, Inc.
Nurse Practitioner Alternatives, Inc.
Columbia, Maryland

Diane C. Seibert, BSN, MS, CRNP
Assistant Professor
Graduate School of Nursing
Uniformed Services University of the Health Sciences
Bethesda, Maryland

Janet S. Selway, MS, CANP, CPNP
Adult and Pediatric Nurse Practitioner
Private Practice
Cockeysville, Maryland

Leslie K. Serchuck, MD
Seniro Clinical Investigator
HIV and AIDS Malignancy Branch
National Cancer Institute
National Institutes of Health
Providence, Rhode Island

Amy B. Sharron, MS, RN, CS, GNP
Nurse Practitioner
Blood and Marrow Transplant Unit
Roger Williams Medical Center
Providence, Rhode Island

Laura E. Shay, MS, CANP
Nurse Practitioner
National Institutes of Health
Internal Medicine Consultation Service
Bethesda, Maryland

Donna M. Thompson, RN, MS, APRN
Assistant Professor, High Acuity Nursing
Department of Health Sciences
Salt Lake Community College
Salt Lake City, Utah

Laura Keiler Topper, RN, MS, NP
Adult and Geriatric Nurse Practitioner
Wilkens Medical Center
MedStar Physician Partners
Baltimore, Maryland

Jan Wemmer, MS, CRNP
Nurse Practitioner
Johns Hopkins Hospital
Baltimore, Maryland

Inez Wendel, MS, CRNP
Clinical Instructor, School of Nursing
Geriatric Nurse Practitioner
School of Medicine
Division of Geriatric Medicine and Gerontology
Johns Hopkins University
Baltimore, Maryland

David S. Wing, BBP, MSc
Consultant Pharmacist
Calgary, Alberta; Canada

Theresa Pluth Yeo, MSN, MPH, CRNP
Instructor
School of Nursing
The Johns Hopkins University
Baltimore, Maryland

Linda R. Young, PharmD
Assistant Professor
Director, Drug Information Center
College of Pharmacy
Pharmacy Practice and Pharmacoeconomics Department
University of Tennessee
Memphis, Tennessee

Contributors

Victoria L. Anderson, MSN, FNP
Laboratory of Host Defenses
National Institute of Allergy and Infectious Diseases
National Institutes of Health
Bethesda, Maryland
Chapter 69 Antiretrovirals

Christine M. Betzold, MSN, NP, IBCLC
Chapter 8 Special Populations: Pregnant and Nursing Women

Bonnie R. Bock, RN, MS, CRNP
Clinical Instructor
Department of Family and Community Health Nursing
University of Maryland School of Nursing
Baltimore, Maryland
Chapter 16 Upper Respiratory Agents
Chapter 75 Complementary and Alternative Medicine

Linda L. Bransgrove, PharmD, BCPS
Clinical Pharmacy Specialist
Amarillo VA Medical Center
Amarillo, Texas
Chapter 56 Hormone Replacement Therapy

James Cawley, MPH, PA-C
Associate Professor
School of Medicine and Health Sciences
The George Washington University
Washington, DC
Chapter 3 Prescriptive Authority and the Physician Assistant

Sandra L. Cotton, MS, RN, C-ANP
Director, Faculty Practice
West Virginia University School of Nursing
Morgantown, West Virginia
Chapter 33 Diuretics

Christy L. Crowther, MS, ANP
Chesapeake Orthopedic and Sports Medicine Center
Glen Burnie, Maryland
Chapter 39 Gout Medications

Margaret Dean, RN, CS, GNP, MSN
Instructor, West Texas A&M University
Canyon, Texas
Chapter 56 Hormone Replacement Therapy

Jan DiSantostefano, MS, NP
Family Nurse Practitioner
Women's Health Nurse Practitioner, SAS Institute, Inc.
Cary, North Carolina
Chapter 40 Osteoporosis Treatment

Courtney D. Eckhoff, PharmD
Pharmacy Practice Resident
Clinical Associate, University of Illinois at Chicago
Chicago, Illinois
Chapter 25 Antihyperlipidemic Agents

Marilyn Winterton Edmunds, PhD, ANP/GNP
Adjunct Faculty
Johns Hopkins University, School of Nursing
Baltimore, Maryland
Chapter 1 Prescriptive Authority and Role Implementation: Tradition vs. Change
Chapter 2 Prescriptive Authority: The Role of the NP, CNM, CRNA, and CNS
Chapter 5 General Pharmacokinetic and Pharmacodynamic Principles
Chapter 7 Special Populations: Pediatrics
Chapter 9 Over-the-Counter Medications
Chapter 10 Compliance and the Therapeutic Experiment
Chapter 11 Practical Tips on Writing Prescriptions
Chapter 12 Making Treatment Decisions
Chapter 13 Design and Implementation of Patient Education

James D. Hoehns, PharmD, BCPS
Assistant Professor (Clinical)
University of Iowa College of Pharmacy
Clinical Pharmacist, Northeast Iowa Family Practice
Iowa City, Iowa
Chapter 25 Antihyperlipidemic Agents

Jann Keenan, EdS
President, The Keenan Group
Ellicott City, Maryland
Chapter 13 Design and Implementation of Patient Education

Karen MacKay, MD
Associate Professor of Medicine
Section of Nephrology, West Virginia University
Morgantown, West Virginia
Chapter 33 Diuretics

Maren Stewart Mayhew, MS, ANP/GNP
Nurse Practitioner,
Private Practice
Bethesda, Maryland
Chapter 14 Dermatologic Agents
Chapter 15 Eye, Ear, Throat, and Mouth Agents
Chapter 18 Hypertension and Miscellaneous Antihypertensive Medications
Chapter 19 Coronary Artery Disease and Nitrates
Chapter 20 Chronic Heart Failure and Digoxin
Chapter 21 β-Blockers
Chapter 22 Calcium Channel Blockers
Chapter 23 ACE Inhibitors and Angiotensin Receptor Blockers
Chapter 24 Antiarrhythmic Agents
Chapter 27 Antacids
Chapter 28 Histamine-2 Blockers and Proton Pump Inhibitors
Chapter 29 Laxatives
Chapter 30 Antidiarrheals
Chapter 31 Antiemetics
Chapter 32 Other Gastrointestinal Agents

Chapter 34 Male Genitourinary Agents
Chapter 35 Other Renal/Genitourinary Agents
Chapter 36 Acetaminophen
Chapter 37 Aspirin and Nonsteroidal Antiinflammatory Drugs
Chapter 38 Disease-Modifying Antirheumatic Drugs and Immune Modulators
Chapter 41 Muscle Relaxants
Chapter 45 Migraine Medications
Chapter 48 Antidepressants
Chapter 49 Antianxiety and Insomnia Agents
Chapter 50 Antipsychotics
Chapter 51 Substance Abuse
Chapter 54 Diabetes Mellitus Agents
Chapter 55 Contraceptives
Chapter 56 Hormone Replacement Therapy
Chapter 57 Other Gynecologic Agents
Chapter 58 Principles for Prescribing Antiinfectives
Chapter 59 Treatment of Specific Infections and Miscellaneous Antibiotics
Chapter 60 Penicillins
Chapter 62 Tetracyclines
Chapter 63 Macrolides
Chapter 64 Fluoroquinolones
Chapter 65 Aminoglycosides
Chapter 66 Sulfonamides
Chapter 67 Antitubercular Agents
Chapter 68 Antifungals
Chapter 70 Antivirals and Antiprotozoal Agents
Chapter 72 Weight Management
Chapter 73 Smoking Cessation
Chapter 74 Vitamins and Minerals

Susan D. McConnell, MSN, ANP, GNP
Emory University School of Medicine
Atlanta, Georgia
Chapter 52 Glucocorticoids
Chapter 53 Thyroid Medications

Elizabeth Monsen, MS, CRNP
University of Maryland Medical Center
Division of Cardiology
Baltimore, Maryland
Chapter 24 Antiarrhythmic Agents

Sandra M. Nettina, MSN, APRN,BC, ANP
Nurse Practitioner and Clinical Instructor
Johns Hopkins University School of Nursing
Baltimore, Maryland
Chapter 17 Asthma and COPD Medications

Susan Orsega, CDR, USPHS, MSN, CRNP
Family Nurse Practitioner
National Institutes of Health
Clinical Center Nursing
Bethesda, Maryland
Chapter 69 Antiretrovirals

Barbara E. Pokorny, MSN, RN, CS
Family Nurse Practitioner
Community Health Center of New London
New London, Connecticut
Chapter 52 Glucocorticoids

Barbara Resnick, PhD, CRNP, FAAN, FAANP
University of Maryland School of Nursing
Associate Professor, Nurse Practitioner, Roland Park Place
Baltimore, Maryland
Chapter 6 Special Populations: Geriatrics

Cheryl Pandolf Schenk, MN, RN,CS, CDE
Nurse Practitioner/Certified Diabetes Educator
Veterans Administration Medical Center
Decatur, Georgia
Chapter 54 Diabetes Mellitus Agents

Laurie Scudder, MS, PNP
Private Practice
Nurse Practitioner Alternatives, Inc.
Columbia, Maryland
Chapter 61 Cephalosporins
Chapter 71 Immunizations and Biologicals

Laura E. Shay, MS, C-ANP
United States Public Health Service
Washington, DC
Chapter 4 Economic Foundations of Prescriptive Authority

V. Inez Wendel, MS, ANP, GNP
Johns Hopkins University, School of Medicine
Division of Geriatric Medicine and Gerontology
Baltimore, MD
Chapter 42 Overview of the Nervous System
Chapter 43 Central Nervous System Stimulants and Cognitive Function Drugs
Chapter 44 Analgesics
Chapter 46 Anticonvulsants
Chapter 47 Antiparkinson Agents

Theresa Pluth Yeo, MPH, MSN, CRNP
Assistant Professor
The Johns Hopkins University School of Nursing and
Sydney Kimmel Comprehensive Cancer Care Center at Hopkins
Baltimore, Maryland
Chapter 26 Agents that Act on Blood

Reviewers

Barbara J. Burgel, RN, MS, COHNS, ANP, FAAN
Clinical Professor, Adult Nurse Practitioner
Occupational and Environmental Health Nursing Program
The University of California at San Francisco
School of Nursing
San Francisco, California

Doris Denison, MSN, RN, NP, CCRN, ACNP
Instructor Clinical and Adult Health
Wayne State University, College of Nursing
Detroit, Michigan

Lorrie N. Hegstad, PhD, APRN, BC, ANP/GNP
Associate Professor
Director, Adult & Gerontological Nurse Practitioner
The University of Texas at Arlington, School of Nursing
Arlington, Texas

Melina L. Jenkins, PhD, APRN, BC, C-FNP
Assistant Professor, Columbia University
School of Nursing
New York, New York

Jean E. Lee, MSN, FNP-BC, ANP-C
Kansas City Department of Veteran Affairs Medical Center
Kansas City, Missouri

Margaret A. Lynch, MSN, FNP
The Cambridge Hospital, Department of Family Practice
Cambridge, Massachusetts

Preface

As the title proclaims, this is a text written for all types of primary care providers: nurse practitioners, physician assistants, physicians, nurses, and others. Our goals are to present comprehensive information on the drugs most commonly prescribed in primary care practice, and to do it in a concise and easily digested manner.

As in the first edition of *Pharmacology for the Primary Care Provider,* the second edition assumes that the reader has a strong grasp of biochemical principles and clinical practice, and it therefore focuses on the basic information that every prescriber must know. It does not attempt to cover every drug, nor every facet of the drugs included. Rather, it relies heavily on the most important basic concepts, often applying those concepts to a drug prototype for that category of drugs. All other drugs in the category are then compared with the prototype, and only the information that is new, different, or very important is presented for additional discussion. When the beginning primary care provider masters basic information about the drug category and the drug prototype, it is then easier to discern when other drugs would be more appropriate.

Many features are included here to aid the practitioner in decision making and practice:

- Drug tables at the beginning of each chapter outline the classifications of the drugs discussed.
- Complete discussions on drug action and drug treatment principles are presented for every drug category.
- Clinical Alerts, highlighted by the icon, impart essential information that primary care providers must remember in order to avoid serious problems. The Alerts include cautions for prescribing, information about drug interactions, or warnings about particularly ominous adverse effects.
- Clinical guidelines and algorithms directing clinical decision-making are based on a variety of sources, using evidence-based medicine and expert recommendations.
- The top two hundred drugs prescribed in the United States are identified by the icon. Information distinguishing them from their respective prototypes is presented.
- Patient Education sections in every chapter provide effective patient teaching about medications to help ensure patient compliance.
- Patient Variables sections alert the provider to special considerations based on age, pregnancy, race and other factors.

No part of the health care delivery system changes faster than the pharmacologic component. New information is discovered every day; for example, there is an explosion of new information daily about how cytochrome P450 affects specific drug interactions. New products go on the market almost daily. What we know or don't know about these products affects our care. Clinicians must rely on new information if they are to give safe and effective care.

Using the most recent information is not the exclusive domain of research-based academicians, but the foundation of accepted health care practice for all primary care practitioners. To help the clinician stay current, several continuously updated sources are provided, free of charge, with purchase of this text. In addition to the resources listed in the back of each chapter, instructors and students purchasing the text will receive access to Evolve Learning Resources to Accompany Pharmacology for the Primary Care Provider, second edition. This website is an invaluable resource for continuing education, containing the following:

- Bonus tables providing enrichment information not covered in the text
- Over 1100 weblinks arranged by chapter and helpful to both provider and patient
- Basic level access to Mosby's Drug Consult Internet Edition
- A link to the FDA's *Catalog of FDA Approved Drug Products*
- A subscription to the *Mosby/Saunders ePharmacology Update* newsletter, a quarterly e-mail newsletter providing drug updates, offered free of charge.

Of additional interest for the instructor is a free 300-question testbank and *Mosby's Electronic Image Collection for Pharmacology*, offering over 150 full-color illustrations.

The advent of evidence-based medicine has changed how we think about pharmacotherapeutics. It is important to learn what really works as opposed to what has been done traditionally. Research will have a direct impact upon what we do; for example, consider the changes regarding hormone replacement therapy that have been made in the last few years. Therefore, this book teaches how to think about drug use through discussion of evidence-based medicine studies, appraisal of clinical guidelines and protocols, and consideration of role studies examining how professionals actually prescribe medication and how critical decisions can and should be made.

NEW TO THE SECOND EDITION

With five new units and seven new chapters, this second edition reflects the most current thoughts and trends in primary care. New material includes chapters entitled Over-the-Counter Medications (Chapter 9), Compliance and the Therapeutic Experiment (Chapter 10), Overview of the Nervous System (Chapter 42), Substance Abuse (Chapter 51), Treatment of Specific Infections and Miscellaneous Antibiotics (Chapter 59), Weight Management (Chapter 72), and Complementary and Alternative Medicine (Chapter 75). Updated units provide focus on these important areas: Renal/Genitourinary Agents, Psychotropic Agents, Endocrine Agents, Female Reproductive System Drugs, and Health Promotion.

ORGANIZATION

Part One contains chapters on the essential concepts for the prescription of medications.

- Unit 1 describes primary health care providers and the various dimensions of their role. It also covers the legal parameters and professional role implementation of prescriptive authority and explains what we know about different types of primary health care providers and the economic foundations of prescriptive authority.
- Unit 2 is one of the most important in the whole text. It focuses on the pharmacokinetics and the pharmacodynamics of different drugs. Specific factors are considered in prescribing drugs to geriatric, pediatric, and pregnant patients.
- Unit 3 reviews over-the-counter medications and describes the therapeutic relationship between drug prescriber and the patient. Practical tips in writing prescriptions are explored along with a discussion of the principles of evidence-based medicine, clinical guidelines, critical decision-making, and patient education.

Part Two contains 12 discrete units that discuss common drug categories and the common primary care conditions for which they are used. Chapter text and drug monographs are arranged for easy readability and ready reference in this consistent and logical manner:

Drug names
Indications for use
Disease process and physiology
Drug action and effect
Drug treatment principles
How to monitor
Patient variables
Patient education
Specific drugs (beginning with prototype drugs when relevant and then considering different or especially important information about other drugs in the category)
Resources for patients and providers
Bibliography

THE FUTURE

Pharmacology for the Primary Care Provider, second edition, provides that strong basic knowledge of pharmacology that every care provider needs. The text summarizes extremely complex information in a deceptively simple format in a manner that only expert clinicians can do. Students will appreciate the clear and simple explanations. Mastery of these foundational principles, basic protocols, and prototype drug monographs will prepare primary care clinicians for the realities of daily practice. We invite you to enjoy it, learn from it, carry it with you into the clinical area as you begin practice, and use the resources provided to both deepen and expand your pharmacological arsenal.

As you gain experience with this text, we welcome your comments. As you mature and grow in your role as a primary care clinician, we hope you will help us mature and develop in our role as educators. It is a cooperative relationship.

ACKNOWLEDGMENTS

We would like to acknowledge the contributions of authors for the first edition. Their original work is foundational to the changes that were made for edition two. Those original authors include the following:

Susan E. Appling, RN, MS, CRNP; JoAnne T. Baker, RN, MSN, FNP; Elizabeth Blair, MSN, CS-ANP, CDE; Bonnie R. Bock, RN, BSN, MS, CRNP; Alice M. Brazier, MS, CRNP, GNP; James Cawley, MPH, PA-C; Susan E. Childs, RN, MS, CRNP; Sandra L. Cotton, MS, C-ANP; Christy L. Crowther, RN, MS, CRNP; Charles E. Daniels, RPh, PhD, FASHP; George DeMaagd, PharmD, BCPS; Gloria A. Deniz, RN, MS, ARNP; Jan DiSantostefano, MS, CRNP; Susan Waldrop Donckers, RN, EdD, CS, FNP; Michael Dreis, PharmD, MPH; Diane Fatica, RN, MSN, FNP; Kathleen Ryan Fletcher, RN, CS, MSN, GNP; Annette Galassi, RN, MA, CANP, AOCN; Susanne Scharnhorst Gibbons, ANP, GNP, MS; Cynthia Knoll Grandjean, RN, MGA, MSN, NP; Catherine Hagan, MSN, RN, CNS; Major Nancy (Jo) Heisterman, BS, FNP; Linda C. Hersey, MS, CRNP; James D. Hoehns, PharmD, BCPS; Karen Huss, RN, DNSc, CANP, FAAN; Pamela Lynn Jamieson, RNC, MS, NP; Bonnie Kohl, RN, MS, CRNP; M. Lauren Lemieux, MS; Marilyn Little, BS, MS, CS; Jennifer Loud, MSN, CRNP; Karen MacKay, MD; Douglas Matthews, MS, CRNP; Elaine McIntosh, RN, CS, FNP; Patricia C. McMullen, CRNP, MS, JD; Carolyn S. Melby, DNSc, CRNP; Karen L. Minor, RN, MS, CRNP; Maureen Moriarty-Sheehan, RN, MS, CRNP; Candis Morrison, PhD, ACNP; Kathleen Murphy, RN, MS, CRNP; Julie C. Novak, DNSc, RN, CPNP; Katherine M. O'Rourke, MSN, FNP; Katherine M. Pabst, CRNP, MPH; Julianne B. Pinson, PharmD; Stevelynn J. Pogue, MSN, RN, CS, A/GNP, ET; Barbara E. Pokorny, MSN, RN, CS; Jacqueline Rhoads, PhD, RN, CCRN, ACNP, CS; Laurie Scudder, MS, PNP; Diane C. Seibert, BSN, MS, CRNP; Janet S. Selway, MS, CANP, CPNP; Leslie K. Serchuck, MD; Amy B. Sharron, MS, RN, CS, GNP; Laura E. Shay, MS, CANP; Donna M. Thompson, RN, MS, APRN; Laura Keiler Topper, RN, MS, NP; Jan Wemmer, MS, CRNP; Inez Wendel, MS, CRNP; David S. Wing, BBP, MSc; Theresa Pluth Yeo, MSN, MPH, CRNP; Linda R. Young, PharmD.

Additionally, we want to express our appreciation for the personal stimulation we have received from the many nurse practitioners, physician assistants, nurse midwives, nurse anesthetists, PharmD, physicians, and medical students, we have worked with over the course of the past few years. They have asked challenging questions and have been clear about the need for a good text that has basic medical content integrated with pharmacologic principles and nursing approaches. Some of these individuals have been willing to step forward to write that content, and we are grateful for their wisdom, their knowledge, and their assistance.

And finally, we are deeply grateful for the help of the editorial, production, and design staff at Mosby and specifically wish to thank Barbara Nelson Cullen, Lee Henderson, Celia Cruz, Maureen Iannuzzi, and Mary Stueck. As always, none of this work would have been possible without the tolerance and support of our very patient families. Maren wishes especially to thank Bill, Rosemary, and Dad; Marilyn is indebted to Cliff, Mike, Chris, Clark, Megan, and Eddie and her two daughters-in-law, Ali and Cheryl.

Marilyn Winterton Edmunds, PhD, ANP/GNP
Maren Stewart Mayhew, MS, ANP/GNP

A Note to the Student of Primary Care

Begin this text with the chapters in the first unit. Reread the chapter on pharmacokinetics and pharmacodynamics on a regular basis. It is one of the most important chapters in the book, and it is impossible to master these principles in a single reading. Don't expect to memorize everything. This book will be something you want to refer to often in the clinical area as you begin practice. Try to understand the principles being presented and find examples in your own patients that illustrate them.

As you gain experience with this text, we welcome your comments. As you mature and grow in your role as a primary care clinician, we hope you will help us mature and develop in our role as educators. It is a cooperative relationship.

Contents

UNIT 1

Foundations of Prescriptive Authority

CHAPTER 1

Prescriptive Authority and Role Implementation: Tradition vs. Change

INCREASED FOCUS ON PRIMARY CARE

Primary care as a concept involves the provision of integrated, accessible health care services by clinicians who are accountable for addressing "personal health care needs, developing a sustained partnership with patients, and practicing in the context of family and community" (Vaneslow, Donaldson & Yorday, 1995). It is generally agreed that providing health care includes one or more of the following functions: assessing health status, promoting healthy lifestyles, identifying/diagnosing normal and abnormal conditions, determining the causes of abnormal conditions, providing referral to health care specialists, selecting appropriate therapeutic measures, implementing treatment, and supervising or monitoring the patient on an ongoing basis. These tasks are commonly referred to as *prevention, diagnosis, prescription,* and *treatment.* They describe professional behavior used in deciding what is wrong with a patient and then choosing among available therapeutic options to prescribe and implement a course of treatment. Traditionally, these behaviors have been the exclusive domain of the physician and, to a lesser extent, the dentist, until the past 30 years when other nonphysician provider roles have emerged.

TRADITIONAL PROVISION OF PRIMARY CARE

States first began enacting medical practice acts in the 1920s to protect the public safety. Before that time, the quality of medical education and the competency of physicians were quite variable. Medical practice acts granted title protection to those individuals who called themselves physicians and identified what requirements must be met for that title to be given. Although other categories of health care professionals were certainly in existence at that time, physicians were the first health care practitioners to gain legislative recognition of their practice (Starr, 1982). The statutory definitions initially created by physicians for the scope of their practice were extremely broad. In an exhaustive study of regulatory restrictions on new types of health care providers, Safreit (1992) provided an example (NC Gen. Stat No. 90-18 [1983]) of one state's definition of physician or surgeon as

> Any person . . . who shall diagnose or attempt to diagnose, treat or attempt to treat, operate or attempt to operate on, or prescribe for or administer to, or profess to treat any human ailment, physical or mental, or any physical injury to or deformity of another person.

Because of the way in which the medical practice acts were written, physicians emerged with an exclusive right to practice that gave them a preeminent position in a hierarchy of healing occupations. Designating physicians as the only providers with diagnostic and treatment authority was intended to protect the public. However, the breadth of the medical practice acts, combined with provisions making it illegal for anyone not licensed as a physician to carry out any acts included in the definition, made it difficult for other health care workers to describe their contributions. All other health care providers, including groups such as nurses and nurse midwives, had to redefine their tasks or functions as separate from the all-encompassing medical scope of practice. They then had to seek legislative recognition of their own professional roles, no matter how traditional or longstanding their activities might have been (Safreit, 1992).

Dominance of the physician in the health care hierarchy created a virtual monopoly in health care. The medical sociology and professionalization literature is filled with extensive analyses of the factors that led to the development of the cultural, economic, political, and social authority and dominance of the physician, and especially the growth and power of organized medicine (Freidson, 1970a, 1970b; Starr, 1982).

Having obtained the exclusive right to practice, however, physicians also recognized their need for the services of other practitioners of healing, who were "useful to the physician and necessary to his practice" (Safreit, 1992), even if it required giving up some of their monopolistic control. A noted medical sociologist who has traced the professionalization of physicians notes that to solve this dilemma, physicians extended their right to practice to a right from the state to control the activities of other occupations, "so as to limit what they could do and to supervise or direct their activities" (Freidson, 1970a). In doing so, the profession was able to establish organizational structures that preserved a distinct sphere of professional dominance and autonomy (Safreit, 1992).

The role of the physician has changed dramatically during the past 50 years. Driven by new technology, new procedures, and new medications, physicians have been attracted into specialty practice in greater numbers, leaving primary care positions vacant. Medicare reimbursement has fueled the growth of tertiary care.

The emergence of nonphysicians who claimed preparation for and desire to provide primary care services came at a time when there was a shortage of primary care services. The emergence of this new group challenged the professional dominance of physicians, the organizations that have consolidated their authority, and the legislation designed to protect and preserve that position.

Beginning in 1992, the Physician Payment Review Commission recommended radical changes in Medicare reimbursement methodology. This shift directly increased financial reimbursement to clinicians providing primary care and thus indirectly created an incentive to attract more providers into primary care. The hope was to more evenly align the numbers and types of providers with the numbers and types of patients requiring health care.

Medical schools began placing greater emphasis on preparing primary care clinicians. Teaching methodologies shifted from the acute care model to include a greater focus on primary care. The hospitalist emerged as a specialty, thus relieving the primary care physician of the need to provide in-hospital care. Reimbursement began to reward the general practitioner. All of these changes have been a qualified success, bringing increased credibility and recognition of primary care providers, although there remains a disproportionate number of specialists.

Notwithstanding the longstanding precedent for physicians to provide primary care, there remained a disparity in the ability of physicians to meet the primary care needs of the populace. Nonphysician providers began to fill that niche with increasing success. The nonphysician providers who emerged during the 1960s and 1970s were well accepted by their patients; delivered high-quality, cost-effective care; and generally increased the access of patients to health care (Office Technology Assessment, 1986). These providers continued to work cooperatively with physician providers, most often in joint practices. By the 1990s, as they grew in experience, many of these new providers became increasingly restless in a dependent role and desired fewer formal restrictions on their autonomy from physicians.

IMPORTANCE OF PRESCRIPTIVE AUTHORITY IN HEALTH CARE DELIVERY

Research on the practices of nonphysician providers has demonstrated conclusively that they are qualified to provide primary care (see Chapters 2 and 3). Although physicians have a broader education than other types of health care providers such as nurse practitioners or physician assistants, the extent of education required to provide primary care services is not clear. It appears that many physicians may be overeducated to provide primary care, and other clinicians might be just as competent in delivering primary care (Safreit, 1992), leaving physicians to care for patients with more complicated conditions that clearly require an extensive breadth of education.

Although nonphysician providers demonstrate competency in providing primary care services, restrictive regulations in the language of the original medical practice acts unnecessarily prevent these providers from delivering primary care services. One of the restrictions has been on who might prescribe medications.

Because the medical practice acts of different states subsumed prescriptive authority for physicians, other professionals desiring prescriptive authority have had to seek legislative redefinition or delegated authority from the physicians to write prescriptions. Nonphysician health care providers have crafted rules and regulations in every state, resulting in prescriptive authority with very different permutations. Sometimes the authority granted to nonphysicians is liberal; sometimes it is very conservative. With the increasing effectiveness of drugs in treating many chronic diseases, limiting prescriptive authority for some qualified providers limits their ability to meet patient needs. With the high mobility of today's providers, the state-to-state variability of prescriptive authority for nonphysician providers is recognized as a barrier to practice.

Medications are powerful weapons against disease. Pharmaceutical companies added 32 new drugs and 8 biological agents to the nation's pharmacopoeia in 2001, including 5 for heart disease, the leading cause of death in the United States, and three new treatments for cancer, the second leading killer of Americans. Other newly approved medicines include five drugs for infectious diseases; two each for arthritis, glaucoma, migraine headache, and hepatitis; and one each for human immunodeficiency virus infection/acquired immune deficiency syndrome (AIDS), schizophrenia, and Alzheimer's disease. Thousands of new drugs are in the research and development pipeline, including many new drugs for children and providing a new armamentarium for clinicians to use in treating patients with chronic disease (PhRMA www.pharma.org, January 25, 2002). Other newly approved medications include two new drugs for Parkinson's disease, a protease inhibitor to treat children with AIDS, three new drugs for diabetes, and a new drug to help prevent osteoporosis.

Because of the importance of medications in treating primary care problems and in providing the full scope of health care services required by the typical primary care patient, all providers must be able to prescribe medications. This is especially true in rural areas, where there may be only one provider. However, it is just as true where there are many competing providers, with each trying to make a living. If meeting patients' needs is the primary focus in the provision of primary care services, then providers should not be artificially restricted from meeting as many needs as possible (Safreit, 1992).

RESEARCH ON PRESCRIPTIVE PRACTICE OF PHYSICIANS

Physicians and dentists are the professional roles that have traditionally been given the undisputed right to prescriptive authority. The prescriptive practice of physicians in primary care practice has been thoroughly documented by the pharmaceutical industry. What medications physicians order and how many prescriptions are written are closely monitored. Studies have not only evaluated basic prescribing practices but also analyzed the effects multiple variables have on prescribing habits. Some of the key findings are briefly presented.

The National Ambulatory Medical Care Survey (Cheery et al, 2003) collected data on drugs most frequently used in office-based practice and found that 61.1% of all office visits resulted in the generation of at least one prescription. The top five categories of prescriptions were cardiovascular-renal preparations (14.7%), drugs used for the relief of pain (12.1%), respiratory tract drugs (11.6%), hormones and agents affecting hormonal mechanisms (10.8%), and central nervous system drugs (8.7%). During the past 20 years, these categories have remained relatively consistent, although antimicrobial drugs have now fallen from the top five. In the 2000 National Ambulatory Medical Care Survey (Cherry & Woodwell, 2002), researchers examined physician prescribing in general and family practice. They found that for those patients who made an office visit, 33.9% did not receive any prescription; 28.0% received one prescription, 16.1% received two, 8.8% received three, 4.9% received four, 3.2% received five, and 5.3% received six. The percent of visits involving medications ranged from 78.8% for internists to 29.9% for general surgeons. General and family practice physicians deal with medications in 76.3% of visits.

Many more studies have examined the types of medications prescribed, and over the years patterns have changed. Stolley and Lasagna (1969) found that 95% of all physicians prescribed one or more medications to a patient with a common cold, and more than 60% of these prescriptions were for antibiotics. In 1972, a computerized retrieval system examined 20,000 prescriptions and found that antibiotics topped the list of most frequently prescribed medications, followed by tranquilizers, nonnarcotic analgesics, oral contraceptives, and antitussives (Stolley et al, 1972b). In 1974, researchers found sedatives and hypnotics heading the list (21%) with antibiotics (15%), antihistamines (8%), dermatologic preparations (6.6%), and cardiovascular drugs (6.5%) accounting for the top five classifications (Rosenberg et al, 1974). As the years progressed, sedatives, tranquilizers, and hypnotics began to decline in popularity (Rossiter, 1983; DeNuzzo, 1981; Knoben & Wertheimer, 1976). The 2000 National Ambulatory Medical Care Survey: released by the Centers for Disease Control and Prevention (Cherry & Woodwell, 2002) shows the top categories of drugs by category to be very similar to those reported 20 years earlier. However, antibiotic categories have become antimicrobial, accounting for the change in prescribing due to AIDS. The most frequently prescribed drug in 2000 was Claritin, followed by Lipitor, Synthroid, Premarin, and amoxicillin. Acetaminophen was the generic substance most frequently prescribed. The survey documented a 21% increase over the past several years in the percent of office visits where a cardiovascular-renal drug, such as angiotensin-converting enzyme inhibitors, beta blockers, or antihypertensive medications was prescribed. Between 1997 and 2000, there was a 25% increase in the percent of visits where a hormone was prescribed, whereas the increase in the percent of metabolic/nutrient drug visits rose by 41%. The report suggested that these changes reflect the drug use patterns of the health-conscious baby boomers and the growing number of seniors whose chronic conditions can be treated by the wide variety of medications on the market today.

Less research has been conducted on the appropriateness of physician prescriptive practices, although there is some literature that suggests that physicians write prescriptions for problems that might well respond to many nonpharmacologic treatments (Avorn et al, 1991).

The pharmaceutical industry has expended considerable research dollars to try to determine how to influence prescribers to adopt their drug. When a new drug product is developed, research suggests the rate of adoption by prescribers may de divided into five profiles: innovators, early adopters, early majority, late majority, and laggards. Although the speed at which prescribers adopt the drug varies, the individuals within each profile all go through a four-step process: awareness of the new drug, interest, evaluation, and trial—leading to adoption.

Denig & Haaijer-Ruskamp (1992) described an "evoked set" that includes a small number of possible treatments (typically containing all therapies, including nondrug therapies) that a physician might consider for a specific condition. Clearly, if a therapy is unfamiliar or unknown, it will not be included in the physician's evoked set. The evoked set for all possible medical problems makes up the "total drug repertoire" or "therapeutic armamentarium" and, on average, includes 144 drug preparations per physician. Research concluded that in a 12-month period, physicians write 5.4% prescriptions for new drugs, and that 42% of the time, this product replaces a drug that was previously part of the repertoire. "Once a product is part of the evoked set, it has a propensity to be prescribed through habit rather than through active problem-solving" (Groves, Flanagan & MacKinnon, 2002). So prescribers both adopt and relinquish drugs in their therapeutic armamentarium. This change in the product choice comes as innovation is diffused or communicated through certain channels over time among the members of a social system. Burban, Link, and Doucette (2001) suggested the factors that influenced new drug adoption were the perceived attributes of the innovations, communication channels used to discuss these attributes, nature of the social system, and physician characteristics.

Other studies over the years have attempted to predict what variables most affect prescribing habits. Younger physicians and specialists tend to prescribe more appropriately and prescribe fewer medications (Stolley et al, 1972a, 1972b: Miles & Roland, 1975; National Center for Health Statistics, 1983a). Stolley et al (1972b) also noted that generally the more appropriate prescriber was one who was in a large group practice and who used physician consultants and journal articles to guide pharmacologic decision making. Miller (1973, 1974), Smith (1977), and Stolley & Lasagne (1969) found multiple variables influencing drug prescribing. Colleagues, phamaceutical representatives, journal articles, the *Physicians' Desk Reference,* medical meetings, and journal advertising were the primary sources of information about medications and therapeutic regimens.

In a summary of recent literature, it has been suggested that financial ties to drug companies may influence physicians' prescribing judgments. One study found that physicians who requested specific additions to a hospital pharmacy were substantially more likely to have met with drug company representatives or accepted money from the drug companies. However, physicians may not recognize the potential influence of drug companies on their behavior. One study of primary care physicians said that they placed little weight on drug advertisements (68%), pharmaceutical representatives (54%), or patient preference (74%) and that they relied heavily on academic sources for drug information. Yet the study found that commercial rather than scientific sources of drug information dominated their drug information reading.

Guidelines issued by the US Food and Drug Administration in 2001 prompted the American Medical Association and the Pharmaceutical Manufacturers and Researchers of America to issue ethical guidelines that clarify the appropriate relationship between pharmaceutical companies and drug prescribers. These guidelines forbid pharmaceutical companies from giving non–patient care–related items exceeding $100 value to prescribers as well as clarifying the role that the companies can and cannot play in continuing education of provider groups.

PROBLEMS IN THE PRESCRIBING PRACTICE OF PHYSICIANS

Difficulties documented over the years in prescribing have been remarkably consistent. The conclusions of numerous studies suggest the following.

1. **Problems created because of physician failure to keep abreast of changes.** Information about new products and new research findings diffuse slowly into practice. Typically many physicians have been wary about suggestions for change in their practices until they have seen evidence of the safety and utility, especially for medications. Physicians in solo or isolated practice often fail to realize that they are out of step with other general practice because they may not have opportunity for the daily critical debate and exchange among colleagues. Few physicians have had sufficient time to keep up to date on new materials, relying on drug advertisements and pharmaceutical representatives. Most information in pharmacology textbooks is outdated before it is printed. New methods of staying up to date on information will be required to practice safely. Use of the Internet, medical journals on CD-ROM, evidence-based medicine reports, and the ability to obtain specialist consultations through Telehealth will dramatically affect how providers obtain and use information and whether it will make a difference in their practice.
2. **Pharmaceutical company influence on practice and drug samples.** When the bulk of information coming to a physician is provided through biased marketing sources, physicians have had a difficult time evaluating the relative merits of competitive products (Smith, 1977; So, 1998). Intervention by the FDA over the years has limited the amount and types of pressure that drug detail men could exert directly on physicians to encourage them to use their products. Requirements for more balanced presentations of information about diagnostic and treatment methods has helped upgrade the quality of valid information given to physicians.
3. **Lack of time has become a major factor in all medical practices.** The emphasis on making money in many health maintenance organizations has led to decreased time for patient encounters, leading to inadequate history-taking, failure to clearly define the problem, and an overreliance on drug therapy (Avorn et al, 1991; Munroe et al, 1982; Ramsey et al, 1998).
4. **Consumer pressure to prescribe medications.** Although consumer interest in their health care is usually a positive step, the demand of patients on the physician to "do something" has translated into an increased insistence by the consumer on being given a prescription. Giving in to these pressures has resulted not only in the appearance of a society that takes a pill for everything but also in the widespread overuse of antibiotics, thus contributing to the problems caused by drug-resistant organisms.
5. **Illegibility of prescriptions.** Pharmacists report great difficulty in accurately reading the writing of many physicians. This has led to major errors in dispensing of medications as they try to determine what the physician might have written. Use of preprinted prescription pads, fax machines, and computer-generated forms will help decrease these problems.
6. **Failure to detect or anticipate drug interactions.** Modern research on the liver has revealed the presence of the cytochrome P450 enzyme system. Lack of provider awareness about the influence of different drugs on these pathways has made many medications ineffective.

Five million times last year, one of the nation's largest real-time computer systems alerted American pharmacists that prescribed drug combinations could trigger potentially lethal drug interactions. The prescription warning system issues 45 million alerts annually. Many warnings are for drug interactions that have been well described in the professional literature.

CONCLUSION

Because physicians and dentists have been the only major health care providers with prescriptive authority, all of what we know about prescriptive behavior is based on their behavior. Thus the practice characteristics of other health care practitioners will inevitably be compared with the physician. However, this is not to suggest that physician prescriptive practices represent the gold standard. They have been the only standard, by default. Rigorous methodologies have not yet been implemented to examine whether physician performance consistently correlates to approved therapeutic practice. As additional health care providers enter the system, their prescriptive practice should not be compared with physicians. All providers should be held to a standard of approved therapeutic practice. These standards of care are just beginning to be defined and are being driven from the concepts of evidence-based medicine.

The bulk of primary care medicines will continue to be prescribed by physicians. What physicians prescribe, and how effective they are in determining the appropriate medication will continue to be important information shared by all prescribers with prescriptive authority. The challenge for new health care providers is to learn from the experience of the traditional health care prescribers. How nonphysician prescribers bring their own talents and philosophies in the prescriptive processes will surely provide new solutions and new dilemmas to those already encountered by physicians.

RESOURCES FOR PATIENTS AND PROVIDERS

Top drugs: www.rxlist.com

Lists the top 200 drugs prescribed in the United States each year, with a detailed database on prescriptions.

REFERENCES

Avorn G, Everitt DE, Baker MW: The neglected medical history and therapeutics: choices for abdominal pain: a nationwide study of 799 physicians and 151 nurses, *Arch Intern Med* 151:694-698, 1991.

Burban GM, Link BK, Doucette WR: Influences on oncologists' adoption of new agents in adjuvant chemotherapy of breast cancer, *J Clin Oncol* 19:954-959, 2001.

Cherry DK, Burt CW, Woodwell DA: *National Ambulatory Medical Care Survey: 2001 summary,* US Dept HHS, CDC, NCHS, Advance Data, Number 337, Aug 11, 2003.

Cherry DK, Woodwell DA: *National Ambulatory Medical Care Survey: 2000 summary,* US Dept HHS, CDC, NCHS, Advance Data, Number 328, June 5, 2002.

Denig P, Haaijer-Ruskamp FM: *Therapeutic decision making of physicians,* Pharmaceutisch Weekblad Scientific Edition. 14:9-15, 1992.

DeNuzzo R: *25th annual prescription survey. Medical marketing and the media,* New York, 1981, Albany College of Pharmacy of Union University.

Freidson E: *Profession of medicine: a study of the sociology of applied knowledge,* New York, 1970a, Harper and Row.

Freidson E: *Professional dominance: The social structure of medical care,* Chicago, 1970b, Aldine.

Freidson E: *The professions and their prospects,* Beverly Hills, 1971, Sage Publications.

Groves KEM, Flanagan PS, MacKinnon NJ: Why physicians start or stop prescribing a drug: literature review and formulary implications, *Formulary* 37:186-194, 2002.

Knoben S, Wertheimer A: Physician prescribing patterns—therapeutic categories and age considerations, *Drug Intell Clin Pharm* 10:398-400, 1976.

Mahoney DF: Nurse practitioners as prescribers: past research trends and future study needs, *Nurse Practitioner* 17:44, 47-48, 50-51, 1992.

Mahoney DF: Appropriateness of geriatric prescribing decisions made by nurse practitioners and physicians, *IMAGE J Nurs Scholarship* 26:41-46, 1994.

Miles D, Roland D: Prescribing patterns in a rural community, *Drugs Health Care* 2:187-194, Summer, 1975.

Miller R: Prescribing habits of physicians—a review of studies on prescribing of drugs. Parts IV-VI, *Drug Intell Clin Pharm* 7:557-564, 1973.

Miller R: Prescribing habits of physicians—a review of studies on prescribing of drugs. Parts VII-VIII, *Drug Intell Clin Pharm* 8:81-91, 1974.

Munroe D et al: Prescribing patterns of nurse practitioners, *Am J Nurs* 82:1538-1542, 1982.

National Center for Health Statistics: *Drug utilization in general and family practice by characteristics of physicians and office visits, National Ambulatory Medical Care Survey, 1980,* Hyattsville, MD, March 18, 1983a, US Public Health Service, No. 87 DHHS Pub. No (PHS) 83-1250.

National Center for Health Statistics: *Drugs most frequently used in office-based practice: National Ambulatory Medical Care Survey, 1981,* Hyattsville, MD, April 1983b, US Public Health Service, No. DHHS Pub. No. (PHS) 83-250.

Office Technology Assessment: *Nurse practitioners, physician's assistants, and nurse midwives: a policy assessment,* Washington DC, 1986, Office Technology Assessment, US Congress, Health Technology Assessment Report No. 37.

Ramsey PG et al: History-taking and preventive medicine skills among primary care physicians: an assessment using standardized patients, *Am J Med* 104:152-158, 1998.

Rosenberg S et al: Prescribing patterns in the New York City Medicaid Program, *Medical Care* 12:138-151, 1974.

Rossiter L: Prescribed medicines: findings from the National Medical Care Expenditure Survey, *Am J Public Health* 73:1312-1315, 1983.

Safreit B: Health care dollars and regulatory sense: the role of advanced practice nursing, *Yale J Regul* 99:417-488, Summer, 1992.

Smith M: Drug product advertising and prescribing: a review of the evidence, *Am J Hosp Pharm* 34:1208-1224, 1977.

So AD: Free gifts: redundancy or conundrum? *J Gen Intern Med* 13:213-215, 1998.

Starr P: *The social transformation of American medicine,* New York, 1982, Basic.

Stolley P et al: The relationship between physician characteristics and prescribing appropriateness, *Medical Care* 10:17-28, 1972a.

Stolley P et al: Drug prescribing and use in an American community, *Ann Intern Med* 76:537-540, 1972b.

Stolley P, Lasagna L: Prescribing patterns of physicians, *J Chronic Dis* 22:395-405, 1969.

Top drugs: Available at www.rxlist.com (Lists the top 200 drugs prescribed each year, with a detailed database on prescriptions).

Vanselow NA, Donaldson MS, Yorday KD: From the Institute of Medicine, *JAMA* 273:192, 1995.

Woodwell DA: *National Ambulatory Medical Care Survey: 1996 Summary,* Washington, DC, December 17, 1997, US Dept HHS, CDC, NCHS, Advance Data, No. 295.

CHAPTER 2

Prescriptive Authority: The Role of the NP, CNM, CRNA, and CNS

OVERVIEW

For many years, the boundaries of nursing practice have been carefully constrained by state nurse practice acts that maintained that "nurses do not treat, diagnose, nor prescribe" (Kelly, 1974). However, the 1960s saw a critical mass of bored, talented nurse clinicians, whose substantial scientific education had been underused and whose ideas about making changes in their role were spurred on by the consciousness raising of the feminist movement. This happened at a time when other health care personnel were being pulled into the Vietnam War, and there was a concern about how primary health care could be delivered (Edmunds, 1978).

This time was formative for the nurse practitioner (NP) movement. Although some educators decried the NP movement as designed to encourage nurses to leave nursing to become handmaidens to physicians (Rogers, 1972), many nurses and some nursing leaders believed that this role breathed new life into the profession of nursing (Ford, 1979).

The expanded role of the nurse did not begin with NPs. Certified nurse-midwives (CNMs) and certified registered nurse anesthetists (CRNAs) had already established their own, very clearly defined roles several decades earlier. The clinical nurse specialist (CNS) trend in educational preparation grew out of increased utilization of registered nurses in the high-technology cardiac units, intensive care units, and dialysis units in hospitals at about the same time the NP role was being initiated in the primary care setting. What all of these roles had in common was that, in each role, nurses assumed some of the functions traditionally reserved for physicians. As such, they came to be known as advanced practice roles.

CHANGES IN ROLES FOR NURSES: WHEN AND WHY

Advanced practice nurses (APNs) were called by a variety of titles, the most lasting of which were *midlevel providers, non-physician providers,* or *physician extenders.* The educational programs for these new roles had varying names and different curricula, awarded different credit, and prepared graduates with varying skills and competencies.

Unlike NPs with their primary care focus, CNSs were educated for and practiced primarily in acute inpatient settings and specialty units. As such, although their practice was certainly advanced, they were not responsible for initiating the medical diagnosis and treatment of patients but were true experts in nursing care (Lewis, 1970). They provided advanced consultation, education, teaching, and research about specific patient problems. This group was frequently the most highly educated of the advanced practice nursing groups, with a master's degree almost mandatory for entry into the role. However, because they do not directly generate revenue, their role has been difficult to maintain.

Initially, it was unclear if there would be jobs for any of these nurses with advanced diagnostic and therapeutic training. It was also unclear if they could legally perform some of the tasks that they were educated to perform. However, the educational programs that were eventually established were highly selective of their students and demanding in their requirements. Students were not allowed to graduate unless they could demonstrate a high degree of competence. The students were typically experienced nurses who were determined to practice nursing in a different way and wanted to make a difference. They were assertive and creative, and they were risk takers (Edmunds, 1978). Because of this combination of experience, competence, and assertiveness, these nurses earned support from patients and grudging acceptance from their physician colleagues.

Although all expanded nursing roles enjoyed an uneasy relationship with medicine during the early phase of their professional development, many physicians assisted in role development by teaching in educational programs and hiring the new types of providers. These physicians clearly came to respect and support the accomplishments of nurses in these new functions. Early antagonism changed to tolerance or acceptance. Then, in the 1990s, new sources of hostility developed among physicians who had once been supportive. The American Medical Association began urging physicians to consciously limit further "erosions of their turf" legislatively and professionally and to view nurses with expanded roles who wanted direct reimbursement for their services as true competitors for patient loyalty and money (Safreit, 1992).

Because of growth in acceptance of the NP role and passage of legal authorization for expanded nursing practice, educational programs thrived. The certificate programs that developed to prepare NPs gave way to university programs with the understanding that NP education should be at the graduate level if it was going to withstand the criticism of medicine. Over time, universities felt the demand from more students seeking entry into NP programs. This led to the development of a multitude of master's degree programs with varying curricula, different standards, and questionable competencies. By 1995, with sudden media attention growing out of health care reform debates, congressional recognition of the NP role, and increased professional visibility for NPs, many other graduate nursing programs were emptying as students rushed to become NPs. This included many of those nurses with preparation as CNSs, who were now seeking retraining as NPs. Capitalizing on increased demand, many faculties lowered their admission standards to take advantage of the growing number of NP applicants, some of whom had never even practiced as nurses before electing to enter this new role. This action ignored the market's limited ability to both teach and hire the increased number of NP students.

In 1996, the American Association of Colleges of Nursing (AACN) released a document called *The Essentials of Master's Education for Advanced Practice Nurses*. The discussion and acceptance of recommendations in the *Master's Essentials* curriculum led to the notion that almost all nurses with a master's degree were APNs. Thus the term *advanced practice nurse* lost its ability to denote the CNS, CRNA, CNM, or NP whose role overlapped so much with traditional physician practice. To distinguish themselves from the now generic title of *advanced practice nurse* used by all nurses with master's degrees, those who assumed tasks usually performed by physicians began referring to themselves as "nurses with diagnosing and prescribing authority."

Clearly, all of these expanded practice roles have survived for more than 40 years because the clinicians practicing within them were competent (Brown & Grimes, 1995; Office of Technology Assessment, 1986). Patients liked the blend of nursing and expanded assessment and treatment skills of the new providers. The weight of the evidence indicates that, "within their areas of competence, NPs . . . and CNMs provide care whose quality is equivalent to that of care provided by physicians. Moreover, NPs and CNMs are more adept than physicians at providing services that depend on communication with patients and preventive actions . . . Patients are generally satisfied with the quality of care provided by NPs . . . and CNMs, particularly with the interpersonal aspects of care" (Office of Technology Assessment, 1986).

These new providers offered access to care that was acceptable, increased access to care, increased productivity, and offered cost-effective alternatives (Office of Technology Assessment, 1986). These behaviors, combined with successful legislative efforts within each state to legally authorize the expanded practice of nurses, ensured survival and growth of the role.

One component of role function, however, with which each of these groups had to grapple was prescriptive authority. Most NPs thought they could not fully implement their role or provide services that patients required without being able to prescribe medications (Safreit, 1992). The need for CRNAs and CNMs to have prescriptive authority was less clear. Additionally, some CNS practice began to move away from hospital-based acute care services and looked increasingly like NP primary care practice. These nurses also desired prescriptive authority. So, these groups of nurses were required to amend the nurse practice acts in all 50 states to give broader authority to them in their new roles and to gain specific authorization to "treat, diagnose, and prescribe." Every state has since addressed this issue, with great variability in the legislation passed.

LEGAL FOUNDATION OF PRESCRIPTIVE AUTHORITY FOR NURSES IN ADVANCED PRACTICE ROLES

Federal and state statutes and administrative law determine control of drugs, including the act of prescribing. How these three elements work together to protect the public has evolved over time. Early regulatory precedents gave primary prescriptive authority to physicians. These became a barrier to change for those new health care providers seeking the prescriptive authority (Safreit, 1992; Sutliff, 1996).

Role of the Federal Government

Before the turn of the century, there were no laws governing drugs. A myriad of elixirs, tonics, and pills, containing any combination of drugs including opium and cocaine, were sold freely to anyone willing to pay the price. It was not until 1906 that the federal government enacted the first law, the Food and Drug Act, prohibiting adulterated or misbranded food or drugs from interstate commerce (Nielsen, 1992).

However, true drug safety was not effectively addressed until 1938, when the US Congress passed the Food, Drug, and Cosmetic Act (21 U.S.C. 301 et seq.) requiring drugs to be appropriately tested for safety and labeled with adequate directions for use. However, the explosion of new drug development in the 1940s made the labeling provision difficult to achieve. Thus the Durham-Humphrey Amendment of 1951 was implemented, creating a separate category of drugs: *legend drugs*. Drugs were considered to be legend drugs if they bore the legend "Caution: Federal law prohibits dispensing without a prescription" (21 U.S.C. 353). These drugs did not require specific package labeling but instead required medical supervision for their sale and use. This act also instituted the process of the pharmacist dispensing legend drugs after first obtaining a written prescription from an authorized prescriber (Nielsen, 1992).

The other major piece of federal legislation affecting drug regulation was the Comprehensive Drug Abuse Prevention and Control Act of 1970. This act limited prescribing, dispensing, manufacturing, and distribution to only those individuals registered with the Drug Enforcement Administration (DEA), an agency of the Department of Justice. It also classified narcotics and other drugs such as depressants and stimulants by their abuse potential with differing levels of control for each class (Nielsen, 1992). Thus some legend drugs were further categorized as controlled substances (see Chapter 11 for a classification of controlled substances) and had additional restrictions placed on them.

As noted, the DEA *will* register individuals who may prescribe narcotics and other controlled substances. However, registration depends on state authority to prescribe controlled substances. Only health care providers who are granted authority to prescribe controlled substances may be registered by the DEA and receive a DEA number. Consequently, only nurses working in states that grant authority to prescribe controlled substances may receive a federal DEA number.

State Control of Prescriptive Privileges

Although the federal government has broad control over drug regulation, it has no control over who may prescribe, dispense, or administer drugs (Buppert, 1999). This role belongs solely to the states and is generally addressed in the statutes, rules, and regulations outlining the licensure and scope of practice of specific health care providers. The state law that enables nurses to practice nursing is a legal statute entitled the Nurse

Practice Act. Nurses are individually licensed by each state in which they practice.

In their efforts to protect a vulnerable and possibly ill-informed public receiving health care, every state has enacted licensing laws for health care providers. If people do not have the information or the ability to make safe judgments about the qualifications and abilities of providers, the state serves as a proxy to gather this information through licensing. Although the state establishes a list of minimum requirements one must meet to be licensed within that state, meeting these requirements does not necessarily guarantee that the provider is competent. Thus licensure as a mechanism to protect the public has not been conclusively demonstrated (Bullough, 1980).

Boards of nursing have been somewhat perplexed about how to make certain they are protecting the public safety when the nursing role has changed so dramatically over time. In 1985, the National Council of State Boards of Nursing (NCSBN) adopted a position paper on advanced clinical practice calling for regulations to be adopted within each state that mandate a minimum of master's preparation in a clinical nursing practice specialty to serve as the basis for advanced clinical nursing practice. NCSBN also mandates recognition of national certification to identify nurses for advanced clinical nursing practice. However, it is clear that using a national certification examination (established to provide professional recognition) to obtain a license to practice within a state has its own problems (Edmunds, 1992).

Whether traditional registered nurse licensure adequately protects the public when a nurse moves into an expanded role has been debated for years (Edmunds, 1992). Discussion about second licensure for APNs is ongoing, with no resolution in sight. Nurses with advanced education want legislative parity with physicians, who are not required to obtain additional licenses if they are professionally credentialed in another specialty.

As a result of all these factors, there is wide variability among states relative to who may prescribe and under what conditions prescriptive authority is granted. In addition, the degree of prescriptive autonomy and authority constantly evolves as new laws are passed and regulations are promulgated.

Fink (1975) and, later, Trandel-Korenchuk and Trandel-Korenchuk (1978) attempted to categorize the variations in prescriptive authority allowed in different states as they related to NPs. Essentially, two types of prescriptive authority are afforded to NPs. These are delegable authority and authority legislated by nursing statues or regulations. *Delegable authority* requires the nurse to perform under the direction of a physician, mandates the initial physician-patient relationship, and is legally based in medical practice acts. Delegable prescriptive authority can be further delineated into three subtypes: (1) physician determination of patient-specific medications and authorization of the nurse to prescribe accordingly for that patient, (2) standing order/protocols serving as instructions for prescribing, and (3) renewal of prescriptions by the nurse, based on prescriptions initially ordered by the physician. Without delegated authority, the nurse cannot legally prescribe medications under any circumstances except for recommendations for nonprescription medications.

Prescriptive authority legislated by the state nurse practice act or by rules and regulations proposed by state boards of nursing and, at times, medical and pharmacy boards, also developed. Two types of prescriptive authority are permitted in nursing legislation. The first type, *dependent authority*, requires that the physician retain ultimate authority by countersignature of prescriptions and/or by a written agreement between the NP and physician, outlining the need for NP chart review, discussion, etc., with the physician collaborator (Bell, 1980). This mode is similar to the delegated authority concept described previously and is practiced in many states. Conversely, *independent authority* allows the NP alone to prescribe. Independent authority may still be restricted, for example, excluding controlled substances or limiting drugs to those listed in a formulary.

AN OVERVIEW OF THE DIAGNOSING AND PRESCRIBING NURSES AND THEIR ROLES

Clinical Nurse Specialists

Definition and Scope of Practice. The clinical specialist in nursing practice is a nurse who, through study and supervised clinical practice at the graduate level (master's or doctorate), has become expert in a defined area of knowledge and practices in a selected clinical area of nursing (American Nurses Association, 1980).

The CNS's role is a unique combination of tasks. The specialist is prepared to serve as an expert in clinical practice, an educator, a consultant, a researcher, and, often, an administrator. "The boundaries of the specialty are defined by the phenomena of interest to the CNS. These phenomena may change, reflecting the needs of society, and may therefore cause the boundaries to expand" (American Nurses Association, 1986; Sparacino, et al, 1990).

Educational Preparation and Certification. CNSs are a diverse group of nurses whose main commonality is having a master's degree. Almost all other components of their program title, curriculum, specialty area, extent of clinical practice, and competency vary according to the philosophy of the university, individual strengths of the faculty, and practice site.

Originally perceived as experts in nursing who would both provide direct clinical services to patients in tertiary settings and help other nurses develop skills in caring for patients with specific problems, the role has been variously interpreted and varyingly accepted (Riehl & McVay, 1973). West Coast hospitals generally interpreted the CNS role as providing direct one-on-one specialty care to patients and teaching other nurses how to do the same. These nursing roles often became integral to meeting the needs of the institution. East Coast CNSs more frequently define the role as advocating for a particular specialty, such as geriatric or diabetic patients, or providing administrative, educational, consultative, or research services within an acute care setting. Because many of the important contributions CNSs made to patient care were not billable services for the hospital, CNSs were not revenue generators. However, they often commanded some of the highest salaries. This made them vulnerable to staffing cuts (Edmunds, 1992). Thus this role was often perceived as a luxury for an institution and often was the first position to be eliminated during times of fiscal austerity.

Many CNSs have had growing difficulty in finding employment using their expertise and education. Their excellent contributions to increasing the quality of nursing care have often been undervalued. Lack of job security and lack of recognition coupled with the growing employment demand for NPs have driven many CNSs into the NP role. This has resulted in virtual NP cannibalization of the CNS role in some geographic areas (Breuninger, 1996; Carr, 1996). However, because of their critical care background, these CNS-NPs have begun to return to the hospital in the developing acute care NP roles.

Certification for CNSs has always been optional. The nurses who electively sit for national certification in a specialty most closely resemble their physician colleagues, who become board-certified in a particular specialty. This type of certification professionally recognizes the nurse as an expert. This differs from other nursing groups like NPs, who are often required by states to obtain national certification to be licensed for entry into practice.

Status of Prescriptive Authority. CNSs who were hospital based had no need for prescriptive authority. However, as CNSs left the acute care area to take specialty practice into the home or community, there was increasing desire for them to be able to write prescriptions if they were to meet the needs of their patients. Currently, CNSs have some form of prescriptive authority in 30 states; in 8 of these states, the authority is restricted to those clinical specialists in psychomental health.

In almost all of the states in which CNSs have obtained prescriptive authority, it has been because they (1) formed coalitions with other APNs and (2) were granted prescriptive authority because of that coalition. In many states, CRNAs, CNMs, NPs, and CNSs are all defined by legislative statute as APNs, and the legislation is written to grant prescriptive authority to APNs, not to the individual titles within that category. Because of this, many CNSs acknowledge that they have piggybacked on the efforts of other advanced practice nursing groups within the state to obtain prescriptive authority. There are no states in which CNSs obtained prescriptive authority while other nurses were denied those privileges (Pearson, 1998). This is a trend that is likely to continue.

There are no identifiable research studies that focus on CNS prescribing practices. Without research documenting the safety and accuracy of CNSs with prescriptive authority, few conclusions may be drawn about their practices.

Certified Registered Nurse Anesthetists

Definition and Scope of Practice. The CRNA is a licensed registered nurse with advanced specialty education in anesthesia who, in collaboration with appropriate health care professionals, provides preoperative, intraoperative, and postoperative care to patients and assists in the management and resuscitation of critical patients in intensive care, coronary care, and emergency situations. Nurse anesthetists are certified after the successful completion of credentials and state licensure review and a national examination directed by the Council on Certification of Nurse Anesthetists (CCNA) (1998). They develop their specialty in anesthesia by taking a graduate curriculum, emphasizing development of critical judgment and critical thinking. "They are qualified to make independent judgments relative to all aspects of anesthesia care based on their education, licensure, and certification. As clinicians, they are legally responsible for the anesthesia care they provide" (American Association of Nurse Anesthetists, 1992; American Association of Nurse Anesthetists website, 1998).

Nurse anesthetists have been providing anesthesia services in this country for more than a century. Working in conjunction with anesthesiologists, surgeons, and, where authorized, podiatrists, dentists, and other health care providers, nurse anesthetists administer approximately 65% of all anesthetics given each year in the United States. They are found in every setting in which anesthesia is provided and work with every age group and type of patient. They use the full gamut of anesthesia techniques, drugs, and technology and are the sole anesthesia providers in more than 70% of rural hospitals (American Association of Nurse Anesthetists website, 1998).

Educational Preparation and Certification. Early nurse anesthetists faced a challenge to the legality of their practice when they were charged with illegally practicing medicine in Kentucky (1917) and California (1936). Landmark decisions in these cases established that CRNAs were practicing nursing and not medicine. Today, there are more than 27,000 CRNAs practicing in all 50 states (American Association of Nurse Anesthetists website, 2002).

The common denominator for all CRNAs is that they are "anesthesia specialists with a generic foundation in professional nursing" (American Association of Nurse Anesthetists, 1990). Accredited programs throughout the United States and Puerto Rico have gradually moved to master's degree graduate level education, with half of the programs located within schools of nursing. Some CRNAs continue to see themselves as nurses, whereas many believe that they have "left nursing" to become specialists in administering anesthesia.

The Council of Accreditation (COA) of Nurse Anesthesia Educational Programs establishes program curricula and accreditation standards for all programs. The educational curriculum ranges from 24 to 36 months in an integrated program of academic and clinical study, with COA requiring at least 30 credit hours of formalized graduate study in advanced anatomy, physiology, pathophysiology, biochemistry, physics related to anesthesia, advanced pharmacology, research methodology and statistical analysis, and principles of anesthesia practice. It should be noted that most programs require 45 to 65 credit hours, not 30, in science courses (American Association of Nurse Anesthetists, 1997).

Students also gain clinical experience through residencies where they are closely supervised as they learn anesthesia techniques, provide anesthesia care to patients, and begin to apply knowledge to clinical problems. COA requires each student to complete a minimum of 450 cases, with most programs providing about 1000 hours of hands-on clinical experience (American Association of Nurse Anesthetists, 1997).

Graduates of accredited nurse anesthesia educational programs must meet all requirements prescribed by the COA to take the national examination for certification. Passage of this rigorous examination qualifies the graduate for certification as

BOX 2-1

CRNA RECERTIFICATION TEST AREAS IN PHARMACOLOGY

1. General principles
   a. Pharmacodynamics
   b. Pharmacokinetics
   c. Anaphylaxis
   d. Drug interactions
2. Inhalation anesthetics
3. Intravenous anesthetics
   a. Barbiturates
   b. Opioids (agonists/antagonists)
   c. Benzodiazepines
   d. Other
4. Local anesthetics
   a. Esters
   b. Amides
5. Muscle relaxants/antagonists
6. Autonomic and cardiovascular drugs
7. Others
   a. Central nervous system drugs
   b. Diuretics
   c. Autocoids

a nurse anesthetist. Every 2 years the CRNA must meet certain practice and continuing education requirements for recertification (American Association of Nurse Anesthetists, 1997). As a group, CRNAs are the highest paid of all expanded practice roles with nursing preparation.

The American Association of Nurse Anesthetists (AANA) is the only professional association for nurse anesthetists. Organizationally separate, the COA exerts a powerful role over all nurse anesthetist programs through its program accreditation process. However, although there are rigid standards that must be met, there is wide variability in the ways in which programs meet curricular standards. As a result, there is no universal curriculum for what the nurse anesthetist student will learn about pharmacology. Various AANA documents concerning scope and standards for nurse anesthesia practice and guidelines for clinical privileges contain some general objectives that mention medications.

For example, AANA (1996) maintains that the CRNA scope of practice includes, among other things:

- Performing and documenting a preanesthetic assessment and evaluation of the patient, including requesting consultations and diagnostic studies; selecting, obtaining, ordering, and administering preanesthetic medications and fluids; and obtaining informed consent for anesthesia
- Developing and implementing an anesthesia plan
- Selecting, obtaining, and administering the anesthetics, adjuvant and accessory drugs, and fluids necessary to manage the anesthetic
- Facilitating emergency and recovery from anesthesia by selecting, obtaining, ordering and administering medications, fluids, and ventilatory support
- Implementing acute and chronic pain management modalities
- Responding to emergency situations by providing airway management, administration of emergency fluids and drugs, and using basic or advanced cardiac life support techniques (American Association of Nurse Anesthetists, 1996b)

The CCNA's 1998 recertification handbook provides the content outline for examination questions used in the national examination (Box 2-1). Approximately 30% of the total questions on the examination are in the area of basic sciences and pharmacology (CCNA, 1998). Some nurse anesthetist programs teach content around the topics on the examination; other programs require students to take more general pharmacology courses to prepare them for anesthesia duties and work in pain clinics. They may take these more general courses with medical students or with other graduate nursing students to obtain a more general pharmacology preparation that helps them deal with patients who have diabetes, cardiovascular problems, or another comorbidity that may influence their anesthesia plans.

Status of Prescriptive Authority for CRNAs. The primary care focus of this text might suggest to some that CRNAs should be excluded from discussion. However, the increasing use of CRNAs in chronic pain clinics and hospice sites has raised the question as to whether some CRNAs need prescriptive authority. Whether they are providing primary care or not, the CRNAs have been, often by default, included in state legislative efforts for other nursing groups seeking to gain prescriptive authority.

The federal definition of *prescription* means an order for medication, which is dispensed to or for an ultimate user, but does not include an order for medication that is dispensed for immediate administration to the ultimate user. Therefore an order to dispense a drug to a patient in bed for immediate administration in a hospital is *not* a prescription (21 CFR 1306.02).

Because of this definition, the traditional practice of nurse anesthetists, which involves ordering and directly administering controlled substances preoperatively, intraoperatively, and postoperatively, does not constitute "prescribing" under federal law. Therefore CRNAs engaged in traditional practice do not need prescriptive authority or a DEA registration number to do so (Tobin, 1991).

CRNAs engaged in traditional anesthesia practice have no need for a DEA number. However, if the state grants prescriptive authority to CRNAs, and they elect to use prescriptive authority in their practice, they then become subject to DEA registration requirements.

In some states, CRNAs thought that restrictions might be placed on implementation of their role without full prescriptive authority. Generally, CRNAs attempt to choose policy or legislative solutions that have the least potential to restrict their practice. Therefore CRNA groups attempting to determine if they needed prescriptive authority within their states often summarize the arguments thus:

Possible Benefits to CRNAs. Acquiring prescriptive authority may enhance professional autonomy and independence, may reduce fears of surgeons about their liability for CRNA practice, may open up future opportunities in pain management clinics, may help reduce bureaucratic red tape, and may resolve issues related to the need for co-signatures.

Possible Disadvantages to Seeking Prescriptive Authority. If lack of prescriptive authority is not really a problem, why raise the issue in other people's minds? If CRNAs introduce legislation for prescriptive authority and the legislation does not pass, does it diminish the implicit authority or perceived competency of CRNAs in the minds of legislators? Is it possible to get legislation passed without making some other compromises that would be troublesome, such as restrictive protocols?

The American Society of Anesthesiologists oppose CRNAs having prescriptive authority, and it has been suggested that they may galvanize other groups against CRNA incursion into this area (Tobin, 1998).

The official position of AANA has been that, whether CRNAs need prescriptive authority or not, independent prescriptive authority enhances the role and so is desirable. It also alleviates confusion about the exact nature of the authority of the CRNA. However, prescriptive authority is not viewed as an essential component without which they cannot practice (Tobin, 1998). State CRNA chapters vary in their perceived need for prescriptive authority and on their evaluation of the political and professional environment that might make seeking such authority successful.

Currently five states grant independent prescriptive authority to CRNAs (Alaska, New Hampshire, Wyoming, Montana, and Washington). Eighteen other states and the District of Columbia have some type of prescriptive authority linked to physician control (Tobin, 1998).

Certified Nurse-Midwives

Definition and Scope of Practice. Nurse-midwifery practice is the independent management of women's health, focusing particularly on pregnancy, childbirth, the postpartum period, care of the newborn, and the family planning and gynecologic needs of women. The CNM practices within a health care system that provides for consultation, collaborative management, or referral as indicated by the health status of the client. Certification requires education at the postgraduate level in nursing or an allied professional health care field (American College of Nurse Midwives, 1992).

The philosophy of the American College of Nurse Midwives (ACNM) (1989) clearly emphasizes the focus of the midwife on the needs of the individual and family for care; physical, emotional, and social support and involvement of significant others in this care according to their cultural values and personal preferences. The practice of nurse-midwifery is delivered throughout the life span, advocating nonintervention in normal processes of reproduction and development and health education for women throughout the childbearing cycle. Midwifery has also expanded to include gynecologic care of well women throughout the life cycle. Nurse-midwives provide this comprehensive health care most frequently in collaboration with other members of the health care team.

Women have always taken responsibility for the delivery of children. With the passage of the first medical practice acts in the 1920s, midwives suddenly found themselves directly opposed by obstetricians and legally outside the laws that physicians had crafted. This led to the expansion of formal academic midwifery programs and the requirement for midwives to obtain legal authorization for their services.

In 1963 there were only 275 practicing nurse-midwives in the United States. By 2002, that number has increased to more than 7000 CNMs (American College of Nurse Midwives website, 2002). Traditionally, CNMs find most of their clients among the indigent, who both fear and cannot afford hospital-based obstetric care. Many of these clients have used lay midwives and view birthing as a natural process that should be under the supervision of women. This varies dramatically from the existing medical philosophy. While continuing to provide care to underserved populations, CNM care is now sought by women from all cross sections of the country (American College of Nurse Midwives, 1997).

The number of CNM-attended births has increased every year since 1975, the first year that the National Center for Health Statistics began collecting data. In 1998, the most current year for which data are available from the National Center for Health Statistics, there were 277,811 CNM-attended births in the United States, accounting for 9% of all vaginal births that year (American College of Nurse Midwives website, 2002).

CNMs practice in every type of setting. In addition to more traditional health care settings, some CNMs choose to provide home birth services or work in birthing centers with other CNMs. A collaborative team of CNMs and physicians offers women a combination of primary and preventive care, with specialized services as needed. The degree of collaboration with physicians depends on the medical needs of the individual woman and the practice setting. Of all visits to CNMs, 90% are for primary, preventive care (70% for care during pregnancy and after birth and 20% for care outside of the maternity cycle). Nurse-midwives on average devote about 10% of their time to direct care of birthing women and their newborns (American College of Nurse Midwives, 1997).

Since the formal inception of the CNM role, extensive research has documented their positive contributions to maternal and fetal care (American College of Nurse Midwives, 1998; Bell & Mill, 1989; Butler et al, 1993; Capan et al, 1993; Clark, Martin & Taffel, 1997; Davis et al, 1994; Hueston & Rudy, 1993; Knedle-Murray et al, 1993; MacDorman & Singh, 1998; Oakley et al, 1995; Rosenblatt, 1997).

After controlling for a wide variety of social and medical risk factors, the risk of experiencing an infant death was 19% lower for births attended by CNMs than for births attended by physicians; the risk of neonatal mortality (an infant death occurring in the first 28 days of life) was 33% lower, and the risk of delivering a low birth weight infant was 31% lower. Mean birth weight was 37 g heavier for the CNM-attended births than for the physician-attended births. At the same time, CNMs attended a greater proportion of women who are at higher risk for poor birth outcome: African Americans, Native Americans, teenagers, unmarried women, and those with less than a high-school education (MacDorman & Singh, 1998).

CNMs were less likely to use continuous fetal monitoring, induce or augment labor, use epidurals, or perform episiotomies. The patients of CNMs also had cesarean section rates of only 8.8% compared with 13.6% for obstetricians and 15.1% for family physicians. As a result, CNMs used 12.2% fewer resources than did their physician colleagues (Rosenblatt, 1997).

Educational Preparation and Certification. The ACNM, as the sole professional organization representing CNMs, has crafted the professional direction for midwives. They issued professional standards, program accreditation, certification standards; commissioned research; and lobbied legislatively on behalf of CNMs.

The ACNM Certification Council oversees the quality and content of nurse-midwifery education programs. The ACNM document *Core Competencies for Basic Nurse-Midwifery Practice* (1997) sets up the basic clinical competencies of every beginning nurse-midwife, regardless of educational program. Students seeking to become midwives who are not already registered nurses but who possess a bachelor's degree in an allied field may attend graduate level midwifery programs and become credentialed as a certified midwife (CM). ACNM has defended its policy for accepting nonnurses into their programs based on internal research demonstrating that differences in the educational backgrounds of nurses versus nonnurses have not resulted in a difference in certification test results. Analysis of certification examination results demonstrates that degrees do not enhance the clinical competence of a midwife and reflect the ability of both types of programs to prepare competent beginning midwife practitioners. The pursuit of higher degrees by nurse-midwives is encouraged for the purpose of preparing educators, researchers, and theoreticians, as these roles are important for advancing the profession. The ACNM therefore supports certificate as well as degree programs in midwifery and opposes mandatory degree requirements for state licensure (American College of Nurse Midwives, 1992.)

The ACNM Division of Accreditation establishes the criteria for accreditation of educational programs in nurse-midwifery. All accredited programs are required to provide curriculum as defined in ACNM's *Core Competencies for Basic Nurse-Midwifery Practice.* These core competencies delineate the fundamental knowledge, skills, and practices expected of a new graduate. Every 5 years the core competencies are extensively evaluated and revised to ensure that CNMs have the skills to provide care needed by women today. All ACNM DOA-accredited education programs are affiliated with an accredited university, college, or another institution of higher learning.

There are currently 47 ACNM accredited nurse-midwifery education programs in the United States. Most of these programs offer a master's degree. Approximately 68% of CNMs have a master's degree, and 4% have a doctoral degree (American College of Nurse Midwives website, 2002).

Midwifery practice is based on three documents: *Core Competencies for Basic Nurse-Midwifery Practice, The Standards for the Practice of Nurse-Midwifery,* and the *Code of Ethics* promulgated by the ACNM. The core competencies (May, 1997) not only are important in the accreditation process but also constitute the basic requisites for graduates of all nurse-midwifery and midwifery education programs accredited by the ACNM. Midwifery education is based on a strong health science foundation and includes clinical preparation to use the knowledge, judgment, and skills necessary to provide primary care and independent management of women and newborns. This care is delivered within a health care system that provides for medical consultation, collaborative management, or referral as appropriate. Each education program may develop its unique identity and may choose to extend beyond the core competencies into other areas of health care. In addition, each graduate is responsible for complying with the laws of the jurisdiction where the practice of midwifery is conducted (American College of Nurse Midwives, 1997). Midwives who have been certified by the ACNM Certification Council, Inc. (ACC) assume responsibility and accountability for their practice as primary care providers (American College of Nurse Midwives, 1997). As such, CNMs assume responsibility for the provision of and referral for appropriate services within a defined scope of practice.

Because of the unique way in which each midwifery program is designed, content may vary, as long as students learn the basic competencies. For example, the content taught in pharmacology may differ significantly, depending on the emphasis of the program. Box 2-2 lists the core competencies in the area of pharmacology that were extracted from the total list of core competencies of the CNM (American College of Nurse Midwives, 1997).

Status of Prescriptive Authority for CNMs. Laws and regulations governing the practice of nurse-midwifery are rapidly changing. CNMs are regulated on the state level; therefore how these professionals practice and interact with other health care professionals, such as physicians, can vary from state to state (American College of Nurse Midwives, 1997).

Certified nurse-midwives have legislatively authorized practice in all 50 states and United States territories. In most states, the regulatory agency for the practice of nurse-midwifery is the state board of nursing. Reed (1997) provides an overview of trends and changes to state laws and regulations governing the practice of nurse midwifery in the United States from 1995 to 1997 and includes tables documenting many components of midwifery practice.

As of October 2002, 48 states, the District of Columbia, American Samoa, and Guam granted prescriptive authority to nurse-midwives in statutes or regulations governing practice. Although some states granted independent authority for the full scope of prescribing privileges, 8 states have limited prescribing authority, 11 states place a restriction on prescribing controlled substances, and 7 states consider prescribing by nurse-midwives to be a delegated medical act (American College of Nurse Midwives, 1998; Pearson, 1998).

Nurse Practitioners

Definition and Scope of Practice. Although use of the term *nurse practitioner* has been debated and criticized because of its similarity to the term *licensed practical nurse,* this title has earned a high degree of acceptability among legislators, educators, and researchers, who now recognize a different type of nursing service provided by this group of nurses. Nurse practitioner refers to those registered nurses who have obtained advanced education, usually through a graduate master's degree or post-master's certificate program, that prepares them to assume responsibility for the primary health care needs of individuals. This responsibility includes the assessment of client status, diagnosis of common acute and chronic problems, and management of care. The definition implies a con-

BOX 2-2

CNM CORE COMPETENCIES RELATED TO PHARMACOLOGY

Applies knowledge of midwifery practice in the antepartum, intrapartum, and postpartum periods that includes, but is not limited to the following:

1. Management techniques and therapeutics, including complementary therapies, to facilitate
   a. Healthy pregnancy and outcome
   b. Normal labor progress
   c. Healthy puerperium
   d. Neonatal period
   e. Health
   f. Treatment of common health problems of essentially healthy women
   g. Common gynecologic problems and family planning needs
   h. Alleviation of the common discomforts that accompany aging
2. Pharmacokinetics and pharmacotherapeutics of medications commonly used
   a. During pregnancy
   b. During labor and birth
   c. During the puerperium
   d. For immunizations
   e. For common health problems
   f. For family planning and gynecologic care
   g. For the perimenopausal and menopausal woman
3. Postpartum self-care, infant care, contraception, and family relationships
4. Management of discomfort during the puerperium
5. Methods to facilitate adaptation to extrauterine life including stabilization at birth, resuscitation, and emergency management

American College of Nurse Midwives: *Core competencies for basic nurse-midwifery practice,* Education Section, Division of Education, Washington, DC, May 31, 1997, American College of Nurse Midwives.

tinuing health care relationship over an extended period of time, as the nurse listens, teaches, and negotiates with the patient on how to maintain health. The NP is part of the larger health care team and works collaboratively with other health care providers in providing care.

The primary care focus of the NP clearly dictates the curriculum, skills, and focus of the practitioner. The scope of practice for the NP has been limited to the provision of primary care for the age groups (pediatrics, geriatrics, adult) or specialty (women's health) for which the NP was prepared. Only in the past decade has a role emerged for an acute care NP.

Education and Certification. The first NP program began as a pilot study at the University of Colorado. It was the brainchild of Dr. Loretta Ford, RN, and a physician colleague, Dr. Henry Silver. They believed that specially trained masters-prepared nurses could deliver much of the care in pediatric primary care. Their success was touted in many journal articles but was only a step ahead of other nurses in the country who were, at the same time, seeking to expand their practice. Nurses responded quickly to this new concept. Nurses who felt their skills and knowledge had been underused, as well as those who were dismayed by the lack of recognition, pay, and authority of the registered nurse role, flocked to continuing education programs that were set up almost overnight to accommodate their demand. New programs to educate NPs varied from 1 week to 18 months. They were all unique in design but all depended heavily on physician teachers and preceptors. The continuing education programs provided a way for talented nurses from diploma and associate's degree programs to receive this preparation (as they were excluded from participating in the master's programs that were slower to develop.) The first 10 years of the NP movement included so much diversity that it caused a great deal of confusion in both the nursing and medical communities. From the turmoil, it eventually became clear that nursing had once again created problems for itself by having two different educational entry levels—the continuing education certificate and the master's degree. This caused conflict within the nursing community and made the new role vulnerable to charges from other disciplines that some clinicians were not as well prepared as others. This educational schism has only been recently mended with the agreement by accrediting agencies that all NPs should be master's prepared.

Moves to Standardize Curricular Content. As NP programs became more widely established, it was clear that greater consistency among educational programs was mandatory if the role was to survive. More careful scrutiny of the preparation of NPs and criticism of that preparation by physicians and legislators propelled discussions among faculty about what must be done.

In 1988, the National Organization of Nurse Practitioner Faculties (NONPF) published *Guidelines for Family Nurse Practitioner Curricular Planning.* This was followed in 1990 by their *Advanced Nursing Practice: Nurse Practitioner Curriculum Guidelines* to identify essential curriculum content for all NP educational programs. This work was expanded in 1993 and 1994 with the documents *Primary Care Nurse Practitioner Graduate Outcomes* and *Model Program Standards for Nurse Practitioner Programs.* All of these documents circulated within educational groups but did not have significant impact on the exploding number of curricula. There was no accreditation of NP programs apart from that granted every 8 years by the National League for Nursing, as part of general school of nursing accreditation. In 1995, NONPF issued their *Advanced Nursing Practice: Curriculum Guidelines and Program Standards for Nurse Practitioner Education.* This document finally began to attract attention.

That same year, the AACN began a 2-year effort to establish and define appropriate graduate level nursing curricula.

Working in conjunction with NONPF and including many of their recommendations for NP education, AACN issued *The Essentials of Master's Education for Advanced Practice Nursing* (AACN, 1996). All of these documents were written in an attempt to promote standardization of educational requirements essential for the preparation of fully qualified NPs. In April 2002, *Nurse Practitioner Primary Care Competencies in Specialty Areas: Adult, Family, Gerontological, Pediatric, and Women's Health,* (USHHS, 2002) was published, and it continued efforts to define and standardize primary care competencies for NPs.

Family Nurse Practitioner Pharmacology Curriculum Recommendations. Concurrent with attempts to standardize the general NP curriculum, an NONPF task force developed the *Curriculum Guidelines and Criteria for Evaluation of Pharmacology Content to Prepare Family Nurse Practitioners for Prescriptive Authority and Managing Pharmacotherapeutics in Primary Care* (NONPF, 1997). The pharmacotherapeutic preparation of NPs had been among some of the most variable components of curricula. A few programs accepted whatever courses nurses had taken in their undergraduate program, whereas some other programs required 6 to 7 hours of biochemistry and advanced pharmacology taken with medical students. With more states passing legislation for NP prescriptive authority, NPs wanted to be well prepared for the legal and professional responsibility associated with writing prescriptions. The move to more clearly specify content in the area of pharmacotherapy was intended to help dispel any criticisms that NPs might not have adequate preparation to prescribe (see Box 2-3 for a summary of the pharmacology content recommendations).

Credentialing. As each state determines the requirements for recognizing NPs, considerable differences are seen among the states. All states either have enacted new legislation, have more broadly interpreted their nurse practice acts, or have instituted more clarity of the NP role through written rules and regulations. Some states require a second license for all those in the diagnosing and prescribing roles; some states also have required nurses to pass a national certification examination in their area of specialty to obtain state licensure as advanced practice clinicians (Buppert, 1999).

Certification examinations in other health care disciplines are constructed to provide professional recognition to outstanding clinicians. Thus NP certification examinations may not be appropriate for use as a method for determining entry into practice (Bosma, 1997). Certification examinations may be calibrated to a higher or lower level of difficulty and a broader or narrower scope of subject matter than would otherwise be appropriate for regulation. From a management perspective, they also may not be constructed psychometrically in a manner appropriate for legal regulation (Edmunds, 1992).

From a regulatory point, a specific concern about advanced practice certification is that not all states require national certification as a minimal requirement for authorization to practice in an advanced practice role. The American Nurses Credentialing Center (ANCC) and the American Academy of Nurse Practitioners (AANP) have developed certification examinations across several specialties, and over the years, there is greater cooperation among these certifying groups to develop psychometrically equivalent examinations (Edmunds, 1992; Robinson, McKenzie & Niemer, 1996). Other certifying bodies limit their examinations to a selected group of professionals. Each certifying agency evaluates each NP program curriculum to establish the eligibility of the applicant to sit for a national examination. These reviews are not uniform and range from formal to informal program evaluation.

Unlike PAs, CNSs, CRNAs, and CNMs, NPs have not had a single major professional organization to take the lead in establishing standards, policy, and certification requirements. During early role development, NPs were unable to come together under the umbrella of the American Nurses Association and so had fractured into different specialty groups. Each group looked after their own interests. By 1994 there were 14 major professional organizations for NPs, with 5 groups offering certification examinations and no groups offering program accreditation. Variability in the perceived quality of the certification examinations caused the NCSBN to express concern about whether they should step forward with a national examination (Robinson, McKenzie & Niemer, 1996).

Currently, there is no national policy on NP certification or second licensure. In those states where national certification is not required, there is no way to compel graduates to take the examination. For those who have passed the examination, its meaning is unclear (Bosma, 1997; Robinson, McKenzie & Niemer, 1996; Sharp, 1997). Movement by the NCSBN to set up an interstate compact whereby states agree to recognize RNs and APNs licensed in other participating states may lead to more uniform requirements over time and decrease the disparity in obligations and privileges for nurses moving among states.

Status of Prescriptive Authority for NPs. Over the past three decades NPs have steadily gained prescriptive authority on a state-by-state basis through legislative and/or administrative changes in the laws governing their practice. The annual state survey of NP regulation clearly illustrates the wide variation among states (Pearson, 2002).

All states and the District of Columbia now grant some form of prescriptive authority to NPs. Currently, 12 states and the District of Columbia (26%) allow full independent prescriptive authority for all classifications of medications, including controlled substances; thus there is no physician-mandated involvement in the prescriptive process. Thirty-two states (62%) grant NPs prescriptive authority for all medications, including narcotics, but require some degree of physician involvement or delegation of prescription writing. Six additional states exclude prescriptive authority for controlled substances and require physician involvement in the prescriptive process (Pearson, 2002).

Variability within these categories also exists. The degree of physician involvement may range from a loose collaborative practice agreement with limited oversight to strict physician supervision and review of prescriptive practices. Educational requirements for prescriptive practice also vary widely, with some states requiring only graduation from an approved educational program and/or passage of a certifying examination,

BOX 2-3

RECOMMENDED COURSE CONTENT AND PROGRAM COMPETENCIES IN PHARMACOTHERAPEUTICS FOR FAMILY NURSE PRACTITIONER (FNP) PROGRAMS

RECOMMENDED PHARMACOLOGY COURSE CONTENT

1. Basic principles
   a. Pharmacokinetics—Absorption, distribution, metabolism (biotransformation), excretion, bioequivalence, volume of distribution, clearance, half-life, steady state, dosing considerations, therapeutic drug monitoring
   b. Pharmacodynamics—Dose-response relationships/therapeutic index, structure-activity relationships, receptors, agonists/antagonists, signaling mechanisms
   c. Adverse drug reactions
   d. Drug interactions—Drug–drug; drug–food; drug–disease
   e. Special populations—Pregnant mothers, nursing mothers, neonates/children, elderly
   f. Special considerations—Self-treatments, alternative therapies, cost, cultural influences, gender, illness, poisoning, abuse, dependence, proper drug administration, genetic and racial effects
   g. Professional roles
   h. Other sources of drug information, evaluation of information, evaluation of drug production/promotion; clinical investigational drug research; patient education, adherence and participation; monitoring drug effects
2. Prescription writing
   a. Legal considerations
   b. Ethical considerations
   c. Modes of transmitting prescriptions
   d. Minimizing errors
   e. Controlled substances
3. Pharmacotherapeutics of drug groups
   a. Drugs used to manage bacterial, fungal, parasitic, and protozoal infections—Cell wall–cell membrane inhibitors, protein synthesis inhibitors, nucleic acid synthesis inhibitors, immunizations, other antiinfective agents
   b. Drugs used to manage cardiovascular conditions—Diuretics, angiotensin-converting enzyme inhibitors, centrally acting antihypertensives, adrenergic inhibitors, beta blockers, alpha blockers, vasodilators, calcium channel blockers, nitrates and nitrites, cardiac glycosides (digoxin), antiarrhythmics, antihyperlipidemics
   c. Drugs used to manage blood conditions—Iron preparations, vitamin B_{12}, folic acid, erythropoietin, anticoagulant agents, antiplatelet agents
   d. Drugs used to manage neuropsychiatric conditions—Antiseizure agents, antiparkinsonian agents, antipsychotic agents, mood stabilizers, anxiolytics, hypnotics, dementia drugs, psychostimulants, antidepressants, appetite suppressants, autonomic nervous system drugs
   e. Drugs used to manage pain and inflammatory conditions—Opioids, nonsteroidal antiinflammatory drugs, other agents used to treat pain, anti-gout drugs, muscle relaxants, antimigraine drugs, local and topical anesthetics, nonnarcotic analgesics
   f. Drugs used to manage respiratory conditions—Bronchodilators, nonsteroidal antiinflammatory drugs, corticosteroids, mast cell inhibitors, antihistamines, decongestants, antitussives, antibacterial agents
   g. Drugs used to manage gastrointestinal conditions—H_2 blockers, proton pump inhibitors, antacids, cytoprotectants, antimicrobial agents, anticholinergic agents, laxatives, antidiarrheals, antiemetics, colorectal treatments, stool softeners, prokinetic agents, prostaglandin analog, antiflatulents, emetics
   h. Drugs used to manage endocrine conditions—Antithyroid agents, thyroid agents, gonadal hormones, contraceptive agents, pancreatic hormones, diabetic agents, glucocorticoids, antiosteoporosis agents
   i. Drugs used to manage genitourinary conditions—Bladder inhibitors, bladder stimulants, prostatic agents, antibacterial agents
   j. Drugs used to manage dermatologic conditions—Antibacterials, antifungals, antivirals, ectoparasiticides, sunscreen agents, acne preparations, antiinflammatory agents, antipruritics, prohirsutics, emollients, astringents
   k. Drugs used to manage electrolyte and nutritional conditions—Vitamins, minerals, electrolytes, appetite stimulants
   l. Drugs used to manage substance abuse and dependency—Smoking-cessation aids, alcohol and other drug deterrents

END-OF-PROGRAM COMPETENCY REQUIRED OF FNP GRADUATE

1. Integrates knowledge of pharmacokinetic processes of absorption, distribution, metabolism, and excretion, and factors that alter pharmacokinetics into drug, dosage, and route selection
2. Integrates knowledge of drug interactions in safe prescribing and monitoring practice
3. Detects actual and potential significant drug reactions and intervenes appropriately
4. Incorporates bioavailability and bioequivalence principles into drug selection
5. Prescribes based upon appropriate indications for pharmacotherapeutic agents
6. Prescribes therapeutic agents to treat individuals with specific conditions based on factors such as pharmacokinetics, cost, genetic characteristics, etc
7. Analyzes the relationship between pharmacologic agents and physiologic/pathologic response when prescribing drugs
8. Educates clients about expected effects, potential adverse effects, proper administration, and costs of medication
9. Selects/prescribes correct dosages, routes, and frequencies of medications based on relevant individual client characteristics (e.g., illness, age, culture, gender, and illness)
10. Monitors appropriate parameters for specific drugs
11. Writes and transmits proper prescriptions that minimize risk of errors
12. Adheres to ethical and legal standards of pharmacotherapeutics
13. Incorporates strategies to improve client adherence to prescribed regimens
14. Consults appropriately when she or he recognizes limitations in knowledge of pharmacotherapeutics
15. Applies current drug information to pharmacotherapeutics
16. Involves client in decision-making process concerning therapeutic intervention, including self-treatment

From National Council of State Boards of Nursing et al (National Organization of Nurse Practitioner Faculties): *Curriculum guidelines and regulatory criteria for family nurse practitioners seeking prescriptive authority to manage pharmacotherapeutics in primary care, summary report, 1998,* HRSA 98-41, Washington, DC, 1998, US Department of Health and Human Services.

whereas others may mandate attending yearly continuing education courses or passage of a required pharmacology course (Pearson, 2002).

The use of protocols, formularies, guidelines, and algorithms developed by various regulatory boards, including the boards of nursing, medicine, and pharmacy, also control the prescriptive practices of NPs in different states. Finally, freedom to prescribe controlled substances varies not only across states but also across the various schedules of controlled substances (Buppert, 1999).

Prescriptive authority within the United States is primarily controlled and regulated by state legislatures and regulatory bodies. They determine the types of drugs to be prescribed, the degree of prescriptive authority, the regulatory bodies involved in controlling prescriptive practice, and the educational standards needed to obtain prescriptive privileges (Bosma, 1997). Changes to prescriptive practices occur through the coordinated efforts of health care providers and other interested groups working with legislators (Sharp, 1997). Over the years, all 50 states have required consumer, health care provider, legislator, and regulatory body interactions to craft a prescriptive practice environment designed to meet the needs of consumers. How well this has been done, and how well the resultant regulations address the concerns of all, is quite variable. The primary differences among states are the degree of professional autonomy or independence recognized by each state and the range of drugs from which NPs are permitted to select.

Safreit, in her exploration of the NP literature from a legal and regulatory vantage point (1992), concluded that

> Organized medicine has played a central role in shaping the states' current provisions for APN prescriptive authority. Consistently, individual physicians and medical associations have lobbied against any legislative efforts to acknowledge prescriptive authority as part of the APN's scope of practice. Organized medicine's position on this issue is reflected in the recently adopted AMA state model legislation on the "Regulation of Prescription-Writing Authority of Nurse Practitioners." . . . [In effect] the model legislation envisions direct physician supervision of the NP, as well as limitations upon the types of drugs the NP may select and the types of patients the NP may prescribe for.
>
> (Safreit, 1992)

PRESCRIBING CONTROLLED SUBSTANCES

Federal policy establishes that only health care providers who are granted prescriptive authority to prescribe controlled substances by the state can be registered by the DEA to obtain DEA numbers. Controversy surrounding the ability of NPs to obtain DEA numbers came to the forefront in 1991, when the DEA published proposed rules and regulations requiring health care providers to have "plenary" (defined as independent) authority to prescribe controlled substances. NPs lacking plenary authority would be defined as *affiliated practitioners* and be required to use the DEA number of their physician supervisor with a suffix attached indicating their affiliated status.

As a result, NPs in many states found that the statutes and regulations governing their practice did not grant independent authority to prescribe controlled substances. For instance, states that allowed NPs to prescribe controlled substances but required them to use protocols or establish a written agreement with a physician were considered to have derived or dependent authority as delegated by physicians and were not considered to have independent authority. According to the DEA, those NPs could not obtain their own federal DEA number.

The DEA's action created barriers to practice. For instance, the DEA recommendation that an NP share the DEA number of his or her collaborating physician posed a legal dilemma. NPs who worked with more than one physician also faced logistical issues. In states where NPs were found to lack independent authority, efforts to change these proposed DEA regulations or to establish independent authority within state statutes/regulations were initiated (Buppert, 1999). For example, Maryland NPs responded by writing letters of opposition to the DEA, requested a state attorney general's opinion regarding the status of independent prescriptive authority for NPs practicing in the state, and, finally, supported efforts to clarify statutory language in Maryland regarding independent NP practice.

In response to these and other efforts, the DEA amended the proposed rules and, in June 1993, presented a final rule titled *Definition and Registration of Mid-Level Practitioners (MLPs)* (21 CFR Parts 1301 and 1304 or 58 FR 31171). The specific wording is found in the June 1, 1993, *Federal Register* and it amends Title 21 of the Code of Federal Regulations Parts 1301 and 1304. This rule provided for the registration of all midlevel practitioners (MLPs), including NPs who were authorized by state law to prescribe controlled substances. To differentiate MLPs from other registered providers, the letter *M* precedes any DEA numbers issued to MLPs. In doing so, the DEA has set NPs and other MLPs apart from traditional DEA registrants such as physicians. The DEA considered this necessary because

> . . . the controlled substance authority granted to MLPs varies not only from state to state, but often from MLP to MLP within a state at the discretion of the board or of a collaborating physician. The different format registration number serves as an indicator to pharmacists and wholesalers to be alert to the probability that the MLP's controlled substance authority may be subject to specific state restrictions.
>
> (58 *Federal Register* 31171)

The publication of this rule did not address two ongoing issues in many states related to the inappropriate use of DEA numbers. First, selected insurance companies require all prescriptions to include the prescriber's DEA number as a unique identifier for tracking and billing. Second, some pharmaceutical companies require providers to include their DEA numbers when accepting drug samples. These instances of inappropriate DEA number use have frustrated providers who normally would not find it necessary to obtain a DEA number because their practices did not require controlled substance prescribing.

DISPENSING PRIVILEGES

Traditionally, pharmacists dispense medication based on a prescription from an authorized prescriber. Federal law addresses

TABLE 2-1 Summary of Pharmacology Preparation and Status of Prescriptive Authority for Diagnosing and Prescribing Nurses

	Nurse Practitioners (NPs)	Certified Nurse Midwives (CNMs)	Certified Registered Nurse Anesthetists (CRNAs)	Clinical Nurse Specialists (CNSs)
Pharmacology preparation	Pharmacology included in various nursing certificate and master's degree programs; move to require all NPs to have MS degree; NONPF has guidelines for standard NP curriculum; recommendations for FNP pharmacology course content; *Master's Essentials* document specifies advanced pharmacology course; certification exams have pharmacology content but many exams available and they vary in quality; exams are not mandatory for all NPs; programs not preaccredited; nursing programs accredited every 8 years by NLN as part of general nursing school reaccreditation	Pharmacology included in various nursing and non-nursing graduate and certificate programs; core competencies described but programs left to determine the content and format of pharmacology content; certification exam has pharmacology content but exam is not mandatory; all programs must be ACNM accredited credited before students may be admitted and reaccredited on a regular basis; faculty must ensure that students meet competencies for program to retain accreditation	Pharmacology included in various nursing and non-nursing programs; standards and guidelines for accreditation of NA programs describe expectations regarding use of pharmacology in practice but individual programs are free to determine how to meet those standards; certification exam has pharmacology content and most graduates take exam; programs must be accredited by AANA before students may be admitted and reaccredited or a regular basis; faculty must ensure that students meet competencies for program to retain accreditation	Pharmacology taught in various nursing master's degree programs; nursing programs accredited every 8 years by NLN as part of general school reaccreditation; advanced pharmacology course recommended by Master's Essentials document; content varies widely in practice and by program and specialty; some pharmacology on national certification exams but exam is elective
Status of prescriptive authority	Fifty states and DC with prescriptive authority with varying levels of restriction	Forty-seven states with prescriptive authority, with varying levels of restriction	Four states with independent authority; 18 states and DC with dependent authority	Thirty states with prescriptive authority with varying levels of restriction; in 8 states, authority limited to psych–mental health CNS

the labeling and packaging requirements to be followed. It does not exclude specific prescribers from dispensing medication. Currently NPs in all states may receive and/or dispense pharmaceutical samples. However, dispensing is often limited to specific sites or circumstances (Pearson, 1999). For instance, in some states, NPs may only be able to dispense samples of medications or may be limited to dispensing in sites located far from pharmacies or within specific types of clinics. Only a few states, such as New Mexico and Arizona, allow unrestricted dispensing of medications.

Prescriptive issues still remain. The question of whether a prescription written by an NP can be filled by a central distribution pharmacy located in a state other than the one in which the NP is licensed had not come up at the time current laws governing pharmacy and pharmacists were written. Therefore no laws specifically address the issue. The Food and Drug Administration (FDA) has issued but not enforced guidelines stating that if a state recognizes a licensed prescriber and there is no specific regulation against it, pharmacists in other states should recognize as legal and fill an out-of-state prescription. However, many of these mail order pharmacies refuse to recognize the legitimacy of an NP prescription. As more and more health plans direct their members to use online or out-of-state mail order pharmacies to fill prescriptions, this is a major problem when the pharmacies refuse to recognize NP prescriptions and delay NP's patients from receiving needed medications. A search of relevant regulations suggest that only Texas pharmacy law may have some restrictions on whether they may fill an out-of-state prescription. NPs as individuals and as groups are petitioning both the FDA and the Federal Trade Commission (FTC) for support in requiring pharmacies to follow the previously established regulations and guidelines (see Table 2-1 for nursing summary).

RESEARCH ON THE PRESCRIPTIVE PRACTICES OF NURSES IN THE DIAGNOSING AND PRESCRIBING ROLES: NPs, CNMs, CRNAs, AND CNSs

Limitations on prescriptive practice can effectively restrict the public's access to affordable and comprehensive primary care delivered by diagnosing and prescribing nurses. Yet, despite the impact prescriptive privileges can have on access to care, a paucity of research exists on prescriptive practice. What research has been collected has been mostly on NPs who most strongly thought that not having prescriptive authority restricted their ability to deliver needed care.

The first studies of NP prescriptive practices were performed in the early 1980s. One of the largest studies was undertaken by the state of California in 1981 in an effort to guide future legislative initiatives surrounding prescriptive authority for NPs and other midlevel providers. After evaluating the prescriptive practices of over 400 providers in 261 ambulatory practice sites in many underserved areas, results revealed overwhelming support for prescriptive authority for NPs and other MLPs. All supervising physicians thought that the providers were competent prescribers, and 99% thought they made correct diagnoses. Patient acceptance was also high at 97%. Cost-effectiveness was evaluated as well, and it was found that $2.5 to $3 million more would be necessary to provide the same level of patient services if additional time had to be purchased from traditional providers such as physicians. Furthermore, clinic administrators believed that medical services would either be sharply curtailed or completely eliminated to significant population groups should prescriptive privileges be denied (Houghland, 1982).

An extension of the Houghland study examined the types and numbers of prescriptions written and the effect NP and patient demographics had on prescribing practices. More than 1700 prescriptions from 18 NPs who prescribed to a relatively young healthy female population were evaluated. Prescribing was guided by a formulary with physician and pharmacy consultation available as needed. Results showed a low prescribing rate, with 26% of the patients seen receiving prescriptions, and physician consultation required for only 5% of all prescribing encounters. Drugs prescribed were those commonly used in treatment of self-limiting health problems, including antibiotics, cough and cold preparations, vitamins, and topical applications (Rosenaur et al, 1984).

An earlier study similar to that of Rosenaur et al was conducted in 1982 by Monroe et al examining the prescribing practices of six master's-prepared NPs working in an urban ambulatory care facility and providing wellness-focused care to predominantly healthy women. Prescribing was again guided by a formulary, physician consultation was available, and similar findings were reported. Only one third of patients received a prescription; most prescriptions were for antibiotics and other commonly prescribed medications; prescriptions were appropriate, safe, and congruent with protocols; and physician consultation occurred for 8% of all medications prescribed.

Batey and Holland extended the study of prescriptive practices in their two studies (1983 and 1985) by analyzing the impact of prescriptive autonomy as revealed in state statutes and regulations on prescriptive practices. They compared prescriptive practices of NPs in states with relatively broad prescriptive authority with those with restrictive authority. They found that prescriptive practices were similar across diverse regulatory environments and physician consultation rates remained constant despite more stringent physician oversight requirements in the less-autonomous states. Across all settings, 48% of patients were given a prescription, and of those who received a prescription, 1.3 prescriptions were generated. The prescribing rate was affected by the degree of physician supervision, with the lowest rate of prescribing occurring in practice sites without a physician on staff. Additionally, the authors found that in states with statutes mandating prescribing by formulary, NPs prescribed essentially the same number of different medications as NPs in less restrictive states. Finally, nearly three fourths of all prescriptions generated were for antibiotics, respiratory preparations, analgesics, and hormones, specifically oral contraceptives.

In 1985, and again in 1994, studies examining NP prescriptive practices in Maryland were conducted using a methodology similar to that of Batey and Holland. These studies were unique in that they examined prescriptive practice of NPs both before and after NPs obtained prescriptive authority. Appling (1985) surveyed all NPs in Maryland, asking respondents to estimate the frequency and types of drugs prescribed and/or recommended. Unlike the findings in the previous studies, the 153 respondents (representing nearly 50% of the NP population) were active prescribers, generating at least one prescription for 56% of their patients. Of those patients receiving a prescription, usually two prescriptions were generated. These rates are higher than most previous NP studies and were generally thought to result from differing patient populations, that is, an older and presumably sicker patient group. Indeed, the prescriptive practices of the sample more closely resembled physician prescribing patterns (National Center for Health Statistics, 1983). Moreover, the NPs in this study prescribed more cardiovascular preparations, diuretics, and immunizations/vaccines. This resulted, again, from a differing population group.

The methods used by NPs in the Appling study to obtain medications for their patients included a variety of mechanisms because prescriptive authority was not yet available to NPs in the state. However, nearly 75% of all NPs used physician co-signature when prescribing. Presigned prescription pads and calling the pharmacy with a medication order were other methods used by NPs to obtain medication for their patients. The rate of physician consultation was also higher in this study, with NPs requesting advice for almost one fifth of all prescriptive events. Finally, practice specialty and employment site help account for these prescriptive practices, with the NP sample dominated by adult and women's health NPs. NPs working in health maintenance organizations and clinics prescribed most frequently.

Nearly a decade later the Appling study was replicated. During the ensuing years, enabling legislation was passed granting NPs in Maryland the ability to prescribe medications pursuant to a written agreement with a collaborating physician. Within these guidelines, most NPs had broad prescriptive authority, usually prescribing all categories of medications without specific protocols, formularies, or physician countersignature, and consulting with the collaborating physician only on an as-needed basis. Results from the replication study by Hoover (1994) demonstrated one major effect of the legislative change—a significant decrease in the number of NPs who prescribed using a physician countersignature, falling from 75% to 15%. Additionally, the frequency of physician consultation decreased from 18.6% to 7.6% in the later study. Yet in most other ways, NPs in 1990s prescribed very similarly to those in the 1980s despite broader prescriptive authority. They remained active prescribers, generating prescriptions for one third of patients seen; of those who received prescriptions, an average of three were written. Categories of drugs most frequently prescribed changed slightly, with antibiotics, contraceptives, nonsteroidal antiinflammatory drugs, cardiovascular agents, immunizations/vaccinations, respiratory drugs, and analgesics accounting for nearly three fourths of all prescriptions. NP specialty and practice sites continued to influence the types and numbers of prescriptions written, as in the previous study.

In 1988, Sullivan surveyed pharmacists in the state of Maryland to identify concerns among pharmacists on the issue of prescription writing by NPs. Using the concept of territorial defense, she demonstrated that pharmacists who had worked with NPs or who were aware of new legislative statutes granting prescriptive authority to NPs were more likely to be in agreement with the law. Even among those agreeing that NPs could have prescriptive authority, 97% wanted to see prescriptive privileges limited to specific drug categories such as over-the-counter, antihistamines/decongestants, nonsteroidal antiinflammatory drugs, and oral contraceptives. More than 90% of pharmacists thought that NPs should not be prescribing scheduled analgesics, psychotropic agents, and anginal/antiarrhythmics. Seventy percent of pharmacists thought physician collaboration in the prescribing process was necessary. However, pharmacists thought that if NPs had prescriptive authority, the possible benefits might include the following:

- Better access to the health care system
- Decreased waiting time for physician to see and examine patients
- Lowered cost to patients, as NPs generally prescribe fewer medications
- Greater responsibility and authority given to NPs
- Better handwriting than physicians
- Fewer errors than physicians

Some pharmacists felt just the opposite, that potential problems might develop if NPs had prescriptive authority. They expressed the following thoughts:

- Concern over insufficient knowledge of NPs
- Possibility that NPs might make more errors
- Possibility that NPs might increase the numbers of drugs prescribed and thus increase patient costs

Although most pharmacists were aware that NPs within Maryland had been given prescriptive authority, the majority were unclear if they had ever filled a prescription written by an NP and thus could not document any real problems with their performance.

In 1986, Harris and associates collected data for a national study on the appropriateness of prescribing decisions made by NPs and physicians. Both groups were given a hypothetical vignette and asked to make diagnostic and treatment decisions about the cases. A multidisciplinary panel of experts scored their anonymous responses. The NP group averaged higher scores rating appropriateness of prescribing decisions and ordered fewer drugs than physicians (1.7 versus 2.7 per patient).

In unpublished doctoral research, Slate (1996) used a computer encounter record to accurately document the practice patterns of a national sample of NPs from different states. Among the data collected were information showing that antibiotics were the most frequently prescribed type of medication, with 27.4% of visits resulting in a prescription for an antibiotic. Respiratory medications were the second most frequent prescriptions, with 17.7% of visits resulting in a prescription for one of these products. Analgesics and antipyretics accounted for 13.3% of visits. Other categories of medications were prescribed 3% to 10% of the time. Antimigraine and dermatologic medications were the least frequently prescribed in this study. These data were appropriately correlated with the diagnoses of patients seen, which were highly skewed toward respiratory infections. Data showed no statistically significant differences between the NPs practicing in states with more legislative restrictions on prescriptive practice and those in less legislatively restrictive environments with respect to medication-prescribing behaviors. The Slate research is unique in that all components of the patient encounter were recorded at the time the patient was seen, rather than relying on estimates of behavior or recall so common in other research studies of this topic.

TABLE 2-2 Medication Categories Prescribed by NPs (N = 1399)

Medication Category	Number	Percentage*
Antiinfectives	1139	81.4
Diuretics and cardiac agents	851	60.8
Respiratory	998	71.3
CNS	585	41.8
Gastrointestinal	979	70.0
Hormones, including OCPs	825	59.0
Antiinflammatories, analgesics, antipyretics, steroids	1120	80.1
Topicals	1040	74.3
Antineoplastic	64	4.6
Vitamins, nutritional	837	59.8

*Note: percents do not total 100 because each NP had multiple responses.
From Edmunds MW, Scudder LC: *Annual descriptive survey of prescriptive practices of nurse practitioners,* National Conference for Nurse Practitioners, Washington DC, 1996–1998, NPA, Inc.

Edmunds and Scudder (1996, 1997, 1998) collected data from a national sample of NP attendees at national NP conferences. Their most recent data, based on a sample of 1399, shows the medications currently ordered by this sample of NPs to be fairly consistent with other studies of prescriptive practice (Woodwell, 1997). However, because of their systematic annual data collection, they have been able to document a significant drop in percentage of prescriptions written for medications in all categories each year (Table 2-2).

In the 1998 study, 2.6% of NPs reported writing five or fewer prescriptions in a clinical day, whereas 17.3% reported writing more than 20 prescriptions per day. The majority of NPs (64.8%) wrote 11 to 20 prescriptions per day. The top 25 drugs prescribed by this sample include (in descending order) Bactrim, ibuprofen, amoxicillin, albuterol, hydrocortisone, naproxen, cephalexin, Augmentin, azithromycin, Lotrimin, ranitidine, metronidazole, erythromycin, ciprofloxacin, immunizations, Claritin, beclomethasone, Synthroid, Biaxin, Prilosec, estrogen, Cortisporin, fluconazole, Zoloft, and Zovirax.

The Edmunds and Scudder data also demonstrate that NPs frequently recommend over-the-counter products. A total of 47.6% of the NPs recommend 5 to 10 over-the-counter preparations a day, 17% recommend 10 to 20 over-the-counter preparations a day, and 35% recommend less than 5 over-the-counter preparations a day. Thirty-three percent of the sample had their own DEA number, 25.8% used a physician's DEA number, and 41.0% do not prescribe drugs requiring DEA numbers. (The annual trend is for more NPs to have their own DEA number. The relatively large numbers of NPs who do not prescribe drugs requiring DEA numbers is not to be interpreted as meaning that those NPs cannot obtain DEA numbers. A large number of NPs working in employee health, occupational health, or pediatric clinics report that they have relatively low requirements for controlled substances or may be in the military or US Public Health Service and be exempt from DEA registration.) More than 63% of NPs were free to order any drugs they wished, without restriction to an institutional, state, federal, or Medicaid formulary. Seventy-seven percent of patients were managed with little or no NP consultation with physicians.

These several studies conducted over the years are remarkably consistent in their findings. NPs tend to order medications appropriate to their preparation as primary care providers and for patients across the age span. NPs consistently order fewer prescriptions than do physicians. These conclusions seem to dispel the concerns expressed by some physicians and pharmacists that, if NPs were given prescriptive authority, they would have no restraints on what they might order (Sullivan, 1988).

A synthesis of the data supplied by Batey and Holland (1985), Appling (1985), Hoover (1994), and Slate (1996) suggests that the degree of prescriptive autonomy granted by legislative statutes and administrative regulations has little impact on the overall prescriptive practice of NPs. The types and numbers of prescriptions remain relatively stable across regulatory environments, with only the methodology used to generate a prescription varying significantly. Thus it is difficult to justify imposing strict regulatory limitations on NP prescribing (Safreit, 1992). This conclusion has been shared by an increasing number of state legislative bodies despite consistent attempts by the medical profession to block legislative advances in prescriptive authority.

BARRIERS TO PRACTICE FOR NURSES IN THE DIAGNOSING AND PRESCRIBING ROLES

Four major problems have persisted that prevent the full implementation of APN roles:

1. Regulatory irregularity among the states authorizing practice continues to be a major problem for a profession that is fairly mobile. The differences in definitions, standards, scope of practice, and restrictions defined by a nurse practice act vary from state to state and impose difficulties on health professionals as they move to a new state, practice in neighboring states, or provide services over the Internet. The NCSBN has instituted an interstate nursing compact that would help solve some of these problems. A multistate license would allow a nurse to practice in all states that sign on to an agreement, so that the nurse would not require separate licensure in each state (Sharp, 1997). Requirements for a second license for APNs has been discussed for years (Edmunds, 1992) and continues to remain an issue (Robinson, McKenzie & Niemer, 1996; Sharp, 1997).
2. There has developed increased antagonism from organized medical groups competing with APNs for patients. There is now a fairly large group of very talented CNMs and NPs, some with 30 years of experience. These nurses are ready to be more independent and want to receive direct reimbursement for the care they provide and not just remain as salaried employees of the physician. They are aware that they have made major financial contributions to many hospitals and practices, but most of them have not participated in the rewards. NP salaries have not risen much higher than those of traditional nurses. Lack of direct reimbursement to NPs for their services has been tied to a fight over who is designated as a primary care provider. For many years NPs were designated as primary care providers for Medicaid patients (the poor) and in school-based clinics (children). However, with recent Medicare reimbursement and managed care panel status being tied to the primary care provider designation, physicians are rethinking whether NPs should be able to get direct reimbursement rather than having all reimbursement money go through them.
3. The growing number of NP graduates is of great concern to those NPs already in clinical practice. The profusion of NP programs, many with inexperienced or unqualified faculty, and the fight to obtain adequate clinical experiences for all the students, raises questions not only about the quantity but about the quality and competency of student educational preparation. With a dwindling employment base, NPs are already facing shrinking finances as new graduates drive down annual salaries, cannot find employment, or take jobs away from more experienced (and more costly) NPs.
4. Finally, lack of a mechanism to require programs to comply with NONPF and AACN curricular guidelines *hurts* NPs. Standardized program accreditation procedures, consistent state licensing requirements, and comparable certification examinations should be mandatory to ensure the high standard of quality practice essential for NP role survival in a health care arena that is increasingly competitive. Movement in all these areas is beginning as professional groups tackle these issues.

SUMMARY

The diversity among the advanced diagnosing and prescribing nurses has proved to be a limitation in obtaining uniform prescriptive authority. Although data suggest their clinical practice is accepted, safe, and effective, legislative and reimbursement barriers continue to limit their full utilization in health care.

RESOURCES FOR PATIENTS AND PROVIDERS

http://www. aana.com
Contains basic information and facts as well as links to many state chapter web sites.

American College of Nurse-Midwives, http://acnm.org
Includes a summary of the most up-to-date information on all components of midwifery practice.

American College of Nurse Practitioners, http://www.nurse.org/acnp/
Has fact sheets for review on many components of nurse practitioner practice.

Nurse Practitioner Alternatives, Inc., http://www.npedu.com
A company providing continuing professional education for NPs. Supports an interactive forum and "Frequently Asked Questions (FAQs) about NPs," including an annotated bibliography of key articles and research about NPs.

REFERENCES

American Association of Colleges of Nursing: *The essentials of master's education for advanced practice nursing,* Washington, DC, 1996, 1998, American Association of Colleges of Nursing.

American Association of Nurse Anesthetists: *Guidelines for clinical privileges,* Park Ridge, IL, 1996a, American Association of Nurse Anesthetists.

American Association of Nurse Anesthetists: *Scope and standards for nurse anesthesia practice,* Park Ridge, IL, 1996b, American Association of Nurse Anesthetists.

American Association of Nurse Anesthetists: *Qualifications and capabilities of the certified registered nurse anesthetist,* Park Ridge, IL, 1992, American Association of Nurse Anesthetists.

American Association of Nurse Anesthetists: *Nurse anesthetists: providing anesthesia into the next century: executive summary,* Park Ridge, IL, 1998, American Association of Nurse Anesthetists.

American Association of Nurse Anesthetists: Annual Committee Reports of the AANA, 1989-1990, AANA News Bull 44(10)(Suppl):37-38, 1990.

American College of Nurse Midwives: *Accreditation of education programs,* Washington, DC, 1992, American College of Nurse Midwives.

American College of Nurse Midwives: *Code of ethics,* Washington, DC, 1997, American College of Nurse Midwives.

American College of Nurse Midwives: *Core competencies for basic nurse-midwifery,* Washington, DC, 1997, American College of Nurse Midwives.

American College of Nurse Midwives: *Philosophy,* Washington, DC, 1989, American College of Nurse Midwives.

American College of Nurse Midwives: *Standards for the practice of nurse-midwifery,* Washington, DC, 1992, American College of Nurse Midwives.

American College of Nurse Midwives: *Nurse midwifery today; handbook on state legislation,* Washington, DC, 1997, American College of Nurse Midwives.

American College of Nurse Midwives: *Midwifery education,* Washington, DC, 1997, American College of Nurse Midwives.

American Nurses Association: *Nursing: a social policy statement,* Kansas City, MO, 1980, American Nurses Association.

American Nurses Association: *The role of the clinical nurse specialist,* Kansas City, MO, 1986, American Nurses Association.

Appling S: *Prescriptive practices of nurse practitioners in Maryland,* unpublished master's thesis, Baltimore, MD, 1985, University of Maryland at Baltimore.

Batey M, Holland J: Impact of structural autonomy accorded through state regulatory policies on nurses' prescribing patterns, *IMAGE J Nurs Scholar* 15:84-89, 1983.

Batey M, Holland J: Prescribing practices among nurse practitioners in adult and family health, *Am J Pub Health* 75:258-260, 1985.

Bell D: Writing of prescriptions through delegation, *Minn Med* 63:337-338, 1980.

Bell K, Mill JI: CNM effectiveness in the health maintenance organization obstetric team, *Obstet Gynecol* 74:112-116, 1989.

Bosma J: Using nurse practitioner certification for state nursing regulation: an update, *Nurse Pract* 22:213, 1997.

Breuninger K: CNS and NP role merger? *Nurse Pract* 21:12, 1996.

Brown SA, Grimes DE: A meta-analysis of nurse practitioners and nurse-midwives in primary care, *Nurs Res* 44:332-339, 1995.

Bullough B: *The law and the expanding nursing role,* ed 2, New York, 1980, Appleton-Century-Crofts.

Buppert C: *Nurse practitioner's business practice and legal guide,* Gaithersburg, MD, 1999, Aspen Publishers.

Butler J et al: Supportive nurse-midwife care is associated with a reduced incidence of cesarean section, *Am J Obstet Gynecol* 168:1407-1413, 1993.

Capan P et al: Nurse-managed clinics provide access and improved health care, *Nurse Pract* 18:500-505, 1993.

Carr M: Merging advanced practice roles, *Nurse Pract* 21:160, 1996.

Clark S, Martin JA, Taffel SM: Trends and characteristics of births attended by midwives, *Statistical Bulletin,* Jan-Feb, 78:1, NY, 1997, Metropolitan Life Insurance Co.

Council on Certification of Nurse Anesthetists: *1998 Recertification candidate handbook,* Park Ridge, IL, 1998, Council on Certification of Nurse Anesthetists.

Davis LG et al: Cesarean section rates in low-risk private patients managed by CNMs and obstetricians, *J Nurs Midwifery* 39:91-97, 1994.

Edmunds MW: Council's pursuit of national standardization for advanced practice nursing meets with resistance, *Nurse Pract* 17:81-83, 1992.

Edmunds MW: Evaluation of nurse practitioner effectiveness: an overview of the literature, *Evaluation Health Professions* 1:69-82, Spring, 1978.

Edmunds MW: Should clinical nurse specialists cost out nursing services? *Clin Specialist* 12:12, 1992 (guest editorial).

Edmunds MW, Scudder LC: *Annual descriptive survey of prescriptive practices of nurse practitioners,* National Conference for Nurse Practitioners, Washington, DC, 1996, 1997, 1998, NPA, Inc.

Fink JL: Drug prescribing by physician extenders, *Drugs Health Care* 2:195-199, 1975.

Ford LC: A nurse for all settings: the nurse practitioner, *Nurs Outlook* 27:516-521, 1979.

Harris L: *Nurse practitioners and physicians,* Study No. 851025, New York, 1986, Louis Harris and Associates.

Hoover A: *Prescriptive practices of nurse practitioners in Maryland,* unpublished master's thesis, Baltimore, MD, 1994, University of Maryland.

Horton B, Jordan LM: Profile of nurse anesthesia programs, *J Am Assoc Nurs Anesthetists* 62:400-404, 1994.

Houghland D: *Final report to the legislature and the Healing Arts Licensing Boards: prescribing and dispensing pilot projects,* Office of Statewide Health Planning and Development: Division of Health Profession Development, State of California, 1982.

Hueston WJ, Rudy MA: A comparison of labor and delivery management between CNMs and family physicians, *J Fam Prac* 375:449-454, 1993.

Kelly LY: Nursing practice acts, *Am J Nurs* 74:1311-1319, 1974.

Knedle-Murray ME et al: Production process substitution in maternity care: issues of cost, quality, and outcomes by nurse-midwives and physician providers, *Med Care Rev* 50:91-112, 1993.

Lewis EP, editor: *The clinical nurse specialist,* New York, 1970, American Journal of Nursing.

MacDorman MF, Singh GK: Midwifery care, social and medical risk factors and birth outcomes in the USA, *J Epidemiol Community Health,* May, 1998.

Monroe D et al: Prescribing patterns of nurse practitioners, *Am J Nurs* 82:1538-1542, 1982.

National Center for Health Statistics: *Drugs most frequently used in office-based practice: National Ambulatory Medical Care Survey, 1981,* No. DHHS Pub. No. (PHS) 83-1250, Hyattsville, MD, April, 1983, US Public Health Service.

National Council of State Boards of Nursing et al (National Organization of Nurse Practitioner Faculties): *Curriculum guidelines and regulatory criteria for family nurse practitioners seeking prescriptive authority to manage pharmacotherapeutics in primary care, summary report, 1998,* HRSA 98-41, Washington, DC, 1998, US DHHS.

National Organization of Nurse Practitioner Faculties: *Advanced nursing practice: curriculum guidelines and program standards for nurse practitioner education,* Washington, DC, 1995, National Organization of Nurse Practitioner Faculties.

National Organization of Nurse Practitioner Faculties: *Guidelines for family nurse practitioner curricular planning,* Washington, DC, 1980, National Organization of Nurse Practitioner Faculties.

National Organization of Nurse Practitioner Faculties: *Advanced nursing practice: nurse practitioner curriculum guidelines,* Washington, DC, 1990, National Organization of Nurse Practitioner Faculties.

National Organization of Nurse Practitioner Faculties: *Primary care nurse practitioner graduate outcomes,* Washington, DC, 1993, National Organization of Nurse Practitioner Faculties.

National Organization of Nurse Practitioner Faculties: *Curriculum guidelines and criteria for evaluation of pharmacology content to prepare family nurse practitioners for prescriptive authority and managing pharmacotherapeutics in primary care,* Washington, DC, 1996, National Organization of Nurse Practitioner Faculties.

National Organization of Nurse Practitioner Faculties: *Model program standards for nurse practitioner programs,* Washington, DC, 1994, National Organization of Nurse Practitioner Faculties.

Nielsen JR: *Handbook of federal drug law,* ed 2, Philadelphia, 1992, Lea & Febiger.

Oakley D et al: Processes of care: comparisons of CNM and obstetricians, *J Nurs Midwifery* 40:399-409, 1995.

Office of Technology Assessment, US Congress: *Nurse practitioners, physician assistants, and certified nurse midwives: a policy analysis,* Health technology case study 37, Washington, DC, 1986, Office of Technology Assessment.

Pearson L: Annual update of how each state stands on legislative issues affecting advanced nursing practice, *Nurs Pract* 24:16-83, 1999.

Pearson L: Annual update of how each state stands on legislative issues affecting advanced nursing practice, *Nurs Pract* 27:10-52, 2002.

Reed A: Trends in state laws and regulations affecting nurse-midwives: 1995-1997, *J Nurs Midwifery* 42:421, 1997.

Riehl JP, McVay JW: *The clinical nurse specialist: interpretations,* New York, 1973, Appleton-Century-Crofts.

Robinson DL, McKenzie C, Niemer L: Second licensure for advanced practice: current status, *Nurs Pract* 21:71, 1996.

Rogers M: Nursing: to be or not to be? *Nurs Outlook* 20:42-46, 1972.

Rosenaur J et al: Prescribing behaviors of primary care nurse practitioners, *Am J Public Health* 74:10-13, 1984.

Rosenblatt RA: Interspecialty differences in the obstetric care of low-risk women, *Am J Public Health* 87:344-351, 1997.

Safriet B: Health care dollars and regulatory sense: the role of advanced practice nursing, *Yale J Regulation* 9:417-488, Summer, 1992.

Sharp N: Regional or multistate licensure: is it coming soon? *Nurs Pract* 22:170, 1997.

Slate AC: *A comparison of activities of primary care nurse practitioner practice in legislatively more restrictive versus less restrictive regions using an author-constructed encounter information system,* unpublished doctoral dissertation, Baltimore, MD, 1996, University of Maryland at Baltimore School of Nursing.

Sparacino PSA, Cooper DM, Minarik PA, editors: *The clinical nurse specialist: implementation and impact,* Norwalk, CT, 1990, Appleton & Lange.

Sullivan D: *Prescriptive privileges for nurse practitioners: a survey of pharmacists in Maryland,* master's thesis, Baltimore, MD, 1988, University of Maryland at Baltimore School of Nursing.

Sutliff LS: Myth, mystique, and monopoly in the prescription of medicine, *Nurs Pract* 21:15, 1996.

Tobin MH: *Nurse anesthetists and prescriptive authority: what is it and do you need it?* Presentation at Fall Assembly of States, American Association of Nurse Anesthetists, 1991.

Tobin MH: Personal telephone interview by MW Edmunds on prescriptive status of CRNAs with American Association of Nurse Anesthetists Director of State Government Affairs, January 26, 1998.

Trandel-Korenchuk D, Trandel-Korenchuk K: How state laws recognize advanced nursing practice, *Nurs Outlook* 26:613-619, 1978.

USHHS, Health Resources and Services Administration, Agency for Health Care Policy and Research: *Curriculum guidelines & regulatory criteria for family nurse practitioners seeking prescriptive authority to manage pharmacotherapeutics in primary care: summary report, 1998.* Washington, DC, 1998, US Government Printing Office, HRSA 98-41.

USHHS, Health Resources and Services Administration, Bureau of Health Professions, Division of Nursing: *Nurse practitioner primary care competencies in specialty areas: adult, family, gerontological, pediatric, and women's health.* Washington, DC, April 2002, US Government Printing Office, HRSA 00-0532 [p].

Woodwell DA: *National Ambulatory Medical Care Survey: 1996 summary. Advance data from vital and health statistics,* No. 295, Hyattsville, MD, 1997, National Center for Health Statistics.

CHAPTER 3

Prescriptive Authority and the Physician Assistant

James Cawley

In over 35 years of clinical practice, physician assistants (PAs) have gained considerable legitimacy as a profession in the American health care system. New state health occupations regulatory acts were necessary with the introduction of PAs and nurse practitioners (NPs) in 1965 to allow them to perform tasks that were traditionally in the domain of medicine. Legislative and regulatory changes in state medical practice acts to accommodate PA practice included defining the required qualifications for occupational licensure or certification, defining scope of practice, developing supervisory stipulations, establishing board representation and governance policies, creating professional disciplinary standards, and granting prescribing authority.

Acceptance of PAs by US physicians, patients, and other health professions has grown steadily. PAs have proved to be safe and effective health care providers (Office Technology Assessment, 1986). PAs demonstrate versatility across clinical practice settings and are employed in private medical offices, teaching and community hospitals, managed care delivery systems, and other health care settings. The medical generalist orientation of PAs allows them to assume functions effectively not only in primary care roles but also in inpatient care services and medical specialty practices.

Prescribing authority for PAs was won through legal and political maneuvering on a state-by-state basis over the past three decades. It has been a long but successful trip to increased recognition of the skills and contributions of the PA role.

OVERVIEW OF PA ROLE

PAs are health professionals who practice medicine under physician supervision. As members of the health care team, PAs provide a broad range of medical diagnostic, therapeutic, and preventive care services. PAs are qualified by formal education and authorized by national certification to exercise a designated level of autonomy in performing clinical responsibilities within their scope of practice and supervisory relationship. PA clinical practice spans both primary care and specialty care roles in a wide range of medical practice settings in rural and urban areas. In addition to their clinical roles, PA professional responsibilities may include providing health services that complement physician services, such as health promotion and disease prevention and/or assuming educational, research, and/or administrative duties (Jones & Cawley, 1994; Cawley, 2002).

Qualifications

All states have specific requirements for the PA seeking entry into practice. Typically, individuals must be graduates of a PA educational program accredited by the Accreditation Review Committee Physician Assistant (ARC-PA) of the Commission on Accreditation of Allied Health Educational Programs (CAAHEP) and most states require they pass the Physician Assistant National Certifying Examination (PANCE).

Education

PA educational programs comprise intensive 2- to 3-year biomedical-based curricula emphasizing a primary care/medical generalist approach. Nationally, PA educational programs do not award a single academic credential. The competency-based model of PA qualification for medical practice is demonstrated by completion of an approved educational program and receiving national board certification, rather than by a process tied to a specific academic degree. This format has gained acceptance among medical licensing boards and occupations regulators, although pressure for a standard academic degree awarded for PA education will continue to increase in the future (Cawley & Jones, 1997). Thus a PA may have an AA, a BA, a BS, or an MS degree. There were 134 ARC-PA–accredited PA educational programs in 2002, an increase from 107 in 1998. More than 65 programs now award the master's degree, all of which have been implemented since 1988. The remaining programs (55) award either the bachelor's degree or a certificate or associate's degree. PA programs are sponsored by universities, academic health centers, medical schools, teaching hospitals, and colleges and graduate approximately 5000 students annually (American Academy of Physician Assistants, 1998).

PA academic training usually comprises 10 to 12 months of didactic course work with instruction in (1) the basic sciences—anatomy, physiology, biochemistry, microbiology, pathology, and pharmacology—and (2) the basic clinical sciences—history-taking and physical examination, behavioral science, clinical medicine, and diagnosis, including pharmacologic aspects of patient management.

Because a knowledge of pharmacology is a required component of practice for a PA, ARC-PA–accredited PA programs must include formal course instruction in basic and clinical pharmacology. ARC-PA standards mandate that PA programs teach "the principles of clinical pharmacology and medical therapeutics appropriate to the medical therapy for common problems in clinical practice" (Standards for Accreditation of Education Programs for PA, 2000).

During the second academic year, PA students obtain clinical training and experience by rotating through inpatient and outpatient settings. Required rotations typically include inpatient medicine, outpatient medicine, surgery, pediatrics, obstetrics/gynecology, emergency medicine, and psychiatry, followed by several clinical electives and, commonly, a final preceptorship in primary care. The contents of PA clinical rotations and preceptorships stress the appropriate use of drugs and medications as part of patient care management.

The American Academy of Physician Assistants (AAPA) estimates that the typical PA student receives 105 to 110 weeks of required medical instruction (academic and clinical experiences); medical students receive about 153 weeks of analogous instruction. Pharmacology and medical therapeutics are part of the core requirements of every PA program. Of 55 PA programs surveyed in 1990, 49 averaged 66 hours of instruction in pharmacology, with a range of 28 to 128 hours. It is anticipated that a model clinical therapeutics curriculum developed at the University of Utah will be adopted by a majority of PA programs.

Certification

The national certifying examination for PAs, the PANCE, comprises both written and practical components, with test item content and scoring standards being developed by the National Board of Medical Examiners (NBME). The National Commission on Certification of Physician Assistants (NCCPA) has administered this examination since 1973, and NCCPA certification is required for PA qualification in 47 states. More than 92% of the 45,000 PAs in active clinical practice in 2002 hold NCCPA certification (American Academy of Physician Assistants, 2001).

PANCE question item content assumes that PAs possess academic and clinical training in patient pharmacologic management. On any given PANCE administration, 32% to 38% of the examination items relate to pharmaceutical aspects of patient care (National Commission on Certification of Physician Assistants, 1994). To meet requirements for continuing certification, NCCPA requires PAs to obtain 100 hours of continuing medical education (CME) hours annually and to recertify by formal examination (the Physician Assistant National Recertifying Examination [PANRE]) every 6 years. Nineteen states require PAs to maintain ongoing NCCPA certification, and a number of states have similar CME requirements for PAs for them to maintain state licensure (American Academy of Physician Assistants, 1998).

LEGAL FOUNDATION OF PA PRESCRIPTIVE AUTHORITY

Working with supervising physicians, PAs perform a wide range of delegated medical diagnostic and patient management tasks required in primary care and specialty practice settings, including prescribing medications. Although their clinical practice duties overlap considerably with those of physicians, PAs work in a dependent practice mode.

Initial PA statutes took either a delegatory or regulatory direction. Some states passed PA statutes that were quite broad in nature. On a fundamental level, they simply affirmed the notion of physician task delegation without any specific delineation of the performance of those tasks (delegatory model). Other states enacted laws that accepted the principle of physician task delegation as the basis of PA practice but went further in placing certain stipulations on PA scope of practice and medical task performance (regulatory model). The current trend among a majority of states is toward the regulatory model (Gara, 1990). State regulatory agencies now tend to recognize prescribing activities within circumscribed boundaries by PAs as an essential component of their modern practice roles (Hansen, 1992; Sekscenski et al, 1994).

In a recent comparative analysis of state regulatory experiences and policy approaches in authorizing PA prescribing, Cohen (1996) found that experiences and policy varied widely. Approval of PA prescribing authority has been controversial in some states. Prescribing has been a particularly troublesome barrier to PA practice effectiveness in Maryland and Ohio. A key determinant in the outcome of whether prescriptive authority would be granted was the position of the involved stakeholder groups (medical societies, nursing groups) (Group Health Association of America, 1992).

One major aspect of treatment that has limited PA practice is lack of full prescriptive authority. When legally authorized, the privilege of prescribing is usually a restricted one. Because medication is the most frequently employed treatment in medical care, the absence of this privilege limits the scope of medical practice; it restricts where and how PAs can practice. With few exceptions, the legal right to prescribe is still largely the exclusive domain of the physician. Consequently, the issue of prescribing privilege is a significant concern of the PA profession. It is also an issue among managers, administrators, and policy makers in the larger health care community because PAs appear to be less costly substitutes for physicians in a variety of clinical situations (Cohen, 1996).

Statutes authorizing state medical and health occupation boards to regulate medical practitioners constitute the legal basis of PA prescribing activities. Typical state regulatory acts establish PAs as the agents of their supervising physicians, and PAs maintain direct liability for the services they render to patients. Supervising physicians define the broad parameters of PA practice activities and the standard to which PA services are held and are vicariously liable for services performed by their PAs.

The legal basis of PA practice is predicated on the doctrine of *respondeat superior,* which affirms and defines the authority of a licensed physician to delegate medical tasks to a qualified health professional working in that practice. A key stipulation is that the physician must appropriately supervise PA practice activities and assume liability for any adverse actions (Hooker & Cawley, 1997).

State health occupations regulatory policy emanating from this tenet has evolved with the stipulation that physician-PA practices should be required to appropriately define the clinical role activities, prescribing activities, and terms of supervision of the PAs they employ (Gara, 1989).

Most states in which PAs are legally authorized to prescribe have constraints on their prescribing. Such constraints may include the following:

- A physician co-signature is required on an order within a given timeframe for inpatient medical or therapeutic orders.
- Limitations are placed on the categories of medications that may be prescribed, that is, drugs delineated in a specific formulary or medication list.
- FDA Schedule II agents (i.e., those defined by the Controlled Substances Act as having the potential for abuse) are excluded from prescriptive authority.
- Prescribing authorization is granted only when drug treatment protocols are used.

BOX 3-1

COMMON STATE REQUIREMENTS FOR PA PRESCRIPTIVE AUTHORITY

- Cosignature requirements
- Restriction to formulary; exclusionary formulary
- Controlled substances (Schedule II medications)
- Restriction by practice setting
- Required practice guidelines/management protocols
- Educational requirements
  - Minimum academic degree
  - Continuing medical education

- Limitation is placed on the quantities of drugs that may be prescribed by PAs; a few states have limited prescribing authority to specific medical practice settings (Ohio, Maryland) or to an outpatient or nonhospital setting.

Box 3-1 lists common state requirements imposed on PAs seeking prescriptive authority (American Academy of Physician Assistants, 1997).

Among the states with prescribing regulations in place, only a few grant PAs prescribing privileges for Schedule II through Schedule IV drugs in addition to "prescription legend" drug preparations. Schedule I drugs are not relevant to this discussion because it is illegal for licensed practitioners in the United States to prescribe these drugs. The prescribing privilege for Schedule II drugs is a limited one in about six states. In the other states, the prescribing privilege applies to Schedule III through Schedule V drugs, including prescription legend drugs, with some restrictions by various states on prescribing Schedule III drugs.

Drug preparations referred to as "prescription legend" drugs can be prescribed by PAs with prescribing privileges. PAs may also prescribe over-the-counter medications or drug preparations that do not, by law, require the written order of a licensed prescriber.

HISTORY OF PA PRESCRIPTIVE AUTHORITY AMONG STATES

The first statute authorizing prescribing privileges for PAs was passed in Colorado in 1969. That statute stipulated that graduates of the University of Colorado Child Health Associate Program (one of the first academic health center–based PA programs offering a focus in pediatrics) could prescribe medications without immediate consultation from a supervising physician, provided that the latter subsequently approved the prescription. New York authorized PA prescribing privileges in 1972; later, Maine, New Mexico, North Carolina, Oklahoma, and Kansas followed. By 1979, PA prescribing privileges existed in 11 states (Weston, 1980).

Currently, PAs are recognized as health care practitioners authorized to perform physician-delegated medical diagnostic and therapeutic tasks (diagnosis, testing, treating, and follow-up of patients) by professional licensing boards in all 50 states and the District of Columbia. Mississippi was the last state to formally recognize PA practice.

All except three states (Indiana, Louisiana, and Ohio) authorize the supervising physician to delegate prescriptive responsibility to PAs, and 40 states include controlled substances in that authorization. Although some states initially required that PAs use the supervising physician's Drug Enforcement Administration (DEA) registration number when prescribing controlled medications,[8] all states that allow PA prescribing of controlled substances now authorize PAs to obtain DEA registration. PAs are authorized by statute or regulation to prescribe in the aforementioned states, as well as Guam, the District of Columbia, and in most federal facilities, including the military, state, and federal correctional institutions and the Veterans' Administration. Table 3-1 lists the details on prescriptive authority among the different states.

PAs prescribe in a wide variety of settings, yet there have been only a small amount of empirical data on how and when PAs prescribe. Studies of patient expectations and satisfaction levels affirm the notion that PAs are expected to perform prescribing activities as part of their roles in patient management. One survey administered to PAs working in states with prescriptive authority found that 90% of PAs included prescriptive authority as part of their authorized clinical duties (Willis, 1990).

Nationwide, PAs are estimated to have over 150 million patient visits and to write 165 million prescriptions. This amounts to about 8% of all prescriptions written annually (American Academy of Physician Assistants, 1996). Among the medications most commonly prescribed by PAs were antihypertensives, cholesterol-lowering agents, bronchodilators/respiratory therapy agents, agents to treat diabetes, gastrointestinal medications, and oral contraceptives. According to data from a national survey of medical staffs of health maintenance organizations, 60% of PAs versus 74% of advanced practice nurses held prescribing credentials (Group Health Association of America, 1992; Cawley, 1995).

Sixty percent or more of the PAs reported prescribing urinary/vaginal agents, upper respiratory medications, gastrointestinal agents, antiarthritic anti-gout agents, and analgesics. The mean number of prescriptions written by each PA was 50 per week (American Academy of Physician Assistants, 1997).

In 2002, the 47 states with PA prescribing privileges encompass over three fourths of the practicing US PAs, covering approximately 75% of the total US population. New York has long permitted physicians to delegate prescribing privilege to the PAs they supervise. In New York, outpatient prescribing is restricted to nonscheduled drugs. A randomized sample of New York PAs surveyed regarding their prescribing activities revealed that the most frequently prescribed drugs were, in order, oral antibiotics, antihistamine/decongestants, topical antibiotics, pain/fever medications, and otic/ophthalmologic preparations. Prescribing PAs reported recommending over-the-counter preparations an average of nine times a day. Aspirin and other pain medications, cold and allergy products, cough preparations, and antacids were among the most frequently recommended medications. PAs in nonhospital settings, representing about half of the respondents, reported writing an average of 17 outpatient prescriptions per day. Eighty-eight percent of PAs agreed with the statement that "the average patient does not feel

TABLE 3-1 PA Prescriptive Authority Status among States

State	Authority	Restrictions Including Controlled Substances
AL	X	Noncontrolled from board formulary
AK	X	Physician name and DEA number required on prescription Sch III-V
AZ	X	No refills: DEA registration required; Sch II-III limited to 72-hr supply; Sch IV-V, 34-day supply
AR		
CA	X	Must have patient-specific order from MD
CO	X	Written protocol on case-by-case and per-patient-visit basis required: MD countersign on charts required within 3 days; controlled
CT	X	Sch IV-V
DE	X	Therapeutics approved by physician and board
D.C.	X	Noncontrolled only
FL	X	Board formulary
GA	X	Delegation by physician, Sch III-V; limited to 30-day supply; maintenance drugs limited to 90-day supply
HI	X	
ID	X	Board formulary
IL		
IN		
IA	X	Must be ordered by physician in written protocol or in an emergency; Sch III-V orally, Sch II orally in emergency
KY	X	
LA		
ME	X	DEA registration; Sch III-V
MD		Medical order writing in hospitals, correctional systems, public health clinics
MA	X	Sch II-V
MI	X	Noncontrolled only
MN	X	NCCPA-certified required; excludes anesthetics, other than local
MS		
MO	X	
MT	X	Delegation by physician, Sch II-V; limited Sch II to 34-day supply
NE	X	Physician authorization required; meds include 72-hour supply, Sch II
NV	X	Board approval and pharmacy registration required; controlled; limited to supervising physician's prescriptive authority
NH	X	Pharmacy law exam required; controlled
NJ		
NM	X	Board formulary; Sch II-V
NY	X	Noncontrolled only
NC	X	Pharmacy board approval required; Sch II-V; Sch II-III limited to 7-day supply
ND	X	Sch III-V
OH		
OK	X	Noncontrolled on board formulary
OR	X	Physician and board approval and DEA registration required; Sch III-V
PA	X	Formulary drugs, except Sch I-II and parenterals (except insulin and allergy kits)

From The American Academy of Physician Assistants and the Intergovernmental Health Policy Project, Washington, DC, 1998, The George Washington University.

TABLE 3-1 PA Prescriptive Authority Status among States—cont'd

State	Authority	Restrictions Including Controlled Substances
RI	X	State drug control office and DEA registration required; Sch V
SC	X	Sch V
SD	X	Sch II-V; Sch II limited to 48-hour supply
TN	X	Noncontrolled only
TX	X	Limited to underserved areas, practices with high rates of indigent patients, physician's primary practice site, hospital, or other site; individually determined dangerous drug prescriptions limited to physician's primary practice site
UT	X	Sch IV-V (7-day supply)
VT	X	Physician authorization required; individually determined
VA	X	Noncontrolled on board formulary
WA	X	DEA number required; Sch II-V
WV	X	Two years of experience; board-approved pharmacology course and NCCPA; board formulary; DEA required; Sch III-V
WI	X	With written protocols and consultation with physician; controlled
WY	X	DEA number required; Sch III-V

treated without getting a prescription." Seventy-one percent agreed that pharmaceutical companies regularly calling on PAs are "those whose products the PA will tend to prescribe." Pharmaceutical sales representatives were mentioned by PAs as one of the five factors that most influenced their selection of drug products (Mittman & Mirotznik, 1984).

PA professional practice activities, including prescribing activities, tend to be closely regulated by health occupations licensing agencies, most commonly boards of medicine. In some instances, PA and other health occupations regulation is assigned to boards of professional regulation, education, or the healing arts. In 11 states, there are specific PA licensing boards.

During the past few years, there has been a tremendous effort by state PA chapters to revamp and modernize state enabling legislation. The advent of managed care has made the issue of licensure an important one in regard to reimbursement and credentialing. Most managed care organizations will not deal with someone who is not a licensed provider. A number of states certify or register PAs, and this has led to problems when managed care organizations began contracting with physicians and groups. There also is difficulty with a number of unlicensed personnel performing functions similar to those of PAs and NPs and requesting payment. This has led payers to deny payment for services unless a physician provided them. Several states have been successful in converting from certification or registration to licensure. They have been successful in removing restrictive language from their acts and loosening up the scope of practice as well.

Organized medicine has also played a pivotal role in state regulation of PA practice. Physicians wrote many of the early PA laws because there were no PAs to write them. As the profession grew, there was predictable strife over how PAs would fit into the health care system. In some states, organized medicine was the state PA chapter's strongest ally; in others, it was their most significant opponent.

In many states, the state medical society is regarded as the voice of medicine. As state legislators considered bills that modified PA regulation and delegated scope of practice, they commonly asked, "What's the medical society's position on this bill?" During the past decade, state medical societies have shown an increased willingness to work as colleagues with PA state societies on health law issues. Today, 42 state PA organizations have sustained relationships with their respective state medical societies (Davis, 2002). This increased level of communication has had a positive impact on the development of state laws and regulations governing PA practice.

The policies of organized medicine on the national level have also played a significant role in state regulation of PA practice over the past 10 years, the result of stable and productive relationships with physician leaders. In 1995, the AMA issued guidelines that offered a framework for physician-PA practice; these were adopted as policy by many state medical societies and used as a default position by others (Davis, 2002).

RESEARCH ON PRESCRIPTIVE PRACTICES OF PAs

PA employers have long expected PAs to possess clinical skills in drug management. PA competency, safety, and effectiveness in discharging prescribing activities in medical practices are well established over three decades of clinical experience. Safety, in this context, refers to prescribing activity that minimizes the risk of an adverse consequence. Effectiveness is the contribution of the drug prescribed to the outcome of treatment. PA competence has been demonstrated in numerous health services research studies, as summarized in the following brief overview of the prescriptive practice literature.

Large proportions of PAs work in outpatient primary care settings. The quality of care provided by PAs in US Air Force primary medicine clinics was assessed in an Institute of Medicine report on the VA hospital system (IOM, 1992). PAs assumed a considerable portion of the care formerly provided by physicians. Quality of care judgments were based on diagnostic, therapeutic, and disposition criteria. Therapeutic criteria included desirable actions (e.g., prescribing the appropriate class of antibiotic for infectious otitis media at the first visit) and undesirable actions (e.g., prescribing an antibiotic for viral syndrome with gastroenteritis). On five of six such criteria identifying desirable therapeutic actions, PAs performed as well as physicians. For all eight criteria identifying undesirable actions, PAs performed as well as or better than physicians.

Kane et al (1978) compared the quality of care performance of Medex-trained PAs to that of their supervising physicians. One criterion of quality evaluated was whether medication was ordered for specific diagnoses. The study found that PAs were less likely than physicians to use antibiotics for fevers of undetermined origin or for upper respiratory tract infections and somewhat less likely to use systemic steroids for contact dermatitis and asthma. These data concluded that PA prescribing decisions for these morbidities were as good or better than those of physicians.

Other studies evaluating PA care in 14 rural primary care settings concluded that PAs were competent, in both diagnostic and therapeutic skills, for the three following practice patterns: (1) when all patients were initially seen by the PA and then by the physician, (2) when patients (not preselected) were managed concurrently by physicians and PAs, and (3) when patients with specific problems were assigned to PAs (Hooker & Cawley, 1997).

Another early 1977 study investigated how physicians and PAs at two different clinics managed patients medically with acute respiratory illnesses. The PAs used clinical algorithms to guide their choices of diagnostic tests and treatment. The findings showed that the PAs did not prescribe antibiotics needlessly or more than internists for conditions not generally requiring an antibiotic and prescribed antibiotics similarly for treatable bacterial conditions. Internists had the highest medical care costs per patient. Care provided by the PAs was as effective as, and less costly than, the care provided by physicians (Thompkins et al, 1977).

Kane and colleagues (Kane, Olson & Castle, 1978) also compared functional outcomes, patient satisfaction, outcome, and mean costs per episode of care among family practice residents, faculty, and Medex-trained PAs at two university-associated family practice training centers. PAs performed as well or better than other providers on each assessed clinical measure.

In the Kaiser Permanente HMO system, Record (1981) examined the performance of PAs, NPs, and physicians in handling episodes of four specific primary care morbidities: strep throat, upper respiratory infection (URI), bursitis, and bronchitis. One outcome criterion was safety, as measured by the rate of adverse effects from antibiotics and other drugs provided in the treatment of upper respiratory infection. No differences in rates were observed between PA and physician clinical measures.

An Iowa study reported that 95% of physicians and 93% of PAs believed that practicing PAs were qualified to prescribe medication with little or no supervision by the physician (Ekwo et al, 1979). Similarly, all 29 Montana physicians responding to a 1989 survey expressed confidence in the ability of the PAs they were supervising to prescribe therapeutic agents, with 40% having no reservations regarding PAs prescribing any agent (Willis & Reid, 1990).

A stratified sample of 19.6% of Wisconsin pharmacists was surveyed about their attitudes toward PA prescribing. The survey was conducted 8 months after PAs were authorized to prescribe nonschedule prescription drugs with the physician supervisor required to co-sign the patient's medical record. Of the 47% of those responding, over half of the 392 pharmacists reported dispensing prescriptions written by PAs. At the time of the survey, Wisconsin PAs were prescribing an average of 27 prescriptions per month, or about 1 per day. The findings indicated that pharmacists found PA prescriptions "completed appropriately and legibly prepared." They were confident in "filling a prescription from a PA." Nevertheless, Wisconsin pharmacists expressed little support for expanded prescribing authority for PAs (Willis, 1993).

Hooker and Cawley (2002) determined the extent of prescribing by adult primary care PAs and NPs to be 15% of the prescriptions in the department of internal medicine and family practice while staffing the departments at 20% full-time equivalent personnel.

PA PRACTICE IN RURAL STATES

Geographic practice isolation in rural and frontier settings may by necessity result in varying degrees of off-site physician supervision and require the PA to exercise autonomy in clinical judgment and selection of therapeutic management approaches. This is particularly true when the PA is the only available on-site clinical provider in a medical practice. Regulatory agency reluctance to support such physician-PA relationships in satellite and remote clinical settings restricts the ability of PAs to provide services that are well within their scope of practice (Hansen, 1992).

The presence of prescribing authority can have a profound effect on the utilization of PAs, at least in rural states. This finding is illustrated by experiences observed in several Western states (Willis & Reid, 1990). For example, the Montana legislature amended the state's medical practice act to permit PA prescribing within specific but typical parameters. In 1988, there were 26 PAs practicing in Montana; in 1991, 43; and in 1995, 130 (Willis & Reid, 1990).

Another example of the impact of PA prescribing authority on practice utilization was observed in Texas in the early 1990s following the passage of a PA prescribing bill. At that time, Texas had 26 federally certified rural health clinics. Less than 5% of the state's PA clinicians were in practice in small rural communities (less than 10,000 population). Texas PA practice regulations permitted neither prescribing of medications nor off-site practice supervision, despite the fact that the state had more than 70 counties either partially or fully designated as provider shortage areas. Shortly after the passage of PA prescribing regulations in 1991, there was a marked increase in the number of PAs employed in rural health clinics. In 1992, the number of PAs had nearly quadrupled to 99, and the percentage practicing in rural communities had tripled from 5% to 15% (Hooker & Cawley, 2003). In 1998, about 34% of all PAs worked in communities of less than 50,000 population (American Academy of Physician Assistants, 2001).

A consistent finding of most research studies on the prescriptive practices of PAs appears to be that when PAs are given prescriptive authority, through either delegated power or protocols to guide them in specified clinical situations, they do at least as well as physicians in writing prescriptions, ordering drug treatment, and producing "good" processes of care. Although the evidence is not sufficient to generalize to all PA prescribing, it does appear that PA performance is generally adequate for all aspects of acute episodes of illness in office-based primary care.

BARRIERS TO PA PRACTICE

Overly restrictive legal stipulations on prescriptive authority have kept PAs from completely implementing their roles in many settings. Barriers to prescriptive authority increase the costs associated with PA utilization if a physician must also be consulted and may deter PAs from practicing in certain states and/or serving medically needy populations. Inconsistency in state medical practice acts, lack of prescriptive authority, and the absence of Medicare and private third-party reimbursement affecting many rural ambulatory practice settings have been shown to restrict PA utilization (Hansen, 1992; Henderson & Choban, 1994). The AAPA has developed model guidelines for state practice acts governing PA practice and prescribing activities to try to increase PA practice flexibility and standardization among states (AAPA, 1997).

On the public policy level, barriers to practice do exist. It may be noted that there are medical, legal, and economic factors that directly or indirectly present obstacles to PAs in performing the full range of clinical tasks for which they are both educated and certified (Henderson & Choban, 1994). States, through their health occupations licensing boards, have considerable control over the qualification requirements and practice activities of PAs, as well as those of physician and other nonphysician health providers such as NPs. State authority in regulating PA and NP health providers permits boards to define provider scope of practice, determine physician supervisory requirements, authorize prescribing activities, and establish and enforce standards of professional conduct and disciplinary procedures.

A number of clinical practice factors have been identified where PAs could be better used in health service delivery (Hansen, 1992). For example, with the growing need for more providers to care for geriatric and nursing home care patients, nonphysicians were viewed as playing an increasingly important role in service delivery. However, a recent review of the PA and nonphysician literature on their utilization in geriatric care settings shows that they are not being used as anticipated, because of the many legal and regulatory barriers that limit what nonphysician providers can do, including restrictions on prescribing authority (Sekscenski et al, 1994).

The symbolic and political weight of PA prescribing has other practical implications for the physician. For example, prescribing a drug demonstrates to the patient that the physician is concerned and is trying to help. A prescription may substitute for real communication with the patient. Delegation of prescribing authority to PAs has been viewed by some physicians as empowering PAs in establishing patient relationships and reducing the power of the physician in that same relationship (Hooker & Cawley, 1997).

Whether this desire to retain the sole privilege of prescriptive authority arises from the traditional power of the role or from economic or political factors, physicians have been reluctant to share this prescriptive prerogative with newcomers to health care. Regardless of the preparation of the new providers, it is difficult to make changes in the status quo. That so many states have been willing to permit delegation of this authority to PAs and other nonphysician providers attests to the success nonphysicians have had in drug prescribing. In fact, there is no suggestion in the research literature that nonphysicians do not perform well in meeting the medication requirements of patients (OTA, 1986).

A number of reasons have been advanced as to why state regulatory agencies have limited the prescribing privilege of PAs. One reason, cited early in the development of the PA role, is that PAs were not sufficiently trained to be competent prescribers. Further, because the agencies regulating PA practice have historically been comprised largely of physicians, there has been concern about the potential of increased legal liability of supervising physicians because of the practice of PA. Physician reluctance can also come from various cultural and/or gender biases. Another possible reason for these agencies limiting or denying prescribing privileges to PAs is the opposition of other health professionals (namely nurses and pharmacists) (Cohen, 1996).

Another possible reason for limiting prescribing privilege is largely economic. The initial purpose for developing the PA role was to alleviate a shortage of physician services. In more recent years, and with the advent of a more abundant supply of physician services, the distinction between whether PAs complement physician services or are alternatives for physician services is less clear. The latter quandary over role function implies that PAs are currently viewed as being in competition with physicians for patients (Grumbach & Coffman, 1998).

The opposition to prescribing privileges for PAs from other health professionals, such as pharmacists, is basically confined to attempts to influence regulatory agencies and state legislatures through testimony and lobbying efforts (Cohen, 1996).

SUMMARY

As originally envisioned, the role of the PA was that of a medical generalist, a role that would encompass the PA working with the physician and span the full range of clinical practice settings: private office, clinic, hospital, nursing home, surgical suite, or the patient's home. PAs were, literally, conceived of as assistants to the physician. PA laws in many states were written to give the physician-PA team a wide practice scope, whereby the supervising physician would delegate to the PA a broad range of medical tasks. Latitude in task delegation requires PAs to exercise some clinical judgment and autonomy in decision-making within the parameters of the state scope of practice regulations and the supervisory relationship. As the PA role has matured, greater movement from close physician supervision has been increasingly seen.

The reality of modern clinical practice demands that PAs possess a strong working knowledge of pharmacology and therapeutic management. States have increasingly recognized this necessity and have adopted regulations to codify this role preparation.

ACKNOWLEDGMENTS

The author acknowledges the contributions of Howard Cohen, JD, MA, Roderick Hooker, MBA, PA, David Mittman, PA-C, and Nicole Gara for critical review and editorial assistance in the preparation of this chapter.

REFERENCES

Accreditation Review Committee Physician Assistants: Standards for accreditation of educational programs for physician assistants, 2000, AAPA.

Alexander BJ, Lipscomb J, Institute of Medicine: *Physician staffing for the VA, vol II, supplementary papers, nonphysician panel report,* Alexandria, VA, 1992, National Academy Press.

American Academy of Physician Assistants: *Physician assistant prescribing and dispensing,* Alexandria, VA, 2000, American Academy of Physician Assistants.

American Academy of Physician Assistants: *Physician assistants: state laws and regulations,* 8th ed, Alexandria, VA, 2000, American Academy of Physician Assistants.

American Academy of Physician Assistants: *Annual census on PAs,* Alexandria, VA, 2001, American Academy of Physician Assistants.

Cawley JF: The profession in 2002 and beyond, *J Acad Physician Assist* 10:7-15, 2002.

Cawley JF: The possibility of an impending health professions glut, *Am Acad Physician Assist* 10:80-92, 1997.

Cawley JF (principal author): *Physician assistants in the health workforce, 1994, Report of the Advisory Group on Physician Assistants and the Workforce to the Council on Graduate Medical Education, Bureau of Health Professions, Health Resources and Services Administration,* Rockville, MD, 1995, Department of Health and Human Services.

Cohen H: *Physician assistant pursuit of prescribing authority: a five-state analysis,* master's thesis, Baltimore, MD, 1996, The Johns Hopkins University.

Davis A: Putting state legislative issues in context, *J Am Acad Physician Assist* 10:27-32, 2002.

Ekwo E et al: The physician assistant in rural primary care practices: physician assistant activities and physician supervision at satellite and non-satellite practice sites, *Med Care* 17:787-795, 1979.

Gara N: State laws for physician assistants, *J Am Acad Physician Assist* 2:303-313, 1989.

Gara N: Regulation of physician assistant prescribing, *J Am Acad Physician Assist* 3:71-78, 1990.

Group Health Association of America: *A survey of clinical staffing of HMOs,* Washington, DC, 1992, Group Health Association of America.

Grumbach K, Coffman J: Physicians and nonphysician clinicians: complements or competitors? *JAMA* 280:285-286, 1998.

Hansen C: *Access to rural health care: barriers to practice for nonphysician providers,* Bureau of Health Professions, Health Resources and Services Administration (HRSA-240-89-0037), Rockville, MD, November, 1992, Department of Health and Human Services.

Henderson T, Choban M: *Removing practice barriers of nonphysician providers: efforts by states to improve access to primary care,* Intergovernmental Health Policy Project, Washington, DC, 1994, The George Washington University.

Hooker RS, Cawley JF: *Physician assistants in American medicine,* ed 2, New York, 2002, Churchill-Livingstone.

Jones PE, Cawley JF: Physician assistants and health care reform, *JAMA* 271:1266-1272, 1994.

Kane RL et al: Differences in the outcomes of acute episodes of care provided by various types of family practitioners, *J Fam Pract* 6:133-138, 1978.

Kane RL, Olson DM, Castle CH: Effects of adding a Medex in practice costs and productivity, *J Community Health* 3:216-226, 1978.

Mittman D, Mirotznik J: PA prescribing behavior and attitudes: a profile, *Physician Assist* 3:15, 16, 21-24, 1984.

National Commission on Certification of Physician Assistants: *PANCE content blueprint,* Atlanta, GA, 1998, The Commission.

Office Technology Assessment, United States Congress: *Nurse practitioners, physician assistants, and certified nurse midwives: a policy assessment,* Health Technology Assessment Report No. 37, Washington DC, 1986.

Record JC: The productivity of new health practitioners. In Record JC: *Staffing primary care in 1990: physician replacement and cost savings,* New York, 1981, Springer Publishing.

Sekscenski E et al: State practice environments and the supply of physician assistants, nurse practitioners, and certified nurse midwives, *N Engl J Med* 331:2366-2371, 1994.

Thompkins R et al: The effectiveness and cost of acute respiratory illness medical care provided by physicians and algorithm assisted physician's [sic] assistants, *Med Care* 15:991-1003, 1977.

Weston JL: Distribution of nurse practitioners and physician assistants: implications of legal constraints and reimbursement, *Public Health Reports* 95:253-256, 1980.

Willis JB: Barriers to PA practice in primary care and rural medically underserved areas, *J Am Acad Physician Assist* 6:418-422, 1993.

Willis JB: Prescriptive practice patterns of physician assistants, *J Am Acad Physician Assist* 3:39-56, 1990.

Willis JB, Reid J: Montana physician's survey, *J Am Acad Physician Assist* 3:57-60, 1990.

CHAPTER 4

Economic Foundations of Prescriptive Authority

Laura E. Shay

Advances made in health care have decreased morbidity and mortality rates, increasing productivity and adding to the gross domestic product (Richards, 1995). However, the cost of health care is rising at a faster rate than the consumer price index for all items and represents an increasingly larger share of the gross domestic product. The Health Care Financing Agency projected that by 2002, national health expenditures would total $2.1 trillion—an estimated 16.6% of the gross domestic product. In general, the most expensive medical conditions are diabetes, asthma and allergic diseases, chronic obstructive pulmonary disease, hypertension, skeletal muscular problems, depression, cardiovascular diseases, and maternity. Of health care costs, preventable illness makes up approximately 70% of the burden of illness and the associated costs and account for eight of the nine leading categories of death—980,000 deaths per year.

Increasing health care costs result from many factors, including increases in and aging of the population, inflation, increased utilization of services and facilities, increased government participation in health care, advances in technology, increase in consumer demand, broader managed care networks, provider consolidation, and health care labor pressures. The costs for medications are imbedded in several of these factors. *The total pharmaceutical portion of health care costs is significant, with more than $65 billion spent at the retail level for drugs and pharmaceutical services in 1992, representing 8.9% of the nation's personal health care bill* (Inglehart, 1999).

Third party payment has been considered a mechanism for solving the high cost of health care. However, third party payment does not reduce the cost; instead, it spreads the cost over a larger population. In reality, third party payment may increase health care costs because administrative costs and increased utilization are inherent in these programs. Third party payers are obligated to ensure the delivery of cost-effective services to their subscribers. Concern over increasing personal health care costs stimulated the development of various alternative prepaid health delivery systems, particularly managed care programs. These systems include health maintenance organizations (HMOs), preferred provider organizations (PPOs), and administrative service organizations (ASOs). All of the managed care programs have the objective of providing quality health services while concurrently attempting to reduce the rate of increase in health care costs. Because of managed care programs, the cost-containment objectives of increased competition has ensured that only the most cost-effective providers are employed.

In the past, providers often paid little attention to health care costs. The primary focus of the provider was to provide the best available treatment to the patient regardless of cost. However, as the numbers of individuals grew who could not afford health care, there was growing recognition that the best health care is of little benefit if a significant proportion of the population cannot pay for it.

RETAIL DRUG COSTS

Expenditures for prescription drugs are increasing more rapidly than other components of health care spending. Prescription drugs represent approximately 10% of the total national personal health care spending, but these prescription drug costs have been increasing in double-digit percentages since 1995. Newer, higher cost drugs and increasing utilization are the drivers behind these higher costs. The average retail price of prescription drugs has increased two to three times as fast as the general inflation rate in recent years. The cost of newer, more expensive therapies and increasing use of those therapies contribute significantly to the dramatic rise in average retail price and expenditures. Prices for prescriptions for brand-name drugs are more than triple those for generic drugs.

Additionally, prescription utilization is increasing rapidly. Per capita prescription use increased by more than two prescriptions per year in the past decade. Increased utilization by patients is due to age, insurance coverage, and the number and scope of drugs available. New, more expensive drugs in the product mix outpace the increase in the percentage of generic prescriptions, resulting in a decrease in the proportional sales of generic drugs. One study forecasted a 15.5% increase in drug expenditures in 2002 for hospitals and clinics and an 18.5% increase for outpatient care settings (Shah, Vermfulen & Santell, 2002).

At the same time, pharmaceutical companies claim that their costs have escalated due to increased spending on research and development (R&D), increased spending on promotion, including increased direct-to-consumer (DTC) advertising, and declining consumer out-of-pocket expenses. As a result, analysts expect that insurers will be forced to increase health premiums even more over the next few years to overcome the rising costs of covered services. The Centers for Medicaid and Medicare Services (CMS, formerly the Health Care Financing Administration [HCFA]) project that outpatient prescription and over-the-counter drug costs for their programs will increase by 21% from 2002 through 2010.

The public wonders why drug prices are so high. The industry has a standard response: research costs are high. US companies have researched and developed new drugs at a remarkable rate compared with companies from other

TABLE 4-1 Preclinical Trials

Approximately 2-3 Years Development		
Approximately 20-30 Remaining Substances Screening	**Approximately 18 Remaining Substances (Phase I)**	**Approximately 12 Remaining Substances (Phase II)**
Basic pharmacologic and biochemical screening Patent application	Acute toxicity with single administration to 12 animal species Detailed pharmacologic studies (main effect, side effects, duration of effects, etc.) Analysis of active substance Stability of active substance	Pharmacokinetics Absorption Distribution Metabolism Elimination Subchronic toxicity: repeated administration (medium term) to two animal species Reproduction-toxicologic studies Fertility Teratogenicity Perinatal and postnatal toxicity Mutagenicity Synthesis of active substance on technical scale Development of final dosage form Analytical evaluation of final dosage form Stability of final dosage form Production of clinical samples

Data from Bartling D, Hadamik H: *Development of a drug. It's a long way from laboratory to patient,* Darmstadt, Germany, 1982, Rhone-Poulenc.

countries. The proportion of the US gross national product from prescriptions has remained small and constant for the past 25 years. The price of a new drug product depends on numerous factors. In addition to the cost of R&D, drug-related factors include the extent to which the marketing strategy can differentiate the product from competitors, estimates of sales, duration of the product's patent protection, value of benefit from product use, cost of alternative treatments, prospect of competing therapies coming to market, cost of any free product distribution to needy people (a public relations strategy used successfully by several companies), and the anticipated public response to the proposed price or what the market will bear.

Other factors influencing the price for a product are probably related to general conditions within the company. Some of these additional factors include prospects for gaining marketing approval of other drugs with large sales potential, patent life of products that generate substantial cash flow, estimates of future operating costs, and profitability. Company policy changes, and unforeseen delays may also profoundly influence drug development and pricing.

DRUG TESTING

Before 1938, a pharmaceutical company was not required to submit to the federal government any evidence of efficacy or safety of any drug product it proposed to market (Troetel, 1986). In 1938, more than 100 children died from ingesting ethylene glycol, a toxic solvent used to solubilize a sulfa drug. Congress reacted almost immediately and passed the Food, Drug and Cosmetic (FD&C) Act of 1938, requiring any new drug to be evaluated for safety for the labeled use by its manufacturer before marketing. It was not until 1962 when the Kefauver-Harris Amendments were passed that companies were required to prove efficacy for the labeled indication, in addition to safety, before product approval would be granted by the Food and Drug Administration (FDA) for marketing.

In the United States, bringing a drug from discovery and synthesis in the laboratory through preclinical and clinical trials to eventual appearance in the marketplace is a costly, time-consuming, and complex procedure (Bartling & Hadamik, 1982; Katz, 1995; United States Pharmacopeia, 1998) (Tables 4-1, 4-2, and 4-3). For legal sale, new drugs have to pass through a rigorous system of approval specified by the FD&C Act and supervised by the FDA. Ideally, drug development proceeds in an orderly, planned sequence. Each phase of development generates and provides, without serious interruption, the data necessary for the intelligent conduct of the next phase. This sequence continues until all the required data have been accumulated to support a complete NDA (New Drug Application) that can be reviewed within the legislated time interval. This scenario is not only ideal, it is rare. The development of a drug is usually marked by surprises that derail even the most detailed planning. Each study often raises new and unexpected questions. These questions must be addressed to better understand the capacity of a drug to induce benefit or cause harm.

There has been general consensus for years that drug development takes too long. However, gaining a relatively complete understanding of a drug's properties is necessary before a drug is made available to the general public. Ensuring the safety of subjects during premarketing testing is also necessary and may take a substantial amount of time that cannot be shortened. It also takes the cooperative efforts of a fully staffed FDA and a

TABLE 4-2 Clinical Trials

Approximately 3-4 Years Development		
Approximately 4-5 Remaining Substances Clinical Testing (Phase I)	**Approximately 2-3 Remaining Substances Clinical Testing (Phase II)**	**1 Remaining Substance Clinical Testing (Phase III)**
Tolerability in healthy volunteers Highest tolerated dose Smallest effective dose Dose-effect relationship Duration of effect Side effects Pharmacokinetics in humans Subchronic toxicity (other animal species) Supplementary animal pharmacology	First controlled trials on efficacy in the patient Chronic toxicity with repeated administration (long term) Carcinogenicity trials Supplementary animal pharmacology	Therapeutic large-scale trial at several trial centers for final establishment of therapeutic profile Indications Dosage and types of administration Contraindications Side effects Precautionary measures Proof of efficacy and safety in long-term administration Demonstration of therapeutic advantages Clarification of any interactions with concomitant medication

Data from Bartling D, Hadamik H: *Development of a drug. It's a long way from laboratory to patient*, Darmstadt, Germany, 1982, Rhone-Poulenc.

TABLE 4-3 Registration, Launch, and Sales

Approximately 2-3 Years Development	
1 Remaining Substance, Registration with Health Authorities	**Launch and Sales**
Documentation of all relevant data for application for registration Expert opinion on clinical trials Expert opinion on pharmacologic trials Expert opinion on toxicologic trials Expert opinion on analytic-pharmaceutical trials Preparation for launch Marketing plan Training of sales force Information for Physicians Pharmacists Wholesalers Preparation of packaging materials Dispatch of samples and products for introduction	Production of final dosage form and packaging Quality control of production

Data from Bartling D, Hadamik H: *Development of a drug. It's a long way from laboratory to patient*, Darmstadt, Germany, 1982, Rhone-Poulenc; and Phillips PJ: Regulatory approval process, *ASAOP J* 43:881-882, 1997.

dedicated pharmacology industry for safe and effective drugs to be marketed in the shortest possible time.

Box 4-1 illustrates the flow of activities involved in the development of a pharmacologically active substance from its first preparation in the laboratory to its market launch (Bartling & Hadamik, 1982). In pharmaceutical research, the earliest stage of activity generally takes many years. It is during this time period that the particular disease is scientifically investigated, and research programs are devised to examine various pharmacologic solutions. Stage I starts only after this expensive, time-consuming, and often frustrating investigative stage.

The scientific rate of success for new drugs is approximately 1:8000 to 10,000. Clearly, many new products are not economic successes for the firm concerned. Assuming that every other new product is economically successful, the economic chance of success is 1:16,000 to 20,000 (Novarro, 1997).

DRUGS OF A DIFFERENT CLASS

Investigational New Drug

Investigational new drugs (INDs) are drugs that have not been approved by the FDA in the United States for general use but (as implied by the name) are under investigation according to strict study protocols (Anonymous, 1991a). These drugs may be on the market in other countries. A manufacturer in the United States must receive clearance from the FDA for a drug to receive investigational status.

Before an investigation of the use of a new drug entity in humans can start, the sponsor must submit to the FDA an IND application. A clinical investigator–sponsored IND is

BOX 4-1

STAGES INVOLVED IN BRINGING A NEW DRUG TO MARKET

- Research concept and discovery of active substances: approximately 1 to 2 years development; approximately 8000 to 10,000 potential substances
- Research target
  Research planning
- Medical target
- Sales target
- Chemical structures planning
- Literature search
- Patent search
- Selection of structure
- Synthesis planning
  Synthesis of active substance
  Synthesis of active substance on laboratory scale
  Determination of animal models
  Chances of success: 1:8000 to 10,000
  Development period: 8 to 10 years
  Cost: $100 million
  Sales and profit:?

Modified from Bartling D, Hadamik H: *Development of a drug. It's a long way from laboratory to patient*, Darmstadt, Germany, 1982, Rhone-Poulenc.

usually intended to permit use of the drug in early clinical patient trials to advance scientific knowledge. A pharmaceutical company–sponsored IND is generated to support an application for the drug to be marketed for specific approved uses. Clinical investigator–sponsored INDs are three to four times more common than are drug company–sponsored INDs. However, the drug company–sponsored IND is much more comprehensively treated and includes the entire clinical program to develop the drug for marketing. For example, chemical composition of the drug, results of all preclinical investigations (including animal safety studies), a protocol for the proposed clinical investigation, information on the experience of clinical investigators, arrangements and procedures for protecting the rights and safety of human subjects developed in accordance with the requirements of human subjects protection committees (institutional review boards), and an agreement to submit annual progress reports must all be provided.

After the IND has been submitted to the FDA, the agency legally has 30 days to review the proposed clinical study for safety issues. The sponsor of the IND may proceed with the planned studies in humans after notification of approval or absence of comment from the FDA within the 30-day review period.

New Drug Application

To market a new drug for human use in interstate commerce, a manufacturer must have a new drug application (NDA) approved by the FDA (United States Pharmacopeia, 1994). The NDA is a compilation of all information obtained on the new drug during the IND program (Troetel, 1986). When the IND sponsor believes that the data are sufficient to fulfill the requirements for FDA drug approval, an NDA is filed. From 4 to 6 years is often required in the IND phase to complete controlled trials necessary for an acceptable FDA application. By statute, the FDA must review the NDA within 180 days. Usually, additional information and/or clarification is requested by the FDA, and at least 1 to 3 years is needed to review and approve an NDA (Commission on Federal Drug Approval Process, 1982). With growing criticism from clinicians, patients, and legislators about the time involved in getting new and needed drugs on the market, new legislation was introduced in 1997 to reduce the time for FDA review and approval (Anonymous, 1993, 1998; Cimmons, 1997, Miller, 1998; Phillips, 1997; Reh, 1998). This has shortened the review time for all drugs, not just those selected for fast-track approval.

Supplemental New Drug Application

After a new drug has been marketed, the FDA requires further clinical proof of safety and efficacy if new or additional labeling indications or statements are desired for a product. A supplemental NDA is required for any changes in approved use of a product. Generally, whether new claims are added to the official label depends on whether the pharmaceutical company has sufficient interest to initiate and follow the procedures necessary to obtain a supplemental NDA (Cote, 1997). The process of approval for a supplemental NDA, although less demanding than the initial NDA, still requires considerable time before the new claim can appear on the official labeling.

Abbreviated New Drug Application

The Drug Price Competition and Patent Term Restoration Act of 1984 (the Waxman-Hatch Amendments) provides the opportunity to extend patents on drug products. This is to encourage the development of new drugs as well as to amend the FD&C Act to expand the universe of drugs for which the FDA may accept abbreviated new drug applications (ANDAs) (Fink & Simonsmeier, 1995). Before enactment of this new law, ANDAs were required only for duplicates (i.e., generic versions of drug products first approved between 1938 and 1962). Copies of pre-1938 drugs (e.g., digoxin, phenobarbital) may be marketed without FDA approval. The law now provides for the submission of ANDAs for duplicates of any previously approved drug product, including post-1962 drug products. Additionally, this law permits generic drug products to become available more quickly. This law is currently targeted for federal change to further speed up the process.

Before passage of this law, all drugs approved on or after October 10, 1962 could be handled by an administrative process known as the "Paper NDA" or literature-supported NDA, regardless of patent status. Because the new drug approval process has already been satisfactorily completed (either by the same or a different manufacturer), the clinical investigations for safety and efficacy need not be repeated. However, the manufacturer must demonstrate that the proposed formulation meets United States Pharmacopeia standards for identity, strength, quality, and purity if it is an official drug. If it is a nonofficial drug, the manufacturer's standards must be acceptable to the FDA, but the FDA has no uniform standards that apply equally to all manufacturers of the drug. Bioequivalence testing is required for each active ingredient (Troetel, 1986). Since the 1984 amendments went into effect, generic versions have been introduced for several hundred drugs previously available only as brand-name (innovator or pioneer) products.

An ANDA may be granted to a generic manufacturer after submitting pharmaceutical, manufacturing, and bioequivalence data (Troetel, 1986). The bioequivalence study may cost about $150,000 and take 6 months to complete. The time required for approval ranges between 9 months and 2 years. There is little difference between the manufacturing data required of an innovator compared with those for a generic manufacturer.

Drugs for Life-Threatening Illnesses: Accelerated Approval Process and Treatment

Investigational New Drug Application (Treatment IND). In October 1988, the FDA issued interim regulatory procedures to hasten the availability of new therapies to treat persons with life-threatening or severely debilitating illnesses, especially when no satisfactory alternatives exist (Anonymous, 1988). Under the new regulation, a drug is made available more rapidly by the elimination of Phase III clinical trials. The FDA and drug sponsors meet at the end of Phase I to design Phase II controlled clinical trials that will provide sufficient safety and efficacy data to support a decision on the limited approvability of the drug for marketing. Furthermore, when reviewing marketing applications for drugs to treat life-threatening and severely debilitating illnesses, the FDA will consider whether the benefits of the drug outweigh the known and potential risks and also consider the absence of satisfactory alternative therapies. When granting approval of a drug, FDA may seek agreement from the sponsor to conduct postmarketing studies to obtain additional information about the drug's risks, benefits, and optimal use.

The most common way for a physician to obtain a treatment investigational new drug (IND) is through direct contact with the sponsor (usually a pharmaceutical manufacturer) who has already obtained FDA approval of the treatment protocol. The sponsor will make the drug available to the physician and provide a brochure containing technical information about the drug and describing the conditions of use allowed under the treatment protocol.

Compassionate Use (Compassionate IND). *Compassionate use* describes an approval requested from the FDA by a specialist physician to use a drug for a single patient, usually in a desperate situation when there is no response to other therapies or in which no approved or generally recognized treatment is available. Approval for compassionate use might be sought in the following situations:

- When an IND is in effect, but the drug is not sufficiently advanced in the testing process to be used as part of approved treatment
- When an IND is in effect, but the physician needs the drug for purposes not described in the IND protocol
- When a drug has FDA approval, but it is not marketed
- When a drug had FDA approval, but it has been withdrawn from the market, usually because of questions regarding safety
- When a drug is being investigated or marketed abroad, but no IND is in effect in the United States

Usually specialists are involved in seeking this type of approval, and the individual physician must contact the review division of the FDA responsible for the drug or disease in question. In these situations, the FDA often will permit the proposed use under a commercial sponsor's IND or under a new IND filed by the patient's physician for an identified patient. In such cases, the FDA requires that the physician provide a report on the efficacy and any adverse reactions observed with the drug.

Orphan Drugs. The Orphan Drug Act defines an *orphan drug* (Anonymous, 1991b; Benzi et al, 1997; McNamee, 1996; Thamer et al, 1998) as a drug or biologic product for the diagnosis, treatment, or prevention of a rare disease or condition (Anonymous, 1991b). A rare disease is one that affects fewer than 200,000 persons in the United States, or one that affects more than 200,000 persons but for which there is no reasonable expectation that the cost of developing the drug and making it available will be recovered from sales of that drug in the United States.

Rare diseases have always been a dilemma for the medical profession because of the difficulty of diagnosis, the lack of treatment options, and, sometimes, the ethical considerations that may arise from counseling, genetic advice, and prognosis. Only in the last decade have citizens and advocacy groups drawn the attention of Congress to the fact that there were few or no drugs commercially available for treatment of rare diseases. The federal government, medical profession, academia, industry, private foundations, and organizations representing patients have finally combined in a joint effort to facilitate the research, development, and marketing of such products.

It is estimated that the majority of approximately 5000 rare diseases remain untreated because potentially useful products have not been developed. Often knowledge of the underlying pathophysiology of rare diseases is insufficient to devise meaningful therapies. Potential treatments for these diseases are usually of limited commercial value. The drug approval process has become more complex and costly because of regulations requiring the demonstration of a drug's safety and efficacy. For an orphan drug, the situation is even more complicated because it may not be patentable, the number of patients requiring the drug is limited, and the production costs may be prohibitive. In addition, evaluating effectiveness and assessing drug risk-benefit ratios in patients with rare diseases is difficult because of the small number of patients available for statistical analysis.

The FDA Office of Orphan Products Development (OPD) provides an information package that includes an overview of the FDA's Orphan Drug Program, a brief description of the Orphan Products Grant Program, and a current list of designated orphan products. OPD's information package also contains a directory listing sources of information about the treatment of rare diseases, patient organizations, and the availability of orphan drugs. Requests for the Rare Disease

Information Directory or the entire Orphan Drug Information Package may be made by contacting the office at

Office of Orphan Products Development (BF-35)
5600 Fishers Land
Rockville, Maryland 20857
(301) 443-2043

Drugs for Unlabeled Uses. Drugs used for nonapproved indications or at doses not included in the FDA-approved labeling are defined as *unlabeled uses*. Use in other patient populations or via a route of administration that is not covered by FDA-approved labeling are additional examples of unlabeled uses (ASHP, 1992). Other terms used to describe unlabeled use include *off-label use, out-of-label use, usage outside of labeling,* and *unapproved use*. The term *unapproved use* is a misnomer because it implies that the FDA regulates prescribing and dispensing. The FDA cannot approve or disapprove particular provider prescribing practices of legal drugs on the market. The FDA does regulate what manufacturers may recommend about uses in their product labeling and what can be included in advertising and promotion.

Standards differentiating between experimental and established practices will probably always be lacking because of constant advances and the dynamic nature of health care practice. The evolving nature of various drug therapies (e.g., biotechnology, cancer chemotherapy, AIDS treatments) makes it difficult for regulatory agencies to review scientific data and develop standards that are current. To revise FDA-approved labeling, additional documentation must be submitted by the manufacturer to support additional indications and/or doses. Manufacturers are aware that unlabeled uses are permitted. With the added time-consuming and expensive process required, some manufacturers have chosen not to change their product labeling. Consequently, product information sometimes lags behind accepted medical practices.

GENERIC VERSUS BRAND-NAME DRUGS

Effect of Patents

Drug products considered to be identical with respect to their active ingredients are *generic equivalents*. Brand-name drugs are usually more expensive than generic drugs because the manufacturer of the brand-name drug is attempting to recoup the money invested to research and develop the drug. The generic market is expected to grow substantially by 2005, with an estimated $35 billion in patent expirations. However, newer brand-name drugs and changing treatment patterns may limit the potential cost reductions associated with these brand-to-generic shifts unless major health policy requires generic drugs to be used in Medicare and Medicaid programs.

After a new drug enters the market, a patent protects the financial interest of the drug developer for some time (United States Pharmacopeia, 1994). The traditional protection period is 17 years, but the actual period is much less because of the extended time required to gain approval before marketing. In addition to a patent granted by the US Patent and Trademark Office, a drug may be further protected from generic competition through patent extensions (sometimes called market exclusivity provisions). The Drug Price Competition and Patent Term Restoration Act of 1984 permits patent extensions on certain drugs whose patents were shortened by the time required for FDA review and approval (Hogan, 1985). The act allows the FDA to add the NDA review time to the original expiration date of the patent (Troetel, 1986). The Waxman-Hatch Amendment granted the innovator 5 years' exclusivity on every NDA approved by the FDA (i.e., the innovator will have at least 5 years of exclusivity regardless of the amount of time left on the life of the patent). New legislative proposals under discussion seek to place limits on the number of times that pharmaceutical companies may extend the life of the patent to speed up the appearance of more generic products.

Generic manufacturers may submit ANDAs, and tentative FDA approval may be granted pending patent or market exclusivity protection. However, no generic product may be marketed until both the patent term and market exclusivity have expired. Following the ANDA, the applicant must show that its product is bioequivalent to the innovator's product (*United States Pharmacopeia*, 1994). The extensive testing performed by the innovator does not have to be repeated, but comparative testing between products is required to ensure they are therapeutically equivalent.

Drug purchase prices usually decline when generic products compete with the innovator product (Ensor, 1992). The expiration of a single patent on a brand-name product does not necessarily lead to commercial availability of a competitive generic product. Multiple factors influence generic product development and marketing. It is not uncommon for manufacturers to hold separate patents on a single drug, the method of manufacture, and the dosage form. Manufacturers may introduce a new dosage form (e.g., extended release) to protect market share of a drug whose patent is about to expire. The product may be complicated to manufacture or the raw ingredients difficult to obtain, which may also delay market entry of a generic product. Patent terms are often challenged and must be verified in court, sometimes taking years to resolve.

Bioequivalence and the *Blue Book*

In the 1970s, there was little information on bioequivalence among drug products. Such information was necessary for rational drug product selection. The lack of bioequivalence data led to the formation in early 1974 of the Drug Bioequivalence Study Panel of the Office of Technology Assessment (OTA). The panel was to determine whether it was technologically possible to ensure that drug products with the same physical and chemical composition would produce comparable therapeutic effects. In July 1974, the panel concluded that although bioequivalence is important, not all products have bioequivalence issues and that it is therefore unnecessary to perform in vivo bioequivalence testing on all products. The panel recommended the rapid creation of an official list of interchangeable drug products and the distinction between two classes of drugs: those in which bioequivalence is not essential and those in which it is critical.

One result of the OTA panel's recommendations was the FDA's release in 1975 of proposed regulations with criteria for determining whether a drug would be subject to a bioequivalence requirement. The regulations were finalized and published in January 1977. In January 1976, the FDA published

Holders of Approved Drug Applications for Drugs Presenting Actual or Potential Bioequivalence Problems. This list (referred to as the *Blue Book*) identified drugs thought to have bioequivalence problems, but it did not indicate which companies had demonstrated the bioequivalence of their products.

Therapeutic Equivalence and the *Orange Book*

In most cases, generic products have the same effect as the brand-name product. However, different effects are possible (e.g., differences in the nonactive ingredients may cause side effects in some patients). At about the same time as the *Blue Book* was being created, New York State requested the FDA's assistance in 1977 to evaluate the therapeutic equivalence of products for the state's drug product selection list. The FDA responded with equivalence recommendations, and other states began to request assistance with their lists. The FDA recognized that providing a single product selection list based on common policies and usable in all states would be preferable to evaluating drug products with differing definitions and criteria in various state laws. In May 1978, the Commissioner of Food and Drugs announced the FDA's intention to prepare a national list. The FDA list would include all marketed prescription drug products that had been approved for safety and effectiveness by the FDA.

Drafted in January 1979 and first published in October 1980, the *Orange Book* (officially known as *Approved Drug Products with Therapeutic Equivalence Evaluations*) is generally considered the most reliable reference in the United States for determining which products are therapeutically equivalent (Knoben, Scott & Tonelli, 1990). The FDA considers generic products with the same ingredients that have the same therapeutic effect to be "therapeutically equivalent."

The origin of the *Orange Book* can be traced to the late 1960s, when the Department of Health and Human Services convened the Task Force on Prescription Drugs to study the problems of including prescription drug costs under Medicare. From proposals of the task force, the department created the Maximum Allowable Cost-Estimated Acquisition Cost (MAC-EAC) program in 1973, which took effect in August 1976, to establish upper reimbursement limits. When the MAC-EAC program was proposed, any state with antisubstitution drug laws would be excluded. The MAC-EAC proposal set the stage for the repeal of antisubstitution legislation that existed in many states. By 1978, some 40 states had generic drug product selection laws. Today, all states have some form of selection law, which generally allows substitution of products.

As used in the *Orange Book,* the concept of therapeutic equivalence applies only to products containing the same active ingredients. The FDA classifies as therapeutically equivalent those products that meet the following outlined criteria:

- They are approved as both safe and effective.
- They are pharmaceutical equivalents, in that they (1) contain identical amounts of the same active ingredients in the same dosage form and route of administration and (2) meet compendia or other applicable standards of strength, quality, purity, and identity.
- They are bioequivalent, in that (1) they do not present a known or potential bioequivalence problem and they meet acceptable in vitro standards and (2) if they do present a known or potential problem, they are shown to meet an appropriate bioequivalence standard.
- They are adequately labeled.
- They are manufactured in compliance with FDA's Good Manufacturing Practice regulations

The *Orange Book* contains public information and advice. It is not an official national compendium. The therapeutic equivalence recommendations result from scientific and medical judgments based on data submitted to the FDA. Exclusion of a drug product from the list does not necessarily mean that the drug product violates the FD&C Act or that such a product is not safe or effective or not therapeutically equivalent to other drug products. Instead, the exclusion is based on the FDA not having evaluated the safety, effectiveness, and quality of the drug product. Although the list is widely used, product selection is a professional activity that is based largely on social and economic policies administered at the state level to minimize drug costs. Health professionals and states are not required to accept the therapeutic equivalence recommendations in the *Orange Book,* and the FDA takes no official position on state regulation of drug product selection.

Needy Patient Assistance Programs

Many pharmaceutical companies recognize that patients may need medications that they cannot afford. For a variety of reasons, both economic and altruistic, these companies have established patient assistance programs to enable individuals to receive their products. NeedyMeds is an Internet site located at http://www.needymeds.com that contains information on patient assistance programs offered by pharmaceutical manufacturers. They have information on over 125 companies and over 800 drugs. An alert service was recently added so that users will know whenever changes are made to the database.

Occasionally a provider will desire to contact a pharmaceutical company directly about a product. Pharmacology reference books such as *Drug Facts and Comparisons* or *Mosby's Drug Reference* lists telephone numbers for providers to use in querying pharmaceutical companies about products. **evolve** This information can also be found on the Evolve website.

Application of Pharmacoeconomic Theory

The economic consequences of medication choice for patients have become increasingly important. A wide range of therapeutic options exists for treatment of many diseases, and the costs associated with those options vary widely because of factors often not obvious to either patient or clinician. For the health care prescriber, the most important goal is to identify the drug or drugs that will meet the therapeutic objective for a specific patient. Use of a drug that is not likely to accomplish the therapeutic goal will not be a good choice, regardless of the economic implications. Sound economic decision-making rests on recognition of this fact.

The information most frequently required by prescribers to make cost-effective decisions answers the following questions:

- Which drugs are effective for the specific disease?
- What is the relative total cost of the various drug options?
- Who pays for what?

Finding answers to these questions provides information that the prescriber may use to identify the best set of options from an economic perspective.

GENERAL ECONOMIC PRINCIPLES APPLIED TO DRUG THERAPY

Economics is a scientific way of thinking. It uses theory to predict outcome. The test of a theory is how well it predicts what really happens. The following economic principles are part of the economic theory suggesting how the health care system works (Bootman, Townsend & McGhan, 1996; Gwartney & Stroup, 1996; Walley et al, 1997):

- *All scarce goods have a cost.* "There are no free lunches" is a common slogan in economics. This means that if people choose to spend their money on one thing, they probably do not have enough money for something else. In many homes, the choice may be between health care and food. Thus many people with reduced incomes go without needed health care. Some people find money to see a health care provider only to realize that they do not also have enough money to purchase needed medications. Many highly effective drugs are available only with a prescription written by an authorized health care provider, but many individuals do not have either access to health care providers or the money to pay for expensive prescriptions. Thus medications are a good example of *scarce economic goods* (when there is less of a good that is freely available than consumers would like).
- *Decision-makers choose purposefully.* People economize by gaining what they want at the least possible cost. This also means that when choosing among items of equal cost, individuals will choose the option that yields the greatest benefit. This is clearly seen when patients choose herbal or over-the-counter drugs rather than going to the health care provider for prescription products. This process is also clearly demonstrated in the strength of the generic drug market, where both individuals and companies profit from use of the lower cost generic products if the results are the same as the more expensive brand-name products.
- *Incentives matter.* Human choice is influenced in a predictable way by changes in economic incentives. As the personal benefits from choosing an option increase, other things being equal, a human decision-maker will be more likely to choose the option. (For example, people who are positive for human immunodeficiency virus [HIV] infection may be willing to take complicated drug regimens to help reduce their chances of developing HIV disease.) In contrast, as the costs associated with the choice of an item increase, a person will be less likely to choose the option. (So, if the cost for the HIV medications is so high that other things must be forgone, people may decide not to continue taking the medication.)
- *Economic thinking is marginal thinking.* Most economic decisions are concerned with the effects produced by a very small change. For example, how much are individuals willing to spend to maintain health or prevent disease? They may be willing to have a yearly Pap smear or prostate examination. Are they also willing to spend more money to have a mammogram, a PSA test, a blood sugar measurement, and a TB test? How much do people need to spend to feel that they are getting their money's worth? How much is too much? How much are patients with hypertension willing to do to get their blood pressure down to the recommended limits? Go on a restricted diet? Lose weight? How many new medications will they take? How many side effects of drugs will they tolerate?
- *Information, like other resources, is scarce.* Therefore even purposeful decision-makers will not have perfect knowledge about the future when they make choices. There is a cost in time, money, effort, and sometimes education to collect the information needed to make informed decisions. It is unreasonable to believe that patients will be able to have enough information about drugs to determine which product is best or to learn about new products as they come on the market.
- *Secondary effects should be remembered.* Economic actions often generate additional or secondary effects in addition to their immediate effects. Some secondary effects are positive; for example, taking antidiabetic drugs may help preserve a patient's vision or renal function, or taking antihypertensive medications may reduce the incidence of atherosclerotic heart disease or myocardial infarction. However, some secondary effects may be negative, such as the impotence experienced by some patients when taking those same antihypertensive medications.
- *A negative relationship exists between the price of a good and the amount of it buyers are willing to purchase (the law of demand).* Thus, when medication costs are low, one may expect that more patients will choose to purchase the drug and take it. When the price is high, fewer patients will choose to purchase the drug.
- *A positive relationship exists between the price of a good and the amount of it offered for sale by sellers (the law of supply).* When the cost of a drug is very high, more manufacturers are interested in selling the product, and the supply increases.
- *The highest valued benefit that must be sacrificed or forgone as the result of choosing an alternative is called the opportunity cost.* Thus the opportunity costs may be too high if people have to give up food or shelter to purchase health care.

ECONOMIC ANALYSIS APPLIED TO HEALTH CARE

Some critics have questioned the applicability of economics to the study of health care services for two reasons. First, they question the accuracy of the assumptions underlying economic behavior of consumers and health care providers. Second, they challenge the implicit values, such as consumer control and rights, that influence the goal to be achieved: consumer satisfaction and increased health. For example, critics have claimed that it is inaccurate to assume that the patient receiving health care is rational and that he or she has sufficient information when deciding on use of services (Johannesson et al, 1998). In fact, sick patients may not be rational at all. Unlike some industries where spending more money gets you more of what you want, there is not a direct relationship between health care services, or health care spending, and perfect health. This means that doing more and spending more may not necessarily bring a patient any closer to better health. Critics also claim that the purchaser of medical services is not the consumer, as in nonmedical markets, but may be the physician or some other health care provider, who also has a financial interest in the services to be purchased (Fox, 1995).

Clearly, some market factors are distorted when patients have health insurance that pays for the immediate costs of health care or medications. In seeking to maximize their options, patients paying out of pocket for services would be reluctant to spend money for health care or drugs unless these were not vitally needed. However, with insurance coverage, out-of-pocket costs are separated from the purchase and thus may not deter the use of services or purchases. Therefore the usual cost barriers may be ineffective. This is particularly true when an employer rather than the patient is paying for the health insurance, further removing the patient from directly feeling the cost of any purchases made (D'Errico, 1998).

With regard to economists' traditional assumptions about providers of health care services, critics claim that the traditional analysis of market economics is also distorted. They claim that these health care providers are organized more as nonprofit organizations and therefore do not have the same motivations as for-profit firms in other industries (Gwartney & Stroup, 1996). Further, because incompetent providers may irreparably harm consumers, more stringent controls must be exercised over the provision of medical services than over non-medical goods and services. Finally, such critics may also claim that access to health care service is considered a right by society and its distribution cannot be left solely to the ups and downs of the marketplace (D'Errico, 1998). However, to the extent that economic analysis can clarify the cost of alternatives and make the values underlying those alternatives explicit, it remains a useful approach to the study of medical care.

Increased FDA regulation of the drug industry has increased the safety and effectiveness of drugs entering the market, although these tightened regulations have also resulted in fewer drugs being approved (*USP DI*, 1997). However, some unique dynamics in the health care market make this increased protection to patients very important. Unlike when someone purchases a car or buys a television set, patients generally do not have the ability to obtain or understand the complex information they need to make an accurate choice about the safety or efficacy of a particular drug. They must rely on the knowledge of their providers. Prescribers also face a constant challenge in keeping up with the vast scientific literature about drugs and their best use.

Patients who are ill expect good health care and that includes the best drugs to help treat their problems. However, there are no perfect drugs—even the best drugs produce adverse effects in some individuals. Health care prescribers, drug manufacturers, and federal regulators all try to balance the difficult process of using drugs that are the safest for most patients while eliminating the drugs that would provide an unacceptable risk. Researchers are familiar with this struggle when they try to balance the incidence of Type I error (the probability of being wrong, that is, of having introduced a drug that should not have been introduced) against the possibility of Type II error (the probability of not introducing new drugs when they should have been introduced). In each type of error, patients may experience adverse consequences. Thus these struggles illustrate that, for every benefit, there is a cost (D'Errico, 1998).

PHARMACOECONOMIC METHODS

Economists generally describe four different varieties of comparative analyses to aid in decision-making about a given course of action (Bootman, Townsend & McGhan, 1996): (1) cost-benefit analysis (CBA), (2) cost-effectiveness analysis (CEA), (3) cost-minimization analysis (CMA), and (4) humanistic (cost-utility) analysis (CUA).

CBA is used to evaluate the impact of an intervention, activity, or program on general society. It relies on such concepts as the economic value of a life or the economic value of added productive years. It is most frequently considered as an aid in policy development and decision-making. The critical measure for this type of analysis is the benefit-cost ratio. The ratio defines the economic relationship between a dollar of benefit from the program and a dollar invested to fund it. The ratio thus ends up as:

$$\text{Benefit-cost ratio} = \frac{\text{Dollars of economic benefit}}{\text{Dollar cost of the program}}$$

This type of analysis might be used, for example, in deciding whether the federal government should provide peritoneal dialysis, home hemodialysis, or outpatient hemodialysis in a program for patients with end-stage renal disease.

A positive benefit-cost ratio suggests that more than a dollar of benefit is gained for each dollar spent. This type of analysis is most valuable when comparing two or more non-like programs, that is programs with non-like objectives. Comparison of the benefit-cost ratio of funding early childhood education programs compared with public prenatal care clinics would be an example of the use of CBA.

CEA is used to compare two activities with similar objectives. An example of this may be the improvement in survival of patients with breast cancer. In CEA, two different programs are compared by creating a common outcome, such as years of added life. The CEA measure may, for example, compare an "alternative medicine" approach to treatment of breast cancer with a traditional medical protocol (combination of surgery, drugs, radiation, and so forth). The CEA analysis is often reported in terms of dollars per year-of-life, or *quality-adjusted life year.* The cost of the two different programs may then be compared to find the cost to add 1 year of life. CEA can be applied at the health-system level and may affect what types of programs will be developed and supported by a funding agency.

CMA is actually a special type of CEA in which the outcomes are determined to be directly comparable and clearly measurable. Examples of this might be otitis media cure, hypertension control, or pain management. CMA usually does not emphasize the relative effects but presumes them to be essentially equivalent. This type of analysis is most frequently applicable when a provider is comparing relevant costs of drug therapy decisions.

CUA incorporates nonmonetary measures such as quality of life into decision-making. It is not regularly used in medication selection decision-making at this time. However, it may become an important component of future drug selection algorithms.

In applying economic principles to drug prescribing, CEA/CMA are the most applicable types of analysis for the individual or group of prescribers (Bootman, Townsend & McGhan, 1996).

COSTS OF THERAPY

One of the most challenging aspects of pharmacoeconomic analysis is determining what needs to be included when thinking about drug costs. Drug therapy costs fall into two general categories: the primary costs of the drug itself (including the supplies required to use the drug) and the secondary costs that are associated with use of that drug. These secondary costs include such things as the cost of medication administration (if not self-administered), laboratory drug-level monitoring costs, and the cost of follow-up for routine, nonroutine, or emergency visits. The cost of retreat, or rescue therapy after treatment failures, must be included in the later category (Marwick, 1994).

The essence of the economic decision is based on identification of relevant costs and the probability of each outcome. In various combinations, prescribers, patients, and payers will all complete their economic decision based on the relevant combination of primary and secondary costs in the decision probability model. Thus from the scientific knowledge of disease process, treatment options, and likely outcome, it may be cost effective to start a new diabetic patient on insulin. However, certain patients may be reluctant to take insulin, knowing they will have to purchase needles, syringes, alcohol wipes, blood glucose testing machines, and so forth out of pocket when they can scarcely meet current rent and food bills. Furthermore, the inconvenience and discomfort associated with blood testing and insulin injections negatively affect those patients' quality of life. Therefore a cost-effective therapy may be an unacceptable choice for an individual within the same disease cohort. This is important to recognize and should serve as the basis for education and negotiation with the patient if a cooperative relationship is to develop between provider and patient (Bootman, Townsend & McGhan, 1996).

Development of a Decision Probability Model

A comprehensive analysis of the best drug to order from an economic point of view requires the development of a probability (decision tree) model for the disease being treated. This is a substantive process in a formal academic analysis. For the prescriber, the development of this model may be simple, but it is still required to best evaluate the pharmacoeconomics underlying the decision. The decision probability model attempts to determine the possible options associated with a particular disease treatment and the likelihood of their occurrence. Figure 4-1 demonstrates a simple decision tree format. In the decision probability model, the prescriber needs to be aware of the probability of success in meeting the therapeutic objectives for each likely therapeutic choice. For example, the model might be used in choosing an antibiotic, an antiretroviral product, a topical product for vaginal candidiasis, or an asthma medication. Filling in the different drugs and estimating their safety or risk of adverse effects may help determine the best drug to prescribe. These types of models are at the core of some disease-management programs.

Pharmacoeconomic Cost Equation

The following equation may be applied to summarize cost-related factors relevant to the prescribing decision:

$$\text{Total cost} = \begin{array}{l} \text{Supply costs} \\ + \text{Monitoring laboratory costs} \\ + \text{Cost of follow-up care} \end{array}$$

Supply costs include drug costs and cost of supplies used to administer or prepare drugs. *Cost of follow-up care* includes cost of clinic visits, emergency department visits, retreatment

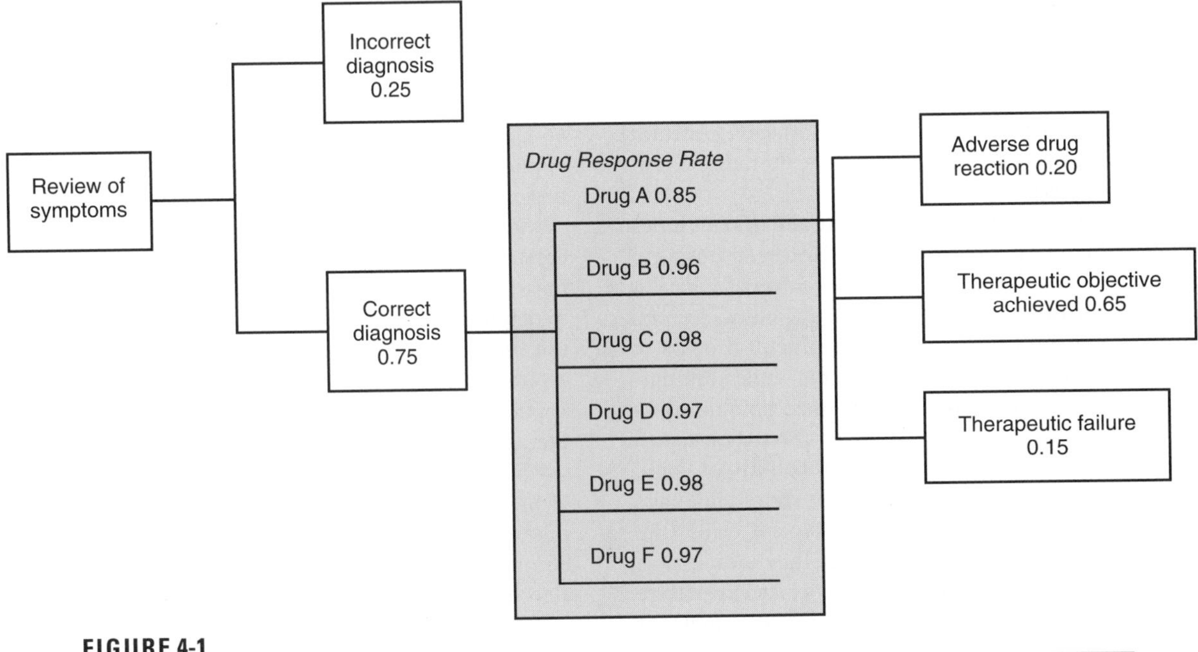

FIGURE 4-1

Decision probability model.

of failure cases, etc. Do not, however, substitute patient charges for costs. Patient charges typically include other elements of the price and revenue program that are not relevant to cost finding for pharmacoeconomic purposes.

Determination of a complete total cost equation relies on an understanding of the course of a disease under the best circumstances as well as cases where success does not come quickly after initial therapy. A sound pharmacoeconomic decision will use the results of this equation in conjunction with clinical and other relevant factors in making a final decision about the medication to prescribe.

How It Works. The following outline provides a generic format for evaluation of most agents used in routine short-term medication therapy. Antiinfective agents are a therapy for which this evaluation is relevant, but other agents for which a limited-time course of therapy is used will work in a similar way:

Determine the Costs

- *Identify the drug and supply cost for a typical course of therapy based on the disease and the drug.* If drug A is used 3 times daily for 10 days (30 doses) and drug B is used once daily for 3 days (3 doses), then the drug cost of 30 doses should be compared with the cost of 3 doses, respectively. In most cases with oral agents, the overall supply cost will be identical to the drug cost.
- *Identify the cost per follow-up visit to clinic or emergency department.* In this example, $200 will be used.
- *Use data, as available, to identify the failure rate of the initial drug therapy that results in retreatment or secondary intervention (e.g., surgical procedure)*

  Retreatment costs = Costs to treat once with statistically improved alternative therapy × Failure rate of initial therapy

- *Do the math.* Once the individual cost information has been determined, the evaluation is simply a matter of mathematical analysis of the total cost equation for each agent. (See Table 4-4 for an example of total cost calculation for different drugs.)
- *Compare the results.* Based on this example, the pharmacoeconomic preference would be drug C, with a total cost per treatment of $29.91. It is noteworthy that the lowest cost drug based on drug cost alone ends up only one-third least expensive if all the added costs are included. Also important to note is the fact that a change in any of the factors (drug cost, failure rate, cost of follow-up visit, and so forth) can quickly change the total cost of the therapy. For instance, development of antimicrobial resistance would quickly change the failure rate following initial treatment. If the failure rate of drug C goes from the present 2% to 5%, the total costs increase to $63.00 and drug E then becomes the economically preferred agent.

This example shows the incorrect decision that may result from failure to correctly identify all components of the cost equation. Because of the dynamic nature of the factors involved in the cost calculation, the lowest cost option today may not be so in the next week. When any of the factors in the equation change in value, the outcome may also quickly change.

Other Considerations. In the case of diseases requiring long-term therapy, a similar analysis can be conducted based on a probability chart and relevant cost components.

Drugs are often selected for hospital or health plan formularies based on cost minimization calculations. In many cases, the products that have demonstrated cost-effectiveness are given priority for use. Some high-cost options may be unavailable or restricted by the formulary process. This is often true for new drugs for which little information is available (Johannesson et al, 1998; Pausjenssen et al, 1998).

Many patients must still purchase medications where there is no formulary to provide guidance. Because the total cost equation requires inclusion of components that can vary widely (e.g., cost of follow-up visit, co-pay, and so forth), the best selection for one payment plan may not be recommended for self-pay patients.

A cost-conscious drug selection process is important to both the patient and the health care system. Inclusion of the economic factor in medication selection is part of correct prescribing practice. In an era when cost limitations may affect how much care will be provided to a given patient, efforts by individual prescribers to evaluate the impact of the health care dollar is wise. Cost-effectiveness or cost-minimization studies are most relevant for individual prescribing decisions. The total cost of prescribing includes much more than the simple cost per course of therapy or drug cost per month. A "total cost" decision will incorporate all of the relevant costs that impact on the prescribing decision (Marwick, 1994).

It is also important to note that there is surprising variability of charges for the same medications both throughout

TABLE 4-4 Comparison of Total Costs for Different Drug Treatment Options

Drug	Supply Cost	Failure/Retreatment Rate	Follow-up or ER Costs	Retreatment Costs	Total Costs
A	$2.90	15%	$30.00	$3.83	$36.73
B	$55.00	4%	$8.00	$1.02	$64.02
C	$25.40	2%	$4.00	$0.51	$29.91
D	$57.00	3%	$6.00	$0.77	$63.77
E	$25.75	2%	$4.00	$0.51	$30.26
F	$53.70	3%	$6.00	$0.77	$60.47

different geographical areas of the country and at different pharmacies in the same area. Where patients have their prescriptions filled may be limited by prescription plans. Patients often assume that medications will cost a lot of money and that they have no choice. However, it is often possible for them to save money on prescriptions by asking for advice from their pharmacist. Large pharmacy chains that buy in bulk and are affiliated with many prescription reimbursement plans are able to sell medications at a low cost but still make money through volume repeat sales. Thus they are willing to offer lower charges on many medications that they know will be filled multiple times. By shopping at one pharmacy, the patient is also able to increase the probability that drug duplications and interactions will be identified.

Some insurance companies direct patients to mail their prescriptions to out-of-state pharmacies that will provide medications at a discounted rate. In filling prescriptions, pharmacists are directed under FDA rules to adhere to both the state law that governs the prescriber's authority to prescribe and the state law that governs the pharmacist's authority to dispense. Thus if prescribers transmitting prescriptions are authorized to prescribe the particular medications in the states where they are licensed and receiving pharmacists are not prohibited from dispensing them in the states where they are licensed, it should be expected under federal rules that such prescriptions will be filled. Despite these regulations, many nonphysician prescribers find that out-of-state pharmacies refuse to fill their prescriptions.

GENERIC VERSUS TRADE MEDICATIONS

One recurrent question in medication product selection is what to do about the use of generic medications when they are available. Generic drugs have decreased the cost of medication therapy in almost every case where they have entered the market. For example, the 1997 *Drug Topics Red Book* listed the average wholesale price for the brand-name drug lorazepam (e.g., Ativan) 0.5 mg at $68.45 per 100 tablets, whereas a major generic drug manufacturer offers the nonbrand (generic) product for $16.55.

The lower cost of most generic drugs allows many patients who must pay for their own medication to obtain required medication when they would not otherwise be able to afford the trade name product. For cost-management objectives, most third party payers provide positive or negative incentives so that generics are used preferentially when available. In some cases, direct patient incentives are used through reduced co-pays to individuals who will voluntarily accept a generic substitute. In other cases, trade name products will not be covered by insurance or reimbursement provided an approved generic product is available.

Strong cases have been made both for and against the use of generic drugs. Some of these arguments are data based, but many are not. It may be important to note that recall of drugs for quality problems happens regularly to both generic and brand-name pharmaceutical manufacturers. Do not automatically assume that the trade or brand name products have a higher quality level. The FDA maintains a list of generic products with bioequivalence information for all products that have been reviewed and approved for commercial use. Although this source provides a documented basis for decision-making, it has several limitations. In some cases, generic products are manufactured by the innovator of the product but sold under a generic line (e.g., cimetidine). Who actually makes a specific generic product is one of the most complex issues in the generic quality controversy. Some generic vendors simply buy and repackage from other manufacturers. Several large hospital purchasing groups have addressed this issue by specifying that the actual manufacturer of the drug will not change over the life of an awarded contract (Schulman & Linas, 1997).

Health care prescribers may need to collect more information about specific generic products by talking to local pharmacists. They should seek advice on which generic drugs suppliers' pharmacists use for specific drugs and whether they are considered to be bioequivalent by the FDA. If this information is not readily available, pharmacists should be asked if they are willing to research the question and offer an answer at a later time. Some institutional drug information centers may also be willing to provide this information.

There is not one single generic-versus-trade medication question that is appropriate to ask in all circumstances. Some critical questions to consider are:

- *How stable is the patient on the currently prescribed medication?* Patients who have been difficult to manage or unstable because of other medical conditions may be risky candidates for changes in drug products. This does not always preclude the use of a generic product but suggests that changes from one supplier to another should be done with caution. Concerns about changing drug sources are best addressed by determining where patients have their prescriptions filled and calling the pharmacy to request that the manufacturer of a dispensed medication not be changed without advising the health care prescriber. This may also be communicated to the pharmacist on the prescription.
- *How narrow is the therapeutic index for the specific drug?* Those drugs that have a narrow therapeutic index, such as warfarin or digoxin, have historically posed higher risks for the patient in switching from manufacturer to manufacturer. For this reason, once a patient has been stabilized on one product, changes should be done only with careful monitoring of laboratory or other relevant information.
- *Is the high price of a brand-name product likely to prevent the patient from using the medication in the optimal way?* Some patients create imaginative ways of taking their medications to save money. They may cut each pill into two or more pieces, skip doses, or not take their medications 1 or more days a week. Patient compliance failure confounds even the best treatment and product selection plans. There is a clear place for use of generic products in the cost-focused environment of today's health care system. Care should be taken in evaluating both patients and drugs to determine those patients who might encounter difficulty if their medication is produced by different manufacturers. The help of the pharmacist may need to be included in implementing the therapeutic plan for patients using some types of medications.

FORMULARY RESTRICTIONS

The inclusion or exclusion of certain agents on "restricted" formulary status is now common practice in most institutions and pharmacy benefits programs as a way of decreasing drug costs. Most formularies rely heavily on generic drugs. Many private health insurance programs, the United States military, and many state Medicaid programs all have formularies for drugs for which reimbursement is provided. Some programs preclude the pharmacist from filling a prescription for a nonformulary drug without obtaining a prospective override; some require pharmaceutical companies to give a discount to the program to have their products included on a formulary. Increased co-pay or failure to cover outpatient prescriptions for nonauthorized drugs is another approach to enforcing restriction policies (Stewart, 1998).

Unfortunately, it is patients who are most inconvenienced if they take the prescription to the pharmacy only to have to pay out of pocket or to experience a delay in getting the medication because they must get authorization or have the prescriber called for an alternate medication. It is also patients who suffer when insurance does not cover newer proprietary drugs that are more effective in treating their conditions than traditional, generic, less-expensive drugs.

USE OF DRUG SAMPLES

Pharmaceutical companies often provide drug samples for distribution to patients. Drug sampling is primarily a marketing technique by the manufacturer to draw attention to the product. Giving health care providers drug samples was historically the major way companies had of introducing new products into the market. Arguments in favor of sample use include the opportunity for the provider to try a different medication without asking the patient to pay for a trial course or to give the patient a few doses until a prescription can be filled.

However, there are inherent problems with the use of medication samples and the practice has increasingly fallen into disfavor by many professionals. Samples in clinic areas are often not stored under ideal conditions to protect them from dust, heat, and humidity. Demand for certain types of medications may vary, leading some products to remain in storage until long after their expiration date or until packages have clear signs of deterioration. Of additional concern is that the casual oversight of most medications may place them in the hands of staff or providers for whom they were not intended and for use that is not supervised or authorized. In some cases this leads to misuse or abuse of the medications. Accrediting agencies usually carefully check the process for sample storage and documentation of distribution. For these reasons, many institutions have elected to eliminate the use of samples in their facilities.

Fraud and misbranding of sample products have also led to strict federal regulations on distribution of samples from manufacturer to prescriber. To keep drug samples out of the hands of unauthorized individuals, regulations have also been passed by many states about who may sign for receipt of drug samples. This has caused professional tensions in some states when physician assistants and nurse practitioners are authorized to prescribe medications but are not allowed by ill-informed pharmaceutical company representatives to receive samples. Because of strict enforcement of these laws, many manufacturers have ended the practice of providing product samples.

Attitudes about giving samples to patients have also gradually changed over time. FDA regulation has reduced the flagrant courtship of physicians by drug companies by instituting many policies about what companies can offer to potential prescribers of their products and when (D'Errico, 1998). The Pharmaceutical Researchers and Manufacturers Association and the Accreditation Council Continuing Medical Education have both issues guidelines designed to eliminate unethical behavior from pharmaceutical companies in influencing prescribers through gifts or biased continuing education programs. However, there is also growing recognition of some of the more subtle psychological pressures that are associated with sampling. Using the theory of "gift giving," research has shown that a provider who accepts samples from a pharmaceutical representative often feels a subtle sense of obligation to that company, which may affect prescribing behavior. In turn, patients may feel a sense of obligation to the provider who gives them free drug samples, which in turn may affect their behavior. For example, patients may feel more reluctant to report adverse effects or that they are not feeling better when they take a drug sample (Poe, 1977).

If the health care provider plans to distribute drug samples to patients, the following list of suggestions should be considered:

- Be familiar with and follow any applicable state laws on sample acquisition and distribution.
- Determine if there are any clinic or institutional policies related to sample use and follow them every time a sample is provided to a patient.
- Keep a readily retrievable list of the patients who have received drug samples. Record the lot numbers for each sample given in case the company recalls the medication.
- Be certain to give the patient a clear set of written instructions with the sample as well as providing any verbal instructions and warnings.

SUMMARY

The growing trend to evaluate the costs of new drugs as part of clinical trials and the increased emphasis on pharmacoeconomics are here to stay. Health care providers need to understand basic economic principles and how they influence prescribing practice and drug use. Those who do will be more adequately prepared to develop strategies that meet therapeutic objectives and assist patients in coping with increased costs and payment requirements.

REFERENCES

American Society of Hospital Pharmacists (ASHP): ASHP statement on the use of medications for unlabeled uses, *Am J Hosp Pharm* 49:2006, 1992.

Anonymous: Drug-approval pace remains brisk in 1997, *Am J Health Sys Pharm* 55:336-337, 1998.

Anonymous: FDA issues regulations on accelerated drug-approval process, *Clin Pharm* 12:253-254, 1993.

Anonymous: Investigational new drug, antibiotic, and biological drug product regulations; procedures for drugs intended to treat life-threatening and severely debilitating illnesses, *Fed Reg* 53:41516-41524, 1988.

Anonymous: Prescription practices and regulatory agencies. In Bennett DR, editor: *Drug evaluations, annual 1992,* Chicago, 1991a, American Medical Association.

Anonymous: Orphan drugs. In Bennett DR, editor: *Drug evaluations, annual 1992,* Chicago, 1991b, American Medical Association.

Bartling D, Hadamik H: *Development of a drug. It's a long way from laboratory to patient,* Darmstadt, Germany, 1982, Rhone-Poulenc.

Benzi G et al: Drugs trying to get to the parents: there will be incentives for the European scientific community to develop research in the field of the orphan drugs, *Pharmacol Res* 35:89-93, 1997.

Bootman JL, Townsend RJ, McGhan WF: *Principles of pharmacoeconomics,* ed 2, Cincinnati, OH, 1996, Harvey Whitney Books.

Cimmons M: Moving closer to FDA reform, *Nat Med* 3:940, 1997.

Commission on Federal Drug Approval Process: *Final report,* Washington, DC, March 31, 1982.

Cote CJ: Unapproved uses of approved drugs, *Paediatr Anaesth* 7:91-92, 1997.

Data JL: Potential stifling effects of pharmacoeconomics and regulatory policies, *Am J Cardiol* 81:34F-35F, April 1998.

D'Errico CC: Pharmacoeconomics analysis in a pediatric population, *Ann Thorac Surg* 65(6 Suppl):S52-S54, 1998.

Ensor PA: Projecting future drug expenditures 1992, *Am J Hosp Pharm* 49:140-145, 1992.

FDA's approved drug products with therapeutic equivalence evaluations. United States Pharmaceutical Drug Information, Rockville, MD, 1997, Food and Drug Administration.

Fink JL III, Simonsmeier LM: Laws governing pharmacy. In Gennaro AR, editor: *Remington: the science and practice of pharmacy,* ed 19, Easton, PA, 1995, Mack Publishing.

Fox JL: Pharmacoeconomics: drug pricing's new guise, *Biotechnology* 13:435-436, May 1995.

Gwartney JD, Stroup R: *Microeconomics: private and public choice,* ed 8, New York, 1996, Academic Press.

Hogan GF: Repercussions on the Drug Price Competition and Patent Term Restoration Act of 1984, *Am J Hosp Pharm* 42:849-851, 1985.

Inglehart JK: The American health care system—expenditures, *N Engl J Med* 340:January 7, 1999.

Johannesson M et al: Economics, pharmaceuticals, and pharmacoeconomics, *Med Decis Making* 18(2 Suppl):S1-S3, 1998.

Katz R: The introduction of new drugs. In Gennaro AR, editor: *Remington: the science and practice of pharmacy,* ed 19, Easton, PA, 1995, Mack Publishing.

Knoben JE, Scott GR, Tonelli RJ: An overview of the FDA publication Approved Drug Products with Therapeutic Equivalence Evaluations, *Am J Hosp Pharm* 47:269-270, 1990.

Marwick C: Pharmacoeconomics: is a drug worth its cost? *JAMA* 272:1395, November 9, 1994.

McNamee D: Different kind of drug-company freebie, *Lancet* 348:695, 1996.

Miller HI: FDA "reform"? *Science* 279:158-159, 1998.

Novarro L: Drugs and money: in the high-stakes hunt for blockbuster pharmaceuticals, companies are pouring billions each year into research and development with no guarantee that their products will ultimately pass FDA scrutiny, *Hosp Health Network* 71:54-56, 1997.

Pausjenssen AM et al: Guidelines for measuring the costs and consequences of adopting new pharmaceutical products: are they on track? *Med Decis Making* 18(2 Suppl):S19-S22, 1998.

Phillips PJ: Regulatory approval process, *ASAOP J* 43:881-882, 1997.

Poe DB: The giving of gifts: anthropological data and social psychological theory, *Cornell J Soc Relations* 12:47-63, 1977.

Reh M: Changes at FDA may speed drug approval process and increase off-label use, *J Natl Cancer Inst* 90:805-807, 1998.

Richards JW: Community pharmacy economics and management. In Gennaro AR, editor: *Remington: the science and practice of pharmacy,* ed 19, Easton, PA 1995, Mack Publishing.

Schulman KA, Linas BP: Pharmacoeconomics: state of the art in 1997, *Annu Rev Public Health* 18:529-548, 1997.

Shah ND, Vermfulen MS, Santell JP, Projecting future drug expenditures—2002, *Am J Health Syst Pharm* 59:131-142, 2002.

Stewart A: Choosing an antidepressant: effectiveness based pharmacoeconomics, *J Affect Disord* 48:125-133, 1998.

Thamer M et al: A cross-national comparison of orphan drug policies: implications for the US orphan drug act, *J Health Polit Policy Law* 23:265-290, 1998.

Troetel WM: How new drugs win FDA approval, *US Pharmacist* 54-66, November 1986.

United States Pharmacopeia: *Complete drug reference,* Maryland, 1998, St Martin's Press.

Walley T et al: Pharmacoeconomics: basic concepts and terminology, *Br J Clin Pharmacol* 43:343-348, 1997.

UNIT 2

Pharmacokinetics and Pharmacodynamics

CHAPTER 5

General Pharmacokinetic and Pharmacodynamic Principles

A *drug* is any substance that is used in the diagnosis, cure, treatment, or prevention of a disease or condition (McKenry & Salerno, 2002). This is a very general definition that is not very useful because of the great diversity in the characteristics and actions of drugs. To be more precise, *pharmacokinetics* is the study of the action of drugs in the body, including the processes of absorption, distribution, metabolism, and biotransformation. It may be thought of as what the body does to the drug. *Pharmacodynamics* is the study of the biochemical and physiologic effects of drugs on the function of living organisms and of their component parts (Hardman et al, 2001). It includes consideration of the mechanisms of drug action and may be viewed as what the drug does to the body.

These concepts are essential to the understanding of the prescribing role. Although many readers of this text may have had extensive prior experience in administering drugs, mastery of the content in this chapter is mandatory for moving to the more advanced role of drug prescriber. This chapter therefore is one of the most important in the book and presumes an extensive understanding of scientific principles of biochemistry, anatomy, physiology, and pathophysiology. The information in this chapter is necessary for the provider to progress from memorization of drug names (an increasing impossible task) to understanding the process of drug utilization and being able to generalize from basic principles. It will be important to read this chapter more than once and to try to apply the principles to specific drugs. Not everything can be absorbed in one sitting.

A good understanding of physiology is necessary to understanding the mechanisms of drug actions. The reader may find it useful to review relevant physiology before undertaking the study of a class of drugs. This chapter attempts to express clearly and simply some of the more complex principles of pharmacokinetics. Definitions or concepts that are important in the understanding of pharmacotherapeutics are emphasized. It is written at a deceptively simple level to help clinicians clearly understand major concepts that are commonly overlooked or skimmed quickly but never really mastered.

Goodman & Gilman's Pharmacological Basis of Therapeutics (now edited by Hardman et al, 2001) is the classic reference for the study of pharmacotherapeutics, or the use of drugs in the treatment of disease. As a comprehensive source of information, or where contradictory material is found in the literature, this is the source that may usually be depended on to have factual information. However, for everyday reference, it may be somewhat difficult to retrieve information from this text, and it is certainly not a book that can easily be carried around.

DRUG NOMENCLATURE

Drugs have three names: chemical name, generic name, and trade, or brand, name. The *chemical name* describes the drug's chemical composition and molecular structure. The *generic name,* or *nonproprietary name,* is the official name assigned by the manufacturer with the approval of the US Adopted Name Council (USAN) and is the name listed in pharmacology reference books (McKenry & Salerno, 2002). The *trade name* is the patent name given to the medicine by the company marketing the drug. If more than one company manufactures the drug, then the drug will have more than one trade name, thus adding to the confusion. Trade names are usually simpler and easier to remember than generic names, because drug companies want you to remember their name and to use their drug. However, providers should learn drugs by their generic names and refer to drugs by their generic names when communicating with patients and other health care providers. This is very important in over-the-counter (OTC) medications because the contents of trade name products may change.

PHARMACOKINETICS

Pharmacokinetics focuses on the processes concerned with absorption, distribution, biotransformation (metabolism), and excretion (elimination) of drugs (Figure 5-1).

Absorption

Absorption describes how much of the drug and how fast the drug leaves its site of administration. The bioavailability of the product is what is most important clinically. *Bioavailability* is how much of the drug that is administered reaches its site of action (Hardman et al, 2001). The fraction of the drug that reaches the systemic circulation is called the *f value.* After the oral ingestion of a solid or liquid drug, the drug must break up (disintegrate) and then become soluble in body fluids (dissolution) before the process of pharmacokinetic absorption begins (Stringer, 2000).

Bioequivalence is an issue in generic versus trade drugs. *Bioequivalence* means that two drug products (1) contain the same active ingredients; (2) are identical in strength or concentration, dosage form, and route of administration; and (3) have essentially the same rate and extent of bioavailability (Hardman et al, 2001). Although a generic drug may have the same amount of drug, because of variabilities in the way the medication is manufactured, it may have slightly more or less drug bioavailability. Legally the drug must be ±20% of the proprietary drug. This variance becomes a concern in certain drugs, especially where there is a narrow therapeutic window (e.g., Lanoxin versus digoxin). Avoiding variation and complying with preferred drug formularies are the major reasons for ordering "Dispense as written" trade name prescriptions.

Factors that Affect Absorption. Four primary factors must be considered in evaluating drug absorption: drug

	Absorption	Distribution	Biotransformation	Elimination
SITES	Gut ⟶ Plasma	Plasma ⟶ Tissue	Liver	Kidney
CONCEPTS	Bioavailability	Volume of distribution	Enzyme inhibition/ induction First-pass effect	Clearance Half-life Steady state Linear/nonlinear kinetics
	Factors: Drug characteristics Blood flow Cell membrane	Phases: 1. Blood flow from site of administration 2. Delivery of drug into tissues at site of drug action	Phase 1: Oxidation Cytochrome P450 Phase 2: Glucuronidation	

FIGURE 5-1

The process of pharmacokinetics.

characteristics, routes of administration, blood flow, and cell membrane characteristics.

Drug Characteristics. The following list includes some general drug characteristics relevant to all routes of administration. (Other factors are discussed under the specific route of administration.)

- *Formulation of the drug*—Influences dissolution rate of solid form of drug.
- *Concentration of the drug*—The higher the concentration, the more quickly the drug is absorbed.
- *Lipophilic drug formulations are more readily absorbable*—Nonionized drugs are more lipid soluble and may readily diffuse across cell membranes. Ionized drugs are lipid insoluble and nondiffusible.
- *Acidic drugs become nonionized in the acidity of the stomach and then diffuse across membranes*—Basic drugs (alkaloids) tend to ionize in the stomach, are not well absorbed in the stomach, but may be better absorbed in the small intestine. A change in the pH of the stomach will affect the absorption of many drugs (Katzung, 2000).

Routes of Administration. The complexity of routes of administration and delivery systems has increased greatly. The most common routes for giving medications include oral (PO), topical (TOP, TD), subcutaneous (SQ), intramuscular (IM), intravenous (IV), and rectal (PR). Other less common routes used include intradermal (ID), sublingual (SL), buccal, intra-articular, inhalation, intravaginally, ophthalmic, and aural.

Oral ingestion is the most common method of drug administration. It is the most convenient, economical, and safest. However, disadvantages of oral administration include the following:

- Poor gastrointestinal absorption may occur because of the physical characteristics of the drug.
- Irritation to the gastrointestinal mucosa may result in ulceration or emesis.
- Destruction of drugs may occur because of digestive enzymes and low gastric pH.
- Interactions may occur between the drug and food or other substances in the gastrointestinal tract.

There are many variations in oral drug formulations (listed in order from the fastest absorption rate to the slowest absorption rate): liquids, elixirs, syrups, suspensions, solutions, powders, capsules, tablets, coated tablets, enteric-coated tablets, and slow-release formulations (Hardman et al, 2001; Katzung, 2000).

Oral. Controlled-release preparations are designed to provide slow, uniform absorption of a drug (usually with a short half-life) over a long period of time, usually 8 to 12 hours. These work with varying degrees of success. Some formulations come in a wax matrix that is not absorbed but is excreted in the feces (Hardman et al, 2001). Patients may become concerned about the appearance of this substance in the feces unless they are warned.

Sublingual Preparations. Some drugs that are nonionic and have high lipid solubility are readily absorbed by the oral mucosa. A major advantage to this route is that it avoids the hepatic first-pass metabolism. When drugs are absorbed orally, they immediately pass through the liver before being distributed to the rest of the body. Many drugs are extensively metabolized on this first pass, allowing little of the drug to remain active. Drugs absorbed sublingually bypass the first-pass phenomenon; therefore smaller doses may be used effectively. Sublingual nitroglycerin is an example of this type of medication.

Topical. Few drugs easily penetrate intact skin. Lipid-soluble drugs may not be absorbed because the skin acts as a lipid barrier. However, many other types of solutions may be absorbed. Skin that is not intact will absorb drugs more readily. Thus it is important to apply topical medications to intact, healthy skin to ensure the correct absorption. Other drugs are readily absorbed though mucous membranes, which absorb drugs more readily than intact skin because of increased vascularity. Topical administration has the same advantage of avoiding the first-pass metabolism of the drug through the liver (Hardman et al, 2001).

Rectal. Medications that cannot be given orally can often be given rectally. Rectal medications are usually given when the patient is vomiting or unconscious. One advantage is that there is less first-pass metabolism of the drug through the liver for rectal than for oral preparations. However, rectal absorption tends to be more inconsistent and less complete than oral absorption, and many drugs can cause rectal irritation. It is not always necessary to have a specially formulated rectal preparation (Edmunds, 2003). For example, oral time-release morphine tablets will be absorbed rectally and are useful when the patient is unable to take an occasional oral dose of pain medicine.

Inhalation. Drugs can be given by nasal spray for local topical absorption through mucous membranes or by inhaler or nebulizer for pulmonary absorption. Pulmonary absorption uses a large surface area, making absorption rapid. This also avoids first-pass metabolism in the liver. Inhalation delivers the medication directly to the desired site of action, forcing particles of drugs down into the pulmonary system. The disadvantages of inhalation therapy are in regulating the exact dosage and the difficulty many patients have in self-administering a drug via inhaler.

Ophthalmic. Drops or ointments may be prescribed for the eye. These should be instilled into the pouch of the lower eyelid and not applied directly to the eye surface itself (Edmunds, 2003). Anything formulated for use on the eye can be used anywhere else in the body.

Blood Flow. Circulation at the site of administration is important in the drug absorption process. Decreased circulation (as seen in congestive heart failure) will result in decreased drug absorption (Katzung, 2000). For example, insulin injected into a thigh muscle, followed by exercise, will produce more rapid absorption of the insulin than without exercise.

Cell Membrane Characteristics. When drugs are absorbed, they pass through cells, not between them; therefore the drug must pass through the cellular wall or membrane. The structure of the cell membrane influences this process (Figure 5-2). The cell membrane is composed of a two-molecule layer of lipids containing protein molecules between the lipids. It also contains carbohydrate molecules that are attached to the outer surface of the membrane. The proteins can be either integral (in which case they go through the membrane) or peripheral (in which case they are attached to the surface of the membrane) (McCance & Huether, 2001). Integral proteins act as structural channels for the transportation of water-soluble substances (ions) or as carrier proteins in active transport. Peripheral proteins are enzymes. Glycoproteins may be antigenic sites in immune reactions or drug receptors. The pores permit the passage of small water-soluble substances such as water, electrolytes, urea, and alcohol (Hardman et al, 2001).

Drugs cross membranes via either passive diffusion or active transport. *Passive diffusion* involves the random movement of drug molecules from high to low concentrations. *Active transport* moves molecules that are moderate sized, water soluble, or ionic across cell membranes. In active transport, these molecules form complexes with carriers for transport through the membrane and then dissociate from them. Active transport requires expenditure of energy and can occur against the concentration gradient (Stringer, 2000) (Figure 5-3).

In passive diffusion, the drug molecule penetrates along a concentration gradient as a result of its solubility in the lipid layer of the membrane (Figure 5-4). The transfer is in proportion to the magnitude of the concentration gradient across the membrane. The higher the concentration, the more rapid is the diffusion across the membrane. If the drug is not an electrolyte, a steady state is attained when the concentration of the free drug is the same on both sides of the membrane. If the drug is an ionic compound, the steady-state concentration will depend on the difference in the pH across the membrane (Hardman et al, 2001).

Whether the drug is lipophilic or hydrophilic affects absorption across cell membranes. Lipids pass through membranes better than do hydrophilic molecules. However, most cell membranes are permeable to water, either by diffusion or by hydrostatic or osmotic differences across the membrane (Stringer, 2000). The water may carry with it small water-soluble substances such as urea.

The pH of a drug also affects absorption. Nonionized drugs are more lipid soluble and may readily diffuse across cell membranes. Ionized drugs are lipid insoluble and nondiffusible. Acidic drugs such as aspirin become nonionized in the acid environment of the stomach and thus can diffuse across the membranes (DiPiro et al, 2002; Stringer, 2000). A change in the acidity of the stomach, as occurs with antacids, will affect absorption of drugs. Basic drugs such as alkaloids ionize in the stomach and are not well absorbed. These drugs are better absorbed in a less acid environment such as the small intestine.

Distribution

Distribution is the transport of a drug in body fluids from the bloodstream (at the site of absorption) to various tissues in the body. The pattern of distribution depends on the pharmacokinetic activity of different types of tissue and the different physiochemical properties of drugs (Hardman et al, 2001). Drugs vary in their ability to move into various body compartments (brain, fat, lung, eye, and so forth). The best way to know how much of a given drug gets into a particular body compartment

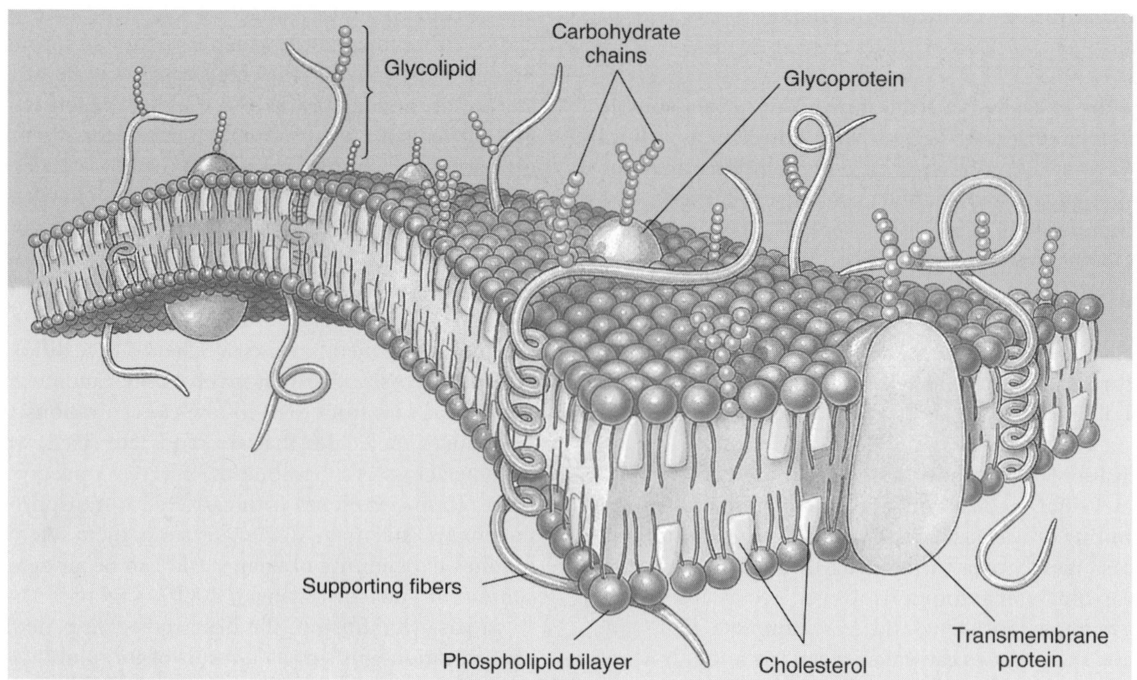

FIGURE 5-2

Cell membrane structure. The lipid bilayer provides the basic structure and serves as a relatively impermeable barrier to most water-soluble molecules. (Modified from Thibodeau GA, Patton KI: *Structure and function of the human body*, ed 11, St Louis, 2000, Mosby.)

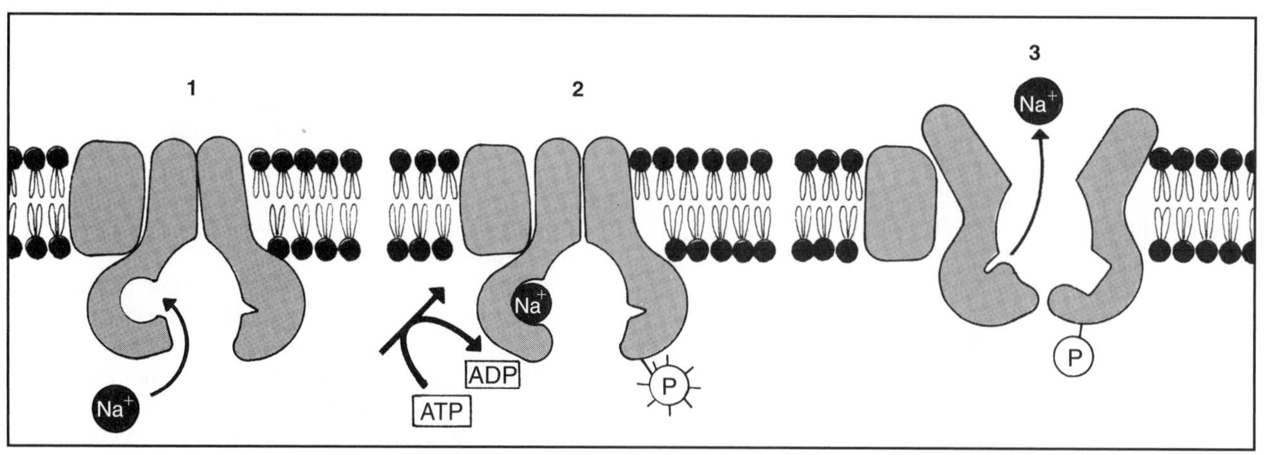

FIGURE 5-3

Active mediated transport. Metabolic energy is necessary for the active transport of many substances, including Na^+. (Modified from Alberts B et al, editors: *Molecular biology of the cell*, ed 3, New York, 1994, Garland.)

is to consult standard reference texts. Because blood is an easily accessible body fluid, blood concentrations are often studied to determine how they relate to drug concentrations in other body compartments. The dose-related effects of a drug are then correlated with a given blood concentration or range of concentration. Once a relationship has been established, blood concentrations can then be used to monitor therapy.

There are two phases of distribution. The first involves movement from the site of administration into the bloodstream. Delivery of the drug into the tissue at the site of action is the second phase of distribution (Katzung, 2000).

The volume of distribution (Vd) is a concept useful in understanding where the drug goes once it is absorbed. *Volume of distribution* is a description of the amount of space into which a drug can be spread. It is the calculated volume or size of a compartment necessary to account for the total amount of drug in the body if it were present throughout the body at the same concentration found in the plasma (Hardman et al,

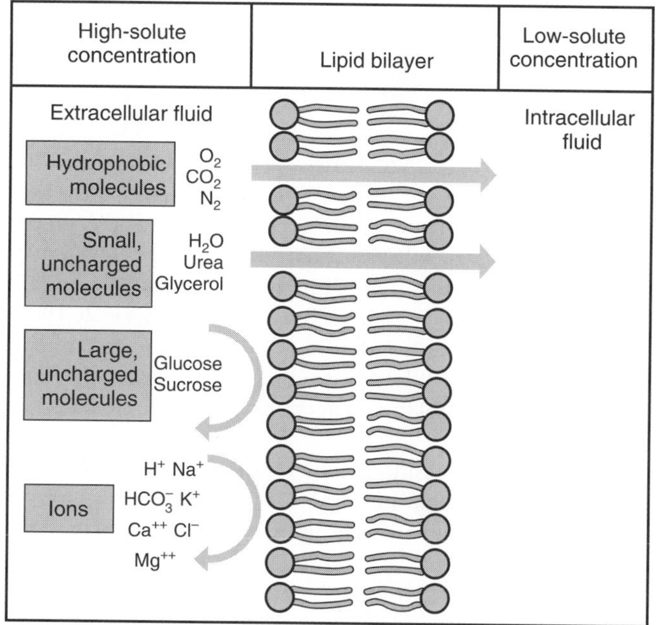

FIGURE 5-4

Passive diffusion. Oxygen, nitrogen, water, urea, glycerol, and carbon dioxide can diffuse readily down the concentration gradient. Macromolecules are too large to diffuse through pores in the plasma membrane. Ions may be repelled if the pores contain substances with identical charges. (From McCance KL, Huether SE: *Pathophysiology: the biologic basis of disease in infants and children,* ed 4, St Louis, 2001, Mosby.)

2001). Because most drugs are not equally distributed, this is a theoretical concept and not a real volume. It is, however, useful in predicting drug concentrations, understanding how well a drug is absorbed into tissues, and understanding whether it will be accumulated in the tissues. If a drug has a small volume of distribution, it means it stays in the central compartment and is not widely distributed. If the drug has a large volume of distribution, it means it is widely found throughout the body. The larger the Vd, the more drug is in the tissue. Because we are able to measure the amount of drug in the bloodstream only through serum levels, calculation of the volume of distribution allows us to estimate or predict the concentration of the drug in the tissue (Stringer, 2000).

The Vd may be calculated by examining the following relationships:

If

$$\text{Concentration of drug in blood} = \frac{\text{Amount of drug in body}}{\text{Vd}}$$

then

$$\text{Vd} = \frac{\text{Amount of drug in body}}{\text{Concentration}}$$

This means that the Vd is equal to the amount of drug in the body divided by the concentration in the blood (Hardman et al, 2001).

Water-soluble drugs have a Vd similar to the plasma volume because they are distributed into the blood. The plasma volume for a normal adult is about 3 to 5 liters. Lipophilic drugs have a larger Vd. The total fluid volume in the body is about 40 liters for a 70-kg (150-lb) person. Because the Vd of a lipophilic drug can exceed this volume, it is important to remember that this calculation is of a hypothetical volume, not a real volume. It is the volume that would be required to contain the entire drug in the body if the drug were distributed in the same concentration as in the blood or plasma (Hardman et al, 2001).

Factors that affect the volume of distribution include plasma protein binding, obesity, edema, and tissue binding. Therefore the Vd for a given drug can change as a function of the patient's age, gender, disease, and body composition.

Drugs that are highly protein bound (>90%) have a volume of distribution about the same as the amount of plasma. This is a small volume of distribution. An example would be the thyroid hormones. If the patient has a decreased serum albumin, protein-bound drugs will then have more active drug available. If there are two protein-bound drugs, the most tightly protein-bound drug will tend to displace the other. Examples of these drugs are furosemide and cephalosporins (DiPiro et al, 2002; Hardman et al, 2001).

Any alteration in the normal muscle-to-fat ratio will change the Vd of a drug. For example, in obesity, lipophilic drugs distribute into adipose tissue and tend to accumulate. Thus less drug will be available elsewhere to have an effect. For example, phenobarbital is fat soluble. The drug may become trapped in the fatty tissue, causing low blood levels of phenobarbital. The fat-soluble drugs are slowly released from the fat into the bloodstream, so they have a longer duration of action. This factor may also prolong duration of side effects or affect dosing schedules.

Geriatric patients often have relatively less muscle and more fat, placing them at risk for accumulation of lipophilic drugs in the adipose tissue. If these patients lose weight and take the same dose, they could become toxic. This can be a particular problem with lipophilic benzodiazepines. In these patients, water-soluble drugs have a smaller Vd, resulting in increased blood concentrations. This effect is even greater if the patient is dehydrated. An example of a drug producing this situation is gentamicin.

In addition, excess fluid in the interstitial spaces, such as is seen with edema, will affect the distribution of water-soluble drugs.

Some drugs have an affinity for specific tissues. This affinity becomes useful in treating certain infections. For example, ciprofloxacin and tetracycline have an affinity for bone.

It is not generally necessary to calculate Vd when using drugs. However, it is an important concept to understand when administering a drug and may influence the dosage or choice of a drug. Always consider where the drug will go and how much will get to the target organ or tissue.

The distribution of drugs from the bloodstream to the central nervous system is different than that through other cell membranes. The endothelial cells of the brain capillaries do not have intercellular pores and vesicles. Passive distribution of hydrophilic drugs is restricted. However, lipophilic drugs will easily pass the blood-brain barrier, limited only by cerebral blood flow (Hardman et al, 2001). Highly fat-soluble drugs also cross the blood-brain barrier easily and are more likely to cause central nervous system side effects such as confusion and drowsiness.

Biotransformation (Metabolism)

Biotransformation is the chemical inactivation of a drug through conversion to a more water-soluble compound that can be excreted from the body. Biotransformation occurs primarily in the liver, but also in the lungs and GI tract. It involves two major steps in enzyme activity. Phase I is *oxidation,* making the drug more hydrophilic. Minor changes in the structure of the drug make it more hydrophilic but allow it to maintain all or part of its pharmacologic activity. The cytochrome P450 enzyme system is a part of phase I. Phase II is called *glucuronidation.* It involves *conjugation,* or attaching particles to the molecule, making it a highly water-soluble substance with little or no pharmacologic activity (Honkakoski & Negishi, 1997). If there is decreased blood flow to the liver, drugs will be more slowly metabolized, leading to a longer duration of action.

Lipophilic drugs pass easily through membranes, including renal tubules, making them difficult to excrete. Biotransformation changes a lipophilic drug that is active and transforms it into a hydrophilic inactive compound that is readily excreted. However, metabolites occasionally have biologic activity or toxic properties (Figure 5-5).

Phase I: Oxidation or Reduction of Drugs. Phase I involves oxidation or reduction, hydrolysis reactions that make drugs more water soluble so that they can be excreted. During this phase, perhaps as many as 40 different P450 enzymes present in the liver may be available to participate as catalysts in oxidization of drugs. It appears that the metabolism of most drugs can be accounted for by a relatively small subset of these enzymes, with probably half attributed to CYP 3A4. The information about the P450 enzyme system is a field of rapidly expanding attention, with new information becoming available constantly.

The cytochrome P450 enzyme system operates throughout the body. It is concentrated in the liver, intestine, and lungs. The P450 enzyme system resides in the ribosomes, which are sacs in the endoplasmic reticulum. It is named P450 because this is the length of the wave of light that these enzymes absorb. Chemically, the enzymes are glycoproteins or a sugar plus a protein. Many of the proteins contain heme, hence the name *chrome.* This family of enzymes is divided into groups according to similarity. There are 40 major groups that have been identified in humans so far. The major groups named 1, 2, 3, and 4 are known to be involved in drug interactions. These major groups are further divided into groups by their chemical structure, named A, B, and C. The A, B, and C groups are then divided into subgroups named 1, 2, 3, etc. The groups most important in human drug interactions are as follows: CYP 2D6, CYP 3A3/4, CYP 1A2, CYP 2C9/10, and CYP 2C19. In the groups with 3/4 and 9/10, the two are so close in structure that they are hard to differentiate and have very similar actions (Adedoyin et al, 1998; Guengerich, 1997; Honkakoski & Negishi, 1997).

Technology has resulted in an explosion of information concerning the cytochrome P450 isoenzymes and increased awareness of life-threatening interactions with such commonly prescribed drugs as cisapride and some antihistamines. Knowledge of the substrates, inhibitors, and inducers of these enzymes assists in predicting clinically significant drug interactions.

The P450 enzyme system is not the same in every individual. Each person receives genetic material that determines individual variations in the enzyme system; this is called *genetic polymorphism.* Thus there may be individual differences as well as racial and gender differences. These are not yet well known or understood. Patients express their enzyme system in different ways. This explains why different patients react differently to a drug. For example, some patients metabolize codeine (CYP 2D6) quickly and need larger doses, whereas other patients metabolize it slowly and need less.

The essential facts to master about the P450 enzyme system are that there are six primary enzymes that account for the metabolism of nearly all clinically important drugs and that two of these systems are critically important for drug metabolism.

CYP 3A4 is an enzyme needed to metabolism antihistamines, antibiotics, lipid-lowering drugs, antihypertensives, protease inhibitors, and antifungals. This system is used in the metabolism of about 50% of all clinically useful medications. These enzymes are the most abundant and clinically signifi-

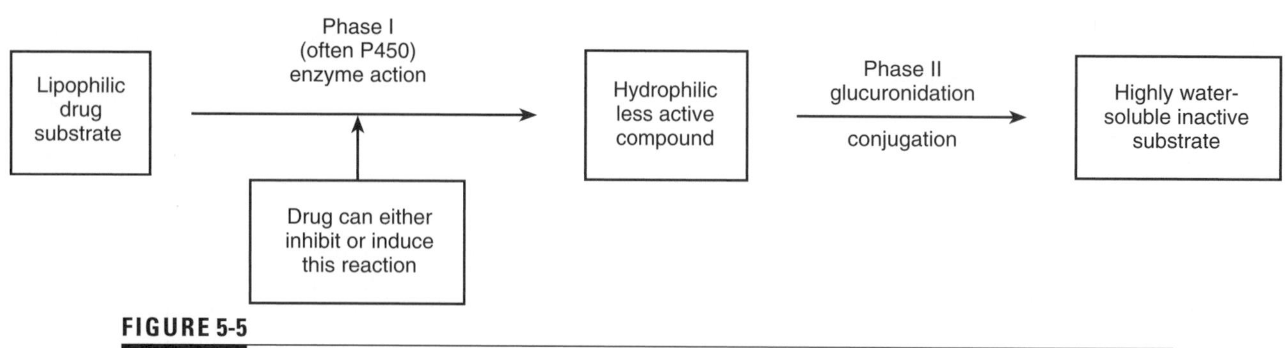

FIGURE 5-5

Processes involved in biotransformation.

cant. (In CYP 3A4, the notation CYP indicates that the property is part of the cytochrome P450 system; 3 indicates the family; A indicates the subfamily; and 4 indicates that it is the fourth enzyme in that subsystem.)

The CYP 2D6 enzyme looks different and is different. It metabolizes selective serotonin reuptake inhibitors (SSRIs), pain relievers, beta-blockers, and other drugs. This enzyme metabolizes about 30% of all clinically useful medications, is the second most abundant, and participates in converting codeine to morphine.

Of the other four enzymes, the most notable features of each are as follows:

- CYP 2C19—Metabolizes proton pump inhibitors, nonsteroidal antiinflammatory drugs (NSAIDs), and beta blockers
- CYP 2C9—Metabolizes sulfonylureas, NSAIDs, (S)-warfarin, and sildenafil citrate (Viagra)
- CYP 1A2—Metabolizes acetaminophen, (*R*)-warfarin, theophylline, caffeine, diazepam (Valium), and verapamil
- CYP 2E1—Metabolizes acetaminophen, ethanol, inactivation of toxins, and dextramorphan (Michalets, 1998)

A drug can be a *substrate* or one that is affected by alteration in its enzyme metabolism. A drug can also be the one that causes the alteration in the enzyme metabolism of another drug by being an *inhibitor* or an *inducer*. The cytochrome P450 enzyme system may speed up a reaction because it causes the drug to change to a more hydrophilic substance. Any drug that causes the enzyme to metabolize more slowly, or decreases the capacity of the enzyme pathway, is called an *inhibitor.* For example, if a patient on fluoxetine (Prozac) takes acetaminophen with codeine, the fluoxetine inhibits the P450 enzyme system from converting codeine to the active form. Thus the patient would have less pain relief from the medication. A drug that causes the enzymes to metabolize the substrate more quickly is called an *inducer.* Any drug can be involved in this process in two ways. It can be the drug or substrate that is being acted upon, or it can be the inhibitor or inducer that is acting on the enzyme to increase or decrease enzyme conversion of the substrate drug into an inactive compound. The same drug can be both a substrate and an inducer or inhibitor (Hardman et al, 2001). For example, carbamazepine is an autoinducer—it induces its own metabolism. It is the enzyme system, *not* the drug that is being induced or inhibited (see Figure 5-5 to examine these relationships).

A drug can inhibit an enzyme pathway by two mechanisms. The first is competition. This is not usually a problem. If it occurs, it occurs immediately. Most inhibition is metabolic. The inhibitor drug decreases the production of the enzyme. It shrinks the enzyme pathway. This is not an immediate reaction; it will take from 24 hours to a week to see the effect, depending on the half-life of the drug (Hardman et al, 2001). From a pharmacokinetic standpoint, the major effects of drug–drug interactions can be understood in terms of causing a high or low plasma and tissue level of the drug.

Enzyme induction is much less common than inhibition. These drugs make the pathway work quickly, causing the substrate drug to be deactivated more rapidly. This will lower the level of the drug in the body. The clinically important inducers are anticonvulsants. All anticonvulsants should be considered as possible inducers. Evaluation of these drugs is particularly important when adding them to a patient's medication regimen.

In addition to cytochrome P450, oxidation of drugs and other xenobiotics can also be mediated by non-P450 enzymes, the most significant of which are flavin monooxygenase, monoamine oxidase, alcohol dehydrogenase, aldehyde dehydrogenase, aldehyde oxidase, and xanthine oxidase. Drug oxidation catalyzed by some of these enzymes may often produce the same metabolites as those generated by P450, and thus drug interactions may be difficult to predict without a clear knowledge of the underlying enzymology. Although oxidation catalyzed by non-P450 enzymes can lead to drug inactivation, oxidation may be essential for the generation of active metabolites that create drug action (Beedham, 1997).

Phase II: Biotransformation. Phase II biotransformation consists of conjugate reactions in which a compound is added to the drug. These reactions bind a chemical group on to the drug compound via a covalent linkage. The chemical groups added to the drug are generally highly polar, or ionized. This makes them water soluble and generally inactive. However, a few of these conjugate compounds are active (Hardman et al, 2001).

First-Pass Effect. When a medication is taken orally, it passes from the intestine directly to the liver by way of the hepatic portal blood flow. Certain drugs are extensively metabolized to inert compounds when they first pass through the liver, such as, nitroglycerin and estrogen. Because of this, very large amounts of the drug must be given to have a sufficient dose remain after the first pass through the liver. This is known as the first-pass effect (Stringer, 2000). It is why these drugs are often given via an alternative. route, such as sublingual or topical, to avoid the liver on the first pass. Alternative route dosing also makes it possible to give a smaller amount of the drug and have it be effective.

Prodrug. A *prodrug* is a chemical that is pharmacologically inactive. It is biotransformed into a biologically active metabolite in the body. The angiotensin-converting enzyme inhibitor enalapril is an example of a medication that is transformed from a prodrug into a biologically active metabolite (Hardman et al, 2001). This activity may be reduced in congestive heart failure if the liver is congested, thus delaying treatment of the heart failure.

Elimination

Elimination is the process by which drugs and their metabolites are removed from the body. The liver and the kidney are the two major organs responsible for elimination.

The majority of elimination occurs through excretion by the kidneys. The processes involved in renal elimination are glomerular filtration, tubular secretion, and partial reabsorption. In glomerular filtration, the drug enters the renal tubule by filtration. This depends on the amount of protein binding

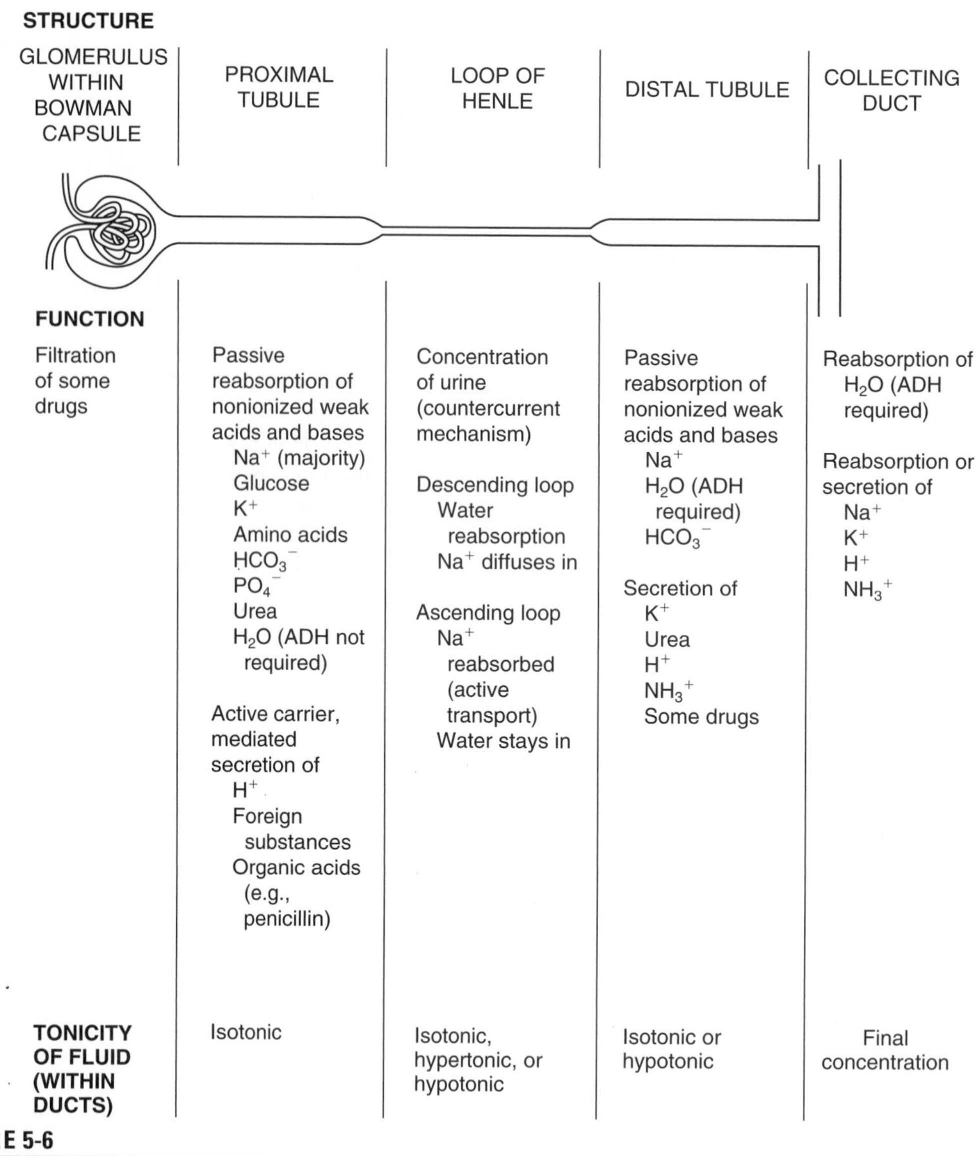

FIGURE 5-6

Drug elimination by the kidney. (Modified from Wong DL: *Whaley and Wong's nursing care of infants and children,* ed 6, St Louis, 1998, Mosby.)

because a drug does not filter into the tubule if it is bound to a protein. This action also depends on the rate of glomerular filtration, which in turn depends on the kidney function and cardiovascular status of the patient (Figure 5-6).

Active, carrier-mediated tubular secretion is responsible for adding some organic anion and cation molecules to the proximal renal tubule. The carrier systems are fairly nonselective and organic ions compete for transport. Thus two drugs may compete for the same active transport carriers and their excretion will be slowed (Hardman et al, 2001). Although it may be difficult to predict the result, a drug can be both secreted and actively reabsorbed. Penicillin is an important example.

Once the drug is excreted via active transport in the proximal tubule, weakly acidic or alkaline molecules may undergo passive reabsorption. How much is reabsorbed depends on the pH of the urine. Alkalinization of the urine will increase the excretion of acidic molecules. Acidification of the urine will increase the excretion of basic molecules. Clinical alteration of the pH of urine is used to hasten the excretion of some drugs, as in the case of drug poisoning or drug toxicity (DiPiro et al, 2002).

If there is a decreased glomerular filtration rate in the kidneys, the drug remains in the blood longer. In patients with kidney damage, it is necessary to determine the creatinine clearance to modify the dosage of medication necessary. This may be calculated with the following:

$$\text{Creatinine clearance} = \frac{\text{Weight (kg*)} \times (140 - \text{Age [in years]})}{72 \times \text{Serum creatinine (mg/dl)} (\times 0.85)\dagger}$$

Other routes by which drugs and their metabolites are excreted are fecal, respiratory, through breast milk, and other miscellaneous ways. The fecal route is often clinically significant. Drugs are metabolized in the liver, and the metabolites are excreted in the bile. These metabolites are reabsorbed into the blood and then excreted in the urine or, less commonly, simply excreted in the feces. Excretion from the liver into the bile is accomplished by active transport systems, which are limited in the quantity of metabolites they can excrete (Stringer, 2000). Different drugs may compete for transport. This competition may slow down the excretion of certain drugs; steroids provide an example of competition that slows excretion.

The respiratory route is an important route of excretion in anesthetic gases. Excretion in breast milk is important, not for the quantity excreted, but because of the effect it may have on a nursing infant. Other routes such as perspiration, saliva, tears, hair, and skin are not usually clinically significant.

Clearance is loosely defined as a measure of the rate at which the drug is removed from the body (Stringer, 2000). The body can eliminate the drug only if the drug is in contact with the eliminating organ. If a drug is being stored in adipose tissue, it cannot be cleared from the body. Thus volume of distribution affects the clearance of a drug and hence the half-life.

Specifically, clearance is defined as the volume of plasma from which all drug is removed in a given time. It is measured in volume divided by time:

$$\text{Clearance} = \frac{\text{Rate of removal of drug (mg/min)}}{\text{Plasma concentration of drug (mg/ml)}}$$

*Lean body weight may reflect creatinine production more accurately.
†In females, multiply value × 0.85.

This formula gives milliliters of plasma that has had the drug removed from it in the specified amount of time (1 minute). *Total body clearance* is the sum of the clearances from the various metabolizing and eliminating organs (Stringer, 2000).

Steady state means there is a stable concentration of the drug, or the drug is being administered at the same rate at which it is being eliminated. This is fairly simple with a continuous infusion of drugs. In intermittent administration of medication, the frequency and amount of the drug must be adjusted to achieve steady state. Parkinson's medications such as carbidopa/levodopa (Sinemet) often require adjustment for both the amount and the interval of dosing to achieve therapeutic levels without reaching toxic levels. Patients who are eliminating drugs more slowly than normal will need smaller doses of a drug than will patients who eliminate the drug normally.

Plasma Concentration-Time Curve. The plasma concentration-time curve (Figure 5-7) illustrates what happens when a single dose of a drug is given. The time between when the drug is given and when it first takes effect is the *latent period. Onset of action* is the time it first takes effect. When the drug no longer has an effect, this is known as *termination of action*. The *duration of action* is the period of time in which the drug has its effect. The *minimal effective concentration* is the lowest level of concentration that produces the drug effect. The *peak plasma level* is the highest level the drug reaches. If the concentration is high enough to cause adverse drug reactions, this level is known as the *toxic level*. The *therapeutic range* is the area between the minimal effective concentration and the toxic concentration.

First-Order/Linear Kinetics. The concept of *half-life* is an important one to understand. The half-life of a drug is the amount of time required for the amount of drug in the body to decrease by one half. This is a significant factor in

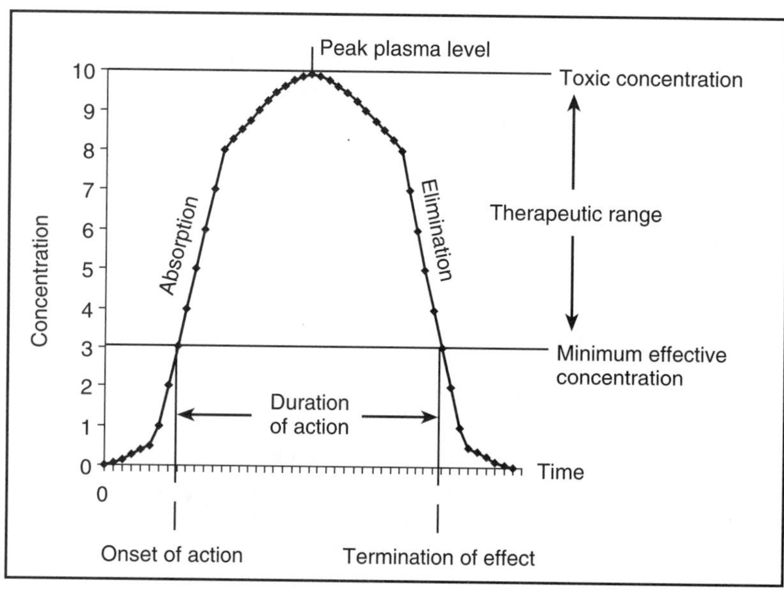

FIGURE 5-7

Plasma concentration time curve with single dose of drug.

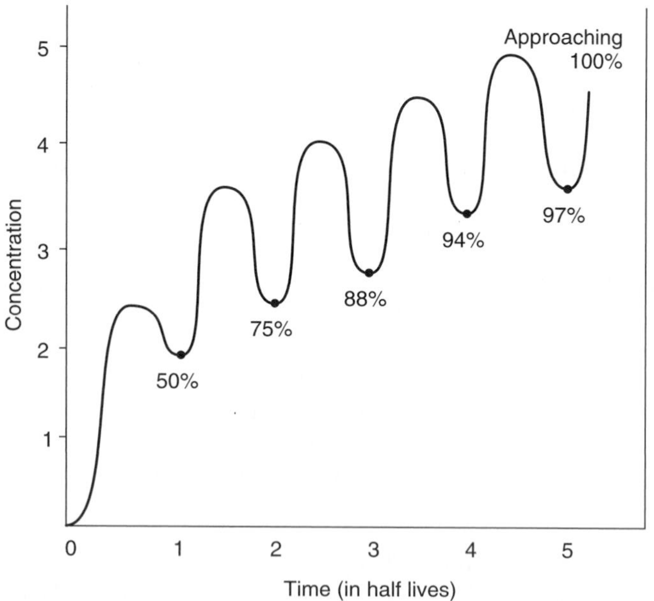

FIGURE 5-8

Drug accumulation time to steady state. The line shows concentration of drugs in the body. (Modified from Hardman JG, Limbird LW et al, editors: *Goodman and Gilman's pharmacological basis of therapeutics*, ed 10, New York, 2001, McGraw-Hill.)

accumulation and elimination of drugs. It depends on clearance and volume of distribution. When a patient is given a drug on a regular schedule, the drug will continue to accumulate until the steady state is achieved (Stringer, 2000) (Figure 5-8). The half-life of a drug listed in reference books is an approximation of what the most likely or usual half-life will be in a normal, healthy adult. However, there is much individual variation based on factors that affect volume of distribution and elimination. Half-life is useful to estimate the amount of time it takes to reach a steady state of a drug after a dosage regimen is started. Steady state is reached after 4 to 5 half-lives, which will be 94% to 97% of the eventual steady state. Half-life can also be used to estimate the amount of time to eliminate a drug from the body after it has been discontinued. Again, after 4 to 5 half-lives, about 94% to 97% of the drug will have been eliminated from the body (Hardman et al, 2001). Of course, there is always a difference between the absolute (or theoretical) steady state and what is seen in fact for each patient.

Some drugs with short half-lives are ibuprofen and the benzodiazepine lorazepam. Examples of some drugs with long half-lives are anticoagulants, diazepam, digoxin, and fluoxetine (Prozac). Drugs with long half-lives need to be closely monitored because toxic effects or adverse reactions may last a long time.

In linear or first-order kinetics, drug concentration is increased or decreased in a linear fashion, depending on dosage, clearance, volume of distribution, and half-life. The drugs appear and disappear from plasma, depending on concentration. However, the percent of drug eliminated is constant.

Average concentration when the steady state is attained during intermittent drug administration may be calculated as follows:

$$\text{Concentration} = \frac{\text{Drug availability} \times \text{Dose}}{\text{Clearance} \times \text{Time}}$$

Nonlinear Kinetics. Nonlinear kinetics, or zero-order kinetics, is more complicated. In this case, elimination does not depend on the dose or concentration of a drug. The amount of drug eliminated is constant. The drug is removed by saturation of a function, such as protein binding (limiting the amount of protein available for binding), hepatic metabolism (limiting the amount of enzyme causing metabolism), and active renal transport (limiting the amount of carrier). The half-life of the drug depends on the concentration (DiPiro et al, 2002; Stringer, 2000).

Phenytoin is a clinically important example of nonlinear kinetics because of both protein binding and hepatic metabolism. As phenytoin is absorbed, it is bound to plasma protein. When a regimen is started, most of the drug is bound to protein, leaving little free drug. However, as the proteins reach saturation, suddenly there is a much greater percentage of the absorbed drug that is not protein bound and is free drug. When the proteins are saturated, suddenly the free drug, measured as a serum drug level, will rise rapidly. A narrow therapeutic window makes toxicity a frequent problem. When the amount of drug concentration exceeds the ability of the liver to metabolize the drug, nonlinear kinetics occur (DiPiro et al, 2002). Again, the body has a finite ability to produce enzymes that metabolize the drug. Once the body is working at capacity, any additional drug will accumulate and cause toxicity. Another example of a drug that follows nonlinear kinetic principles is theophylline. Drugs that follow nonlinear kinetics are far more difficult to maintain in the therapeutic range and must be monitored more closely for toxicity.

PHARMACODYNAMICS

Pharmacodynamics is the study of biochemical and physiologic effects of drugs and the mechanisms of their action (Hardman et al, 2001). A concise definition of pharmacodynamics to remember is "the effect of the drug on the body."

Mechanisms of Drug Action

Most drugs act on the body by chemical reactions with some large molecular component of the organism. The drug alters the function of the component, thereby causing biochemical and physiologic changes that are characteristic of the response to the particular drug. The drug interacts with a chemical receptor (Katzung, 2000). The concept of drug receptors explains the mechanisms of action.

Drug Receptors. A *receptor* is the component of the organism with which the drug binds or interacts to change a function within the body. Receptors or ligands are molecules occurring naturally in the body that react to form a complex with another molecule (Stringer, 2000). An example is a hormone molecule. Figure 5-9 shows three types of cellular receptors. Drugs generally do not create an effect by themselves but through a receptor. The site at which a drug acts depends on the

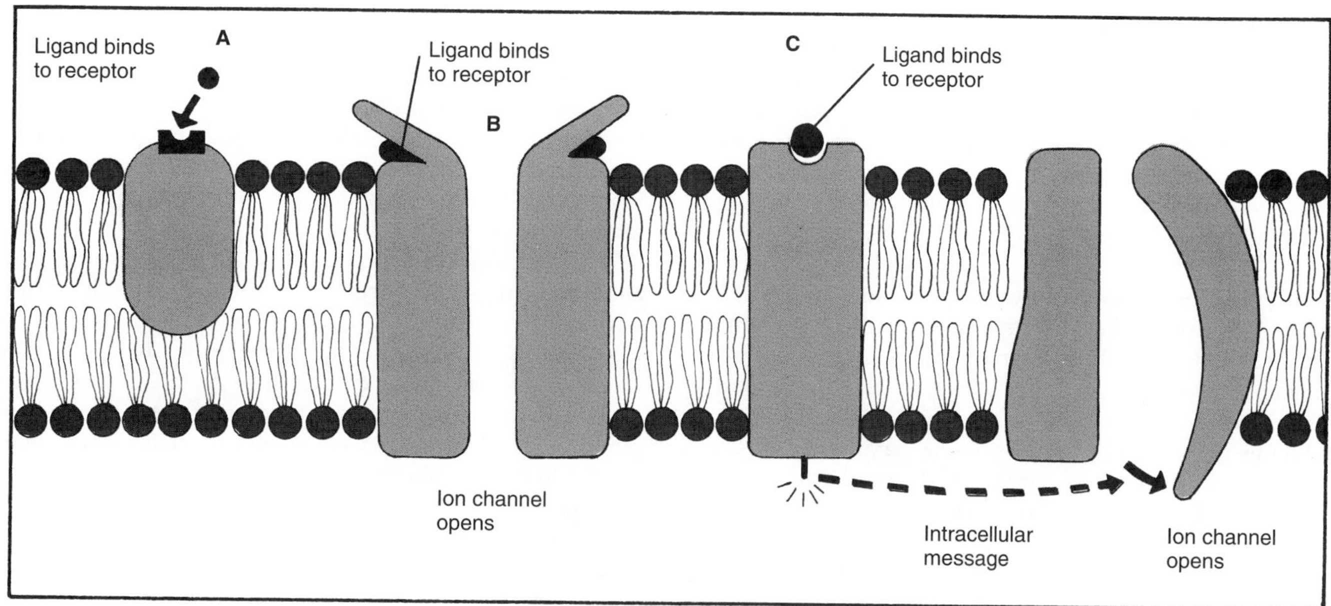

FIGURE 5-9

Cellular receptors. **A**, Plasma membrane receptor for a ligand on the surface of an integral protein. **B** and **C**, A neurotransmitter can exert its effect on a postsynaptic cell by means of two fundamentally different types of receptor proteins: channel-linked receptors and non–channel-linked receptors. Channel-linked receptors are also known as ligand-gated channels. (A is from Huether SE, McCance KL: *Understanding pathophysiology,* ed 4, St Louis, 2001, Mosby. B and C are modified from Alberts B et al, editors: *Molecular biology of the cell,* ed 3, New York, 1994, Garland.)

localization of the specific receptors (McCance & Huether, 2001). This concept sounds obvious, but it is important to understand how drugs accomplish what they do.

Most drug receptors are proteins. Some of the most clinically important receptors are cellular proteins, whose normal functions are to be receptors for bodily (endogenous) regulatory molecules (McCance & Huether, 2001). Examples of such molecules are hormones and neurotransmitters. Receptors can be enzymes that are chemical in nature (making it easy for reactions to occur) but that are not totally used up in the reaction. Enzymes free themselves and then continue being available for reactions with other substrates.

The lock-and-key model of drug–receptor interaction states that the drug molecule must fit into a receptor like a key fits into a lock (Figure 5-10). *Drug affinity* is the propensity of a drug to bind or attach itself to a given receptor site. There are two types of drug receptor interactions: agonist and antagonist. An *agonist* is a drug that has affinity for and stimulates physiologic activity at cell receptors normally activated by naturally occurring substances. An *antagonist* is a drug that inhibits or counteracts effects produced by other drugs or eliminates undesired physiologic effects caused by illness. An antagonist may work competitively, with an affinity for the same receptor site as an agonist; or it may be noncompetitive, in which it inactivates the receptor so that the agonist cannot be effective at any concentration.

Actions of Drugs Not Mediated by Receptors. Some drugs interact with small molecules or ions that are found in the

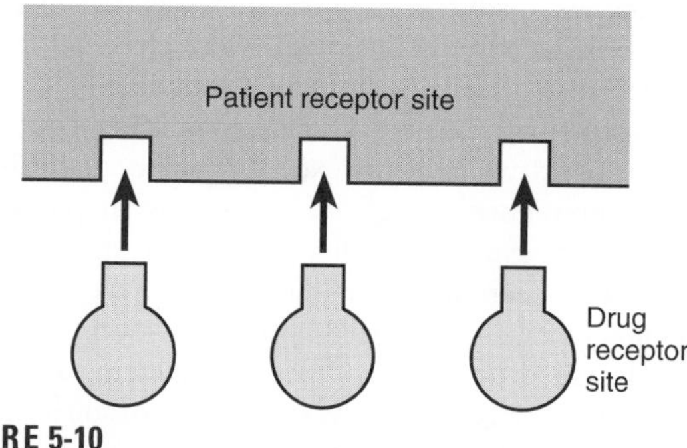

Drug receptor sites
Agonist: Chemical fits receptor site well; chemical response is usually good.
Antagonist: Drug attaches at drug receptor site but then remains chemically inactive; no chemical drug response is produced.
Partial agonist: Drug attaches at drug receptor site but only a slight chemical action is produced.
Patient receptor site
Drug receptor site

FIGURE 5-10

Drug receptor sites. (From Edmunds MW: *Introduction to clinical pharmacology,* ed 4, St Louis, 2003, Mosby.)

body. For example, antacids neutralize the gastric acid in the stomach. Other drugs have structures close enough to normal biologic chemicals that the body may incorporate them into cellular components, which then alters function. Examples of this type of activity include purines that are incorporated into nucleic acids and are useful in treating cancer and viruses. Recombinant DNA may also serve in this manner, working with new drugs or being used in new treatment regimens.

Quantifying the Drug–Receptor Interaction. Attempts to quantify the drug–receptor interaction involve calculating the concentration of drug–response relationships. Agonist drug interactions with a receptor are reversible. The amount of effect depends on how many receptors are occupied or being acted on by the drug. Efficacy reflects the maximal response a drug can produce (Stringer, 2000). *Free drug* is the amount of drug in the body that is NOT bound to a receptor site. *Potency* is the dependency of effect on its concentration. A drug is more potent if it takes less drug to achieve the desired effect. An antagonist will bind to a receptor to inhibit the action of a drug but has no intrinsic action of its own. Inhibition is competitive if it can be overcome by the increased concentration of the agonist. A noncompetitive antagonist prevents the action of the agonist at any concentration.

Adverse Drug Reactions and Side Effects

An *adverse event* is any undesirable experience associated with the use of a drug or medical product in a patient. Adverse reactions include any response to a drug that is unfavorable or unintended and that occurs at doses used in humans for prophylaxis, diagnosis, or therapy of disease or for the modification of physiologic function (Food and Drug Administration, 1990). This is different from a *side effect*, which is an additional effect, desirable or undesirable, of a drug that is not the primary purpose of giving the drug. For example, an adverse reaction could be the development of a pancytopenia from taking chloramphenicol. A side effect might include photosensitivity caused by tetracycline taken for acne. An unfavorable reaction would be one that is noxious, hurtful, not wholesome, or damaging to tissue. These types of reactions may occur immediately or take weeks or months to develop, such as the hirsutism, "buffalo-hump," and gynecomastia seen after long-term steroid use.

The incidence of adverse drug reactions has been estimated at around 28%, accounting for about 3% to 6% of all hospital admissions (Lipsy, 1998). Adverse reactions may be classified into three distinctive type of reactions: (1) an inherent pharmacologic effect of a drug, either an excessive degree of the desired effect or an unintended side effect, for example, hypoglycemia seen with insulin use; (2) an allergic reaction, manifested by typical signs and symptoms of an immunologic response; or (3) a local irritant effect characterized by inflammation.

Most adverse drug reactions are nonallergic. They may result from overdosage, if there is impaired biotransformation or excretion of normal doses or an excess intake of medication. They might be a side effect reflecting an unavoidable nontherapeutic effect of the drug. A paradoxical effect or an effect opposite to those expected may develop. Drug interactions may occur. Or an idiosyncratic reaction may result from unusual resistance to large doses or unexpected responses to ordinary or even low doses (Stringer, 2000).

Many significant drug–drug interactions can be understood in terms of cytochrome P450 reactions. However, drug–drug interactions are more complex for at least two reasons. First, some drug–drug interactions can be attributed to pharmacokinetic differences resulting from other enzymes such as monoamine oxidases, flavin-containing monooxygenases, UDP-glucuronosyl transferases, and sulfotransferases. These and other drug-metabolizing enzymes also show the characteristics of induction and inhibition by drugs that are associated with P450s although most have not yet been studied as extensively (Honkakoski & Negishi, 1997). The other aspect of drug–drug interactions is that some of these are probably pharmacodynamic instead of pharmacokinetic; this is when drugs compete for binding to a receptor directly related to the pharmacologic response.

Common drug interactions may be described as summative (when the combined effects of two drugs produce a result that equals the sum of the individual effects of each agent, such as is seen with colestipol plus lovastatin); synergistic (when the combined effect of two drugs is greater than the sum of each individual agent acting independently as seen with HCTZ with angiotensin-converting enzyme inhibitor); or potentiating (when one drug increases the effect of the other drug, such as probenecid inhibiting the clearance of penicillin from the body, thereby increasing its effect). These effects may occur rapidly (within 24 hours) or be delayed for days or weeks (Honkakoski & Negishi, 1997).

The clinician should always evaluate the risk versus benefit of any possible combination of drugs. The first evaluation is the possibility of a serious drug–drug interaction. Only approximately 5% of all drug interactions are clinically significant. Is the possible reaction serious, such as death or pregnancy? Is it reversible? Second, the therapeutic window of the drug in question is important. If the drug has a narrow therapeutic window, the chances of a drug interaction are increased. Third, consider the time course of the drugs involved. A drug with a long half-life will cause a longer adverse reaction than one with a short half-life. Multiply the half-life of the drug being affected by 4 to 5 times, and this will tell you when you achieve a new steady state drug level. Fourth, the age of the patient is important. Although most of the research has been done on adults, they are the least likely to have drug interactions. Extremes of age, either old or young, predispose a patient to adverse reactions. Fifth, coexisting morbidity is also an important factor. Patients with a seizure disorder, cardiovascular disease, or HIV or other infection are at risk for drug interactions. Patients with cardiovascular disease are at an extra risk because they often have poor perfusion of their liver, which will affect the enzyme action. Also, they are usually on several drugs that may have P450 interactions, such as antiarrhythmics and calcium channel blockers (DiPiro et al, 2002).

In general, if in doubt, assume that the new drug will interact with the drugs the patient is already taking. Consult recent literature about the possibility of P450 enzyme activity. Usually it is only necessary to closely monitor for drug interactions by checking for signs and symptoms or by monitoring serum drug levels. On occasion, it is wise to adjust the dosage of one medicine when another is added (Hardman et al, 2001). This is a very complicated clinical decision that is difficult to make. A good candidate for extra caution would be an elderly patient with cardiovascular disease who is taking a very toxic drug with a narrow therapeutic window, particularly when adding a new drug that is a known inhibitor of metabolism of the toxic drug currently being taken.

Certain categories of medications are more likely to be involved in important P450–drug interactions. Some of the most important drug categories involved in drug–drug interactions because of the P450 system are the following:

- Many antibiotics present a risk. Erythromycin is both a substrate and an inhibitor. Many newer quinolones are inhibitors. For example, these antibiotics may inhibit metabolism of theophylline.
- The azole antifungals are inhibitors.
- Drugs for HIV metabolism are susceptible to induction and inhibition.
- The nonsedating antihistamines are inhibitors. Terfenadine was a very potent inhibitor and was taken off the market because of interactions with several antiinfectives. The other antihistamines have much less inhibitor effects.
- The anticonvulsants can be inducers.
- The metabolism of oral contraceptives can be induced. By induction, the oral contraceptive is metabolized more quickly, leaving less drug in the system and causing the patient to be at higher risk for pregnancy. If a woman on birth control pills takes an antibiotic, she should use a barrier contraceptive for that month.
- Many antidepressants, such as fluoxetine and nefazodone, are inhibitors and substrates.
- Among the cardiovascular drugs, antiarrhythmics may be inhibitors and substrates. Calcium channel blockers are both inhibitors and substrates. Several beta blockers are substrates. All statins are either substrates or inhibitors. For example, losartan is a substrate.
- Codeine is a substrate whose metabolism may be induced/inhibited.
- Warfarin is a substrate drug whose metabolism is induced/inhibited by many drugs. It has a very narrow therapeutic window with serious side effects. Extensive information should be collected about any drug added to a patient on a warfarin regimen. Prothrombin times should also be followed.
- Cimetidine is an inhibitor of several isoenzyme pathways.
- Cyclosporine is a substrate whose metabolism can be inhibited by many drugs.
- The benzodiazepines can be a substrate whose metabolism is induced or inhibited.
- Caffeine is a substrate.
- Grapefruit juice inhibits the cytochrome P450 enzyme system in the intestine, allowing more absorption of a drug. So drinking grapefruit juice may increase the level of a drug up to three-fold. The cause and mechanism of this are unknown. It can allow a patient to take a lower dose of a very expensive drug such as cyclosporine for transplantation. The problem is that this effect is not consistent.
- The effect of herbal medicines is unknown. There is anecdotal evidence of drug interactions but no scientific evidence. To be safe, assume that herbal medicines are active in the enzyme system and discourage their use in a patient with risk factors for drug interactions.
- Vitamins, including the antioxidants, are not significant inducers or inhibitors.
- In the future, new immunostimulation therapy will probably affect the P450 enzyme system, generally acting as inhibitors.

See Box 5-1 for a complete listing of known reactions related to the P450 system.

Finally, the activity of specific metabolizing enzymes is selectively affected in individuals with liver disease. The enzyme CYP 2C19 is more sensitive than CYP 2D6. Any recommendations for modification in drug dosage in the presence of liver disease should be based on knowledge of the particular enzyme involved in metabolism of the drug. Much of this information has yet to emerge from ongoing studies (Honkakoski & Negishi, 1997).

For the clinician to conclude that a patient is having an adverse reaction to a drug, causality must be demonstrated. This may be done sequentially by (1) examining the chronologic relationship between the adverse reaction and the drug administration, (2) seeing resolution of the adverse reaction once dose is decreased or discontinued (dechallenge), and (3) seeing recurrence of symptoms after readministration of the agent (rechallenge). A patient should be rechallenged to confirm causality only when it is imperative to use that particular drug (Food and Drug Administration, 1990). It is obvious that most clinicians must balance the strict documentation of causality with what is practical. This is often determined by how essential the drug is for patient therapy.

In most cases, an adverse reaction is confirmed less strictly because the adverse reaction is a known response pattern of the drug or may be measured by physiologic effects (that is, blood pressure, laboratory abnormality, serum drug concentration). Occasionally, a patient reaction will be classified as an adverse reaction if it seems unrelated to the patient's concomitant diseases, clinical status, or other therapies (past or present).

Adverse reactions may also be classified by severity. With mild reactions, the patient may experience signs or symptoms, but they are easily tolerated. They often do not require treatment. Moderate reactions produce enough discomfort to interfere with usual activity and require treatment. Severe adverse reactions may incapacitate the patient or interfere with the ability to work or complete activities of daily living. They may even be life-threatening or contribute to the death of the patient. Although the rate of severe drug reactions may be 5% to 10% of all those reported, Food and Drug Administration (FDA) records show that the elderly have an increased risk for severe adverse reactions, with patients over 60 years of age accounting for nearly half of adverse drug reaction–associated deaths (Lipsy, 1998). These types of reactions often require hospitalization, intensive medical care, and more than 15 days for recovery. Severe adverse reactions may also be associated with production of congenital anomalies. See

BOX 5-1

KNOWN CYTOCHROME P450 ENZYME REACTIONS WITH DRUGS

CYTOCHROME 1A2 ISOENZYMES

Substrates	Inhibitors	Inducers
amitriptyline	cimetidine	phenobarbital
caffeine	ciprofloxacin	phenytoin
clomipramine	clarithromycin	rifampin
clozapine	enoxacin	ritonavir
cyclobenzaprine	erythromycin	**SMOKING/POLYCYCLIC AROMATIC HYDROCARBONS**
desipramine	fluvoxamine (potent)	
diazepam	Grapefruit juice	
haloperidol	isoniazid	
imipramine	ketoconazole	
(*R*)-warfarin	levofloxacin	
tacrine	norfloxacin	
theophylline	omeprazole?	
zileuton	paroxetine	

CYTOCHROME 2C ISOENZYME

Substrates	Inhibitors	Inducers
amitriptyline	amiodarone 2C9	carbamazepine
clomipramine	chloramphenicol 2C9	phenobarbital
diazepam 2C9	cimetidine 2C9	phenytoin
imipramine	fluconazole	rifampin
losartan 2C9	fluoxetine	
omeprazole	fluvastatin	
phenytoin 2C9	fluvoxamine 2C9, potent	
(*S*)-warfarin 2C9	isoniazid	
tolbutamide	ketoconazole (weak)	
topiramate 2C9	omeprazole 2C9, 2C19	
	sertraline	
	topiramate 2C19	
	zafirlukast 2C9	

CYTOCHROME 2D6 ISOENZYMES

Substrates		Inhibitors	Inducers
amitriptyline	maprotiline	carbamazepine	amiodarone
bisoprolol	meperidine	phenobarbital	cimetidine
chlorpromazine	methadone	phenytoin	clomipramine
clomipramine	methamphetamine	rifampin	desipramine
clozapine	metoprolol	ritonavir	fluoxetine
codeine	mexiletine		fluphenazine
cyclobenzaprine	morphine		haloperidol
desipramine	nortriptyline		mibefradil
dexfenfluramine	oxycodone		paroxetine
dextromethorphan	paroxetine		propafenone
donepezil	perphenazine		quinidine
doxepin	propafenone		ritonavir
fenfluramine	propranolol		sertraline
flecainide	risperidone		thioridazine
fluphenazine	thioridazine		
fluoxetine	timolol		
haloperidol	tramadol		
hydrocodone	trazodone		
imipramine	venlafaxine		

From Michalets EL: Clinically significant cytochrome P-450 drug interactions, *Pharmacotherapy* 18:84-112, 1998.

BOX 5-1

KNOWN CYTOCHROME P450 ENZYME REACTIONS WITH DRUGS—cont'd

CYTOCHROME 3A4 ISOENZYMES

Substrates

alfentanil
alprazolam
amitriptyline
amlodipine
astemizole
atorvastatin
busulfan
Cannabinoids
carbamazepine
cisapride
clindamycin
clomipramine
clonazepam
cocaine
cyclobenzaprine
cyclophosphamide
cyclosporine
dapsone
dexamethasone
dextromethorphan
diazepam (minor)
diltiazem
disopyramide
donepezil
doxorubicin
dronabinol
erythromycin
Estrogens, OBC
ethosuximide
etoposide
felodipine
fentanyl
fexofenadine
ifosfamide
imipramine
indinavir
isradipine
ketoconazole
lansoprazole (minor)
lidocaine
losartan
lovastatin
mibefradil
miconazole
midazolam
navelbine
nefazodone
nelfinavir
nicardipine
nifedipine
nimodipine
nisoldipine
ondansetron
paclitaxel
pravastatin
prednisone
quinidine
quinine
rifampin
ritonavir
(*R*)-warfarin
saquinavir
sertraline
tacrolimus
tamoxifen
temazepam
terfenadine
testosterone
triazolam
verapamil
vinblastine
vincristine
zileuton

Inhibitors

amiodarone
Cannabinoids
clarithromycin
erythromycin
fluconazole
fluoxetine
fluvoxamine
Grapefruit juice
indinavir
itraconazole
ketoconazole
omeprazole (slight)
metronidazole
mibefradil
miconazole
nefazodone
nelfinavir
norfloxacin
quinine
ritonavir
saquinavir
sertraline
troleandomycin
zafirlukast

Inducers

carbamazepine
dexamethasone
ethosuximide
phenobarbital
phenytoin
primidone
rifabutin
rifampin
troglitazone

Box 5-2 for some of the drugs commonly implicated in serious adverse effects.

Serious adverse reactions should be voluntarily reported to the FDA Medical Products MedWatch Reporting Program by calling 1 (800) FDA-1088 [or 1 (800) 4USP PRN] or Faxing to 1 (800) FDA-0178 [or (301) 816-8532]. The FDA uses reports from health professionals and manufacturers to identify problems in products already on the market. The agency evaluates the seriousness of the health hazard, takes corrective action, and communicates those actions to the health professional community. The corrective actions may include the FDA requiring manufacturers to add new information to the labeling of a product. If a serious warning is required to ensure the continued safe use of a product, the FDA may require the warning to be displayed in heavy type and boxed text at the beginning of the package insert (the "Black Box"). Finally, the FDA may require a manufacturer to recall or withdraw a product because of a serious problem. Product withdrawals can mean that marketing of the product may be stopped permanently (Food and Drug Administration, 1990).

BOX 5-2

DRUGS ASSOCIATED WITH SERIOUS ADVERSE EFFECTS

Hepatotoxic Drugs
acetaminophen
4-aminoquinolines
amiodarone
Anabolic steroid agents
Antithyroid agents
asparaginase
azlocillin
carbamazepine
carmustine
Contraceptives (estrogen)
dantrolene
daunorubicin
disulfiram
divalproex
erythromycin
estrogen DES, conjugated
etretinate
gold compounds
halothane
isoniazid
ketoconazole
mercaptopurine
methotrexate
methyldopa
mezlocillin
naltrexone
phenothiazine
phenytoin
piperacillin
plicamycin
rifampin
sulfonamides
tetracycline
valproic acid

Nephrotoxic Drugs
acyclovir
aminoglycoside antibiotics
amphotericin B
analgesic combinations
capreomycin
captopril
cisplatin
cyclosporine
demeclocycline
edetate calcium disodium
enalapril
gold compounds
lithium
methotrexate
methoxyflurane
neomycin
NSAIDs
penicillamine
pentamidine
plicamycin
rifampin
streptozocin
sulfonamides
tetracyclines
vancomycin

Other Toxicities
Anaphylaxis: penicillins, heparin, aspirin, parenteral iron, dextran
Asthma: aspirin, ibuprofen
Blood dyscrasias: chloramphenicol, anticonvulsants, penicillins, hydralazine, sulfonamides, anticancer drugs
Damage to eighth cranial nerve: furosemide, aspirin and other salicylates, vibramycin, gentamicin
Eye damage: topical corticosteroids, ethambutol, thorazine, chloroquine
Peripheral neuritis: isoniazid, vincristine, hydralazine, ethambutol

Modified from McKenry LM, Salerno E: *Mosby's pharmacology in nursing,* ed 22, St Louis, 2002, Mosby; Hardman JG, Limbird LW et al, editors: *Goodman and Gilman's pharmacological basis of therapeutics,* ed 10, New York, 2001, McGraw-Hill; and Katzung BG: *Basic and clinical pharmacology,* ed 8, Norwalk, Conn, 2000, Appleton & Lange.

Drug Interactions

Food and Drug Interactions. Because many medications are administered orally, the potential for interaction with food is high. Taken together, food and drugs may alter the body's ability to utilize a particular food or drug. Part of these interactions may result from activation of the P450 enzyme system or competition with receptor sites. Monoamine oxidase inhibitors (MAOIs) are some of the drugs most noted for drug–food interactions, because they cannot be taken with aged cheese or many processed foods. Because both OTC and prescription drugs may interact with food, some principles that are important to stress with every patient include the following:

- Cigarettes can diminish the effectiveness of medication or create other problems with particular drugs by increasing metabolism.
- Caffeine, found in coffee, tea, soft drinks, chocolate, and some medications, can also affect the action of some drugs.
- Medication should never be taken during pregnancy without the advice of the health care provider (see Chapter 9).
- Patients should know that if they have any problem related to medication, they should call their health care provider or pharmacist immediately.

See Table 5-1 for specific materials concerning food–drug interactions that should be communicated to patients.

TABLE 5-1 Common Food–Drug Interactions

Medication Category	Common Medication Examples	Interactions and Instructions to Patients
ANTIINFECTIVES		
Penicillins: used to treat a wide variety of infections	amoxicillin (Trimox, Amoxil); ampicillin (Principen, Omnipen); penicillin V (Veetids)	Amoxicillin and bacampicillin may be taken with food; however, absorption of other types of penicillins is reduced when taken with food. Avoid acidic fruit juices, citrus fruits, or acidic beverages, such as cola drinks. The antibiotics are acid labile (reduce absorption). Take drug 1 hr AC or 2 hr PC.
Cephalosporins	cefaclor (Ceclor, Ceclor CD); cefadroxil (Duricef); cefixime (Suprax); cefprozil (Cefzil); cephalexin (Keflex, Keftab)	Take on an empty stomach 1 hr before or 2 hr after meals. Can be taken with food if severe GI upset.
tetracyclines: used to treat a wide variety of infections	tetracycline HCl (Achromycin V, Sumycin), doxycycline (Vibramycin); minocycline (Minocin)	These drugs should not be taken within 2 hr of eating dairy products such as milk, ice cream, yogurt, or cheese or of taking calcium or iron supplements. Calcium forms complex with the drug, resulting in reduced absorption of the antibiotic. Take 1 hr AC or 2 hr PC.
erythromycin or macrolides: used in treating skin, ear infections	erythromycin (E-Mycin, Ery-Tab, ERYC); erythromycin and sulfisoxazole (Pediazole); azithromycin (Zithromax); clarithromycin (Biaxin)	Erythromycins vary in their reactions with food. Avoid meals, acidic fruit juices, citrus fruits, or acidic beverages, such as cola drinks. The antibiotics are acid labile (reduce absorption). Take drug 1 hr AC or 2 hr PC.
Sulfonamides: used to treat stomach and urinary infections	sulfamethoxazole and trimethoprim (Bactrim, Septra)	Avoid alcohol because the combination may cause nausea. Take on an empty stomach if possible.
ANTIFUNGALS	fluconazole (Diflucan); griseofulvin (Grifulvir V); ketoconazole (Nizoral); itraconazole (Sporanox)	Avoid taking these medications with dairy products or antacids. Avoid drinking alcohol or using medications or food that contain alcohol for at least 2 days after taking ketoconazole. It may produce a disulfiram-type reaction.
methenamine: used in treating urinary tract infections	methenamine (Mandelamine, Urex)	Cranberries, plums, prunes, and their juices help the action of this drug. Avoid citrus fruits and citrus juices. Eat foods with protein but avoid dairy products.
nitroimidazole: used to treat intestinal and genital infections caused by bacteria and parasites	metronidazole (Flagyl)	Do not take alcohol while using this drug; it will cause stomach pain, nausea, vomiting, headache, flushing, or redness of the face.
Quinolones	ciprofloxacin (Cipro); levofloxacin (Levaquin); floxacin (Floxin); trovafloxacin (Trovan)	Take on an empty stomach 1 hr before or 2 hr after meals. Can be taken with food if severe GI upset. Avoid calcium-containing products and vitamins and minerals containing iron and antacids because they significantly decrease drug concentrations. Taking with caffeine products may increase caffeine levels and produce excitability and nervousness.
CARDIOVASCULAR DRUGS		
Diuretics: eliminate water, sodium, and chloride	furosemide (Lasix); triamterene-hydrochlorothiazide (HCTZ) (Dyazide, Maxzide); triamterene (Dyrenium); bumetanide (Bumex); metolazone (Zaroxolyn); HCTZ (Esidrix, HydroDIURIL)	Diuretics vary in their interactions with nutrients. Loss of potassium, calcium, and magnesium occurs with some diuretics. May require potassium supplement. With some diuretics, potassium loss is less significant.
Nitrates: relax veins and/or arteries to reduce work of the heart	nitroglycerin (Nitro, Nitro-Dur, Transderm-Nitro); isosorbide dinitrate (Isordil, Sorbitrate)	Use of sodium (salt) should be restricted for medication to be effective. Use with alcohol may drastically lower blood pressure. Check labels on food packages for sodium.
Antihypertensives: relax blood vessels, increase the supply of blood and oxygen to the heart and lessen its workload; may regulate heartbeat	β-Blockers: atenolol (Tenormin); metoprolol (Lopressor); propranolol (Inderal); nadolol (Corgard); ACE inhibitors: captopril (Capoten); enalapril (Vasotec); lisinopril (Prinivil, Zestril); quinapril (Accupril); moexipril (Univasc)	Use of sodium (salt) should be restricted for medications to be effective. Check labels on food packages for sodium. Alcohol and propranolol combination may dramatically lower blood pressure. ACE inhibitors: food can decrease absorption. ACE inhibitors may increase the amount of potassium. Avoid eating large amounts of foods high in potassium.

Modified from National Consumers' League: *Food drug interactions*, Washington, DC, 1999, National Consumers League; McKenry LM, Salerno E: *Mosby's pharmacology in nursing*, ed 22, St Louis, MO, 2002, Mosby.

Continued

TABLE 5-1 Common Food–Drug Interactions—cont'd

Medication Category	Common Medication Examples	Interactions and Instructions to Patients
CARDIOVASCULAR DRUGS—cont'd		
Anticoagulants: prolong clotting of the blood	warfarin (Coumadin)	Moderation in consumption of foods high in vitamin K is recommended because vitamin K produces blood-clotting substances. Such foods include beef liver; green leafy vegetables such as spinach, cabbage, cauliflower, and Brussels sprouts; potatoes; vegetable oil; and egg yolk. High doses of vitamin E (400 IU or more) may prolong clotting time.
Antihyperlipidemics: HMG/CoA reductase inhibitors or "statins" lower cholesterol	atorvastatin (Lipitor); fluvastatin (Lescol); lovastatin (Mevacor); pravastatin (Pravachol); simvastatin (Zocor)	Mevacor should be taken with the evening meal to enhance absorption. Avoid large amounts of alcohol as it may increase risk of liver damage.
CENTRAL NERVOUS SYSTEM DRUGS		
Analgesics/antipyretics	acetaminophen (Tylenol, Tempra)	Take on an empty stomach for more rapid relief as food may slow the body's absorption of the drug. Concurrent use with alcohol can increase the risk of liver damage or GI bleeding.
Antianxiety drugs	lorazepam (Ativan); diazepam (Valium); alprazolam (Xanax)	Use with caffeine may cause excitability, nervousness, and hyperactivity and lessen the antianxiety effect. Use with alcohol may impair mental and motor functions.
Antidepressants	paroxetine (Paxil); sertraline (Zoloft); fluoxetine (Prozac)	Avoid concurrent use with alcohol. These medications can be taken with or without food.
Analgesics/narcotics	codeine with acetaminophen (Tylenol No. 2, 3, 4); morphine (Roxanol, MS Contin); oxycodone with acetaminophen (Percocet, Roxicet); meperidine (Demerol); hydrocodone with acetaminophen (Vicodin, Lorcet)	Avoid concurrent use with alcohol because of the sedative effects. Use caution when motor skills are required.
lithium carbonate: regulates changes in chemical levels in the brain	Various names	Follow the dietary and fluid intake instructions of health care provider to avoid very serious toxic reactions.
MAO inhibitors: act as antidepressant	phenelzine (Nardil); tranylcypromine (Parnate)	A very dangerous, potentially fatal interaction can occur with foods containing tyramine, a chemical in alcoholic beverages, particularly wine, and in many foods such as hard cheeses, chocolate, beef or chicken livers, sour cream, yogurt, raisins, bananas, avocados, soy sauce, yeast extract, meat tenderizers, sausages, and anchovies. Patient may develop severe headache, nosebleed, chest pain, photosensitivity, or severe hypertension with hypertensive crisis.
Sedative-hypnotics	Various names	Do not use alcohol with any sleep medications. Oversedation occurs.
GASTROINTESTINAL DRUGS		
Antacids, antiulcer medications, histamine blockers: work to reduce acid in the stomach	cimetidine (Tagamet); famotidine (Pepcid); ranitidine (Zantac); nizatidine (Axid)	Follow specific diets given by health care provider. Avoid large amounts of caffeine; dairy products such as milk or cream may increase acid secretion. If calcium carbonate is used as a calcium supplement, avoid concurrent administration of bran and whole-grain breads or cereals that reduce absorption of calcium.
Laxatives: stimulate intestine, soften stool, add bulk or fluid to stool	Various names	Excessive use of laxatives can cause loss of essential vitamins and minerals and may require replenishment of potassium, sodium, and other nutrients through diet. Mineral oil can cause poor absorption of vitamins A, D, E, and K and calcium. Take 2 hr before eating food.
MUSCULOSKELETAL DRUGS		
aspirin: used to reduce pain, fever, and inflammation*	aspirin (Bayer, Ecotrin)	Because aspirin can cause stomach irritation, avoid alcohol. To avoid stomach upset, take with food. Do not take with fruit juice. Buffered or enteric-coated aspirin may also reduce GI bleeding.
NSAIDs: used to relieve pain and reduce inflammation and fever	ibuprofen (Advil, Motrin); naproxen (Anaprox, Aleve, Naprosyn); ketoprofen (Orudis); nabumetone (Relafen)	These drugs should be taken with food or milk because they can irritate the stomach. Avoid taking with the kinds of foods or alcoholic beverages that tend to irritate stomach.

*Many over-the-counter cold remedies contain aspirin in combination with other active ingredients.

TABLE 5-1 Common Food–Drug Interactions—cont'd

Medication Category	Common Medication Examples	Interactions and Instructions to Patients
MUSCULOSKELETAL DRUGS—cont'd		
indomethacin: used to reduce pain, swelling, joint pain, and fever in certain types of arthritis and gout	indocin	This drug should be taken with food because it can irritate the stomach. Avoid taking with the kinds of foods or alcoholic beverages that tend to irritate the stomach.
piroxicam: used to reduce pain, swelling, stiffness, joint pain and fever in certain types of arthritis	feldene	This medication should be taken with a light snack because it can cause stomach irritation. Avoid alcohol because it can add to the possibility of stomach upset.
Corticosteroids: used to provide relief to inflamed areas; lessen swelling, redness, itching, and allergic reactions	methylprednisolone (Medrol); prednisone (Deltasone); prednisolone (Pediapred, Prelone); cortisone acetate (Cortef)	Take with food or milk to decrease GI distress. Avoid alcohol because both alcohol and corticosteroids can cause stomach irritation. Also avoid foods high in sodium (salt). Check labels on food packages for sodium. Take with food to prevent stomach upset.
Codeine narcotic: used to suppress cough and relieve pain; often with ASA or acetaminophen	aspirin with codeine, Tylenol with codeine	Do not drink alcohol with this medication as it increases the sedative effect. Take with meals, small snacks, or milk because this medication may cause stomach upset.
RESPIRATORY DRUGS		
Antihistamines: used to relieve or prevent symptoms of colds, hay fever, and other types of allergy; act to limit or block histamine	brompheniramine (Dimetane, Bromphen); chlorpheniramine (Chlor-Trimeton); Teldrin; diphenhydramine (Benadryl, Banophen); clemastine (Tavist); fexofenadine (Allegra); loratadine (Claritin); cetirizine (Zyrtec); astemizole (Hismanal)	Avoid taking with alcoholic beverages because antihistamines combined with alcohol may cause drowsiness and slowed reactions. Take prescription antihistamines on an empty stomach to increase their effectiveness.
Bronchodilators: used to treat the symptoms of bronchial asthma, chronic bronchitis, and emphysema; these medicines relieve wheezing, shortness of breath, dyspnea; they work by opening the air passages of the lungs	theophylline (Slo-bid, Theo-Dur, Theo-Dur 24, Uniphyl); albuterol (Ventolin, Proventil, Combivent); epinephrine (Primatene Mist)	Avoid eating or drinking large amounts of foods or beverages that contain caffeine because both bronchodilators and caffeine stimulate the central nervous system. High-fat meals may increase the amount of theophylline in the body, while high-carbohydrate meals may decrease it. The effect of food on theophylline in the body, while high-carbohydrate meals may decrease it. The effect of food on theophylline products varies.

Alcohol–Medication Interactions. Alcohol is another product with vast potential for interactions with drugs. In an alert distributed by the National Institute of Alcohol Abuse and Alcoholism (1995), it was estimated that alcohol–medication interactions may be a factor in at least 25% of all emergency department admissions (Holder, 1992). An unknown number of less serious interactions go unrecognized and unrecorded.

It has been estimated that approximately 70% of the adult population consumes alcohol at least occasionally, and up to 10% of people may drink daily (Midanik & Room, 1992). Research also suggests that about 60% of men and 30% of women have had one or more adverse alcohol-related life events (American Psychiatric Association, 1994). These figures together with the facts concerning the substantial numbers of people who take medications suggest that some concurrent use of alcohol and medications is inevitable (Seppala et al, 1995).

One segment of the population at particular risk for alcohol–drug interactions are the elderly, who take 25% to 30% of all prescription medications (Gomberg, 1990). Elderly individuals are more likely to experience medication side effects than are younger persons, and these effects tend to be more severe with advancing age (Gomberg, 1990). Among persons aged 60 years or older, 10% of those in the community and 40% of those in nursing homes fulfill criteria for alcohol abuse (Egbert, 1993).

How Alcohol and Drugs Interact. Both drugs and alcohol travel through the bloodstream to exert the desired effects on the body. With alcohol, the site of action is the brain, causing intoxication until the alcohol is finally metabolized and eliminated, principally by the liver.

The extent to which an administered dose of a drug reaches its site of action is described in terms of its availability. Alcohol can influence the effectiveness of a drug by altering its availability (National Institute for Alcohol Abuse and Alcoholism, 1995). Typical alcohol-drug interactions include the following (Lieber, 1992; DiPadova, 1992):

- An acute dose of alcohol (a single drink or several drinks over several hours) may inhibit a drug's metabolism by competing with the drug for the same set of metabolizing enzymes. This interaction prolongs and enhances the drug's availability, potentially increasing the patient's risk of experiencing harmful side effects from the drug (Fraser et al, 1992; Shoaf and Linnoila, 1991).

TABLE 5-2 Specific Drug–Alcohol Interactions

Drug Interaction	Physiologic Result
Anesthetics	Chronic alcohol consumption increases the dose of propofol (Diprivan) required to induce loss of consciousness. Chronic alcohol consumption increases the risk of liver damage that may be caused by the anesthetic gases enflurane (Ethrane) and halothane (Fluothane).
Antibiotics	With acute alcohol consumption, some may cause nausea, vomiting, headache, and possibly convulsions; among these antibiotics are furazolidone (Furoxone), griseofulvin (Grisactin and others), metronidazole (Flagyl), and the antimalarial quinacrine (Atabrine). Acute alcohol consumption decreases the availability of isoniazid in the bloodstream, whereas chronic alcohol use decreases the availability of rifampin.
Anticoagulants	Acute alcohol use enhances warfarin's availability, increasing the patient's risk for life-threatening hemorrhages. Chronic alcohol consumption reduces warfarin's availability, lessening protection in blood-clotting disorders.
Antidepressants	Alcoholism and depression are frequently associated, leading to a high potential for alcohol–antidepressant interactions. Alcohol increases the sedative effect of tricyclic antidepressants, such as amitriptyline, impairing mental skills required for driving. Acute alcohol consumption increases the availability of some tricyclics, potentially increasing their sedative effects; chronic alcohol use may increase availability of some tricyclics and decreases the availability of others. A chemical called tyramine, found in some beers and wine, interacts with some antidepressants, such as monoamine oxidase inhibitors, and one drink may produce a dangerous rise in blood pressure.
Antidiabetic medications	Acute alcohol use prolongs and chronic alcohol consumption decreases the availability of tolbutamide (Orinase). With other drugs, antidiabetic medications may also produce symptoms of nausea and headache such as those described for metronidazole.
Antihistamines	Alcohol may intensify the sedation caused by some antihistamines or cause excessive dizziness and sedation in older persons.
Antipsychotic medications	Acute alcohol use increases the sedative effect of these drugs, resulting in impaired coordination and potentially fatal breathing difficulties and may result in liver damage.
Antiseizure medications	Acute alcohol increases availability of phenytoin (Dilantin) and the risk of side effects. Chronic drinking may decrease phenytoin availability, significantly reducing the patient's protection against epileptic seizures, even during a period of abstinence.
Antiulcer medications	cimetidine (Tagamet) and ranitidine (Zantac) may increase the availability of a low dose of alcohol under some circumstances.
Cardiovascular medications	Acute alcohol use interacts with some drugs to cause dizziness or fainting on standing up. These drugs include nitroglycerin, reserpine, methyldopa, hydralazine, and guanethidine. Chronic alcohol use decreases the availability of propranolol, potentially reducing its therapeutic effect.
Narcotic pain relievers	The combination of opiates and alcohol enhances the sedative effect of both substances, increasing the risk of death from overdose. A single dose of alcohol can increase the availability of propoxyphene, potentially increasing its sedative side effects.
Nonnarcotic pain relievers	Some of these drugs cause stomach bleeding, particularly in the elderly, and inhibit blood clotting; alcohol can exacerbate these effects. Aspirin may increase the availability of alcohol, heightening the effects of a given dose of alcohol. Chronic alcohol use activates enzymes that transform acetaminophen into chemicals that can cause liver damage, even when used in small amounts.
Sedatives and hypnotics	Benzodiazepines that are sedating may cause severe drowsiness with alcohol, increasing the risk of all accidents, especially in the elderly. Low doses of flurazepam (Dalmane) interact with low doses of alcohol to impair driving ability, even when alcohol is ingested in the morning. Alcohol and lorazepam may result in depressed heart and breathing functions. Acute alcohol consumption increases the availability of barbiturates, prolonging their sedative effect. Chronic alcohol consumption decreases barbiturate availability through enzyme activation. In addition, acute or chronic alcohol consumption enhances the sedative effect of barbiturates at their site of action in the brain, sometimes leading to coma or fatal respiratory depression.

From Institute of Alcohol Abuse and Alcoholism: *Alert on alcohol and medication interactions*, No. 27 PH355, Washington, DC, January, 1995, Institute of Alcohol Abuse and Alcoholism.

- In contrast, chronic (long-term) alcohol ingestion may activate drug-metabolizing enzymes, thus decreasing the drug's availability and diminishing its effects. After these enzymes have been activated, they remain so even in the absence of alcohol, affecting the metabolism of certain drugs for several weeks after cessation of drinking (Guram, Howden & Holt, 1992). Thus a recently abstinent chronic drinker may need higher doses of medications than those required by nondrinkers to achieve therapeutic levels of certain drugs.
- Enzymes activated by chronic alcohol consumption transform some drugs into toxic chemicals that can damage the liver or other organs.
- Alcohol can magnify the inhibitory effects of sedative and narcotic drugs at their sites of action in the brain.
- To add to the complexity of these interactions, some drugs affect the metabolism of alcohol, thus altering its potential for intoxication and the adverse effects associated with alcohol consumption (Dufour et al, 1992; Lieber, 1992).

The Institute for Alcohol Abuse and Alcoholism Alert is especially precise in summarizing common drug–alcohol interactions. See Table 5-2 for these interactions.

Over-the-Counter Drug Interactions with Prescription Drugs. When patients are taking prescription medications, the additional use of OTC products may become a problem. Although specific drugs should be evaluated for their potential OTC interactions, it is important to be aware of common interactions (Table 5-3). Patients should always read the label of OTC products because common drug interactions are listed in the "warning" section on those labels. Patients who experience a side effect after taking an OTC medicine for a common ailment should discontinue the product at once and consult a health care provider for guidance.

Precipitation of Genetic Disorders. Each person has a specific genetic composition that may be activated in the P450 enzyme system during metabolism. However, there are other underlying genetic disorders that may be precipitated by medications. Specific metabolic defects in genetic disorders have been discovered, and the increased availability of laboratory studies necessary to make a specific diagnosis has made it possible to be more specific in diagnosis. More widespread exposure of populations to drugs has revealed hitherto unsuspected errors of metabolism. New knowledge has indicated how certain genetic disorders may be treated by drugs and also expanded the list of medications that might precipitate problems. See Table 5-4 for a list of medications implicated in precipitating or exacerbating genetic disorders (McKenry & Salerno, 2002). Research has also clarified that individual variation in how individuals handle some medications (requiring larger or smaller doses) is probably related to the P450 enzyme system and not other hidden genetic defects.

Drug Effects on Laboratory Tests and Blood Substances. Although medications exert a therapeutic effect, they may also have unintended consequences on other natural sub-

TABLE 5-3 Common OTC Drug Interactions with Prescription Products

Type of OTC Product	Prescription Interactions
Acid reduces (H_2 agonists)	May interact with theophylline, warfarin, phenytoin
Antacids	If antacid contains aluminum, calcium, or magnesium, it has high potential for drug interactions.
Antiemetics	Do not use with sedatives or tranquilizers. May also be a problem in patients with asthma, glaucoma, or enlarged prostate gland.
Antihistamines	May interact with antidepressants, alcoholic beverages, sedatives, tranquilizers
Cough products	If product contains dextromethorphan, must not be taken with a monoamine oxidase inhibitor (MAOI).
Nasal decongestants	Do not use with monoamine oxidase inhibitor (MAOI), sedatives, tranquilizers, products with diphenhydramine. If patient is taking antihypertensives or antidepressants, they should not take a nasal decongestant without provider consultation.
Menstrual products	For products containing caffeine, limit the use of foods or beverages containing caffeine. If product contains ammonium chloride, do not use in patients with kidney or liver disease.
Nicotine replacement products	May interact with antidepressants or asthma medications, requiring dosage adjustments.
Pain relievers	If product contains aspirin or salicylate, do not use with anticoagulants. Use care if patient has diabetes, gout, or arthritis. Limit alcohol to less than three drinks per day.
Sleep aids	Avoid sedatives, tranquilizers, MAOIs. Avoid alcoholic beverages.
Weight control aids	Do not use with cough/cold or allergy medication containing any form of phenylpropanolamine. This ingredient also should not be used in patients under treatment for high blood pressure, eating disorders, depression, heart disease, diabetes, or thyroid disease.

Modified from National Consumers League: *Food drug interactions*, developed jointly by the American Pharmaceutical Association, Food and Drug Administration, Food Marketing Institute, and National Consumers League, 1989.

TABLE 5-4 Medications Implicated in the Precipitation of Genetic Disorders

Medication or Drug	Genetic Disorder Stimulated
Anesthetic agents	Sickle cell anemia (hemoglobin S)
atropine, homatropine, ephedrine, other mydriatics or anticholinergics	Angle-closure glaucoma
Barbiturates, aminopyrine, sulfonamides, griseofulvin, hexachlorobenzene, meprobamate, chlordiazepoxide	Acute intermittent porphyria
Corticosteroids	Primary open-angle glaucoma
levodopa	Huntington chorea
Oral contraceptives	Dubin-Johnson syndrome
primaquine, other oxidant drugs	Glucose-6-phosphate dehydrogenase (G6PD) deficiency
Salicylates, menthol, corticosteroids	Crigler-Najjar syndrome
Sulfonamides, nitrites, acetanilid	Erythrocyte diaphorase deficiency
Sulfonamides, sulfones	Hemoglobin H, hemoglobin Zurich

Information from DiPiro JT, et al, editors: *Pharmacotherapy: a pathophysiologic approach*, ed 5, Norwalk, Conn, 2002, Appleton & Lange; Hardman JG et al, editors: *Goodman and Gilman's pharmacological basis of therapeutics*, ed 10, New York, 2001, McGraw-Hill; and Katzung BG: *Basic and clinical pharmacology*, ed 8, Norwalk, Conn, 2000, Appleton & Lange.

stances in the blood or may alter various laboratory tests. The clinician should be aware of these changes as they interpret laboratory values and attempt to monitor drug action. Tables 5-5 and 5-6 describe some of these common chemical interactions. Medications may also dramatically change the color of urine or feces. These changes are so startling that the patient should be warned to expect them. In most cases, the color changes are otherwise insignificant (McKenry & Salerno, 2002).

Chronotherapy. Research has demonstrated the increased efficacy of certain treatment regimens when correlated with the circadian rhythm. The circadian clock controls rhythms in endocrine gland secretion, metabolic processes, and behavioral activity. Cyclic variations caused by these processes are often demonstrated by normal temperature changes throughout the day. Certain diseases, such as asthma, angina, diabetes mellitus, and hypertension, fluctuate according to the circadian cycle. Chronotherapy attempts to correlate the peak of drug activity with when it is needed by the body. Some drugs are particularly affected by circadian rhythm, such as coumadin, growth hormone, antibiotics, theophylline, antianginals, vasoactive drugs, immunologic drugs, antihistamines, hypnotics, and analeptic drugs. Clinicians are just beginning to understand that when a drug is administered makes a great deal of difference in its action. For example, secretion of catecholamines increases early in the morning as the patient awakens. Catecholamines cause an increase in heart rate, contractile force, cardiac output, and systolic blood pressure, which places stress on the heart (Berne & Levy, 1998). It is important that any

TABLE 5-5 Selected Drug Interference with Laboratory Tests

Drug	Test	Method	Possible Result
acetaminophen	Blood glucose Pancreatic function testing Serum uric acid	Glucose oxidase/peroxidase Bentiromide Phosphotungstate uric acid test	False decrease False increase False increase
Anticonvulsants	Thyroid tests	Protein-bound iodine (PBI)	False decrease
Antihistamines	Skin testing	Allergen extracts	False negatives
Antimuscarinic, atropine	Urine test	Phenolsulfophthalein (PSP) excretion test	False decrease
ascorbic acid (megadoses)	Occult blood in stool Liver test, LDH and serum transaminases Urine glucose	 Autoanalyzer Glucose oxidase test	False negative Interference False decrease
Cephalosporins	Blood glucose Antiglobulin test Urine glucose Bleeding time (coagulation)	Ferricyanide test Coombs' test, direct Copper sulfate test (Benedict's or Fehling's) Prothrombin time (PT)	False negative with cefuroxime False positive in neonates when mother received before delivery False positive or negative Increase or prolonged time
Coffee, tea, cola drinks, chocolate, acetaminophen	Theophylline test for patients taking aminophylline, oxtriphylline, theophyline	Spectrophotometric	False increase
NSAIDs	Urinary bile Urinary 5-hydroxyindoleacetic acid (5-HIAA) and urinary steroid determinations	Diazo tablets Various assays	False positive with Ponstel False increase

Modified form McKenry LM, Salerno E: *Mosby's pharmacology in nursing*, ed 21, revised reprint, St Louis, 2002, Mosby.

TABLE 5-6 Selected Drug Effects on Specific Blood Substances

Drug	Effect on Blood Chemicals
All drugs	Possible increase in SGOT, SGPT
aminoglycoside	Possible increase in SGOT/SGPT, BUN, bilirubin; possible decrease in K^+, Na^+
Anticonvulsants	Possible increase in glucose
Antidepressants	Possible increase or decrease in glucose
β-Blockers	Possible increase in K^+, SGOT/SGPT, uric acid, BUN
carbamazepine	Possible increase in SGOT/SGPT, BUN, bilirubin
carbidopa/levodopa	Possible increase in SGOT/SGPT, BUN, bilirubin
Cephalosporins	Possible increase in PT, increase in SGOT/SGPT
cinoxacin	Possible increase in SGOT/SGPT, SUN
cisplatin	Possible increase in uric acid, BUN; possible decrease in K^+
diflunisal	Possible decrease in uric acid
Diuretics (loop)	Possible increase in glucose, uric acid, BUN; possible decrease in K^+, Na^+
Diuretics (thiazide)	Possible increase in glucose, uric acid, bilirubin; possible decrease in K^+, Na^+
Diuretics (potassium sparing)	Possible increase in glucose, K^+, uric acid, BUN; possible decrease in Na^+
mefenamic acid	Possible increase in PT
methyldopa	Possible increase in K^+, Na^+, SGOT/SGPT, uric acid, BUN, bilirubin
norfloxacin	Possible increase in SGOT/SGPT, BUN
NSAIDs	Possible decrease in glucose
propoxyphene	Possible increase in SGOT/SGPT
penicillin G-K	Possible increase in K^+
Injectable	Almost all increase SGOT/SGPT
azlocillin	Possible increase in Na^+, bilirubin; possible decrease in uric acid
carbenicillin	Possible increase in Na^+
mezlocillin	Possible increase in Na^+, bilirubin
piperacillin	Possible increase in Na^+, bilirubin
ticarcillin	Possible increase in Na^+, bilirubin; possible decrease in uric acid
prazosin	Possible increase in Na^+
rifampin	Possible increase in SGOT/SGPT, uric acid, BUN, bilirubin
trimethoprim	Possible increase in SGOT/SGPT, BUN, bilirubin
tetracycline	Possible increase in BUN (excepted doxycycline, minocycline), bilirubin
valproic acid	Possible increase in SGOT/SGPT, bilirubin

Modified from McKenry LM, Salerno E: *Mosby's pharmacology in nursing,* ed 22, St. Louis, 2002, Mosby.

antihypertensive medication is still at a therapeutic level during this period of time. If a nitroglycerin patch is removed at bedtime, it leaves the patient with low drug levels in the morning at a time the heart is at increased risk for an anginal episode.

Toxicities and Overdosage

Although changes in patient health, compliance factors, and overaggressive therapy may occasionally lead to overdosage, the most frequent cause of drug toxicity is accidental overdosage. Patients who repeat doses because they cannot remember whether they took their medications, because of confusion over proper dosages, or because of failure to make needed modifications may all lead to drug toxicity, particularly with those medications with narrow therapeutic margins. Patients at either end of the age spectrum are particularly susceptible to high accumulation of medications because of their relative distribution of muscle, bone, and adipose tissue (McKenry & Salerno, 2002). With OTC products such as ibuprofen and acetaminophen, the dosage for small infants, children, and adults varies dramatically. The suggested amount may not always seem logical; however, the wrong drug dosage may prove lethal. Additionally,

BOX 5-3

POISON CONTROL CENTERS

American Association of Poison Control Centers Certified Regional Poison Centers provides a list of centers with routine and emergency telephone numbers. There is frequent change in these listings. Contact the American Association of Poison Control Centers at (202) 362-7217 for updated information.

even well-maintained patients may become intolerant of their medications if they become dehydrated.

Some of the earliest signs of toxicity may be subtle. For example, the first signs of digoxin toxicity may be feelings of extreme fatigue and heaviness of the legs. Malaise, slight confusion, lack of appetite, inability to concentrate, mild weakness, and changes in sleeping patterns are all easy to overlook unless the clinician has some index of suspicion that toxicity may be a factor.

Unfortunately, a relatively high number of cases of overdosage or poisoning are the result of children inadvertently taking medication when unsupervised. Little children may open pill containers left at bedsides or in bathroom cupboards and confuse the pills with candy. Even vitamins and iron may prove lethal to small children. Despite a national campaign to safety-proof homes, the number of children who die each year as a result of drug overdosages is far too high.

It also cannot be ignored that some patients, for a variety of reasons, deliberately overdose on medications. Some of these episodes are true suicide attempts; others represent actions occurring because of alcoholic confusion or attempts to gain chemical "highs" that go wrong.

A study by the faculty at the University of California San Francisco finds medication overdose treatment advice in the *Physicians' Desk Reference* (a source frequently consulted for overdosage information) to be "inadequate, incorrect, outdated, and incomplete and could threaten patients' lives." Therefore an immediate call to the pharmacist at the local or regional Poison Control Center (Box 5-3) will provide superior information for clinicians seeking to respond to possible or confirmed cases of drug overdosage. Other information may be obtained by consulting the pharmaceutical manufacturer of the drug.

Risk-Benefit Ratio

Every type of drug therapy carries a risk that may be worth taking if the benefits far exceed the predictable morbidity and mortality rates of the therapy itself. This is fairly simple to determine for short-term therapy where results are quickly seen or the therapy can be terminated if toxicity becomes evident. Risks and benefits are more complicated to calculate for long-term therapy because the results may not be seen until months or years of treatment. With long-term care, it is more difficult for the clinician to determine if therapies should be terminated if some toxicities develop because the amount of good that is sacrificed is not always clear, especially to the patient. For example, methotrexate is an agent highly toxic to the bone marrow and the liver but offers substantial hope in preventing joint destruction in rheumatoid arthritis patients. When properly administered and closely monitored, the risk is slight compared with the potential for joint preservation (DiPiro et al, 2002). However, vitamin D therapy for rheumatoid arthritis is not recommended because the morbidity is far greater than any modest expected benefits.

Unsuccessful and even dangerous therapies existed for decades before the medical profession realized that they did more harm than good. Increasingly, information summarized from research studies that underlie the practice of evidence-based medicine will help to define benefit and risk more clearly in the future. Large-scale randomized controlled trials of drugs will continue to provide data about whether drugs should be used and what degree of risk the patient might be facing with their prescription.

The risk-benefit ratio expresses the amount of "acceptable" risk of adverse reaction or treatment failure that a patient might have in taking a drug versus the calculation of the potential benefit. It is generally estimated for each drug. The patient and provider together must determine the degree of risk that will be tolerated. This will probably depend on the severity of the disease being treated.

Design and Optimization of Dosage Regimens

Calculating the Therapeutic Index. A decision to use pharmacologic therapy requires the clinician to determine what degree of drug effect is desirable and achievable. If some effect of the drug can easily be measured (e.g., blood pressure for an antihypertensive medication), it can guide dosage. The medication can be adjusted up or down to achieve the optimal dosage in both a practical and sensible manner. However, it is often not possible to measure drug effect so simply. The clinician will need to establish some decision rules about how often to change dosage and by how much. Alternatively, some drugs have very little dose-related toxicity, and maximum efficacy is usually desired. For these drugs, doses well in excess of the average required will both ensure efficacy and prolong drug action.

The therapeutic index is a measure of drug safety and is calculated by the toxic dose divided by the therapeutic dose:

$$\text{Therapeutic index} = \frac{\text{Toxic dose}}{\text{Therapeutic dose}}$$

Response of the patient to the drug may be increased by factors that cause higher blood concentrations of a drug or by factors that make the patient more sensitive to a given blood concentration.

The therapeutic response is monitored by examining the index of therapeutic effect to determine if the therapeutic goal is attained (e.g., an infection is suppressed). It should be discriminating and should be practical to measure. The index of toxic effect may also be measured. Again the measurement should discriminate, it should be sensitive to detect toxicity promptly, and it should be practical to measure.

The concept of therapeutic window is not the same as the therapeutic index. The therapeutic window describes the range between the lowest therapeutic concentration and the beginning of toxicity (Figure 5-11). Some drugs have a very narrow therapeutic window, making patient monitoring especially important.

There are several different strategies in determining how much medication to use. These include determining a target level, maintenance dosing, loading dose, individualizing therapy, and performing therapeutic drug monitoring.

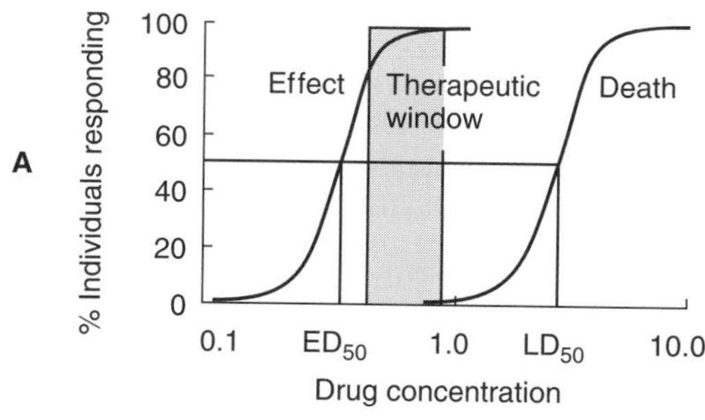

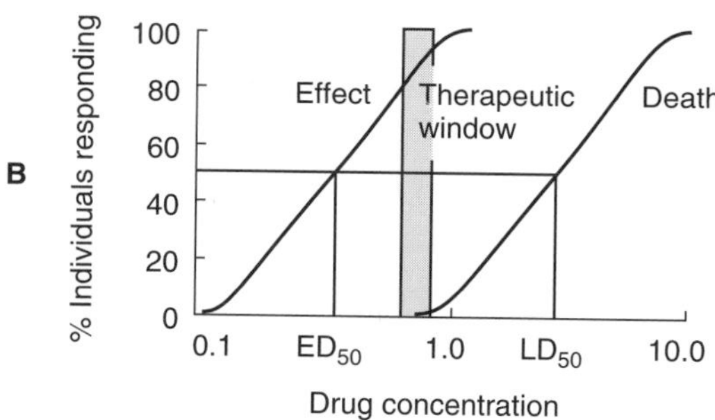

FIGURE 5-11

Therapeutic window. The therapeutic window compares the range of effective drug concentration to the safety of the drug. Notice that the drug in A has a much wider therapeutic window than the drug in B, even though both drugs have the same therapeutic index. *ED*, Effective dose; *LD*, lethal dose. (From Stringer JL: *Basic concepts in pharmacology*, ed 2, New York, 2000, McGraw-Hill.)

Target Level. In target level dosing, a desired or target steady-state concentration of the drug (usually in plasma) is identified, and a dosage is computed that is expected to achieve this value. Drug concentrations are subsequently measured, and dosage is adjusted if necessary to approximate the target more closely. This type of dosing is advisable when the effects of a drug are difficult to measure (or if the drug is given for prophylaxis). Target level dosing is also seen when toxicity and lack of efficacy are potential problems, or when the therapeutic window is very narrow. All of these situations require careful titration of dosages (DiPiro et al, 2002; Hardman et al, 2001).

In using target-level dosing strategy, the therapeutic objective must relate to an established blood serum therapeutic range, such as that seen with theophylline or digoxin levels. The lower limit of the therapeutic range appears to be approximately equal to the drug concentration that produces about half of the greatest possible therapeutic effect. The upper limit of the therapeutic range is fixed by toxicity, not by efficacy. Usually the upper limit of the therapeutic range is such that no more than 5% to 10% of patients will experience a toxic effect (DiPiro et al, 2002). These figures are highly variable; however, the target is usually chosen as the center of this therapeutic range.

Maintenance Dose. Most drugs are administered either as a continuous infusion or as a series of doses, designed to maintain steady-state concentration of the drug in plasma and to keep it within a given therapeutic range. To achieve the maintenance dose, the rate of drug administration is adjusted such that the rate of input equals the rate of loss. If the clinician knows the clearance and availability for that drug in a particular patient, the appropriate dose and dosing interval may be calculated to achieve the desired concentration of drug in the plasma (Hardman et al, 2001).

Loading Dose. If the target concentration of a dose must be met rapidly, a "loading dose" is one dose or a series of doses that are given at the onset of therapy. This may be desirable if the time required to attain steady state by the administration of the drug at a constant rate (four to five elimination half-lives) is long relative to demands of the condition being treated. This is commonly seen with antiarrhythmic drugs when the effect of the drug is required immediately. Because loading doses tend to be large and are often given parenterally and rapidly, they can be particularly dangerous if toxic effects occur as a result of actions of the drug. An overly sensitive individual may be exposed abruptly to a toxic concentration of a drug. If the drug involved has a long half-life, it may also take a long time for the concentration to fall if the level achieved is excessive (Hardman et al, 2001).

Individualizing Dose. Information about the patient also helps tailor the dosage. Calculation of the glomerular filtration rate and creatinine clearance may be required to determine dosage in individuals with kidney disease. Adjustments in dosage to compensate for liver damage may also be necessary. Comorbidity and the concurrent use of other medications, food, or alcohol may also require dosage modifications to achieve the desired level in the patient.

Therapeutic Drug Monitoring. Therapeutic drug monitoring involves measuring serum drug levels in patients receiving drugs with a narrow therapeutic window to maximize efficacy and minimize toxicity (Hardman et al, 2001; Katzung, 2000; Postelnick, 1995). Some of the most common drugs that must be closely monitored with serum blood levels include theophylline, phenytoin, carbamazepine, digoxin, and aminoglycoside antibiotics.

In monitoring serum drug levels, it is important to consider the time of sampling of the drug concentration. If intermittent dosing is used, a concentration of drug measured in a sample taken at virtually anytime during the dosing interval will provide information about drug toxicity and may be used to confirm other clinical findings that suggest toxicity (DiPiro et al, 2002; Katzung, 2000). However, serum drug levels used to measure drug concentration for the purposes of adjusting the dosage regimens must be taken at specified times to reflect accurate levels.

Drug levels vary dramatically throughout the dosing cycle, because the blood level rises and falls throughout the day, as in a trough. If a blood sample is taken shortly after administration of the drug, the level may be uninformative or even misleading. The levels may be very high but not reflective of toxicity; conversely, levels may be low because distribution is delayed relative to changes in plasma concentration (Hardman et al, 2001; Katzung, 2000). When the goal of measurement is adjustment of dosage, the sample should be taken well after the previous dose. As a rule of thumb test just before the next

TABLE 5-7 Therapeutic Ranges of Serum Drug Concentrations for Selected Drugs

Drug	Serum Concentration (Therapeutic Level, µg/ml unless otherwise indicated)	Time to Draw Blood Samples (Hours After Last Dose)
ANTIBIOTICS		
amikacin (Amikin)	15-25	Obtain peak and trough levels: draw peak 15-30 min after IV dose or 1 hr after IM dose; trough 15 min before next dose
gentamicin (Garamycin)	4-10	
netilmicin (Netromycin)	6-10	
tobramycin (Nebcin)	4-10	
ANTICONVULSANTS		
carbamazepine (Tegretol)	4-12	Steady state 1-2 weeks
ethosuximide	10-100	Steady state 10-30 days
phenobarbital	10-40	Steady state 1-2 weeks
phenytoin (Dilantin)	10-20	Steady state 2-3 days
primidone (Mysoline)	5-12	Steady state 1-2 days
valproic acid (Depakene, Depakote)	50-100	Steady state 1-2 days; then draw sample before next dose
ANTIDEPRESSANTS		
lithium	0.6-1.4 mEq/L	Steady state 3 weeks; draw before next dose
CARDIOVASCULAR		
digoxin (Lanoxin)	0.9-2 ng/nl	Steady state 1 week; draw before next dose, at least 6 hr after last dose
lidocaine (Xylocaine)	1.5-5	Steady state 6-12 hr; draw any time during infusion
procainamide (Pronestyl)	4-10	Steady state 12-24 hr; draw before next dose
quinidine (various)	3-6	Steady state 1.5 days; draw before next dose
RESPIRATORY		
theophylline (various)	10-20	Steady state in 1-2 days in adults; up to 1 week in neonates; IV: draw any time; oral; draw before next dose

From McKenry LM, Salerno E: *Mosby's pharmacology in nursing,* ed 21, revised reprint, St Louis, 2002, Mosby.

planned dose, when the concentration is at its minimum level. This, of course, would not provide relevant information about drugs that are nearly completely eliminated between doses. For individuals with renal failure, in whom concerns about drug accumulation are high, determination of both maximal and minimal concentrations is recommended.

It is also important to consider whether the patient has reached steady-state concentrations before taking a serum sample. Steady state is usually achieved after four to five half-lives have passed. If a sample is obtained too soon after dosage is started, it will not accurately reflect clearance. Yet, for toxic drugs, if one waits until the drug is at steady state, the level may already be at a toxic range. The protocol in Hardman et al (2001) suggests that when it is important to maintain careful control of concentrations, one may take the first sample after two half-lives (as calculated and expected for the patient), assuming no loading dose has been given. If the concentration already exceeds 90% of the eventual expected mean steady-state concentration, the dosage rate should be halved, another sample obtained in another two half-lives, and the dosage halved again if this sample exceeds the target. If the first concentration is not too high, one proceeds with the initial rate of dosage. Even if the concentration is lower than expected, one usually can wait until steady state is achieved in another two half-lives and then proceed to adjust dosage. (Computer programs are available for management of particularly difficult drug level calculations.) Table 5-7 shows the best time to draw blood levels for several different medications.

PRACTICAL APPLICATION OF PHARMACOKINETICS AND PHARMACODYNAMICS TO DRUG PRESCRIBING

Using the underlying scientific principles inherent in pharmacokinetics and pharmacodynamics, some very practical suggestions might be made for rational drug therapy:

- *Always try nonpharmacologic therapy first.* Continue it even after starting a medication.
- *Use a drug only when clearly indicated for a specific purpose.* It may be difficult for a provider to resist prescribing a medication for every symptom that annoys the patient, particularly when the patient is demanding resolution or relief. Well-directed advice and sound instructions often substitute for medication.
- *Use only one drug whenever possible.* Many patients with chronic disease who take numerous medications may need to have drugs stopped and reevaluated. Elderly patients, in particular, may have been on drugs almost forever, and nobody has ever thought to stop them. They may have had an acute illness that required additional medications or higher dosages that are no longer required. Some patients become very attached to particular drugs and do not want to stop them.
- *Use lowest effective dose.* If dosage is titrated up to a higher level and no additional benefit is seen, titrate it down to previous dose. This saves money and decreases the risk of adverse effects. Drug reactions are often dose-related and may be prompted by the philosophy that if a little bit is good, an added amount will do no harm and may ensure success.

TABLE 5-8 Electronic Media Sources with Current Drug Information

Title	Address	Description
FDA Human Drugs Page	www.fda.gov/ www.fda.gov/cder/drug.htm www.fda.gov/cder/regguide.htm	Extensive library of information specific to drugs; regulatory guidance
Food-Drug Interactions	www.babybag.com/articles/fdadrugs.htm	Extensive discussion of interaction between food and different medications
HealthGate	www.healthgate.com/	Extensive pharmacology information, consumer information, and links to other medical databases
Martindale's Health Science Guide '97	www.sci.lib.uci.edu/-martindale/pharmacy.html	Crosslinks to other good sources
Med Files	www.geocities.com/HotSprings/2255/drugs.html	Comprehensive listing of medical-pharmaceutical information
Rx List	www.rxlist.com/	Top 200 drugs; detailed database on prescriptions
Virtual Hospital	vh.radiology.uiowa.edu/	Wide variety of information regarding medical-pharmacology
Pharmacy Page	www.virtual Library: 157.142.72.77/pharmacy/company.html	Information about a wide variety of domestic and foreign pharmacy companies with links to their websites

- *Start low and go slow.*
- Usually, change dosage by no more than 50% and no more often than every three to four half-lives. This usually means no change for 1 to 2 weeks after starting a dose.
- *Simplify the regimen whenever possible.* Give the fewest doses and at the most convenient hours of the day to improve compliance.
- *If possible, use the side effect profile of one drug to treat other symptoms.* For example, if a patient has depression and insomnia, use trazodone or mertazepine, which may be sedating, instead of sertraline (Zoloft) or fluoxetine (Prozac), which are most commonly associated with insomnia.
- *Monitor closely for therapeutic effects.* Although drug levels may be evaluated as appropriate, trust your observation of the patient's clinical response more than the blood level. For example, the therapeutic level of phenytoin is usually between 10 and 20 μg/ml. However, elderly patients often do best on a drug level of 8 μg/ml. Drugs that are given over prolonged periods of time are more apt to produce adverse reactions; thus the dosage must be carefully monitored and reduced at the first sign of difficulty.
- *Keep good patient records.* A history of allergy, recent hepatitis, renal insufficiency, smoking, alcoholism, or other comorbidity all help alert the health care provider that the patient may be at greater risk for developing adverse reactions or drug–drug interactions.
- *Be particularly careful with some drugs that are highly associated with adverse effects.* Insulin, steroids, and many drugs used in chemotherapy and AIDS treatment are good examples. Prescription of these drugs mandates that the health care provider offer extensive education to the patient and the family if the drugs are to be used safely.
- *Always keep drug interactions and adverse effects in mind when evaluating the patient.* They are the rule rather than the exception. When using drugs with a great potential for adverse reactions, careful monitoring may prevent more serious problems. Pancytopenia need not occur if leukopenia is detected early; deafness will not result if signs of eighth nerve impairment are promptly investigated. It is not just luck that allows the health care provider to help the patient avoid problems with drug therapy.
- *Finally, stay up to date.* Many journals hold articles for 6 to 12 months before publication; most textbooks are more than a year in production after they are submitted for publication. Thus these sources of information may be outdated before they are even printed. New research findings should constantly be consulted and evaluated; valid findings should be incorporated into practice. In the age of electronic information dissemination, the standards of practice may be expected to shift to incorporate more new knowledge than ever before. Thus it is imperative for clinicians to find ways to update their knowledge on a regular basis.

Many publishers of pharmaceutical information have realized that information about new products and new recommendations have to reach health care providers in a more timely manner. Several of the most comprehensive drug texts have developed methods for accomplishing this. *Facts and Comparisons* (J. B. Lippincott) allows readers to subscribe to a monthly update service for their text, as well as providing content on disk and CD-ROM. Mosby's *DrugConsult* also comes in electronic form.

The Internet is becoming the biggest source for online in-formation about drugs. Electronic databases, linked to either universities or pharmaceutical companies, contain the latest information about drugs receiving FDA approval and being marketed. Table 5-8 lists some of the best and most user-friendly sites currently available to update drug information. evolve A list of pharmaceutical company websites can be found on the Evolve Learning Resources website.

SUMMARY

Current drugs provide health care providers many options in medications they may use, alone or in combination. These drugs represent real opportunities to cure disease, resolve symptoms, and improve the quality of life for patients. More information about how the agents work, how to increase their effectiveness, and the risks inherent in their use is discovered every day. Used wisely and thoughtfully, medications are wonderful assets to the health care provider's treatment armamentarium; used unwisely, they may cause even greater difficulties and distress for both the patient and the provider.

RESOURCES FOR PATIENTS AND PROVIDERS

Internet resources

Drug information, www.babybag.com/articles/fdadrugs.htm
FDA list of food/drug interactions.

Pharmacology data base, www.rxlist.com
Provides detailed information on top 200 prescribed medications.

USDA Food and Nutrition Information Center, www.nal.usda.gov/fnic, 10301 Baltimore Ave #304, Beltsville, MD 20705, (301) 504-5719.

General resources

Facts and Comparisons
Facts and Comparisons Drug Newsletter
American Drug Index, 1998
Drug Interaction Facts
Facts and Comparisons (CD-ROM, hardcover, base plus monthly updates)
Nurses Drug Information Service
Patient Drug Information
Professional's Guide to Patient Drug Facts (drug facts in patient language)

The Medical Letter, Vol 30 1988 to Vol 39 December 1997.
Available on CD-Rom or subscription: 1000 Main Street, New Rochelle, NY 10801-7537; 1 (800) 211-2769.

National Consumers League, 815 15th Street NW, Suite 928-N, Washington, DC 20005.
Patient education publications in English and Spanish on drug safety include:
When Medications Don't Mix: Preventing Drug Interactions
Guide to Warning Labels on Nonprescription Medications

National Technical Information Service (NTIS), Springfield, VA 22161; (703) 487-4650.

General Publishing Office (GPO); (202) 512-1800 for prices and ordering information.

U.S. Pharmacopeia, 12601 Twinbrook Parkway, Rockville, MD 20852.

USP DI
Volume I, *Drug Information for the Health Care Professional*
Volume II, *Advice for the Patient*
Volume III, *Approved Drug Products and Legal Requirements*

USP DI Customized Patient Education Leaflets
Every Woman's Guide to Prescription and Nonprescription Drugs
The USP Guide to Medicine
The USP Guide to Heart Medicines
The USP Guide to Vitamins and Minerals

USP Practitioners' Reporting Network (USP PRN)
To report problems, obtain reporting forms, or request information about adverse drug effects, contact:
MedWatch or USP Practitioners' Reporting Network, 12601 Twinbrook Parkway, Rockville, MD 20852 USA. Telephone 1 (800) 4USP PRN (1-800-487-7776), Fax (301) 816-8532.

REFERENCES

Adedoyin A et al: Selective effect of liver disease on the activities of specific metabolizing enzymes: investigation of cytochromes P450 2C19 and 2D6, *Clin Pharmacol Ther* 64:8-17, 1998.

American Psychiatric Association: *Diagnostic and statistical manual of mental disorders,* ed 4, Washington, DC, 2000, The Association.

Beedham C: The role of non-P450 enzymes in drug oxidation, *Pharm World Sci* 19:255-263, 1997.

Berne RM, Levy MN: *Physiology,* ed 4, St Louis, 1998, Mosby.

DiPadova C et al: Effects of ranitidine on blood alcohol levels after ethanol ingestion: comparison with other H2-receptor antagonists, *JAMA* 267:83-86, 1992.

DiPiro JT et al, editors: *Pharmocotherapy: a pathophysiologic approach,* ed 5, Norwalk, CT, 2002, McGraw-Hill/Appleton & Lange.

Dufour MC et al: Alcohol and the elderly, *Clin Geriatr Med* 8:127-141, 1992.

Edmunds MW: *Introduction to clinical pharmacology*, ed 4, St Louis, 2003, Mosby.

Egbert AM: The older alcoholic: recognizing the subtle clinical clues, *Geriatrics* 48:63-69, 1993.

Food and Drug Administration: *MedWatch Drug Reporting Program,* Washington, DC, 1990.

Fraser AG et al: Ranitidine, cimetidine, famotidine have no effect on postprandial absorption of ethanol 0.8 g/kg taken after an evening meal, *Aliment Pharmacol Ther* 6:693-700, 1992.

Gomberg ESL: Drugs, alcohol, and aging. In Kozlowski LT et al, editors: *Research advances in alcohol and drug problems,* vol 10, New York, 1990, Plenum Press.

Guengerich FP: Role of cytochrome P450 enzymes in drug-drug interactions, *Adv Pharmacol* 43:7-35, 1997.

Guram MS, Howden CW, Holt S: Alcohol and drug interactions, *Pract Gastroenterol* 16:47, 50-54, 1992.

Hardman JG et al, editors: *Goodman and Gilman's pharmacological basis of therapeutics,* ed 10, New York, 2001, McGraw-Hill.

Holder H: *Effects of alcohol, alone and in combination with medications,* Walnut Creek, CA, 1992, Prevention Research Center.

Honkakoski P, Negishi M: The structure, function, and regulation of cytochrome P450 2A enzymes, *Drug Metab Rev* 29(4):977-996, 1997.

Institute of Alcohol Abuse and Alcoholism: *Alert on alcohol and medication interactions,* No. 27, PH 355, Washington, DC, January, 1995, The Institute.

Katzung BG: *Basic and clinical pharmacology,* ed 8, Norwalk, Conn, 2000, Appleton & Lange.

Lieber CS: Interaction of ethanol with other drugs. In Lieber CS, editor: *Medical and nutritional complications of alcoholism: mechanisms and management,* New York, 1992, Plenum.

Lipsy RJ: Adverse drug reactions. In Green HL, Johnston WP, Lemchke D, editors: *Decision-making in medicine,* ed 2, St Louis, 1998, Mosby.

McCance KL, Huether SE: *Pathophysiology,* ed 4, St Louis, 2001, Mosby.

McKenry LM, Salerno E: *Mosby's pharmacology in nursing,* ed 22, St Louis, 2002, Mosby.

Michalets EL: Clinically significant cytochrome P-450 drug interactions, *Pharmacotherapy* 18:84-112, 1998.

Midanik LT, Room R: The epidemiology of alcohol consumption, *Alcohol Health Res World* 16:183-190, 1992.

National Institute for Alcohol Abuse and Alcoholism: *Alert on alcohol and medication interactions*, No 27, PH 355, Washington, DC, January 1995, The Institute.

Postelnick M: Therapeutic drug monitoring: where have we been and where are we going? *J Pharm Pract* 8:1, 1995.

Seppala T et al: Drugs, alcohol and driving, *Drugs* 17:389-408, 1979.

Shoaf SE, Linnoila M: Interaction of ethanol and smoking on the pharmacokinetics and pharmacodynamics of psychotropic medications, *Psychopharmacol Bull* 27:577-594, 1991.

Stringer JL: *Basic concepts in pharmacology,* ed 2, New York, 2000, McGraw-Hill/Appleton & Lange.

CHAPTER 6

Special Populations: Geriatrics

Barbara Resnick

Over the past century, the number of older adults has increased more than tenfold. In 2000 there were approximately 35 million people age 65 or older (National Center for Health Statistics, 2002), and the population of older adults increases each year. Women who reach age 65 can expect to live an additional 19 years, and men at age 65 can expect to live an additional 16 years. This growth is in part due to improved medical care, increased use of preventive health services, public health efforts, and healthier lifestyles. There has been a decline in number of deaths due to heart disease and stroke, although this continues to be a major cause of death in older adults. In 2000, heart disease, stroke, and cancer actually accounted for 60% of all deaths among people age 65 and older. The death rates for cancer and for chronic lower respiratory disease have increased, as has the death rate for diabetes. Although there is an increase in the length of life, older adults are living longer with chronic illnesses (Kovner, 2002). Specifically, nearly 60% of older African American adults have high blood pressure and a growing share of elderly African Americans, Hispanics, and Native Americans have diabetes.

Older adults account for 30% of medication expenditures, and up to 82% are on at least one drug (Kaufman et al, 2002). The most common drug classes used are cardiovascular, analgesic, and central nervous system drugs (Rathmore et al, 1998). Elderly patients are more often victims of polypharmacy, both because they see multiple prescribers and because of self-treatment with over-the-counter (OTC) medications. It is estimated that greater than 40% of OTC drugs are purchased by people in this same age group. Despite the fact that older adults are a major group of drug users, most drug studies are performed on individuals 55 years of age or younger. Due to a variety of issues, including limited knowledge of the impact of specific drugs on older adults, multiple medication use, and normal age- and disease-associated changes, older adults are at increased risk of experiencing drug reactions (Bourne, 2001). It is essential to consider these issues before prescribing medications for this population.

PHARMACOKINETIC CHANGES THAT AFFECT DRUG THERAPY

Pharmacokinetics refers to the way drugs are absorbed, metabolized, distributed, and eliminated from the body. Although variable from patient to patient, the aging patient undergoes changes in some of these areas that may significantly affect the way a drug is handled by the body. Consideration of each of these processes when prescribing drug therapy in the elderly can prevent inappropriate dosing and prevent adverse drug reactions (ADRs) and their complications in patient care.

Absorption

The overall significance of changes in the absorption of drugs with aging is not completely clear. There appears to be little, if any, significance in the amount of drug absorbed in drugs that are passively absorbed. There is, however, some reduced absorption in older adults for some compounds that are actively absorbed such as galactose, calcium, thiamin, and iron (Bourne, 2001). Physiologic changes that affect the gastrointestinal tract include a reduction in acid output and subsequent alkaline environment. These changes affect drugs such as B_{12} that require an acid medium for absorption, although this is not well documented. Reductions in blood flow, enzyme activity, gastric emptying, and bowel motility may support the delay in absorption of some drugs, although such reductions probably have minimal, if any, effect on the extent of absorption. Further support for the insignificance of these physiologic changes is based on the fact that most drugs are absorbed via passive diffusion. Because the gastrointestinal tract has such a large surface area, the extent of absorption of most drugs is not affected. Nonionized forms of a drug (i.e., those that are more lipid soluble) are more readily absorbed than those in the ionized forms. If a drug such as an antacid is administered, the gastrointestinal pH will be raised and the absorption of acidic drugs may be delayed or decreased. Table 6-1 provides some examples of this alteration when certain drugs or dietary products are given concurrently. Compounds such as iron, calcium, or certain vitamins that depend on active transport mechanisms and thus the delivery of oxygen for absorption may be affected by decreased blood flow in the aging patient's gastrointestinal tract (Evans, 1992).

There can also be a change in the rate of absorption due to alterations in the motility and rate of gastric emptying. Cathartics can increase gastrointestinal motility and thereby increase the rate at which another drug passes through the gastrointestinal tract. This can be a problem for enteric-coated products. Similarly, anticholinergics decrease motility and metoclopramide stimulates motility, thereby altering the rate of drug absorption with some medications (e.g., ethanol, levodopa, tetracycline, acetaminophen). Food can also delay or reduce the absorption of certain drugs, particularly antibiotics.

Distribution

The distribution of drugs in the body, which is dependent on the chemical composition of the agent involved, may be affected by the aging process. As individuals age, the decline in total body water and lean body mass may affect drugs that are distributed into these areas (Box 6-1). The changes in total body water and lean body mass may result in less distribution

TABLE 6-1 Drug Absorption Challenges

Drug	Issues with Concurrent Administration
tetracycline Antacids, iron, calcium	tetracycline, with the exception of doxycycline and minocycline, are influenced when given with foods high in iron or calcium, antacids, or direct supplements. The drugs will be less well absorbed and should be given 2 hr apart from dietary intake or supplements.
cholestyramine and colestipol Thyroid hormone, digoxin, and warfarin	cholestyramine and colestipol will bind with these drugs in the gastrointestinal tract, thereby decreasing absorption. Drugs should be given 2 hr apart.
Antidiarrheal mixtures and antacids All medications	Antidiarrheals and antacids can absorb certain medications and decrease absorption. There is no comprehensive list of drugs in which this occurs; therefore patients should be instructed to take antidiarrheals and antacids 2 hr before or after other medications.

BOX 6-1

DRUGS THAT DISTRIBUTE INTO BODY WATER OR LEAN BODY MASS

digoxin
lithium
meperidine
theophylline
cimetidine
gentamicin
phenytoin

Data compiled from Abrams WB et al: Clinical pharmacology in an aging population, *Clin Pharmacol Ther* 63:281-284, 1998; Evans WE: General principles of applied pharmacokinetics. In Evans WE et al, editors: *Applied pharmacokinetics: principles of therapeutic drug monitoring,* ed 3, Vancouver, WA, 1991, Applied Therapeutics; and Mayersohn MB: Special pharmacokinetic considerations in the elderly. In Evans WE et al, editors: *Applied pharmacokinetics: principles of therapeutic drug monitoring,* ed 3, Vancouver, WA, 1991, Applied Therapeutics..

of drugs into these areas. Unadjusted dosing can result in greater serum concentrations, leading to a greater effect or toxicity.

Specifically, as we age, the decrease in lean body mass is usually coupled with an increase in total body fat. Changes in body fat are reported as increasing from 18% to 36% in males and 33% to 48% in females from the ages of 15 to 60. The increase in body fat can result in an increase in the volume of distribution of lipid-soluble drugs, leading to drug accumulation and the potential for toxicity. For example, certain drugs such as diazepam and chlordiazepoxide have a higher volume of distribution than do other anxiolytics such as lorazepam and oxazepam because of the lipid soluability of the former two drugs. Box 6-2 lists additional examples of lipid-soluble drugs that may require downward adjustments in doses and slowly titrated increases if used in the elderly. The risk of accumulation and toxicity is a real concern with high doses of these agents in the elderly (Abrams et al, 1998; Evans, 1992; Mayersohn, 1992).

Another common age change that effects distribution of drugs in older adults is a decrease in serum albumin. Albumin concentrations decrease slightly with age in most elderly patients, although significant changes that may affect drug therapy may be seen in the chronically ill or malnourished elderly patient (Bourne, 2001). Albumin is the most common protein that binds to various acidic drugs. Significant decreases in albumin may result in a greater free concentration of highly protein-bound drugs. Box 6-3 lists some drugs that have significant protein binding, which may result in greater free concentrations when albumin is significantly reduced. Generally, drugs that are highly protein bound to albumin should be pre-

BOX 6-2

EXAMPLES OF LIPID-SOLUBLE DRUGS

diazepam
chlordiazepoxide
flurazepam
thiopental
Antipsychotics
Antidepressants

Data compiled from Evans WE: General principles of applied pharmacokinetics. In Evans WE et al, editors: *Applied pharmacokinetics: principles of therapeutic drug monitoring,* ed 3, Vancouver, WA, 1991, Applied Therapeutics; and Jinks MJ, Fuerst RH: Geriatric drug use and rehabilitation. In Young LY, Koda-Kimble MA, editors: *Applied therapeutics: the clinical use of drugs,* Vancouver, WA, 1995, Applied Therapeutics.

BOX 6-3

DRUGS WITH HIGH BINDING AFFINITY TO ALBUMIN

phenytoin
warfarin
naproxen
theophylline
phenobarbital
Antidepressants

Data compiled from Evans WE: General principles of applied pharmacokinetics. In Evans WE et al, editors: *Applied pharmacokinetics: principles of therapeutic drug monitoring,* ed 3, Vancouver, WA, 1991, Applied Therapeutics; and Jinks MJ, Fuerst RH: Geriatric drug use and rehabilitation. In Young LY, Koda-Kimble MA, editors: *Applied therapeutics: the clinical use of drugs,* Vancouver, WA, 1995, Applied Therapeutics.

scribed in reduced doses in patients with low serum albumin values (Bourne, 2001). A practical example of the clinical significance of this relationship can be described with the anticonvulsant phenytoin. In an elderly patient with a low serum albumin concentration (normal, 3.5 to 5 mg/dl), the phenytoin level reported from the laboratory will reflect both the bound and free concentrations and, in a hypoalbuminemic individual, may appear normal or even subtherapeutic. This is because of the greater free amounts of phenytoin getting into the tissue and acting at the receptor level but not portrayed in the total serum level. The actual level may be much higher or even in the toxic range. Treatment decisions with older adults should not be based solely on drug levels. Treatment decisions must be based on consideration of the patient characteristics as well as drug levels.

Other protein changes may also have an influence on drug therapy. Patients with acute disease, such as a myocardial infarction, respiratory distress, or infectious insult, for example, may experience increases in alpha-1-glycoprotein, an acute phase reactant protein. This may result in the increased binding of weakly basic drugs, including propranolol or lidocaine, and a less-than-normal response to therapy. Data are lacking concerning the real significance of changes in alpha-1-glycoprotein and drug therapy in the elderly (Abrams et al, 1998).

BOX 6-4

DRUGS WITH HIGH LIVER EXTRACTION RATIOS OR FIRST-PASS EFFECT

lidocaine
meperidine
morphine
propranolol
metoprolol
verapamil
Estrogens
Nitrates
Barbiturates (e.g., phenobarbital)

Data compiled from Evans WE: General principles of applied pharmacokinetics. In Evans WE et al, editors: *Applied pharmacokinetics: principles of therapeutic drug monitoring,* ed 3, Vancouver, WA, 1991, Applied Therapeutics; Jinks MJ, Fuerst RH: Geriatric drug use and rehabilitation. In Young LY, Koda-Kimble MA, editors: *Applied therapeutics: the clinical use of drugs,* Vancouver, WA, 1995, Applied Therapeutics; Mayersohn MB: Special pharmacokinetic considerations in the elderly. In Evans WE et al, editors: *Applied pharmacokinetics: principles of therapeutic drug monitoring,* ed 3, Vancouver, WA, 1991, Applied Therapeutics; and Wynne HA, Cope LH, Mutch E, et al: The effect of age upon liver volume and apparent liver blood flow in healthy men, *Hepatology* 9:297-301, 1989.

Biotransformation (Metabolism)

Numerous age-related changes in hepatic structure and function have been described, although liver function seems to be quite well maintained in old age. Few consistent and reproducible observations and a lack of correlation between structural and functional data characterize the present state of our knowledge. In contrast to renal clearance, no equally reliable method exists to estimate hepatic drug clearance. The contribution of age to altered drug clearance in the elderly is difficult to assess because drug interactions, numbers and types of drugs taken at a time, underlying disease, and increased interindividual variability are superimposed on the aging process. A decline in liver volume and blood flow and a reduction in *in vitro* and *in vivo* metabolic capacity have been shown in older subjects, and explain the physiologic basis of reduced hepatic drug clearance in this age group.

The significance of hepatic blood flow changes may be seen with drugs that have a high extraction ratio or a high first-pass metabolism in the liver. These drugs are considered to have flow-limiting metabolism. When flow is reduced as may occur with aging, less drug is metabolized and increased amounts may be present in active form in the blood. When prescribing drugs with high extraction ratios in the elderly, lower doses may be necessary. Examples of drugs that have high extraction ratios are listed in Box 6-4 (Abrams et al, 1998; Evans, 1992; Mayersohn, 1992).

Other hepatic changes occurring with age that may affect the metabolism of drugs include changes in specific pathways or types of metabolism. The purpose of drug metabolism is generally to make drugs more water-soluble for elimination. Phase I metabolism can be described as preparatory processes where minor molecular modifications are made to drugs. Phase I includes oxidation reductions, demethylation, and hydroxylation. Phase I metabolism is more likely to decrease with age than phase II metabolism. Drugs that are metabolized by phase I metabolic pathways, including CYP450 enzyme systems, may accumulate in the older adult. Such drugs should be used cautiously and at lower doses in the elderly. Examples of drugs that undergo phase I metabolism include lidocaine, phenytoin, propranolol, and theophylline. If possible, the use of alternative agents within a class of drugs that are metabolized differently (e.g., phase II) should be considered. If these drugs are prescribed in the elderly, lower doses should be used and patients monitored for adverse effects. Examples of drugs whose clearance depends on phase I metabolism are listed in Box 6-5. Drugs that are metabolized by phase II metabolic processes, including conjugation, acetylation, sulfonation, and glucuronidation, have no reported change in clearance with aging (Evans, 1992; Mayersohn, 1992).

Drugs that are metabolized by the liver may have reduced metabolism with aging because of changes within the liver itself or changes resulting from other disease states. Aging influences associated with declining liver mass, decreased hepatic blood flow, altered nutritional status, other physiologic changes, and diseases such as congestive heart failure may result in a loss of hepatic reserve. Consequently, these patients are at increased risk of adverse effects because of competition for the same metabolic enzymes when drugs are added to the existing regimen (Abrams et al, 1998; Mayersohn, 1992). Drug substances that are metabolized and excreted by the liver should be used at a starting dose that is 30% to 40% less than the average dose used in middle-aged adults (Zeeh & Platt, 2002).

BOX 6-5

SAMPLE DRUGS THAT UNDERGO PHASE I METABOLISM

diazepam
flurazepam
chlordiazepoxide
piroxicam
quinidine
Barbiturates

Data compiled from Evans WE: General principles of applied pharmacokinetics. In Evans WE et al, editors: *Applied pharmacokinetics: principles of therapeutic drug monitoring,* ed 3, Vancouver, WA, 1991, Applied Therapeutics; Greenblatt DJ, et al: Kinetics and clinical effects of flurazepam in young and elderly noninsomniacs, *Clin Pharmacol Ther* 4:475-486, 1986; Jinks MJ, Fuerst RH: Geriatric drug use and rehabilitation. In Young LY, Koda-Kimble MA, editors: *Applied therapeutics: the clinical use of drugs,* Vancouver, WA, 1995, Applied Therapeutics; Mayersohn MB: Special pharmacokinetic considerations in the elderly. In Evans WE et al, editors: *Applied pharmacokinetics: principles of therapeutic drug monitoring,* ed 3, Vancouver, WA, 1991, Applied Therapeutics.

Elimination

Longitudinal studies reflect a great degree of variability in renal function changes with aging. Age-related changes in renal function are the single most important physiologic factor resulting in ADRs. Biologic changes that occur in the aging kidney include decreases in the number of nephrons; decreases in renal blood flow, glomerular filtration rate, and tubular secretion rate; and increases in the number of sclerosed glomeruli. In addition, atherosclerotic changes and declining cardiac output decrease renal perfusion by 40% to 50% between ages 25 and 65. The end result of these changes is a decrease in creatinine clearance, which is reported to decrease 10% for each decade after age 40 (Abrams et al, 1998).

In addition to the normal reduction that may occur in renal function with aging, chronic diseases, including congestive heart failure, liver disease, and conditions leading to dehydration, can also affect renal function and further complicate the required dosing. Creatinine is a muscle byproduct and is almost exclusively removed by the kidney, making it an excellent marker to measure renal clearance. Daily creatinine is related to age and serum creatinine concentrations. A drug's clearance is the amount of blood from which a drug is cleared per unit time. Although creatinine clearance is used to measure renal function, it is important to note that it is only an estimated value. Numerous formulas are available that can calculate the creatinine clearance values, many of which may overestimate or underestimate the patient's true creatinine clearance. Creatinine clearance is measured by collecting urine for 24 hours. This, unfortunately, may not be practical in many institutions, therefore we calculate estimated creatinine clearance. In older adults, creatinine clearance calculations may be especially inaccurate as these individuals have very little muscle mass and produce very little creatinine. This patient's serum creatinine may be reported as low for example, 0.5 (normal, 0.6 to 1.2 mg/dl), thus reflecting good excretion of creatinine. This can be very deceptive and will often result in overestimation of renal function when used in the various formulas available. When prescribing renally excreted drugs in the elderly, calculated creatinine clearance should be used to estimate renal function. Lower drug doses or longer intervals between dosing should be used when there is evidence of renal impairment. Table 6-2 lists drugs that depend on the kidneys for elimination and therefore may require dose adjustments in the elderly (Mayersohn, 1992).

TABLE 6-2 Drugs that May Require Dose Adjustments in the Elderly Because of Renal Impairment

Drug Class	Drug Names
Antibiotics	aminoglycosides, e.g., gentamicin, tobramycin, amikacin sulfamethoxazole, trimethoprim β-Lactams: cephalosporins (most), imipenem, ticarcillin tetracycline vancomycin aztreonam ciprofloxacin, norfloxacin nitrofurantoin
Antivirals	amantadine, rimantadine
Antineoplastics	methotrexate, bleomycin, nitrosourea, cisplatin
Antifungals	amphotericin B, fluconazole acyclovir, famciclovir
Analgesics	Opiate analgesics, e.g., meperidine, morphine
Cardiac medications	β-Blockers, e.g., atenolol, nadolol digoxin procainamide, bretylium Angiotensin-converting enzyme inhibitors, e.g., captopril, lisinopril, and others Other antihypertensives, e.g., clonidine Diuretics, e.g., thiazides, furosemide, spironolactone
Ulcer medications	$Histamine_2$ blockers: cimetidine, ranitidine, famotidine
Psychoactive medications	lithium
Other agents	allopurinol, acetazolamide, chlorpropamide, gold sodium thiomalate, metoclopramide

Data compiled from Jinks MJ, Fuerst RH: Geriatric drug use and rehabilitation. In Young LY, Koda-Kimble MA, editors: *Applied therapeutics: the clinical use of drugs,* Vancouver, WA, 1995, Applied Therapeutics; Mayersohn MB: Special pharmacokinetic considerations in the elderly. In Evans WE et al, editors: *Applied pharmacokinetics: principles of therapeutic drug monitoring,* ed 3, Vancouver, WA, 1991, Applied Therapeutics; O'Connell MB, Dwinell Am, Bannick M: Predictive performance of equations to estimate creatinine clearance in hospitalized elderly patients, *Ann Pharmacother* 26:627-635, 1992; and Smythe M et al: Estimating creatinine clearance in elderly patients with low serum creatinine concentrations, *Am J Hosp Pharm* 51:198-204, 1994.

A common formula used to calculate the estimated creatinine clearance is the Cockcroft-Gault equation. Unfortunately, the Cockcroft-Gault equation is noted to overpredict glomerular filtration rate. A simple modification of the Cockcroft-Gault equation has been recommended (Oo & Hill, 2002). This substitutes serum creatinine with 1 mg/dl if the value is less than 1 mg/dl.

TABLE 6-3 Age-Related Changes Influencing Drug Response

Age-Related Changes	Drugs Affected by Changes or the Exacerbate Changes
Orthostatic hypotension	Phenothiazines, tricyclic antidepressants
Bowel and bladder problems: Urinary retention, constipation, prostatic hypertrophy	Anticholinergics
Impaired thermoregulation	Phenothiazines, alcohol, aspirin
Reduced cognitive function	Any psychoactive medication
Postural stability impaired	Alcohol, diuretics, anticholinergics, antihypertensives
Glucose intolerance	Glucocorticoids, insulin

$$\text{Men: } \frac{\text{Creatinine}}{\text{clearance}} = \frac{\text{Weight (kg*)} \times (140 - \text{Age in years})}{72 \times \text{Serum creatinine (mg/dl)}}$$

$$\text{Women: } \frac{\text{Creatinine}}{\text{clearance}} = \frac{\text{Weight (kg*)} \times (140 - \text{Age in years})}{72 \times \text{Serum creatinine (mg/dl)}} (\times 0.85)\dagger$$

Creatinine clearance can also be estimated by using a computer program. This is done using programs such as the USC PACK PC (Jelliffe, 2002). Other kidney changes that occur with aging include a decrease in renal concentrating ability and renal sodium conservation, which may be a factor in patients on high-dose diuretics.

In summary, it is recommended that when prescribing drugs for older adults, a lower dose than normally indicated should be the starting dosage and the dosage should be titrated up slowly (Bourne, 2001; Evans, 1992; Mayersohn, 1992).

PHARMACODYNAMIC CHANGES IN THE ELDERLY THAT MAY AFFECT DRUG THERAPY

Pharmacodynamic changes are defined loosely as changes in concentration-response relationships or receptor sensitivity. Pharmacodynamic changes in the elderly may be due to changes in receptor affinity or number or to changes in hormonal levels. The impact of drugs affecting the central nervous system (benzodiazepines, anesthetics, metoclopramide, or narcotics) and the cardiovascular system (beta-blockers, calcium channel blockers, or diuretics) is frequently altered in older adults. The physiologic changes associated with aging and the altered homeostatic mechanisms in the elderly may cause an increased sensitivity to specific drugs. Table 6-3 lists the common age-associated changes and the medications that are affected by them. This increase in sensitivity may be the result of changes in the drug receptors with aging or may possibly be caused by a reduced reserve capacity in the aged patient. The results of these receptor changes include greater sensitivity or intensity to drug action in addition to a greater duration of drug action (Bourne, 2001).

The body system most significantly affected by increased receptor sensitivity is the central nervous system, wherein increased sensitivity to numerous drugs is evident (Davis & Mathew, 1998). Factors that may contribute to this greater sensitivity include a decrease in neuronal numbers, decrease in cerebral blood flow, and an increased permeability of the blood-brain barrier. In the central nervous system, inhibitory and excitatory pathways are delicately balanced to modulate cognition. With aging, there is a selective decline in some pathways and the preservation of others (Davis & Mathew, 1998).

*Lean body weight; may reflect creatinine production more accurately.
†In women, multiply value × 0.85.

TABLE 6-4 Categories of Anticholinergic Drugs that Can Cause Adverse Effects in Elderly Patients

Drug Class	Drug Names
Antispasmodics	belladonna, dicyclomine, propantheline
Antiparkinson agents	benztropine, trihexyphenidyl
Antihistamines	diphenhydramine, chlorpheniramine, hydroxyzine
Antidepressants	amitriptyline, imipramine
Antiarrhythmics	quinidine, disopyramide
Neuroleptics	thioridazine, chlorpromazine
Over-the-counter agents	Cold remedy products, antidiarrheals, doxylamine

Data compiled from Feinberg M: The problems of anticholinergic adverse effects in older patients, *Drugs Aging* 3:335-348, 1993; Jinks MJ, Fuerst RH: Geriatric drug use and rehabilitation. In Young LY, Koda-Kimble MA, editors: *Applied therapeutics: the clinical use of drugs*, Vancouver, WA, 1995, Applied Therapeutics.

Drugs with anticholinergic side effect profiles are often used in the elderly (Table 6-4), and these drugs are commonly associated with central and peripheral adverse effects. Commonly reported adverse side effects include sedation, confusion, constipation, dry mouth, urinary retention, tachycardia, and blurred vision (Bourne, 2001; Feinberg, 1993). The increased incidence of these with aging may be the result of a decrease in the neurotransmitter acetylcholine associated with the aging process (Gales & Menard, 1995). This greater sensitivity to anticholinergic side effects includes a greater risk of dizziness and subsequent falls and fractures, along with loss of cognitive performance (Bourne, 2001; Sloan, 1992). Drugs with anticholinergic effects should be avoided if at all possible in the elderly. If they are used, consider using doses corresponding to roughly half the normal dose (Bourne, 2001; Feinberg, 1993).

Benzodiazepines, including diazepam, alprazolam (Xanax), flurazepam, lorazepam, and others, have an increased pharmacodynamic effect in elderly patients. Benzodiazepine-induced psychomotor impairment may include ataxia, delayed reaction time, increased body sway, and decreased proprioception (Bourne, 2001).

Changes in responsiveness to other parts of the central nervous system can also affect the response to drug therapy. A decline in the neurotransmitters norepinephrine and dopamine has been reported in the elderly. The decline in dopamine may lead to an increased sensitivity to dopamine-blocking agents (e.g., neuroleptic agents and structurally similar agents, including metoclopramide) (Bourne, 2001).

The cardiovascular system is another body system where pharmacodynamic changes can result in a greater sensitivity (Bourne, 2001) or, in a few cases, loss in sensitivity to cardioactive drugs. Orthostatic hypotension occurs more commonly in the elderly because of the loss of baroreceptor response and a failure of cerebral blood flow autoregulation; it can also be aggravated by drugs with sympatholytic activity (Box 6-6). The consequences of orthostatic hypertension in the elderly are dizziness and an increased risk of falls and fractures. Medications that cause orthostatic changes should probably be used with caution in the elderly, and lower doses should be prescribed.

Other cardiovascular changes that occur in the aging patient that may be influenced by drug therapy include a decrease in resting heart rate and a decrease in cardiac output in response to exercise. Drugs that can affect cardiac output include calcium channel blockers and β-blockers; their use should be monitored carefully, especially in patients with a history of severe systolic dysfunction (Flockhart & Tanus-Santos, 2002). Positive inotropic agents such as digoxin have an increased effect in the elderly because of their greater sensitivity to the drug, predisposing them to a greater risk of toxicity.

Although many drugs have a reported greater response in the elderly, a few have a decreased response. β-blockers are reported to have a lesser response in the elderly, suggesting changes within the receptors themselves or a response to elevated plasma norepinephrine levels with age. Although not well documented, a lack of effect of β-blockers in reducing blood pressure in the elderly may exist (Sloan, 1992; White & Leenen, 1994).

Anticoagulant drugs may produce a greater response or effect in the elderly are those reflecting an intrinsic, age-related change in receptor sensitivity. Drugs such as warfarin and heparin may produce an exaggerated response in the elderly patient, possibly because of a decrease in clotting factors with age or because of protein-binding changes (Bourne, 2001). These agents should initially be dosed lower in the elderly patient and monitored carefully for an appropriate response.

BOX 6-6

DRUGS THAT MAY CAUSE ORTHOSTATIC HYPOTENSION IN THE ELDERLY

Antihypertensives
Anticholinergics
guanethidine
reserpine
Phenothiazines
Antidepressants (e.g., amitriptyline, trazodone)
Diuretics
Vasodilators (e.g., nitrates, alcohol)

Data compiled from Davis KM, Mathew E: Pharmacologic management of depression in the elderly, *Nurs Pract* 23:16-45, 1998; Jinks MJ, Fuerst RH: Geriatric drug use and rehabilitation. In Young LY, Koda-Kimble MA, editors: *Applied therapeutics: the clinical use of drugs*, Vancouver, WA, 1995, Applied Therapeutics; and Lipsitz LA: Orthostatic hypotension in the older patients, *N Engl J Med* 321:952-957, 1989.

COMMON CONCERNS RELATED TO MEDICATION USE IN OLDER ADULTS: ADVERSE DRUG REACTIONS, POLYPHARMACY, COMPLIANCE, AND COSTS

Adverse Drug Reactions

An ADR is any response that is unintended and undesired and that occurs at normal recommended dosages. The reaction may be idiosyncratic or pharmacologically predictable. Cumulative side effects of medications taken concurrently increase the risk for adverse reactions. ADRs are more common in older adults, and it is anticipated that many of these reactions are left unidentified by older adults who assume the problems are normal age changes. Medication use in elderly patients increases their risk for ADRs and potentially serious consequences, including falls and subsequent fractures. (Falls are a leading cause of death in the United States in adults over 65 years of age and contribute to 40% of nursing home admissions.) The rate of ADRs in the elderly is higher than that in younger adults (Anderson & Wahler, 2002; Lien et al, 2002). The body systems most associated with ADRs in the elderly are cardiovascular and CNS.

The most important class of drug interactions involves the cytochrome P450 microsomal enzyme system, which handles a variety of xenobiotic substances (Flockhart & Tanus-Santos, 2002). A potential for interactions with these enzymes exists with calcium channel blockers, beta-adrenergic blocking agents, angiotensin-converting enzyme inhibitors, and angiotensin receptor blockers. There are no interactions with diuretic antihypertensives as these drugs are renally eliminated and more vulnerable to drug interactions that occur in the kidney.

Adverse reactions are associated with medications with different degrees of certainty (Table 6-5). The certainty with

TABLE 6-5 Certainty of Association between Drug and Adverse Reaction

Degree of Certainty	Description
Causative	The drug concentration has been established by toxicologic examination of the tissue and found to be in the generally acceptable range recognized as toxic. Definite temporal relationship was established.
Probable	Reasonable temporal relationship was established, and the response has been previously reported.
Possible	A reasonable temporal relationship was established, and the reaction resembles previously reported experiences with the suspected drug. However, nondrug and/or other drug causes cannot be ruled out.
Coincidental	There are no previous reports of similar reactions with the suspected age, but it is possible that there was a relationship between drug use and reaction.
Negative	The temporal relationship, disease pattern, pathologic studies, or specific analytical laboratory findings clearly eliminate the possibility of a drug-induced reaction.

which this is determined is important as it helps providers know which drugs must be stopped and/or avoided in older individuals and which drugs may be used, albeit with caution. There are many factors that put older adults at risk for developing ADRs (Table 6-6). These reactions may be from actions by the prescriber, the pharmacist, or the patient.

A trial that examined drug prescribing in community-dwelling elderly patients (Atkin et al, 1999) concluded that nearly 25% were receiving inappropriate medications, which placed them at increased risk for ADRs. ADRs can mimic many clinical syndromes in the geriatric patient. The importance of monitoring for ADRs cannot be overemphasized. ADRs may be associated with drug interactions, which is a preventable drug-related problem in patients on multiple drugs. Drug reactions occur in up to 24% of institutionalized elderly patients and may be even higher in community-dwelling elderly patients, who often self-medicate with numerous OTC drugs. Drug interactions and ADRs can have serious consequences in the elderly and can increase both morbidity and mortality in this most vulnerable population (Wilcox, Himmelstein & Woolhandler, 1994).

There are certain drugs that commonly result in ADRs in the elderly, and these drugs should be used with caution. These drugs include digoxin, nonsteroidal antiinflammatory agents, systemic corticosteroids, diuretics, β-blockers, methyldopa, clonidine, benzodiazepines, calcium channel blockers, and sedative-hypnotics. Table 6-7 describes the ADRs that are most likely to occur when these drugs are used. Newer drugs and drug groups must likewise be used cautiously in older adults.

Specifically, the treatment of depression with selective serotonin reuptake inhibitors (SSRIs) is common among older adults (Spina & Scordo, 2002). When using these drugs, clinicians should consider the possibility of the serotonin syndrome. These drugs have a high potential for pharmacokinetic interactions because of their selective effects on CYP isoenzymes. Therefore these agents should be closely monitored or avoided in elderly patients treated with substrates of these isoforms, especially those with a narrow therapeutic index. On the other hand, citalopram and sertraline have a low inhibitory activity on different drug-metabolizing enzymes and appear particularly suitable in an elderly population. Among other newer antidepressants, nefazodone is a potent inhibitor of CYP 3A4 and its combination with substrates of this isoform should be avoided.

TABLE 6-6 Risk Factors for Developing Adverse Drug Reactions

Provider	Activities that Increase Risk of Drug Reactions
Prescriber	Duplication of medications Unclear directions Incomplete drug history Inappropriate dosing (no age adjustments) No follow-up
Pharmacist	Automatic refills Prescription errors Failure to review medication profile Lack of appropriate patient education
Patient	Use of over-the-counter drugs Incomplete knowledge of drug history Use of alcohol Use of multiple pharmacies with no coordination of drugs Use of multiple providers Poor compliance: drug overuse or underuse

Polypharmacy

Many older adults need to take a variety of medications (Anderson & Wahler, 2002). The highest prevalence of medication use is among older women 65 years of age and above. Among a national sample of 2950 older adults, 12% took 10 medications daily and 23% took 5 prescription medications (Kauffman et al, 2002). In general, older adults comprise 13% to 14% of the total population and use one fourth of OTC drugs and up to one third of the prescribed medications. The average older adults uses 4.5 prescription medications each day and two OTC medications. In addition, these individuals may add supplements, vitamins, and various home remedies to the regimen. Moreover, many of these drugs are inappropriately prescribed (Sloane et al, 2002; Linjakumpu et al, 2002; Hanlon et al, 2002). Those who are 85 years of age or older are at even

TABLE 6-7 Adverse Drug Reactions Commonly Caused in Older Adults

Drug	Likely Adverse Reaction
Tricyclic antidepressants	Urinary incontinence
Antiparkinsonian agents Diuretics Sedative-hypnotics Antihistamines	Urinary retention
Antianxiety agents β-Blockers Antihypertensives: methyldopa, clonidine, reserpine digoxin	Depression
diuretics Sedative-hypnotics Benzodiazepines Nonsteroidal antiinflammatory drugs cimetidine Narcotics Alcohol	Delirium
Sedative-hypnotics Alcohol Antihypertensives Antiparkinsonian agents Narcotics Nitrates Diuretics Neuroleptics	Increased risk for falls
Tricyclic antidepressants quinidine Antihistamines bethanechol propantheline	Constipation

greater risk of polypharmacy (Linjakumpu, 2002). Use of multiple medications increasing the risk of drug–drug interactions, adverse reactions, and potential exacerbation of medical problems. In a study of older adults admitted into acute care facilities with congestive heart failure (Lien et al, 2002), polypharmacy was reported to be one of the direct causes of disease exacerbation.

Complementary and alternative medicine (CAM) use is increasing in popularity in the United States. These products are not rigidly regulated, and it is therefore difficult to assess the likelihood of drug–drug interactions, toxic effects, or side effects. Moreover, these interactions/reactions to CAM are not anticipated by many individuals. In a study (Wren et al, 2002) of older adults undergoing preoperative screening, it was noted that almost half (42.7%) used CAMs, 20% used CAMs that resulted in anticoagulation, 14% used CAMS that altered blood pressure, and 7% used CAMs that had other cardiac effects. Older adults need to be educated about the potential drug interactions and side effects of CAMs, and providers need to be alert to the prevalent use of these products among this population.

To help decrease the risk of multiple medication use, there are software programs to help older adults monitor their medication regimens for possible interactions (Neafsey, 2002). The specific outcomes of these types of interventions to decrease the risk of polypharmacy are being evaluated. The trend, however, is to continue to encourage both older adults and their health care providers to consider the potential risk of multiple medications and to use only those medications that are necessary.

Compliance with Drug Regimen

Compliance is defined as the extent to which a patient adheres with a provider's planned medical regimen. Drug noncompliance takes many forms including: deliberate omission of a medication, unintentional and intentional overdosing, errors in dosing frequency, use of medications other than provider intended, incorrect mode of administration, and using drugs prescribed for another individual. Noncompliance may be deliberate or unintentional. It is essential to explore with the older individual what he or she is actually doing with regard to daily medication use and then compare this against the "prescribed" medication regimen. Patients should bring all medicines with them to office visits. Allow and encourage the individual to explain reasons for any deviations and provide clarification if there has been some confusion about how to take a specific medication. Box 6-7 provides a listing of some of the commonly identified reasons for drug noncompliance. Address each of these potential reasons and help the patient come up with a reasonable solution to facilitate future compliance. Simple techniques such as writing out, in large print, daily medications; filling daily medication boxes for those with cognitive impairment; and/or changing to a generic (i.e., less expensive) drug option may resolve problems with compliance.

Costs of Medications

Prescription drugs are a significant out-of-pocket cost for older adults. Over 15% of the older adults who use prescription medications are unable to pay for them. All prescription medications are not a covered service under Medicare, although there are some private insurers and health maintenance organizations that do provide some coverage. Medicaid does cover prescription drugs listed on state Preferred Drug Formularies for those individuals who qualify. In addition, pharmacy assistance, a state-run program to provide prescription drug services for those who do not qualify for Medicaid, is available in some states. Box 6-8 provides some examples of ways in which drug costs can be controlled.

It is essential to consider the cost benefit for drugs prescribed using findings from randomized clinical trials and sophisticated cost analyses. Gaspoz et al (2002) considered the cost benefit to the use of aspirin and clopidogrel to reduce the rate of cardiovascular events in patients with coronary heart disease. The findings indicated that increased prescription of aspirin for secondary prevention of coronary heart disease is attractive from a cost-effectiveness perspective. Clopidogrel, however, is more costly and is not cost-effective unless its use is restricted to patients who are ineligible for aspirin. Nyman et al (2002) considered the cost effectiveness of gemfibrozil, an agent that raised high density lipoprotein cholesterol levels, lowered triglyceride levels, and reduced major cardiovascular events in male coronary heart disease patients in a randomized controlled multicenter trial. This cost analysis indicated that there would be a cost saving at an annual drug cost of $100 or less in 1998 dollars. Even at the higher drug prices represented

BOX 6-7

COMMON REASONS FOR DRUG NONCOMPLIANCE

- Cost of medications
- Complicated schedule
- Unrealistic schedule
- Impaired cognition and judgment
- Unpleasant side effects
- Lack of knowledge related to NEED and purpose of medication
- Denial of problem for which treatment is being prescribed
- Fear of drug side effects or exacerbation of other problems
- No perceived response/effect for drug treatment

BOX 6-8

TECHNIQUES TO DECREASE COSTS FOR PRESCRIPTION MEDICATIONS

- Check on drug costs before prescribing, and search for the lowest cost alternative within drug groups.
- Use generics when possible.
- Start with small quantities of new prescriptions (starter dosings with 1-week supplies).
- Use the lowest dose necessary for the desired effect.
- Eliminate all unnecessary medications.

by the average wholesale price in the United States, the cost of a life-year saved is well below the threshold that would be deemed cost-effective. However, the age of the patient is a big factor in looking at cost savings. Huse et al (2002) considered the economic benefits of early discharge of patients treated for DVT with LMWH using data pooled from multiple healthcare plans. Data sources were integrated medical and pharmacy claims paid by 37 US health plans (the PharMetrics Integrated Outcomes Database, PharMetrics, Inc., Watertown, MA). Outpatient anticoagulation therapy for DVT with enoxaparin and warfarin is associated with earlier hospital discharge, fewer readmissions, and lower total DVT-related costs compared with warfarin monotherapy. Findings such as these can then be used to guide providers in prescriptive practices and to focus on those drugs that are not only clinically effective but also cost effective for patients.

RESOURCES FOR PATIENTS AND PROVIDERS

Administration on Aging, www.aoa.dhhs.gov/
Content for both health care providers and patients maintained by the US Department of Health and Human Services. For practitioners there is information about advocacy groups for the elderly, welfare programs, and managed care issues. The patients' section provides a collection of links to many other web sites and provides educational information pertaining to the elderly. The site also provides other annotated web resources grouped by topics.

Agency for Health Care Policy and Research, www.ahcpr.gov/
Clinical practice guidelines and patient education material in full-text versions, quick-reference versions, or patient guides in English or Spanish.

American Geriatrics Society, www.americangeriatrics.org/
Information on membership, professional publications, and abstracts or full-text version of certain articles of their journals.

Gerontological Society of America, www.geron.org/
Professionals will find general information about the society, links to publications, a calendar of conferences, career development information, legislative and policy updates, and information on grants and fellowships.

Geriatric Education, www.med.ufl.edu/medinfo/geri/
Maintained by the College of Medicine of the University of Florida; offers geriatric teaching cases. Each module includes an outline of the major geriatric topics covered and a list of the drugs used in the case.

Health Care Financing Administration, www.hcfa.gov/
Maintained by the US government agency that oversees the federal Medicare program, this site has a great deal of information of interest to clinicians as well as to their elderly patients or their families. Provides telephone numbers, organized by state, insurance counseling, and other information. Also offers 21 manuals, such as the Hospital Manual, Home Health Agency Manual, and Hospice Manual, and can be downloaded in full-text version.

Healthy Seniors/Seniors Health Medical Information, www.healthyseniors.com/ or http://www.mediconsult.com/senior/
This site gives users the chance to retrieve medical news, self-help material, and other information on 15 chronic conditions and illnesses.

Mosby's Gerontological Nursing, www.mosby.com/
Periodicals/Nursing/GN/ Full-text version of articles, complete abstracts, and continuing education units in gerontology.

NACDA Data Archive, www.icpsr.umich.edu/NACDA/archive.html/
The National Archive of Computerized Data on Aging is a database searchable by topic or researcher and maintained by the Inter-University Consortium for Political and Social Research at the University of Michigan, Ann Arbor. Contains data on demographics, social characteristics, economics, psychologic characteristics, and health care needs of older adults in the United States.

National Institute on Aging, www.nia.nih.gov/
Maintained by a division of the National Institutes of Health with information on research and funding opportunities and issues pertaining to aging research. Also offers online publications for professionals and patients.

Federal government's web site for older adults, www.Seniors.gov.

Official web site for the US Administration on Aging, www.aoa.gov.

Main web site for the Centers for Disease Control and Prevention, www.cdc.gov.

Rural Elderly, www.iml.umkc.edu/cas/nrc.htm/
Site for rural practitioners in aging.

General internet sites of interest to older adults

American Association of Retired Persons, www.aarp.org.

AARP Guide to Internet Resources Related to Aging, www.aarp.org/cyberguide1.htm.

Achoo, www.achoo.com.

Age of Reason, www.ageofreason.com.

Age Pages, www.nih.gov/nia/health/pubpub/pubpub.htm.

Andrus Foundation, www.andrus.org.

Bringing the Future to Senior Citizens, www.si.umich.edu/-jbrob/si723.

Caregiver Alliance, www.caregiver.org.

ChronicNet, www.chronicnet.org.

Directory of Web and Gopher Sites on Aging, www.aoa.dhhs.gov/aoa/webres/craig.htm.

Elderhostel, www.elderhostel.org.

ElderPage: Information for Older Persons and Families, www.aoa.dhhs.gov/elderpage.html/%Generations United: www.gu.org.

GriefNet, www.rivendell.org.

Health A to Z, www.healthatoz.com.

Internet Development for the Aging Network: Online Resources, www.aoa.dhhs.gov/aoa/pages/guidrev.html.

Life Expectancy Calculator, www.retireweb.com/death.html.

National Aging Information Center, www.aoa.dhhs.gov/naic.

National Council on Aging, www.ncoa.org.

REFERENCES

Abrams WB et al: Clinical pharmacology in an aging population, *Clin Pharmacol Ther* 63:281-284, 1998.

Ahronheim J: Practical pharmacology for older patients: avoiding adverse drug effects, *Mt Sinai J Med* 60:497-501, 1993.

Atkin PA et al: The epidemiology of serious adverse drug reactions among the elderly, *Drugs Aging* 14:141-152, 1999.

Bourne D: A First Course in Pharmacokinetics and Biopharmaceutics (2001). Available at www.boomer.org/c/pl/index.html.

Calkins E, Ford AB, Kaltz P, editors: *Practice of geriatrics,* Philadelphia, 1992, WB Saunders.

Carlson JE: Perils of polypharmacy: 10 steps to prudent prescribing, *Geriatrics* 51:26-30, 1996.

Davis KM, Mathew E: Pharmacologic management of depression in the elderly, *Nurs Pract* 23:16-45, 1998.

DeMaagd GD: High-risk drugs in the elderly population, *Geriatr Nurs* 16:198-207, 1995.

DeMaagd GD: The pharmacological causes of delirium in the elderly, *Consult Pharm* 10:461-474, 1995.

Evans WE: General principles of applied pharmacokinetics. In Evans WE et al, editors: *Applied pharmacokinetics: principles of therapeutic drug monitoring,* ed 3, Vancouver, WA, 1991, Applied Therapeutics.

Feinberg M: The problems of anticholinergic adverse effects in older patients, *Drugs Aging* 3:335-348, 1993.

Flockhart DA, Tanus-Santos JE: Implications of cytochrome P450 interactions when prescribing medication for hypertension, *Arch Intern Med* 162:405-412, 2002.

Gales BJ, Menard SM: Relationship between the administration of selected medications and falls in hospitalized elderly patients, *Ann Pharmacol* 29:354-358, 1995.

Gaspoz JM et al: Cost effectiveness of aspirin, clopidogrel, or both for secondary prevention of coronary heart disease, *N Engl J Med* 346:1800-1806, 2002.

Hanlon J et al: Use of inappropriate prescription drugs by older people, *J Am Geriatr Soc* 50:26-34, 2002.

Huse DM et al: Outpatient treatment of venous thromboembolism with low-molecular-weight heparin: an economic evaluation, *Am J Managed Care* 8(1 Suppl):S10-S16, 2002.

Jeliffe R: Estimation of creatinine clearance in patients with unstable renal function, *Am J Nephrol* 22:320-324, 2002.

Jinks MJ, Fuerst RH: Geriatric drug use and rehabilitation. In Young LY, Koda-Kimble MA, editors: *Applied therapeutics: the clinical use of drugs,* Vancouver, WA, 1995, Applied Therapeutics.

Kaufman D et al: Recent patterns of medication use in the ambulatory adult population of the United States: the Slone survey, *JAMA* 287:1804-1805, 2002.

Kovner CT, Mezey M, Harrington C: Who cares for older adults? Workforce implications of an aging society, *Health Aff (Millwood)* 21:78-89, 2002.

Lien C et al: Heart failure in frail elderly patients: diagnostic difficulties, co-morbidities, polypharmacy and treatment dilemmas, *Eur J Heart Fail* 4:91-98, 2002.

Linjakumpu T et al: Psychotropics among the home-dwelling elderly-increasing trends, *Int J Geriatr Psychiatry* 17:874-883, 2002.

MacKichan JJ: Influence of protein binding and use of unbound (free) drug concentrations. In Evans WE et al, editors: *Applied pharmacokinetics: principles of therapeutic drug monitoring,* ed 3, Vancouver, WA, 1992, Applied Therapeutics.

Mayersohn MB: Special pharmacokinetic considerations in the elderly. In Evans WE et al, editors: *Applied pharmacokinetics: principles of therapeutic drug monitoring,* ed 3, Vancouver, WA, 1992, Applied Therapeutics.

Meuleman JR: Walking the tightrope: the challenge of elderly care, *J Am Geriatr Soc* 44:1466-1468, 1996.

Michocki RJ et al: Drug prescribing for the elderly, *Arch Fam Med* 2:441-444, 1993.

National Center for Health Statistics (2002). Available at www.cdc.gov/nchs

Neafsey P, Shellman J: Misconceptions of older adults with hypertension concerning OTC medications and alcohol. *Home Health Nurse* 20:300-306, 2002.

Nyman JA et al, The VA-HIT Study Group: Cost-effectiveness of gemfibrozil for coronary heart disease patients with low levels of high-density lipoprotein cholesterol: the Department of Veterans Affairs High-Density Lipoprotein Cholesterol Intervention Trial, *Arch Intern Med* 162:177-182, 2002.

O'Connell MB, Johnson JF: Evaluation of medication knowledge in elderly patients, *Ann Pharmacotherapeu* 26:919-921, 1992.

O'Connell MB, Dwinell AM, Bannick M: Predictive performance of equations to estimate creatinine clearance in hospitalized elderly patients, *Ann Pharmacother* 26:627-635, 1992.

Oo C, Hill G: Change in creatinine clearance with advancing age, *J Am Geriatr Soc* 50:1603, 2002.

Rathmore S et al: Prescription medication use in older Americans: a national report card on prescribing, *Fam Med* 30:733-739, 1998.

Semla TP, Beizer SL, Higbee MD: *Geriatric dosage handbook,* ed 2, Hudson, OH, 1995-1996, Lexi-Comp.

Sloan RW: Principles of drug therapy in geriatric patients, *Am Fam Phys* 45:2709-2718, 1992.

Sloane P et al: Inappropriate medication prescribing in residential care/assisted living facilities, *J Am Geriatr Soc* 50:1001-1011, 2002.

Smythe M et al: Estimating creatinine clearance in elderly patients with low serum creatinine concentrations, *Am J Hosp Pharm* 51:198-204, 1994.

Spina E, Scordo M: Clinically significant drug interactions with antidepressants in the elderly, *Drugs Aging* 19:299-320, 2002.

Stewart RB et al: Polypharmacy in the aged: practical solutions, *Drugs Aging* 4:449-461, 1994.

Swan SK, Bennett WM: Drug dosing guidelines in patients with renal failure, *West J Med* 56:633-638, 1992.

Thomas DR, Brahan R, Haywood BP: Inpatient community-based geriatric assessment reduces subsequent mortality, *J Am Geriatr Soc* 41:101-104, 1993.

US Bureau of the Census: *Decennial census of population 1900-1983L, a projection of the population of the U.S. 1982-2050,* Pub. No. 922 Washington, DC, 1982, US Bureau of the Census.

Vestal RE: Aging and pharmacology, *Cancer* 80:1302-1310, 1997.

Walley T et al: Prescribing in the elderly, *Postgrad Med J* 71:466-471, 1995.

Wallsten SM et al: Medication-taking behaviors in the high- and low-functioning elderly: MacArthur field studies of successful aging, *Ann Pharmacol* 29:359-364, 1995.

White M, Leenen FHH: Aging and cardiovascular responsiveness to B-agonist in humans: role of changes in B-receptor responses versus baroreflex activity, *Clin Pharmacol Ther* 56:543-553, 1994.

Wilcox SM, Himmelstein DU, Woolhandler S: Inappropriate drug prescribing for the community dwelling elderly, *JAMA* 272:292-296, 1994.

Wren K, Kimbrall S, Norred C: Use of complementary and alternative medications by surgical patients, *J Perianesth Nurs* 17:170-177, 2002.

Zal HM: Depression in the elderly: differing presentations, wide choice of therapies, *Consultant* 3:355-366, 1994.

Zaleon CR, Guthrie SK: Antipsychotic drug use in older adults, *Am J Hosp Pharm* 51:2917-2943, 1994.

Zeeh J, Platt D: The aging liver: structural and functional changes and their consequences for drug treatment in old age. *Gerontology* 48:121-127, 2002.

CHAPTER 7

Special Populations: Pediatrics

The dramatic decrease in infant mortality rates throughout the twentieth century has paralleled the development of improvements in the prevention, diagnosis, and treatment of pediatric problems, the introduction of better technology, and the increasingly effective use of pharmacologic products. Because children may be subject to many of the same diseases as adults, they are sometimes treated with the same drugs and biologic products as adults.

The production of valid and generalizable knowledge about drug use in children has been problematic at best. Few clinicians want to experiment with children; few parents would knowingly allow their infants or small children to participate in research studies that would entail risk of any kind. As a result, many drugs are currently labeled with the comment, "Safety and efficiency not established for children." Much of the initial data about drug use in children were based on first-hand observations by clinicians who tried drugs even when there were no guidelines to assist them. What these clinicians quickly determined was that children are not just small adults who require smaller doses. Those who have that very cavalier attitude are likely to create trouble for their patients.

PHARMACOKINETICS OF DRUG THERAPY IN INFANTS AND CHILDREN

Determining how to give medications to children involves having an especially good understanding of the various physiologic factors that may be affected by these drugs. The growing but immature child is a dynamic and changing entity whose unique characteristics must be understood if errors are to be avoided. The practitioner must remember that information must be mastered for each of the age groups that comprise the pediatric category: preterm infants (gestational age younger than 36 weeks), neonates (30 days old and younger), infants (1 to 12 months), toddlers (1 to 4 years), children (5 to 12 years), and adolescents (12 years and older). Fundamental to this understanding is a knowledge of the unique pharmacokinetic variables that may be encountered in pediatric dosing for each of these groups. In recognizing the maturational disparities among children of the same age, developmental differences are further compounded by the same qualities that affect therapeutic response in adults, such as disease, environment, and genetic traits. Consequently, when compared with adults, a wider range of responses to a particular drug treatment can be expected in a population of children; in fact, the same child's response to a regimen can change rapidly during a single treatment course.

Experts generally agree that devising a therapeutic regimen is most difficult for the youngest patients, particularly neonates. Signs of efficacy or toxicity are difficult to recognize and newborns are the least able to withstand adverse effects. Neonates often experience the greatest number of therapeutic errors.

Drug Absorption

Many expect drug absorption in infants and children to follow the same basic principles as in adults. However, three factors tend to be especially important in children. First, the physiologic status of the infant or child determines the blood flow at the site of parenteral drug administration. Factors that may reduce blood flow to muscular or subcutaneous tissues include cardiovascular shock, vasoconstriction caused by sympathomimetic agents, and heart failure. Under these conditions, there would be reduced absorption of any medications injected into intramuscular or subcutaneous tissues. In premature infants with little muscle mass, perfusion to these areas and the resulting absorption is extremely irregular. In larger children, there is more rapid absorption from the deltoid muscle than from the vastus lateralis muscle, whereas medications are absorbed the slowest from the gluteal muscles (American Academy of Pediatrics, 1997). Peripheral vasomotor instability, thermal instability, and reduced muscular contractions in premature infants compared with other children and adults also influence drug absorption from intramuscular sites. Toxic drug concentrations may be provoked if perfusion to intramuscular or subcutaneous tissues suddenly increases, promoting greater absorption of medication and increasing the amount of the drug entering the circulation. Drugs that have narrow therapeutic margins, such as anticonvulsants, cardiac glycosides, or aminoglycoside antibiotics, are particularly good examples of drugs where toxicity might be encountered when absorption is variable (Berlin, 1999).

Second, for neonates, another factor in absorption is the changing status of gastrointestinal (GI) function. In the first weeks of life, the intestine is very permeable and premature babies may absorb substances that cannot penetrate the more mature intestine. The presence of amniotic fluid in the stomach ensures an alkaline pH during the days after birth. (Although neonates quickly develop an acidic gastric environment, they do not produce normal levels of gastric acid until somewhere between the ages of 3 and 7 years.) During the neonatal period, the absorption of orally administered members of the penicillin family is enhanced, as is the absorption of carbamazepine suspension, diazepam, and digoxin. Both increased production of gastric acid and slow or varying peristalsis through the GI tract create situations where orally administered drugs may be partially or totally inactivated by the low pH of gastric contents.

Acid-labile drugs, such as ampicillin, nafcillin, and penicillin, develop higher serum concentrations in the presence of higher gastric acid, whereas lower serum concentrations may be found with phenobarbital, phenytoin, and acetaminophen (Besunder, Reed & Blumer, 1988; Levine, Poon & Walson, 2000). Drug absorption may also be either delayed or increased more than anticipated because of the absence of intestinal flora, reduced enzyme function, delays in gastric emptying, deficient transport mechanisms across neonatal intestinal membranes, or slow GI transit. The stomach begins emptying more quickly once the infant is 6 to 8 months old. At that time, GI transit may become faster and more unpredictable. Low concentrations of bile acids and lipase may decrease the absorption of lipid-soluble drugs. The activity of pancreatic enzymes is decreased in neonates and infants up to 4 months of age (Koren & Cohen, 2000). These factors are particularly important to remember when contemplating the administration of a sustained-release agent. If the drug passes through the GI tract rapidly, absorption will be insufficient and a subtherapeutic dose will be delivered. Rectal suppositories should generally be avoided for drug administration, primarily because children may not retain the dosage form long enough to receive the entire dose.

Because so little research has been conducted on oral versus intravenous administration, differences in bioavailability of drugs from different routes of administration in premature infants are poorly understood. If a drug is poorly absorbed from the GI tract of an adult, the absorption may be much more efficient in a premature child because of the delayed emptying. The one common finding of most studies is that drug absorption varies widely; the younger the child, the more erratic may be the absorption (Besunder, Reed & Blumer, 1988).

Third, the skin of premature and newborn infants has a greater ability to absorb some chemicals because of increased hydration and increased permeability, resulting from underdevelopment of the stratum corneum in the epidermal barrier. The transdermal route may be used therapeutically in selected infants to reduce the unpredictability of some oral and intramuscularly administered medications, such as theophylline (Evans et al, 1985). However, commercially available transdermal dosage forms are not intended for pediatric patients and would deliver doses much higher than needed for infants and children. Rubbing the drug into the skin, incorporating the drug in an oily vehicle, and using an occlusive dressing sometimes by wrapping the infant in plastic wrap may increase cutaneous absorption of topical products (Edmunds, 2003). Children have the potential for increased absorption through the skin because their skin is thinner and more sensitive—thus allowing for greater penetration—particularly if the skin is damaged or an occlusive dressing (even a diaper) is applied over the medication. Factors that increase transdermal drug absorption also increase the risk to the infant of toxic effects following topical use of drugs, as well as such items as hexachlorophene soaps, boric acid, powders, or rubbing alcohol (Gilman, 1990; Tyrala et al, 1977). Both clinicians and parents should remember that small children can ingest a topical drug by sucking or licking it off of an accessible patch of skin.

DRUG DISTRIBUTION IN THE PEDIATRIC PATIENT

Drug distribution as a process is determined by two factors: (1) the physiochemical properties of the drug itself (i.e., the molecular weight, etc.), which do not vary, and (2) the physiologic factors specific for the patient, including total body water, extracellular water, protein-binding, and pathologic conditions modifying physiologic function, all of which vary widely in different patient populations (Nahata, 2002).

The distribution volumes of drugs vary in the child as the body composition changes through growth and development. The neonate has a higher proportion of its body weight in the form of water than does the adult, who has 50% to 60% of body weight in water. Small premature neonates may have 85% of their body weight as water, with 40% of that amount as extracellular water, whereas the normal full-term neonate usually has only about 70% body weight as water. Because many drugs are distributed throughout the extracellular water space, the volume or size of the extracellular water compartment may be important in determining the concentration of drug at the receptor sites. This is an especially important consideration because many neonates diuresis heavily in the first 24 to 48 hours of life, and many important drugs are water soluble (Koren & Cohen, 2000; Nahata et al, 1984). Water-soluble drugs, such as the aminoglycoside antibiotic gentamicin, will be distributed more widely in the body, resulting in lower serum levels. To compensate, a higher dosage is necessary.

Another variable that affects drug distribution in premature infants is a reduced percentage of fat. Premature infants may have 1% of body weight in fat compared with 15% in normal full-term infants (Yaffe, 1992). Organs that would ordinarily accumulate high concentrations of lipid-soluble drugs in adults and older children may not accumulate as much in more immature infants. Early on, when the proportion of body fat is small, lipid-soluble drugs such as vitamins A and E do not distribute as well, provoking higher drug concentrations in the serum. In such cases, the dosage may have to be reduced to avoid toxicity. In older children, the alterations of body fat associated with obesity and extreme emaciation obviously affect fat storage of drugs just as they do in adults.

In addition to fat, selected drugs are also stored to a smaller extent in other tissues. For example, the tetracyclines chelate with calcium and so have a high affinity for the rapidly growing teeth and bones of infants and young children (Behrman, 2000).

Drugs are not distributed uniformly throughout the body. For example, drug distribution to the central nervous system is small, and movement through the brain's rich blood supply is unique. Drugs must move from the bloodstream across the blood-brain barrier. Because certain drugs, such as highly lipid-soluble drugs (e.g., tetracycline and diazepam), readily penetrate the central nervous system, there is no absolute barrier. However, the blood-brain barrier is encountered when drugs moving from the blood across the capillary endothelium are restricted by the close approximation of the glial cells with the capillary endothelium. Also, drug access to the cerebrospinal fluid is limited by the epithelium of the choroid plexus (Behrman, 2000).

In premature infants, incomplete glial development enhances permeability of the blood-brain barrier and permits drugs and bilirubin to more readily enter the central nervous system. Poorly lipid-soluble drugs such as gentamicin and penicillin may then cross the blood-brain barrier when administered in large doses, when administered via rapid intravenous infusion, or when they are administered to neonates with renal failure. The permeability of the blood-brain barrier in infants and children of all ages is increased in meningitis, brain tumors, and cranial trauma. In these conditions, drugs that do not ordinarily enter the central nervous system may do so without difficulty (Yaffe, 1992).

Some drugs are reversibly bound to plasma proteins (usually albumin), fat, bone, or other tissues. Drugs such as diazepam, digoxin, furosemide, and warfarin are examples of drugs that are highly bound to plasma albumin. When bound, these tissue-bound drugs are not free to gain access to receptor sites and thus are pharmacologically inactive. Some tissue-bound drugs are released when plasma concentrations fall; thus these tissues are said to act as drug storage depots (Besunder, 1988).

Plasma protein binding in neonates is comparatively low because of the decreased plasma protein concentration, lower binding capacity of protein, decreased affinity of proteins for drug binding, and competition for certain binding sites by endogenous compounds. Because of this, the concentration of free drug in plasma is increased and exerts powerful pharmacologic effects that can result in greater drug effect or toxicity (Nottarianni, 1990). Acidosis, cold stress, and hypoglycemia in the neonate may produce free fatty acids that act to displace drugs from plasma albumin-binding sites (Hardman & Limbird, 2001). However, because drugs bound to plasma proteins cannot be eliminated by the kidneys, an increase in free drug concentration may also increase its clearance (Nahata, 2002).

In the neonate, bilirubin, maternal hormones, and other endogenous substances also occupy available plasma protein-binding sites. Sulfonamides, furosemide, large doses of vitamin K, and sodium benzoate given to the mother during labor, delivery, or passed to the baby through breastfeeding may compete with serum bilirubin for binding to albumin. If these drugs are given to a neonate with jaundice, they can displace bilirubin from albumin. Because of the greater permeability of the neonatal blood-brain barrier, substantial amounts of bilirubin could then enter the brain and cause kernicterus. Additionally, as the serum bilirubin rises for physiologic reasons or because of a blood group incompatibility, bilirubin displacement of a drug from albumin can substantially raise the free drug concentration. This might occur without altering the total drug concentration and would result in a greater therapeutic effect or toxicity at normal concentrations (Drug toxicity in the newborn, 1985; Koren & Cohen, 2000).

The decreased capacity for plasma protein binding of drugs can increase their apparent volumes of distribution. The clinical implications of this action are that to obtain a therapeutic serum concentration of many drugs, premature infants will require a larger loading dose than that for older children and adults (Roberts, 1984).

Finally, certain drugs distributed in the breast milk of breastfeeding mothers may pose problems for infants. Drugs should be avoided by the mother during pregnancy and breastfeeding if at all possible. The American Academy of Pediatrics has issued a list of major drugs and their effect on infants (see Chapter 8). Drugs that are absolutely contraindicated during breastfeeding include bromocriptine, cimetidine, clemastine, cyclophosphamide, ergotamine, gold salts, methimazole, phenindione, and thiouracil (American Academy of Pediatrics, 1994).

Drug Metabolism

The biotransformation of drugs in the body into usable substances involves chemical reactions that convert a drug to an inactive or a less active compound. These metabolic reactions usually produce less lipid-soluble metabolites that are more readily eliminated than are highly lipid-soluble compounds. Not all metabolites are pharmacologically inactive. Active metabolites are either excreted unchanged or undergo further metabolic reactions. Poorly absorbed lipid-soluble drugs, such as the penicillins, are not metabolized but are excreted unchanged (Hardman & Limbird, 2001).

In general, drug metabolism in infants is substantially slower than that in older children and adults. The newborn's kidneys are immature, and because most drug metabolism takes place in the liver, the fact that the P450-dependent mixed-function oxidases and the conjugating enzymes of infants are only 50% to 70% of adult values is an important consideration in treatment of children (Leeder, 1997). There are varying amounts of the different enzymes, but the capacity to increase production of all enzymes continues until the third or fourth year of life. For example, the glucuronidation pathway is undeveloped in infants, but the sulfation pathway is relatively well developed and may compensate for deficits in the other pathway in the presence of some drugs (Gupta & Waldhauser, 1997; Rane, 1992).

Given neonates' decreased ability to metabolize drugs, they may be at increased risk for adverse effects because of slow clearance rates and prolonged half-lives, particularly in drugs given over long periods. One of the earliest cases in which serious adverse events were observed in neonates following administration of a drug that had not been adequately studied in pediatric patients was the development of "gray baby syndrome" after treatment with the antibiotic chloramphenicol (Powell, 1982). After 23 deaths in neonates, it was determined that the immature livers of these infants were unable to clear chloramphenicol from the body, allowing toxic doses of the drug to accumulate (Levine, Poon & Walson, 2000). These facts make it essential to consider the maturation of the infant when evaluating whether to administer drugs metabolized in the liver. Conversely, some drugs that a mother might take would induce the fetal hepatic enzymes to mature early. This would result in faster metabolism of certain drugs, with less therapeutic effect and lower plasma drug concentrations. One of the drugs that might cause this action is phenobarbital (Koren & Cohen, 2000). By the first birthday, the liver's metabolic capabilities are not only mature, but more vigorous than those of an adult, probably because the child's liver has a greater volume per kilogram of body weight. Although this phenomenon is probably most apparent between the ages of 2 and 6 years, it continues until approximately 10 to 12 years of age so that certain drugs may need to be given in higher dosage or more often. An example of this is theophylline. A child between 1 and 9 years of age with asthma might require markedly higher doses of theophylline on a weight basis compared with an adult (Hardman & Limbird, 2001).

Although most drug metabolic reactions occur in the liver, the GI tract, kidney, and plasma may also biotransform some drugs. The extent of the use of these alternate forms of metabolism is usually identified in pharmacokinetic tables and accounts for only a small percentage of drug metabolism.

Excretion

As with metabolism, the growth and maturity of the child's organs have a significant effect on the elimination of drugs. Difficulties excreting drugs that result from incomplete development of the fetal renal excretion system, including reduction in glomerular filtration, tubular secretion, and tubular reabsorption, are gradually resolved with increased gestational age but may still be markedly decreased at birth and only slowly develop to capacity over the first year of life.

For the first few days of life, the glomerular filtration rate (GFR) of a neonate may be at only 30% to 40% of the adult rate. This rate may be even lower in premature babies. As the child grows and matures, the clearance rate improves, even during the first week of life. By the end of the third week of life, GFR is usually 50% to 60% of the adult value and may reach adult values by 6 months (Hardman & Limbird, 2001).

This developmental process has implications for drug clearance, particularly for common drugs such as penicillin, aminoglycosides, and digoxin, where rates may fall to 17% to 34% of the adult clearance rate. If a child is ill enough to require these drugs, its GFR may not improve as predicted during the first weeks and months of life. This will necessitate adjustments in dosage and dosing schedules. The child will also require more vigilant monitoring, and appropriate dosages should be calculated based on plasma drug concentrations determined at intervals throughout the course of therapy (Koren & Cohen, 2000).

Changes in urinary pH may also affect the rate at which a drug is excreted. Ammonium chloride, ascorbic acid, or other drugs that acidify the urine increase the rate at which pseudoephedrine, meperidine, quinidine, and other weak bases are excreted. Sodium bicarbonate and other drugs that alkalinize the urine increase the rate at which phenobarbital, aspirin, nitrofurantoin, and other weak acids are excreted. Although increasing the rate at which a drug is excreted shortens its effect, decreasing urinary excretion increases the drug's duration of action (Yaffe, 1992).

EFFECT OF DISEASE ON DRUG PROCESSES IN CHILDREN

Drugs generally produce their effects by combining with an enzyme, cell membrane, or other cellular component. The cellular component, or receptor, with which the drug combines has a chemical or structural affinity for a highly specific drug. Investigators have reported that receptors are present and functional in young children, and the degree of receptor response appears to correlate with birth weight (Yaffe, 1992). However, requirements for larger doses of medications such as digoxin for infants and children has been attributed to a greater affinity of the child's developing myocardial digoxin receptors for digitalis derivatives (Hardman & Limbird, 2001). Other examples include the increased sensitivity of neonates to curare and atropine and the heightened resistance to succinylcholine, secondary to immature development of receptors for these drugs.

The liver and kidney play major roles in the metabolism and excretion of drugs. Thus diseases of either of these organs often affect drug action. Drug metabolism is a complex function of the liver and varies because of modifications in hepatic blood flow, extraction capacity of the drug from the blood, and serum drug binding. Both type and severity of liver disease may alter all of these factors. Shifts to different metabolic pathways within a diseased liver may sometimes compensate for damage to one part; therefore it is sometimes difficult to predict how drug metabolism will be altered in illness.

Feinstein and Miles (1985) suggest that drugs can be divided into two categories on the basis of hepatic extraction characteristics. The first category consists of drugs with a high hepatic extraction ratio (>0.7), whose clearance will be affected by blood flow. Drugs such as lidocaine, morphine, and propranolol have high extraction ratios, and, if given to patients with cirrhosis and congestive heart failure, the clearance of such drugs is decreased. The second category includes drugs with a lower extraction ratio (<0.2) and a low affinity for plasma proteins. The action of these drugs would be influenced more by hepatocellular function and less by changes in hepatic blood flow or plasma protein binding. Examples of these drugs include acetaminophen and theophylline. Most of the information about the effect of liver damage on drug metabolism comes from studies on adults; how it relates to children is unclear. What has been determined is the need for careful monitoring to avoid toxic reactions in children with liver damage.

In cases of renal failure, again, the major information on drug clearance comes from studies on adults. Renal clearance of drugs is directly proportional to the GFR as measured by endogenous creatinine clearance tests. The increased numbers of fatty acids associated with renal impairment may also displace drugs from protein binding sites. The decrease in plasma albumin that accompanies the nephrotic syndrome reduces the number of available binding sites; consequently, extensively bound drugs would achieve higher plasma concentrations (Hardman & Limbird, 2001). Attention to the pharmacokinetic data on drugs eliminated by the kidney is required in children, particularly for those drugs with narrow therapeutic margins and for drugs that produce few observable, measurable clinical responses.

Other disease conditions may also affect drugs. Cystic fibrosis appears to be associated with a requirement for increased doses of drugs (Editorial, 1995). Cases of hypoxemia, critically ill patients with severe head trauma, and those with a variety of GI diseases may all require dosage adjustments for a variety of medications (Behrman, 2000). Again, the adjustments required have often been based on clinical anecdotes and have not been confirmed by valid research studies.

CHOOSING A DRUG REGIMEN

The goal of pediatric drug therapy is to provide the desired therapeutic response without adverse effects. Although most drugs are not labeled for pediatric use, few are absolutely contraindicated. When children become critically ill, medications perhaps considered risky for use may be required. Case studies of these treatment decisions provide important information for clinicians. Some of the drugs avoided in children include the following:

- Tetracycline—stains the permanent teeth when administered to children younger than 9 years
- Codeine and dextromethorphan—poor antitussives for infants who are vulnerable to respiratory depression. CYP 2D6 converts codeine to morphine and this enzyme is not developed in very young babies
- Aspirin—Associated with Reye syndrome
- Valproic acid—Higher incidence of liver toxicity in children younger than 2 years

ADVERSE DRUG REACTIONS IN CHILDREN

The potential for drug–drug interactions and adverse effects is increased in very ill children and infants. Children may be exposed to drugs likely to provide adverse reactions in three major ways: transplacentally, when the drug is administered to the mother during pregnancy and delivery; by direct administration of the drug to the child; and by ingestion of the drug in breast milk after administration of the drug to a nursing mother (American Academy of Pediatrics, 1995). These three periods are the only stages in life in which one is exposed to and affected by drugs administered to another person, the mother (Gupta & Waldhauser, 1997).

The incidence of adverse reactions in pediatric patients is unknown. Because of the fragility of young children and the complexity of their illnesses, their pharmacotherapy is frequently complicated with misadventure and adverse drug reactions that are unavoidable or difficult to assess. However, studies have generally found the rate of adverse reactions to equal those in adults. This rate may be as high as 5.8% of drugs administered to children, although the rate is higher if the child is hospitalized rather than ambulatory (Hansten & Horn, 2001). Because of their differences in morphology and disease process and treatments, young children experience a different range of adverse drug reactions. These reactions may not necessarily be predictable from the adult experience. Adverse drug reactions may have profound immediate, delayed, and long-term implications for children's neurologic and somatic development (Gupta & Waldhauser, 1997).

The drugs affecting the fetus transplacentally are discussed in detail in Chapter 8 on pregnant and breast-feeding women. The effects of adverse reactions from drugs administered during labor and delivery are usually easily noted and short-lived. Central nervous system depression in the newborn may result from analgesics or anesthetics. Excess uterine stimulants are associated with anoxic encephalopathy, whereas excess intravenous fluids may cause convulsions or electrolyte disturbances (Hardman & Limbird, 2001). Any drugs given to a premature infant or neonate while the liver is immature may potentially cause adverse reactions. The persistence of maternal hormones and drugs in the newborn's bloodstream increases the risk of such interactions. (See section on metabolism in Chapter 5 on pharmacokinetics).

With younger children, it may be difficult to distinguish whether the child is having an adverse reaction or just experiencing symptoms of the underlying illness (Gupta & Waldhauser, 1997) or having a paradoxical reaction to a drug (such as hyperactive behavior with antihistamines or chloral hydrate and sleepiness with stimulants like Ritalin). Over-the-counter preparations (particularly antihistamines and adrenergic drugs found in various cough syrups, cold remedies, decongestants, and nose drops) may also provoke adverse reactions in pediatric patients. A broad spectrum of reactions may be seen, varying from minor hypersensitivity reactions to more serious problems with alterations in growth, damage of anatomic or physiologic systems, and numerous other problems (Hansten & Horn, 2001). A list of adverse effects associated with commonly prescribed drugs is found in Table 7-1.

CALCULATION OF PEDIATRIC DOSAGES

Simple approximated reduction in the adult dose may not be adequate to determine a safe and effective pediatric dose because of differences in pharmacokinetics in infants and children. The package insert provided by the manufacturer is the best source for pediatric dose recommendations. If that information is not available, the proper dosage is calculated based on weight, age, or surface area. These rules for calculating pediatric dosages are not precise and should never be used if the manufacturer of the drug provides a recommended pediatric dose. Usually manufacturer recommendations are stated in milligrams per kilogram or per pound.

A variety of formulas are used to calculate pediatric dosages (Edmunds, 2003). Some of these formulas include:

Pediatric Dosage Rules Based on Age

- Young's rule is used for children ages 2 to 12:

$$\frac{\text{Adult dose} \times \text{Child's age (years)}}{\text{Child's age} + 12} = \text{Child's dose}$$

- Fried's rule is used for infants and children under age 2:

$$\frac{\text{Infant's age in months}}{150} \times \text{Adult dose} = \text{Infant's dose}$$

All children of the same age are not the same size. If the pediatric patient is approximately normal size for his or her age, these rules may be used. If the child is unusually sized for his or her age, it is better to use a weight calculation.

Pediatric Dosage Rules Based on Weight (Clark's Rule)

$$\text{Adult dose} \times \frac{\text{Weight (kg)}}{70} = \text{Child's dose}$$

or

$$\text{Adult dose} \times \frac{\text{Weight (lb)}}{150} = \text{Child's dose}$$

As shown, this formulation remains the same whether the weight is calculated in pounds or in kilograms. Clark's rule using weight is usually more accurate than a rule based on age.

Calculations of dosage based on age or weight are conservative and tend to underestimate the required dose. A technique that more closely approximates the recommended dosages is based on body surface area (BSA). If manufacturers recommend using BSA for calculating the medication dosage,

TABLE 7-1 Drugs Associated with Specific Adverse Effects in Infants and Children

Drug	Adverse Effect
iodides, corticosteroids	Acne
Penicillins, heparin, aspirin, parenteral iron, dextran preparations	Anaphylaxis
aspirin, bethanechol, Mucomyst inhalation, epinephrine inhalation	Asthma
Barbiturates, minocycline, phenytoin, amikacin, streptomycin	Ataxia
chloramphenicol, anticonvulsants, penicillins, hydralazine, sulfonamides, anticancer drugs	Blood dyscrasias
Penicillins (especially ampicillin), allopurinol, anticonvulsants, nitrofurantoin, sulfonamides, phenobarbital, anticancer drugs	Cutaneous eruptions
furosemide, aspirin and other salicylates, vibramycin, gentamicin	Damage to the eighth cranial nerve (auditory and vestibular)
Sodium and potassium penicillin salts; diuretics, salicylates, ammonium chloride, sodium bicarbonate, potassium chloride	Electrolyte disturbances
tetracycline, hexachlorophene, phenothiazine	Exaggerated sunburn
Topical corticosteroids, ethambutol, thorazine, chloroquine	Eye damage
Antihistamines, atropine, and other anticholinergic agents	Hallucinations
atropine, bulk-forming laxatives, diphenoxylate	Ileus, intestinal obstruction
isoniazid, rifampin, erythromycin estolate, acetaminophen, sulfonamides, methyldopa, chlorpromazine	Liver damage
penicillamine, trimethadione, probenecid	Nephrotic syndrome
isoniazid, vincristine, hydralazine, ethambutol	Peripheral neuritis
Penicillins, lead, salicylates, outdated tetracyclines, cephaloridine, anticonvulsants, gentamicin, streptomycin, amikacin, neomycin, kanamycin	Renal damage
Antihistamines, nasal decongestants, bronchodilators, central nervous system stimulants	Restlessness, agitation, insomnia, excessive crying
Anabolic steroids, adrenocorticosteroids, psychotropic drugs, central nervous stimulants, vitamins given in excess	Suppression of growth
Tetracyclines in children under 8 years	Temporary suppression of bone growth
carbenicillin, clindamycin, clofibrate, gold preparations, griseofulvin, iron	Unpleasant taste, altered taste sensation

Modified from Russell H: *Pediatric drugs and nursing interventions*, New York, 1980, McGraw-Hill.

a nomogram for calculating a child's BSA (Fig. 7.1) may be included in the package. Nomograms are also available in standard pediatric textbooks. The reliability of the BSA method rests on the accuracy with which the body surface area is calculated. Critics of the method maintain that the errors inherent in determining BSA make this method less reliable than dosage based on accurate weights.

When the prescribed drug has a wide therapeutic index and is dosed on a per-kilogram basis, weight can be estimated within 10% of the patient's actual weight without greatly influencing the final dosage. Once a patient weighs 40 to 50 kg (88 to 110 lb), it is time to switch to an adult dose. It is mandatory to look at your weight-based dosage calculations repeatedly. If the calculated dosage exceeds the usual adult dosage, recheck your numbers. Remember, sometimes a child's dosage will exceed an adult's because of their faster metabolic rate.

Another common source of error in children's dosage is failure to divide the total daily per-kilogram dose by the number or doses to be given in a day—mistaking it for an individual dose that needs to be repeated.

PEDIATRIC VARIABLES AND DOSAGE FORMULATION

The form in which a drug is manufactured and the way in which the parent gives the drug to the child determines the actual dose administered. Most oral drugs in soluble solutions are readily absorbed from the GI tract. Solid oral dosage forms (tablets, capsules, powders) cannot cross the GI membrane until they have been dissolved in the GI fluids. If dissolution is extremely slow, a portion of the drug will be lost in the feces (Gupta & Waldhauser, 1997). A slow dissolution rate increases drug exposure to gastric acid, thereby increasing the risk of degradation. Some drugs, such as erythromycin estolate, are esters that cannot be absorbed until they have been converted by intestinal enzymes. Infants with immature intestinal

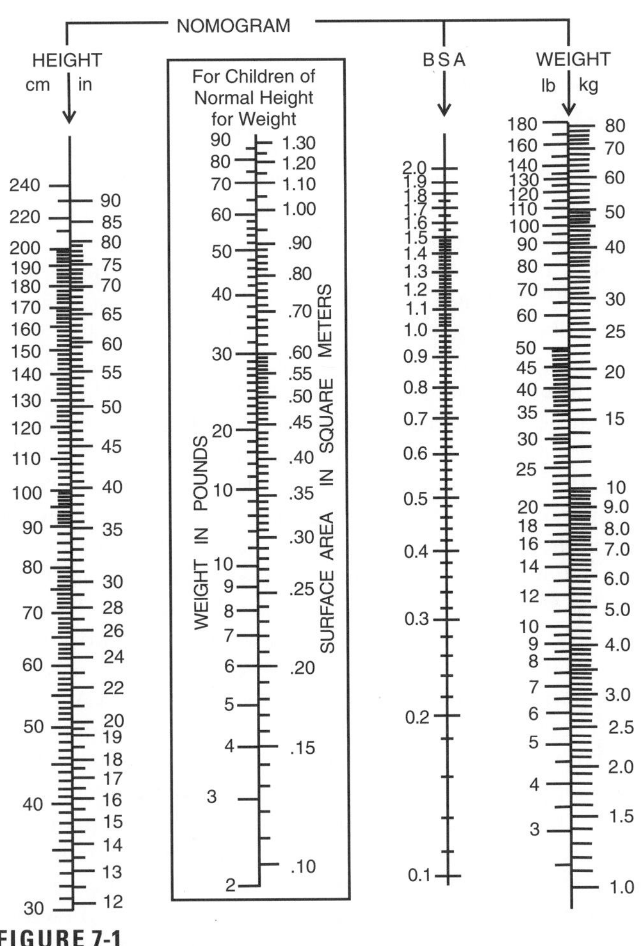

FIGURE 7-1

BSA is indicated where the straight line that connects height (on the left) and weight (on the right) intersects the BSA column or, if client is above average size, from weight alone (enclosed area). (From McKenry LM, Salerno E: *Mosby's Pharmacology in Nursing*, ed 21 revised and updated, St. Louis, 2003, Mosby.)

enzyme function may be unable to convert these drugs; thus they may be lost in the feces (Hardman & Limbird, 2001).

Many drug preparations for children are in the form of elixirs or suspensions. Elixirs are alcoholic solutions in which the drug molecules are dissolved and evenly distributed. No shaking is required, and unless some of the vehicle has evaporated, the first dose from the bottle and the last dose should contain equivalent amounts of drug (McKenry & Salerno, 2002).

Suspensions contain nondissolved particles of drug that must be distributed throughout the vehicle by shaking. If shaking is not thorough each time a dose is given, the first doses from the bottle may contain less drug than the last doses, with the result that less than the expected plasma concentration of the drug may be achieved early in the course of therapy. This will result in decreased drug effectiveness. Conversely, toxicity may occur late in the course of therapy, when unexpectedly high doses are given. This uneven distribution is a potential cause of inefficacy or toxicity in children taking phenytoin suspensions (Edmunds, 2003).

Health care personnel or parents who crush or mix medication with other products may increase drug palatability but make changes that affect the pharmacokinetic properties of the drug. It is particularly common for parents to mix medication with infant cereal, applesauce, or even formula. Thus it is essential that the prescriber know the form in which the drug will be dispensed and provide proper instructions to the pharmacist and patient or parent (McKenry & Salerno, 2002).

Timed-release oral drugs are specially formulated to promote slow absorption over a period of several hours, when a prolonged duration of action is desirable. Some Dilantin capsules and antihistamine combination products come as time-released products for children. There is evidence that these products are often erratically absorbed and may be quite susceptible to changes in gastric pH and GI motility (McKenry & Salerno, 2002).

The difficulties in intramuscular absorption because of decreased muscle mass and poor blood flow have already been discussed; however, it should also be mentioned that drugs in aqueous vehicles are rapidly absorbed from the muscle. Other drugs in poorly soluble vehicles that are incompletely absorbed include digoxin, diazepam, and phenytoin. In fact, some of these drugs not only are painful when administered intramuscularly but often precipitate at the injection site and are either gradually redissolved or removed by phagocytosis. Other poorly absorbed drugs include ampicillin, cephradine, and dicloxacillin (Yaffe, 1992).

Administration of medications by buccal and sublingual routes avoids drug destruction by GI fluids and the liver. However, the effectiveness of this form of delivery depends on whether the child is old enough to keep the drug in contact with the absorbing membrane and if he or she can refrain from swallowing or chewing the tablet until it is completely dissolved. Because most drugs administered by these routes produce an unpleasant taste and mild irritation (Edmunds, 2003), even older children may not be able to cooperate with this route of administration.

Pediatric suppositories and rectal solutions are common forms of drug administration, particularly for neonates. However, the absorption in older children is very slow and highly unreliable and may produce substantial bowel irritation. Although it is difficult to control the amount of medication actually absorbed, this route avoids destruction of the medication by GI products and the liver. The presence of feces in the bowel limits absorption, presumably by limiting drug access to the absorbing membrane. Drug absorption is terminated if the child defecates (Edmunds, 2003). Additional research on rectal administration suggests that aminophylline retention enemas permit better dosage control than administering the same drug as a rectal suppository and that inflammation of the colon increases the amount of hydrocortisone absorbed as a retention enema (McKenry & Salerno, 2002).

The pulmonary epithelium and respiratory tract mucosa allow rapid passage of volatile liquids, gases, aerosol preparations, and isoproterenol. Although pulmonary dosage is irritating to the mucosa and difficult to regulate, the rich blood supply, extensive absorbing surface area, and high permeability of the respiratory tract aid in the absorption of large amounts of medication. If the child is able to hold his or her breath after aerosol nebulization, effective dosage may be achieved. Otherwise, medication may be lost when it goes into the mouth, is swallowed, and excreted (Edmunds, 2003).

Many drugs used in pediatric patients are not available except in injectable form. Drugs such as atropine, digoxin, epinephrine, morphine, phenobarbital, and phenytoin must be diluted and a dosage used that is smaller than that intended for adult patients. Dilution of some productions may alter the bioavailability or compatibility of the drugs. If multiple drugs are administered through the same site, additional problems of drug interactions may be seen. Children may also develop toxicity from some ingredients used in drug preservatives or stabilizers (Edmunds, 2003). Errors that occur in the calculation of the parenteral dosage, the dilution of the product, or even the administration of very small dosages, may produce errors with potentially dangerous consequences.

Ophthalmic absorption of medication is promoted by measures that increase the amount of drug the eye can retain and that increase the length of time the drug is in contact with the absorbing membrane. Thus ointments that cover the eye with an oily film provide higher dosages than ophthalmic drops (Edmunds, 2003). Little children are usually very intolerant of eye drops, and trying to get them to hold their head back during installation, to close their eyes, or to refrain from blinking is rarely successful. Ocular inflammation or injury decreases the blood–aqueous humor barrier, thereby increasing absorption of many ophthalmic drugs (Hardman & Limbird, 2001). Ophthalmic absorption is so great that in premature babies the extent of absorption could potentially lead to systemic toxicity.

Nasal solutions are often well absorbed across the nasal and sinus mucosa. However, infants and young children are likely to swallow these preparations, even when the child's head is held in the lateral head low position.

STATUS OF DRUG DOSING AND POLICY REGARDING CHILDREN

According to the American Academy of Pediatrics (1995), only a small proportion of all drugs and biologic products marketed in the United States have had clinical trials performed in pediatric patients, and a majority of marketed drugs are not labeled for use in pediatric patients or for use in specific pediatric age groups. A recent Food and Drug Administration (FDA) survey similarly concluded that most products that are indicated for diseases occurring in both adults and children have very little information about pediatric use in their labeling (Pina, 1998). For vaccines and antibiotics, pediatric use information is generally adequate, but many drugs used in the treatment of both common childhood illnesses and more serious conditions carry little information about use in pediatric patients. Data on the pharmacokinetics, pharmacodynamics, efficacy, and safety of drugs in infants and children are even more difficult to find. For example, a recent report from the FDA demonstrates that less than half the drugs approved for treatment of human immunodeficiency virus (HIV) infection or accompanying opportunistic infections carry any pediatric safety or effectiveness information. Of drugs that do have pediatric information, the data are often incomplete and limited to certain pediatric age groups. Pediatric labeling is also particularly inadequate for such drug classes as antidepressants, antihypertensives, antirheumatic drugs, medications to treat GI problems, steroids, prescription pain medications, and drugs to treat ulcerative colitis (Witt, 1995).

Many of the drugs and biologic products most widely used in pediatric patients carry disclaimers stating that safety and effectiveness in pediatric patients have not been established (Cote, 1996; Pina, 1998). Clearly, the term *children* used in much of the pharmaceutical literature refers to a group with widely differing members. Thus safety and effectiveness information about some of these group members may not be valid for other group members, and attempting to generalize from one category to another may result in drug errors. The unique differences in neonatal, as opposed to adolescent, drug response is obvious, but subtle changes in the response to drugs occur throughout the total growth and developmental cycle.

An evaluation of available pharmacologic recommendations for children documents that for some pediatric age groups, information is particularly sparse. For example, there is almost no information on use in patients under 2 years of age for most drug classes (Pina, 1998). The FDA compiled a list of the 10 drugs that were most widely prescribed for pediatric patients, on an outpatient basis, based on 1994 data from IMS America, Ltd, a research firm that provides data on prescription drug use. These drugs included albuterol inhalation solution, Phenergan, ampicillin injections, Auralgan otic solution, Lotrisone cream, Prozac, Intal, Zoloft, Ritalin, and Alupent syrup. In each case, the drug label lacked any use information for the age group to which the drug was prescribed, or the information was inadequate. These 10 drugs were prescribed over 5 million times in 1 year for pediatric patients in age groups for which the label carried a disclaimer or lacked adequate use information (Witt, 1995). evolve For information on the ten most widely prescribed drugs for pediatric patients, see the Evolve website.

The absence of pediatric labeling information may sometimes require the physician caring for children to choose between prescribing drugs without well-founded dosing and safety information and using other potentially less effective therapy. Inadequate pediatric labeling thus exposes children to the risk of unexpected adverse reactions or lack of optimal treatment. Even after a drug has been used in pediatric patients for some time and there has been substantial clinical experience with the drug, directions for safe and effective use in pediatric patients are not provided on the label (Witt, 1995).

Children were formerly viewed as a population entirely distinct from adults, in whom the safety and effectiveness of a drug had to be established entirely independently. It has become increasingly accepted, however, that children may be considered a demographic subpopulation with many similarities to the adult population. In some cases, drugs and biologic products behave similarly in the demographic subgroups, including age and gender subgroups, even though there may be some variations in pharmacokinetics (Witt, 1995). As the FDA has already stated in the *Federal Register* (59 FR 64240, December 13, 1994), adequate and well-controlled trials may not be needed in children to establish pediatric use information (Witt, 1995).

Clearly, there are difficulties associated with the testing

of drugs in the pediatric population. These include, among others, ethical issues surrounding the difficulty in recruiting study patients, obtaining informed consent for tests not directly of benefit to the child, use of placebo controls in a vulnerable population, and the possible discomfort and risk to the child. Because of these problems, research that includes children has had difficulty receiving approval from many institutional review committees (Nahata, 2002). Failure to conduct pediatric testing may therefore deprive pediatric patients, in some cases, of significant therapeutic advances. Shirkey coined the term *therapeutic orphans* to refer drugs that lack sponsorship for use in children. Unfortunately, this problem is even greater now than it was in 1975 when the term was coined (Cote, 1996).

Although use of a particular drug in children is no longer considered a new indication (with the exception of specific pediatric indications), the development of additional information in pediatric patients is needed to provide appropriate dosing recommendations. The correct pediatric dose cannot necessarily be extrapolated from adult dosing information using an equivalence based either on weight milligrams per kilogram (mg/kg) or body surface area (mg/square meter [m^2]). Because potentially significant differences in pharmacokinetics may alter a drug's effect in pediatric patients, dosing is much less precise.

The effects of growth and development of various organs, maturation of the immune system, alterations in metabolism throughout infancy and childhood, changes in body proportions, and other developmental changes may result in significant differences in the doses needed by pediatric patients and adults (Nahata, 2002). For example, studies have shown that fentanyl, a potent opioid widely used in the anesthetic management of infants and small children but not labeled for use in pediatric patients under 2 years of age, demonstrates differences in clearance between the neonatal period and 2 or more months of age, resulting from improving hepatic blood flow and hepatic microsomal maturation (Koren, 1990). Comparable doses in adults and neonates (calculated on a μg/kg basis) produce a twofold to threefold higher plasma concentration in neonates. Again, the gray baby syndrome after the administration of chloramphenicol to infants with immature livers was directly related to a decreased metabolism of this drug by the glucuronyl transferase that could convert it to the inactive glucuronide metabolite (Kuhn et al, 1986). Pharmacokinetic differences of this kind demonstrate the importance of studying the pharmacokinetics of a drug in pediatric patients or in different ages before they are widely exposed to it.

Inadequate dosing information may expose pediatric patients to dangerously high doses or to ineffective treatment. This dramatically increases the probability of adverse reactions. Cases in which inadequately studied drugs have resulted in serious adverse effects in pediatric patients include teeth staining from tetracycline, kernicterus from sulfa drugs, withdrawal symptoms following prolonged administration of fentanyl in infants and small children, seizures and cardiac arrest caused by bupivacaine toxicity, development of colonic strictures in pediatric cystic fibrosis patients after exposure to high-dose pancreatic enzymes, and hazardous interactions between erythromycin and midazolam (Agarwal et al, 1992; Editorial, 1995; Kauffman, 1991; McCloskey et al, 1992; Mevorach et al, 1993; Nathan et al, 2003; Olkkola et al, 1993; Rieder, 1997).

Other factors may also interfere with the appropriate drug dosing of children. Many drugs widely prescribed for infants and children are not available in a suitable dosage form for children. Examples include phenobarbital, acetazolamide, and rifampin. When these products are altered to give to children through either dilution or reformulation, questions must be raised about their stability and compatibility. The problems associated with intravenous infusion of medications are compounded by the need for low fluid volumes and the limited access to intravenous sites (Nahata, 2002). Failure to develop a pediatric formulation may also deny pediatric patients access to important therapeutic advances or require pediatric patients to take the drug in homemade or poorly bioavailable formulation (Witt, 1995).

The absence of pediatric testing may thus result in less-than-optimal treatment for many pediatric patients (American Academy of Pediatrics, 1997; Witt, 1995). Although significant progress has been made in the area of pediatric pharmacokinetics over the last several decades, few studies have correlated pharmacokinetics with pharmacodynamics (Kearns et al, 1997).

In late 1994, the FDA amended its regulations governing the content and format on labeling for human prescription drug products. The final rule revised the current "Pediatric Use" subsection of the professional labeling requirements for prescription drugs to provide for the inclusion of more complete information about the use of a drug in the pediatric population (ages birth to 16 years). The final rule, which applies to prescription drug products, including biologicals, recognized several methods of establishing substantial evidence to support pediatric labeling claims. This includes, in certain cases, relying on studies carried out in adults. This final rule also requires that if there is not substantial evidence to support any pediatric use or use in a particular pediatric population, the labeling shall state this. Drug company sponsors are required to reexamine existing data on their products to determine whether the "Pediatric Use" subsection of the labeling for drugs already being marketed can be modified based on already adequate and well-controlled studies in adults. In such cases, the FDA will have concluded that the course of the disease and the positive and negative effects of the drug are sufficiently similar in the pediatric and adult populations to allow extrapolation from the adult efficacy data to pediatric patients. Other information supporting pediatric use must ordinarily include data on the pharmacokinetics of the drug in the pediatric population for determination of appropriate dosage. In some cases, companies will be required to submit a supplemental application to comply with new drug labeling requirements, to show that the drug can be used safely and effectively in pediatric patients (Newman, 1997).

The specific labeling required by the FDA under the "Pediatric Use" subsection of the labeling says

> The safety and effectiveness of (drug name) have been established in the age groups to (note any limitations [e.g., no data for pediatric patients under 2, or only applicable to certain indications approved in adults]). Use of (drug name)

in these age groups is supported by evidence from adequate and well-controlled studies of (drug name) in adults with additional data (insert wording that accurately describes the data submitted to support a finding of substantial evidence of effectiveness in the pediatric population)

(FDA, 1994).

If appropriate, under the Clinical Pharmacology, Contradictions, Warnings, Precautions, and Dosage and Administration sections, additional and specific information might be provided as a "Pediatric Use" subsection.

A list of drugs for which additional pediatric information could produce health benefits in the pediatric population is being compiled by the FDA by looking at all drugs with at least 50,000 prescriptions/year used in pediatric patients. Drugs with "meaningful therapeutic benefit" over existing treatments, or when a product is to be widely used in pediatric populations, will now be required to have specific pediatric studies completed by the drug manufacturing company before it may be marketed (Food and Drug Administration, 1994). The new rules for testing were designed to provide more pediatric use information in the labeling of drugs. This should help practitioners to have reliable information on which to base a decision to prescribe a drug for use in their pediatric patients. It is not intended to limit the manner in which a practitioner may prescribe an approved drug.

SPECIAL COMPLIANCE PROBLEMS IN CHILDREN

Compliance may be more difficult to achieve in pediatric patients than other individuals because it involves not only the parent's conscientious effort to follow directions but also such practical matters as measuring errors, spilling, and spitting out. For example, because the measured volume of "teaspoons" ranges from 2.5 to 7.8 ml (Hardman & Limbird, 2001), the parents should obtain a calibrated medicine spoon or syringe from the pharmacy for dosing small children. These devices improve the accuracy of dose measurements and simplify administration of drugs to children.

When evaluating compliance, it is often helpful to ask if an attempt was made to give another dose of medicine after the child spilled part of what was offered. The parents may not always be able to say with confidence how much of a dose the child actually received. The parents must be told whether to wake the baby for its every-6-hour dose day or night. These matters should be discussed and made clear, and no assumptions should be made about what the parents may or may not do. Compliance problems frequently occur when antibiotics are prescribed to treat otitis media or urinary tract infections and the child feels well after a few days of therapy. The parents may also feel the child is well and stop giving the medicine, even though it was prescribed for 10 or 14 days. This common situation should be anticipated so the parents can be told why it is important to continue the medicine for the prescribed period even if the child seems to be "cured."

Practical and convenient dosage forms and dosing schedule should be chosen to the extent possible. The easier it is to administer and take the medicine and the easier the dosing schedule is to follow, the more likely it is that compliance will be achieved.

Consistent with their ability to comprehend and cooperate, children should also be given some responsibility for their own health care and for taking medications. This should be discussed in appropriate terms both with the child and the parents. This is particularly true with chronic problems such as asthma, diabetes, and arthritis. Possible adverse effects and drug interactions with over-the-counter medicines or food should also be discussed. Whenever a drug does not achieve its therapeutic effect, the possibility of noncompliance should be considered. There is ample evidence that when noncompliance with the prescribed regimen is a big factor in a child not getting well, parents' or children's reports about their compliance may be grossly inaccurate. Random measurement of serum concentrations and pill count may help disclose noncompliance (Bailey, 1997). The use of computerized pill containers, which record each lid opening, have been shown to be very effective in measuring compliance.

CONCLUSION

Working with children is a rewarding experience. However, the responsibility for accuracy and careful monitoring and record-keeping is even greater with children. Their physical and developmental immaturity often presents a vulnerability and risk that gives little margin for error.

RESOURCES FOR PATIENTS AND PROVIDERS

Internet Resources

ABCs of Safe and Healthy Child Care, www.cdc.gov/ncidod/hip/abc/abcorder.htm.

American Academy of Family Physicians, www.aafp.org/ American Academy of Pediatrics www.aap.org/.

Ask the WebDoctor, www.parentsplace.com/genobject.cgi/readroom/dr answers.html.

Healthfinder, www.healthfinder.gov.

The Informed Parent, www.informedparent.com/currentissuerightframe.html.

Kids' Health and Fitness, www.ced.appstate.edu/whs/goals2000/projects/fitness.htm.

KidsHealth (Nemours Foundation), www.kidshealth.org/nf/ncbc/index.html.

Parenting Q&A, www.parenting-qa.com/parentqa/qanda/.

ParentsPlace-Childrens Health Center, www.parentsplace.com/.

Pediatric News at your Desktop (free but must register), www.medconnect.com.

Pediatric Database (PEDBASE), www.gretmar.com/Webdoctor/pedbase.html.

Points of Pediatric Interest, www.med.jhu.edu/peds/neonatology/poi3.html#Misc/%.

United States Consumer Product Safety (Healthtouch), www.healthtouch.com/level1/leaflets/cpsc/Other resources.

Mosby's pediatric patient teaching guides, St Louis, 1996, Mosby.

REFERENCES

Agarwal R et al: Seizures occurring in pediatric patients receiving continuous infusion of bupivacaine, *Anesth Analgesia* 75:284-286, 1992.

American Academy of Pediatrics, Committee on Drugs: Alternative routes of drug administration advantages and disadvantages (subject review), *Pediatrics* 100:143-152, 1997.

American Academy of Pediatrics, Committee on Drugs: Guidelines for the ethical conduct of studies to evaluate drugs in pediatric populations, *Pediatrics* 95:286-294, 1995.

American Academy of Pediatrics, Committee on Drugs: The transfer of drugs and other chemicals into human milk, *Pediatrics* 93:137-150, 1994.

Bailey B et al: Noninvasive methods for drug measurement in pediatrics, *Pediatr Clin North Am* 44:15-26, 1997.

Behrman N et al: *Nelson's textbook of pediatrics,* ed 16, Philadelphia, 2000, WB Saunders.

Berlin CM Jr: Advances in pediatric pharmacology, toxicology, and therapeutics. *Adv Pediatr* 46:507-538, 1999.

Besunder FA et al: Principles of drug biodisposition in the neonate: a critical evaluation of the pharmacokinetic-pharmacodynamic interface (two parts), *Clin Pharmacokinet* 14:189, 1988.

Cote CJ et al: Is the therapeutic orphan about to be adopted? *Pediatrics* 98:118-123, 1996.

Drug toxicity in the newborn (Symposium), *Fed Proc* 44:2301, 1985.

Editorial: Cystic fibrosis and colonic strictures, *J Clin Gastroenterol* 21:2-5, 1995.

Edmunds MW: *Introduction to clinical pharmacology,* ed 4, St Louis, 2003, Mosby.

Evans NJ et al: Percutaneous administration of theophylline in the preterm infant, *J Pediatr* 107:307-311, 1985.

Food and Drug Administration: *Specific requirements on content and format of labeling for human prescription drugs: Revision of Pediatric Use subsection in the labeling: final rule,* Health and Human Services, Food and Drug Administration, 21 CFR Part 201, December 13, 1994.

Feinstein RA, Miles MV: The effect of acute viral hepatitis on theophylline clearance, *Clin Pediatr* 24:357-358, 1985.

Gilman JT: Therapeutic drug monitoring in the neonate and paediatric age group: problems and clinical pharmacokinetic implications, *Clin Pharmacokinet* 19:1, 1990.

Gupta A, Waldhauser LK: Adverse drug reactions from birth to early childhood, *Pediatr Clin North Am* 44:79-92, 1997.

Hansten PD, Horn JR: *The top 100 drug interactions: a guide to patient management,* ed 9, New York, 2001, H & H Publications.

Hardman JG, et al, editors: *Goodman & Gilman's the pharmacologic basis of therapeutics,* ed 10, New York, 2001, McGraw-Hill.

Kauffman RE: Fentanyl, fads, and folly: who will adopt the therapeutic orphans? *J Pediatr* 119:588-589, 1991.

Kearns GL et al: Immediate action needed to improve labeling of prescription drugs for pediatric patients, *Ann Pharmacother* 31:249-251, 1997.

Koren G: *Maternal-fetal toxicology: a clinician's guide,* New York, 1990, Marcel Dekker.

Koren G, Cohen MS: Special aspects of perinatal and pediatric pharmacology. In Katzung BM: *Basic and clinical pharmacology,* ed 8, Norwalk, CT, 2000, McGraw-Hill/Appleton & Lange.

Kuhn R et al: Netilmicin pharmacokinetics in newborn infants, *Eur J Clin Pharmacol* 29:635-637, 1986.

Leeder JS et al: Pharmacogenetics in pediatrics: implications for practice, *Pediatr Clin North Am* 44:55-77, 1997.

Levine S, Poon CY, Walson PD: The essentials in pediatric dosing, *Patient Care Nurse Pract.* 48-75, 2000.

McCloskey JJ et al: Bupivacaine toxicity secondary to continuous caudal epidural infusion in pediatric patients, *Anesth Analg* 75:287-290, 1992.

McKenry LM, Salerno E: *Mosby's pharmacology in nursing,* ed 22, St Louis, 2002, Mosby.

Nahata MC: Pediatrics. In DiPiro JT et al, editors: *Pharmacotherapy: a pathophysiologic approach,* ed 5, Norwalk, CT, 2002, McGraw-Hill/Appleton & Lange.

Nahata MC et al: Effect of gestational age and birth weight on tobramycin kinetics in newborn infants, *J Antimicrob Chemother* 14:59-65, 1984.

Nathan DG, Oski FA et al: *Hematology of infancy and childhood,* ed 6, Philadelphia, 2003, JB Lippincott.

Newman C et al: Comment: regulations for pediatric labeling of prescription drugs, *Ann Pharmacother* 31:1092-1093, 1997.

Nottarianni LJ: Plasma protein binding of drugs in pregnancy and in neonates, *Clin Pharmacokinet* 18:20, 1990.

Olkkola KT et al: A potentially hazardous interaction between erythromycin and midazolam, *Clin Pharmacol Therapeu* 53:298-305, 1993.

Pina LM: *Drugs widely used off label in pediatrics. Report of the pediatric use survey working group of the pediatric subcommittee,* Washington, DC, 1998, Federal Drug Administration, US Government Printing Office.

Powell DA et al: Chloramphenicol: new perspectives on an old drug, *Drug Intell Clin Pharm* 16:295-300, 1982.

Rane A: Basic principles of drug disposition and action in infants and children. In Yaffe JF, editor: *Pediatric pharmacology: therapeutic principles in practice,* Philadelphia, 1992, WB Saunders.

Rieder MJ: In vivo and in vitro testing for adverse drug reactions, *Pediatr Clin North Am* 44:93-111, 1997.

Roberts RJ: Drug therapy in infants: pharmacologic principles and clinical experience, Philadelphia, 1984, WB Saunders.

Russell H: *Pediatric drugs and nursing interventions,* New York, 1980, McGraw-Hill.

Silver HK, Kempe CH, Bruyn HB: *Handbook of pediatrics,* ed 16, East Norwalk, CT, 1991, McGraw-Hill/Appleton & Lange.

Tyrala FF et al: Clinical pharmacology of hexachlorophene in newborn infants, *J Pediatr* 93:481-486, 1977.

Witt AM: *Supplemental information. Content and format of labeling for human prescription drugs; revision of pediatric use,* Washington, DC, January, 1995, Health and Human Services, Food and Drug Administration.

Yaffe S: *Pediatric pharmacology,* Philadelphia, 1992, WB Saunders.

CHAPTER 8

Special Populations: Pregnant and Nursing Women

Christine M. Betzold

Providing drug therapy to pregnant or lactating women poses a unique challenge for health care practitioners. Because they represent a state of duality, the clinician who prescribes a drug for them must always consider the impact of that treatment on the developing fetus or infant. Hence the benefit of any drug to a pregnant patient must be carefully weighed against the potential teratogenic risk to the fetus. Alternatively in the lactating mother, the choices between premature weaning (weaning before the age of 1 year), temporarily interrupting breast-feeding or breast-feeding while taking medication, must be carefully weighed while keeping in mind the numerous benefits of breast-feeding and deleterious effects of early weaning for both the mother and child (Spencer, Gonzales & Barnhart, 2001; American Academy of Family Physicians, 2002).

During pregnancy, the clinician must be aware of the changing physiologic characteristics of the patient throughout gestation as well as those of the growing fetus. Additionally, although multiple factors affect the teratogenicity of a drug, one of the most important is the timing of the drug exposure. Three stages of development are generally considered when assessing the teratogenic potential of a drug (Dicke, 1989; Koren & Cohen, 1994): the 2 weeks after conception and before implantation (the *preimplantation phase*), the embryonic period (weeks 3 through 8), and the fetal period (weeks 9 through delivery). In the past, clinicians have overestimated the ability of the placenta to protect the fetus and in fact, the term *placental barrier* is a misnomer, as the placenta allows crossing of most drugs and dietary substances.

In the breastfed infant, the provider must understand the dynamics between the mechanisms of the drug entry into mother's milk and what happens once the infant ingests it, taking into account the infant's age, health status, and ability to metabolize and excrete the medication. Primarily, medication transfers into human milk through a concentration gradient that allows passive diffusion of free (non–protein-bound) and nonionized medication. Different choices and greater caution may be needed in infants less than 1 week old, premature infants, or compromised infants with health problems as they may have a lessened ability to tolerate, metabolize, or excrete medications. Finally, more medication transfers occur during the early postpartum period due to the large gaps between the mammary alveolar cells, but less transfers occur during the weaning process due to a decrease in the milk supply from nursings that are shorter or fewer (Spencer, Gonzales & Barnhart, 2001).

Overall, what the mother consumes is also consumed by the fetus or infant, with the exception of large organic ions such as heparin and insulin. In fact, virtually all (99%) of drugs cross the placenta and most medications penetrate human milk to some degree (Hollingsworth, 1988; Hale, 2002). Ideally, the pregnant or lactating woman should take as few drugs as possible, although the exposure is usually more significant for the developing fetus than for the breast-feeding infant. Usually breast-feeding infants have less exposure because the concentrations of most medications in human milk are extraordinarily low and with few exceptions the dose delivered to the nursing infant is subclinical (Hale, 2002). Frequently, however, some form of drug therapy is necessary to treat the physiologic and hormonal changes that occur during pregnancy and postpartum, the symptoms produced by the expanding uterus or functioning breast, and/or concomitant illnesses such as asthma, upper respiratory infections, epilepsy or diabetes mellitus. Clinicians in the primary care setting should anticipate such complaints and be prepared to treat them appropriately.

Unfortunately, despite the obvious need for drug therapy and the prevailing apprehension about using drugs in these special populations, limited information exists for clinicians to make astute clinical decisions. Moreover, due to the medicolegal implications of treating pregnant women or infants, this lack of data is further confounded by the ethical constraints in testing these populations. Notably, during pregnancy very few drugs have Food and Drug Administration (FDA) approval for use, and lactation is presently not even categorized. Thus drugs for pregnant or lactating patients must be selected and based on safety data derived from animal research and clinical data generated from case reports, retrospective case-control trials, and personal experience. What's more, during lactation the care given mothers is further confounded by inadequate training about sustaining breast-feeding, a bounty of breast-feeding misinformation, the misperception that formula-feeding versus breast-feeding is virtually equivalent, as well as, a dearth of high-quality studies. These confounders have all led to numerous unsound recommendations to prematurely wean (American Academy of Family Physicians, 2002; Spencer, Gonzales & Barnhart, 2001). Consequently, to provide the most astute and contemporary care, those treating the breastfed infant or pregnant mother may need to consult the most accurate and up-to-date resources available. This includes using both telephone consultations and Internet resources for assistance in choosing the most appropriate medication (Box 8-1). evolve Please also see the supplemental tables on the Evolve Learning Resources website.

DRUGS IN PREGNANT WOMEN

Incidence

Although the ideal condition may be the avoidance of any medications or chemicals during pregnancy, research has demonstrated that 90% of pregnant women have or develop medical

BOX 8-1

RESOURCES

The National Women's Health Information Center (NWHIC). Available at www.4woman.gov/

eMedicine. Available at www.emedicine.com

AAP Policy Statements on breastfeeding, use of psychotropics, transfer of drugs into human milk, and other statements. Available at www.aap.org/

SOURCES OF INFORMATION ON POTENTIAL TERATOGENS

Computerized Databases

American Academy of Pediatrics. Available at www.aap.org.

The Organization of Teratology Information Services (OTIS). Available at www.otispregnancy.org

Repro-Tox, Columbia Women's Hospital, Washington, DC (202) 293-5138

Teratology Information System (TERIS), Department of Pediatrics, University of Washington, Seattle, Washington

TOXLINE, National Library of Medicine, Bethesda, Maryland

Current Pregnancy Exposure Registries

www.fda.gov/womens/registries/registries.html

Textbooks

Briggs GG, Freeman RG: *Drugs in pregnancy and lactation,* Baltimore, 1989, Johns Hopkins University Press

Gilstrap LC, Little BB, Brent RL: *Drugs and pregnancy,* New York, 1997, Chapman

Karen G: *Maternal fetal toxicology,* New York, 1994, Marcel Dekker

Neibyl JR: *Drug use in pregnancy,* Philadelphia, 1988, Lea & Febiger

Schardein JL: *Chemically induced birth defects,* New York, 1993, Marcel Dekker

Shepherd TH: *Catalogue of teratogenic agents,* Baltimore, 1989, Johns Hopkins University Press

During Lactation

Breastfeeding and drugs information, University of California San Diego (900) 226-7536

Hale T: *Medications in mothers' milk*, Amarillo, 2002, Pharmasoft

Tom Hale's lactation registry:
http://neonatal.ttuhsc.edu/lact/html/drug_entry.html
http://neonatal.ama.ttuhsc.edu/lact/
http://neonatal.ama.ttuhsc.edu/lact/html/lactation_registry.html

www.ibreastfeeding.com

Lawrence R: *Breastfeeding: a guide for the medical professional*, St Louis, 1999, Mosby

Newman J, Pitman T: *Dr. Jack Newman's guide to breastfeeding*, Toronto, 2000, Harper Collins Publishing

Depression

Pregnancy and depression information. Available at www.pregnancyanddepression.com

Registry for buproprion exposure. Available at www.pregnancyregistry.gsk.com/bupreg.pdf

problems that require them to take more than one prescription drug during pregnancy (Hollingsworth, 1988). Studies have shown that the average patient uses 5 to 9 different drugs during pregnancy; 4% of pregnant women take more than 10 drugs during pregnancy; and 65% of women admit to self-administration of drugs during pregnancy. Additional research has demonstrated that the extent of fetal exposure to drugs may be vastly underestimated; patient medical charts identify less than one fourth of the drugs actually consumed by the patient (Briggs, 1995; Koren, 1994).

PRINCIPLES OF TERATOLOGY: INCIDENCE AND TYPES OF MALFORMATIONS

The desire for a healthy baby is universal. Mothers cannot help but worry about the health of the unborn child and fear the worst. But regardless of the wishes of the mother, many factors not under her control may influence the outcome of the pregnancy. Information about the thalidomide tragedy in the early 1960s, fueled by regulatory agencies, lawyers, and the public, has stimulated an intense search for the etiology, prevention, and treatment of congenital malformations (Dicke, 1989). But, although there has been heightened vigilance in this area, most knowledge about the effect of different drugs on the fetus comes from the experience and observation of clinicians, not scientific research.

There are many different forms of congenital malformations and their incidence varies widely. The incidence of major malformations in the general population is usually quoted as 2% to 3%, or 20 to 30 per 1000 live births (Blake & Niebyl, 1988; Schardein, 1993). This translates into 200,000 birth defects annually (Schardein, 1993). Major malformations are those that are incompatible with survival (e.g., anencephaly) or require major surgery for correction (e.g., cleft palate, congenital heart disease). If minor malformations are included (e.g., ear tags, extra digits), the rate may be as high as 10% (Blake & Niebyl, 1988). Congenital malformations account for about 14% of all infant deaths. Problems arising during fetal development or within 1 month after birth account for two thirds of all infant mortality in this country (Schardein, 1993).

Although much attention has been paid to the causes of obvious physical deformities, growing research suggests that concern should also extend to events beyond the narrow limit of congenital anatomic malformations. Evidence exists that the future intellectual, social and functional development of the unborn child also can be adversely affected. In particular, toxic manifestations of intrauterine exposure to drugs may be subtle, unexpected, and delayed.

Common lore blames drug exposure by the pregnant mother for any type of fetal damage. However, less than 5% of congenital malformations are probably related to drugs (Briggs & Freeman, 1980. Only 19 drugs or groups of drugs have now been established as probably teratogenic agents in humans (Table 8-1). This is in contrast to the almost 800 identifiable teratogens found for laboratory animals (Schardein, 1993).

TABLE 8-1 Drugs Considered to Be Teratogenic in Humans

Drug	Date Discovered	Major Defects	Approximate No. of Cases
Antihyroid compounds	1903	Hypothyroidism, goiter	140
Aminoglycoside antibiotics	1950	Ototoxicity, eighth nerve	60
Anticancer agents	1952	Polymorphic	50
Androgenic hormones	1953	Masculinization	250
Tetracyclines	1956	Teeth (staining)	Thousands
thalidomide	1961	Limb, ear	7700
phenytoin	1963	Craniofacial, appendicular, cardiac, and skeletal, motor, and mental deficiency	Hundreds
Hypervitaminosis A	1965	CNS, ear, cardiac, palate	20
Coumarin anticoagulants	1966	Nose, skeleton, CNS	55
Alcohol	1967	Facial, microcephaly, mental retardation	Thousands
Methadone anticonvulsants	1970	Facial, cardiac, urogenital, mental, and speech impairment	40
lithium	1970	Heart	25
diethylstilbestrol (DES)	1970	Uterine adenosis, cancer in females, accessory gonadal lesions in males	Hundreds
penicillamine	1971	Skin hyperelasticity	5
primidone	1976	Microcephaly, cardiac, facial, mental deficiency	25
valproic acid	1982	Facial, spina bifida	100
Vitamin A analogues	1983	Craniofacial, cardiac, CNS, thymic, mental retardation	115
cocaine	1987	Cardiovascular, CNS, neurologic defects	Hundreds
carbamazepine	1988	Craniofacial, digital	70

From Schardein JL: *Chemically induced birth defects*, ed 2, New York, 1993, Marcel Dekker.

This public misperception probably grew from the media attention surrounding the extreme fetal deformities resulting as part of the thalidomide tragedy of the 1960s.

Thalidomide

Thalidomide was a central nervous system depressant used as a sedative-hypnotic agent and also for the nausea and vomiting of pregnancy. Perhaps as many as 10,000 deformed children were reported to have resulted from the drug in as many as 30 countries, although the confirmed number is closer to 8000. The thalidomide episode focused the attention of both the scientific and the lay community on the question of safe drug use in pregnant women. This drug was said to increase the rate of dysmelia by 80%, up to a rate of about 3:1000 to 5:1000 births. The reported malformations resulted when thalidomide was taken on days 21 to 36 after conception (days 34 to 50 postmenses). The risk of a woman having a malformed child following thalidomide ingestion has been estimated to range from 2% to 25%, and retrospective analysis suggests there was a mortality rate of 45%. Today there is much controversy over thalidomide research in women affected by human immunodeficiency virus and rheumatoid arthritis.

Determinants of Teratogenicity

The most important determinant of the teratogenicity of an agent is the timing of the drug exposure (Figure 8-1). Exposure to drugs during the preimplantation phase results in an all-or-none effect: the affected cells either die or are undifferentiated, or *totipotential*, meaning that if one cell is damaged, another can assume its function (Dicke, 1989; Gilstrap, Little & Brent, 1997; McCombs, 1993). Therefore during this period, no malformations can be induced, because there is no cell differentiation to allow any selective toxic reaction. Exposure to a teratogen either is lethal to the ovum, or the ovum regenerates completely after exposure to a sublethal dose. Thus exposure during this time may kill the conceptus and the patient may not realize she is pregnant, but, if the pregnancy continues, there is no increased risk of congenital anomalies (Briggs, 1995).

The most critical period in which to avoid drug exposure is the *embryonic period* (weeks 3 through 8), during which major organogenesis occurs and the risk of inducing major malformations is greatest. The damage induced by a drug administered during this period will depend on what organ systems were forming during the time of exposure. Because many organ systems form in parallel, multiple congenital defects are possible from one drug exposure. The classic teratogenic period in humans lasts from 31 days after the last menstrual period through 10 weeks from the last menstrual period (Blake & Niebyl, 1988), which corresponds to the period of organogenesis (14 to 56 days).

After embryogenesis occurs, the organ structures continue to grow and mature physiologically during the *fetal period* (weeks 9 through term). During the fetal period (57 days to term) major malformations are not likely to occur, yet organ systems formed during the embryonic period may be damaged by exposure in the second or third trimester (Gilstrap, Little & Brent, 1997) and anomalies are more likely to involve functional aspects such as mental development and reproduction or fetal growth. Thus exposure to a teratogen during this period may result in intrauterine growth retardation and because the central nervous system continues to develop throughout gestation exposure may cause mental retardation or subtle, delayed behavioral effects.

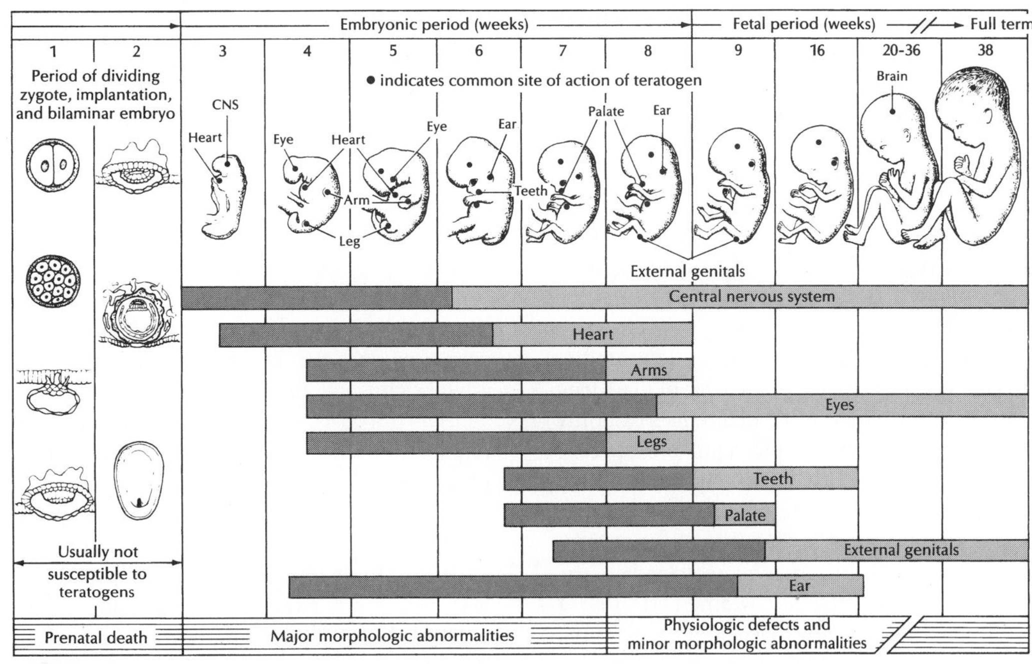

FIGURE 8-1

Critical periods in human development. The periods most susceptible to teratogenesis are indicated in black; less sensitive stages are shown in white. (From Moore K: *Before we are born: basic embryology and birth defects*, ed 5, Philadelphia, 1998, WB Saunders.)

The placenta plays an important role in determining the teratogenic potential of a drug, primarily by allowing drugs to reach the fetus but perhaps also by allowing for the biotransformation of drugs before they reach the fetal circulation. The surface area of the placenta increases during gestation, while placental thickness decreases. Both of these structural changes favor the transfer of chemicals to the fetus (Briggs, 1995). And in fact, as stated earlier, nearly all drugs readily cross the placenta, reaching fetal concentrations 50% to 100% of those in the maternal circulation (McCombs, 1993). Primarily, the physiologic processes that govern passage of drugs across the placenta are the same that apply to the passage of drugs across any lipid membrane. Once the drug has crossed the placenta, it is in the fetal circulation. Several other physicochemical properties affect the rate and/or extent of placental transfer, including lipid solubility, protein binding, and pH of the mother and fetus (Szeto, 1993). Currently, little is known about the contribution of the placenta to the metabolism of drugs passing through it. However, metabolic inactivation of drugs by the placenta appears to be of less clinical concern than the potential for the placenta to metabolize less active compounds to toxic metabolites (Simone, Derewlany & Koren, 1995).

Several other factors that illustrate the principles of teratology include the following (Dicke, 1989):

- *Maternal-fetal genotype*—Maternal absorption, metabolism, distribution, placental transfer, and fetal metabolism characteristics unique to each maternal-fetal pair as a result of genetic heterogeneity influence the fetal susceptibility to a potential teratogen. This is easy to understand when clinicians observe that for the same teratogen, some individuals will prove especially susceptible, whereas others will be unusually resistant.
- *Dose-response relationships*—The amount of medication taken often correlates with the observed response. Aberrant development may range from no effect at low doses to organ-specific malformations at intermediate doses to embryo-fetal toxicity at high doses. The extent of damage is also influenced by the stage of development, and route of administration.
- *Specificity of agent*—The extent of adverse environmental influences on developing tissues depends heavily on the agent involved. Some agents have greater teratogenic potential than others, resulting in part from factors such as the drug dosage, maternal metabolism, and placental transfer.
- *Drug interactions*—Two teratogens administered separately may have a very different effect when given together. Induction or inhibition of enzyme systems and competition for binding sites caused by the two drugs may influence levels of unbound and active teratogen.

Finally, the response of the fetus to an administered medication tends to differ from that of the mother. This may result from increased blood-brain permeability and the immaturity of the liver enzymes in the fetus.

Determining Teratogenic Potential of Drugs

In general, animal models predict poorly whether a drug or chemical is a human teratogen, and it is usually impossible to extrapolate findings in animals directly to pregnant women (Gilstrap, Little & Brent, 1997). As clinicians gain experience with a drug, case reports may provide the first evidence that an agent is teratogenic in humans. Although human investigations are necessary to demonstrate that an agent is teratogenic, such studies are not informative until the agent has already damaged many children (Gilstrap, Little & Brent, 1997). For the best sources of information on potential teratogens, to report or investigate an exposure, or for a list of current pregnancy exposure registries, see Box 8-1.

Counseling Pregnant Patients about Drug Use

The safe use of a drug in a single pregnancy or even in a large number of pregnancies does not ensure that the drug is safe in all pregnancies (Briggs, 1995). Very few drugs can be declared "safe in pregnancy." In fact, less than 10 drugs are specifically indicated for use in pregnancy (McCombs, 1993). The present state of knowledge does not allow prediction with any degree of certainty as to when a particular drug will prove teratogenic to a particular fetus. References can only describe relative risks for a specific population, not specific risks for specific patients (Briggs, 1995). To help quantify the measure of risk a drug presents to the fetus, the FDA in 1979 prepared a list of risk factors that are assigned to all new drugs and in 1980 developed a classification scheme to aid in the selection of drug therapy for pregnant women (Little & Gilstrap, 1992). All drugs marketed after December 1983 must be labeled with a FDA Pregnancy Category Rating (Table 8-2). This system has some flaws, and since 1997, the FDA has been developing a new regulation called the Pregnancy Labeling Initiative that will revamp the pregnancy labeling system. The initiative's goal is to provide a label that effectively conveys the information necessary to counsel and prescribe for lactating and/or pregnant patients (see http://www.fda.gov/cder/present/dia1-2001/dkennedy/tsld004.htm, October, 2002).The current letter categories will be replaced with more detailed, narrative descriptions, and information on fertility, pregnancy, and breast-feeding will be included.

Additionally, several textbooks and computer online services are available to aid clinicians in determining the teratogenic potential of a drug. Several sources of information can help determine whether an agent has known teratogenic potential. However, for most drugs, there is insufficient information to make such a determination. Ultimately, the decision to prescribe a drug to a pregnant woman should be made only after a thorough discussion between the patient and her health care provider. The benefits of the drug to the mother must be weighed against the risk potential to the developing fetus.

The ideal time to counsel women regarding drug use during pregnancy is preconceptually because the critical time for problems occurs before the woman knows she is pregnant. More and more women seek information from their health care providers before conception, hoping to prevent possible adverse effects. Clinicians should stress medication use for preventive purposes, as medically indicated, and only for those medications thought to be safe for continued use during the pregnancy.

When a clinician discovers that a pregnant woman has been exposed to a dangerous drug, it is important to provide the patient with as much information as possible. First determine if the fetus was exposed during organogenesis; if so, refer for a detailed ultrasonogram and to a perinatologist. If the exposure was outside organogenesis, then ordering an ultrasonogram to reassure the mother is an option. With drugs that have a high potential for fetal damage, the patient should be encouraged to make a thoughtful decision regarding whether to continue the pregnancy (Gilstrap, Little & Brent, 1997) (Box 8-2).

COMMON CONDITIONS REQUIRING TREATMENT DURING PREGNANCY

Physiologic Changes

The physiology of pregnancy differs substantially from what is thought of as normal and profound changes occur throughout gestation. As the uterus grows from the beginning of gestation to the end of pregnancy, it progressively occupies more room

TABLE 8-2 Pregnancy Category Ratings

Category	Description
A	Adequate, well-controlled studies in pregnant women have not shown an increased risk of fetal abnormalities. The possibility of fetal harm appears remote.
B	Animal studies have revealed no evidence of harm to the fetus; however, there are no adequate and well-controlled studies in pregnant women. *or* Animal studies have shown an adverse effect, but adequate and well-controlled studies in pregnant women have failed to demonstrate a risk to the fetus.
C	Animal studies have shown an adverse effect, and there are no adequate and well-controlled studies in pregnant women. *or* No animal studies have been conducted, and there are no adequate and well-controlled studies in pregnant women. Give drugs only if the potential benefit justifies the potential risk to the fetus.
D	Studies, adequate well-controlled or observational, in pregnant women have demonstrated a risk to the fetus. However, the benefits of therapy may outweigh the potential risk. Given only if the drug is needed for a life-threatening situation or a serious disease for which safer drugs cannot be used or are ineffective.
X	Studies, adequate well-controlled or observational, in animals or pregnant women have demonstrated positive evidence of fetal abnormalities. The use of the product is contraindicated in women who are or may become pregnant.

From Meadows M: Pregnancy and the drug dilemma, *FDA Consumer magazine*, 2001.
Available at www.fda.gov/fdac/features/2001/301_preg.html#categories, accessed November 2002.

BOX 8-2

COUNSELING PREGNANT PATIENTS WHO HAVE INGESTED MEDICATIONS OR CHEMICALS

INFORMATION TO OBTAIN FROM THE PATIENT

- Name(s) of the drug(s) or chemical(s) involved.
- Exact exposure date(s).
- Exact date of the first day of the last menstrual period, to determine what organs were being formed during exposure(s).
- Exact amount(s) to which the patient was exposed.

INFORMATION TO GIVE TO THE PATIENT

- From 2% to 3% of all pregnancies result in major malformations the expected natural incidence.
- Drugs or chemicals may cause 4% to 5% of major malformations. Caffeine, nicotine, and alcohol in substantial quantities may be harmful and their use should be stopped.
- From 20% to 25% of all pregnancies are spontaneously terminated by completely undetermined factors.
- Abortions are rarely indicated following exposure to drugs, chemicals, or environmental pollutants.

Data from Gilstrap LC, Little BB, Brent RL: *Drugs and pregnancy,* New York, 1997, Chapman; and Rubin PC: Prescribing in pregnancy, *Br Med J* 293 (6559):1415–1417, 1986.

in the abdomen, pressing the digestive organs and diaphragm up toward the lungs.

Maternal blood volume increases 30% to 40% (500 to 1800 ml) to support the requirements of the developing fetus. This may lead to decreased plasma concentrations of some drugs. Renal function improves during gestation as the renal plasma flow increases 30%, and the glomerular filtration rate (GFR) increases as much as 50%. Because of this improved renal filtration, serum urea, creatinine, and uric acid levels are usually decreased in pregnancy. Cardiac output increases as much as 32% because of an increased heart rate (up 10 to 15 bpm) and increased stroke volume (McCombs, 1993).

Not all changes in the system are positive to the mother. During pregnancy, a hypercoagulable state develops, with increased levels of fibrinogen and factors VII, VIII, IX, and X. And, because bowel tone and gastrointestinal peristalsis decrease, pregnant women often have constipation. Pregnant women also have a high incidence of heartburn because of decreased gastrointestinal motility, increased estrogen and progesterone that decreases lower esophageal sphincter tone, and the increased pressure of the growing uterus on the abdomen (McCombs, 1993).

Nausea and Vomiting

Nausea and vomiting in pregnancy (NVP) affects more than 50% of pregnancies, and almost 90% of pregnancies are associated with nausea (Baron, Ramirez & Richter, 1993). NVP is self-limiting, typically starting 2 to 3 weeks after a missed menstrual period and continuing from the 8th to the 12th weeks of pregnancy. It is usually worse in the morning before getting out of bed. Although uncertain, the etiology may result from increased levels of human chorionic gonadotropin (hCG) and/or increased levels of progesterone associated with decreased gastric emptying (Baron, Ramirez & Richter, 1993).

When NVP becomes severe and intractable, it is referred to as *hyperemesis gravidarum.* This condition, affecting 3.5 of 1000 deliveries, is debilitating and can result in significant weight loss, electrolyte imbalance, ketosis, dehydration, and malnutrition (Baron, Ramirez & Richter, 1993). More recently, *H. pylori* infection has been implicated as an etiology for hyperemesis, and treatment sometimes relieves symptoms (Frigo et al, 1998). Such patients often require hospitalization for the administration of intravenous fluids and electrolytes, antiemetics, and sedation. Additionally, treatment with corticosteriods has been found to be effective (Safari et al, 1998) (see Figure 8-2).

Bendectin (10 mg doxylamine/10 mg pyridoxine) was used for NVP in an estimated 10% to 25% pregnant women in the United States from 1958 to 1983. In the 1960s, numerous birth defects (limb deformities, cleft palate, pyloric stenosis) associated with the use of Bendectin were reported worldwide (Gilstrap, Little & Brent, 1997). However, it has now received a pregnancy category rating of A. Although in 1983 the company voluntarily removed the drug from the market, the active ingredients are still available in nonprescription products (e.g., Unisom nightime sleep aid and vitamin B_6) or it can be prescribed and compounded.

Management of mild-to-moderate NVP begins with nonpharmacologic steps, such as those listed in Figure 8-2, before proceeding to medication use. Table 8-3 contains a list of common antiemetics and other drugs used during pregnancy.

Urinary Tract Infection

Bacterial infections of the urinary tract comprise the most common medical complication of pregnancy (McNeeley, 1988; Gordon & Hankins, 1989). Pregnancy itself does not cause a major increase in the acquisition of bacteria, but it sets the stage for the urinary colonization established before pregnancy to lead to symptomatic infection and subsequent invasion of the kidney.

Factors that increase the incidence of urinary tract infections in all women compound the normal physiologic changes in the pregnant woman and increase the potential for infection. Some of these factors include history of previous urinary tract infection, structural abnormalities in the urinary tract, and long periods of inactivity or sitting.

For women at risk for recurrent urinary tract infections, prevention and treatment begin with nonpharmacologic therapy: forcing fluids, wearing cotton underpants, avoiding bubble baths and pantyhose, and taking frequent breaks from sedentary activities to walk around. Choice of an antibiotic agent in pregnancy must be influenced by the potential for the agent to injure the mother and/or her developing fetus. The agents considered safe and thus most widely used in pregnancy are the penicillins and cephalosporins. The sulfonamides may displace bilirubin from albumin-binding sites and consequently have been associated with hyperbilirubinemia when administered near term. Nitrofurantoin is contraindicated near term due to the risk of hemolytic anemia. The sulfonamides and nitrofurantoin, however, have been used safely in

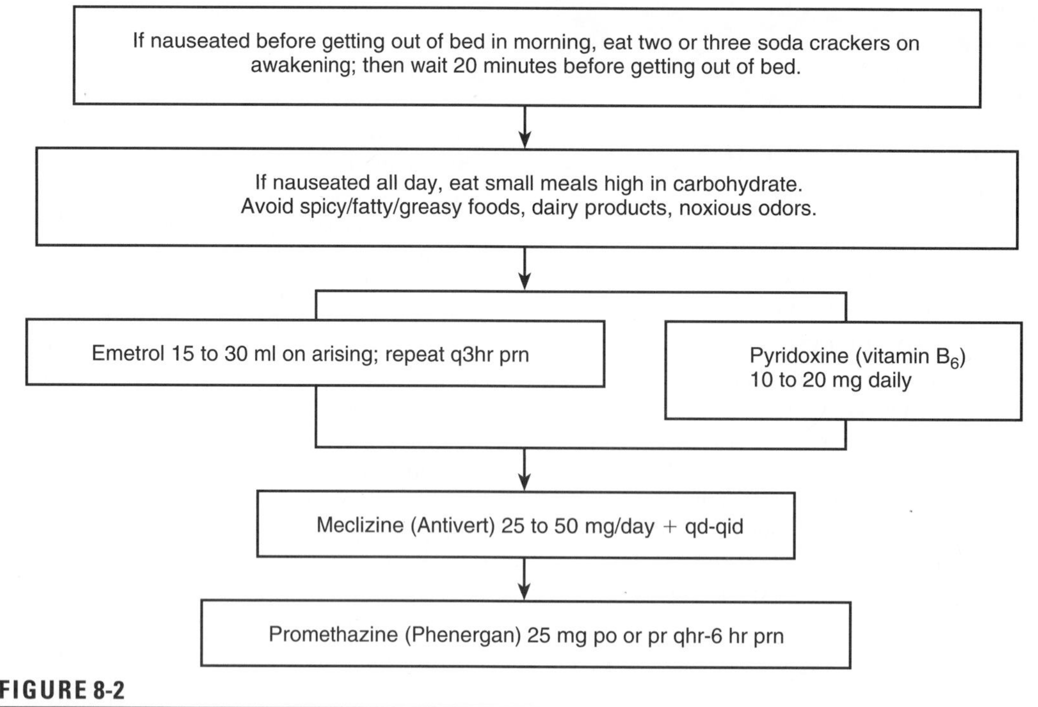

FIGURE 8-2

Suggested management of mild-to-moderate nausea and vomiting in pregnancy. (From Briggs GG, Freeman RD, editors: *Drugs in pregnancy and lactation,* ed 5, Baltimore, 1998, Williams & Wilkins.)

pregnancy when precaution is taken to discontinue before 36 weeks.

Asthma

Retrospective studies suggest that in about one third of women with asthma, asthma becomes worse during pregnancy; in one third, it becomes better, and in one third, it remains unchanged (National Institutes of Health, 1993). In women whose asthma becomes worse during pregnancy, peak severity occurs at 29 to 36 weeks of gestation. Asthma becomes less severe during the last 4 weeks of pregnancy. Wheezing during labor and delivery is uncommon, occurring in only 10% of women and usually responding to inhaled bronchodilator therapy. The change in the severity of asthma during pregnancy is sometime dramatic and tends to be consistent in subsequent pregnancies.

Poorly controlled asthma has been shown to have an adverse effect on the fetus, resulting in perinatal mortality, increased prematurity, intrauterine growth retardation, low birth weight, and neonatal hypoxia. Risks to the mother of uncontrolled asthma during pregnancy include preeclampsia, gestational hypertension, hyperemesis gravidarum, vaginal hemorrhage, and preterm labor. However, when asthma is well controlled, no increased risk of poor outcome is apparent (National Institutes of Health, 1993).

To date, there have been minimal fetal effects following extensive clinical experience with asthma medications (as opposed to controlled clinical trials). To date, no asthma medications have been proved to be teratogenic, and it is clear that the greater risk to the fetus is uncontrolled asthma (National Institutes of Health, 1993). Thus the pregnant patient who is asthmatic may continue taking the same asthma medications she was taking before she became pregnant. Although the fetus may evidence physiologic response to the medications, in most cases, the effect on the developing fetus is negligible. The primary care practitioner should examine the risk category of the different medications to maximize the risk-benefit ratio.

Upper Respiratory Tract Infections

When possible, mothers should forgo treatment with medications and treat symptoms with tincture of time, nasal saline spray, humidifiers, rest, and fluids. Pregnant patients with cough or cold symptoms requiring additional treatment may be managed with topical decongestants or pseudoephedrine and, when necessary, antibiotics (Mandell, Douglas & Bennett, 1995). See Table 8-3 for an evaluation of different medications that may be used.

Epilepsy

During pregnancy, seizure activity increases in 40% of women, decreases in 10%, and does not change in 50% of women (McCombs, 1993; Waters, 1994). While the management of epilepsy during pregnancy is beyond the expertise of the primary care provider, there is some risk-benefit and other information that the clinician may want to be aware of and/or use to provide anticipatory guidance to women of childbearing age.

First, anticonvulsant use during pregnancy has resulted in several "syndromes" and is associated with an increased incidence of malformations at two times the normal rate (Spencer, 2002; Lindhout, 1994; Schardein, 1993). Therefore 8 to 12 months before conception, a referral to a neurologist is warranted to discuss a 6-month or longer drug-free trial versus monotherapy at the lowest effective dose to minimize teratogenicity. Once pregnant (planned or unplanned), the

TABLE 8-3 Recommended Drugs for Common Problems During Pregnancy

Clinical Condition	Recommended Drugs
Nausea and vomiting	Antihistamines
	dimenhydrinate (Dramamine)
	diphenhydramine (Benadryl)
	meclizine (Antivert, Bonine)
	Phenothiazines
	promethazine (Phenergan)
	prochlorperazine (Compazine)
	doxylamine
	metoclopramide (Reglan D)
	phosphorated carbohydrate solution (Emetrol G)
	pyridoxine (vitamin B_6)
Infections	Penicillins
	Cephalosporins
	erythromycin (except estolate)
Cardiovascular	Alpha-adrenergic receptor agonists
	methyldopa (Aldomet)—B: Usually safe but benefits must outweigh the risks.
	labetalol (Normodyne, Trandate)—C: Safety for use during pregnancy has not been established.
	pindolol (Visken)—B: Usually safe but benefits must outweigh the risks.
	metoprolol (Lopressor, Toprol XL)—C: Safety for use during pregnancy has not been established.
	atenolol (Tenormin)—D: Unsafe in pregnancy
	Calcium channel blockers
	nifedipine (Adalat, Procardia)—C: Safety for use during pregnancy has not been established.
	Centrally acting alpha-adrenergic agonists
	clonidine (Catapres)—C: Safety for use during pregnancy has not been established.
	Diuretics
	hydrochlorothiazide (Esidrix, HydroDIURIL)—C: Safety for use during pregnancy has not been established.
	furosemide (Lasix)—C: Safety for use during pregnancy has not been established.
	Vasodilators—Decrease peripheral resistance by inducing vasodilation
	nitroprusside (Nitropress)—C: Safety for use during pregnancy has not been established.
	hydralazine (Apresoline)—B: Usually safe but benefits must outweigh the risks.
Anticonvulsant (for eclampsia)	Anticonvulsants—Administered to prevent seizures in severe preeclampsia or eclampsia
	phenytoin (Dilantin)—C: Safety for use during pregnancy has not been established.
	magnesium sulfate (Bilagog)—A: Safe in pregnancy
Acne	Topical benzoyl peroxide—C
	Topical clindamycin or erythromycin—B
Constipation	Bulk-forming laxatives (e.g., Metamucil, Citrucel, Perdiem)—C; Colace (docusate)—C
Heartburn/gastroesophageal reflux disease	MgAl combination antacids PRN (Milk of Magnesia)
	H_2 antagonists—B
Lice, head lice	permethrin 1% cream rinse (Nix)—B
Pubic lice	permethrin 1% cream rinse (Nix) or pyrethrins with piperonyl butoxide—B
Scabies	permethrin 5% cream (Elimite)—B

Data from Briggs GG, Freeman RG, editors: *Drugs in pregnancy and lactation*, ed 5, Baltimore, Williams & Wilkins; Baron TH, Ramirez B, Richter JE: Gastrointestinal motility disorders during pregnancy, *Ann Intern Med* 118:366-375, 1993; Kastrup et al, editors: *Facts and comparisons*, St Louis, 1998, Facts and Comparisons; McCombs J: Therapeutic considerations during pregnancy and lactation. In Dipiro JT et al, editors: *Pharmacotherapy: a pathophysiologic approach*, ed 2, Norwalk, Conn, Appleton & Lange; MMWR: Sexually transmitted diseases treatment guidelines, *MMWR Mollo Matal Wky Rep* 51:No. RR-6, 2002; ePocrates 6.0 [Computer software], 2002, available at http:www.epocrates.com/

benefit-risk ratio favors continued use of the woman's current anticonvulsant(s). Changing her medication at this point is contraindicated because it is usually too late to prevent teratogenicity and seizure control is imperative (Spencer, 2002). During pregnancy an increase in medication may be needed; therefore drug levels should be monitored frequently both during pregnancy and for 2 to 3 months postpartum, when the need may decrease (Spencer, 2002). Failure to adequately control seizures may lead to status epilepticus, which is associated with 33% maternal and 50% fetal mortality rates.

Second, maternal folic acid deficiency is induced by anticonvulsants (especially valproic acid, phenytoin, and phenobarbital), which reduce gastrointestinal absorption or increase hepatic metabolism of the vitamins with consequent increased risk of neural tube defects. Therefore folic acid supplementation is crucial; the recommendations vary from 1 to 5 mg/day (Spencer, 2002; Briggs, 1995; McCombs, 1993).

Finally, anticonvulsant use (especially phenobarbital and phenytoin) is also associated with hemorrhagic disease of the newborn. This may be caused by decreased vitamin

K–dependent clotting factors (Briggs & Freeman, 1998). Maternal prophylactic oral vitamin K (10 to 20 mg/day) beginning at 36 weeks and newborn prophylaxis with the routine 1 mg given immediately following delivery have been recommended to counteract these effects (American Academy of Pediatrics, 2000; Spencer, 2002). Postpartum breast-feeding is generally not contraindicated and may prevent withdrawal symptoms (Spencer, 2002; Lawrence & Lawrence, 1999). Risks and benefits should be discussed with each mother. Further information about managing women with epilepsy can be found in the American Academy of Neurology's 1998 practice parameters.

Diabetes

Diabetes occurs in 4% of U.S. pregnancies, of which 3% are insulin resistant (i.e., adult-onset) and 90% are gestational diabetes mellitus (GDM) (Moore, 2002). The strong correlation between the level of maternal hyperglycemia and adverse pregnancy outcome has been well established. Therefore the major imperative in management of diabetes in pregnancy is to decrease the glucose level to near normoglycemic values (Langer & Hod, 1996). Achieving normoglycemic values during pregnancy requires close surveillance and meticulous care, which is paramount to achieving optimal mother-infant outcomes.

During pregnancy the mean percentage increase in insulin requirement throughout pregnancy is 114%, compared with a 50% increase in insulin levels in normal pregnancy. It is influenced by prepregnancy maternal weight, weight gain at 20 to 29 weeks, and duration and type of diabetes. During the postpartum period, a precipitous decrease in insulin requirements occurs, and thereafter the insulin requirements gradually increase to prepregnancy levels or slightly higher in the next 5 to 7 days. From 35% to 50% of women with gestational DM will develop non–insulin-dependent diabetes mellitus within 15 years after delivery. Breast-feeding lowers insulin requirements with some mothers, with some even experiencing a complete remission that may last throughout lactation and/or for several years, delaying or reducing the risk of subsequent diabetes (Moore, 2002; Lawrence & Lawrence, 1999).

Pregnant women with diabetes mellitus should be treated with insulin (pregnancy category B), exercise, and diet. Gestational diabetics should be treated with diet and exercise with the addition of insulin as needed. Although oral agents are available, some are pregnancy category D, and while those that are category B are being researched, there is not enough evidence to support their use during pregnancy. Hence today, diet, exercise, and insulin therapy as needed remain the gold standard of care.

Hypertension

Hypertensive disorders during pregnancy are a major cause of maternal morbidity and mortality; again, while there is some pertinent information that the primary care provider may be able to use, it is best managed by the specialist. The National High Blood Pressure Education Program Working Group on High Blood Pressure in Pregnancy (National Heart, Lung, and Blood Institute, 1990) recommends that it be classified into four categories: chronic hypertension, preeclampsia-eclampsia, preeclampsia superimposed on chronic hypertension, and gestational hypertension (transient hypertension of pregnancy or chronic hypertension identified in the latter half of pregnancy). Because these terms are more precise they are preferred over the older but widely used term *pregnancy-induced hypertension*, or PIH (Gibson, 2002).

Hypertension due to preeclampsia complicates about 5% of all pregnancies, 10% of first pregnancies, and at least 20% of pregnancies in women with a history of chronic hypertension. It is the third leading cause of maternal mortality (Gibson, 2002). It is characterized by: visual disturbances such as scintillations and scotomata, headache, and epigastric pain due to hepatic inflammation and swelling; quickly increasing or nondependent edema may be a signal of emergent preeclampsia. However, the signal theory of edema was removed from most diagnostic criteria for preeclampsia (Gibson, 2002). The symptoms appear only during pregnancy or early puerperium. It most frequently appears during the 20th to 24th weeks of gestation and disappears within 40 days postpartum.

Preconceptually choosing a medication that is first line during pregnancy may be wise. Interestingly, in the first trimester some mothers experience a lowering of blood pressure and are able to discontinue their medication (Gibson, 2002). If, however, diastolic blood pressure is greater than 110 mm Hg or systolic blood pressure is greater than 160 mm Hg, regardless of the type of hypertension, treatment is imperative as these values have been associated with an increased risk of intrauterine growth restriction and placental abruption. Finally, patients should be closely monitored for adequacy of treatment to decrease risk to both mother and fetus (Gibson, 2002).

Sexually Transmitted Diseases

Prenatal testing may reveal the presence of one or more sexually transmitted diseases. Adequate treatment of these diseases is important not only for the mother's health but also to reduce the risk to the fetus.

Depression

Mothers with depression are at risk of harming themselves and/or their infant; this, of course, includes suicide and infanticide. Additionally, parenting and infant development are known to be adversely affected by maternal depression (Spencer, Gonzales & Barnhart, 2001). In a 1998 review of prospective controlled studies, both the tricyclic antidepressants and selective serotonin reuptake inhibitors were found to be potentially associated with the risk of minor physical anomalies, neonatal complications, and prematurity yet relatively safe during pregnancy (Austin & Mitchell, 1998). Subsequently, in 2000 a meta-analytical review of epidemiologic studies found that fluoxetine was not associated with the risk of any measurable teratogenic effects in during the first trimester of pregnancy (Addis & Koren, 2000). Research is ongoing in this area, and further assistance in determining the risk-benefit ratio may be found at the "Pregnancy and Depression" website, which lists many past and current studies. A final resource is the American Academy of Pediatric 2000 statement that outlines the risks of several psychotropic medications used during pregnancy for depression as well as other psychiatric illnesses. Although each case should be assessed individually and the risk-benefit ratio should be thoroughly discussed with the mother, it seems that generally the benefits of these medications outweigh the risks, particularly if the mother's disease is severe or she relapses with discontinuation of medication (Austin & Mitchell, 1998). When medication is necessary, it is prudent to prescribe the minimum effective dose. And because withdrawal syndromes have been observed in nonbreastfed infants postpartum (especially with tricyclic antidepressants), consider encouraging breast-feeding or halving the dose 1 week before delivery (Austin & Mitchell, 1998).

During lactation, sertraline (Zoloft), paroxetine (Paxil), and tricyclic antidepressants (Elavil, Pamelor, Norpramin) are a few preferred agents; fluoxetine must be used prudently, if at all, due to its long half-life (Spencer, Gonzales & Barnhart, 2001; Ito, 2000). The tricyclic antidepressants have more maternal side effects, especially drowsiness, but no side effects have been reported in their infants and after a moderate dose of 75 mg, it was essentially undetectable in the infant's serum (Hale, 2002). Several studies of sertraline generally confirm that the transfer of it or its metabolite is minimal and attainment of significant plasma levels in infants is remote when the maternal dose is less than 150 mg. Furthermore, only one ostensible infant side effect has been reported, benign neonatal sleep, which resolved independently (Hale, 2002). Studies of paroxetine generally conclude that infant serum levels are generally undetectable, and no infant side effects have been reported. (Hale, 2002). It has been suggested that mothers' treated with fluoxetine during pregnancy be transitioned to sertraline or paroxetine after delivery (Spencer, Gonzales & Barnhart, 2001). To limit exposure to fluoxetine in this scenario, one strategy would be discontinue fluoxetine 1 week before delivery and then switch her to sertraline or paroxetine shortly after delivery. Alternatively, the mother could be continued on fluoxetine while closely observing the infant and, at about 6 weeks, measuring infant serum levels of fluoxetine and norfluoxetine (Spencer, Gonzales & Barnhart, 2001).

Other Disorders

Pregnant or lactating women have the same problems as nonpregnant women. When symptoms are mild, treatment may be forgone. However, alternative treatment is not always effective, and pharmacologic preparations may be required.

KNOWN HAZARDS TO MOTHERS AND THEIR CHILDREN

Most medical literature supports a negative effect on people from use of alcohol, nicotine, caffeine, cocaine, and marijuana. However, increasing attention has been paid to these and other products and their effect on pregnancy, the unborn fetus, the neonate, and the breastfed infant. Emerging research suggests that the negative effect during pregnancy is more extensive than commonly believed. Effects on the breastfed infant from maternal use of these substances vary from minimal or none to significant morbidity, making them contraindicated during breast-feeding. The following sections outline what is known about these common substances.

Isotretinoin (Accutane)

Isotretinoin, which is used to treat severe recalcitrant nodular acne, is commonly prescribed in the United States. It can only be prescribed under SMART *(System to Manage Accutane Related Teratogenicity)*. To determine if a woman is a candidate for isotretinoin, the clinician must determine that the woman is not breast-feeding or pregnant, reliable in understanding and implementing instructions, able to understand how to prevent pregnancy, and, if currently or potentially sexually active, able to comply with using two types of contraception. A keystone to this program is the use of yellow stickers, which indicate that the woman had an initial negative pregnancy test along with a second negative test taken on the fifth day of the first menses after isotretinoin treatment has begun and thereafter ongoing negative monthly pregnancy tests. Before prescribing and to obtain the yellow stickers, the prescriber must obtain and read the SMART booklet entitled "Guide to Best Practices" and complete the letter of understanding. Isotretinoin is contraindicated during lactation because it is likely significantly secreted in human milk with the subsequent potential treatment risks.

Vaccinations

The rubella vaccine is a commonly prescribed potential teratogen. In the sexually active woman with a negative rubella titer, it is prudent to administer while on the menses and with a negative pregnancy test or immediately postpartum. She should not become pregnant for at least 2 months (Lawrence & Lawrence, 1999). When indicated, the high-risk breastfeeding mother should be vaccinated for rubella regardless of the age of the infant (Hale, 2002). Otherwise, lactating mothers of normal healthy infants may receive the immunization when the child is 1 year or older.

Caffeine

In 1980 the FDA removed caffeine from the list of compounds generally regarded as safe, citing animal evidence that caffeine caused birth defects, fetal death, and decreased birth weight. High doses (25 to 30 cups of coffee in humans) in rats caused skeletal defects, missing digits, and growth retardation. Smaller amounts (two or three cups of coffee in humans) caused delayed bone development (Oyemade, 1994).

Since then, additional studies have refuted the reported association between caffeine and birth defects. At least 15 studies have been published associating the consumption of caffeine-containing beverages during pregnancy with reproductive outcomes (Schardein, 1993). Although caffeine does not appear to be teratogenic in humans, whether it causes spontaneous abortion or low birth weight remains controversial, largely because of limitations in the studies performed to date (Oyemade, 1994).

What is known about the effects of caffeine? The amount of caffeine in an average cup of coffee (about 1.4 to 2.1 mg/kg) is safely below that inducing congenital defect in animals. Quantities in tea and soft drinks are even less. At present, there is no evidence to suggest that pregnant women should avoid caffeine completely. However, they should be encouraged to limit their intake to moderate use (about two to four caffeine-containing beverages per day) because caffeine may exert a small, but measurable, effect on fetal growth (Oyemade, 1994).

Breast-feeding mothers are encouraged to limit their intake to the equivalent of less than five cups of coffee or less than 16 oz per day of chocolate (theobromine) because although the milk levels are low, it can accumulate in the infant, causing symptoms of caffeine excess (Lawrence & Lawrence, 1999; American Academy of Pediatrics, 2001).

Alcohol

Alcohol is a known teratogen, and its use is contraindicated during pregnancy (Little & Streissguth, 1981). It is estimated that 65% of mothers in the United States continue to drink alcohol during pregnancy, exposing their fetus. The result is that as many as 5% of all congenital anomalies may be attributed to prenatal alcohol exposure (Schardein, 1993). Drinking rates during pregnancy are significantly higher among lower socioeconomic status women, those using other illicit drugs, and teenagers.

Among alcoholic women who drink during pregnancy, about 30% to 40% of their offspring will have fetal alcohol syndrome (FAS) (Briggs & Freeman, 1998; Wiemann, 1994). This syndrome is associated with altered morphogenesis, growth deficiency, and mental retardation. FAS has existed for years but has often been overlooked.

In the United States, FAS is generally estimated to occur in 1:1000 to 3:1000 live births. The incidence for children born with only partial expression of FAS may be as high as 3:1000 to 5:1000. The average IQ of children with FAS is 68, or mildly retarded (Little & Steissguth, 1981). FAS now surpasses Down syndrome and spina bifida as the leading cause of mental retardation in the United States (Lewis & Wegingold, 1985; Oyemade, 1994; McGann, 1997). Many other children will show milder effects, including growth retardation and neurologic defects. Significantly higher perinatal mortality, lower birth weight, and lower IQ, not necessarily concurrent with the full syndrome, have all been reported from studies of children of alcoholic mothers (Camilli, 1994; Day, 1993).

The quantity and chronicity of exposure are correlated with increased damage to the fetus. FAS is associated with the mother consuming the equivalent of 90 ml of absolute alcohol/day (six mixed drinks, six 4-oz glasses of wine, or six 12-oz beers) throughout pregnancy. The incidence of infants with lower birth weights occurs with as little as 30 ml absolute alcohol daily (Dicke, 1989). However, infants born to mothers who consumed an average of fewer than two drinks daily have the same rate of malformations as those born to abstinent mothers. The impact of a single drinking binge is unknown (Little & Streissguth, 1981). Despite this research, a specific safe level of alcohol consumption has not been established.

During lactation, occasional moderate use (a drink or two) is acceptable and on the American Academy of Pediatrics list of usually compatible drugs (American Academy of Pediatrics, 2001). Ideally to prevent or minimize alcohol exposure, the mother will breastfeed her infant just before drinking, drink with a meal to slow absorption, and then wait at least 2 to 3 hours to breastfeed again. Heavy or daily ingestion of more than two drinks daily has been associated with psychomotor delay and decreased linear growth (Hale, 2002; Lawrence & Lawrence, 1999). The possible risks of frequent or heavy ingestion should be discussed with the mother. If she is unable to abstain from daily or heavy ingestion, then a discussion about minimizing infant exposure and/or weaning is necessary (Hale, 2002; Lawrence & Lawrence, 1999). While intoxicated, breastfeeding should be delayed until the euphoric effects have dissipated. For each missed feeding during this period, the mother should pump and discard to remain comfortable and maintain milk supply.

Nicotine and Smoking

Cigarette use by pregnant women in urban regions generally has been found to range from 22% to 28% (Fried, 1993, McGann, 1997). Because of the significant numbers of women who smoke during pregnancy, smoking is among the most widely researched topics in teratology. Smoking has not been linked to congenital malformations but is associated with physical and intellectual growth retardation (Camilli, 1994; McGann, 1997; Wiemann, 1994).

How do clinicians help the mother who smokes? First, it is important to assess the level of risk. Clearly, the effects are dose related to the number of cigarettes smoked per day; therefore a reduction in smoking will decrease the risk of fetal retardation.

Several studies have reported that the more pronounced effects of smoking on fetal growth occur after the second trimester. Most recent studies, but not all, have reported a significant relationship between lowered birth weight and the amount of second-hand smoke to which the pregnant nonsmoking woman may be subjected.

Studies indicate that if pregnant smokers also regularly consume at least one alcoholic drink per day and consume high quantities of caffeine (five cups of coffee per day), the risk of retarded fetal growth is considerably increased (Camilli, 1994; McGann, 1997; Wiemann, 1994).

An increase in rate of spontaneous abortions in smokers has been documented, with the relative risks ranging from 1.2% to 1.8%. The greater the amount smoked, the higher is the relative risk. This may result from fetal hypoxia caused by decreased uteroplacental perfusion. Smoking during pregnancy also decreases maternal blood pressure for up to 15 minutes per cigarette smoked, thus decreasing the flow of oxygenated blood from the uterus to the placenta (Camilli, 1994; McGann, 1997; Wiemann, 1994).

Cocaine

Unlike some products with a questionable effect on mother or fetus, cocaine is a known danger to both. National estimates of fetal cocaine exposure range from 91,500 to 240,000 (about 4.5% prevalence). Cocaine and its metabolites readily cross the placenta, exposing the fetus (Bell & Lau, 1995). Many of the adverse fetal outcomes may be blamed on the powerful vasoconstrictor and hypertensive actions of cocaine. Although cocaine use is not confined to any socioeconomic group, lack of prenatal care compounds the risk to the fetus and has traditionally been a hallmark of the maternal cocaine abuser (Hutchins, 1997).

A large number of studies suggest that there are congenital defects and fetal vascular accident defects associated with the use of cocaine in pregnancy. Overall, the risk for teratogenicity for the cocaine-exposed fetus is small but still greater than the overall population. Congenital defects observed include decreased APGAR scores; strokes; congenital heart defects; and genitourinary, limb, facial, and gastrointestinal defects (Day, 1993; Hutchins, 1997; McGann, 1997; Wiemann, 1994). One consistent finding is small head circumference at birth in a fetus exposed to cocaine, which often correlates with a small brain (Bell & Lau, 1995). Other fetal risks associated with cocaine use during pregnancy include intrauterine growth retardation, prematurity, spontaneous abortion, premature rupture of membranes, placenta previa, pregnancy-induced hypertension, abruptio placentae, bradycardia, and neurobehavioral problems.

Several case reports document that infants exposed via breast-feeding experience typical adverse effects; therefore it is contraindicated during lactation. With a one-time exposure, a minimum period of 24 hours of pumping and discarding milk must occur before resuming breast-feeding (Hale, 2002).

Marijuana

The numbers of women reported to use marijuana during pregnancy ranges from 9.5% to 27% (Bell & Lau, 1995). Despite concerns about congenital malformations secondary to marijuana use during pregnancy, a cause-effect relationship has not been established (Day, 1993; Hutchins, 1997; McGann, 1997; Wiemann, 1994). Although marijuana has been found to be teratogenic in animals, maternal marijuana use during pregnancy has not been studied extensively. It has not been conclusively demonstrated that marijuana use has any negative long-term effect on fetal growth. Low birth weight and height may result from impaired fetal oxygenation from high carbon monoxide levels rather than from the marijuana itself (Bell & Lau, 1995). It is contraindicated during lactation as studies show significant absorption and metabolism in infants (Hale, 2002).

DRUGS IN BREAST-FEEDING MOTHERS

The Transfer of Drugs

Regardless of the limitations, research is ongoing in the area of lactation and some data are available for most medications. Most of the available information is derived from measurements of drug concentrations in milk or clinical observations in breast-feeding infants (Briggs, 1995; Elsevier, 1996). Many factors affect the excretion of drugs in breast milk, but most are excreted in subclinical amounts. In fact, medications are usually measured in terms of milligrams per liter (mg/L) or micrograms per liter (μg/L). To provide a prospective, 1 mg/L is the equivalent of 3 drops in 42 gallons, and 1 μg/L is the equivalent of 1 drop in 14,000 gallons (City of Garden Grove, 2000). The average intake of most infants under 6 months is less than 1 liter per day (Lawrence & Lawrence, 1999). Factors or mechanisms that determine the drug entry into breast milk include maternal plasma level (usually the most important factor), amount of protein binding and lipid solubility, molecular weight, oral bioavailability, pK_a of the drug, and half-life. Once the infant has ingested the medicated breast milk, it must evade being destroyed in the infant's gut, be absorbed through the gut wall, and then avoid being metabolized or stored in the liver before it can establish a plasma level and become bioactive in the infant (Hale, 2002; Spencer, Gonzales & Barnhart, 2001). In general these parameters explain the transfer of drugs; however, the absolute dosage the infant receives from the breast milk can really only be determined via research that measures actual milk levels (Hale, 2001).

Assessing Risk Versus Benefit

General considerations to ponder before prescribing and to assist the clinician in determining the optimal drug choice and breast-feeding management plan can be viewed at Box 8-3. Also, both the American Academy of Pediatrics and Dr. Tom Hale have assessed many medications and placed them into risk categories (Boxes 8-4 and 8-5). Keeping these details in mind, most medications (over-the-counter or prescribed) are considered safe for the breastfed infant and do not usually necessitate a disruption in breast-feeding. Moreover, medications that are approved for direct use in the infant's age group, including prednisone (up to 80 mg), fluconazole (Diflucan), inhaled albuterol (Proventil), and acyclovir (Zovirax), are also generally considered safe for use in nursing mothers (Spencer, Gonzales & Barnhart, 2001) (Tables 8-4 to 8-6). Nonetheless, certain exceptions do exist in classes of

TABLE 8-4 First and Alternative Choice Agents Used During Lactation by Maternal Ailment

Problem	First Choice	Alternative Choices
Allergic rhinitis	beclomethasone (Beconase) fluticasone (Flonase) cromolyn (Nasalcrom)	cetirizine (Zyrtec) loratadine (Claritin) Sedating antihistamines
Asthma	cromolyn (Intal) nedocromil (Tilade) albuterol (Proventil) inhaler	fluticasone (Flovent) beclomethasone (Beclovent)
Cardiovascular	hydrochlorothiazide (Oretic) metoprolol tartrate (Lopressor) propranolol (Inderal) labetalol (Normodyne)	nifedipine (Procardia XL) verapamil (Calan SR) Hydralazine (Apresoline)
Contraception	Lactational amenorrhea Barrier methods	Nonhormonal IUD Sterilization
Depression	sertraline (Zoloft) paroxetine (Paxil)	nortriptyline (Pamelor) desipramine (Norpamin) amitriptyline (Elavil)
Diabetes	Insulin glyburide (Micronase) glipizide (Glucotrol)	acarbose (Precose) tolbutamide (Orinase)
Epilepsy	phenytoin (Dilantin) carbamazepine (Tegretol)	ethosuximide (Zarontin) valproic sodium (Depakote)
Pain	ibuprofen (Motrin) morphine/codeine (<30 mg) acetaminophen (Tylenol)	hydrocodone (Vicodan)

Data from Spencer JP, Gonzalez LS, Barnhart DJ: Medications in the breast-feeding mother, *Am Fam Phys* 64:119-126, 2001; Ito S: Drug therapy for breast-feeding women, *N Engl J Med* 343:118-126, 2000; and Hale TW: *Medications in mother's milk*, Amarillo, 2002, Pharmasoft.

TABLE 8-5 Medications for which the Risks of Weaning Normally Outweigh the Risks of Using Medication while Breast-feeding

They are also considered compatible by the AAP, have a Hale rating of L3 (moderately safe), L2 (safer), or L1 (safest), and have had no significant side effects documented to date.

Always watch for applicable side effects. The author provides a foundation based on the current information for making clinical decisions. Each dyad is unique and must be individually assessed with the most up-to-date and current information.

acetaminophen (Tylenol) L1
acyclovir (Zovirax) L2
amoxicillin (Amoxil) L1
carbamazepine (Tegretol) L2
ceftriaxone (Rocephin) L2
cimetidine (Tagament) L2
clindamycin (Cleocin) L2 (vaginal)/L3 (oral)
erythromycin (E-mycin) L1 (one case of pyloric stenosis linked to ingestion through breast milk)
fluconazole (Diflucan) L2 (has an FDA safety profile for neonates ≥1 day old)
hydralazine (Apresoline) L2
ibuprofen (Advil) L1 (preferred NSAID)
labetalol (Normodyne) L2
loratadine (Claritin) L2
methocarbamol (Robaxin) L3 (limited studies)
morphine L3
nifedipine (Procardia) L2
ofloxacin (Floxin) L3 (preferred quinolones use cautiously)
penicillin G L1
prednisone ≤80 mg/day used short term
prednisolone (Prelone) L2 if ≤80 mg/day (for acute use, preferred when dosages of prednisone exceed 20 mg/day)
propranolol (Inderal) L3 (preferred β-blocker)
tetracycline (Terramycin) L2 (avoid long-term exposure)
theophylline (Theo-Dur) L3

TABLE 8-6 Medications for which the Risks of Weaning Normally Outweigh the Risks of Using Medication while Breast-feeding

They have a Hale rating of L3 (moderately safe), L2 (safer), or L1 (safest) and have had no significant side effects or precautions to date, but they have not been reviewed by the AAP.

Always watch for applicable side effects. The author provides a foundation based on the current information for making clinical decisions. Each dyad must be individually assessed with the most up-to-date and current information.

acarbose (Precose) L3
albuterol (Proventil) inhaler L1 (inhaled therapy unlikely to cause side effects)
amoxicillin with clavulanate (Augmentin) L1
azithromycin (Zithromax) L2
beclomethasone (Vanceril Inhaler) L2
cephalexin (Keflex) L1
cetirizine (Zyrtec) L2
chlorpheniramine (Chlor-Trimeton) L3
cromolyn sodium (Intal) L1
clotrimazole (Lotrimin) L1
gabapentin (Neurontin) L3 (limited data)
gentamicin (Garamycin) L2
dextromethorphan (DM) L1
dimenhydrinate (Dramanine) L2
diphenhydramine (Benadryl) L2
famciclovir (Famvir) L2 (acyclovir preferred)
famotidine (Pepcid) L2 (preferred due to low secretion)
guaifenesin (Robitussin) L2
insulin L1
lansoprazole (Prevacid) L3
meclizine (Antivert) L3
miconazole (Monistat) L2
montelukast (Singulair) L3
nedocromil sodium (Tilade) L2
nystatin (Mycostatin) L1
omeprazole (Prilosec) L2 (limited studies)
permethrin 5% (Nix) L2
prochlorperazine (Compazine) L3 (use with caution)
promethazine (Phenergan) L2 (preferred)
ranitidine (Zantac) L2
salmeterol (Serevent) L2 (limited studies)
tobramycin (Tobrex) L3
tretinoin (Retin-A) (topical) L3
valacyclovir (Valtrex) (prodrug of acyclovir) L1
zafirlukast (Accolate) L3 (>99% protein bound and poorly absorbed with food)

Data from American Academy of Pediatrics Policy Statement: Use of psychoactive medication during pregnancy and possible effects on the fetus and newborn, *Pediatrics* 110: 1035-1039, 1997; Ito S: Drug therapy for breast-feeding women, *N Engl J Med* 343:118-126, 2000; Hale TW: *Medications in mother's milk*, Amarillo, 2002, Pharmasoft; Lawrence RA, Lawrence RM: *Breastfeeding: a guide for the medical profession*, ed. 5, St Louis, 1999, Mosby.

medications, particularly among the antidepressants, immunosuppressants, and cardiovascular medications (Spencer, Gonzales and Barnhart, 2001).

Conversely, exposure to radioactive isotopes, antimetabolites, cancer chemotherapy agents, and a minute number of other medications do necessitate a temporary or permanent interruption in breast-feeding. Drugs of abuse—amphetamines, cocaine, heroin, marijuana, and phencyclidine—are all contraindicated during breast-feeding because they are hazardous to the health of both the nursing infant and the mother. Therefore the mother must choose between breast-feeding and the drug. Smoking and alcohol are special circumstances discussed previously under the section on known hazards to mothers and their children.

Overall, even though the available information is limited and there may be risks, it is important to preserve the breast-feeding relationship except for the rare previously mentioned exceptions. See Boxes 8-3 to 8-5.

BOX 8-3

CONSIDERATIONS FOR USE OF DRUGS DURING BREAST-FEEDING

1. Avoid using medication where possible but when indicated, evaluate the infant dose and perform individual risk assessment.
2. Preferred drugs are those for which there are breast-feeding data. Check for alternatives and use the safest drug.
3. For many drugs, a relative infant dose of <10% is considered safe.
4. With dangerous or radioactive compounds wait four to five half-lives before resuming breast-feeding (see http://neonatal.ama.ttuhsc.edu/lact/html/radio.html). Discontinuing breast-feeding for some hours/days may be required, particularly with radioactive compounds. To maintain a full milk supply, mothers should pump both their breasts 8 to 10 times for 15 to 20 minutes with an effective pump and discard milk. When possible, suggest she store up expressed breast milk in advance.
5. Be more cautious during the newborn period as it is generally agreed that medications penetrate milk more during the neonatal period than in mature milk production. This is particularly true for the first 10 days of life when there are large gaps between the mother's alveolar cells, which permit enhanced access for immunoglobulins and most drugs as well.
6. Choose drugs with short half-lives, high protein binding, low oral bioavailability, or high molecular weight. Be cautious with drugs that have active metabolites with longer half-lives or have long pediatric half-lives. Maternal plasma level in conjunction with degree of protein binding are usually the most important determinates of milk concentration. Only that which is "freely soluble" in the plasma can transfer into milk.
7. If there is a possibility that a drug may present a risk to the infant, consider measuring blood concentrations in the nursing infant. Exposure of the infant may be reduced by timing the dosing to occur just after feedings and/or before sleep periods in conjunction with striving to time feedings just prior to dosing or outside the peak. Using expressed breast milk from an earlier strategic pumping or substituting formula (as a last resort) for selected feedings are additional alternatives.
8. Be more cautious with preterm, low birth weight, and ill infants, especially those with liver or kidney disease.
9. Consider the side effects mostly likely to occur in the infant, and educate the mother to watch for them. Changes in feeding, stooling, mental status, behavioral changes, or weakness are the primary side effects that may forewarn of problems.
10. Many drugs are safe in breast-feeding and benefits of breast-feeding often outweigh the risks to the infant's well-being.

Modified from Hale, 2002, www.neonatal.ttuhsc.edu/lact/html/drug_entry.html; Hale, 2002, www.neonatal.ama.ttuhsc.edu/lact/html/radio.html; American Academy of Pediatrics Committee on Drugs: The transfer of drugs and other chemicals into human milk, *Pediatrics* 93:137-150, 1994; Czeizel AE, Toth M: Birthweight, gestational age, and medications during pregnancy, *Int Gynecol Obstet* 60:245-249, 1998; McCombs J: Therapeutic considerations during pregnancy and lactation. In Dipiro JT et al, editors: *Pharmacotherapy: a pathophysiologic approach,* ed 2, Norwalk, Conn, Appleton & Lange.

BOX 8-4

HALE'S LACTATION RISK CATEGORIES

L1: SAFEST

Drug that has been taken by a large number of breast-feeding mothers without any observed increase in adverse effects in the infant. Controlled studies in breast-feeding women fail to demonstrate a risk to the infant and the possibility of harm to the breast-feeding infant is remote; or the product is not orally bioavailable in an infant.

L2: SAFER

Drug that has been studied in a limited number of breast-feeding woman without an increase in adverse effects in the infant. And/or the evidence of a demonstrated risk that is likely to follow use of this medication in a breast-feeding woman is remote.

L3: MODERATELY SAFE

There are no controlled studies in breast-feeding women, however, the risk of untoward effects to a breastfed infant is possible; or, controlled studies show only minimal nonthreatening adverse effects. Drugs should be given only if the potential benefit justifies the potential risk to the infant.

L4: POSSIBLY HAZARDOUS

There is positive evidence of risk to the breastfed infant or to breast milk production but the benefits from use in breast-feeding mothers may be acceptable despite the risk to the infant (e.g., if the drug is needed in a life-threatening situation or for a serious disease for which safer drugs cannot be used or are ineffective).

L5: CONTRAINDICATED

Studies in breast-feeding mothers have demonstrated that there is significant and documented risk to the infant based on human experience, or it is a medication that has a high risk of causing significant damage to an infant. The risk of using the drug in breast-feeding women clearly outweighs any possible benefit from breast-feeding. The drug is contraindicated in women who are breast-feeding an infant.

NR: NOT REVIEWED

Milk Levels

These values are averages and may change and different studies report varying results. Consult Dr. Hale's book for more detailed information.

THEORETICAL INFANT DOSE

This is the maximum infant dose per kilogram based on current documented milk levels.

BOX 8-5

AMERICAN ACADEMY OF PEDIATRICS RISK CATEGORIES

Compatible—Maternal medication usually compatible with breast-feeding

Concern—Drugs for which the effect on nursing infants is unknown but may be of concern

Caution/Side Effects—Drugs that have been associated with significant effects on some nursing infants and should be given to nursing mothers with caution

Cessation/Temporary—Radioactive compounds that require temporary cessation of breast-feeding

Cytotoxic—Cytotoxic drugs that may interfere with cellular metabolism of the nursing infant

NR—Not reviewed

Management of Interruption or Weaning

> "Even a temporary interruption in breast-feeding carries the risk of premature weaning, with the subsequent risks of long-term artificial feeding."
>
> (American Academy of Family Physicians, 2002)

> "Any recommendation to interrupt breast-feeding or recommending weaning must clearly outweigh the benefits conferred by nursing."
>
> (Ito, page 118, 2000).

The American Academy of Pediatrics Committee on Drugs periodically publishes a policy statement regarding the transfer of drugs and other chemicals into human milk but it is a limited resource due to infrequent updates, omissions, and inadequate detail on the medications (Spencer, Gonzales & Barnhart, 2001). To assist in the furthering of knowledge in this field, a lactation registry exists to document the effects of a wide variety of medications in exposed infants and their impact on maternal lactation, in addition to, registering mothers with certain health conditions including breast-feeding related problems (see Box 8-3).

REFERENCES

Addis A, Koren G: Safety of fluoxetine during the first trimester of pregnancy: a meta-analytical review of epidemiological studies, *Psychol Med* 30:89-94, 2000.

American Academy of Family Physicians Policy Statement on Breastfeeding, 2002. Available at www.aafp.org/x6633.xml

American Academy of Pediatrics Committee on Drugs: The transfer of drugs and other chemicals into human milk, *Pediatrics* 108:776-789, 2001.

American Academy of Pediatrics Policy Statement: Breastfeeding and the use of human milk, *Pediatrics* 100:1035-1039, 1997.

American Academy of Pediatrics: Policy Statement: Use of psychoactive medication during pregnancy and possible effects on the fetus and newborn, *Pediatrics* 105:880-887, 2000.

American Diabetes Association: Clinical practice recommendations, *Diabetes Care* 20:1044-1045, 1997.

Austin MV, Mitchell PB: Psychotropic medications in pregnant women: treatment dilemmas, *Med J Austral* 169:428-431, 1998.

Baron TH, Ramirez B, Richter JE: Gastrointestinal motility disorders during pregnancy, *Ann Intern Med* 118:366-375, 1993.

Bell GL, Lau K: Perinatal and neonatal issues of substance abuse, *Pediatr Clin North Am* 42:261-281, 1995.

Blake DA, Niebyl JR: Requirements and limitations in reproductive and teratogenic risk assessment. In Niebyl JR, editor: *Drug use in pregnancy*, ed 2, Philadelphia, 1988, Lea & Febiger.

Briggs GG: Drugs in pregnancy and lactation. In Young LL, Koda-Kimball MM, editors: *Applied therapeutics: the clinical use of drugs*, ed 6, Vancouver WA, 1995, Applied Therapeutics.

Briggs GG, Freeman RG, editors: *Drugs in pregnancy and lactation*, ed 5, Baltimore, 1998, Williams & Wilkins.

Camilli AE et al: Smoking and pregnancy: a comparison of Mexican-American and non-Hispanic white women, *Obstet Gynecol* 84:1033-1037, 1994.

Centers for Disease Control and Prevention: 2002 Sexually transmitted diseases treatment guidelines, *MMWR* 51(RR-6), 2002.

Chantry CJ, Howard CR, Auinger P: Breastfeeding fully for six months versus four months decreases risk of respiratory tract infection, *Abstr ABM News Views* 8:20-21, 2002.

City of Garden Grove: 2000 Water quality report, Public Works Department—Water Service Division, 13802 Newhope Street, Garden Grove, CA 92843.

Collaborative Group on Hormonal Factors in Breast Cancer: Breast cancer and breastfeeding: collaborative reanalysis of individual data from 47 epidemiological studies in 30 countries, including 50 302 women with breast cancer and 96 973 women without the disease, *Lancet* 360:187-195, 2002.

Cunningham AS: Breast-feeding and morbidity in industrialized countries: an update. In Jelliffe DB, Jelliffe EFP, editors. *Advances in international maternal and child health*, Oxford, England, 1981, Oxford University Press.

Czeizel AE, Toth M: Birthweight, gestational age, and medications during pregnancy, *Int Gynecol Obstet* 60:245-249, 1998.

Day NL et al: The epidemiology of alcohol, marijuana, and cocaine use among women of childbearing age and pregnant women, *Clin Obstet Gynecol* 36:237-245, 1993.

Dicke JM: Teratology: principles and practice, *Med Clin North Am* 73:567-582, 1989.

Drugs and human lactation: a comprehensive guide to content and consequences of drugs, micronutrients, radiopharmaceuticals, and environmental and occupational chemicals in human milk, New York, 1996, Elsevier Science.

ePocrates 6.0 [computer software], 2002. Available at www.epocrates.com

Expert Panel Report 2: *Guidelines for the diagnosis and management of asthma*, Bethesda, MD, April 1997, National Asthma Education and Prevention Program, National Institutes of Health, National Heart, Lung, and Blood Institute (No. 97-4051).

Forste R, Weiss J, Lippincott E: The decision to breastfeed in the United States: does race matter? *Pediatrics* 108:291-296, 2001.

Fried PA: Prenatal exposure to tobacco and marijuana: effects during pregnancy, infancy, and early childhood, *Clin Obstet Gynecol* 36:319-337, 1993.

Frigo P et al: Hyperemesis gravidarum associated with *Helicobacter pylori* seropositivity, *Obstet Gynecol* 91:615-617, 1998.

Gibson P. Hypertension and pregnancy, June 14, 2002. Available at www.emedicine.com/med/topic3250.htm.

Gilstrap LC, Little BB, Brent RL: *Drugs and pregnancy*, New York, 1997, Chapman.

Gordon MC, Hankins GD: Urinary tract infections and pregnancy, *Compr Ther* 15:52-58, 1989.

Hale T, Ilett K: *Drug therapy and breastfeeding: from theory to clinical practice*, Boca Raton, FL, 2002, Parthenon Publishing Group.

Hale TW: *Drug entry into human milk*, 2001. Available at www.neonatal.ttuhsc.edu/lact/html/drug_entry.htnl

Hale TW: *Medications in mothers' milk*, ed 10, Amarillo, 2002, Pharmasoft.

Hod M, Langer O: Fuel metabolism in deviant fetal growth in offspring of diabetic women, *Obstet Gynecol Clin North Am* 23:259-277, 1996.

Hollingsworth DR: Drugs and reproduction: maternal and fetal risks. In Gilstrap LC, Little BB, editors: *Drugs and pregnancy*, New York, 1988, Elsevier.

Hutchins E et al: Psychosocial risk factors associated with cocaine use during pregnancy: a case-control study, *Obstet Gynecol* 90:142-147, 1997.

Ito S: Drug therapy for breast-feeding women, *N Engl J Med* 343:118-126, 2000.

Kastrup EK et al, editors: *Drug facts and comparisons,* St Louis, 2003, Facts and Comparisons.

Koren G, Cohen MS: Special aspects of perinatal and pediatric pharmacology. In Katzung BG, editor: *Basic and clinical pharmacology,* ed 6, Norwalk, Conn, 1994, Appleton & Lange.

Langer O, Hod M: Management of gestational diabetes mellitus, *Obstet Gynecol Clin North Am* 23:137-159, 1996.

Lawrence RA, Lawrence RM: *Breastfeeding: a guide for the medical profession,* ed 5, St. Louis, 1999, Mosby.

Lewis DD, Woods SE: Fetal alcohol syndrome, *Am Fam Phys* 50:1025-1032, 1994.

Lewis JH, Weingold AB: The use of gastrointestinal drugs during pregnancy and lactation, *Am J Gastroenterol* 80:912-921, 1985.

Lindhout D et al: Teratogenic effects of antieleptic drugs: implications for the management of epilepsy in women of child-bearing age, *Epilepsia* 35(suppl 4):519-528, 1994.

Little BB, Gilstrap LC: In Gilstrap LC, Little BB, editors: *Drugs and pregnancy,* New York, 1992, Elsevier.

Little RE, Streissguth AP: Effects of alcohol on the fetus: impact and prevention, *Can Med J* 125:159-164, 1981.

Mandell GL, Douglas RG, Bennett JR, editors: *Principles and practice of infectious diseases,* ed 4, New York, 1995, Churchill-Livingstone.

McCombs J: Therapeutic considerations during pregnancy and lactation. In Dipiro JT et al, editors: *Pharmacotherapy: a pathophysiologic approach,* ed 2, Norwalk, Conn, 1993, Appleton & Lange.

McGann KP et al: Alcohol, tobacco and illicit drug use among women, *Primary Care* 24:113-122, 1997.

McNeeley SG: Treatment of urinary tract infections during pregnancy, *Clin Obstet Gynecol* 31:480-487, 1988.

Meadows M: Pregnancy and the drug dilemma, *FDA Consumer Magazine,* 2001. Available at www.fda.gov/fdac/features/2001/301_preg.html# categories

Moore TR: Diabetes mellitus and pregnancy. Available at www.emedicine.com/MED/topic3249.htm

Moreland J, Coombs J: Promoting and supporting breast-feeding, *Am Fam Physician* 61:2093-2100, 2103-2104, 2000.

Mortenson EL et al: The association between duration of breastfeeding and adult intelligence, *JAMA* 287:2365-2371, 2002.

National Institutes of Health, National Heart, Lung, and Blood Institute, National Asthma Education Program: *Report of the working group on asthma and pregnancy: executive summary: management of asthma during pregnancy*, Bethesda, MD, March 1993, National Institutes of Health (No. 93-3279A), pp. 1-20.

Niebyl JR: Drug therapy during pregnancy, *Curr Opin Obstet Gynecol* 4:43-47, 1992.

Oyemade UJ et al: Prenatal substance abuse and pregnancy outcomes among African-American women, *J Nutr* 124(6 suppl):9945-9995, 1994.

Pinson JB: Management of urinary tract infections in pregnancy, *Pharm Perspect Ambulatory Care* 3:103-109, 1991.

Pregnancy Labeling Initiative, October 2002. Available at www.fda.gov/cder/present/dial-2001/dkennedy/tsld004.htm

Report of the National High Blood Pressure Education Program Working Group on high blood pressure in pregnancy, *Am J Obstet Gynecol* 183(1):S1-S22, 2000.

Rubin PC: Prescribing in pregnancy, London, 1986, British Medical Journal Publishing.

Safari HR et al: Experience with oral methylprednisolone in the treatment of refractory hyperemesis gravidarum, *Am J Obstet Gynecol* 178:1054-1058, 1998.

Schardein JL: *Chemically induced birth defects,* ed 2, New York, 1993, Marcel Dekker.

Simone C, Derewlany LO, Koren G: Drug transfer across the placenta: considerations in treatment and research, *Clin Perinatol* 21:463-481, 1995.

Sobel JD, Kaye D: Urinary tract infections. In Mandell GL, Douglas RG, Bennett JR, editors: *Principles and practice of infectious disease,* ed 5, New York, 2000, Churchill Livingstone.

Spencer D: Women's health and epilepsy, April 19, 2002. Available www.emedicine.com/neuro/topic613.htm

Spencer JP, Gonzales LS, Barnhart DJ: Medications in the breast-feeding mother, *Am Fam Physician* 64:119-126, 2001.

Szeto HH: Kinetics of drug transfer to the fetus, *Clin Obstet Gynecol* 36:246-254, 1993.

U.S. Preventive Services Task Force: *Screening for gestational diabetes mellitus: recommendations and rationale,* Rockville, MD, February 2003, Agency for Healthcare Research and Quality (originally in *Obstet Gynecol* 101:393-395, 2003). Available at www.ahrq.gov/clinic/3rduspstf/gdm/gdmrr.htm

Waters CH et al: Outcomes of pregnancy associated with antiepileptic drugs, *Arch Neurol* 53:250-253, 1994.

Wiemann CM et al: Tobacco, alcohol and illicit drug use among pregnant women: age and racial/ethnic differences, *J Repro Med* 39:769-776, 1994.

UNIT 3

The Therapeutic Experiment

CHAPTER 9

Over-the-Counter Medications

Consumers are more educated about health maintenance recommendations and more likely to pursue OTC self-treatment remedies than ever before. Client-initiated health care remedies with over-the-counter (OTC) medications were a booming business in the United States in 2001, with Americans spending $17.8 billion (excluding Wal-Mart sales) on nonprescription remedies (Consumer Health Care Products Association, 2003). Since 1976, 73 ingredients, dosages, or indications have been considered safe enough to be "switched" from prescription to OTC status (Consumer Health Care Products Association, 2003). As a result, most pharmaceutical prescriptions are only part of the drug armamentarium that clients use to improve well-being or treat maladies and illnesses.

EXTENT OF OTC MEDICATION USE

The OTC business in the United States is so large, with more than 300,000 OTC products available in the marketplace (Consumer Health Care Products Association, 2003), that it has been reported that people would rather choose a new car than be faced with the task of determining which OTC they should buy for a particular ailment. The role of OTCs in today's health care is growing because of a more educated consumer and an active self-care movement.

The Nonprescription Drug Manufacturers Association (NDMA) estimates that more than 100,000 products are now available on an OTC basis—200 of these were once available only by prescription. These products contain one or more of about 700 active ingredients and are available in a variety of dosage forms, sizes, and strengths. OTC sales total more than $20 billion a year. The top selling categories of OTCs include cough/cold remedies ($3009 million) and headache remedies ($2045 million) (Consumer Health Care Products Association, 2003). It has been estimated that 77% of Americans take an OTC product to treat common everyday ailments, with adults 65 years and older consuming 33% of all OTC medicines sold in the United States (Consumer Health Care Products Association, 2003).

Nonprescription medications, or OTCs, are defined as drugs considered to be safe and effective without professional supervision, providing the required label directions and warnings are followed. OTC products differ from prescription medications in the following ways (APC, 1998):

- There is a wider margin of safety because most of these drugs have undergone rigorous testing before marketing and have undergone further refinement by years of OTC use by consumers.
- OTCs are advertised directly to the consumer. (This characteristic is no longer exclusive to OTC products, however, as competition for larger markets has induced the pharmaceutical industry to advertise prescription medications, urging consumers to ask their health care provider about them.)
- The distribution of OTCs makes them much more widely available than prescription drugs.

The most common categories of OTCs parallel the products available by prescription, essentially providing the public access to medications without a health care provider's intervention. These include laxatives, acid-peptic disorder products (antacids, H_2-receptor antagonists), analgesics, cough/cold products (antihistamines, decongestants, expectorants, antitussives), vaginal antifungals, smoking cessation products, and topical steroids.

OTCs are sold in pharmacies, grocery stores, gas stations, and many other outlets. Probably less than half of all OTC products are sold in pharmacies. Because there are so many different names and reformulations of products, it is important to learn the drug name, not the product name. In addition, many of these products have multiple ingredients. The cost of buying multiple-ingredient products can be more than buying the ingredients singly, so it is important to check out commonly used products for price.

Surveys show that women are the family members most likely to purchase OTC products and are also more likely to read labels on medicines before taking them than are men. The Food and Drug Administration requires OTC product labels to present all-important information in a manner that a typical consumer can read and understand. Plans are under way to establish a standardized labeling format for all nonprescription drugs marketed in the United States. Key information, beginning with active ingredients, followed by purpose(s), uses, warnings, and directions, would be placed in the same order on all OTC packages in a more readable format.

Nonprescription drug labels have more information than prescription drugs. In May 2002, a new consumer-friendly label was introduced for many OTC products, with all categories of OTC products using the new label by 2005. The new label is based on FDA research that concluded that many consumers could not read the small print on labels, could not understand some of the complex words, and could not discern what information was the most important to them because there was no standardized format. The new format has simple language, easier-to-read type, and a standardized format that lists all active ingredients first, uses next, and warnings and directions for dosage in clearly marked sections.

One of the most important things in reading labels for OTC products is to determine the presence of additional ingredients in a product that might pose some risk to some patients. These hidden ingredients are included for different purposes and may be in the form of preservatives, color additives, delivery, or stabilizing products. If someone has an allergy or intolerance to even small doses of these products, they may not be aware of the risk unless they read the label. Table 9-1 lists common ingredients present in OTC products.

Health care providers should discuss some basic principles about OTC products with patients. Many providers share this through patient information handouts because it is so important for patients to have this information. Whether given verbally or in writing, the following are some basic principles patients should learn:

- Always read label instructions.
- Do not take OTC medicine in higher dosages or for a longer time than indicated on the label.
- If a symptom persists, stop self-treatment and talk with a health care professional.
- Side effects from OTCs are relatively uncommon but know what the potential side effects of the medicine may be.
- Every person is different, and reactions to medicine may also differ.
- All medicines have the potential to interact with other medicines, with food, or with preexisting conditions.
- If you do not understand label instructions, check with a pharmacist to have any questions answered.
- Discard medications after the expiration date.

Parents, in particular, should be aware of special information about using OTCs for children:

- Never guess at the amount of medicine to give a child. Half an adult dose may be too much or not enough to be effective. This is especially true of medicines such as Tylenol or Advil, where several overdoses may actually lead to poisoning, liver destruction, or coma.
- Avoid making conversions. If the label says two teaspoons and you are using a dosing cup with ounces only, get another measuring device.
- Always follow the age-limit recommendations. If the label says not to give a medicine to a child under 2, do not do it.
- Always use the child-resistant cap and relock the cap after use.
- Throw away old, discolored, or expired medicines or medicines that have lost their label instructions.
- Do not give medicines containing alcohol to children.

Trends to watch in the OTC category are (1) the movement of pharmacists to become providers of pharmaceutical care as well as dispensers and (2) the development of a third class of drugs that could only be purchased after talking to a pharmacist.

ADVANTAGES AND DISADVANTAGES TO OTC USE

Buying OTC products from a variety of sources means that most consumers are not talking to health care providers about their symptoms. Patients may be selecting OTC products without giving full consideration as to how these products interact with other medications or what are their side effects. However, consumers have also taken to the Internet and other media outlets to learn more about common ailments and have become more informed regarding their bodies and ways to promote good health. As informed consumers, they are able to make better decisions about OTC products and using them safely.

The rate of products switching from prescription to OTC status appears to be increasing. From the mid 1980s to the mid 1990s, approximately one drug was switched annually. A flurry of activity began in 1995, with the reclassification of several drug classes, including H_2-receptor antagonists for heartburn, nicotine gum and patches, pediatric analgesics, and hair-growth formulations.

Formerly, prescription-only drugs that were granted OTC approval were intended to treat acute or episodic conditions with recognizable symptoms. OTC products were not designed for chronic conditions or diseases that required laboratory tests for either diagnosis or monitoring. Now, many OTC drugs are being used for chronic conditions. This movement gained popularity because of research demonstrating that chronic health conditions are highly undertreated because many Americans lack health insurance. Proponents argue that if drugs to treat many conditions were available over the counter, they might be more widely used. Opponents suggest that many patients

TABLE 9-1 Hidden Ingredients in Over-the-Counter Products

Hidden Drug	OTC Class that May Contain Drug
alcohol (ethanol)	Cough syrups/cold preparations; mouthwashes
Antihistamines	Analgesics, asthma products, cold/allergy products, dermatologic preparations; menstrual products, motion sickness products, antiemetics, sleep aids, topical decongestants
Antimuscarinic agents	Antidiarrheals, cold/cough/allergy preparations, hemorrhoidal products
aspirin and other salicylates	Analgesics, antidiarrheals, cold/allergy preparations, menstrual products, sleep aids
caffeine	Analgesics, cold/allergy products, menstrual or diuretic products, stimulants, weight control products
Estrogens	Hair creams
Local anesthetics (usually benzocaine)	Antitussives; dermatologic preparations; hemorrhoidal products; lozenges; toothache, cold sore, and teething products; weight loss products
Sodium	Analgesics, antacids, cough syrups, laxatives
Sympathomimetics	Analgesics, asthma products, cold/allergy preparations, cough syrups, hemorrhoidal products, lozenges, menstrual products, topical decongestants, weight control products

Modified from Katzung BG: *Basic and clinical pharmacology*, ed. 8, Norwalk, Conn, 2000, Appleton & Lange.

who self-diagnose themselves may go from undertreatment to inappropriate or harmful self-treatment or that patients' conditions will worsen because of inaccurate treatment. Emergency contraception, antimicrobials, and statins are all drugs for which there is great debate about the safety of moving them to OTC products.

The National Council on Patient Information and Education sponsored a survey in which one third of the sample reported that they take more than the recommended dose of nonprescription medicine, believing it will increase the effectiveness of the product. The survey also found that one third said that they are likely to combine OTC medications when they have multiple symptoms. About half of the respondents got their information about the drugs from the mass media and the other half from health professionals (New Drug Facts Label to Help Consumers, 2002).

Some products in OTC medications have fallen into disfavor over time. Phenylpropanolamine and ephedra alkaloids (such as ephedrine) are stimulants (sympathomimetic agents). As stimulants, they have a hypertensive effect that puts some patients at increased risk of heart attack or stroke, especially those with a history of cardiac and hypertensive disease. These adverse effects were the basis for the Food and Drug Administration requiring these agents be removed from products on the market.

Primary care providers should focus on some important principles guiding OTC use, including the following:

- Collect a good database based on a comprehensive drug history.
- Recommend nondrug therapies first, such as exercise, diet, fluids, and rest.
- Look at specific symptoms and treat each separately.
- Select the product that is simplest in formulation with regard to ingredients and dosage. Generally, single-ingredient formulations are preferred.
- Select products that contain therapeutically effective dosing. Watch out for combination products that may contain therapeutic doses of one ingredient and subtherapeutic doses of others.
- Read labels carefully. Products can change names and change the doses of one or more ingredients. Many products contain extended-release properties that may or may not be of benefit to the patient.
- Be wary of advertising claiming the superiority of new products that are, in reality, only the old product in new packaging at higher prices.
- Watch for differences in prices and recommend generic products when available.

VITAMINS AND MINERALS

A major category of client-initiated and -controlled therapy are the vitamin and minerals. Clients frequently decide that they need vitamins. They may or may not seek consultation from a health care provider or pharmacist about what to take. Many products are on the market, and the price varies markedly for the same product. What is fact and what is fiction about the use of vitamins and minerals?

Vitamania has swept the country, with sales of vitamins and minerals soaring to record highs. Americans are using vitamins to fend off cancer, to enhance immunity, to cope with stress, to get stronger bones, and to increase a sense of well-being. The marketing industry has suggested that natural products are better than synthetic vitamins. Not all claims for vitamins have been proved. Costs for some products have greatly increased based on product claims. But does *better* necessarily mean *more expensive?*

What is known is that vitamin and mineral supplements are useful when there are deficiencies, such as in young women and the elderly. Benefits to the average healthy individual who consumes a variety of foods have not been proved. However, some health care groups are suggesting that individuals might benefit from a daily vitamin because of the generally poor nutrition of many Americans. Vitamins are probably the same, whether they are natural or synthetic, costly or cheap. In fact, natural vitamins may contain other products or impurities that may make them less effective than synthetic or more standardized products. However, some preparations dissolve better than others or are in amounts that facilitate the absorption of other coadministered vitamins and minerals.

National surveys have shown that those who least need supplements are the most likely to take them, such as individuals who eat right, exercise, and do not smoke. There is no evidence that clients who take vitamins live longer or have fewer cancers.

There are known dangers to vitamin use, especially high-dose use. Megadoses of vitamins are rapidly excreted into the urine, with no additional benefit to the client. Occasionally, large doses of vitamin A may be stored in the tissues, producing a yellow hue to the skin. Most vitamin products can be toxic to children, and iron supplements can be deadly to small children. Folic acid can react adversely with anticancer treatment medications and mask signs of vitamin B_{12} deficiency. Sometimes the body becomes dependent on large doses of vitamin C when it is taken over a prolonged period of time; a period of deficiency may be noted with a return to normal doses. Clients with increased colon transit times may excrete some vitamin and mineral products unchanged in the stool.

Large amounts of calcium can limit the absorption of iron and other trace elements. They can also cause constipation and impair kidney function. Calcium is needed primarily in menopausal women and older men, particularly those who are at risk for bone loss.

Antioxidant vitamins occupy a large niche in the current literature on nutritional supplements. The major vitamin antioxidants are vitamin E or alpha-tocopherol, beta-carotene or provitamin (precursor to vitamin A), vitamin C or ascorbic acid, and selenium. All of these are found in fruits and vegetables. Many research studies are in the process of studying the mechanism of action of antioxidants. Current research suggests that when low-density lipoprotein (LDL) cholesterol is oxidized, incomplete oxidation often takes place, producing free radicals that are conducive to atherosclerotic plaques. (The analogy has been made to wood that burns incompletely in a fireplace and "pops," sending sparks against the screen.) It is thought that antioxidants retard or prevent LDL oxidation because they are preferentially oxidized over LDL. This slows or eliminates the progression of atherosclerosis. It is also believed that antioxidants slow the process that predisposes cells to cancer. This has resulted in a large market for antioxidants to decrease cardiovascular disease and cancer.

Although many major research studies have looked at antioxidants retrospectively and have suggested major benefits from increased utilization for many disease states, there are at present no intervention studies that determine conclusively that antioxidants prevent cancer. Epidemiologic evidence does indicate that those who eat fruits and vegetables regularly have a decreased risk of cancer. There is no conclusive evidence that this is the result of antioxidants. Therefore supplementation with vitamin antioxidants may be beneficial, but, in certain populations, such as smokers, it may actually be harmful (see Chapter 74 for information on vitamins).

Supplements cannot make up for a poor diet or other unhealthful lifestyle practices such as smoking or lack of exercise. If patients do not eat a well-balanced diet and eat large amounts of high-fat or empty calorie foods, they may want to consider taking a multivitamin/mineral. If patients cannot tolerate certain foods (dairy products, for example), they may need to supplement their diet to ensure they are getting the nutrients provided by that food group.

Most women in the United States age 20 or older consume about 1673 calories a day. Women who diet may eat fewer calories and must work harder to get the Recommended Dietary Allowances for essential vitamins and minerals. The Food Guide Pyramid chart reminds people to balance what they are eating. Balance is important not only to ensure consumption of essential nutrients daily but to take advantage of the positive interactions among the different food groups. For example, vitamin C aids in iron absorption, so a slice of tomato on a turkey sandwich does more than look nice.

There is, however, a growing body of research that suggests intakes of specific nutrients may be helpful in protecting against conditions such as osteoporosis, birth defects, heart disease, stroke, infectious disease, macular degeneration, and cataracts. These products are clearly prescribed for health promotion. Prominent among these products are the supplements discussed in the following sections.

Calcium

In 1993 the FDA approved a health claim to appear on food and supplement labels recognizing the role of calcium in reducing the risk of osteoporosis and the need for calcium supplements by people who fail to obtain adequate levels of calcium from their diets. The current recommendation calls for people over the age of 50 to consume at least 1200 mg of calcium daily. More than three glasses of low-fat milk per day would be required to provide this much calcium. Calcium-fortified products such as orange juice, sardines, salmon, tofu, and other dairy products help meet the daily requirements. The calcium citrate malate, found in fortified orange juice, is one of the best forms of calcium supplement because it tends to be absorbed better than other types. The calcium carbonate found in Tums and other antacids is also acceptable. Vitamin D is important for calcium absorption. It is available in multivitamins, from exposure to the sun, and from fortified milk. Some calcium products also come with a small amount of magnesium, which also facilitates calcium absorption. Calcium supplements are best absorbed when taken with food because food slows down the passage of nutrients through the large intestine.

Folic Acid, Vitamin B_6, and Vitamin B_{12}

There are a great deal of scientific data showing that increased consumption of foods containing folate (citrus fruits, cereals, leafy greens, and whole grains) or taking a multivitamin containing folic acid protects against birth defects such as neural tube defect, spina bifida, and anencephaly and may also reduce the risk of heart disease and stroke. The neural tube of the fetus is formed within the first 28 days of pregnancy, before many women know they are pregnant. However, the scientific evidence of the benefit of folic acid in preventing neural tube defects is so strong that the U.S. Public Health Service issued an official recommendation that "all women of childbearing age in the United States who are capable of becoming pregnant should consume 0.4 mg of folic acid per day for the purpose of reducing their risk of having a pregnancy affected with spina bifida or other neural tube defects." This recommendation should continue for women throughout their childbearing years.

Scientific studies have also shown that modestly elevated homocysteine levels in the blood are a risk factor for heart disease. Folic acid and vitamins B_6 and B_{12} have been shown to reduce homocysteine levels. Intake of these three B vitamins, found primarily in vegetables and legumes, has been shown to be low in the United States, particularly in the elderly. Vitamin B_{12} is found in meat and fish but is not absorbed as readily by people as they age. Some experts are suggesting that enough research has shown that those at risk for heart disease should take a supplement that contains folic acid and vitamins B_6 and B_{12}. Folic acid may be more readily absorbed from supplements and enriched foods than from other sources.

Iron

Iron supplements have long been known to be necessary for those who have anemia resulting from blood loss. Hence young women of childbearing age are often placed on iron supplements. Iron supplements for those not experiencing blood loss have not been shown to be needed or desirable. High levels of iron in the blood can result in heart disease, cancer, and serious infection. Most menopausal women probably could take a multivitamin containing 10 milligrams of iron or less.Vitamins for senior citizens do not contain iron. Iron and calcium supplements should be taken at different times because these two minerals compete for absorption.

Aspirin

The benefits of aspirin use in patients with prior occlusive cardiovascular disease are clear. In both men and women with a wide range of prior cardiovascular disease from a past heart attack or occlusive stroke to angina, coronary bypass surgery, or angioplasty, data from randomized trials demonstrate clear benefits of long-term aspirin therapy. For those in the acute phase of an evolving heart attack, the net benefits of aspirin use are also clear: immediate treatment of all such patients with aspirin will save lives as well as reduce the risk of experiencing another heart attack or a stroke. For those individuals without prior occlusive vascular disease, the side effects of aspirin are the same as for those who have had occlusive vascular events. Thus research has not conclusively determined whether any benefits of aspirin for these individuals outweigh the risks, which include an increased tendency to bleed. One large-scale randomized trial, the Physicians' Health Study, showed conclusively that low-dose aspirin reduced the risk of a first heart attack by 44% in apparently healthy men. There is one ongoing long term study of aspirin use among apparently healthy women but the findings are not yet available. Moreover, even the data in men from the Physicians' Health Study are inconclusive regarding the effect of aspirin on stroke and cardiovascular deaths. These are crucial questions to answer because there is concern that any drug that decreases the tendency to clot might increase the tendency to bleed and contribute to higher risks of hemorrhagic stroke (see Chapter 30).

SUMMARY

OTC preparations, including vitamin and mineral products, constitute a vast proportion of health care products and health care expenditures for individuals of many nations. As the results from research studies become more conclusive, it will continue to be the responsibility of health care providers to communicate to patients about the safety, effectiveness, and dangers inherent in these widely available products.

RESOURCES FOR PATIENTS AND PROVIDERS

Books

Aspen Reference Group: Clinician's handbook of preventive services for primary care physicians. In *Preventive care sourcebook,* Frederick, MD, 1997-1998, 1997, Aspen Publishers.

Labarthe DR: *Epidemiology and prevention of cardiovascular diseases,* Frederick, MD, 1998, Aspen Publishers.

Internet Resources

Food and Drug Administration. Available at www.fda.gov

Provider and consumer information about over-the-counter drugs available at www.ndmainfo.org, nonprofit group whose mission it is to provide better health through responsible self-medication. Site features patient concerns on legal and regulatory issues such as product labeling, industry self-regulation, and relationships with the Food and Drug Administration and making prescription status–to–OTC status switches. Has the latest statistics on OTCs.

Organizations

Food and Drug Administration, Office of Consumer Affairs
HFE 88, 5600 Fishers Lane, Rockville, MD 20857
(301) 827-4420 or (800) 532-4440; www.fda.gov

Consumer Health Care Products Association (formerly Nonprescription Drug Manufacturers Association)
1150 Connecticut Avenue, NW, Suite 1200
Washington, DC 20036
(202) 429-9260; Fax (202) 223-6835; www.ndmainfo.org

The American Geriatrics Society
The Empire State Building
350 Fifth Avenue, Suite 801
New York, NY 10118
(202) 308-1414; americangeriatrics.org

REFERENCES

American Pharmaceutical Council, *Statistics on healthcare,* Washington, DC, 1998, APA.

Consumer Health Care Products Association (CHPA). Available at www.CHPA.org

Katzung BG: *Basic and clinical pharmacology,* ed 8, Norwalk, Conn, 2000, McGraw-Hill/Appleton and Lange.

New drug facts label to help consumers, *Clinician News* July/August, 20, 2002.

Nordenberg T: New drug label spells it out simply, *FDA Consumer Magazine* July-August, 1999 (No. [FDA] 99-3232).

Reynolds T: Switching from prescription to over the counter, *Ann Intern Med* 135:177-180, 2002.

CHAPTER 10

Compliance and the Therapeutic Experiment

"Up to half of all patients with serious chronic illnesses do not take their medication as prescribed and thus fail to derive the expected benefits," says a report, "From Compliance to Concordance: Achieving Shared Goals in Medicine-Taking" (*MarketLetter,* 1997).

How can this finding be true? Whose responsibility is it when patients fail to comply? What role does the provider play either in helping the patient implement the therapeutic regimen or in impeding the process? How can health care providers seek to change this statistic?

Although the health care practices of medicine, nursing, pharmacy, and other related disciplines rest on a scientific foundation, how scientific principles are introduced in the relationship with the patient has everything to do with therapeutic success. Spoken of as the "art" of care, substantial evidence exists that this component of health care is equally as important as the "science" of health care. This dimension of care is behind the admonitions to "treat the patient, not the laboratory numbers" and to "individualize therapy."

The *therapeutic experiment* is a term that has been in vogue in schools of pharmacy for a number of years. The concept of a therapeutic experiment suggests that to have rational use of drug therapy (which implicitly means the right drug, to the right patient, at the right time, in the proper dosage, by the appropriate route of administration, for the right problem), a therapeutic process must take place.

However, the therapeutic experiment is something that should not be limited just to the taking of medications. It is really a concept that may be expanded to apply to the whole gamut of interactions between patient and provider. Basically, what every clinician and every patient wants is to find the best solution for the patient's problems and to establish a cooperative relationship so that the patient will carry out the plan successfully. While this may seem like a simple objective, it is deceptively complicated.

As patient and provider come together, they bring different knowledge, skills, resources, anxieties, and expectations to the relationship. It is not like a chemical reaction, with a predictable product as a result of their interactions. Each patient is so different that, each time therapy is prescribed, it is essentially a therapeutic experiment with that unique patient. It is important to share this attitude of engaging in a therapeutic experiment with the patient at the outset of beginning work together, so that the patient understands the variability of outcomes for each trial.

Patients need to understand that many factors lead to the success of a therapeutic regimen. For example: Two patients with the same problem may both take the same medication but have entirely different outcomes. Thus a continuing relationship with the health care provider is essential in making adjustments to discover the proper therapy for the individual patient.

Pressure was exerted on the faculty of a graduate nursing program by a psychologist who thought all psychologists should gain prescriptive authority. He suggested that all the faculty had to do was to develop some videotapes for psychologists to view that would teach them how to prescribe medications. "It is as simple as following a recipe," he maintained. As he had never written a prescription, clearly, he underestimated both the knowledge base and the interpersonal skills required in the process of working with patients in the prescribing process.

ESTABLISHING THERAPEUTIC RELATIONSHIPS IN TREATMENT

The therapeutic experiment is implemented through the relationship established between the health care provider and the patient. This relationship will be therapeutic if it allows the goals of the treatment to be met. Therefore the major task of patient and provider is to establish a long-term relationship so that treatment, including the use of medications, will be implemented appropriately and effectively. It involves a stepwise process—identify a problem, assess it adequately, identify various potential solutions, examine the variables needed to judge the risk-benefit ratio of the solutions, choose the most appropriate solution, and, finally, identify the effects (both beneficial and adverse) that may result from the implementation of the chosen solution (see Chapter 12 on making clinical decisions).

Several factors are essential to establishing this therapeutic relationship: time, attitude, information, communication, and positive feedback.

Time

Establishing a relationship, particularly with those patients requiring primary care, requires an investment in time. This is especially so with elderly patients. Time is an especially scarce resource in today's managed care environment. But actually time is a wise investment in cost-effective treatment and is required early in the relationship to assess the patient's status accurately, through history taking and listening. Time invested by one consistent provider is also required, with continuity of care essential to collect additional information and to make modifications as the patient evidences response to the initial therapy. Offices with policies that make it easy for patients and providers to have brief follow-up conversations by telephone, whenever either of them requires it, also help make relationships more satisfying and successful.

Attitude

How the clinician uses time with the patient and what the clinician says to the patient reflect a basic attitude. This attitude is expressed in the answer to the question, "Who owns the problem?" If the answer is that the patient owns the problem, then care is delivered with the attitude that the health care provider is there to assist the patient in getting or staying well (Weed, 1975). If the attitude is that the patient has a problem for the provider to solve, then the provider owns the problem and often hastens to solve it. This is an essential concept for clinicians to sort out in their minds because it fundamentally affects how the therapeutic relationship is established and defines the rules for continuing the relationship.

Information

Expert diagnosticians have maintained that the most important part of information gathering comes from the history. Many formats have been established for collecting information needed about a patient. The open-ended questions of medical and nursing school are almost always abbreviated or reduced by the experienced clinician to checklists and forms in day-to-day clinical practice. It is important to obtain a comprehensive database for patients for whom pharmacologic therapy is anticipated, especially in regard to medications. This type of information is often best supplied by having patients fill out preprinted forms regarding their medication experience. Although it would be ideal to have this information before the first visit with the health care provider, the reality is that a comprehensive history may take several visits to acquire collecting a little more information with each visit. Using a history-taking form about medications, such as that illustrated in Figure 10-1, helps standardize the information collected and allows it to be expanded during several succeeding sessions. The information collected should be not only comprehensive but also customized to the patient population (inner-city, migrant, elderly) and to the specific problems under study (cardiovascular, diabetes, etc.). To adequately manage patient medications, an updated medication list should also be part of every chart (Rooney, 2003).

Communication

Real two-way communication between patient and health care provider requires a consistent commitment to respect the other's role in the relationship. It involves more listening than speaking, but a true exchange of information and ideas is essential.

During the course of therapy, the patient's expectations must be fulfilled. *Transference,* or the subconscious redirection to one person of feelings and attitudes toward others (e.g., parents or authority figures), may further influence the patient's relationship with the health care provider in either a positive or negative manner, depending on the patient's previous experiences. All of these factors can help to establish honesty and trust.

Other strategies that have been identified as helpful in establishing a relationship with the patient include the health care provider's friendliness; a positive, confident approach; a thoughtful response to patient complaints; encouraging patient questions; a supportive, nonjudgmental method of eliciting and responding to patient admissions of noncompliance; and encouraging patients to become actively involved in their own care. Techniques that encourage active patient participation as opposed to provider-dominated decisions, negotiating rather than dictating a treatment plan, and identifying and resolving barriers to compliance are also helpful. Finally, attempting to find congruence between patient and provider in their understanding of a problem and its management and efforts to motivate the patient and increase patient satisfaction are also helpful (Heath, 2002; Ibraham, 2002; Lacro et al, 2002; Love, 2002; Nevins, 2002; Swanson, 2003; Taylor, 2002).

Some of the specifics of what is communicated to the patient need to center around discussing the therapeutic goals of treatment. When medications are involved, the nature of the experiment with that particular medication and that particular patient needs to be explored. Clear expectations need to be communicated about mutual decision-making, taking medications as ordered, returning for monitoring of effectiveness of the intervention, and the need to adjust dosages or medications over time.

Health care providers must refine listening and questioning skills. They must focus first on the patient, then the environment, and then themselves. Specifically, the tasks are to learn to judge the patient's verbal or nonverbal cues to see whether the patient is ready to receive information. Providers should attend to the physical environment of the discussion (privacy, freedom from distractions). And, finally, they must pay attention to their own mannerisms, tone of voice, and language. They must use active listening with feedback to ensure that the information sent is the same as the information received (Chessare, 1998)..

After presenting information, the health care provider must elicit the patient's preferences for health and other outcomes. For example, it is not enough to give a family the probability that a child will be left with significant morbidity after a potentially life-sustaining procedure. It is also necessary to have the parents consider what the morbidity may mean to them and their child. This discussion should include the child's somatic and psychological well-being in the context of family life and the financial repercussions for the family of specific clinical decisions (Chessare, 1998). A prudent course must be charted between creating uncontrolled and unfounded anxieties on the one hand and generating a false sense of equally groundless security and reassurance on the other.

To lead discussions of this type, health care providers will need to understand how framing the problem for a decision-maker can affect the decision. Health care providers must know some techniques for helping the patient or family deal with probabilities when making a particularly difficult decision. There are many methods for eliciting preferences from patients and parents regarding the outcomes of medical treatment.

Health care providers also have a societal duty to consider the consequences of decisions by both patients and themselves for the greater good of the community. For example, parents' decision not to provide immunization for their child because

COMPREHENSIVE MEDICATION EVALUATION

Name____________________ Address____________________ Age________

Date____________ Provider__________________________

Updated on:____________________ By____________________

MEDICATION REGIMEN

Record for all OTC products (nonprescription pain relievers, laxatives, vitamins, ear/eye/nose drops, anti-diarrheals, inhalers, breathing medications, creams, ointments, sleeping pills, cough or cold medications, feminine hygiene medications, etc.) and Rx medications.

	Name of Medication	Strength	Dosage Form	Directions	Purpose	Compliance
Med 1						
Med 2						
Med 3						
Med 4						
Med 5						
Med 6						
Med 7						
Med 8						
Med 9						
Med 10						
Med 11						
Med 12						

Which of the above medications has the patient stopped taking? Why? *Put number next to medication.*
(1) per provider's order (2) side effect (3) didn't think it was important (4) couldn't afford it (5) didn't think it was working (6) ran out and couldn't get refill (7) other________________

Does the patient see multiple health care providers? Y N
Does the patient use multiple pharmacies? Y N
Is the patient able to read prescription labels? Y N
Is the patient able to open childproof caps? Y N
Does the patient receive or need assistance with medications? Y N If Yes, describe:________________

History of medication allergy? Y N
If yes, medications involved:____________ ____________ ____________
(1) aspirin (2) sulfas (3) codeine (4) penicillin (5) radioopaque dyes (6) local anesthetics
(7) other (specify)________________
Describe what happened in the allergic reaction(s)________________

Adverse effects (record any major adverse/side effects related to current or past drug therapy):

Medication involved	Description of reaction	Year

FIGURE 10-1

Comprehensive medication evaluation.

SOCIAL HISTORY

What alcoholic beverages does patient drink?

Beverage	How much/day (ounces)?
Wine	________
Beer	________
Hard liquor (whiskey, gin, etc).	________

Does patient smoke tobacco? Y N How many packs/years? ________

How much of the following does the patient drink/day (convert to ounces)?

Beverage	Amount (ounces/day)
Caffeinated coffee	________
Decaffeinated coffee	________
Caffeinated tea	________
Decaffeinated tea	________
Caffeinated sodas	________

Has patient ever used or currently uses any of the following drugs?

	Route	Currently using?	Past user?	Date stopped
Heroin				
Cocaine				
Crack				
Marijuana				
Amphetamines				
Depressants/barbiturates				
Other				

SOURCE/PAYMENT OF MEDICATIONS

How does patient obtain medicines? (1) goes to pharmacy to pick up, (2) caregiver goes to pharmacy, (3) pharmacy delivers to home, (4) pharmacy mails to home, (5) other________

Is it difficult for patient to obtain medicines? Y N Why? (1) can't get out to get them (2) can't get to doctor to get renewed prescriptions (3) can't afford them (4) forget to get them refilled (5) other________
Are prescriptions filled at more than one pharmacy? Y N Unknown

From what type of pharmacy are prescriptions most frequently obtained? (1) chain (2) supermarket chain (3) independent (4) mail order (5) HMO (6) VA pharmacy (7) other________

Name of pharmacy________ Phone # of pharmacy________

Does patient know the pharmacist's name? Y N________
Does pharmacy have a delivery service available? Y N Don't know
Does patient use it? Y N Is there an extra charge? Y N Don't know
Who assists patient in selection of specific OTC products?
(1) health care provider (2) pharmacist (3) friend (4) relative (5) caregiver (6) no one, patient selects them
(7) other________

FIGURE 10-1—cont'd

Comprehensive medication evaluation.

Continued

How are prescription medications paid for? (1) free at the VA (2) medical assistance card (3) pharmacy assistance card (4) prescription insurance card (5) cash
Does patient receive a senior citizen discount? Y N
Does patient have a co-payment per prescription? Y N Amount_______________

ADMINISTRATION

Who gives patient the medications? (1) patient takes them with no assistance (2) patient takes them with assistance (3) spouse gives them to patient (4) professional caregiver gives them to patient (5) other gives them to patient_________

Did patient take medication this morning? Y N Don't know
If not, why not? (1) forgot (2) ran out (3) side effects (4) other_______________
How often does patient NOT take ANY prescription medications? (1) daily (2) once a week (3) less than once a week but more than once a month (4) less than once a month

UNDERSTANDING

Does patient seem to understand purpose of medications?	Fully	Somewhat	Not at all
Does patient understand medication schedule?	Fully	Somewhat	Not at all
Is patient aware of expected side effects?	Fully	Somewhat	Not at all
Does patient have an understanding of what effects to report to health care provider?	Fully	Somewhat	Not at all
Does caregiver understand purpose of medications?	Fully	Somewhat	Not at all
Does caregiver understand medication schedule?	Fully	Somewhat	Not at all
Is caregiver aware of expected side effects?	Fully	Somewhat	Not at all
Does caregiver have an understanding of what effects to report to health care provider?	Fully	Somewhat	Not at all

FIGURE 10-1—cont'd

Comprehensive medication evaluation.

of concerns about adverse reactions places others in the community at risk. When a higher-cost strategy gives no added benefit to the patient, then it is appropriate for the health care provider to use a lower-cost choice. Where there are higher-cost strategies of potential benefit, the health care provider must be able to frame decisions for families such that they understand the expected added benefit (Chessare, 1998). For example, the family of a patient with tuberculosis might be convinced that it is in the interest of public safety for a judge to put the patient in jail until a supervised course of medication therapy can be concluded than to allow the patient to remain noncompliant with drug therapy in the community. Helping the patient learn that there are other factors, in addition to their own preferences, to consider in whether to take a medication for a particular problem is essential.

Implicit in the communication process is the guarantee that, once data about a problem have been presented clearly to a family, health care providers will do their best to provide the best therapy. It is part of the provider's role to avoid strategies that provide no benefit to the patient. Practicing evidence-based medicine leads to cost-effective care because data are sought to validate strategies that lead to the best outcomes.

Providers also do not have the right to withhold effective therapies chosen by the family simply because they are more costly than others. Because managed care is about providing health care within budget constraints, the pressure to contain costs by limiting care is significant in most plans. This is especially true regarding drug therapy. This pressure is strongest in for-profit plans where breaking even is not enough. It is now also seen in Medicaid patients, where drug choices may be severely limited by formularies for less costly, and sometimes less effective, medications. Ethically, providers must refrain from withholding strategies that are marginally superior to others simply because they are too expensive. This is sometimes difficult given the restrictions of some payment plans, but in some situations, to do otherwise is a violation of the patient-provider relationship.

If policies of a managed care organization or other organization would preclude the prescription of recommended therapy, the provider must continue to act as the family's agent and help them obtain the desired care. When the provider cannot support the desires of the [patient], they have a duty to make this clear to the family. If the patient continues to see their desire as appropriate, the provider must assist them in finding another provider (Chessare, 1998).

Not only does communication need to be examined from a philosophical or procedural point of view, but also there is a requirement for specific information to be discussed in the patient encounter. The construction of a diagnostic plan is based on critical decision-making. The problem itself must be clearly defined by some clinically measurable, verifiable means—that is, a lump in the breast can only be defined as a malignant lesion after a pathologic examination. Only known information can be used to define a problem; no assumptions can be accepted in the problem definition.

The provider's assessment of the patient's history and physical and laboratory information will answer the questions, "What etiology?" "Why now?" "How severe?" This step allows for further refinement of the problem and speculation as to the probable causes and potential risk to the patient based on information gathered in the database. "What etiology?" suggests potential treatments of a correctable cause; "why now?" is particularly important in acute exacerbations of chronic disease or detection of immune deficiencies, for it leads to an approach that treats the acute problem as well as preventing further difficulties. "How severe?" leads to decisions on the rapidity and perhaps the nature of treatment (see Chapter 12 on making clinical decisions).

Next, the therapeutic objective must be clearly defined and stated before beginning treatment. The goal or objective should be realistically attainable with available therapeutic agents, must be clearly related to the problem as defined and assessed, and must be measurable.

Finally, the indices of therapeutic effect are determined. These are measures of the therapeutic objective and should be discriminating, identified, and relevant to the therapeutic objective. Identification of discriminating therapeutic indices allows the practitioner to recognize when the therapeutic objective is achieved. It is the identification of those subjective and objective parameters that the practitioner will monitor to determine the degree of therapeutic achievement. These are often suggested from well-established clinical guidelines.

If the patient agrees to drug therapy, the provider must offer specific explanations about what medication the patient is to take and why (see Chapter 12 on making clinical decisions). The selected modality should be as specific for the problem and the therapeutic objective as possible. Evidence-based medicine will provide direction about what has been proved to be effective. In the absence of definitive recommendations, agents or modalities will be selected on the basis of cost, efficacy, lowest toxicity, and other patient and drug variables.

Both patient- and agent-related variables must be considered in the final selection and administration of an agent. *Agent-related variables* are defined as those properties of any agent that are characteristic of that agent and affect its use in a given situation. Examples of this would be chemical properties, formulation, absorption, metabolism and excretion, toxicity, half-life, and bioavailability (see Chapter 5 on pharmacokinetics).

Patient-related variables are defined as those preexisting conditions that in some way alter the expected effects of an agent on the patient, that is, renal function or dysfunction, liver function or dysfunction, age, weight, individual response, concomitant disease, the disease or problem itself, compliance or noncompliance, or allergy. Patient-related variables may also include absolute or relative contraindications for the use of an agent in a given patient. An example would be the use of sympathomimetic amines in a hypertensive patient.

There also must be detailed instructions given to the patient, preferably in writing, about how to take medication (see Chapter 11 on tips in writing prescriptions and Chapter 13 on design and implementation of patient education). One cannot rationally administer an agent without first understanding variables affecting its administration. Patients should understand what they might expect, both positively and negatively, in taking this medication.

And, finally, patients should understand their responsibility to report back to the provider about how the "experiment" is progressing. Direct observation of the chosen indices of effect and toxicity is the final and most important step in the implementation of the therapeutic experiment in the actual situation. This step involves eliciting subjective and objective data as a follow-up to the administration of the agent. Obviously there is no point in establishing a therapeutic objective unless providers will be able to know when the objective has been achieved or when a toxic index is being approached.

From the first discussions of therapy, patients must understand the providers' expectations about having them return for laboratory tests and clinic appointments. Again, whether the report is on what patients have done in handling their problems or whether they report back on the success of the provider's plan depends on the attitude that has been established about who owns the problem.

One example of a realistic expectation might be that the patient will bring all medications (past and present, prescription and OTC, internal and topical, liquid and solids) in a bag with them for follow-up visits. Reviewing the medications together, validating that the medications were taken as ordered, and noting the number of pills left are all important pieces of information for the provider in assessing whether the patient has been compliant.

Positive Feedback

Relationships that acknowledge sacrifice, hard work, and cooperation are likely to thrive. Obstetricians who yell at or scold pregnant women who gain too much weight during their pregnancy finally learned that yelling only drove away the mothers; it did not make them stop eating. Being flexible when possible, accepting occasional lapses in compliance, attempting to understand the patient's point of view, and being appreciative of efforts that are made to change assist in the development of a trusting relationship. Overly critical or rigid clinicians often create a milieu in which it is difficult for patients to tell them the truth about noncompliance. It then becomes impossible to determine whether the medication is working. This dooms the therapeutic experiment.

FAILURES OF THE THERAPEUTIC RELATIONSHIP

The success of the therapeutic relationship will be measured by the compliance of the patient. Patient noncompliance with medications is a major unresolved problem that health care providers must face. Hussar (1975) defines drug noncompliance as the inappropriate self-administration of medications. This also implies that the results of self-administration vary from the health care provider's advice and cannot be equated with therapeutic effectiveness. However, *noncompliance* really is a neutral term, describing one aspect of patient behavior that may be either appropriate or inappropriate to the patient's best interests (Barker, Burton & Zieve, 2002).

How does noncompliance begin? Patients often come to a health care provider almost as a last resort, after having tried a number of remedies for symptoms; consulted family, friends, or other authority figures; and developed half-formed or inaccurate models to explain symptoms and illness. Age, sex, race, ethnic background, family, social class, education, past experience, and place in the world will have affected how the patient views the problem and sees the world in general. Although today's patients are more likely to be better informed about medical care than patients were in the past, they are also more likely to be skeptical of the medical profession. They may have read about successful malpractice suits and medical mistakes, heard about bad experiences in medical care from friends, or have had bad experiences themselves. They may come from a lower socioeconomic class, be less educated, or have different value systems than the health care provider. They may have underlying fears and concerns and certain expectations for the visit but may be reluctant to express them for fear of being thought foolish (Barker, Burton & Zieve, 2002). Direct-to-consumer advertising may have led to self-diagnosis and expectations about therapy.

Although health care providers may make diagnoses and prescribe effective treatments, they may not detect or allay the patients' underlying concerns or meet the patients' expectations for the visit. Providers may make false assumptions that the patients' value systems are like their own.

Noncompliance continues as a growing concern for practicing clinicians. The National Library of Medicine PubMed Database has more than 55,900 articles relating to compliance, representing only a portion of the published literature. The average compliance rate for a prescribed treatment regimen has been estimated at 50%; compliance rates for chronic therapy and asymptomatic diseases were even lower (Swanson, 2003).

If medication is involved in the treatment plan, the provider's goal is simply "to get every patient to purchase, take, continue, report back, identify what helps, and what hinders." Problematic behavior can be exhibited as either overutilization or underutilization of medication. *Overutilization* describes patients who take one or more medications at a higher dose or frequency than prescribed. It also describes patients who take medications from several different providers who are unaware of the other medications the patient is taking, whether prescription drugs or over the counter (McNally & Wertheimer, 1992).

Underutilization includes taking medications at lower doses or at less frequent intervals than prescribed. If a patient does not fill a prescription or stops taking the medication without authorization by the physician, this is considered underutilization. Other examples might include when patients cut their pills in half to stretch out the supply of costly medications. In another scenario, with antibiotic therapy, patients feel better in 3 days and stop taking the medication (McNally & Wertheimer, 1992).

There are no benign consequences of noncompliant behavior. Overutilization of medications places a person at greater risk for adverse effects. Underutilization of medicines may result in therapeutic failures, leading to an increase in disease severity. In either case, a higher rate of hospitalization and increased costs for medical care may result. A metaanalysis of seven research studies demonstrated that an overall hospitalization rate of 5.5% might be attributed to noncompliance. This percentage equals 1.94 million annual hospital admissions, at a cost of $8.5 billion (Sullivan et al, 1990). Noncompliance by cardiovascular disease patients, a particularly prevalent problem, has been estimated to be a factor in 125,000 deaths and several hundred thousand hospitalizations a year. The calculated cost to society is over $1.5 billion in lost earnings, resulting from lost workdays (Burrell & Levy, 1985; Charles et al, 2003; Wang et al, 2002).

Noncompliance with efficacious therapeutic regimens may thwart the goals of both provider and patient in reducing suffering, preventing illness, improving functional status, and increasing longevity. If the extent of the patient's noncompliance is hidden from the provider, poor outcomes may be mistakenly attributed to inadequate dosage, failure of the regimen itself, or incorrect diagnosis. Any of these conclusions could lead to inappropriate action by the health care provider during later patient visits (Barker, Burton & Zieve, 2002).

Most studies of factors associated with compliance are small cross-sectional reports, making inferences of causality subject to error. However, an increasing number are prospective. Most studies of compliance have involved hospital-based patients, leaving questions about their general applicability, but when ambulatory patients have been studied, results tend to be similar. Numerous studies now exist that evaluate the short-term effectiveness of various interventions designed to improve patient compliance. These studies have consistently found that patients are unfamiliar with their prescribed medications and how to take them (Charles, 2003; Durante, 2003; Graney, Bunting & Russell, 2003; Loghman-Adham, 2003; Simpson et al, 2003; Steele & Grauer, 2003) and that patients make errors in taking medications 25% to 59% of the time (Barker, Burton & Zieve, 2002).

The research literature (Love, 2002; Misdrahi et al, 2002; Partridge et al, 2002; Schectman, Nadkarnii & Voss, 2002; Shailansky & Levy, 2002) suggests that there are six major risk factors for noncompliance:

- Noncompliance rates tend to be higher for preventive care than for treatment of established illnesses. It has also been demonstrated that there is better compliance for medications perceived to be important, such as cardiac or diabetic agents, than for those that are seemingly less important, such as antacids or mild analgesics.
- Noncompliance increases in extent with the duration of therapy, such as is seen in chronic diseases such as diabetes, hypertension, epilepsy, and depression.
- Noncompliance is highest for regimens that require significant behavioral change, such as smoking cessation or weight loss.
- Noncompliance often results from a poor understanding of instructions.
- Noncompliance increases with the complexity of the treatment regimen, that is, when many drugs are taken concurrently and/or when drugs must be taken at frequent intervals.
- Noncompliance increases when there are unpleasant side effects.

Clearly, patients who are symptomatic are more likely to be compliant than those who are not, especially if the symptoms are relieved by treatment recommendations. Surprisingly, such sociodemographic variables as sex, race, education, occupation, income, and marital status usually do not correlate with compliance behavior (Charles et al, 2003). People who have a stable support system and stable family situation tend to be more compliant.

Although it is generally accepted that older people are more likely to be noncompliant, the bulk of the early research literature indicates that aging does not affect compliance with prescribed medications. Elderly individuals may have fewer daily distractions in their lives, enabling them to concentrate on their medication regimens. This is in contrast to middle-aged and younger patients who are involved in their careers and other activities, causing them to forget about their medications. Elderly patients, however, have been shown to have difficulty in opening childproof medication containers and may have greater difficulty in reading or understanding instructions (Heft & Mariotti, 2002).

Unfortunately, identifying the noncompliant patient is very difficult. Studies have shown that physicians tend to overestimate patient adherence to treatment regimens (Roth & Caron, 1978). Studies on specific factors related to compliance have found no relationship with sex, socioeconomic status, or education (Haynes, 1976).

So, how can health care providers better identify and improve compliance in their patients? A study by the Royal Pharmaceutical Society of Great Britain and Merck Sharp & Dohme, Ltd., launched in early 1995, claims that the assumption behind the terms *compliance* and *adherence* in medicine-taking suggest patient fault and should be abandoned in favor of the term *concordance*. This term, they suggest, expresses a therapeutic alliance between the prescriber and the patient, describing a negotiated agreement that may even be an agreement to disagree (*MarketLetter*, 1997).

Concordance, as a process, imposes new responsibilities on both parties. Patients must take a more active part in the consultation process, while prescribers must communicate the evidence to enable patients to make an informed decision about diagnosis and treatment, benefit and risk. Prescribers should know and accept patients' choices while continuing to negotiate the treatment as part of a continuing consultation process.

Effective communication practices must extend beyond those used in the patient-provider therapeutic relationship to include the family and the pharmacist.

Primary communication among pharmacist, patient, and provider is through the prescription. At the very least, when pharmacists dispense prescriptions they have the opportunity to detect miscommunications or unfounded expectations, to validate why the medication is being prescribed, and to clarify or reinforce health care prescribers' directions. Reinforcement through repetition is an effective strategy in achieving compliance (Hussar, 1985).

However, pharmacists may assist the provider and patient in many other ways. A growing number of pharmacists use computers to establish and maintain patient profiles. The computer alerts the pharmacist when patients refill their prescriptions too soon, identifying possible overutilization. The pharmacist's regular review of patient profiles also permits identification of underutilization by patients who are not regularly refilling their prescription. Writing complete information on the prescription about how the patient should be taking the medication gives pharmacists valuable information that will assist them in helping the patient be more compliant.

At visits, the clinician should assess whether patients are able to open their medication bottles easily, read the label correctly, and tolerate the dosage. They should detect fears patients have about developing an addiction to the drug, often a particularly insidious but unfounded concern. They also have an opportunity to counsel patients, no matter how well educated, who believe they will "outgrow" their need for insulin, high blood pressure medication, or thyroid medication.

Confusion about therapeutic regimens are frequent following transition times such as discharge from an emergency department, hospital, or long-term care facility. These times are frequently associated with the addition of new prescriptions or a change in prescriptive regimen. One study found that 47% of emergency department visits lead to the prescribing of at least one additional medication, and in 10% of those visits, the new medication adds a potential adverse interaction (Beers et al, 1990). Because health care providers who see patients in these settings are usually not the patients' primary care providers, special care needs to be taken by the primary care provider on the next visit to review prescriptions. Patients may not understand if they are to use the old medications as well as the new ones, to make substitutions in product, or to just make changes in dosage (Kennedy & Erb, 2002; Patel & Zed, 2002).

Another factor that influences compliance is the issue of higher drug prices. The high cost of medication continues to be an important factor in determining if some patients will have a prescription filled. It is difficult for the provider to learn about the cost of these medications, particularly because there may be substantial variability in price, depending on where the prescription is filled. Providers should periodically take the time to contact several community pharmacists for cost information before prescribing new products. And a good relationship with pharmacists will encourage them to alert health care providers to the price differential between new drugs and similar older drugs that may be as effective and much less costly.

SUMMARY

Concordance between provider and patient is the key to therapeutic relationships. In seeking concordance, the problems associated with medicine-taking have been remarkably absent from almost all public discussion about the benefits and expectations of contemporary medicine. Further research is needed into the beliefs that people hold about medicines and about their motivations and reactions to information-giving and to the behavior of health care workers, family members, and friends. Ongoing work on developing interventions to modify medicine-taking behavior should continue.

Efforts to secure appropriate medicine-taking among patients must be based not on manipulation but on strengthening patients' understanding and control over their illnesses and treatment. New medicine may be designed to overcome difficulties posed by noncompliance, for example, combination products, modified (sustained-release) medicine, high-dose short courses, improved tolerability, design features, alternative delivery systems, and linking administration to circadian rhythms.

Providers should consider reevaluating medicines now in use to gauge their robustness in terms of the relationship between dose and effect. Continuing research will be required into the effect of containers, labeling, and other information-giving and how they facilitate or limit medicine-taking (*MarketLetter,* 1997).

Patients want more information on medicines, and giving them more control over treatments received may change compliance. Although establishing a therapeutic relationship is essential, at the other end of the spectrum are all the new electronic and communications media, such as telephone helplines, the development of information materials on the Internet, and use of PDAs and other interactive electronic devices that will increasingly be consulted by patients. The importance of information sources that do not involve face-to-face communication with health care professionals is growing rapidly.

Primary care providers must take care not to focus simply on seeking to achieve better compliance but on empowering patients to take part in concordant partnerships with all health care providers, so that their medicine-taking decisions are as informed as possible by scientific evidence and consonant with their own perceptions and wishes.

REFERENCES

Anderson JG: How the Internet is transforming the physician-patient relationship, *Medscape TechMed* 1(3), 2001.

Barker LR, Burton JR, Zieve PD: *Principles of ambulatory medicine,* ed 6, Baltimore, Lippincott, Williams & Wilkins, 2002.

Beck RS, Daughtridge R, Sloane PD: Physician-patient communication in the primary care office: a systematic review, *J Am Board Fam Pract* 15:25-38, 2002.

Barsky AJ: Forgetting, fabricating, and telescoping: the instability of the medical history. *Arch Intern Med* 162:981-984, 2002.

Bell RA et al: Unsaid but not forgotten: patients' unvoiced desires in office visits, *Arch Intern Med* 161:1977-1984, 2001.

Brach C, Fraser I: Can cultural competency reduce racial and ethnic health disparities? A review and conceptual model, *Med Care Res Rev* 57(suppl 1):181-217, 2000.

Burrell CD, Levy RA: Therapeutic consequences of noncompliance. In *Improving medication compliance,* Reston, VA, 1985, National Pharmaceutical Council.

Charles H et al: Racial differences in adherence to cardiac medications, *J Natl Med Assoc* 95:17-27, 2003.

Chessare JB: Teaching clinical decision-making to pediatric residents in an era of managed care, *Pediatrics* 101(4, pt 2):762-766, 1998.

Cooper-Patrick L et al: Race, gender, and partnership in the patient-physician relationship, *JAMA* 282:583-589, 1999.

Durante AJ et al: Home-based study of anti-HIV drug regimen adherence among HIV-infected women: feasibility and preliminary results, *AIDS Care* 15:103-115, 2003.

el Ibrahim SR: Rates of adherence to pharmacological treatment among children and adolescents with attention deficit hyperactivity disorder, *Hum Psychopharmacol* 17:225-231, 2002.

Gottlieb H: Medication nonadherence: finding solutions to a costly medical problem, *Drug Benefit Trends* 12:57-62, 2000.

Graney MJ et al: HIV/AIDS medication adherence factors: inner-city clinic patient's self-reports, *Tenn Med* 96:73-78, 2003.

Haynes RB: A critical view of the determinants of patient compliance with therapeutic regimens. In Haynes RB, Sackett DL, editors: *Compliance with therapeutic regimens,* Baltimore, MD, 1976, Johns Hopkins University Press.

Heath KV et al: Intentional nonadherence due to adverse symptoms associated with antiretroviral therapy, *J Acquir Immune Defic Syndr* 31:211-217, 2002.

Heft MW, Mariotti AJ: Geriatric pharmacology, *Dent Clin North Am* 46:869-885, 2992.

Hussar DA: Improving patient compliance: the role of the pharmacist. In *Improving medication compliance,* Reston, VA, 1985, National Pharmaceutical Council.

Kennedy J, Erb C: Prescription noncompliance due to cost among adults with disabilities in the United States, *Am J Public Health* 92:1120-1124, 2002.

Lacro JP et al: Prevalence of and risk factors for medication nonadherence in patients with schizophrenia: a comprehensive review of recent literature, *J Clin Psychiatry* 63:892-909, 2002.

Levinson W, et al: A study of patient clues and physician responses in primary care and surgical settings, *JAMA* 284:1021-1027, 2000.

Loghman-Adham M: Medication noncompliance inpatients with chronic disease: issues in dialysis and renal transplantation, *Am J Manag Care* 9:115-171, 2003.

Love RC: Strategies for increasing treatment compliance: the role of long-acting antipsychotics, *Am J Health Syst Pharm* 59(22 suppl 8):S10-S15, 2002.

MarketLetter: *From compliance to concordance,* Washington, DC, March 24, 1997.

McNally DL, Wertheimer D: Strategies to reduce the high cost of patient noncompliance, *Md Med J* 41:223-225, 1992.

Misdrahi D et al: Compliance in schizophrenia: predictive factors, therapeutical considerations and research implications, *Encephale* 23(3 Pt 1):226-272, 2002.

Nevins TE: Non-compliance and its management in teenagers, *Pediatr Transplant* 6:475-479, 2002.

Partridge AH et al: Adherence to therapy with oral antineoplastic agents, *J Natl Cancer Inst* 94:652-662, 2002.

Patel P, Zed PJ: Drug-related visits to the emergency department: how big is the problem? *Pharmacotherapy* 22:915-923, 2002.

Rooney WR: Maintaining a medication list in the chart, *Fam Pract Manag* 10:52-56, 2003.

Roth HP, Caron HS: Accuracy of doctors' estimates and patients' statements on adherence to a drug regimen, *Clin Pharmacol Ther* 23:361, 1978.

Schectman JM, Nadkarni MM, Voss JD: The association between diabetes metabolic control and drug adherence in an indigent population, *Diabetes Care* 25:1015-1021, 2002.

Shalansky SJ, Levy AR: Effect of number of medications on cardiovascular therapy adherence, *Ann Pharmacother* 36:1532-1539, 2002.

Simpson E et al: Drug prescriptions after acute myocardial infarction: dosage, compliance, and persistence, *Am Heart J* 145:438-444, 2003.

Staff: Encouraging patients to assume more responsibility for their health: a key to optimum healthcare, *Drug Ther Perspect* 17:14-15, 2001.

Steele RG, Grauer D: Adherence to antiretroviral therapy for pediatric HIV infection: review of the literature and recommendations for research, *Clin Child Fam Psychol Rev* 6:17-30, 2003.

Sullivan SD et al: Noncompliance with medication regimens and subsequent hospitalizations: a literature analysis and cost of hospitalization estimate, *J Res Pharmaceut Econ* 2:19-23, 1990.

Swanson J: Compliance with stimulants for attention-deficit/hyperactivity disorder: issues and approaches for improvement, *CNS Drugs* 27:117-131, 2003.

Taylor SA, Galbraith SM, Mills RP: Causes of non-compliance with drug regimens in glaucoma patients: a qualitative study, *J Ocul Pharmacol Ther* 18:401-409, 2002.

Weed LL: *Your health care and how to manage it,* Burlington, VT, 1975, University of Vermont.

Wang PS et al: Noncompliance with antihypertensive medications: the impact of depressive symptoms and psychosocial factors, *J Gen Intern Med* 17:504-511, 2002.

CHAPTER 11

Practical Tips on Writing Prescriptions

Many sources describe the importance of prescriptive authority for full implementation of the health provider's role; however, very few texts describe the mechanics and technicalities of the actual process. Students of all disciplines with prescriptive authority admit to extreme anxiety in writing their first prescriptions. They are concerned not only about what they write, but how they write it. However, most clinicians describe learning this process on the job, under the tutelage of another clinician or preceptor, often while under extreme pressure to master other skills. Casual observation of prescriptions submitted to a pharmacy document the wide array of formats used in writing prescriptions some leading to greater chance for errors than others. Research also shows that, like writing a check, the format with which one begins is often the format that persists, even if it is not the best.

WHO MAY WRITE PRESCRIPTIONS?

State law identifies those health care providers authorized to write prescriptions. This fact accounts for the substantial state-by-state variations in prescriptive authority. Traditionally, physicians have had full prescriptive authority, dentists and podiatrists have had prescriptive authority for a more limited formulary, and veterinarians have had the ability to prescribe, dispense, and administer medications. State laws have been amended in every state to provide prescriptive authority to certain other providers, such as doctors of osteopathy (DO), nurse practitioners (NPs), or physician assistants (PAs). This authority may either be granted directly to these providers or indirectly through delegated authority from a physician (see Chapters 1 and 2 on information on nurses and PAs). Each state determines the qualifications and credentials essential for a provider to obtain prescriptive authority; this may include specific courses in pharmacology before receiving prescriptive authority, as well as ongoing requirements for continuing education in pharmacology.

The exact extent of prescriptive authority is also determined by the state. This includes the type of drugs that the provider is authorized to prescribe. Over-the-counter medications require no state authorization. Indeed these medications are often client-initiated and -controlled products. Drugs requiring a prescription include legend drugs and controlled substances. *Legend drugs* include the vast majority of medications, such as those for hypertension, diabetes, or asthma. If a state determines that providers may write prescriptions for controlled substances, they also establish a mechanism for monitoring that activity, either through granting the provider a number or putting the provider on an approved list. Once receiving documentation of this authority from the state, the health care provider is eligible to apply to the federal Drug Enforcement Agency (DEA) for a federal DEA number to be used on all prescriptions for controlled substances.

The federal DEA has oversight of controlled substances. This agency attempts to limit the numbers of professionals who may prescribe controlled substances to those who are authorized and competent to do so and to monitor the activity of such individuals to make certain they are in conformance with federal law. This monitoring is essential because of the potential for misuse and abuse of these substances by both patients and providers. The DEA does not, however, define who is to receive DEA numbers but relies on the states for this information (US Department of Justice, DEA, 1990). Many states issue a state-controlled substance license. This number seems to have little purpose other than to be part of the application process for the federal DEA number.

The health care provider seeking a federal DEA number may obtain an application by calling (202) 307-7255; go to the DEA website at www.DEADiversion.usdoj.gov; or write the Drug Enforcement Administration ODOC Registration Division, Washington, DC 20537, and submit the appropriate information and fees. Fees are sufficiently expensive to deter casual acquisition. Providers must indicate on the application the specific schedules of drugs that they are authorized by the state to prescribe. Nonphysician prescribers are required to fill out a specific addendum to the DEA application validating state authority to engage in the prescription of controlled substances. DEA numbers issued to "midlevel providers" begin with the letter *M*, followed by a number corresponding to the first letter of the last name (i.e., *E* for Edwards) and a computer-generated sequence of numbers. Physician and midlevel practitioners' manuals, available by special request, contain essential rules and regulations related to use or misuse of the DEA number. If applicants meet the DEA requirements, they are issued a number linked to their place of employment. One exception is that military and US Public Health Service physicians are exempted from registration. This number is valid for 3 years and may then be renewed. This federal number is also reported to the state and included in the materials distributed to pharmacists within that state (US Department of Justice, DEA, 1990).

DRUG SCHEDULES

Federal statute establishes five schedules of controlled substances, ranked in order of their abuse potential and in inverse proportion to their medical value. A complete list of controlled substances may be obtained by writing to Superintendent of Documents, US Government Printing Office, Washington, DC 20402. The drugs in these schedules are revised periodically by the DEA as circumstances warrant.

Drugs in Schedule I have the highest potential for abuse and are limited to research protocols, instructional use, or chemical analysis. Ongoing research may eventually establish a medical role for some of these substances under selected circumstances. On the other end of the spectrum, Schedule V drugs are available by prescription or may be sold over the counter in some states, depending on state law (US Department of Justice, DEA, 1990). See Table 11-1 for sample of Schedule of Controlled Drugs.

Controlled drugs often have restrictions on the number of refills permitted. When dispensed to a patient via a prescription, the label of any controlled substance in Schedules II, III, or IV must contain a symbol on the label designating the schedule to which it belongs and the following warning: "Caution: Federal law prohibits the transfer of this drug to any person other than the patient for whom it was prescribed." Internet or mail-order pharmacies may not fill prescriptions for controlled substances.

The classification of drugs into the schedules is flexible. Thus any drug could be placed under control, upgraded or downgraded, or possibly even removed from control over time. For example, new information might cause a change in schedule classification, or epidemic abuse of an uncontrolled drug might cause it to be added to the list.

COMPONENTS OF THE WRITTEN PRESCRIPTION

Although state law may mandate specifics of what is required on a prescription, there is general agreement about some things that should be included, whether required by law or not. Most states insist that the hospital name or the imprinted name of

TABLE 11-1 Federal Schedule of Controlled Drugs

	Substance Characteristics	Type of Restriction	Examples
I	High abuse potential No currently accepted medical use For research, instructional use, or chemical analysis only	Approved protocol necessary	heroin, marijuana, LSD, peyote, mescaline, psilocybin, methylamphetamine, acetylmethadol, fenethylline, tilidine, dihydromorphine, methaqualone
II	High abuse potential Current accepted for medical use as narcotic, stimulant, or depressant drugs May lead to severe psychologic and/or physical dependence	Written prescription only No refills Emergency dispensing without written prescription permitted Container must carry warning label	morphine, codeine, hydromorphone (Dilaudid), methadone, Pantopon, meperidine (Demerol), cocaine, oxycodone (Percodan), oxymorphone (Numorphan), amphetamine (Dexedrine), methamphetamine (Desoxyn), phenmetrazine (Preludin), methylphenidate (Ritalin), amobarbital, phenobarbital, secobarbital, fentanyl (Sublimaze), sufentanil, etorphine hydrochloride, phenylacetone, dronabinol, nabilone
III	Less abuse potential than drugs in Schedules I and II Currently accepted for medical use and includes compounds containing limited quantities of certain narcotic and nonnarcotic drugs May lead to physical dependence or high psychologic dependence	Written or oral prescription required Prescription expires in 6 months No more than 5 prescription refills Container must carry warning label	Derivatives of barbituric acid except those that are listed in another schedule, glutethimide (Doriden), nalorphine, benzphetamine, chlorphentermine, clortermine, phendimetrazine, paregoric and any compound, mixture, preparation or suppository dosage form containing amobarbital, secobarbital, or pentobarbital
IV	Low abuse potential relative to Schedule III substances Currently accepted for medical use May lead to limited physical or psychologic dependence	Written or oral prescription required Prescription expires in 6 months No more than 5 prescription refills Container must carry warning label	barbital, phenobarbital, methylphenobarbital, chloral hydrate, ethchlorvynol (Placidyl), ethinamate (Valmid), meprobamate (Equanil, Miltown), paraldehyde, methohexital, phentermine, chlordiazepoxide (Librium), diazepam (Valium), oxazepam (Serax), clorazepate (Tranxene), flurazepam (Dalmane), clonazepam (Clonopin), prazepam (Verstran), alprazolam (Xanax), halazepam (Paxipam), temazepam (Restoril), triazolam (Halcion), lorazepam (Ativan), midazolam (Versed), quazepam (Dormalin), mebutamate, dextropropoxyphene dosage forms (Darvon), and pentazocine (Talwin-NX)
V	Low abuse potential relative to Schedule IV substances Currently accepted for medical use; consists primarily of preparations of certain narcotic and stimulant drugs generally for antitussive, antidiarrheal, and analgesic purposes Have less potential for physical or psychologic dependence	May require written prescription or be sold over-the-counter Check state law	buprenorphine and propylhexedrine

From US Department of Justice, DEA: *Physician's manual: an information outline of the Controlled Substances Act of 1970*, Washington, DC, March 1990, US Department of Justice.

the prescriber, credentials, address, and telephone number be preprinted on the prescription pad for controlled substances but not for noncontrolled drugs. It is important, however, that the pharmacist be able to easily contact the prescriber. In institutions where there are many prescribers, an institutional prescription pad may allow for the prescriber to use a number rather than have all prescriber names on the pad. Prescriptions must be preprinted, typed, or written in ink and must be signed by an authorized prescriber to be valid. See a sample of a prescription in Figure 11-1.

Is there one correct way to write a prescription? Yes. And it should be followed consistently and without deviation each time a prescription is written (Marek, 1996). It contains the following components.

Top Portion

The top portion of the preprinted prescription form contains the patient's name, address, and age or birth date. The patient's weight may also be included here when relevant. The date on which the prescription is written is required.

- *Name and address of the patient*—Most states require the address if the prescription is written for a controlled substance. It is always a good idea to include the address on a prescription, which will help the pharmacist to make certain that the correct person is picking up the drug.
- *Date that the prescription is written*—By law, a patient usually has up to 120 days to fill a prescription for either a controlled or noncontrolled drug. Medicaid or Medical Assistance prescriptions often must be filled within a shorter period of time, often 10 days, although states may vary on their specific practices. The date on the prescription helps the pharmacist to determine if the patient waited too long to fill the prescription. Some patients hold a prescription in case they need it at another time. This is equivalent to giving patients an inappropriate ability to diagnose and prescribe for themselves in the future.
- *Age and weight of the patient*—This is information the pharmacist needs to help assess the accuracy of the prescription as written. Dosage modifications based on age and weight may be suggested or validated by the pharmacist with this information, particularly for pediatric and geriatric patients.

Middle Portion

The middle portion of the prescription is the part individualized for each patient and contains four main items:

- *Superscription*—The symbol "Rx" from the Latin recipe meaning "take," is included
- *Inscription*—Drug ingredients and their quantities, strength, or concentration are specified.
- *Drug*—The full name of the medication is written clearly and specifically. Do not use abbreviations (Lilly, 1997). If handwriting legibility is an issue, print or type the information required. There must be no question as to meaning of what is written. Some pharmaceutical companies supply preprinted pads for certain prescriptions, reducing the chance for error (and encouraging the prescribing of their product) (Brodell et al, 1997; Winslow et al, 1997).

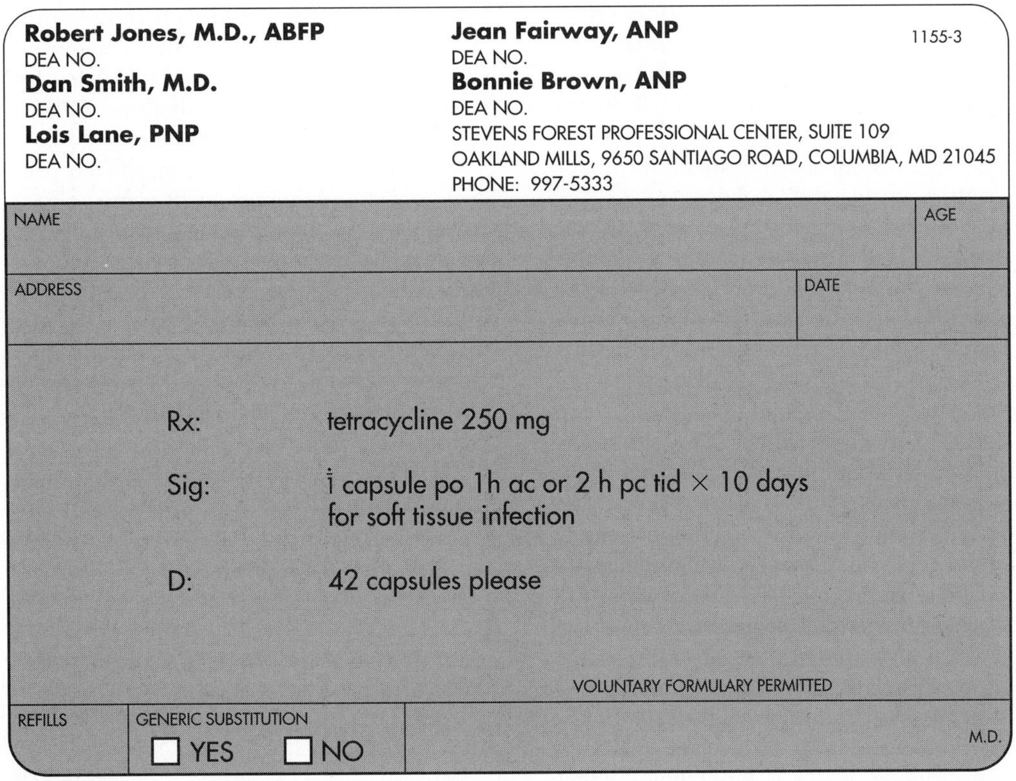

Robert Jones, M.D., ABFP
DEA NO.
Dan Smith, M.D.
DEA NO.
Lois Lane, PNP
DEA NO.

Jean Fairway, ANP
DEA NO.
Bonnie Brown, ANP
DEA NO.
STEVENS FOREST PROFESSIONAL CENTER, SUITE 109
OAKLAND MILLS, 9650 SANTIAGO ROAD, COLUMBIA, MD 21045
PHONE: 997-5333

1155-3

NAME AGE
ADDRESS DATE

Rx: tetracycline 250 mg

Sig: ī capsule po 1h ac or 2 h pc tid × 10 days
for soft tissue infection

D: 42 capsules please

VOLUNTARY FORMULARY PERMITTED

REFILLS GENERIC SUBSTITUTION ☐ YES ☐ NO M.D.

FIGURE 11-1

Common components of the prescription.

- *Strength or concentration*—The dose of the medication to be dispensed is specified.
- *Signature*—This is usually indicated by an "S," representing the Latin *signa*, which means "mark." Other individuals use "Sig." which means, "Write on the label." Thus the signature includes instructions to be put on the outside of the package to direct the patient how and when to take the medicine and in what quantities. The signature component of the prescription should not be confused with the prescriber's signature that is placed at the bottom of the form. It is especially important to be complete in writing instructions for how the medication should be taken.

First, it is important that the patient understands how to take the medication. The prescription should be specific about this and not just indicate "take as directed." Research has shown that failure to write instructions clearly is responsible for many of the medication errors that patients make. Patients often do not understand instructions, become confused over time, or fail to make changes when therapy is modified (Sarriff, 1992). The imprecision of poorly written directions can also influence a patient's ability to comply. To improve patient recall and reduce administration errors, patients require explicit directions. A high percentage of reported administrative errors result from the direct failure of patients to comprehend the directions on the prescription label (Self, 2002, Stein, 1994). If given a prescription for tetracycline 250 mg with the directions, "Take 1 capsule every 6 hours," in one study, only 36% of the 67 participants interpreted the directions to mean around the clock, for a total of 4 doses in 24 hours. Approximately 25% would have been noncompliant by omitting the late-night dose because they would have divided the day into three 6-hour periods while they were awake. Although in this instance the pharmacist has adequate information to counsel the patient, the example demonstrates the importance of prescription writing and labeling.

Second, clarity and precision in writing instructions also help the pharmacist. Federal regulations now mandate that pharmacists must provide education and counseling to patients regarding their medication. Having specific information about why the patient is taking the medication and how the patient should take the medication allows the pharmacist to help reinforce the provider's directions, discover errors in either the writing or the filling of the prescription, or obtain feedback about how patients think they should take the medication (Niederhauser, 1997). Given the growing number of new drugs on the market, the importance of identifying the symptom, indication, or intended effect for which the medication is being prescribed becomes more important and can be added in just a few words, for example, "for nausea," "at headache onset," etc. This additional information allows the pharmacist dispensing the prescription to help assess compliance and reinforce the provider's instructions. An example of this is propranolol, which may be used to treat several different problems. It would be nonsensical for a pharmacist to explain how important it is for a patient to take the medication to control high blood pressure, when the patient is being treated for migraine headaches. Knowing the intent of the treatment will aid the pharmacist in communicating with the patient and providing feedback to the provider (McNally & Wertheimer, 1992).

Finally, specific instructions on the container assists the prescriber in reviewing medications ordered by other prescribers. The patient should always bring all medications they take with them to each office visit. Errors may more easily be detected when instructions on each container are examined. The number of tablets/capsules/teaspoons are designated by small roman numerals, for example: one = *i;* two = *ii,* three = *iii,* etc. Examples of signatures might include: "Take i tablet 1 hour before eating or 2 hours after eating 3 times a day," "Mix i teaspoon in a full glass of orange juice to be taken morning and evening," or "Take ii capsules with food each morning." See Table 11-2 for examples of common abbreviations used in prescribing medications.

- *Subscription*—The pharmacist is instructed on how to compound the medicine. Although there are still compounding pharmacies, the advent of modern pharmaceutical packaging and unit dosing means this component of the prescription is usually met by specifying the dosage form (capsule, tablet, liquid, suspension, cream, ointment) and amount to be dispensed. The prescriber may specify that the product is to be taken PO, IV, IM, etc. The abbreviation "D" preceding the amount to be dispensed, is used to indicate "Give."
- *Quantity or volume*—This indicates how much medication is to be dispensed. Order enough for the standard course of the medication or enough to last until the next scheduled visit. Order standard volumes when writing for liquids. The *Physicians' Drug Reference* or package insert will list standard volumes under "How Supplied." Sometimes the volume or number of doses that may be ordered is limited by how much will be paid for under a prescription-reimbursement plan.

To summarize—In writing this part of the prescription, the first line usually contains the drug name and strength. The second line contains the instructions for taking the drug. The third

TABLE 11-2 Common Abbreviations Used in Prescription Writing

Abbreviation	Meaning
sig	Directions for use
qd	Every day
qAM	Every morning
bid	Two times daily while awake
tid	Three times daily while awake
qid	Four times daily while awake
q8h	Every 8 hours around the clock
ac	Before meals
pc	After meals
hs	At hour of sleep or bedtime
tsp	Teaspoon
prn	As needed

line tells the pharmacist how much and in what form the medication should be dispensed.

Bottom Portion

The bottom portion of the preprinted prescription form contains other standard information. The number of refills and the prescriber's signature and credentials are required. If a controlled substance is prescribed, the federal DEA number is also to be listed. Finally, some prescriptions have a box to check if generic substitution is authorized.

- *Refills*—This section indicates to the pharmacist and patient whether this drug may be refilled. Refills on Schedule II drugs are not permitted. On other scheduled drugs, a maximum of five refills or a 6 months' supply is allowed, whichever comes first. On nonscheduled legend drugs, no limits are placed on the maximum number of refills by law. Medicare, Medical Assistance (Medicaid), or insurance plans often limit the number of medications that may be dispensed per prescription. The prescriber should always indicate the number of refills permitted or to write "NO REFILL" to discourage the patient from entering a number. If it is left blank, the pharmacist will have to contact the prescriber by telephone should a patient request a refill.
- *Provider signature*—Most states require that the prescriber's name must be legibly printed, stamped, or typed following the prescriber signature. Any credentials required by the state should follow the signature.
- *DEA number*—Federal law requires that this number appear on all prescriptions for controlled substances. (This may appear at the top or the bottom of the prescription form, as dictated by state law.) In most states, hospital housestaff who are not licensed within the state may use the hospital DEA number when writing outpatient prescriptions for Schedule III to V drugs. Most states do not recognize a hospital DEA number for Schedule II drugs on outpatient prescriptions. To reduce the exposure of the prescriber's number, DEA numbers should not be used for identification or other purposes and should not be preprinted on the prescription form.
- *Generic substitutions*—The provider may indicate whether the medication ordered may be dispensed with a generic substitution or not. In efforts to decrease cost, this procedure is becoming more common. However, providers must evaluate the bioequivalence of different generic products if substitution is permitted. If you do not wish a generic substitution, be sure to write "Dispense as written" or "Brand medically necessary."

DRUG-PRESCRIBING ETIQUETTE

Many policies for prescription writing came from tradition, commonsense, or institutional practice. A search of the literature produced very few answers about how to handle specific problems or what is universally deemed appropriate. But prescribers encounter these "policies" frequently as they try to care for their patients. Because no written materials could be found on the do's and don'ts of prescription writing, a group of pharmacists were surveyed to describe some acceptable and some less than acceptable behaviors:

- Federal law stipulates that providers may not write prescriptions for narcotics for themselves or their family members. There is no written prohibition against providers writing prescriptions for other nonnarcotic controlled substances for themselves or their family members. However, it is considered a lack of good judgment to do so, unless there are no other providers in the area. A person who is sick enough to require this type of drug probably needs the evaluation of someone besides a family member.
- If a provider consistently writes prescriptions for controlled substances for family members, the pharmacist would probably call to discuss this with the provider. There is no law that requires pharmacists to do so; it would simply be a courtesy to let providers know their behavior does not fit within the norm. However, the DEA, which also closely monitors controlled substance prescription writing, would likely initiate an investigation if prescribing to family came to their attention.
- HMOs, particularly in the western part of the United States, have begun to closely monitor the prescribing practices of their provider employees. Prescriptions written to family members of these plans may not qualify for reimbursement under this more closely restricted supervision. This would particularly be true for providers, such as dentists, who write prescriptions for hormone replacement therapy or oral contraceptives for their wives, or anyone else. This would be perceived as exceeding their scope of authority.
- Prescriptions that are refilled frequently although the patient is not required to return to the provider for evaluation of response stimulate questions in the minds of pharmacists about the therapeutic goal.
- Providers often have large caches of drug samples, some of which they trade or share with other providers who might not ordinarily have access to those products. This practice is on the margin of legality and if known, might prompt an investigation.
- If a friend or family member wants the provider to write a prescription without seeing the patient for a visiting friend from out of town who is ill, it is risky. Remember, providers are legally responsible for whatever they accept responsibility for doing. Friendship should not enter into this very serious professional responsibility. If something seems out of the norm, stay away from it; this is a good rule for a provider to follow, especially if new to the prescribing role.

AVOIDING MISTAKES

It is infrequent that one encounters a provider who approaches writing prescriptions casually. However, concern over not making a mistake is not all that is required to avoid problems. Clearly the most important factor required for safe prescription writing is an adequate knowledge base on the part of the provider (Marek, 1996). Good intentions do not compensate for a lack of knowledge. Because numbers and types of drugs are one of the most frequently changing components of any part of health care, prescribers must keep up to date. Unfortunately, it has been demonstrated in many research studies that prescribers often continue to prescribe the same medications, in the same ways, as when they were students. With the growth in pharmacologic knowledge, this may not only be limiting, but dangerous.

The influx of new drugs places additional demands on the prescriber. Extensive research by pharmaceutical researchers (Denig, 1992; Groves, Flanagan & MacKinnon, 2002; Taylor & Bond, 1991) has demonstrated that most physicians have a "total drug repertoire" with an average of 144 drug preparations. These drugs comprise a number of "evoked sets"—a pooling of different sets containing the small number of possible treatments that a provider might consider for different conditions. The drugs in these "evoked sets" parallel the life cycle of a drug on the market—introduction, growth, maturity, and decline. Marketing firms try to influence rate of the "diffusion" of information about their products as drugs are being developed by sending product information to providers. More recently they have also focused on direct-to-consumer advertising to draw attention to new products. Whether or when a provider adds or drops a drug to his or her "evoked set" depends on whether he or she is an "innovator, early adopter, early majority, late majority, or laggard." Taylor and Bond (1991) found that 5.4% of the new prescriptions written over a 12-month period were for a drug newly adopted by that physician within the previous 12 months. Furthermore, when a new prescription was written, 42% of the time it was to replace a drug that was part of the repertoire.

The 1999 Institute of Medicine report "To Err Is Human" estimated that medication errors account for 7000 deaths per year and led to the House Commerce Subcommittee on Health and Environment February 2000 hearing on this problem (Norton, 2001). The literature is now replete with articles describing errors in health care, what caused them, and what might be done. Virtually every health-related organization has devoted newsletters, websites, or journal articles to the issue of medication errors in their discipline or organization.

Research studies have shown that errors in writing prescriptions are fairly common, varying from 14% to 40% depending on the study and the variables examined (Lesar, Briceland & Stein, 1997; Winslow et al, 1997). In one study of physician behavior, the most frequent errors were ordering of nonformulary drugs and erroneous or unspecified dosage strength. There was no difference in error rate among the physicians with various levels of training. Other studies documented errors in drug use, some of which could be reduced by adding the patient's diagnosis to the prescription to stimulate questions about the appropriateness of the drug selected (Howell & Jones, 1993; Howell et al, 1994). One particularly large study cited specific factors associated with errors such as not noting decline in renal or hepatic function requiring alteration of drug therapy; ignoring patient history of allergy to the same medication class; using the wrong drug name, dosage form, or abbreviation for both brand and generic names; incorrect dosage calculations; and atypical or unusual and critical dosage frequency considerations. In this same study, the most common group of factors associated with errors were those related to knowledge and the application of knowledge related to drug therapy (30%); knowledge and use of knowledge regarding patient factors that affect drug therapy (29.2%); use of calculations, decimal points, or unit and rate expression factors (17.5%); and nomenclature factors (incorrect drug name, dosage form, or abbreviation) (13.4%) (Lesar, Briceland & Stein, 1997).

What we have learned is that medication errors result from single or multiple breakdowns in a system's continuum of diagnosing an ailment, planning a therapeutic regimen, prescribing and dispensing drugs, and administering the drug. Twenty-nine percent of the errors are attributable to the failure to disseminate drug knowledge (Leape, Brennan & Laird, 1991). In another study that evaluated errors, the most common causes were related to drug knowledge (30%), knowledge about the patient (29.2%), the use of calculations and decimal points (17.5%), and nomenclature issues (incorrect drug name, dosage form, or abbreviation) (13.4%) (Lesar, Briceland & Stein, 1997).

What leads to other common errors in prescription writing? One study suggests that there are some conditions that are more likely to produce prescribing errors: those related to work environment (workload, caring for other providers' patients, hurried prescribing), those related to the team (incomplete written communication, verbal orders), and those related to the individual (hunger, tiredness, knowledge deficit). Staffing shortages, poor work environment, low morale, inexperience, excessive tasks, absence of protocols, unhelpful patients, complex diseases, and language or communication problems are also contributing factors (Dean, 2002).

Certainly the failure to write clearly and specifically causes many problems. Analysis has shown that 80% of the errors due to illegible handwriting are caused by only a few providers (Rich, 2001). Pharmacists may inadvertently substitute drugs because of a combination of illegible handwriting on the prescription and the pharmacist's misinterpretation of other clues that might have prevented the errors (Brodell et al, 1997). Individuals who cannot or do not write clearly may want to print in block capital letters rather than use cursive writing. Occasionally, a prescriber's handwriting is so poor that, to avoid problems, they have rubber stamps made or use preprinted pads for the common prescriptions that they write. Increasingly, offices are using computers to electronically transmit prescriptions to pharmacies, thus reducing illegibility problems. E-prescribing has been touted as a way to improve patient safety through generation of legible, accurate prescriptions that have been checked for harmful interactions (Krohn, 2003). These systems are promising, yet widespread enough to currently make a difference.

Many other errors occur through carelessness or inattention, on the part of either the prescriber or the pharmacist (Vitillo & Lesar, 1991). Regulations to restrict the numbers of hours that hospital housestaff practice are aimed at helping health care providers be more alert when they work, including when they are writing prescriptions.

Labeling the prescription with the exact times of day the medication is to be taken, such as 6:00 AM, 12:00 PM, 6:00 PM, and 12:00 AM, may reduce some medication errors. Providers should keep in mind that patients will be more compliant if the regimen complements their daily schedule and if the instructions are easily understood. To improve patient understanding, instructions should be written on the bottle and on an instruction sheet in large enough print for someone who is visually impaired (McNally & Wertheimer, 1992). It is also important to educate each patient aggressively about the names and purposes of all prescription drugs. This helps reduce errors by making the patient a partner in the process.

Using a survey of successful malpractice lawsuits involving medications, Buppert (2000) suggests some specific things that should be done to reduce the potential for problematic prescriptions:

- Write clearly, or invest in an electronic prescription transmission system
- When a patient has disclosed suicidal ideation, write for no more than a 7-day supply of any medication that could be lethal if taken all at once.
- Warn patients of side effects.
- Discontinue a medication when it causes a cautioned side effect.
- Get informed consent when a drug can cause permanent side effects, and there are less risky alternatives available.
- If prescribing differently from the directions on the drug manufacturer's package insert (i.e., "off-label"), document the rationale for deviating from the package insert instructions and be prepared to prove that the standard of care supports the alternative prescribing regimen.
- When a medication is known to cause some adverse effects after long-term use, either avoid using the drug for long-term therapy or monitor carefully for the onset of potential problems.
- Ask, listen, and alter the plan.

Table 11-3 describes some other specific errors and how they might be avoided.

ADMINISTRATIVE CONCERNS

Formularies

In an effort to reduce costs and channel prescriptions to a smaller number of total drugs, a growing number of organizations have established drug formularies. Many managed care

TABLE 11-3 Conmmon Errors Made in Writing Prescriptions

Common Error	Solutions
Patients may fail to recognize that they have two prescriptions for the same medication, especially when some drugs may be listed according to generic name and some according to trade name	Use nonproprietary names when ordering and always use the same drug name in writing a prescription; avoid the chance that the patient may take one "digoxin" tablet per day and one "Lanoxin" tablet per day; add patient diagnosis to prescription
Confusion of look-alike drugs	Watch for drugs that are similar in spelling: acetohexamide vs. acetazolamide hydralazine vs. hydroxyzine Watch for other minor differences: chloroquine HCl vs. chloroquine phosphate quinidine sulfate vs. quinidine gluconate Drug names should never be abbreviated
Errors in dosage strength or concentration	Decimal points may be hard to see: use 50 and not 50.0; use 0.5 and not .5 Solid dosage forms often come in a variety of strengths; liquid preparations, particularly for infants and children, are sometimes available in different concentrations It is dangerous to request a drug by volume without specifying the concentration, particularly for children; order the standard volumes listed in texts or package inserts when writing for liquid antibiotics; for children, have a system of systematic double-checking accuracy of prescriptions Pharmacists may ask patients to turn in old containers when new products are ordered; this provides a double-check on accuracy and what the patient is taking
Patients fail to understand how to take medication	Never write "take as directed"; be specific about what you want the patient to do
Use of misleading abbreviations in writing prescriptions:	
tid vs q8h	Clarify the difference between q8h and tid: tid means while awake
hs: hour of sleep or take at bedtime	What if the patient takes a midday nap or works nights? Clarify sleeping habits
ac or pc: before or after meals	What if patient eats more than three meals/day?
x3d	Does this mean for 3 days or for three doses?
u = units	Avoid using u as an abbreviation for unit; 4u of regular insulin may be read as 40 units
tsp = teaspoonful	The amount of drug varies a good deal depending on the specific teaspoon being used; this is not a good term to use when ordering a drug whose exact dosage is important
prn = as needed	Patients should have a very clear idea as to when they "need" the drug; place limits on the numbers of pills taken, e.g., "take 1 tablet every 4 hours as needed" Do not write "refill prn"; it means *refill indefinitely* and few prescriptions should be given that latitude
Patient altering of prescription to increase number of refills or number of pills	Write "one refill" and not "1 refill" to avoid tempting patients to change it to "4 or 10 refills" Many prescribers draw a tight circle around the number of pills to be dispensed so that patients may not insert a 1 in front of the number, or zeroes after the number or provider may write "ten" instead of 10 to limit tampering with the number.

Data from Aronson J: Confusion over similar drug names: problems and solutions, *Drug Safety* 12:155-160, 1995; Fox GN: Minimizing prescribing errors in infants and children, *Am Fam Phys* 53:1319-1325, 1996; and Vitillo JA, Lesar TS: Preventing medication prescribing errors, *DICP* 25:1388-1394, 1991.

organizations, health maintenance organizations, private insurance plans, and state Medicaid programs, as well as federal Medicare programs, the Veterans Administration, and the military, have created their own formularies to meet the specific needs of their patient population. Although some health care providers object to any limitations being placed on the drugs they may prescribe, this is a growing trend throughout the nation. Pressure is also put on pharmaceutical companies to provide drugs to some programs at a greatly reduced rate if they wish to have their products appear on the approved formulary list. How the formularies are established, how inclusive they are, and how regularly they are updated based on the latest scientific guidelines for care all determine whether the institutional formulary will be an asset or a liability for the provider. A formulary may restrict providers from using those with which they are most comfortable or have the broadest experience. The most frequent complaint against formularies is that they are slow to accept and add new and effective drugs.

As a cost-cutting mechanism, some pharmacies order medications in large doses and then split them. This practice of drug division, either by cutting or weight, leads to inaccuracies in dosage. Prescribers should confirm the pharmacies they work with do not participate in this risky practice (Bachynsky, 2002; Rosenberg, Nathan & Plakogiannis, 2002; Teng et al, 2002).

Medicaid

To write prescriptions for patients on Medicaid (or Medical Assistance, as it is known in many states), the prescriber must be an authorized Medicaid prescriber. Individuals applying to the state will be issued a Medicaid provider number to use on all prescriptions. This number may be different from the Medicaid render number (the number of the person who actually delivers the care to the patient) or the Medicaid reimbursement number (who will receive reimbursement for the service). In some situations, all the numbers will be for the same provider, in some cases, particularly large institutions, the numbers will all be different.

Medicaid prescriptions are filled only from a Medicaid prescription form provided by the state for that purpose. After filling in the authorized prescriber number, the prescriber should check to see if the patient's Medicaid card is up to date before writing the prescription. Each eligible patient must have a separate card.

Because Medicaid is a joint state and federal program, each state has its own specific requirements regarding Medicaid policies. Most states have a Medicaid formulary identifying a circumscribed number of drugs that will be covered under Medicaid. Many new medications, expensive trade name products, or drugs designated as "less than effective" by the FDA have been omitted from these formularies. With the slowing economy and the tremendous financial pressures experienced by states, further cuts were initiated in 2003 by establishing state "Preferred Drug Formulary" lists that reduced the authorized drug lists to around 100 drugs—omitting many of the more expensive trade name drugs. Payment will not be made for drugs outside the formulary unless a waiver stipulating that the treatment is medically necessary or life-sustaining has been obtained before submitting the prescription for filling. Many drugs that have gone from legend to over-the-counter still have some dosages that are available by prescription so that Medicaid or insurance coverage will apply. It is standard among most states that Medicaid prescriptions must be filled within 10 days and the maximum number of refills is two. (Birth control pills often may be filled for a maximum of six cycles—this includes the two refills.) The prescription may usually not be written for more than a 100-day supply of drug. (This includes the initial prescription with two refills.)

Out-of-State Prescriptions

Patients should be cautioned to get prescriptions filled before leaving the state or have it verified that there will not be a problem getting it filled in the state to which they are going. Some states prohibit pharmacists from filling prescriptions written in another state or may have regulations that do not allow them to fill prescriptions if written by a PA or an NP. However, many states have no specific laws regarding the filling of prescriptions written out of state. Regardless of the law, pharmacists may refuse to fill any prescription about which they have suspicions. This is particularly true of prescriptions for controlled substances.

More and more, out-of-state prescriptions are becoming a factor for prescribers to consider. The population is mobile. People both move frequently and travel throughout the country or the world on business. Patients may cross state lines to receive care at the nearest facility. Children may leave home to go to universities in other states. Some prescription plans are centralized, with all prescriptions being filled in a central place in the country and mailed to the enrolled member. Finally, advances in Telehealth may make the distances between prescriber and patient even less important but create the need for different types of licensing, monitoring, and law.

Another recent trend has been for insurance plans to direct their members to send prescriptions to out-of-state mail-order or Internet pharmacies where costs may be less. Many of these large "virtual pharmacies" have refused to recognize legal prescriptions written by providers who are not physicians. The resolution of this problem has been a focus of national NP groups (Edmunds, 2003).

A substantially different problem is for patients to use the Internet to obtain medications without a prescription, or without seeing a physician. This practice is illegal, and any drugs purchased over the Internet, particularly those coming in from outside the country, will be subject to monitoring and seizure by the FDA in conjunction with other federal agencies. Many of the drugs available outside the United States are counterfeit drugs, and there are no guarantees of their purity, safety, or efficacy. Until recently, the United States has been able to limit the use of these drugs through tight federal control. The use of the Internet for ordering makes the control of these products more and more problematic (Edmunds, 2003) (see www.FDA.gov/oc/buyonline).

Prescriptions by Telephone Orders

Except for prescriptions for Schedule I and II drugs, any prescription may be sent via telephone to a pharmacy. Most states provide that in an emergency situation, the pharmacist may dispense a limited amount (usually not more than a 48 hour supply) of a Schedule II drug on the verbal order of a provider. The provider must then make sure that the pharmacy has a written prescription to cover that order within 72 hours.

A common practice in some busy offices is for lay personnel such as receptionists, rather than nurses, to call the pharmacy with a telephone prescription order. This does not remove the provider's legal responsibility for the accuracy of the order. Thus providers who call in their own telephone orders to the pharmacy maintain some control over their liability (West et al, 1994).

Dispensing of Medications

The actual provision of medication to the patient from an office or store supply is termed *dispensing*. This is different from administering medications, the process commonly performed by registered nurses where a pharmacist dispenses the medication and the nurse physically sees that the medication is taken by the patient. Some state laws allow for limited dispensing of medications, usually in the following two situations.

Drug sampling is a type of limited dispensing. Pharmaceutical company field representatives leave medications with health care providers with prescriptive authority who have authorization to receive them. Due to the Pharmaceutical Drug Manufactures Act of 1988, which was passed to decrease provider abuse of sampled drugs, drug field representatives are not authorized to leave samples to any prescriber unless it can be validated that the individual is a legal prescriber. The state boards of medicine give validation companies information about physician prescribers every year and "validate" that they are licensed prescribers. The situation is more complex for nonphysician prescribers. For example, in many states, NPs do not have independent prescriptive authority but have delegated authority established through a collaborative agreement with a physician. In those states, a validation company must not only ensure that the practitioner is a licensed prescriber but also obtain the name of the physician with whom they have a collaborative agreement. This information must come from an authoritative agency, usually the board of nursing. In many states, the boards of nursing cannot or will not give validation companies this information. In attempting to both be compliant with PDMA regulations and provide samples to NPs, companies have attempted to have NPs fill out a form asking for information about their license and collaborating physician. If NPs are willing to fill out the forms, they are being given drug samples. Many NPs refuse to sign the forms, not understanding why they are asked to do so (Esat, 2003).

Medication packets with a few doses, primarily of medications new to the market, are given to providers to encourage them to try the product so they can gain experience with it and then recommend it to their patients. Multiple problems with both the process and the theory behind drug sampling have led to a decline in this process over the years (see the section on drug sampling in Chapter 4).

Limited dispensing of medications is also legal in emergency facilities and is confined to the dispensing of one or two doses of specific medications required in emergency situations. A few doses of narcotic analgesics or antibiotics are the most frequently dispensed drugs in these settings.

Drug Substitution by the Pharmacist

When prescribers write a prescription using a product's trade name, the question of generic substitution arises. In states where generic substitution is automatically allowed or where prescription or insurance plans require generic substitution whenever possible, the pharmacist will need to determine if there is an acceptable generic substitute for an ordered medication. In many situations, pharmacists may dispense the generic substitute without notifying the health care provider. They should, however, notify the patient, pass along cost savings to the patient, and indicate the substituted brand on the original prescription and the prescription drug label. If a prescriber is concerned about the bioequivalence of a particular medication or for patient compliance reasons, the prescriber may write "Do not substitute" or "Dispense as written" on the original prescription if no change is desired from what is written.

PREVENTING PROBLEMS IN DRUG USE

The health care prescriber faces three common problems in the process of providing medications: the abusing patient, the abusing health care provider, and the financially needy patient.

Most health care prescribers will, at some point in their practice, encounter drug-seeking patients. These often include "professional" patients who have become addicted to narcotics or well-intentioned individuals who are misusing drugs. In either case, the provider's index of suspicion should be aroused, particularly about the need for controlled substances, when a patient (1) asks for narcotics by name, indicating that they are the only thing that will relieve the problem; (2) carries copies of abnormal laboratory tests, electrocardiograms documenting a myocardial infarction, or other documents that support subjective complaints of pain; or (3) calls frequently seeking refills or increasingly larger amounts of medication because they lost or spilled their medicine.

Validation of suspicious behavior of a patient may be confirmed in talking with the pharmacist. Attempts to refill prescriptions early, change prescriptions to provide for more drug to be dispensed, and use multiple providers to obtain prescriptions for the same drugs are all indications that the patient has a problem. Sometimes pharmacists have received alerts from other pharmacists or hospitals that a particular patient is in the area telling a particular story. This type of cooperation and sharing of information helps assist health care providers in avoiding traps or being taken in by a scam artist.

Providers who are feeling increasingly uncomfortable about patient drug requests should carefully confront patients about their observations. They should also offer support and assistance if the patient inappropriately relies on medications. They also should not continue to provide prescriptions to the patient. Providers who feel that they cannot continue to meet the needs of a patient have a responsibility to help that patient find another health care provider.

Occasionally a pharmacist or a health care provider will discover that a patient has obtained a prescription pad and is writing his or her own prescriptions. This, or any other, type of illegal behavior must be immediately reported to the police.

The same problems exist when health care providers encounter professional colleagues whose behavior seems inappropriate. When the possibility exists that the health care provider may be involved in drug abuse or misuse, gentle confrontation is essential. These individuals should be referred to the relevant medical, nursing, or pharmacy boards for impaired provider counseling. This is an effective way of acknowledging problems and still remaining in good professional standing so that a license to practice is not permanently sacrificed.

The final type of prescribing problem concerns patients who really need medications but cannot afford to buy them. Many pharmaceutical companies provide medications for people in need, apart from their drug sampling program to providers. NeedyMeds is an Internet site that contains information on patient assistance programs offered by pharmaceutical manufacturers. They have listings on over 125 companies and over 800 drugs. Their site at www.needymeds.com has an alert service so that users will know whenever changes are made to the database.

GOOD COMMUNICATION AND DEVELOPING A POSITIVE RELATIONSHIP WITH THE PHARMACIST

The specialized knowledge and watchful eye of the pharmacist may be an important resource for the primary care provider. Establishing a personal relationship with the pharmacists most likely to fill the prescriber's prescriptions helps to establish a team to eliminate errors and increase patient satisfaction with medications.

Pharmacists are particularly aware of the changing drug formulations in over-the-counter products. Because of this they are able to guide primary care providers in the most effective over-the-counter products to recommend to patients. Pharmacists also tend to be aware of what diseases are endemic in the community and what medications seem to be most effective in controlling them. As pharmacology specialists, they often should be consulted when determining drug therapy for a difficult case. Finally, pharmacists may provide the one centralized source for oversight of the many prescriptions that patients receive from different providers. As such, pharmacists using sophisticated software are often the ones who detect or prevent drug interactions, overdosages, or discover contraindications.

It is true that in the past an adversarial role developed between some pharmacists and new nonphysician prescribers in some states. However, as new prescribers demonstrated their competence and willingness to be part of a responsible health care team, most pharmacists have become very supportive and helpful to these new prescribers. What little research has been conducted in this area demonstrates that very few pharmacists report problems with the prescriptions written by nonphysicians. The most successful prescriber–pharmacist relationships are established on mutual respect for each other's skills and knowledge.

Many primary care providers new to an area or new to the prescriber role would do well to visit their local pharmacies and meet the pharmacists who work there. Providing some written material about who they are and their background, education, credentials, and clinical interests may be important in establishing a positive relationship. Initiating consultation with pharmacists, making time to answer questions, being receptive to suggestions, and expressing appreciation for assistance are essential in establishing a relationship that will provide the best care for the patient. Pharmacists often hear what patients say about their office visits. Thus they may be a valuable source of information about patient understanding and acceptance of the care they have received and their willingness or ability to comply with ordered therapy. All of this feedback is available if there is a good relationship established.

The prescription is a formalized communication between the prescriber and the pharmacist. Although a prescription contains the very formulaic information required by law, there also is no reason why specific directions or concerns for the pharmacist about the medication cannot be written on the prescription. An example might be particular concerns about drug bioequivalence of generic agents and a note asking that the same generic agent be used each time the prescription is filled, or a note for the pharmacist to tell the patient that the prescription cannot be refilled until the patient returns to the provider for further evaluation.

SUMMARY

Writing a prescription may be stressful at first, until the format is ingrained in the student's mind. The most important factors to consider are the accuracy and appropriateness of the prescription, not the format. Working together with the pharmacist, a relationship may be established that will benefit all individuals involved.

REFERENCES

Bachynsky J, Wiens C, Melnychuk K: The practice of splitting tablets: cost and therapeutic aspects, *Pharmacoeconomics* 20:339-346, 2002.

Brodell RT et al: Prescription errors: legibility and drug name confusion, *Arch Fam Med* 6:296-298, 1997.

Buppert C: 8 Ways to prevent malpractice when writing prescriptions, *Gold Sheet*, Annapolis, MD, November 2000.

Dean B et al: Causes of prescribing errors in hospital inpatients: a prospective study, *Lancet* 359L:1373-1378, 2002.

Denig P, Haajer-Ruskamp FM: Therapeutic decision making of physicians, *Pharmaceutisch Weekblad Scientific Ed* 14:9-15; 1992.

Edmunds MW: Advocating for NPs—go and do likewise, *Nurse Pract* 28:56, 2003.

Edmunds MW: Warn patients of imported drug dangers, *Nurse Pract* 28:70, 2003.

Esat A: NP invisibility: validation compliance supports advance practice nurses, *Nurse Pract* 28:52, 2003.

Fox GN: Minimizing prescribing errors in infants and children, *Am Fam Phys* 53:1319-1325, 1996.

Groves KEM, Flanagan PS, MacKinnon NJ: Why physicians start or stop prescribing a drug: literature review and formulary implications, *Formulary* 37:186-194, 2002.

Howell RR et al: Prescription-writing skills questioned, *Fam Med* 26:472-473, 1994.

Howell RR, Jones KW: Prescription-writing errors and markers: the value of knowing the diagnosis, *Fam Med* 25:104-105, 1993.

Ingrim NB et al: Physician noncompliance with prescription-writing requirements, *Am J Hosp Pharm* 40:414-417, 1983.

Krohn R: Making E-prescribing work: a fresh approach, *J Health C Inf Manag* 17:17-19, 2003.

Leape LL et al: The nature of adverse events: I. hospitalized patients. Results of the Harvard Medical Practice Study II, *N Engl J Med* 324:377-384, 1991.

Lesar TS, Briceland L, Stein DS: Factors related to errors in medication prescribing, *JAMA* 277:311-317, 1997.

Lilly LL et al: Look-alike abbreviations: prescriptions for confusion, *Am J Nurs* 97:12, 1997.

Marek CL: Avoiding prescribing errors: a systematic approach, *J Am Dent Assoc* 127:617-623, 1996.

McNally DL, Wertheimer D: Strategies to reduce the high cost of patient noncompliance, *Md Med J* 41:223-225, 1992.

Niederhauser VP: Prescribing for children: issues in pediatric pharmacology, *Nurs Pract* 22:6-18, 1997.

Norton LL: Continuing education: medical and medication errors: a partial summary of reports by the Institute of Medicine and the Quality Interagency Coordination Task Force, *J Manag Care Pharm* 7:62-68, 2001.

Phillips J et al: Retrospective analysis of mortalities associated with medication errors, *Am J Health-Syst Pharm* 58:1824-1829, 2001.

Rich DS: Illegible prescription handwriting; blanket medication orders; "range" medication orders; automatic stop orders, *Hosp Pharmacy* 36:786-789, 2001.

Rosenberg JM, Nathan JP, Plakogiannis F: Weight variability of pharmacist-dispensed split tablets. *J Am Pharm Assoc* 42:200-205, 2002.

Sarriff A et al: A study of patients' self-interpretation of prescription instructions, *J Clin Pharm Ther* 17:125-128, 1992.

Self TH: Prescribing errors: causes—and a plan to "do no harm," *Consultant* 42:1010-1013, 2002.

Stein BE: Avoiding drug reactions: seven steps to writing safe prescriptions, *Geriatrics* 49:28-30, 1994.

Taylor RJ, Bond CM: Change in the established prescribing habits of general practitioners: an analysis of initial prescriptions in general practice, *Br J Gen Pract* 41:244-248, 1991.

Teng J et al: Lack of medication dose uniformity in commonly split tablets, *J Am Pharm Assoc* 42:195-199, 2002.

US Department of Justice, DEA: *Midlevel provider's manual: an informational outline of the Controlled Substances Act of 1970,* Washington, DC, March 1993, US Department of Justice.

US Department of Justice, DEA: *Physician's manual: an informational outline of the Controlled Substances Act of 1970,* Washington, DC, March 1990, US Department of Justice.

Vitillo JA, Lesar TS: Preventing medication prescribing errors, *DICP* 25:1388-1394, 1991.

West DW et al: Pediatric medication order error rates related to the mode of order transmission, *Arch Pediatr Adolesc Med* 148:1322-1326, 1994.

Winslow EH et al: Legibility and completeness of physicians' handwritten medication orders, *Heart Lung* 26:158-164, 1997.

CHAPTER 12

Making Treatment Decisions

CRITICAL DECISION-MAKING

It has been observed that the quality of health care is determined by two main factors: the quality of the decisions that determine what actions are taken and the quality with which those actions are executed—what to do and how to do it. If the wrong actions are chosen, no matter how skillfully they are executed, the quality of care will suffer. Similarly, if the correct actions are chosen but the execution is flawed, the quality of care will suffer (Eddy, 1990). Health care requires clinicians who can make decisions autonomously. It is therefore essential that health care providers consciously strive to develop effective problem-solving and decision-making skills.

How do students learn to make clinical decisions? The traditional educational approach in all health care disciplines has been an implicit apprenticeship model, in which health care providers follow the actions of attending physicians or preceptors with little attention to the mechanics of the diagnostic and treatment strategies. Thus the quality of the learning may be dependent primarily on the skills of the mentor.

Diagnostic reasoning is an important part of the health provider's role. It is not uncommon in the first diagnosis and management class to find students absolutely silent when they hear the first discussions about how to make a diagnosis. Everyone in the room is thinking but no one is saying out loud, "You mean that is how you arrive at a diagnosis? Your best guess?! I must have missed something. It has to be more precise than that."

Clinical decision-making has components of judging and evaluating, but decision-making implies not just contemplation but also action based on choices. Certainly part of the process of decision-making is *critical thinking*, a term that has been in vogue for many years in nursing. However, implicit in the process of decision-making is establishing goals and taking risks beyond what is thought of as critical thinking.

The intrusion of managed care into clinical practice means that resources for health care clinicians are more restricted. Ordering multiple tests to rule in or rule out various disease states is not an option. More than ever before, health care providers need to learn critical thinking skills in making proper clinical judgments. So the question becomes, how to individually and collectively ensure that higher-level thinking is engaged in for health care problem solving.

CRITICAL THINKING

Benjamin S. Bloom's seminal work in 1956 on the original taxonomy of educational objectives for the cognitive domain does not contain the term *decision-making*. However, both of the two higher cognitive domains, synthesis and evaluation, contain verbs that involve planning, composing, designing, constructing, creating, setting up, organizing, appraising, evaluating, comparing, revising, assessing—all components of the decision-making process.

Much of the contemporary research about critical thinking has been conducted by nurses who were required by the National League for Nursing to demonstrate critical thinking outcomes in students for programs seeking accreditation. Many writers agree that critical thinking involves dimensions of logic, problem-solving (Beyer, 1985), and scientific inquiry (Bandman & Bandman, 1995) and might be defined as "careful, deliberate, goal directed thinking based on principles of science and the scientific method" (Bandman & Bandman, 1995). Clearly, the construct of critical thinking is not a set body of knowledge but rather a nonlinear dynamic process (Jacobs et al, 1997; Videbeck, 1997) and not an outcome.

Watson and Glaser (1964) have dominated the literature about critical thinking, arguing that it has two basic components: knowledge and an attitude of inquiry. *Knowledge* includes both knowledge of the domain-specific subject matter and of the specific mental operations or critical thinking skills (Beyer, 1985). *Attitude* denotes frame of mind or an attitude of inquiry, curiosity, and a willingness or desire to examine and explore the problem. This component is uniquely developed in each individual and results from the health care provider's personality and culturally determined behavioral norms.

However, knowledge and an attitude of inquiry alone do not capture true critical thinking. The thinker must critically appraise knowledge. This component of thinking allows the thinker to apply, synthesize, and evaluate what is known and, as such, brings critical thinking into the highest cognitive domain (Hugie, 1992). This process of critical thinking is outlined in Figure 12-1.

As seen from this figure, the clinician's knowledge is key. Clearly, the beginning student or novice will have less knowledge than the expert. However, health care provider students do not have minds as empty as blank pages. They have information from previous courses and experiences. Registered nurses (RNs) returning for nurse practitioner (NP) education may have had years of successful clinical practice. Many older students have had other careers before they turned to health care. All these students have some knowledge but need additional information that is evaluated and then organized so it becomes usable. Some researchers have suggested that the mind might be thought of as a series of matrices in which information is stored. The matrix is entered and information retrieved as the individual recognizes patterns, sees similarities, recognizes what is important, generalizes, and uses common sense (Elstein et al, 1972).

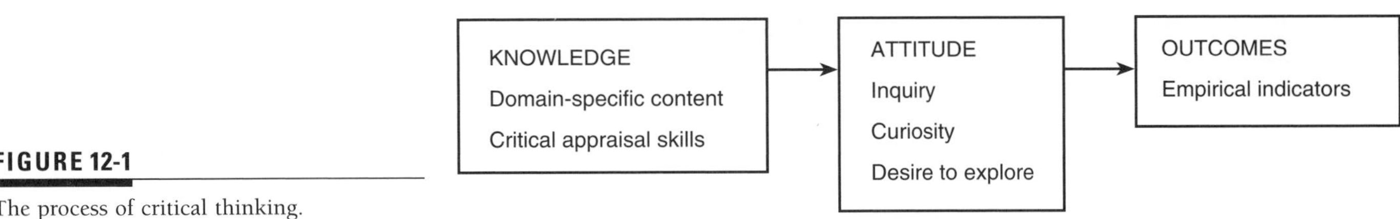

FIGURE 12-1

The process of critical thinking.

Beginners have inconsistent information. Recognition of their lack of knowledge dictates the organization of the curriculum. For example, advanced pharmacology content is wasted in the first semester before students master components of health assessment, physiology, or other basic information about diagnostic or treatment methodologies that will give important context to their drug knowledge.

Research into the critical thinking a clinician uses in diagnostic reasoning and problem-solving suggests two different theories of clinical expertise. The first theory proposes that experts perform better than novices because they have better problem-solving strategies. The alternative theory suggests that experts perform better because they have more knowledge. The current evidence in the literature supports the latter position, that clinical expertise is largely a function of domain-specific knowledge (Benner, 1984; Elstein, Shulman & Sprafka, 1990; Lange et al, 1997). For example, several researchers have found that the diagnostic strategies used by experts and novices are very similar (Newble, Hoare & Baxter, 1982). Norman and colleagues suggest that experts do not possess any innate or learned advantage in problem-solving techniques. Rather, experts solve problems better because they know more in their domains than novices do and that problem-solving expertise generalizes somewhat within a domain of medical knowledge (e.g., rheumatology) but does not necessarily generalize to other domains (e.g., pulmonary or cardiology) (Norman et al, 1985a, 1985b).

There is no ideal way to think. Thinking processes differ for each of us. The literature suggests that it is possible to facilitate the development of cognitive skills in clinical decision-making (Lipman & Deatrick, 1997), but overall there is little information on how the cognitive skills associated with decision-making may be stimulated and, in particular, how the characteristics of critical thinkers may be fostered.

Some examples might prove instructive. In one clinical setting, one wise clinician sends beginning students into the room to begin interviewing the patient and then has them report back after they have obtained only the chief complaint. Then, using the age, sex, and the chief complaint, students are asked to generate a differential of all the things that might be responsible for causing the chief complaint. The faculty member helps students with limited knowledge add to their database of possible differentials by assisting them to stretch their thinking. Students then return to the patient with a systematic plan of questioning, which includes asking about all the possible elements on the differential, to rule them in or rule them out. This is a different way of teaching students to think and to organize information, rather than having them ask all the general questions in a standard comprehensive history. This methodology also teaches students an expectation about broader thinking and systematic questioning.

In other situations, schemata, algorithms, or mental models have been used in decision-making. These are all abstract representations of information gained from experience, and they assist in understanding the world and the reality in which people exist (Howard, 1987). Thiele and colleagues (1986) investigated the effects of teaching cue recognition on a student's ability to make accurate decisions. The works of Benner (1984) and Benner and Tanner (1987) emphasize the place of experience in the quality of thinking. Myrick & Yonge (2002) describe the importance of preceptor questioning in helping students think critically.

Although much of critical thinking and clinical decision-making may be related to natural curiosity and intelligence, there are some attributes (steps or tools) that will tend to make thinking more complete. If clinicians have knowledge, then it is important to observe what they do with that knowledge in order to determine the extent of critical thinking taking place. Some observable behaviors of critical thinkers were identified as the ability to do the following:

- Distinguish between observation and inference and facts and claims
- Determine the reliability of a claim or source
- Determine the accuracy of statements
- Differentiate relevant and irrelevant data
- Differentiate warranted and unwarranted claims
- Recognize ambiguous or equivocal claims/arguments
- Discern inconsistencies in reasoning
- Determine an argument's strength
- Draw inferences

An additional way of determining whether critical thinking has taken place is to look at the outcomes of the critical thinking process. One curriculum that attempted to encourage critical thinking used empirical indicators of critical thinking to measure student performance (Jacobs et al, 1997) (Box 12-1).

Lack of knowledge, problems in attitude, or flaws in critical appraisal result in defective thinking. For example, one may have good knowledge of a subject but may be inflexible or unwilling to consider other options or points of view. Likewise, the individual may have curiosity, motivation, and interest but may lack the knowledge necessary to develop alternatives and to consider options (Eddy, 1990).

DECISION-MAKING

In exploring how people make decisions, nursing has focused almost exclusively on the process of critical thinking, whereas the medical literature is filled with research on diagnostic and clinical decision-making. Reports suggest that in most medical

BOX 12-1

EMPIRICAL INDICATORS OF CRITICAL THINKING

SYNTHESIS OF RELEVANT INFORMATION
Obtains data from all sources
Distinguishes relevant from irrelevant data
Validates data obtained
Identifies missing data

PREDICTION OF OUTCOMES
Predicts multiple outcomes
Recognizes ramification of actions

EXAMINATION OF ASSUMPTIONS
Recognizes assumptions
Detects bias
Identifies unstated assumptions

GENERATION OF OPTIONS
Recognizes relationships of action or inaction
Transfers thoughts and concepts to multiple settings
Develops alternate courses of action

IDENTIFICATION OF PATTERNS
Identifies relationships/patterns
Recognizes logical inconsistencies or fallacies
Determines generalizations
Develops plan of action consistent with a model and/or seeks alternative models

CHOICE OF ACTIONS
Determines a choice of action
Evaluates the effects of own actions
Evaluates the soundness of conclusions
Evaluates worth of action to client/society

From Jacobs PM et al: An approach to defining and operationalizing critical thinking, *J Nurs Educ* 36(1):19-22, 1997.

schools, when clinical reasoning is taught, it is as an add-on and is not continued as an integral component of the rest of the courses. Because of this lack of curricular integration, special courses in clinical reasoning appear to have a marginal effect (Chessare et al, 1996). The general focus of most medical curricula is on acquisition of knowledge; how to search for and critically evaluate evidence is a skill generally addressed superficially, if at all.

In several research studies of RNs, it was suggested that RNs often appear to lack the skills necessary to make effective decisions (Aspinall, 1976; Boney & Baker, 1997). Nurses report receiving little or no education in decision-making during their basic nursing education programs. In several reported studies, RNs demonstrated "a propensity to stereotype, to be influenced by cultural bias and a desire to make rapid decisions, with early or premature closure in decision-making because of a limited knowledge base" (Aspinall, 1976; Lipman & Deatrick, 1997).

Aspinall (1976) concluded that many nurses are action oriented, resulting in a focus on action rather than on analysis of all the data. A study based on NP students found that they often attempted to formulate a diagnosis too early in the decision-making process. Almost all of the NP students had practiced as staff nurses in acute care settings, where rapidly formulating a diagnosis was important. Although that manner of clinical decision-making was successful for experienced clinicians, as inexperienced NP students, formulating hypotheses too early often resulted in incomplete assessments (Lipman & Deatrick, 1997). Thus skills that had helped students as RNs were counterproductive in the new role without a broader knowledge base.

Research suggests that much of the confusion that is seen in some NP students early in their program can be attributed to a reworking of decision-making and critical-thinking skills. The NP program asks them to take their existing domain-specific knowledge, in which they have "expert" skills, and to process information in new ways and to exhibit different behaviors. It appears that asking them to do this temporarily suspends use of their previously learned skills. (Another explanation proposed for this phenomenon is that NPs are inhibited because of the return to intense scrutiny by preceptors/faculty of their performance as they attempt to use newly acquired knowledge and skills [Roberts, Tabloski & Bova, 1997].) What some faculty have begun to accept is that nursing education with medical education may require a paradigm shift for the student, prompting reorganization of existing knowledge and critical thinking skills and not just the addition of new knowledge. In this paradigm shift, NP students must move to a new developmental stage that allows them to recognize the limitations of their existing knowledge and must learn how to acquire needed knowledge to assume increased responsibility for their own judgment and decisions. Simply put, the problem for NP students is probably the result of "taking an expert and asking them to be a novice again" (Roberts, Tabloski & Bova, 1997).

The medical literature abounds with reports on decision-making and development of diagnostic skills (Sox et al, 1988). One of the best to bring together the various theories and ideas is Eddy (1990). He suggests that, in general, the goal of a health care decision-maker is to choose an action that is most likely to deliver the outcomes the patient wants. Eddy goes on to identify the two main steps of making a clinical decision. First, the outcomes of the different options must be estimated; then, the desirability of the outcomes of each option must be compared. "The first step involves collecting and analyzing whatever evidence exists regarding the benefits, harms, and costs of each option. Because the available evidence is virtually never perfect or complete, this step will also involve some subjective judgment" (Eddy, 1990). For example, should a patient with a prostatic mass continue to be monitored, have chemotherapy, or undergo surgery?

The resulting estimates of that analysis then form the basis for the second step. Three types of comparisons are required in the second step: (1) the benefits of a practice must be compared with the harms (e.g., risks, side effects, inconvenience, length of disability, and anxiety), (2) the health outcomes must be compared with any costs, and (3) if it is not possible to do everything because of limited resources, the amount of benefit gained and the resources consumed must be compared with other options to give priority to options that have the highest yield (Eddy, 1990) (Figure 12-2).

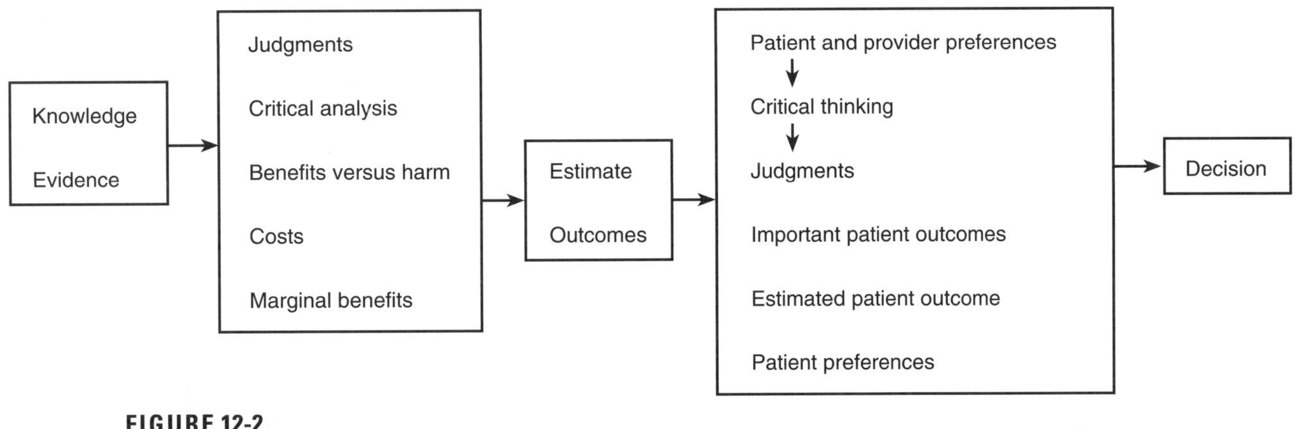

FIGURE 12-2

The two main steps of a decision. (Modified from Eddy DM: Anatomy of a decision, *JAMA* 263:441-443, 1990.)

No matter how explicitly, how consciously, or how correctly each of these steps is performed, these factors must be considered every time a decision is made regarding a health practice. This is true whether the decision is made for an individual clinician, whether a group of health care providers are recommending a guideline for a group of patients, or whether third-party payers are setting policy coverage. To appreciate this, imagine trying to advise a patient regarding the merits of a health practice without considering any evidence of its effects, the magnitude of the benefits or harms of the practice, or of caring whether the benefits outweighed the harms.

Anyone who makes a responsible decision regarding a health practice must have some idea, however uncertain, of the evidence that justifies its use, of its consequences, and of its desirability. It is important to separate the decision process into these two steps for several reasons. Specifically, Eddy's two steps involve different thought processes, have different anchors, and might be performed by different people. In addition, we can expect different degrees of agreement about the results. The first step is a question of facts. The anchor is empirical evidence. The process is a scientific one that involves experiments, analysis of evidence, and forecasting. The required skills are analytic. Finally, assuming there is some evidence to evaluate, it should be possible to get reasonable, open-minded people to agree on the results of this step (Eddy, 1990).

This is where evidence-based medicine (EBM) is to play a role. There are rules of evidence and methods built up from axioms over hundreds of years that can be applied to the evidence. Although there will always be some uncertainty and room for different scientific philosophies or schools of thought, there is at least the prospect that agreement can be reached (Eddy, 1990).

This is where clinical guidelines or decision-making algorithms fit in. It is reasonable to imagine that there is a correct answer out there, and there is a scientific context and language for rational debate and resolution. In short, this is a job for the left side of the brain, and we turn to scientists to do it (Eddy, 1990).

Essentially, this is the *science* of medicine. It is clear that step one, as so clearly articulated by Eddy, resembles very much the model of critical thinking so dominant in the nursing literature. The terminology and the focus may be a little different, but the basic components of domain-specific knowledge and an attitude of evaluation, along with critical analysis of the data, are imbedded in step one of clinical decision-making.

Returning to Eddy's model, the second step is a question not of facts but of personal values or preferences. The move to managed care and the recognition that the patient has rights as a consumer of care with the resulting restriction on resources have served to highlight the necessity of joint decision-making between the patient and clinician. The thought process is not analytic but personal and subjective—an appeal not to the left side of the brain, but to the right side of the brain, or even the gut. Different people can properly have different preferences. There is no single correct answer, and there is no obligation that everyone agree (Eddy, 1990).

Now, we are getting to the *art* of medicine.

To the extent that science is involved in this step at all, it is the science of discovering peoples' preferences—polls, questionnaires, and focus groups. Perhaps most important, the people whose preferences count are the patients, because they are the ones who will have to live (or die) with the outcomes. Others might intervene if an individual's decision is based on inaccurate information (e.g., insistence on antibiotic therapy for a viral upper respiratory tract infection), is illegal (e.g., drug abuse), or harms a public interest (e.g., refusal of control measures for an infectious disease) or when the patient is not competent enough to make a decision. However, assuming these complications do not apply, it is the patient's preferences that should determine the decision (Eddy, 1990).

In one of the classic research studies of how expert clinicians make clinical diagnoses, Elstein and colleagues (1972) proposed that expert physicians generate specific diagnostic hypotheses well before they have gathered most of the data for a particular case. Rather than progressively and systematically converging on a diagnosis through a series of constraining questions, the experienced physicians appear to leap directly to a small array of provisional hypotheses very early in their encounter with the patient. These provisional hypotheses are generated out of the physicians' background knowledge of medicine, including their range of specific experiences, in conjunction with the problematic elements recognized in the early stages of the encounter with the patient.

The physicians in the study by Elstein et al (1972) were considered expert clinicians by their peers. They were not novices but had a substantial body of domain-specific knowledge. In this study, four components of the process of hypothesis generation emerged. Although these are described serially, it is likely that some of them occur together. The components are as follows:

- Attending to initially available cues
- Identifying problematic elements from among these cues and searching long-term memory
- Generating hypotheses and suggestions for further inquiry
- Informally rank-ordering hypotheses according to the physician's subjective estimates

The rank ordering is based on the physician's evaluation of probability (estimates closely approximate the population base rate for a disease), seriousness (life-threatening or incapacitating conditions are ranked higher than their population base rate warrants), treatability (a treatable problem is ranked higher so as not to overlook any treatment that might possibly be helpful), and novelty (uniqueness of the problem keeps the physician interested in the case and ensures that unlikely avenues are explored, thus protecting the patient from the physician's premature closure on a more generally probable hypothesis that, in a particular case, might be in error) (Elstein et al, 1972, 1990).

The work of Benner (1984) remains one of the foremost in describing the passage of a nurse from novice to expert, detailing the ways in which nurses with varying levels of experience function. In addition, the work of Carnevali (1984) in the area of diagnostic reasoning has attempted to address the cognitive domain in relation to decision-making. Benner's (1984) work describes the process of skill acquisition by nurses, indicating a developmental approach to decision-making, commencing with decision analysis and progressing to hypothetical-deductive reasoning, with the eventual emergence of the expert who functions at an intuitive level. Later, with Benner & Tanner (1987), they examine the effects of intuition on an expert nurse's ability to make clinical decisions. They identify the following six key aspects in intuitive judgment:

1. Pattern recognition—Recognition of relationships
2. Similarity recognition—Recognition of relationships despite obvious differences
3. Commonsense understanding—Having a deep understanding of a given entity
4. Skilled know-how—Ability to visualize a situation
5. Sense of salience—Ability to recognize what is important
6. Deliberative rationality—Ability to anticipate events

These six aspects are seen to work in synergy in expert practice and not as solo components of behavior. These aspects are remarkably similar to the reported ways hypotheses were generated by expert physicians (Elstein, 1972).

It is clear, then, that the reality of how both nurses and physician experts make clinical decisions are quite similar and may vary from the model of what might be the ideal proposed by Eddy. Clearly, the extent of knowledge of the clinician makes a difference, as well as the experience of the clinician. However, in view of the switch to a deeper consideration of EBM, the conclusions of the clinicians and their behavior, even if they are experts, will increasingly need to be validated by supporting evidence.

In teaching critical decision-making, the new guiding principle for teacher-learner interactions might be embodied in the question, "What's the evidence?" This new guiding principle must permeate didactic lectures, discussions on rounds, and case-based sessions. New curricula must foster the development of analytic skills in a more purposive manner (Chessare, 1998). Some of the specific competencies that should be taught are summarized in Table 12-1.

It seems clear that diagnostic errors may occur among both experts and novices as a result of inadequate information processing. In Kassirer and Kopelman's important work (1989), diagnostic errors were classified into four major types:

1. Faulty hypothesis triggering
2. Faulty context formulation
3. Faulty information gathering and processing
4. Faulty verification of diagnoses

Faulty hypothesis triggering may occur when the clinician either fails to consider appropriate initial hypotheses or fails to revise hypotheses to reflect new information. *Faulty context formulation* may occur when a clinician has different goals than the patient for a clinical encounter. For instance, a clinician

TABLE 12-1 Specific Curricular Content to Increase Critical Analysis for Problem-Solving

General Content to Include in Curricula	Specific Content
Basic tools of clinical epidemiology	Rates, incidence, prevalence, risk assessment, diagnostic test characteristics, reproducibility of diagnostic information
Rules of evidence and research methodology	Knowledge of research methodology and the assessment of causality, demonstrate knowledge of the hierarchy of research designs to avoid bias and confounding and the strengths and weaknesses of each design
Hypothetical-deductive reasoning process	The science of decision-making, the hypothetical-deductive reasoning process
Biases and heuristics	Learning incumbent biases and mental shortcuts of heuristic thinking
Uncertainty and probabilistic thinking	How to minimize error in judgment and probabilistic thinking
Incorporating the patient's values into medical decisions	Decision analysis
Medicine for populations	Policy analysis, cost-effectiveness analysis

Modified from Chessare JB et al: Impact of a medical school course in clinical epidemiology and health care systems, *Med Teach* 18:233-227, 1996.

could fail to deal with all problems important to the patient when the pressure to see other patients places constraints on the clinician's time. *Faulty gathering and processing of information* may occur when clinicians either fail to order appropriate tests or misinterpret the predictive value of findings or test results. Finally, *faulty verification* may occur when clinicians fail to collect enough evidence to confirm a diagnosis adequately or to rule out competing diagnoses.

It must also be acknowledged that diagnostic errors can result because the information-processing capacities of both experts and novices are limited. Short-term memory capacity of the human information processing system is considerably less than its capacity for long-term memory storage. Thus unstructured inputs of large amounts of information can quickly overload the system. Even in simple medical cases, the range of facts to be considered is quite large compared with the number of items (typically five to seven) about which humans can simultaneously think (Miller, 1956). "Provisional diagnoses or hypotheses formed early in the patient encounter serve as organizers or bases for chunking in data collection, keeping to a manageable number of categories under which information is filed" (Elstein et al, 1972). This strategy of organizing large numbers of facts into smaller numbers of clusters develops automatic, well-learned information management processes (Bower & Gluck, 1984). In diagnostic reasoning, these clusters of information may assume the form of causal models based on pathophysiologic relationships, epidemiologic principles, or schematic algorithms. However, although such heuristics may simplify diagnostic decision-making, they also may lead to diagnostic errors (Kahneman & Tversky, 1974).

The main sources of error in making medical decisions correspond to the two main steps in Eddy's (1990) model; "A decision can be flawed either if there is a misperception of the outcomes or if there is a misperception of the values that patients place on the outcomes." Most misperceptions result from a failure of critical thinking. See Table 12-2 for a summary of common misperceptions that distort clinical decision-making accuracy.

Effective clinical decision-making avoids flaws in either the evaluation of outcomes or patient preferences. Attention to three principles will help. First, decisions should be based on outcomes that are important to all patients. The health outcomes that patients experience and care about are primarily reduction in pain or avoidance of anxiety, disfigurement, disability, and death. These health outcomes are not the same as other outcome measures, such as statistics (e.g., the prevalence of a problem), intermediate biologic outcomes (e.g., the cell type of a cancer), or test results (serum cholesterol level). These other outcome factors may influence the effectiveness of an intervention and may help forecast the health outcomes, but, by themselves, "they cannot be experienced by a patient and should not be the basis for a decision. The logic for this principle is straightforward; the ultimate purpose of all medical practice is to maintain and improve the health of patients. The only way to achieve this is to focus on the outcomes they can experience and care about health outcomes" (Eddy, 1990).

TABLE 12-2 Sources of Error in Clinical Decision-Making

Sources of Error	Examples
Misperception of the outcomes	Important outcome may be ignored. Extraneous outcomes might be included. Available evidence regarding outcome may be incomplete. Existing evidence might be overlooked. Evidence might be misinterpreted. Reasoning might be incorrect. Personal experiences might be given undue weight. Reliance on wishful thinking.
Misperceptions of patients' preferences	Patient might misunderstand outcome. The measure of the effect might be misleading. The outcomes might be presented or framed in different ways, leading to different conclusions. The patient might not be consulted at all. Health care providers might project their own preferences onto the patient.
Logical flaws in thinking and evaluating	
Type of evidence available for determining intervention	"If there is no direct evidence from randomized, controlled trials, intervention should not be used."
Degree of certainty regarding existence of an effect	"The P value is only 0.1, which is not statistically significant. The intervention should not be used."
Seriousness of the outcome	"If the outcome without treatment is very bad, we have to assume the treatment might work."
Need to do something	"This intervention is all that is available."
Novelty or technical appeal of an intervention or treatment	"This machine takes such a pretty picture it must have some use."
Other factors	Pressure from patient, family, the press, the courts; the amount of paperwork; personal financial interests.

Modified from Eddy DM: Anatomy of a decision, *JAMA* 263:441-443, 1990.

Second, the effects of a decision on a patient outcome should be estimated as accurately as possible, given the available evidence. As stated before, the estimates of outcomes should be based on evidence. All the pertinent evidence should be evaluated and critically analyzed with appropriate analytic methods and should not be affected by personal or professional biases. This is the information that clinicians should present to patients in a meaningful and understandable manner (Eddy, 1990).

The third principle is that the preferences assigned to the outcomes of an intervention should reflect as accurately as possible the preferences of the specific person who will receive the outcomes—that is, not just what is generally perceived to be the best outcome but the wishes of the specific patient. This may only be accomplished when the clinician has taken sufficient time to understand the values and wishes of the patient. If a patient chooses to delegate the decision to the provider or someone else, the values of the other person inevitably replace those of the patient and will determine what will happen to the patient. This is a weighty responsibility (Eddy, 1990).

One way to clarify the appropriateness of a decision is to confirm that the goals of the patient and clinician are congruent and appropriately defined (Kassirer & Kopelman, 1989). A goal consists of cognitive expectancies that organize the relationship between perception of the environment and development of the intention to act (Bandura, 1986). On another level, provider goals should not conflict. For NPs, if the dual goals of diagnosing and treating the disease itself and diagnosing and treating the patient's responses to health problems are incongruent, the result may be flawed information processing (Lange, 1997).

Critical Decision-Making Regarding Pharmacologic Therapy

Decision-making is on a higher cognitive plane than critical thinking. Decision-making requires not only critical thought but sometimes a degree of courage to take a position and take action. Both diagnostic and treatment plans arise from the decision that is made.

Not all clinical decisions are critical. In the course of caring for a patient, a multitude of decisions must be made. Some change the course of the patient's health irrevocably, for example, a decision as to whether the patient should undergo chemotherapy or a decision about specific types of surgery. Some of the decisions are clearly those that must be made by the health care provider, for example, tests that are essential. However, most of the decisions should be made by the patient. The effective therapeutic relationship involves negotiation between the health care provider and the patient to arrive at the most acceptable course.

Many systems to organize clinical decision-making into a more simple and systematic process have developed during the past decade. Clinical guidelines, algorithms, and EBM are all designed to specify the critical decisions that must be made with regard to a particular process or procedure.

Some pharmacology texts would suggest that all drug decisions are critical. However, sometimes drugs are virtually identical, and it does not matter what drug is selected. Sometimes patients have preferences for the taste of a certain product, cost may be a factor, the number of doses required per day may be associated with compliance, or patients may be reluctant to make a change. Sometimes decisions that are critical for one patient because of age, comorbidity, or other patient variables are not critical for another patient without those limitations. For example, a drug that produces impotence may be unacceptable to a 40-year-old married man but, for a specific 70-year-old widower, impotence may not be an issue. However, the clinician cannot generalize these preferences.

What decisions are absolutely essential for every patient? Analysis of current pharmacologic texts, journal articles, and contemporary research suggests that for every patient there are at least five critical clinical decisions that must be made by the provider who contemplates drug therapy. Some of these decisions seem obvious. However, they are rarely written down as maxims. They are decisions that are assumed in medicine and often oversimplified in nursing. See the critical decision-making algorithm in Figure 12-3.

Confirm the Diagnosis. This suggestion seems insultingly simple, but failure to do this has led clinicians to prescribe antibiotics before the pathogen is confirmed, leading to the development of antibiotic-resistant organisms. A rush to treat has caused many individuals with swollen, red, painful joints to be placed on colchicine before uric acid crystals were demonstrated from an aspirate. Or in other circumstances, high uric acid levels in asymptomatic patients have led to treatment before a gouty process develops.

Determine whether to continue nonpharmacologic regimens or whether it is time to add pharmacologic intervention. This mandates that providers have the commitment to try nonpharmacologic regimens and do not automatically resort to writing a prescription the first time a patient complains of a problem. Research confirms that this critical decision is often eliminated because of desire by both provider and patient to do something anything even if it is not the right thing (Avorn, 1991).

Determine a Medication Will Be Prescribed and Then Determine How Aggressive the Therapy Is Going to Be. Making these determinations requires the prescriber to define the clinical goal clearly. The goal must also be shared by the patient. Therefore whether the goal is curative, palliative, symptom reduction, or prevention, it must be clearly articulated. Once the goal is specified, then patient and drug variables must be evaluated: age of patient, presence of smoking or allergy, comorbidities (particularly those affecting renal, hepatic, or immunologic systems), other medications being taken, severity of the disease, risk-benefit ratio, and cost of product. All competing options and their projected outcomes must be evaluated and compared.

Select the Drug and Start It. Sometimes there is a standard first-line drug. Sometimes there are many options from which to select. At this point, the patient variables of importance that were listed in making the third critical decision will have ruled in or ruled out some products.

Determine the Effectiveness of the Prescribed Drug Once the Patient Begins Taking the Product. Evaluation of drug effectiveness varies by drug, so the appropriate time interval

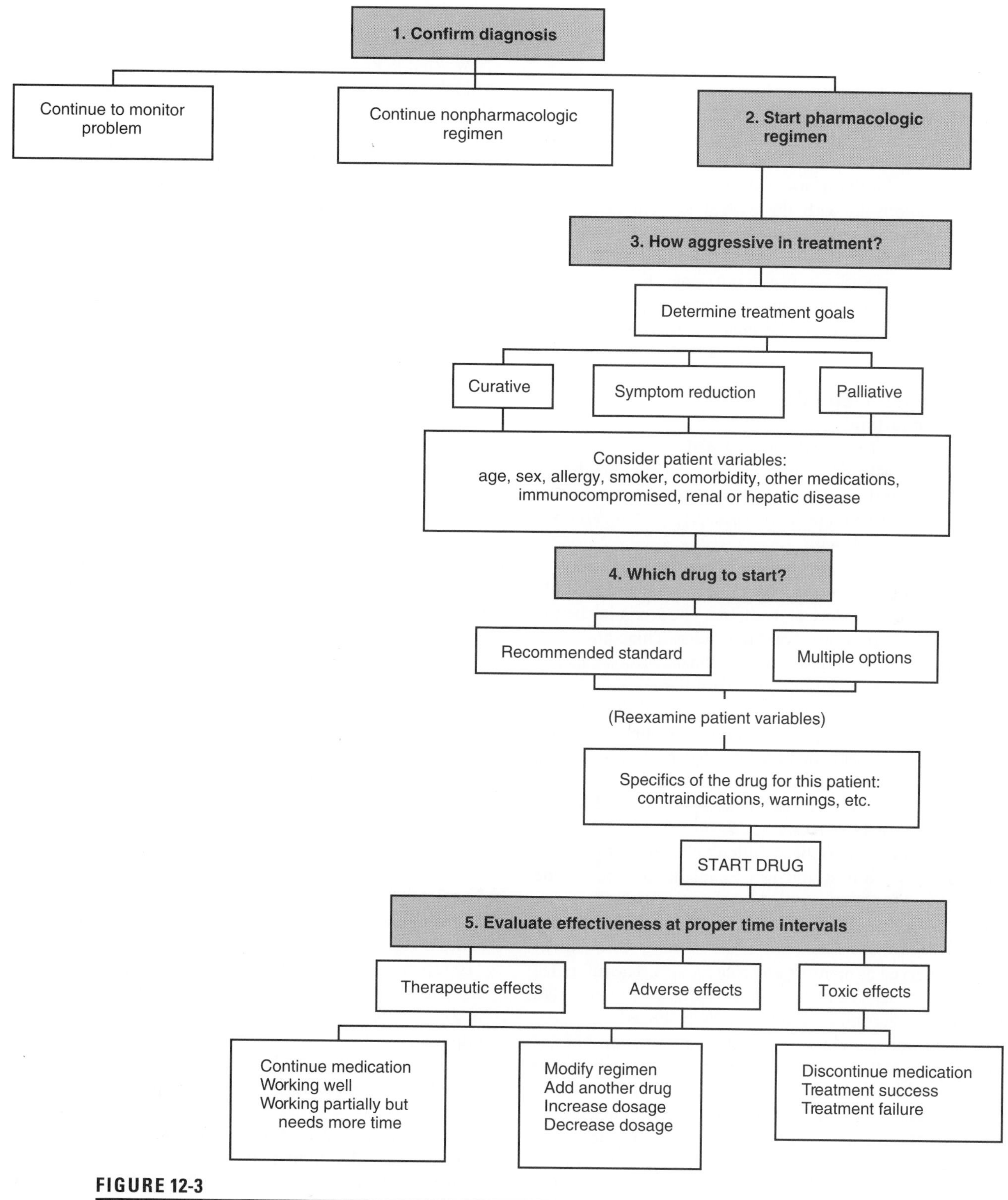

FIGURE 12-3

Critical decision-making algorithm for all patients regarding drug therapy.

must be selected. Selective serotonin reuptake inhibitors (SSRIs) and some antihypertensives may take several weeks for effectiveness to be determined. Antibiotics should probably produce changes in the patient status within 72 hours. The critical elements to look for are not only therapeutic effects but also the presence of adverse or toxic effects. Based on the evaluation of the patient's reaction to the medication, the clinician will decide to (1) continue the medication because it is doing what it should or it is partially working and should be given more time, (2) modify the regimen in some way (another medication added or dosage increased or decreased), or (3) discontinue the medication because the therapeutic objective has been reached and the medication is no longer needed, or the medication was a treatment failure and should be stopped.

The two processes of critical thinking and clinical decision-making converge in the decision to begin the prescription of medication for a patient. How earnestly decision-makers strive to develop their knowledge of drugs, how critically they evaluate the literature, and how attentive they are in developing a therapeutic relationship with the patient to help determine values and preferences will ultimately determine the accuracy of the decisions made. Critical decisions determine, sometimes forever, the course of patients' health outcomes. Focusing adequately on these critical decisions in drug therapy, therefore, is a superior way to achieve the goals of increased patient health outcomes.

EVIDENCE-BASED MEDICINE

Training for Uncertainty

Renée C. Fox, noted medical sociologist, has suggested that one of the major tasks of health care providers as they begin training for their health professional role is training for uncertainty. She suggests that there are two basic types of uncertainty that everyone must deal with.

The first results from incomplete or imperfect mastery of available knowledge. No one can have at his command all skills and all knowledge of the lore of medicine. The second depends on limitations in current medical knowledge. There are innumerable questions to which no physician, however well trained, can as yet provide answers. A third source of uncertainty derives from the first two. This consists of difficulty in distinguishing between personal ignorance or ineptitude and the limitations of present medical knowledge. It is inevitable that every clinician must constantly cope with these forms of uncertainty and that grave consequences may result if he/she is not able to do so (Fox, 1957).

These uncertainties have been difficult challenges for health care providers in the past and will be made more so by the plethora of knowledge now available every day. How does one discover what is known? Formerly, clinicians read textbooks, attended lectures, and learned beside other, more seasoned clinicians, who served as mentors and role models. The influence of these factors established life-long patterns for clinician learning and forever influenced how they practiced.

How does one gain mastery of the information that is known? Although the majority of health care providers take their responsibility to keep current with new research seriously, they simply do not have the time. A study published in a British medical journal estimated that for general medicine alone, clinicians would have to read 19 articles per day, 365 days per year, to stay current. This is an impossible feat; most health care providers have less than an hour per week to devote to reading medical journals.

Today, Fox's two questions have become even more important and even more challenging to answer. Available information about various clinical topics is growing exponentially every day and may have a dramatic impact on how clinicians practice. New research findings that shed light on physiology, pathophysiology, disease management, diagnostic technique, and pharmacology chip away at the "received view," often changing the very foundation of practice. A growing group of scientists are studying the process of information diffusion how what is known becomes communicated to relevant individuals and how it may be translated into usable information. Studies of information diffusion are essential in efforts to assist individuals overwhelmed with the burgeoning knowledge of today. Indeed, one of the major challenges clinicians face today is how to sort through all the information that is available, how to organize it, and how to retrieve the important and valid information essential to their practice.

The Internet has both helped and hindered this process of information retrieval. Large medical databases are being created by many different groups. Depending on their goals, these databases do help organize and retrieve information. However, the quality of data varies widely, and evaluating it is a daunting task. Some of the information is superb; other information is so methodologically flawed that it cannot be accepted as proven. One recent search in the National Library of Medicine PubMed database on the topic of cytochrome P450 metabolism produced 26,980 citations for a restricted 2-year search. Another crucial task today is evaluating the quality of what is reported before it can be incorporated into practice.

Health care practice has changed so profoundly that it can appropriately be called a paradigm shift. A way of looking at the world that defines both legitimate problems and the spectrum of evidence that may bear on their solution is called a *scientific paradigm* (Kuhn, 1970). When limitations or defects in an existing paradigm are widely apparent to such a degree that the paradigm is no longer useful in solving problems, the paradigm is challenged and gradually replaced by a new way of looking at the world.

The new way of looking at health care decision-making has been called EBM. It varies so dramatically from the traditional way of thinking about health care decisions that it may be said to represent a paradigm shift.

The Traditional Decision-Making Paradigm

The details about EBM are most precisely outlined in the article written by the Evidence-Based Medicine Working Group (1992), "Evidence-Based Medicine: A New Approach to Teaching the Practice of Medicine." In this article, components of both the traditional paradigm and the new paradigm were articulated.

As noted, traditional paradigm assumptions about the knowledge required to guide clinical practice have been the following:

- Unsystematic observations from clinical experience are a valid way of building and maintaining one's knowledge about patient prognosis, the value of diagnostic tests, and the efficacy of treatment.
- The study and understanding of basic mechanisms of disease and pathophysiologic principles are sufficient guides for clinical practice.
- The combination of thorough traditional medical training and commonsense is sufficient to allow one to evaluate new tests and treatment.
- Content expertise and clinical experience are a sufficient base from which to generate valid guidelines for clinical practice.

According to this paradigm, clinicians have a number of options in making clinical decisions. They can reflect on their own clinical experience, reflect on the underlying biology, go to a textbook, or ask a local expert. It is clear from examining these assumptions how the notion developed that the best education would be tied to the best teachers in the best schools. Learning at the footstool of good clinicians or experts was important. This paradigm also implies that there are many opportunities for quality learning at these institutions not available to people educated in other institutions.

Additionally, the tradition has been that reading the introduction and discussion sections of a paper could be considered an appropriate way of gaining the relevant information from a current journal. Physicians' research often consisted of flipping through journals and reading the last five sentences of the conclusion of each study, as time permitted.

The traditional paradigm of decision-making puts a high value on traditional scientific authority and adherence to standard approaches. Answers are frequently sought through direct contact with local experts or references to the writings of international experts (Light, 1979).

What Is Evidence-Based Medicine?

EBM is a decision-making framework that facilitates complex decisions across different and sometimes conflicting groups. In EBM, research and other forms of evidence are considered on a routine basis in making health care decisions. Using computer technology to classify, categorize, compare, or analyze content in large databases, the diffusion of knowledge about best practices into clinical care is finally possible.

Researchers and physicians at the Department of Clinical Epidemiology and Biostatistics at McMaster University in Ontario, Canada (www.hiru.mcmaster.ca/ceb) coined the term "evidence-based medicine" (Stevens, 1998). Its core idea is that clinicians should consider the effectiveness and harms of different interventions before they are implemented. The department helped clinicians accomplish that by publishing a series of articles and a textbook and has held annual workshops to teach physicians how to quickly find, evaluate, and extract critical information from medical studies. By now, virtually every major medical school has incorporated EBM into its curriculum to some extent.

Other types of health care providers have been slower than physicians to move to EBM (MacPherson, 1995).

EBM may be defined as the purposeful, conscientious, explicit, and judicious use of the current best evidence in making decisions about the care of individual patients. The key phrase is "making decisions." EBM represents a shift in the way health care providers and researchers use medical research to make decisions. It formalizes some of the critical thinking and clinical decision-making processes that have already been discussed.

In their seminal article, the Evidence-Based Medicine Working Group (1992) specifies the assumptions of the new EBM paradigm:

> Clinical experience and the development of clinical instincts (particularly with respect to diagnosis) are a crucial and necessary part of becoming a competent clinician. Many aspects of clinical practice cannot, or will not, ever be adequately tested. Clinical experience and its lessons are particularly important in these situations. At the same time, systematic attempts to record observations in a reproducible and unbiased fashion markedly increase the confidence one can have in knowledge about patient prognosis, the value of diagnostic tests, and the efficacy of treatment. In the absence of systematic observation one must be cautious in the interpretation of information derived from clinical experience and intuition, for it may at times be misleading.
>
> The study and understanding of basic mechanisms of disease are necessary but insufficient guides for clinical practice. The rationales for diagnosis and treatment, which follow from basic pathophysiologic principles, may in fact be incorrect, leading to inaccurate predictions about the performance of diagnostic tests and the efficacy of treatments.
>
> Understanding certain rules of evidence is necessary to correctly interpret literature on causation, prognosis, diagnostic tests, and treatment strategy.
>
> (Evidence-Based Medicine Working Group, 1992)

It follows from these assumptions that clinicians should regularly consult the original literature. They should be able to critically appraise the methods and results sections to evaluate information important in solving clinical problems and providing optimal patient care. It also follows from a close examination of existing literature that "clinicians must be ready to accept and live with uncertainty and to acknowledge that management decisions are often made in the face of relative ignorance of their true impact" (Evidence-Based Medicine Working Group, 1992).

It is also clear that the new paradigm puts a much lower value on both written and personal authority (Chalmers, 1983). The underlying philosophy of EBM is that health care providers "can gain the skills to make independent assessments of evidence and thus evaluate the credibility of opinions being offered by experts" (Evidence-Based Medicine Working Group, 1992). The decreased reliance on authority does not imply rejection of what can be learned from colleagues and teachers, whose experience has provided with skills and insight into methods of history taking, physical examination, and diagnostic strategies. The knowledge gained from years of practice can never be gained solely from formal scientific investigation. A final corollary of the new paradigm is that providers whose practice is augmented by and based on an understanding of the research will provide superior patient care.

The EBM Working Group (1992) suggests that EBM training focuses primarily on the development of research skills. These include precisely defining a patient problem and what information is required to resolve the problem; conducting an efficient search of the literature; selecting the best of the relevant studies and applying rules of evidence to determine their validity; being able to present to colleagues in a succinct fashion the content of the article and its strengths and weaknesses; and extracting the clinical message and applying it to the patient problem. This process is called the *critical appraisal exercise* (p. 2421).

Closer consideration of EBM as a way of making decisions undermines the assertion of some clinicians that NPs and physician assistants, who do not have the same clinical education as physicians, cannot develop the same clinical database as physicians. NPs and physician assistants may not need the same education as physicians if they have the same skills at retrieval and evaluation of scientific information. In fact, NPs who graduated from master's degree programs may have an advantage over other types of health care providers because they may already have strong research and critical appraisal skills that they developed during the research or thesis component of their programs.

EBM also depends on the clinician having a strong traditional knowledge base. A sound understanding of epidemiology and pathophysiology is necessary to interpret and apply the results of clinical research. The patients for whom clinicians care for may vary substantially from those enrolled in a reported study. Understanding the underlying pathophysiologic processes allows the clinician to better judge whether the research results are applicable to the patient at hand or are not generalizable. Having a strong foundation in science also helps the clinician to conceptualize and remember information about different clinical problems.

EBM emphasizes that research must be a part of every major medical decision. In an attempt to solve the time-constraint problem, EBM provides methodologies, strategies, and technologies that make it possible for health care workers to quickly find the most relevant and reliable research.

At the general research and database level, EBM works by converting complex information from literally thousands of individual studies into user-friendly risk estimates through the following four main steps:

1. Defining a structured question about the target population, outcomes, and intervention or exposure
2. Searching the published literature for sources of data that might answer the question
3. Appraising or evaluating the data for methodologic rigor and relevance to the question
4. Describing and analyzing the resulting data to answer the question posed

In teaching about EBM, criteria may be developed to help evaluate other types of research. Table 12-3 provides criteria helpful in evaluating different types of studies. As learning becomes more sophisticated, additional criteria can be introduced. For example, EBM teaches students to evaluate trials based in part on whether they are randomized. Randomized trials are considered the most reliable. Students must learn to appreciate methodologic merit but not discard all findings if the study is not randomized. Students must learn how to arrive at the strength of inference associated with a clinical decision (Beyea et al, 1998). EBM also has influenced the development of clinical guidelines (Heffner, 1998). Some practice guidelines have begun to be categorized into one of three types. Type A guidelines are supported by randomized trial, type B guidelines are supported by trials other than randomized trials, and type C guidelines are not clearly supported. Teachers can point out instances in which criteria can be violated without reducing the strength of the inference (Hammer, 1997; Stevens, 1998; Zarin, 1997).

TABLE 12-3 Suggested Criteria for Analysis of Diagnosis, Treatment, and Review Articles

Type of Study	Analysis Criteria
Diagnosis studies	Has the diagnostic test been evaluated in a patient sample that included an appropriate spectrum of mild and severe, treated and untreated disease, plus individuals with different but commonly confused disorders? Was there an independent, blind comparison with a "gold standard" of diagnosis?
Treatment studies	Was the assignment of patients to treatments randomized? Were all patients who entered the study accounted for at its conclusion?
Review articles	Were explicit methods used to determine which articles to include in the review?

Modified from Stevens L: Evidence-based medicine, *Med Net* 4:5, 6-11, 1998.

evolve For further information on using evidence-based medicine, see the supplemental tables on the Evolve Learning Resource.

Growth of Evidence-Based Medicine as a Decision-Making Process

In an ideal world, during an actual patient encounter, a health care provider would look up research for use in solving problems on a terminal in the examining room or using a hand-held personal digital assistant (PDA). The most important aspect of EBM is that the research health care providers' review be related to specific problems on which the providers are working and that the review be done quickly and efficiently.

Much of the process of teaching EBM involves helping clinicians hone their computer database search skills. The process of defining the problem, determining the information needed to solve the problem, and selecting the relevant and most reliable research requires skills not previously emphasized in the clinical curricula.

Key to the development and greater use of EBM is the greater availability of computers and use of the Internet. Many articles have been published about EBM with instructions on how to access, evaluate, and interpret the medical literature. Curricular revisions have been suggested for teaching programs. Proposals have been put forward to help clinicians use the principles of clinical epidemiology in everyday clinical practice (Sackett et al, 1991). The format in writing textbooks has begun to change, including rigorous review of available evidence, including the methodologic criteria used to evaluate the validity of the clinical evidence and the quantitative techniques used for summarizing the evidence (Sinclair & Braken, 1992). Several medical journals have revised the abstract format for their articles, incorporating material in the abstract about methods and design to help assist the readers in article evaluation (Haynes et al, 1991). Practice guidelines are now being developed based on rigorous methodologic review of the available evidence (Audet, Greenfield & Field,

1990), and ethical guidelines overseeing professional continuing education suggest greater reliance on EBM in content presentations.

One example of the type of information being developed to facilitate EBM is the Cochrane Collaboration (Stevens, 1998), an international initiative to prepare and disseminate systematic reviews of health care research. The Cochrane Database of Systematic Reviews (CDSR) (www.hcn.net.au/cochrane/) synthesizes studies, making it easier for researchers to review the literature. Abstracts of the reviews are available to the general public on the website, and full text is available for people who have purchased the databases. Using the database, rather than reading 5 or 10 different articles, the health care provider can read one Cochrane review. Other resources include The National Library of Medicine online services (available at www.nlm.gov) and collections of recent publications about research presented on various MEDLINE clinical centers (www.Medscape.com).

Barriers to the Implementation of Evidence-Based Decision-Making

Despite the advantages of EBM touted by some, EBM has not been universally applauded. Both antipathy and skepticism toward EBM may result from doubt about whether EBM can ever truly be applied in day-to-day practice. Some clinicians react negatively to the process because the name implies that what physicians did previously was not evidence based. Other emotional barriers to the acceptance of EBM may include the facts that

- New providers start with rudimentary critical appraisal skills and the topic may be threatening to them.
- People like quick and easy answers. Cookbook medicine has its appeal. Critical appraisal involves additional time and effort and may be perceived as inefficient and distracting from the real goal (to provide optimal care for patients.
- For many clinical questions, high-quality evidence is lacking. If such questions predominate in attempts to introduce critical appraisal, a sense of futility can result.

The concepts of EBM are met with skepticism by many faculty members who are unenthusiastic about modifying their teaching and practice in accordance with its dictates (Evidence-Based Medicine Working Group, 1992).

Based on the experience of the Evidence-Based Medicine Working Group (1992) there are several common misinterpretations of the EBM paradigm, as follows.

Evidence-Based Medicine Ignores Clinical Experience and Clinical Intuition

> On the contrary, it is important to expose learners to exceptional clinicians who have a gift for intuitive diagnosis, a talent for precise observation, and excellent judgment in making difficult management decisions. . . . The more the experienced clinicians can dissect the process they use in diagnosis, and clearly present it to learners, the greater the benefit. Institutional experience can also provide important insights. Diagnostic tests may differ in their accuracy depending on the skill of the practitioner.
>
> (Evidence-Based Medicine Working Group, 1992)

Understanding of Basic Investigation and Pathophysiology Plays No Part in Evidence-Based Medicine

> The dearth of adequate evidence demands that clinical problem-solving must rely on an understanding of underlying pathophysiology. Moreover, a good understanding of pathophysiology is necessary for interpreting clinical observations and for appropriate interpretation of evidence (especially in deciding on its generalizability)
>
> (Evidence-Based Medicine Working Group, 1992)

Evidence-Based Medicine Ignores Standard Aspects of Clinical Training, Such as the Physical Examination

> Careful history taking and physical examination provide much, and often the best, evidence for diagnosis and direct treatment decisions. The clinical teacher of evidence-based medicine must give considerable attention to teaching the methods of history taking and clinical examination, with particular attention to which items have demonstrated validity and to strategies that enhance observer agreement
>
> (Evidence-Based Medicine Working Group, 1992)

It may be observed that there are five factors that go into making a medical decision: (1) the patient's situation, (2) the patient's desires and values, (3) the health care provider's values, (4) the health care provider's experience, and (5) evidence from research. EBM plays a role only in the last factor.

There is clearly a beginning movement toward use of more scientific data that is emerging as a result of the introduction of clinical practice guidelines, the focus on disease management strategies, the application of quality improvement methodologies in health care, and the need to translate clinical trial results into actual practice. Many of these trends are driven by health economic factors. Increasingly, practice guidelines are not written by a group of gray-haired academicians in a room but include EBM data to help clinicians evaluate the reliability of the guidelines.

Does Evidence-Based Medicine Improve Patient Outcomes?

Whether EBM will succeed in becoming the dominant philosophy in clinical decision-making rests on whether patients cared for in this fashion enjoy better health. "This proof is no more achievable for the new paradigm than it is for the old, for no long-term randomized trials of traditional and evidence-based medical education are likely to be carried out" (Evidence-Based Medicine Working Group, 1992). What we do have are a number of short-term studies that confirm that the skills of evidence-based medicine can be taught. Growing research suggests that teaching this way may also help graduates stay up to date.

Health care providers will continue to face a burgeoning volume of literature, increased use of new technologies, deepening concern about escalating health care costs, and growing scrutiny of the quality and outcomes of medical care. In a real sense, whether EBM becomes a mainstream process depends in part on the goals one has for it. The EBM movement has already influenced how practice guidelines and critical pathways are written. Also, health care clinicians in most major U.S. and British Commonwealth professional schools have learned how to distinguish reliable from unreliable studies and how to search medical databases for data that can be used to solve real world medical problems. If nothing else, EBM will complement traditional methods of learning and decision-making by attempting to lighten the load of clinicians, who are trying to keep up with and evaluate published literature in their field.

CLINICAL GUIDELINES

Accepted standards of clinical conduct practice guidelines have proliferated throughout medicine over the last decade. Health care providers are confronted with a plethora of guidelines developed for different purposes by a diverse body of public and private organizations. Practice guidelines that specify how to treat specific medical conditions and perform procedures are published in health care literature. Their use by managed care plans, hospitals, and government programs is expected to affect health care practice substantially in the coming years.

Recommendations for practice in medical textbooks and review articles often do not provide a systematic and careful explanation of the underlying rationale associated with clinical practice guidelines. Review articles often reflect what an author (who may or may not be an expert) believes is proper practice (Eddy, 1990). Readers of medical textbooks or review articles often do not know to what extent the recommendations are based on science or on personal opinion because the author is not required to perform a systematic literature review or to demonstrate how the recommendations are linked to the science, as is expected in a practice guideline (Woolf, 1995).

Clearly, there are differences between agreed-on, normative practice standards and clinical practice guidelines recommended as the "usual" way to treat patients or guide treatment within a particular institution to achieve cost containment or to increase efficiency. However, acceptance of clinical practice guidelines may have other consequences by redefining the scope of practice for the various clinicians involved, serving as a way to pinpoint careless or negligent practice or making it difficult to practice outside of a clinical guideline (Sullivan & Mann, 1994). This is a particular problem if clinicians fail to individualize guidelines for their specific patients. Guidelines that also mandate when procedures may be performed, lengths of hospital stay, and other practices may affect clinical practice dramatically. Aspects of primary care are logical targets for the development of clinical practice guidelines, and primary care clinicians may now frequently be required to comply with them for reimbursement or legal reasons.

What Are Clinical Practice Guidelines?

Official statements that outline how to prevent, diagnose, and treat specific medical conditions or how to perform certain clinical procedures are called *clinical practice guidelines* (Woolf, 1995). (They may also be called *clinical policies, standards, treatment protocols, practice parameters,* or *appropriateness criteria.*) Clinical practice guidelines are frequently issued by government agencies, medical specialty societies, and other health organizations. These guidelines address specific health problems (such as the 19 clinical practice guidelines from the Agency for Health Care Policy and Research [AHCPR]), clinical practices, or groups of clinical practices (e.g., *Guide to Clinical Preventive Services,* U.S. Preventive Services Task Force).

Guideline development has been encouraged over the years by changes in the traditional reimbursement mechanisms that forced health care organizations and providers to seek new ways to control escalating health care costs by reducing practice variances and enhancing the quality of patient care. They are acknowledged methods designed to inform and teach both the seasoned and novice clinician.

MEDLINE searches provide thousands of entries about clinical guidelines. The National Guideline Clearinghouse (NGC) (www.guideline.gov/) is a comprehensive database for thousands of the most up-to-date clinical practice guidelines. Valid guidelines, when appropriately disseminated and implemented, are purported to lead to changes in clinical practice and improvements in patient outcome.

evolve For a list of organizations involved in the development of clinical practice guidelines, see the supplemental tables on the Evolve Learning Resources.

Guidelines are more likely to be valid if they are developed using systematic reviews, national or regional guideline development groups (including representatives of key disciplines), and explicit links between recommendations and scientific evidence. Peer review guidelines are another element of the process that may ensure validity. (See Table 12-4 for factors to consider when evaluating a clinical practice guideline).

Considerable resources are required to develop evidence-linked guidelines, but this investment can be recouped by relatively small changes in the process or outcome of care. Good leadership and technical support are required for the successful development of clinically valid guidelines, which depends on the small-group processes of guideline development panels and the translation of evidence into recommendations. The process of valid guideline development is certainly an area where future research is required (Grimshaw, Eccles & Russell, 1995).

Process For Guideline Development

One of the best analyses of information about clinical guidelines comes from Woolf 1995. His work suggests that current methods for developing practice guidelines include (1) informal consensus development, (2) formal consensus development, (3) evidence-based guideline development, and (4) explicit guideline development.

Informal consensus development is the most common methodology. Experts meet to discuss and decide on the recommendations subjectively, based on their experience and knowledge. Guidelines produced in this manner without explicit decision rules are often of poor quality. They usually do not include adequate documentation of how conclusions were reached. *Formal consensus development* uses a systematic approach to formally assess expert opinion, reach agreement, and make recommendations. This popular 1970s approach often used a modified Delphi method to arrive at recommendations by scoring the opinions of experts (Goodman & Baratz, 1990). Both the informal and formal consensus development methods describe what experts believe is appropriate based on their own knowledge, research, and experience.

TABLE 12-4 Factors to Consider When Evaluating a Clinical Practice Guideline

Factors to Consider	Specific Things to Evaluate
Source	Sponsoring organization, federal agency, panel composition
Appropriateness of methodology	Informal consensus panel, formal consensus panel, evidence-based process, explicit approach
Scientific rigor in evaluation of scientific evidence	Comprehensiveness of literature review, classification of study designs, consideration of sources of bias, methods for synthesizing results
Use of expect opinion/clinical experience	Qualifications of panel as experts
Decision-making	Documentation of rationale, decision rules, link between strength of recommendations and quality of evidence, appropriateness of recommendation language
Public policy issue considerations	Cost-effectiveness considered, recognition of health care system constraints
Feasibility issues	Ability for guideline to be implemented, time, simplicity, medicolegal, reimbursement issue consideration
Peer review	Groups or individuals that reviewed guidelines and provided feedback
Congruence with other practice guidelines	Presence of conflicting guidelines on the same topic, impact on other general or institutional policies
Timeliness	Recent research findings incorporated
Funding	Did funding source introduce bias into guideline development?

Modified from Woolf SH: Practice guidelines: what the family physician should know, *Am Fam Phys* 51(6):1455-1463, 1995.

Evidence-based guideline development first appeared in the 1980s. In this approach, an expert panel follows a systematic research methodology for gathering relevant studies, reviewing the data. Based on the validity of findings, recommendations are linked directly to scientific evidence of effectiveness. In making recommendations, rules of evidence are emphasized over expert opinion.

Finally, *explicit guideline development* more specifically clarifies any recommendations by calculating the potential benefits, harms, and costs of available interventions, estimating the possibility of the outcomes, and comparing the desirability of the outcomes based on patient preferences. These guidelines are based on statistical probability and arise primarily from organizational imperatives.

In both the evidence-based and the explicit approach, the clinician should have a clear understanding of the quality of the evidence on which the recommendations are based and the extent to which the guidelines are based on opinion. Woolf also suggests that there are four essential steps in the development of practice guidelines:

- *Introductory decisions*—This includes the selection of topic and panel members and clarification of purpose of the clinical practice guideline.
- *Assessment of clinical appropriateness*—This is accomplished through review of scientific evidence and expert opinion. An extensive literature review of perhaps thousands of articles may be performed to search for relevant research studies. The research is rigorously critiqued, and data may be supplemented by expert opinion when data are lacking.
- *Assessment of public policy issues*—Resource limitations and feasibility issues are major factors to consider.
- *Guideline document development and evaluation*—This involves drafting of the document, peer review, and pretesting.

A successful example of clinical practice guidelines are those developed by the Mayo Health System as part of their overall approach to disease and health management. One of their first guidelines was for the treatment of cystitis, and it provided very simple and clear guidelines focused on two factors: urine cultures are not necessary to diagnose a urinary tract infection in women ages 10 to 64, and 3-day antibiotic therapy is just as effective as 5-, 7-, or 10-day therapy. They maintain that the guideline has produced practice changes that have reduced cost and antibiotic utilization without compromising outcomes (COR Healthcare Resources, 1997). Working with the Institute for Clinical Systems Integration (ICSI), an independent nonprofit organization funded by Health Partners, the Mayo Health System published an annotated treatment algorithm for hypertension diagnosis and treatment that revolves around three simple factors: recognition and following up on elevated blood pressure, increasing the frequency of the correct classification of blood pressure staging, and control of blood pressure to prevent complications (COR Healthcare Resources, 1997).

Regardless of the care with which clinical guidelines are developed, it is difficult for them to define optimal care (Woolf, 1995). This is partly because science cannot define optimal care with certainty. "Data are often lacking in medicine, and studies often suffer from design flaws that limit internal and external validity. Subtle aspects of clinical judgment cannot always be measured empirically" (Tanenbaum, 1993). Additionally, the process of analyzing evidence and blending it with expert opinion is imprecise.

Techniques used to summarize data, such as metaanalysis and decision analysis, may be inappropriate and so may generate misleading results. Expert panel recommendations may be skewed by panel member biases or distorted by organization politics. "Experts" on the panel may not be representative of all experts on the subject (Woolf, 1995).

Finally, recommendations that may be based on what is best, as defined in guidelines, may not be appropriate for an individual or a local population. Thus the patient's medical history, personal circumstances, coexisting illnesses, patient preferences, and biologic variability may indicate that an individual patient is better served by options other than those recommended in the guidelines (Woolf, 1995). Therefore a central issue that must be addressed in practice guideline development is how to develop guidelines that appropriately allow for variations in clinical populations and practice settings. Despite recognition of this problem, guideline development by its formalistic approach works against incorporating flexibility into recommendations. It is difficult to determine when clinical circumstances vary enough that guideline recommendations should differ, how recommendations should be modified for a specific clinical setting, and whether the benefit associated with such site-specific guidelines justifies the expense of their development. Early research in this area suggests that site-specific guidelines can substantially improve the expected health benefit of the patient and the economic efficiency of practice guidelines (Owens & Nease, 1997).

Limitations in the Use of Clinical Practice Guidelines

There are limitations in clinical practice guidelines. This is not a problem as long as guidelines are worded in such a manner that they recognize limitations. If guidelines are written so rigidly that they overstate the certainty of recommendations, underestimate the complexity of patient care, or use rigid language to define the certainty of optimal care, "cookbook medicine" occurs (Redelmeier & Tversky, 1996). Guidelines that describe treatment without linking it to valid scientific evidence, or that ignore the individuality of patients, restrict the professional intuition of skilled clinicians and mislead students. Thus both sensitivity to these issues and crafting of the language of the guidelines are paramount in evaluating the final product.

Another limitation to practice guidelines is the degree of precision with which they are written. Some guidelines have been criticized because they are too vague. Lack of clarity in the recommendations, particularly for diagnostic testing or monitoring, is commonly seen. However, explicit recommendations can be harmful if they are derived arbitrarily, without supporting evidence, or provide an unreasonable and expensive standard that attorneys, utilization reviewers, insurance companies, or others might insist be met. If good evidence exists for clarity of recommendations, then it is important to be precise; if evidence is inadequate and explicit language is used simply in the interest of clarity, there is a risk that other possibly appropriate treatments may be precluded (Woolf, 1995).

Using Guidelines to Modify Clinical Practice

When a new guideline appears in a professional journal or text, clinicians should be skeptical about its utility until it has been closely evaluated. The same critical analysis used in EBM or that nurse practitioners and physician assistants learn in writing scholarly papers or theses should serve them well in evaluating the scientific rigor on which the guideline is built. The same validity tests and critical thinking that are used by all disciplines in critiquing clinical studies should be applied to analysis of the merits of the clinical guideline.

Gordon Mossler (1997) describes six half-truths about clinical guidelines:

- *Guidelines are cookbook medicine*—Evidence-based guidelines require the application of judgment, assessment, and decision-making in their use and differ from cookbook medicine that dictates elements of care.
- *Guidelines are a legal hazard*—Good guidelines specify good medicine in that they are evidence based and not opinion driven.
- *Guidelines do not work*—Alone, they do not improve care. They must be incorporated into an organized, systematic approach to reduce variations in practice.
- *Time and effort should not be wasted on developing guidelines because they are available from other sources*—Internal guideline development introduces many new people to the improvement process and improves their understanding of problems and solutions.
- *The task of implementing guidelines is the task of getting physicians to use them*—This is only part of the task. A team-oriented attitude is warranted.
- *Guideline use should be validated by outcomes data*—If *outcomes* means results of improvement processes, then this is true. But if *outcomes* refer to individual adverse events, these data are of little value and should not be a routine part of the guideline process.

The validity of the clinical guidelines should be seriously questioned if inadequate information is provided about how the recommendations were derived. As in any research study, the methodology should be clearly specified, and the participants described. The quality of the scientific arguments used in making the recommendations should be weighed. If the recommendations are supported by strong evidence, compliance with the recommendations should be considered. If evidence is equivocal or weak and the recommendations are based primarily on expert opinion, the personal preferences of the provider and the patient should influence the decision. Providers have personal views on the relative importance of science and opinion in making practice decisions. Providers who believe that clinical practice should always be based on science will decide not to follow guidelines that do not meet their standards. Those who have confidence in the opinion of experts might be more willing to follow weaker guidelines.

Patient preferences must also be considered if the evidence is not conclusive because their evaluation of potential benefits and harms can make the same practice acceptable for one patient and inappropriate for another (Barry et al, 1988). Table 14-2 identifies some factors to consider when evaluating a clinical practice guideline. The evaluation of these factors will help clinicians determine if they should or should not change their practice to be in accordance with the recommendations of the guideline.

Clinicians need to look beyond the guidelines to consider who is writing the guideline and whether that group has an agenda. Does the organization have a dominant philosophy that might influence the flavor of a guideline? Are the panel members biased? Who funded the expensive research process that underlies most guideline development? When experts or organizations with an interest in a specific clinical problem develop guidelines, the examination of the topic may be conducted with a narrow focus and little concern for other important health problems. The resulting recommendations may be based on the implicit and mistaken assumption that the provider's attention, time, and other resources can be devoted entirely to that problem. Although such an approach comes naturally to topic-oriented experts, such recommendations may be unreasonable for primary care providers, who are responsible for preventing or treating dozens of health problems in every patient.

Some practice guidelines dictate expensive laboratory testing or are so cumbersome that they become unrealistic, potentially harmful, and costly. "The problem of focused preoccupation groups that develop guidelines has been apparent to primary care providers struggling to provide children with universal hepatitis B vaccination, universal lead screening, and universal hearing screening. Each of these initiatives was recommended by groups concerned only with these problems" (Woolf, 1995).

Primary care clinicians will be faced with growing numbers of guidelines and the need to become more sophisticated consumers of practice guidelines. The guidelines should set criteria for accepting recommendations. Those that lack documented methods should receive less attention than those based primarily on science. Evidence-based guidelines often rate the quality of the supporting evidence (such as "good evidence for . . . ," "insufficient evidence to make recommendation," "good evidence to exclude").

Guidelines may be less biased if an interdisciplinary body that includes multiple perspectives develops them. Recommendations issued by a specialty society or other organization whose members benefit from the practice may reflect the effect of the recommendations on the specialty and its members (Ferrucci, 1993). Occasionally, clinical practice guidelines issued by different organizations have contradictory recommendations. Then the clinician must critique the methods by which the guidelines were developed. If the conflicting groups do not agree on the scientific evidence, the provider should personally examine the critical studies to reach an independent conclusion. If there is no disagreement on the scientific basis for the recommendations, differences in recommendations may be because of differences in panel member opinions, organizational policies, or writing styles. The clinician will have to come to their own conclusions about what should be the recommendations (Woolf, 1995).

Long-Term Consequences of Clinical Guideline Use

Currently, most practice guidelines are developed entirely on the basis of clinical concerns. Although health economics may have played a major role in the surge in guideline development, most current practice guidelines generally do not include analyses of cost-effectiveness although the long-term treatment selected may have considerable financial implications. This is often because the clinical experts on such panels lack expertise in economic issues. When these experts recommend against performing diagnostic tests or treatments, it is often not because of cost considerations but rather because of concerns about potential adverse effects or inadequate evidence of benefit. This may not be true for groups that have a strong business interest in controlling costs, such as payers, employers, and health plans.

The increased use of clinical practice guidelines has implications for both public policy and for litigation. Providers are concerned that the introduction of practice guidelines will reduce their clinical decision-making authority and that the failure to follow clinical practice guidelines will lead to medical liability. Although practice guidelines are an increasing part of medical practice, there has been only limited litigation to determine the extent to which guidelines will be used to set the applicable standard of care.

From a legal perspective, the primary issue is whether guidelines will be used to set the standard of care or will be just one more piece of evidence that a jury would consider in determining medical liability. Some writers have suggested that perhaps the courts should admit guidelines into evidence but that they should not be used as the sole determinant of the standard of care. This approach will surely facilitate health care provider acceptance of guidelines by not imposing liability for the failure to follow guidelines without additional evidence to determine the standard of care (Jacobson, 1997). Several independent legal reviews have also concluded that practice guidelines may be more likely to reduce than to increase malpractice liability (Hirshfeld, 1994).

In theory, it might be assumed that the use of evidence-based guidelines derived from studies of clinical outcomes will improve patient outcomes. However, although interest in clinical guidelines is growing, there is no documentation showing their effectiveness. Few studies have examined whether guidelines change health care provider practices and patients' health. The debate over guideline effectiveness has been hampered by the lack of a rigorous overview. In an examination of 59 published evaluations of clinical guidelines, all except 4 of the studies detected significant improvements in the process of care after the introduction of guidelines, and, in studies that assessed the outcome of care, significant improvements were also found. However, the size of the improvements in performance varied considerably (Grimshaw & Russell, 1993).

To cut through all of the rhetoric written about clinical practice guidelines, it is clear that the development of practice guidelines might both help and harm patients and providers. They might improve clinical decision-making of health care clinicians by assisting in the education of new clinicians, provide current evidence and expert opinion on important clinical topics, and improve the research focus by identifying gaps in the evidence. However, they have the potential to harm patient care if the recommendations are inaccurate and if compliance with flawed recommendations is enforced by organizations or courts. Health care providers who practice outside accepted clinical guidelines may risk losing reimbursement for services, losing precertification for procedures, and sacrificing favorable practice insurance. The extent of pressure on health care providers to comply with guidelines is anticipated to increase and may become a condition for licensure, reimbursement, or avoidance of fines (Woolf, 1995).

Expectations for guidelines remain high because they are one of the only instruments of health care reform that promises to improve the quality of care while reducing overall health care costs. Thus efforts to develop guidelines are likely to continue unabated in the foreseeable future. Additional research comparing different methods of developing and disseminating guidelines is needed (Walker et al, 1994).

REFERENCES

Agency for Health Care Policy and Research: Invitation to submit guidelines to the National Guideline Clearinghouse, *Fed Reg* 63:18027, 1998.

Aspinall MJ: Nursing diagnosis: the weak link, *Nurs Outlook* 24:433-437, 1976.

Audet AM, Greenfield S, Field M: Medical practice guidelines: current activities and future directions, *Ann Intern Med* 113:709-714, 1990.

Avorn J, Evenitt DE, Baker MW: The neglected medical history and therapeutic choices for abdominal pain, *Arch Intern Med* 151:694, 1991.

Bandman EL, Bandman B: *Critical thinking in nursing,* Norwalk, CT, 1995, Appleton & Lange.

Bandura A: *Social foundations of thought and action,* Englewood Cliffs, NJ, 1986, Prentice-Hall.

Barry Y et al: Watchful waiting vs immediate transurethral resection for symptomatic prostatism: the importance of patients' preferences, *JAMA* 259:3010-3017, 1988.

Benner P: *From novice to expert: excellence and power in clinical practice,* Menlo Park, CA, 1984, Addison-Wesley.

Benner P, Tanner C: How expert nurses use intuition, *Am J Nurs* January, 23-31, 1987.

Beyea SC et al: Developing clinical practice guidelines as an approach to evidence-based practice, *AORN J* 67:1037-1038, 1998.

Beyer BK: Critical thinking: what is it? *Soc Educ* 270-276, 1985.

Bloom BS: *Taxonomy of educational objectives for the cognitive domain,* New York, 1956, David McKay.

Bower GH, Gluck MAA: Evaluating an adaptive network model of human learning, *J Memory Lang* 27:166-195, 1984.

Braddock CH 3rd et al: Informed decision-making in outpatient practice: time to get back to basics, *JAMA* 282:2313-2320, 1999.

Carnevali DL et al: *Diagnostic reasoning in nursing,* Philadelphia, 1984, Lippincott.

Carter WB et al: Outcome-based doctor-patient interaction analysis, *Med Care* 20:550-556, 1982.

Cassell EJ: The nature of suffering and the goals of medicine, *N Engl J Med* 306:629-645, 1982.

Chalmers I: Scientific inquiry and authoritarianism in perinatal care and education, *Birth* 10:151-164, 1983.

Chessare JB: Teaching clinical decision-making to pediatric residents in an era of managed care, *Pediatrics* 101(4, pt 2):762-766, 1998.

Chessare JB et al: Impact of a medical school course in clinical epidemiology and health care systems, *Med Teach* 18:223-227, 1996.

COR Healthcare Resources, New York, 1997, Medical Management Network.

Djulbegovic B, Hozo I, Lyman GH: *Linking evidence-based medicine therapeutic summary measures to clinical decision analysis,* MedGenMed, January 13, 2000, Medscape, Inc.

Donald A: Evidence-based medicine: key concepts. *Medscape Psychiatry & Mental Health eJournal* 7(2):2002.

Eddy DM: The challenge, *JAMA* 263:287-290, 1990.

Eddy DM: Anatomy of a decision, *JAMA* 263:441-443, 1990.

Elstein AS et al: Methods and theory in the study of medical inquiry, *J Med Edu* 47:85-92, 1972.

Elstein A, Shulman L, Sprafka S: Medical problem solving: a ten-year retrospective, *Eval Health Prof* 13:5-36, 1990.

Ende J et al: Measuring patients' desire for autonomy: decision-making and information-seeking preferences among medical patients, *J Gen Intern Med* 4:23-30, 1989.

Evidence-Based Medicine Working Group: Evidence-based medicine: a new approach to teaching the practice of medicine, *JAMA* 268:2420-2425, 1992.

Ferrucci JT: Screening for colon cancer: programs of the American College of Radiology, *AJR Am J Roentgenol* 160:999-2003, 1993.

Fox RC: Training for uncertainty. In Merton R, Reader GE, Kendall R, editors: *The student-physician: introductory studies in the sociology of medical education,* Cambridge, MA, 1957, Harvard University Press, pp 207-218, 228-241.

Freed GL et al: Adopting immunization recommendations: a new dissemination model, *Maternal Child Health J* 2:231-239, 1998.

Goodman C, Baratz SR, editors: *Improving consensus development for health care technology assessment: an international perspective,* Washington DC, 1990, Council on Health Care Technology, Institute of Medicine, National Academy Press.

Goolsby MJ: Evaluating and applying clinical practice guidelines, *J Am Acad Nurse Pract* 13:3-6, 2001.

Grimshaw J, Eccles M, Russell I: Developing clinically valid practice guidelines, *J Eval Clin Pract* 1:37048, 1995.

Grimshaw JM, Russell IT: Effect of clinical guidelines on medical practice: a systematic review of rigorous evaluations, *Lancet* 342:1317-1322, 1993.

Guyatt G et al: Users' guides to the medical literature, XXX: evidence-based medicine: principles for applying the users' guides to patient care, *JAMA* 284:1290-1296, 2000.

Hammer A: Evidence based practice, *Physiother Res Int* 2:59, 1997.

Hart YM et al: National general practice study of epilepsy: recurrence after a first seizure, *Lancet* 336:1271-1274, 1990.

Haynes RB: The origins and aspirations of ACP Journal Club, *Ann Intern Med* 114(ACP J Club suppl 1):A18, 1991.

Haynes RB et al: More informative abstracts revisited, *Ann Intern Med* 113:69-76, 1990.

Hayward R et al: User's guides to the medical literature VIII: How to use clinical practice guidelines: Are the recommendations valid? *JAMA,* 274, 570-574, 1005.

Heffner JE: Does evidence-based medicine help the development of clinical practice guidelines? *Chest* 113(3 suppl):172S-178S, 1998.

Hirschfeld EB: Practice parameters versus outcome measurements: how will prospective and retrospective approaches to quality management fit together? *Nutr Clin Pract* 99:207-216, 1994.

Howard RW: *Concepts and schemata: an introduction,* London, 1987, Cassell.

Hugie P: *Teaching strategies to develop students' critical thinking skills in the clinical area,* unpublished master's project, Salt Lake City, 1992, University of Utah.

Hutchinson A: The philosophy of clinical practice guidelines: purposes, problems, practicality and implications, *J Qual Clin Pract* 18:63-73, 1998.

Jacobson PD: Legal and policy considerations in using clinical practice guidelines, *Am J Cardiol* 30:74H-79H, 1997.

Jacobs PM et al: An approach to defining and operationalizing critical thinking, *J Nurs Educ* 36:19-22, 1997.

Johnson E: EBM is dead? I didn't even know it was sick! *Fam Med* 32:720-721, 2000.

Kahneman D, Tversky A: Judgment under uncertainty, *Science* 185:1124-1131, 1974.

Kassirer JP, Kopelman RI: Cognitive errors in diagnosis: instantiation, classification, and consequences, *Am J Med* 86:433-441, 1989.

Kuhn TS: *The structure of scientific revolutions,* Chicago, 1970, The University of Chicago Press.

Lange LL et al: Use of Iliad to improve diagnostic performance of nurse practitioner students, *J Nurs Educ* 36:36-45, 1997.

Light DW: Uncertainty and control in professional training, *J Health Soc Behav* 20:310-322, 1979.

Lipman TH, Deatrick JA: Preparing advanced practice nurses for clinical decision-making in specialty practice, *Nurse Educ* 22:47-50, 1997.

MacPherson DW: Evidence-based medicine, *CMAJ* 152:201-204, 1995.

Mossler G: Half a dozen hobbling half-truths about practice guidelines, *Group Prac J* 46:34-44, 1997.

Myrick F, Yonge O. Preceptor questioning and student critical thinking, *J Prof Nursing* 18:176-181, 2002.

Newble DI, Hoare J, Baxter A: Patient management problems: issues of validity, *J Med Educ* 16:137-142, 1982.

Norman GR et al: Measuring physicians' performances by using simulated patients, *J Med Educ* 60:925-934, 1985a.

Norman GR et al: Knowledge and clinical problem-solving, *J Med Educ* 19:344-356, 1985b.

Owens DK, Nease RF Jr: A normative analytic framework for development of practice guidelines for specific clinical populations, *Med Decis Making* 17:409-426, 1997.

Redelmeier DA, Tversky A: Discrepancy between medical decisions for individual patients and for groups, *N Engl J Med* 332:1162-1164, 1996.

Roberts SJ, Tabloski P, Bova C: Epigenesis of the nurse practitioner role revisited, *J Nurs Educ* 36:67-73, 1997.

Sackett DL et al: *Clinical epidemiology: a basic science for clinical medicine,* ed 2, Boston, 1991, Little Brown.

Shea B et al: A comparison of the quality of Cochrane reviews and systematic reviews published in paper-based journals, *Eval Health Prof* 25:116-129, 2002.

Sinclair JC, Braken MB, editors: *Effective care of the newborn infant,* New York, NY, 1992, Oxford University Press.

Sox HC et al: *Medical decision making,* Stoneham, MA, 1988, Butterworths.

Stevens L: Evidence-based medicine, *Med Net* 4:5, 6-11, 1998.

Sullivan JM, Mann RJ: Clinical practice guidelines: implications for use, *Dermatol Nurs* 6:413-416, 1994.

Tanenbaum SJ: What physicians know, *N Engl J Med* 329:1268-1271, 1993.

Thiele JE et al: An investigation of decision theory: what are the effects of teaching cue recognition? *J Nurs Educ* 25:319-324, 1986.

Videbeck SL: Critical thinking: a model, *J Nurs Educ* 36:1997.

Walker RD et al: Medical practice guidelines, *West J Med* 161:39-44, 1994.

Watson G, Glaser E: *Critical thinking appraisal manual,* New York, 1964, Harcourt & Brace.

Woolf SH: Practice guidelines: what the family physician should know, *Am Fam Phys* 51:1455-1463, 1995.

Zarin DA et al: Evidence-based practice guidelines, *Psychopharmacol Bull* 33:641-646, 1997.

CHAPTER 13

Design and Implementation of Patient Education

Marilyn Winterton Edmunds and Jann Keenan

Practitioners teach patients about their disease, their medications, and how to help improve health. When patients accurately understand their medications, compliance and cooperation are enhanced. However, many patients do not understand materials given them to read because of low health literacy. Less than full understanding of health materials and written medical directions will inevitably decrease the patient's ability to implement the treatment plan. Greater attention and effort should be taken to ensure that patient education materials are designed so that patients really get the message clinicians want to teach.

THE PROCESS OF PATIENT EDUCATION

Many texts describe the different components of the teaching process in depth (see resources section at end of chapter). Experts (Barker, Burton & Zieve, 2002; Carter, 1992; Mullen et al, 1985; Redman, 1993) agree that the essential items to incorporate into teaching include the following:

- Assess patients' specific needs to learn.
  It is beneficial to determine the patient's need to learn. Often the provider wishes to provide information about a new treatment regimen or medication or to respond to the patient's direct questions. Just because a provider knows that a patient needs information does not mean that the patient recognizes that need or, in fact, expects to learn from the provider. Patient education cannot be a one-way dispensing of information.
- Patients must view the proposed patient education as relevant.
  A study that examined the information-seeking behavior of individuals regarding their prescriptions (Morris et al, 1987) concluded that patients exhibited one of four distinct types of behavior about receiving drug information, as summarized in Table 13-1. This study suggests that patients gravitate to the information source they feel is most appropriate or with which they feel most comfortable.
- Assess the patient's motivation *and* ability to learn.
  This requires getting to know patients and questioning them to determine their interest in learning. Educational materials should then be tailored to patients' individual needs, including knowledge, reading ability, beliefs, and experiences.
- Negotiate, together, what needs to be taught.
  Formalize this negotiation by writing specific and measurable objectives with the patient. ("Learn about adverse effects of the medication" is not measurable; "list five possible adverse effects" is considered a measurable and obtainable objective.)
- Select a teaching method.
  Offering verbal instructions, written materials, audiovisual materials, Internet materials, or a combination may all be used. The method and pace of the teaching must be designed for each patient, acknowledging the differences in the way people learn and the rate at which they learn. Different teaching skills may be needed at different times for the same patient. Teaching should be carried out in small segments over several sessions.
- Evaluate learning.
  Ask patients to repeat back, return a demonstration, or follow through on a behavior that illustrates how well they have learned the material also allows the provider to determine the degree of patient understanding or mastery. You may say, "I want to make sure I was clear with my message. In your own words, explain to me how to take this medicine." Feedback enhances learning. It shows patients the extent of their progress and increases confidence they can learn the material.
  Reinforcement provides rewards for a given behavior and may be positive or negative (Morris, Burkhart & Lamy, 1975). Offering verbal praise, congratulations for good compliance, or a change in behavior may be the most effective. Negative reinforcement or fear-arousing may be effective, but it must be used cautiously.
- Reduce barriers to compliance.
  Evaluation of compliance by an experienced clinician may lead to finding ways to eliminate problems with the regimen and facilitate cooperation. You might suggest your patient's use special pill containers, adjust medicine regimen around their activities, or ways to reduce cost.
- Combine several methods of teaching for optimally effective interventions.
  Using multiple types of teaching techniques can accommodate learning abilities or preferences, compensate for low literacy, increase retention of information, and promote reinforcement.

What Should the Patient Be Taught?

The patient's need for information depends on the disease process, the treatment plan, and the patient-provider relationship. When a patient is first diagnosed with a medical problem, education must start with what has gone wrong and what the prognosis might be. It is only when patients understand what has happened to them that they can move on to consideration of what to do about it.

The initiation of new medication therapy requires fairly extensive teaching. It is clearly not possible to provide all information patients might need in one teaching session. Instead, the health care provider needs to have a plan in mind for the things that need to be covered, and this needs to be shared with patients. There is also information that needs to be shared regarding perceptions, expectations, and options (Carter, 1992) (Box 13-1).

TABLE 13-1 Categories of Drug Information–Seeking People

Classification	Percentage	Characteristics
Uninformed	34	This group tended to be older, was less likely to have received provider or pharmacist written or verbal counseling, and did not seem to recognize the consequences of improper drug use.
Physician reliant	40	This group consisted of passive recipients of prescription information from the physician and were most likely to obtain prescriptions from chain pharmacies.
Pharmacist reliant	19	This was the youngest group; they received more counseling at the pharmacy and perceived few barriers to receiving information.
Questioners	7	Those in this group were more likely to receive information from books or magazines. They required clear information that answered specific questions and appeared to be the most difficult group to satisfy.

Modified from Morris LA et al: A segmentational analysis of prescription drug information seeking, *Med Care* 25:953-964, 1987.

BOX 13-1

KEY INFORMATION TO PROVIDE TO PATIENTS ABOUT MEDICATIONS

Drug name (generic and brand)
Intended use and expected action
Route, dosage form, dosage, and specific administration schedule (hours of day to take)
Special directions for storage or preparation of medication
Special directions for administration of medication
Common side effects and serious adverse reactions
What patient should do if there are side effects
Potential drug–drug, drug–food, or drug–alcohol interactions
Prescription refill information
Action to be taken in the event of a missed dose
Special precautions when taking medication (driving, actions requiring alertness)
Other information particular to the patient or drug
When to return to the health care provider
How patients will know that the drug is doing what it should do

From Carter BL: Patient education and chronic disease monitoring. In Herfindal ER, Gourley DR, Hart LL, editors: *Clinical pharmacy and therapeutics,* ed 5, Baltimore, 1992, Williams & Wilkins, and Selby MR: An in-depth study of educational strategies for increased patient compliance with medications, unpublished scholarly paper written to meet graduation requirement, University of Maryland at Baltimore, School of Nursing, 1983.

Additional teaching will be required when therapy is changed, medication dosages or schedules are adjusted, or changes in a patient's condition warrant further modifications in therapy. Teaching, then, becomes individualized to what the patient requires and thus is packaged in quantities that the patient can handle.

The health care provider must be familiar with the legal issues involved. Patients have the right to obtain information about their diagnosis, treatment, and prognosis. Informed consent is a principle implicit in the process of prescribing a medication for a patient. The practitioner has a legal obligation to ensure that patients understand their condition, the treatment proposed, and the risks and benefits of the treatment recommendations. The law requires that the amount and type of information provided to the patient be "reasonable." It is up to the practitioner to determine what is reasonable for each patient to understand. Practitioners are held legally responsible if they fail to advise a patient adequately.

Various studies have found discrepancies between the information that clinicians perceive as important and what information patients desire. Discussions of rare or serious side effects are awkward to discuss. Some health care providers have been reluctant to volunteer in-depth discussion of these topics for fear of frightening patients, believing it may decrease their compliance with treatment. However, Quaid (1990) found that seizure patients wanted to receive specific information on potentially serious side effects associated with carbamazepine. Although the information made the patients perceive the drug as risky, no patient refused treatment, and there was no evidence of a negative reaction after giving patients extensive information. The authors concluded that patients given more information may even be better able to correctly recognize side effects should they occur (Carter, 1992).

Although formal teaching is carefully planned, teaching in the clinical areas is often in response to a patient's question and is implemented on the spur of the moment without adequate preparation, planning, or overall consideration of what the patient needs to know. Using scientific or professional jargon, providing too much technical detail, or being unnecessarily vague all hinder or destroy the teaching process. Although it is impossible to avoid answering impromptu questions (even if they take the provider by surprise), it is essential to have an overall written plan that will cover what will be taught, how it will be taught, and how the clinician will know when the patient has learned the material.

Formalization of the teaching–learning experience begins with the writing of specific objectives. Objectives reflect the blend of patient and provider decisions regarding the treatment philosophy, the use of results from research, learner motivation and need to learn, continuity in learning, sequential arrangement of the behavior to be learned, and the priority of learning. The objectives must outline new behaviors that will occur because of changes in patients' thinking or understanding. The best objectives are precisely stated by describing the important conditions surrounding performance and by specifying the criteria of acceptable performance. These are often based on national recommendations, clinical guidelines, or standard treatment goals for a particular disease or problem (Redman, 1993). Specific goals help clarify for patients what they are to do (Strecher et al, 1994). For example, "Blood pressure will decrease to the diastolic reading of less than 95 mm Hg within 3 months" is specific, measurable, and based on national guidelines. As patients and providers craft objectives together, the provider has a chance to evaluate patients' knowledge, understanding, and general motivation to change behavior.

How Will Patient Education Be Accomplished?

Both the content and the process of patient education are important factors to consider in planning the specific teaching–learning objectives. Many patients are overwhelmed when they first learn that they have a new diagnosis. Fear and anxiety increase the confusion they often feel and interfere with their learning. Address these anxieties directly ("No, you don't have cancer.").

To avoid increasing the stress that patients may feel, teaching should be conducted systematically. It should be provided in a timely manner, in a quiet and unhurried environment that gives patients a chance to ask questions. It is hard to fulfill these criteria in today's busy health care system. Educational research has suggested that people are able to remember three major things that they are taught in any one session. And they generally remember those things in the order in which they are presented. Providers who accept those premises and develop a teaching plan consistent with them can set aside small periods of time to devote to teaching a few, very specific things. Review on subsequent visits will evaluate learning, and then allow the provider to move on to the next phase of information-sharing that has been identified.

In an effort to specifically increase medication compliance, the literature suggests a variety of strategies to provide patients with information about their medications (Barker, Burton & Zieve, 2002; Culbertson et al, 1988; Ley, 1996; Selby, 1983). Some of these strategies include verbal instruction, verbal and written instruction, and/or audiovisual aids. Some CDs, DVDs, or websites on the Internet combine audiovisual and written information in an interactive process.

Verbal education is often one-on-one counseling, particularly when a patient is first diagnosed with a problem and therapy is being implemented. Verbal instruction provides content and then gives the patient a chance to ask questions. Patients with chronic diseases such as diabetes or hypertension who have extensive needs for teaching may come together in small groups for part of their teaching experiences. Group interactions and observation may actually enhance learning because there is more of a context for it.

Written information can include special labels for prescription bottles, patient package inserts, single-page materials that are developed by individual pharmacists or organizations, and booklets. The health care provider, institution, or professional specialty organizations may develop written information. Regardless of the source, it should be provided to meet specific educational needs and not just be information dumped on the patient.

Audiovisual programs may use CDs or videocassettes. The greater availability of these resources and the wider use of VCRs, DVDs, and CDs in the home have led to the development of lending libraries on common topics. Wider availability of personal computers has increased the use of CDs for teaching patients. Use of the Internet to collect information allows patients to select what they want and download it for future reference.

More research attention is now focused on the use of computers, both to assess the needs of patients and in meeting those needs. Research suggests that patients might actually be more comfortable disclosing personal information to a computer than to a human being even though they know the information will be reviewed by a health care professional. Although many educators initially thought that computers would not be appropriate for audiences with poor literacy skills, research findings have revealed the opposite. The use of an audio computer-assisted self-interview system may result in more candid reporting of certain health behaviors and be acceptable to subjects with poor literacy skills (Slater et al, 1994).

All teaching methods, with the possible exception of patient package inserts, have been shown to improve knowledge and information retention (Morris, Burkhart & Lamy, 1975; Mullen et al, 1985). A combination of verbal and written information, or the use of verbal counseling along with audiovisual aids, is generally superior to the use of traditional written material only (Morris, Burkhart & Lamy, 1975). Most patients prefer a combination of written and verbal information, and studies have shown this approach to be the most effective in improving knowledge (Culbertson et al, 1988). Using other criteria (such as efficacy, volume, logistics, and cost) to evaluate the best strategy for providing patient education, the preferred method is still to provide both written and verbal information. This is especially important for new prescriptions (Culbertson et al, 1988). Providing only written information is usually insufficient in achieving patient education.

Reduced Literacy As a Barrier to Patient Education

Functional health literacy is

> "the ability to read, understand, and act on health information. This includes such tasks as reading and comprehending prescription labels, interpreting appointment slips, completing health insurance forms, following instructions for diagnostic tests, and understanding other essential health-related materials required to adequately function as a patient. Functional health literacy varies by context and setting and may be significantly worse than one's general literacy."
>
> (Andrus & Roth, 2002)

An individual may be able to read and understand general materials with familiar content at home or at work but struggle when presented with medical material of the same complexity that contains unfamiliar vocabulary and concepts. This even applies to well-educated patients.

Lack of adequate literacy skills is a major barrier to patients receiving proper health care. People with low reading levels have problems accessing the health care system, understanding recommended treatments and consent forms, and following the instructions of providers. Patients are routinely expected to read and understand labels on medicine containers, appointment slips, informed consent documents, and health education materials (Williams et al, 1995). Thus patients with lower literacy often have poor health outcomes. In the classic 1980 research of literacy experts Doak and Doak, they noted that patients' report of the number of years of school completed was four or five levels higher than their actual reading ability based on the Wide Range Achievement Test (WRAT), a word pronunciation and recognition test.

Many of the health educational materials that have been developed for patients by pharmaceutical companies, professional associations, or institutions are not suitable because there is a serious mismatch between the level at which the patient can read, and the level at which the materials are written. The Educational Testing Service research suggests approximately half of the population struggles with basic reading skills (Educational Testing Service, 1993). A 1998 study by Williams et al at a large urban public hospital found the following:

- 35% of English-speaking patients could not read or understand basic health-related materials (i.e., had inadequate or marginal functional literacy)
- 42% of patients were unable to comprehend direction for taking medication on an empty stomach
- 60% could not understand a standard consent form
- 81% of elderly patients (age >60 years) had inadequate functional literacy

Clearly, literacy problems are very prevalent and so critical that it is understandable that Healthy People 2010 devoted some of the health communication objectives to this issue (U.S. Department of Health and Human Services, 2002).

Notwithstanding the desire of some providers to develop patient teaching materials, there is no lack of prewritten patient educational materials. Many materials are available for sale, although the investment to purchase this information for all patients may become prohibitive. In fact, the problem is not in finding patient education materials but in evaluating their quality, readability, and applicability. Many patient education handouts, such as those available over the Internet, may be modified and customized to the individual patient. However, even a cursory evaluation of these materials will demonstrate that most of them are written at a higher level than essential for most patients. No commercially available handouts should be used for patients without being carefully assessed for readability. Most will require revision to be acceptable no matter how "pretty" they look or how much money was spent to prepare them. Information from drug companies must be carefully screened as they are often more advertisement than information. Keeping sentences short and choosing simple words make it much easier to develop reading materials at a simple and straightforward reading level.

Developing Written Materials Based on Literacy Requirements

The health literacy problem in the United States is extensive. The mean literacy level in the United States is at or below the eighth-grade level (Redman, 1993). One in five adults tested at or below the two lowest levels as determined by the National Adult Literacy survey. These levels are roughly translated to reading at about the fifth-grade reading level. Most health materials are written at the tenth-grade level or above (Kirsch et al, 1993).

To match the learner to the material, teachers must know something about the factors that determine readability. Readability can be predicted in three ways: (1) by the Cloze method in which every fifth word in a reading passage is removed, and the reader is asked to fill in the words based on the meaning of other words in the passage; (2) by the predictability of certain words in reading passages; and (3) by formulas based on the length of words and sentences. The formulas have been validated against reading tests.

Assessing the readability of content that is already commercially prepared, or that is being developed by the clinician, was formerly a very cumbersome process. Redman (1993) explains three of the most common methods used to determine grade level of health care content; all involve counting number and length of sentences and syllables in words. Computer word processing software now almost universally has a program to automatically analyze the reading difficulty of files. However, there has not been good congruence between the computer calculations of readability and those that are done by hand and many literacy specialists frown on the computer calculations.

If clinicians plan to develop their own written materials, they should be familiar with the various readability formulas that are useful for different kinds of text. For example, the FRY Readability Formula requires a graph to determine the level of materials from grades 1 through college; however, the standard FRY formula is not useful with passages of fewer than 300 words. Modified FRY tools and a dictionary of words correlated to grade level have been developed that may be used with shorter passages. The FOG formula uses number of sentences and number of polysyllabic words and is useful for grade 4 through college. The Flesch Formula uses average sentence and word length and is useful for grades 5 through college (see Box 13-2 for an example). The SMOG Formula counts the number of sentences and the number of words with three or more syllables and is useful for grades 5 through college. Meade and Smith have compared readability formulas conducted with the same health education materials and have found that the Flesch, FOG, and Fry formulas correlate highly with each other.

Designing Patient Education Materials

Part of the overall objectives that are written to ensure that patients understand their health conditions, proper administration of their drugs, and general medical instructions should cover what is included in the written material given to patients. Particular attention should be paid to including the essential facts that each patient should know about his or her medications.

If only one handout will be prepared for all patients receiving a given drug, the readability should be below eighth-grade level and preferably at the fifth-grade level (Morrow, Leirer & Sheikh, 1988). (By contrast, most patient leaflets included with medicine are written at a 10th- to 12th-grade level.) In the ideal world, two or three handouts at different ability levels could be prepared for each drug. In some communities, handouts in several languages may be needed.

BOX 13-2

FLESCH READABILITY FORMULA

1. For short pieces, test the entire selection. For longer pieces, test at least three randomly selected samples of 100 words each. Do not use introductory paragraphs. Start each sample at the beginning of a paragraph.
2. Determine the average sentence length (SL) by counting the number of words in the sample and dividing by the number of sentences. Count as a sentence each independent unit of thought that is grammatically independent that is, if its end is punctuated by a period question mark, exclamation point, semicolon, or colon. In dialog, count speech tag (e.g., "he said") as part of the quoted sentence.
3. Determine the word length (WL) by counting all the syllables in the sample as if reading the words aloud. Divide the syllables by the number of words in the sample and multiply by 100.
4. These indices are then applied to the formula to compute the reading ease, RE = 206.835 − 1.015 SL − 0.846 WL, where RE is the reading ease score, SL is the average sentence length in words, and WL is the average word length measured as syllables per 100 words.

INTERPRETATION OF THE FLESCH READING EASE SCORE

Reading Ease	*Grade Level*	*Description of Style*	*No. Syllables/100 Words*	*Average Sentence Length*
90-100	5	Very easy	123	8
80-90	6	Easy	131	11
70-80	7	Fairly easy	139	14
60-70	8-9	Standard	147	17
50-60	10-12	Fairly difficult	155	21
30-50	College	Difficult	167	25
0-30	College graduate	Very difficult	192	29

From Flesch R: *The art of readable writing*, New York, 1974, Harper Collins.

People at all literacy levels prefer simple, attractive materials. Pictures, diagrams, and videotapes help communicate information to patients, especially those with low literacy skills. Most people, even those who read well, rely on visual clues to reinforce learning.

Oral and visual tools help patients absorb new information, which increases learning. Supplementing text with pictures helps when providing self-care or medication instructions to low-literate patients.

Some General Principles to Use in Preparing Patient Education Materials

- The goals of the handout should be stated in the material.
- Limit content to one or two educational objectives. List what the reader will learn and do after reading the information.
- Emphasize the desired behavior rather than the medical facts. Patients find it difficult to relate abstract statistics to their own experience.
- Use clear captions, ample "white space," and photographs or realistic illustrations to attract the reader's attention and reinforce the message. The illustrations should depict the desired behavior you want the patient to follow.
- Always avoid medical jargon, and use common words. Terms should be concrete and familiar to the patient. For example, replace "antithrombotic agent" with "a drug that prevents blood clots."
- The most readable education materials are on no more than one page, front and back. Longer materials can be used as long as they follow basic health literacy principles.
- The material should have sections of bulleted lists in lieu of exclusively using running text in paragraphs. Key items or warnings should be highlighted with bullets or icons.
- The print size should be at least 12 point for body copy for the general public. Use 14-point type face if the material is designed for older adults.
- Written instructions should be interactive. Practitioners can accomplish this by developing materials that ask patients to do, write, say, or show something to demonstrate their understanding of a concept (Weiss & Coyne, 1997).
- Whenever possible, prepare materials in cooperation with patients who have low health literacy skills. Their input results in more culturally sensitive and personally relevant information.

Writing "easy-to-read" goes beyond writing at the fifth-grade reading level or limiting three syllable words. Individuals should develop materials so their patients not only *can* read the materials but also will *want* to read them. A checklist developed by Jann Keenan, EdS, a health literacy specialist and public health educator, to assess written materials appears in Box 13-3.

Using Multimedia for Patient Education

Audiovisual (AV) materials might be reserved for common conditions with lengthy or complex instructions. Some videotapes, audiotapes, or slides are available from pharmaceutical manufacturers for products that have complicated interaction, mixing, or administration features. The patient should be allowed time to view the material in a private or semiprivate area and then be given a chance to ask questions. The provider should reinforce verbally the important points of the videos and provide additional written materials to which the patient might refer.

Intervention studies have examined the feasibility and efficacy of using multimedia presentations of health information

BOX 13-3

CHECKLIST FOR ASSESSING WRITTEN MATERIALS

Check	Items Included in the Written Material
	The text follows a logical order
☐	• The cover lets the reader know exactly what the brochure is about.
☐	• The most important information is provided first.
☐	• Desired behavior is clearly outlined in the opening paragraphs.
☐	• Only three to five main points are covered.
☐	• Headers and subheads contain useful information. They guide the reader and inform them about what will be addressed.
☐	• Important information is repeated or summarized.
	Your writing style is vivid
☐	• The document is written in active voice. The tone is conversational and friendly.
☐	• Action words and descriptive adjectives are used.
☐	• There is little technical or medical jargon. If jargon must be used, it is well explained.
☐	• Limit the number of three syllable words whenever possible. For example, replace "immediately" with "right away," and replace "excessive" with "too much."
☐	• Offer to fill in the blanks, checklists, questions and answers, and testimonies from patients when appropriate to draw readers into the content.

to reach audiences with poor literacy skills. The AMC Cancer Research Center examined the use of an interactive computer program to deliver information regarding breast cancer to women with poor literacy skills. In the formative research stages, women reported that they thought that the computer would be an appropriate channel to deliver such information because they could use it at their own pace and select information that was of most interest to them. In addition, they reported that they would want the computer to be located in a kiosk or private area so that others would not know the material they were studying.

Patient and Provider Use of the Internet for Educational Purposes

The Internet is becoming a source of up-to-date health information not only for providers but also for patients. Many Internet sites meet the needs of both (see Boxes 13-4 and 13-5).

Although many commercial websites provide reliable information, others may be more interested in selling something. Commercial sites are identifiable by "com" near the end of their web addresses. They often scatter ads through their web pages, charge fees or dues, or promote retail-shopping options. The letters "org" denote a nonprofit group, "gov" a government agency, and "edu" an educational entity.

A number of sites offer instructions for navigating the Internet. They range from The Internet Learning Tree and Beginners Central, which emphasize the basics, to the more advanced Internet Web Text Index.

Research on Internet use for health care information concludes that physicians are more enthusiastic about the Internet's value for them than for their patients. In actual practice, even providers who use the Internet regularly for professional purposes prefer more traditional methods of patient education. A survey of online physicians showed that physicians believe that the amount of online consumer/patient-oriented health and medical information available is still too small to warrant attention but have never really checked this out on their own. They believe that most of their patients are not yet online or are not sophisticated enough to evaluate the quality of online consumer health and medical information. They have mixed feelings about patients who come to appointments with Internet printouts (they do not want to spend time to interpret the materials). Some fear that their patients will read online journal articles before they themselves have had a chance to review the information. This is a real possibility because the reality is that many more patients than physicians are using the Internet for health information.

Several studies, including those done by Strecher et al (1994), indicate that computerized health information is equally effective in increasing knowledge compared with face-to-face instructions. Research by Kalichman and colleagues (2001) suggests that knowledge, active coping, information seeking coping, and social support were promoted by HIV/AIDS patients using the Internet. Their preliminary findings suggest an association between using the Internet for health-related information and health benefits among people living with HIV/AIDS.

Patients from many different cultures and demographic backgrounds are using the Internet. Online men are more likely to search for health information about their own problems; online women are more likely to search for information on behalf of someone else. Fully 77% of patients say what they really want is online information from their own health care providers and are dismayed that so few of them have web pages or suggest condition-specific lists of recommended online resources.

Giving patients information on the basic terminology and search engines involved in retrieving health care information (such as those provided in Box 13-6 and Table 13-2) will probably be all that is necessary to dramatically increase use of these resources. You may suggest to your patients that sites ending in .gov, .edu, or .org are generally more acceptable than sites ending in .com. One of the major challenges will be to identify quality patient education online.

EVALUATION OF LEARNING

Patient education in general is designed to change behavior and increase satisfaction. When objectives are written specifically, the outcomes of behavior change are clearly articulated. Thus it should be simple to monitor the extent of learning that has taken place. When blood sugars do not come down and stay down, when blood pressure remains high, when weight is not lost—there is failure somewhere in the process. Sometimes the failure is right at the beginning of the teaching–learning process because the patient does not accept the provider's

BOX 13-4

PROFESSIONAL ORGANIZATIONS

American Academy of Allergy, Asthma, and Immunology, 611 E Wells St, Milwaukee, WI 53202, (414) 272-6071, Fax: (414) 272-6070, www.infoaaaai.org

American Academy of Dermatology, 930 N Meacham Rd, Schaumburg, IL 60173-4965, (847) 330-0230

American Academy of Family Physicians, 8880 Ward Pkwy, Kansas City, MO 64114, (816) 333-9700, Fax: (816) 333-0303, www.aafp.org/familymed

American Academy of Neurology, 1080 Montreal Ave, St. Paul, MN 55116, (612) 695-1940, www.aan.com

American Academy of Nurse Practitioners, Capitol Station LBJ Building, PO Box 78711, Austin, TX 78711, (512) 442-4262, Fax: (512) 442-6469, www.aanp.org

American Academy of Physician Assistants, 950 N Washington St, Alexandria, VA 22314-1552, (703) 836-2272

American Academy of Orthopaedic Surgeons, 6300 N River Rd, Rosemont, IL 60018-4262, (847) 823-7186

American Academy of Pediatrics, 141 Northwest Point Blvd, Elk Grove Village, IL 60007, (847) 228-5005, Fax: (847) 228-5097, www.kidsdocsaap.org; wwwaap.org

American Association of Nurse Anesthetists, 222 South Prospect Ave, Park Ridge, IL 60068, (708) 692-7050

American Cancer Society, 1599 Clifton Rd NE, Atlanta, GA 30329, (404) 320-3333

American College of Chest Physicians, 3300 Dundee Rd, Northbrook, IL 60062-2348, (847) 498-1400, Fax: (847) 498-5460

American College of Emergency Physicians, PO Box 619911, Dallas, TX 75261, (972) 550-0911, Fax: (972) 580-2816, www.acep.org

American College of Gastroenterology, 4900-B S 31st St, Arlington, VA 22206-1656, (703) 820-7400, www.acg.gi.org

American College of Nurse Midwives, 818 Connecticut Ave NW, Ste 900, Washington DC 20005, (202) 408-7050, Fax: (202) 408-0902, www.nurse.org/ACNP/

American College of Nurse Practitioners, 111 19th Street NW, Suite 404, Washington, DC 20036, (202) 559-2190, Fax: (202) 659-2191, www.nurse.org/acnp

American College of Obstetricians and Gynecologists, 409 12th St SW, PO Box 96920, Washington, DC 20090-6920, (202) 638-5577, www.acog-com

American College of Physicians, Independence Mall, W 6th St at Race, Philadelphia, PA 19106-1572, (215) 351-2400, www.acponline.org

American College of Surgeons, 633 St. Clair St, Chicago, IL 60611, (312) 664-4050, Fax: (312) 440-7014, postmaster facs.org; www.facs-org

American Diabetes Association, 1660 Duke St, Alexandria, VA 22314, (703) 549-1500, www.diabetes-org

American Federation of Home Health Agencies, 1320 Fenwick Ln, Ste 100, Silver Spring, MD 20910, (301) 588-1454

American Gastroenterological Association, 7910 Woodmont Ave, 7th Fl, Bethesda, MD 20814-3015, (301) 654-2055, Fax: (301) 654-5920, www.gastro.org

American Geriatrics Society, 770 Lexington Ave, Ste 300, New York, NY 10021, (212) 308-1414, Fax: (212) 832-8646, infoamgeramericangeriatrics.org www.american geriatrics-org

American Heart Association, 7272 Greenville Ave, Dallas, TX 75231-4596, (214) 373-6300 www.americanheart.org

American Hospital Association, One N Franklin, Ste 27, Chicago, IL 60606, (312) 422-3000, www.aha.org

American Lung Association, 1740 Broadway, New York, NY, 10019-4374, (212) 315-8700, www.lungusa.org

American Medical Association, 515 N State St, Chicago, IL 60610, (312) 464-5000, Fax: (312) 464-4623, www.ama-assn.org

American Neurological Association, 5841 Cedar Lake Rd, Ste 204, Minneapolis, MN 55416, (612) 545-6284, Fax: (612) 545-6073, www.lwilkersoncompuserve.com

American Orthopaedic Society, 6300 N River Rd, Ste 727, Rosemont, IL, 60018, (847) 698-1694, Fax: (847) 823-0536

American Psychiatric Association, 1400 K St NW, Washington, DC, 20005, (202) 682-6000, Fax: (202) 682-6114, www.apapsych.org or www.psych.org

American Public Health Association, 1015 15th St NW, 3rd Fl, Washington, DC 20005-2605, (202) 789-5600, Fax: (202) 789-5661, www.apha.org

American Society on Aging, 833 Market St, Ste 511, San Francisco, CA, 94103-1824, (415) 974-9600 or (800) 537-9728, (415) 974-0300

American Society of Internal Medicine, 2011 Pennsylvania Ave NW, Ste 800, Washington, DC 20006, (202) 835-2746

American Thoracic Society, 1740 Broadway New York, NY 10019-4374, (212) 315-8700, Fax: (212) 315-6498, www.thoracic.org

Arthritis Foundation, 1330 W Peachtree St, Atlanta, GA 30309, (404) 872-71010, www.arthritis.org

Association of Reproductive Health Professionals, 2401 Pennsylvania Ave NW, Ste 350, Washington, DC 20037, (202) 466-3825, Fax: (202) 466-3826, www.arhp.org

Asthma and Allergy Foundation of America, 1125 15th St NW, Ste 502, Washington, DC 20005, (202) 466-7643, Fax: (202) 466-8940, www.infoaafa.org

Gerontological Society of America, 1275 K St NW, Ste 350, Washington, DC 20005-4006, (202) 842-1275

Infectious Disease Association of America, 11 Canal Center Plaza, Ste 104, Alexandria, VA 22314, (703) 299-0200, Fax: (703) 299-0204

National Hospice Organization, 1901 N Moore St, Ste 901, Arlington, VA 22209-1714, (703) 243-5900, Fax: (703) 525-5762, www.nho.org

National Organization of Nurse Practitioner Faculties, One Dupont Circle, NW #530, Washington, DC 20036, (202) 452-1405, Fax: (202) 452-1406, www.nonpfaacn.nche.edu

BOX 13-5

TOLL-FREE SELF-HELP NUMBERS FOR PATIENTS AND PROVIDERS

Adoption Center, National (800) 862-3678
Adoption of Special Kids (415) 543-2275
Agent Orange (Veterans Payment Program) (800) 225-4712
AIDS Clearinghouse, National (800) 458-5231
AIDS Clinical Trials Information Service (800) TRIALS-A
AIDS and HIV Hotline, National (800) 342-AIDS, (800) 344-7432 (Spanish)
Al-Anon Family Group Headquarters, Inc. (800) 344-2666
Alcohol and Drug Information, National Clearinghouse for (800) 729-6686, (800) 487-4889
Alcoholism, American Council on (800) 527-5344
Alcoholism and Drug Dependence, National Council on (800) 622-2255
Alzheimer's Association (800) 272-3900
Alzheimer's Disease Education and Referral Center (800) 438-4380
American Liver Association (800) 223-0179
American Red Cross (202) 737-8300
Amyotrophic Lateral Sclerosis Association (800) 782-4747
Anemia Foundation (800) 522-7222
Arthritis Consulting Services (800) 327-3027
Arthritis Foundation (800) 283-7800
Autism Hotline, National (304) 525-8014, (800) 428-8476
Battered Women's Justice Project (800) 903-0111
Blind, American Foundation for the (800) 232-5463
Blind Children's Center (800) 222-3566
Blind and Dyslexic, Recordings for the (800) 221-4792
Blind, Guide Dog Foundation for the (800) 543-4337
Blind, Job Opportunities for the (800) 638-7518
Blind, National Office of the (800) 424-8666
Blinded Veteran's Association (800) 669-7079
Blindness, Foundation Fighting (RP) (800) 683-5555
Blindness (Prevent Blindness America) (800) 331-2020
Brain Injury Association (202) 296-6443
Brain Injury National Foundation (800) 444-6443
Breast Cancer, Y-Me National Organization Hotline (800) 221-2141
Burn Association, American (312) 642-9260
Burn Victim Foundation, National (800) 803-5879
Cancer Foundation, The Candlelighters Childhood (800) 366-2223
Cancer Information and Counseling Line, AMC (800) 525-3777
Cancer Institute, National (Cancer Information Service) (800) 4-CANCER
Cancer Research, American Institute for (800) 843-8114
Cancer Society, American (800) ACS-2345
Cerebral Palsy Association, United (800) 872-5827
Child Abuse and Family Violence, National Council on (800) 222-2000
Child Abuse, National Committee to Prevent (312) 663-3520, (800) 422-4453
Child Protection and Custody, Resource Center on (800) 527-3223
Cleft Palate Foundation (800) 242-5338
Cocaine (Phoenix House Foundation) (800) COCAINE (800), DRUG HELP (800) 262-2463
Craniofacial Association, Children's (800) 535-3643
Crohn's and Colitis Foundation (800) 343-3637
Cystic Fibrosis Foundation (800) FIGHT-CFU (800) 344-4823
Deaf, Captioned Films and Video Programs for the (800) 237-6213
Deafness Research Foundation (800) 535-3323
de Lange Syndrome Foundation (800) 753-2357
Depressive Illness, National Foundation for (800) 248-4344
Depressive and Manic Depressive Association, National (800) 82-NDMDA
Diabetes Association, American (800) DIABETES
Diabetes Foundation, American (800) 232-3472
Diabetes Foundation, Juvenile (800) 223-1138
Domestic Violence, National Coalition Against (303) 839-1852
Domestic Violence, National Hotline (800) 799-SAFE
Domestic Violence, National Resource Center (800) 537-2238
Down Syndrome Congress, National (800) 232-NDSC
Down Syndrome Society, National (800) 221-4602
Drug and Alcohol Treatment Routing Service, National (800) 662-HELP (4357)
Drug Dependence, National Council on Alcoholism (800) 622-2255
Drug Information, National Clearinghouse for Alcohol (800) 729-6686
Dyslexia Society (800) 222-3123
EAR Foundation (800) 545-4327
Easter Seal Society (800) 221-6827
Eldercare Locator Information and Referral Line (800) 677-1116
EMERGE (Counseling and Education to Stop Male Violence) (617) 422-1550
Epilepsy Foundation American (800) 332-1000
Epilepsy Information Service (800) 642-0500
Eye Care Project Helpline, National (800) 222-3937
Facial Disfigurement (800) 332-3223
Facial Reconstruction, National Foundation for (212) 263-6656
Family Violence Helpline, National Council on Child Abuse and (800) 222-2000
Genetic Support Groups, Alliance of (800) 336-GENE
Guillain-Barré Syndrome Foundation, International (610) 667-0131
Headache Foundation, National (800) 843-2256
Hearing Aid Helpline (800) 521-5247
Hearing and Communication Handicaps (800) 327-9355
Hearing, Dial-a- (Screening Test) (800) 222-EARS
Hearing Information Center (800) 622-3277
Hearing Institute, Better (800) 327-9355
Heart Association, American (800) 242-8721
Hemophilia, National Foundation (800) 42-HANDI
Hepatitis Hotline, American (800) 223-0179
High Blood Pressure Line (National Heart, Lung and Blood Institute) (800) 575-WELL
Hospice International, Children's (800) 242-4453

Continued

BOX 13-5

TOLL-FREE SELF-HELP NUMBERS FOR PATIENTS AND PROVIDERS—cont'd

Hospice Organization Helpline, National (800) 658-8898
Huntington's Disease Society (800) 345-HDSA (4372)
Impotence Information Center (800) 843-4315
Incontinence Information Center (800) 543-9632
Incontinence, Simon Foundation for (800) 23-SIMON
Interstitial Cystitis Association (212) 979-6057
Juvenile Diabetes Foundation (800) 533-2873
Kidney Foundation, National (800) 622-9010
Kidney Fund, American (800) 638-8299
Kidney Patients, American Association of (800) 749-2257
Knight-Ridder Information, Inc (800) 334-2564
Leukodystrophy Foundation, United (800) 728-5483
Liver Association, American (800) 223-0179
Lung Association, American (800) LUNG-USA
Lung Line Information Center (National Jewish Center for Immunology and Respiratory Medicine) (800) 222-LUNG
Lupus Foundation of America (800) 558-0121
Lyme Disease Foundation (800) 886-5963
Lymphedema Network, National (800) 541-3259
March of Dimes Birth Defects Foundation (914) 428-7100
Marfan Foundation, National (800) 8-MARFAN
Medicare Hotline (800) 638-6833
Mental Health Association, National (800) 969-6642
Mentally Ill, National Alliance for the (800) 950-NAMI
Healthy Mothers, Healthy Babies Coalition (202) 863-2458
Multiple Sclerosis Association of America (800) 833-4672
Multiple Sclerosis Society, National (800) LEARN-MS, (800) 344-4867
Muscular Dystrophy Association (800) 572-1717
Myasthenia Gravis Foundation (800) 541-5454
National Alliance for the Mentally Ill (800) 950-6264
National Drug and Alcohol Treatment Hotline (800) 662-HELP
National Manic/Depressive Assoc (800) 826-3632
Neurofibromatosis Foundation (800) 323-7938
Obsessive-Compulsive Foundation (203) 878-5669
Optometric Association, American (314) 991-4100
Organ Donation, The Living Bank (800) 528-2971
Organ Donor Hotline (800) 243-6667
Osteoporosis Foundation, National (800) 223-9994
Ostomy Association, United (800) 826-0826
Paget's Disease Foundation (800) 23-PAGET
Panic Disorder Information Helpline (800) 64-PANIC
Paralysis Association, American (800) 225-0292
Parkinson's Disease Association, American (800) 223-APDA (2732)
Parkinson's Disease Foundation (800) 457-6676
Parkinson Foundation, National (800) 327-4545
Planned Parenthood Federation of America (800) 230-7526
Podiatric Medical Association, American (800) FOOT-CARE
Prevent Blindness America (800) 331-2020
Prostate Information Center (800) 543-9632
Psoriasis Foundation, National (503) 297-1545
Radon (Federal Hot Line) (800) 767-7236
Rare Disorders, National Organization for (800) 999-6673
Red Cross, American (202) 737-8300
Rehabilitation Information Center, National (800) 346-2742
Rehabilitation Technology, Center for (800) 726-9119
Respiratory (Lung Line Center) (800) 222-5864
Reyes Syndrome Foundation, National (800) 233-7393
Safety Council, National (800) 621-7619
Scleroderma Foundation, United (800) 722-4673
Sexually Transmitted Disease Hot Line, National (800) 227-8922
Sickle Cell Disease Association of America (800) 421-8453
Skin Cancer Foundation (800) SKIN-490
Sleep Disorders Association, American (507) 287-6006
Social Health Association, American (919) 361-8422
Speech-Language-Hearing Association, American (800) 638-TALK
Spina Bifida Association of America (800) 621-3141
Spinal Cord Injury Association (800) 962-9629
Stroke Association, National (800) 787-6537
Stroke Connection of the AHA (800) 553-6321
Stuttering, National Center for (800) 221-2483
Sudden Infant Death Syndrome (SIDS) Alliance (800) 221-SIDS, (800) 638-7437
Tourette Syndrome Association (800) 237-0717
Trauma (American Trauma Society) (800) 556-7890
Tuberous Sclerosis Association, National (800) 225-NTSA
Victim Assistance, National Organization of (202) 232-6682
Vietnam Veterans and Their Families, National Information System for (800) 922-9234
Vision and Aging, Lighthouse National Center for (800) 334-5497
Visiting Nurse Preferred Care (800) 426-2547
Wegener's Granulomatosis Support Group, Inc (800) 277-9474
WomanKind (612) 924-5775

recommendations for change. The goals that are established are meeting the needs of the provider and not the patient. Sometimes the process breaks down when patients do not understand what to do, cannot afford the treatment plan, or lose confidence in their ability to change. Whatever the problem, the health care provider must attempt to discover where the process went wrong.

It is important that the patient be involved during the teaching process. Active participation in learning facilitates retention. The more active the participation and the more sensory involvement provided, the more effective is the learning that takes place.

Throughout the teaching process, summarize, repeat, and keep it simple. Providers should check for comprehension as they go along. Have patients repeat important points. It is important not to be threatening or intimidating when quizzing patients on information that has been discussed (Barker, Burton & Zieve, 2002). Then document the extent and result

BOX 13-6

FREQUENTLY USED TERMS IN ELECTRONIC COMMUNICATIONS

BBS: Bulletin Board System, allowing users to hold discussions and make announcements that others can read and to which they can respond.

Browser: Software for bringing up and displaying web pages. Examples: Netscape Navigator and Microsoft Internet Explorer.

E-Mail: Electronic messages sent between or among computers. Like an electronic telephone.

HTML (HyperText Markup Language): Web page format coding system.

http (HyperText Transfer Protocol): System of communication rules for the World Wide Web.

Home Page: Website introductory page.

Hypertext: Text that can be linked to other text by clicking with a mouse at designated points.

Internet: A massive worldwide electronic network composed of smaller computer networks that are linked together.

Listserves: Groups of users, usually with a common interest, linked together through the Internet. Facilitates rapid delivery of information to everyone and allows query and responses.

Modem: Accessory connecting computers to telephone lines that allows computers to talk to each other.

Password: Personal letters or numerals to identify an authorized user access to locked systems.

Search engine: Software programs that search databases or documents for key words or phrases.

SMTP (Simple Mail Transfer Protocol): Governs transmission of e-mail through the Internet.

URL (Uniform Resource Locator): Internet address of an Internet page. Like a telephone number, each is unique.

Usenet Newsgroups: Electronic discussion groups organized around topics of mutual interest to participants.

Virus: A destructive program that invades and infects other programs, causing them to malfunction or self-destruct.

www (World Wide Web): Network of electronic sites linked to form a global electronic network for transmitting information in text, graphics, audio, or video formats.

TABLE 13-2 Web Sites that Offer Information for Navigating the Web

Site	URL Address
Beginners Central	www.northernwebs.com/bc
The Help Web	www.imagescape.com/helpweb
The Internet Learning Tree	world.std.com/-walthowe/ilrntree.html
Internet Starter Kit	ss2.mcp.com/resources/geninternet/frameiskm.html
Internet Web Text Index	www.december.com/web/text
Too Old for Computers?	www.portals.pdx.edu/-isidore/tooold.html
Welcome to Folks Online	www.folksonline.com

of education in the patient's chart. List the important topics covered, state what written material was given to the patient, and provide an assessment of the patient's level of comprehension and any evidence of the patient's intention to comply.

Specific things that might also assist in improving compliant medication-taking behavior in general for most patients include developing treatment plans that have frequent provider–patient contacts; use of reminder cards; use of evaluation drug assays; tailoring the therapeutic regimen to the patient's characteristics and environment; providing reinforcement through behavioral feedback that either promotes compliance or discourages noncompliant behavior; and enhancing patient involvement in such activities as taking blood pressures at home or establishing therapeutic contracts with the provider. These strategies should be kept in mind in crafting both objectives for learning and evaluation of the learning process.

SUMMARY

Sufficient research has been conducted to demonstrate that patient education is really not an optional activity for the health care provider. Although long recognized as important, it has often been omitted because of lack of time, lack of reimbursement, and lack of intrinsic valuing. Patient educational needs were often perceived as needs of the patient and not really as a need that had to be met by the health care provider. However, if health care providers are forced to pay attention to the bottom line of health care costs, they can no longer remain so cavalier about a process that may save so much money and bring such great dividends in increased patient awareness. Indeed, providing patient education empowers patients to more fully become partners in establishing and meeting their own health care goals.

RESOURCES FOR PATIENTS AND PROVIDERS

American Society of Health-System Pharmacists: *Medication teaching manual,* ed 7, Bethesda, MD, 1998. American Society of Health-System Pharmacists, (301) 657-3000.

Ball J: *Mosby's handbook of patient teaching,* St Louis, 1998, Mosby.

Deck M: *Instant teaching tools for health care educators,* St Louis, 1995, Mosby.

Deck M: *More instant teaching tools for health care educators,* St. Louis, 1998, Mosby.

Drug Facts and Comparisons: *Patient drug facts,* St Louis, 2003, Drug Facts and Comparisons.

Yearly-quarterly updates or as a software product for PC. (800) 223-0554.

Ferri FF: *Ferri's patient teaching guides,* St Louis, 1999, Mosby.
Griffith HW, Griffith JA, Moore SW: *Griffith's instructions for patients,* ed 6, Philadelphia, 1998, WB Saunders.
Miller SA, McEvers G, Griffith H, editors. *Instructions for obstetric and gynecologic patients,* ed 2, Philadelphia, 1997, WB Saunders.
Mosby's patient teaching guides and *Mosby's patient teaching guides update I and update II,* St Louis, 1996, Mosby.
Available on disk or as a looseleaf notebook for photocopying for patients.
National Health Information Clearing House, Office of Disease Prevention and Health Promotion, US. Department of Health and Human Services, PO Box 1133, Washington, DC 20012-1133, (800) 336-4797.
Pharmaceutical Manufacturing Association, 1100 15th Street NW, Washington, DC 20005, (202) 835-3463.
Has guide booklet to 438 health education materials.
Ragland G: *Instant teaching treasures,* St Louis, 1997, Mosby.
Offers creative ideas and exercises for a more effective learning experience.
Rudd R, Moeykens B, Colton T: *Health and literacy: a review of medical and public health literature,* San Francisco, CA, 2002, Jossey-Bass.
Annual review of adult learning and literacy.
Schmitt B: *Instructions for pediatric patients,* ed 2, Philadelphia, 1997, WB Saunders.
Also available in Spanish.
Sodeman P: *Instructions for geriatric patients,* Philadelphia, 1995, WB Saunders.
Teaching patients with acute conditions, Springhouse, PA, 1992, Springhouse.
Teaching patients with chronic conditions, Springhouse, PA, 1992, Springhouse.
United States Pharmacopeial Convention: *USP DI Advice for the patient,* Vol II, Rockville, MD, 2003, US Pharmacopeia, (800) 227-8772.
Yearly, with monthly updates.
United States Pharmacopeial Convention: *USP DI Patient Education Leaflets,* Rockville, MD, 2003, US Pharmacopeia, (800) 227-8772.
Yearly, with monthly updates or as USP leaflet diskette or a software product.

REFERENCES

Andrus MR, Roth MT: Health literacy: a review, *Pharmacotherapy* 22:282-302, 2002.
Baker DW et al: The health care experience of patients with low literacy, *Arch Fam Med* 5:329-334, 1996.
Baker DW et al: Health literacy and performance on the Mini-Mental State Examination, *Aging Ment Health* 6:22-29, 2002.
Baker DW et al: The relationship of patient reading ability to self-reported health and use of health services, *Am J Public Health* 87:1027-1039, 1997.
Barker LR et al: *Principles of ambulatory medicine,* ed 6, Baltimore, 2002, Lippincott, Williams & Wilkins.
Brez SM, Taylor M: Assessing literacy for patient teaching: perspectives of adults with low literacy skills, *J Adv Nurs* 25:1040-1047, 1997.
Carter BL: Patient education and chronic disease monitoring. In Herfindal ER, Gourley DR, Hart LL, editors: *Clinical pharmacy and therapeutics,* ed 5, Baltimore, 1992, Williams & Wilkins.
Culbertson VL et al: Consumer preferences for verbal and written medication information, *Drug Intell Clin Pharm* 22:390-396, 1988.
Davis T et al: How poor literacy leads to poor health care, *Patient Care* 10:94-127, 1996.
Davis TC et al: Reading ability of parents compared with reading level of pediatric patient education materials, *Pediatrics* 93:460-468, 1994.
David TC et al: Rapid estimate of adult literacy in medicine: a shortened screening instrument, *Fam Med* 25:391-395, 1993.
Doak LG, Doak CC: Patient comprehension profiles: recent findings and strategies, *Patient Educ Counsel* 2:101-106, 1980.
Doak CC, Doak LG, Root JH: *Teaching patients with low literacy skills,* ed 2. St. Louis, 1996, JB Lippincott.
Doak LG, Doak CC, Meade CD: Strategies to improve cancer education materials, *Oncol Nursing Forum* 23:305-312, 1996.
Fisher E: Low literacy levels in adults: implications for patient education, *J Contin Educ Nurs* 30:56-61, 1999.
Gannon W, Hildebrandt E: A winning combination: women, literacy, and participation in health care, *Health Care Women Int* 23:754-760, 2002.
Gausman Benson J, Forman WB: Comprehension of written health care information in an affluent geriatric retirement community: use of the Test of Functional Health Literacy, *Gerontology* 48:93-97, 2002.
Gazmararian JA et al: Health literacy among Medicare enrollees in a managed care organization, *JAMA* 281:545-551, 1999.
Hanson-Divers EC: Developing a medical achievement reading test to evaluate patient literacy skills: a preliminary study, *J Health Care Poor Underserved* 8:56-69, 1997.
Hayes KS: Literacy for health information of adult patients and caregivers in a rural emergency department, *Clin Excel Nurse Pract* 4:35-40, 2000.
Kalichman SC et al: Health-related Internet use, coping, social support, and health indicators in people living with HIV/AIDS: preliminary results from a community survey, *Health Psychol* 22:111-116, 2001.
Kefalides P: Illiteracy: the silent barrier to health care, *Ann Intern Med* 130:333-336, 1999.
Kirsch I et al: Adult literacy in America. A first look at the results of the National Adult Literacy Survey. Educational Testing Service, September 1993. Available at www.nces.ed/gov/nadlits/index.html.
Lee PP: Why literacy matters. Links between reading ability and health, *Arch Ophthalmol* 117:100-103, 1999.
Ley P, Florio T: The use of readability formulas in health care, *Psychol Health Med* 1:351-363, 1996.
Mailloux S et al: How reliable is computerized assessment of readability? *Comput Nurs* 13:221-224, 1995.
Moon RY et al: Parental literacy level and understanding of medical information, *Pediatrics* 102:e25, 1998.
Morris RW, Burkhart VD, Lamy PP: Technical and theoretical aspects of patient counseling using audiovisual aids, *Drug Intell Clin Pharm* 9:485-488, 1975.
Morrow D, Leirer V, Sheikh J: Adherence and medication instructions: review and recommendations, *J Am Geriatr Soc* 36:1147-1160, 1988.
Mullen PD, Green LW, Persinger GS: Clinical trials of patient education for chronic conditions: a comparative meta-analysis of intervention types, *Prev Med* 14:753-781, 1985.
O'Donnell L et al: The effectiveness of video-based interventions in promoting condom acquisition among STD clinical patients, *Sexual Transm Dis* 22:97-103, 1995.
Parker RM et al: The test of functional health literacy in adults: a new instrument for measuring patients' literacy skills, *J Gen Intern Med* 10:537-541, 1995.
Plimpton S, Root J: Materials and strategies that work in low literacy health communication, *Public Health Rep* 109:86-92, 1994.
Quaid KA et al: Informed consent for a prescription drug: impact of disclosed information on patient understanding and medical outcomes, *Patient Educ Counsel* 15:249-250, 1990.
Redman BK: *The process of patient education,* ed 7, St Louis, 1993, Mosby.
Root J, Stableford S: Easy-to-read consumer communications: a missing link in Medicaid managed care, *J Health Politics Policy Law* 24:1-26, 1999.
Rost K, Carter W, Innu T: Introduction of information during the critical medical visit: consequences for patient follow through with physician recommendations for medications, *Soc Sci Med* 28:315, 1989.
Roter D, Rudd R, Comings J. Patient literacy: a barrier to quality of care, *J Gen Intern Med* 13:850-851, 1998.
Selby MR: An in-depth study of educational strategies for increased patient compliance with medications, unpublished scholarly paper written to meet graduation requirement, University of Maryland, School of Nursing, 1983.
Slater MD et al: Hypermedia use by the disadvantaged: assessing a health information program, *Hypermedia* 6:67-86, 1994.

Strecher VJ et al: The effects of computer-tailored smoking cessation messages in family practice settings, *J Fam Pract* 39:262-270, 1994.

US Department of Health and Human Services, *Healthy People*, Washington, DC, 2002.

Weiss BD, Coyne C: Communicating with patients who cannot read, *N Engl J Med* 337:272-274, 1997.

Weiss BD, Hart G, Pust R: The relationship between literacy and health, *J Health Care for Poor Underserved* 1:351-363, 1991.

Williams MV et al: Relationship of functional health literacy to patients' knowledge of their chronic disease: a study of patients with hypertension or diabetes, *Arch Intern Med* 158:166-172, 1998.

Williams MV et al: Inadequate functional health literacy among patients at two public hospitals, *JAMA* 274:1677-1682, 1995.

Williams MV et al: The role of health literacy in patient-physician communication, *Fam Med* 34:383-389, 2002.

Williams-Deane M, Potter LS: Current oral contraceptive use instructions: An analysis of patient package inserts, *Family Planning Perspective* 24L:111-115, 1992.

Wilson FL. Measuring patients' ability to read and comprehend: a first step in patient education, *Nursing Connections* 13:19-27, 2000.

Wilson FL. The suitability of United States Pharmacopeia Dispensory Information psychotropic drug leaflets for urban patients with limited reading skills, *Arch Psychiatr Nurs* 13:204-211, 1999.

UNIT 4

Topical Agents

Unit 4 discusses drugs that are placed directly on the site of action. These drugs are organized by site of application. They are used to treat a wide variety of unrelated conditions. Because of the large numbers of products available, only a selection of those seen most frequently in primary care are presented. The focus of this unit is on the general concepts of topical application, not the individual drugs.

These drugs act directly at the site of application; the effect is not based on systemic absorption. Therefore their mechanism of action is fairly straightforward. Treatment consists of applying the correct agent according to directions and monitoring for effectiveness. Most of these drugs are also given orally for other problems. Their mechanism of action is discussed at length in the chapters covering oral use of the drug.

- **Chapter 14,** Dermatologic Agents, discusses drugs that are placed on the skin. These include topical corticosteroids, topical infectives, acne preparations, and local anesthesia. The diseases discussed are the common primary care problems: fungal infections and acne.
- **Chapter 15** discusses eye, ear, mouth, and throat agents. These are all placed topically. These include anti-infectives, nonsteroidal antiinflammatory agents, mast cell stabilizers, steroids, antiglaucoma preparations, lubricants, topical anesthetics, and diagnostics. The diseases discussed include conjunctivitis and glaucoma.

CHAPTER 14

Dermatologic Agents

Drug Names

Class	Subclass	Generic Name	Trade Name
TOPICAL CORTICOSTEROIDS (see Table 14-2)			
Nonsteroidal antiinflammatories		pimecrolimus	Elidel
ANTIINFECTIVES			
Topical antibiotics		(200) muciprocin	Bactroban
		bacitracin	Bacitracin, Baciguent
		erythromycin	Ilotycin
		gentamycin	Garamycin
		neomycin	Mycostatin
		polymyxin B sulfate	In Polysporin, Neosporin
Topical antifungals	Azoles	econazole	Spectazole
		(P) clotrimazole	Lotrimin, Mycelex
		ketoconazole	Nizoral
		miconazole	Monistat-Derm
	Allylamine/benzylamine derivatives	butenafine	Mentax
		naftifine	Naftin
		terbinafine	Lamisil
	Other	nystatin	Nystatin, Mycostatin
		haloprogin	Halotex
		tolnaftate	Tinactin
		ciclopirox	Penlac, Loprox
		selenium sulfide lotion	2.5% Selsun
Antivirals		acyclovir	Zovirax
		penciclovir	Denavir
Scabicides/pediculicides		crotamiton	Eurax
		malathion	Ovide
		permethrin	Elimite, Nix
		lindane	Kwell, Scabene
ACNE PREPARATIONS			
Antibacterial/keratolytic		benzoyl peroxide	Benzac (prescription), many brands OTC
Topical retinoid		tretinoin	Retin-A, Avita
Oral retinoid		isotretinoin	Accutane
LOCAL ANESTHETICS			
	Short acting	procaine HCl	Novocain
		chloroprocaine	Nesacaine
	Intermediate acting	lidocaine HCl	Xylocaine
		mepivacaine HCl	Carbocaine HCl
		prilocaine HCl	Citanest
	Long acting	bupivacaine HCl	Marcaine, Sensorcaine
		etidocaine	Duranest
		tetracaine HCl	Pontocaine HCl

(200), Top 200 drug; (P), prototype drug.

General Uses

Indications

- Corticosteroid-responsive dermatoses
- Superficial skin infections: bacterial, fungal, viral, and parasitic
- Acne
- Local anesthesia

• • •

This chapter discusses preparations used for skin, nail, and hair problems. These preparations are used for an extremely large array of dermatologic problems. See each section for more specific indications. General issues in topical medications are discussed, and then corticosteroids, antiinfectives, acne medications, and local anesthesia are each discussed in a separate section. The purpose of this chapter is to discuss the most common of the various agents available. It does not attempt to mention all of the preparations or the myriad indications for these agents. This chapter focuses on the topical use of these products. See specific chapters for more information about drugs from specific drug categories.

DISEASE PROCESS

Anatomy and Physiology

The skin is the largest organ of the body, with three distinct layers: epidermis, dermis, and subcutaneous (Figure 14-1). The epidermis is the outer layer of the skin. The thickness of the epidermis ranges from 0.05 mm on the eyelids to 1.5 mm on the palms and soles. Five layers make up the epidermis. Basal cells form a single layer of cells, which make up the innermost layer of the epidermis. The basal cells divide to form keratinocytes. The other layers are formed as keratinocytes change until they migrate to the outer layer to become the major component of the stratum corneum. The stratum corneum provides protection to the skin by acting as a barrier. The thicker the epidermis, the greater is the barrier protection provided.

The dermis, like the epidermis, varies in thickness, ranging from 0.3 mm on the eyelid to 3.0 mm on the back. Three types of connective tissue—collagen, elastic tissue, and reticular fibers—make up the dermis. Unlike the epidermis, the dermis has nerves, blood vessels, hair follicles, and apocrine and eccrine glands.

Subcutaneous tissue is the deepest layer. Distribution is dependent on sex characteristics. Age, heredity, and caloric intake also influence distribution. The subcutaneous tissue provides padding and insulation to the underlying structures.

The primary function of the skin is as a barrier. It also functions to protect and thermoregulate. It is involved in the immune response, biochemical synthesis, and sensory detection. The skin's barrier function is compromised when the skin has been damaged or when inflammation is present.

Pathophysiology

There are three types of primary skin lesions: the macule, the papule, and the vesicle. Variations of these lesions are named according to the size of the lesion. Secondary lesions include erosion, ulcer, fissure, crust, lichenification, atrophy, excoriation, scar, and keloid.

When describing a skin lesion, it is important to accurately name the type of lesion using this terminology. Location on the body and pattern of distribution are important. Timing and course should include whether the onset was acute or insidious. Also note the presence of any systemic signs and symptoms.

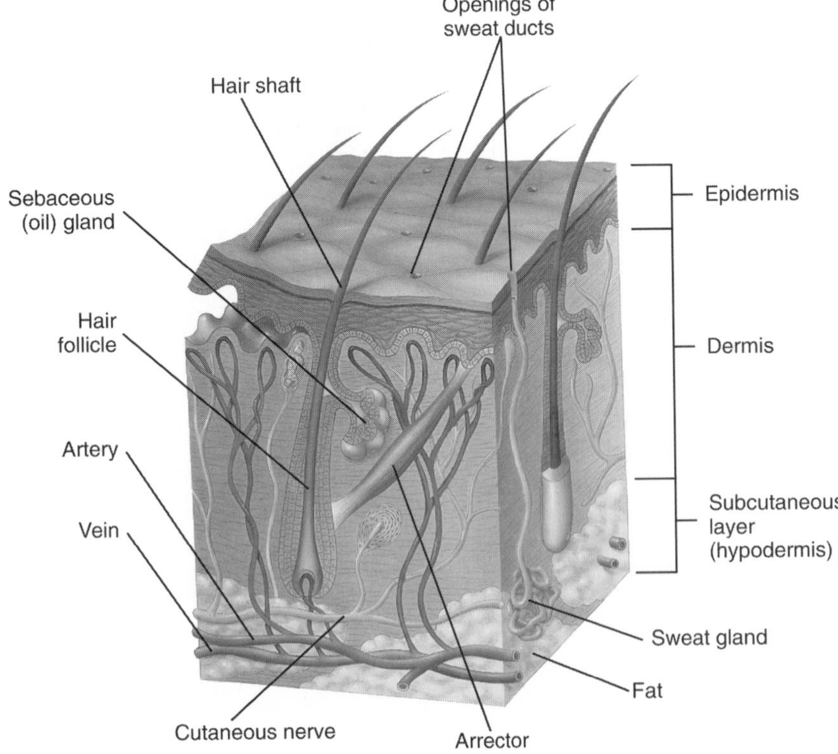

FIGURE 14-1

Structure of the skin. (From Thibodeau G, Patton K: *Anatomy and physiology*, ed 3, St Louis, 1996, Mosby.)

DRUG ACTION AND EFFECTS

Topicals work by being absorbed into the skin. Their effect is local. The specific mechanisms of action are discussed in each separate section.

DRUG TREATMENT PRINCIPLES

There is a bewildering array of topical preparations, including many combination products, different strengths of steroid products, and antiinfectives of every kind. The primary care provider should become familiar with a few products and treatment measures rather than try to master the complete array. Superficial skin infections and acne are commonly treated in primary care. If the patient does not respond to standard care, he or she is referred to dermatology. Primary care providers should be able to identify suspicious lesions and refer promptly to dermatology; such patients frequently require surgical treatment.

Factors Affecting Drug Absorption

Topical therapy is unique because the skin is directly accessible for both diagnosis and therapy. Drugs to treat skin problems can be applied directly to the site. All topical agents can also be absorbed systemically. Consider the adverse effects of the systemic medication when ordering topical agents.

Factors that affect the extent of drug absorption into the skin are the status of the skin, the characteristics of the drug, and the characteristics of the administration vehicle. Absorption is increased if the skin is broken or inflamed. Also, absorption increases if the skin integrity is compromised and where the skin is thinner. Because of the vascular composition, mucous membranes absorb medication in high concentrations. The vehicle or base affects percutaneous absorption (Table 14-1). The vehicle may hydrate the outer layer of the skin by preventing water loss. With improved hydration, the absorption of medication and the depth of penetration are enhanced. Absorption of topical medications is slow and incomplete compared to drugs given orally.

Prescribing the appropriate amount of topical medication is important. Too large a tube may be very costly to the patient, yet a small tube may not be enough to cover the entire area. To estimate the amount to prescribe, the rule of nines can be used (Figure 14-2).

How Topical Agents Are Used

Creams, Ointments, Pastes

1. Take a small amount of cream or ointment into the palm of the hand, and rub the hands together until medication has a thin sheen.
2. Apply a small amount of ointment or cream as a thin layer to the skin. Excess medication will rub off onto clothing and be wasted.

TABLE 14-1 Characteristics of Vehicle of Selected Topical Products

	Creams	Ointments	Gels	Solutions and Lotions	Aerosols
Base	Mixture of several different organic oils and water	Mixture of a limited number of organic compounds consisting primarily of petroleum jelly with little or no water	Greaseless mixtures of propylene glycol, water, and alcohol	Alcohol, water, and some chemicals	Drug suspended in a base and delivered via a propellant (e.g., isobutane, propane)
Color	White, somewhat greasy	Translucent, greasy feeling persists on skin	Clear with a gelatinous consistency	Clear or milky	
Versatility	Most frequent base prescribed, used on nearly all body areas, especially useful in the intertriginous areas (i.e., groin, genital area, axilla)	Greater penetration, useful for drier lesions, enhanced potency	Unpleasant sticky feeling, may be irritating	Most useful for scalp because it penetrates the hair shaft	Useful for applying to scalp via a long probe attached to can
Miscellaneous	Cosmetically more acceptable; can be drying after prolonged use, best used for acute exfoliative dermatitis	Too occlusive for acute exudative eczematous inflammation; too occlusive for intertriginous areas	Alcohol gels feel cool and are drying; useful in acute exudative inflammation (i.e., poison ivy); nonalcoholic gels are more lubricating and can be useful in drying scalp lesions; useful in scalp areas because other vehicles mat hair	May be drying and irritating when used in intertriginous areas	Convenient for patients who lack mobility and have difficulty in reaching lower legs; useful for moist lesions (i.e., poison ivy)

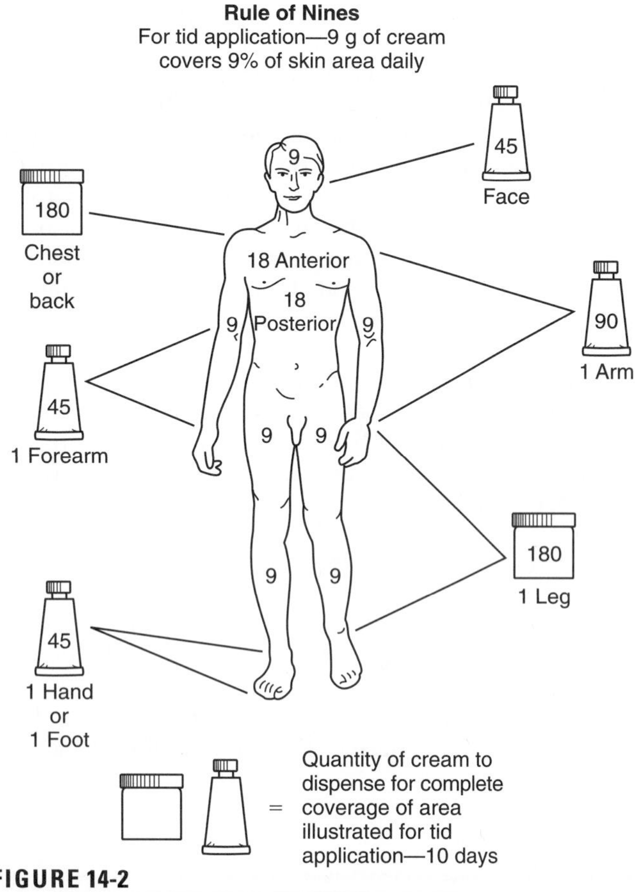

FIGURE 14-2

Rule of nines to calculate quantity of medication to dispense. (From Habif TP: *Clinical dermatology,* ed 4, St Louis, 2004, Mosby.)

3. Apply topical medications with long, downward strokes to the affected areas. Avoid back-and-forth strokes because they may cause irritation of the hair follicles.
4. A tongue blade may be used for the application of topicals in a paste form.

Lotions

1. Instruct the patient to shake the container to mix the suspension well.
2. Carefully pour a small quantity of lotion into the palm of the hand.
3. Apply a thin layer to skin using firm, downward strokes. Avoid using gauze unless the liquid is very thin. The use of a cotton ball should be avoided because it will retain the suspended particles of medication.

Sprays and Aerosols

1. Shake the container well.
2. While holding container upright 6 to 12 inches away from body, direct spray toward the affected body part. Avoid spraying into eyes.

Powders

1. Apply powder lightly to dry skin with gauze or powder puff as needed.

HOW TO MONITOR

- Monitor for therapeutic effect and adverse effects. See specific classes of drugs for details.

PATIENT VARIABLES

- Specifics are discussed under each class of drug.
- Geriatric skin is thinner and absorbs more than that of younger adults.
- Children absorb about three times as much as do adults.
- Pregnant and lactating women need to be especially careful about topical agents being absorbed systemically. Agents known to be harmful to the fetus include tretinoin, lindane, and podophyllum.

PATIENT EDUCATION

Topical medications come in many forms. Each has an effective and appropriate method of application. Topical medications should be applied thinly or lightly. The application of extra amounts usually does not provide increased benefits. Teach the patient the correct method for their particular preparation.

- Apply a small amount to the affected area two to four times a day.
- These products are for external use only. Do not use in the eyes.
- If the condition does not improve in 3 to 5 days, call the health care provider.
- If the condition worsens or if skin reaction develops, discontinue the agent. Wash the affected area and call the health care provider.

Topical Corticosteroids

For a listing, see Table 14-2.

General Uses

Use in cases of inflammatory and pruritic dermatoses that are responsive to corticosteroids, such as psoriasis, eczema, contact dermatitis, and many other dermatoses.

Toxicity to topical corticosteroids, although not common, is the same as that when steroids are given systemically.

The most common complication is the suppression of the hypothalamic-pituitary-adrenal (HPA) axis, which usually is not associated with symptoms until the steroid is stopped.

Other more common adverse effects are atrophy, striae, telangiectasia, purpura, acne, perioral dermatitis, and steroid rosacea. Glaucoma and cataracts may develop after prolonged use of corticosteroids around the eyes. There is an increased risk of side effects when the topical corticosteroids are used over a prolonged time, under occlusion, on the face, and on intertriginous locations.

DRUG ACTION AND EFFECTS

Topical corticosteroids diffuse across cell membranes. They have the same pharmacologic effects as those taken systemi-

TABLE 14-2 Dosage, Administration, and How Supplied for Topical Corticosteroids Ranked by Potency*

Group	Generic Name	Strength (%)	Brand Name
I High	clobetasol propionate	0.05	Temovate cream, ointment
	betamethasone dipropionate	0.05	Diprolene ointment
	diflorasone diacetate	0.05	Psorcon
II High	amcinonide	0.1	Cyclocort ointment
	betamethasone dipropionate	0.05	Diprosone ointment
	halcinonide cream, ung, solution	0.1	Halog cream
	fluocinonide	0.05	Lidex cream, gel, ointment, solution
	betamethasone dipropionate	0.05	Maxivate cream, ointment
III Medium	triamcinolone acetonide	0.05	Aristocort cream, ointment
	amcinonide	0.1	Cyclocort lotion
	triamcinolone acetonide	0.5	Kenalog cream, ointment
	betamethasone dipropionate	0.05	Maxivate lotion
		0.05	Diprosone cream
	mometasone furoate	0.1	Elocon ointment
IV Medium	amcinonide	0.1	Cyclocort cream
	mometasone furoate	0.1	Elocon cream, lotion
	halcinonide	0.025	Halog cream, ointment
	triamcinolone acetonide	0.1	Kenalog ointment
	fluocinolone acetonide	0.025	Synalar ointment
V Medium	tramcinolone acetonide	0.1	Aristocort cream
	triamcinolone valerate	0.1	Kenalog cream, lotion
	triamcinolone acetonide	0.025	Kenalog ointment
	fluocinolone acetonide	0.025	Synalar cream
	hydrocortisone valerate	0.2	Westcort cream, ointment
VI Low	triamcinolone acetonide	0.025	Aristocort cream
		0.025	Kenalog cream, lotion
VII Low	fluocinolone acetonide	0.01	Synalar cream, lotion
	hydrocortisone	1.0, 2.5	Hytone cream, lotion, ointment
		1.0, 2.5	LactiCare lotion
		1.0, 2.5	Synacort cream

*Range: group I (very potent) to group VII (least potent).

cally. Topical corticosteroids inhibit the migration of macrophages and leukocytes into the area by reversing vascular dilation and permeability of the small vessels in the upper dermis. See Chapter 53 for further information.

DRUG TREATMENT PRINCIPLES

Topical corticosteroids are ranked according to potency, with group I as the most potent and group VII as the least potent. It is usually sufficient to divide them into high-, medium-, and low-potency groups. Frequently, weaker strengths are used because they are considered to be safer. However, adequate strength is necessary for a therapeutic response. Weak over-the-counter (OTC) hydrocortisone is not effective against many dermatoses; a medium-strength steroid from class III or IV is often more effective. If the patient does not respond, treatment should be reevaluated.

Potency is the most important variable when choosing a topical steroid. A drug from each potency level should be chosen for the prescriptive needs of the patient. The potency of a steroid is not determined by its strength but by vasoconstrictor assays.

The dose of one steroid does not correlate with the dose of another; that is, diflorasone diacetate (Psorcon) ointment 0.05% is much stronger than hydrocortisone 2.5%.

Vasoconstrictor assays measure skin blanching when an agent is applied to skin under occlusion. There may be a difference in potency between generic and name brand corticosteroid equivalents. Pharmacists are allowed to substitute generic drugs unless the health care provider requests "no substitutions" or "Brand medically necessary."

Use low-potency agents in children, on large areas, for mild conditions, and on body sites that are especially prone to steroid damage such as the face, scrotum, axilla, flexures, and skin folds.

More potent steroids are used on more severe conditions or on a small area.

Reserve high-potency agents for areas and conditions resistant to treatment with milder agents; they may be alternated with milder agents. Short-term intermittent therapy using high-potency agents may be more effective and cause fewer adverse effects than continuous treatment with lower-potency agents. No fluorinated or high-potency steroid should be used on the face.

For all groups, apply product sparingly two to four times a day. Adequate results are usually achieved with a twice-a-day application and a course of therapy of 2 to 6 weeks. Do not discontinue treatment abruptly after long-term use or a potent agent to prevent rebound. Reduce frequency of application or use a lower-potency agent.

When results are not achieved, stop therapy for 4 to 7 days and then resume treatment with a different agent. A more potent steroid may be needed.

Group I

Topical corticosteroids in group I are megapotent. The amount of drug applied to the body per day and the duration of treatment must be carefully monitored. Per week, a maximum of 50 g of cream or ointment should be used. Two weeks is the maximum time a group I drug should be used. A period of a week is needed before a group I topical steroid is used again. This is called *cyclic* or *pulse dosing*. Diflorasone diacetate (Florone) can be used under occlusion; betamethasone dipropionate (Diprolene) cannot. Occlusive dressings should not be used for more than 12 hours at a time. Renal suppression, skin atrophy, and other side effects are possible. Patients using group I topical corticosteroids should be monitored closely for HPA suppression. Prescriptions should limit refills.

Group II

These are also considered high-potency corticosteroids; however, there is less risk of adverse effects.

Groups III through V

These are considered medium-potency preparations. These are the most commonly indicated preparations for skin conditions requiring prescription-strength corticosteroids.

Groups VI and VII

These are the low-potency preparations, useful for covering large areas. Group VII are generally OTC preparations and are not strong enough for many conditions.

HOW TO MONITOR

- Reevaluate after about 10 days to determine if the condition is responding to treatment.
- Monitor for superinfection.
- High-potency topical steroids may require periodic evaluation of the HPA axis suppression by using morning plasma cortisol, urinary free cortisol, and ACTH stimulation tests. If there is evidence of HPA axis suppression, the health care provider should attempt to gradually withdraw the topical corticosteroid. Decrease the number of applications or change to the use of a less-potent steroid to withdraw the steroid from the patient.

PATIENT VARIABLES

Geriatrics

- Geriatric patients are more susceptible to secondary infections when steroids are used.
- They are also more susceptible to the systemic effects of topically applied medications because their skin tends to be thinner.

Pediatrics

- Children, in comparison with adults, have a larger skin surface area–to–body weight ratio. They may be more susceptible to a topical corticosteroid–induced HPA axis suppression and Cushing syndrome. In children, symptoms of HPA may be linear growth retardation, delayed weight gain, and low cortisol levels.
- The least-potent strength compatible with effective treatment should be used.
- Potent corticosteroids should not be used to treat diaper dermatoses.

Pregnancy

- *Category C:* there have not been any reports associating congenital anomalies or adverse effects with the use of corticosteroids during pregnancy.

Lactation

- Effects are not known.
- Corticosteroids absorbed systemically can be detected in breast milk in quantities that are not likely to affect the infant.
- Use with caution.

PATIENT EDUCATION

- Do not use for longer than prescribed.

Specific Drugs

Contraindications

- Allergy to any component in the product
- Primary bacterial infections, such as impetigo, acne, erysipelas, cellulitis, rosacea, or perioral dermatitis
- Treatment of rosacea

Warnings

HPA axis suppression has occurred. Limit amount, potency, and length of treatment.

Precautions

- Very high– or high-potency agents should not be used on the face, under the arms, or in the groin.
- Care should be taken when applying topical corticosteroid to the eyelids or around the eyes because it may get into the eyes.
- With prolonged use, steroids may cause steroid-induced glaucoma or cataracts.

- Local irritation may develop; discontinue use.
- Skin atrophy is common with higher potency and longer duration of treatment.
- Psoriasis: do not use as sole therapy in widespread plaque psoriasis.
- Infections: treating skin infections with topical corticosteroids can worsen the infection.

Pharmacokinetics
- Corticosteroids are absorbed through the skin.
- Time to peak concentration is 12 to 24 hours.
- They are protein bound, metabolized by the liver, and excreted in urine and bile.

Adverse Effects
Local
- Itching, burning, erythema, folliculitis, perioral dermatitis, acneform eruptions, dryness of the skin, allergic contact dermatitis, maceration, secondary infection, skin atrophy striae, and telangiectasia. Using topical corticosteroids under occlusion may cause these adverse effects more frequently.
- With the reduction or discontinuation of potent topical corticosteroids, chronic plaque psoriasis may develop into pustular psoriasis. To prevent rebound effects, long-term or potent topical corticosteroids should be gradually discontinued or the patient switched to a less-potent steroid to facilitate withdrawal.

Systemic
- Reversible HPA axis suppression may be induced by topical steroids.
- Symptoms of Cushing syndrome, hyperglycemia, and glycosuria may also be induced.

Overdosage
- Topical steroids are absorbed systemically in quantities sufficient to produce systemic complications.

Nonsteroidal Antiinflammatory Drugs

Specific Drugs

pimecrolimus (Elidel)

Indications
- Short-term and intermittent long-term treatment of mild to moderate atopic dermatitis in nonimmunocompromised patients who are at least 2 years old

Mechanism of Action
- Blocks production of proinflammatory cytokines by T-lymphocytes and prevents release of inflammatory mediators from cutaneous mast cells and basophils
- Less likely to cause systemic immunosuppression than topical corticosteroids
- Does not cause skin atrophy

Pharmacokinetics
- Minimally absorbed through skin even when applied to large areas of inflamed skin

Adverse Effects
- Transient local irritation with mild to moderate burning, warmth, or stinging.

Dosage and Administration
- Apply twice daily until resolved.

Topical Antiinfectives (Antibiotics)

General Uses

Indications
- Infection prophylaxis in minor cuts, wounds, burns, and skin abrasions; aid to healing.
- Treatment of superficial infections of the skin caused by susceptible organisms amenable to local treatment.

Mupirocin is the only drug in this class used exclusively for topical infections and is the only one discussed in detail. Mupirocin is a major advance because it allows topical treatment of impetigo. Bacitracin is very effective for most topical infections. Triple antibiotic ointments vary in their composition; usually, they contain neomycin, which causes more allergic reactions than other topical agents. See Chapter 59 for more information on other drugs.

DISEASE PROCESS
Most pathogens cultured from infected dermatoses are group A β-hemolytic streptococci, *Staphylococcus aureus, Streptococcus pyogenes,* or any of these pathogens in combination.

Gram-negative infections of the skin are relatively rare.

DRUG ACTION AND EFFECTS
See Chapters 58 through 60 for details.

Mupirocin blocks the protein synthesis of bacteria by binding with the transfer ribonucleic acid (tRNA) synthetase.

DRUG TREATMENT PRINCIPLES
The appropriate drug selection depends on the diagnosis and culture whenever possible.

Systemic antibiotics are needed for diffuse impetigo, cellulitis, or other more-than-superficial infections. Apply gauze dressing if indicated.

Treatment should be reevaluated if there is no improvement in 3 to 5 days (Table 14-3).

! Apply with caution to skin with impaired integrity because this may allow increased systemic absorption of the drug. Combination antibiotic and steroid preparations are not often indicated because topical steroids can impair the body's ability to fight infection.

TABLE 14-3 Important Characteristics of Topical Antibiotics

Antibiotic	Effective Against	Formulation	Administration
mupirocin	Gram positive	2% Ointment	tid
bacitracin	Gram positive	500 U/g ointment	qd-qid
erythromycin	Gram positive	2% Ointment, gel	bid/tid
gentamycin	Gram negative	0.1% Ointment, cream	tid
neomycin	Gram negative	3.5 mg/g ointment, cream	tid
polymyxin	Gram negative	5000 *or* 10,000 U/g cream, ointment	tid

HOW TO MONITOR

- Reevaluate in 3 to 5 days; if no improvement, change treatment.
- Monitor long-term use especially carefully.
- Prolonged use may result in the development of resistant organisms. It may also result in the overgrowth of nonsusceptible organisms, including fungi.
- Neomycin hypersensitivity may manifest as redness, edema, dry scaling, itching, and failure to heal.

PATIENT EDUCATION

- Cover with sterile bandage if needed.

Specific Drugs

See Table 14-3 for dosage and administration recommendations for selected topical antibiotics.

mupirocin (Bactroban)

Indications

Impetigo is caused by *S. aureus*, β-hemolytic streptococci, and *S. pyogenes*.

Mupirocin is a naturally occurring antibiotic. It is structurally different from other topical antibiotics. Mupirocin is the result of fermenting *Pseudomonas fluorescens*. It is useful against infections caused by *S. aureus*, including methicillin-resistant and β-lactamase–producing strains, *Staphylococcus epidermidis, Staphylococcus saprophyticus*, and *S. pyogenes*.

Contraindications

- Prior sensitization to any of the ingredients
- Use in eyes

Warnings

- For external use only
- Deep infections may require systemic antibiotics
- Use with caution in large or deep wounds, animal bites, or serious burns

Precautions

- Mupirocin has not been formulated for use on mucosal surfaces; intranasal use may produce stinging and drying.
- Polyethylene glycol is a component of the base. It can be absorbed systemically through damaged skin. Because polyethylene glycol is excreted via the kidneys, the product should not be used over large areas in patients with renal failure.

Patient Variables

Pregnancy

- *Category B:* Adequate studies on pregnant women have not been performed.

Lactation

- It is not known if mupirocin is excreted in breast milk. While breast-feeding, the use of mupirocin should be temporarily discontinued.

Pharmacokinetics

- There is no measurable systemic absorption.

Adverse Effects

- Local adverse effects consist of burning, stinging, or pain (1.5%), and itching (1%).
- In less than 1%, patients reported rash, nausea, erythema, dry skin, tenderness, swelling, contact dermatitis, and increased drainage.

Dosage and Administration

- A small amount of mupirocin should be applied to the affected area three times a day.
- If no improvement is seen in 3 to 5 days, the treatment should be reevaluated.
- A gauze dressing may be applied over the topical antibiotic.

Other Drugs in Class

Other drugs in this class are similar to the prototype except as follows.

bacitracin (Bacitracin, Baciguent)

- Bacitracin, a polypeptide antibiotic, inhibits streptococci, pneumococci, and staphylococci and other gram-positive organisms.
- Bacitracin is very poorly absorbed through the skin.
- Allergic sensitivity is rare but may develop.

neomycin sulfate (Neomycin, Myciguent) and gentamicin (Gentamicin, G-Myticin, Garamycin)

- Neomycin and gentamicin are aminoglycosides. They are effective against gram-negative organisms such as *Escherichia coli, Proteus, Klebsiella*, and *Enterobacter* species.
- Neomycin is an ingredient in the triple antibiotic ointments.

- Gentamicin is more effective than neomycin against *Pseudomonas aeruginosa,* staphylococci, and groups A β-hemolytic streptococci.
- In a patient in renal failure, the drug may accumulate and lead to nephrotoxicity, neurotoxicity, and ototoxicity.

polymyxin B sulfate

- Polymyxin B is most effective against anaerobic gram-negative organisms, that is, *Pseudomonas aeruginosa, E. coli, Enterobacter*, and *Klebsiella* species.
- Gram-positive organisms and most strains of *Proteus* and *Serratia* are resistant to polymyxin B.
- Polymyxin B–induced toxicity may lead to neurotoxicity and nephrotoxicity.
- Hypersensitivity to polymyxin B rarely occurs.

Antifungals

General Uses

Indications

- Superficial fungal infections (Table 14-4)

Some topical fungal infections are treated topically, others systemically. The systemic antifungals are discussed in Chapter 68. The decision to treat topically or systemically depends on the severity of the infection, the extent of the skin infected, and prior treatment.

DISEASE PROCESS

Fungal, or dermatophyte, infections can affect almost every part of the body. Tinea means *fungal infection*. Dermatophytes infect and live in the dead keratin of the stratum corneum, hair, and nails. They can affect the skin and mucosal surfaces and can become internal infections. *Candida* species are yeastlike fungi. The most common cause of candidiasis is *Candida albicans*, which causes infections in skinfolds and groin, with red skin and satellite lesions.

Fungal infections are classified by body region. *Tinea capitis* is a seborrheic-like scaling of the hair region of the head. It is commonly caused by *Trichophyton tonsurans* or *Microsporum audouini*. *T. tonsurans* does not fluoresce under Wood's lamp. A negative potassium hydroxide (KOH) test does not rule out tinea. Diagnosis is made by the brush method of culturing.

Tinea corporis presents as ring-shaped lesions or scaly patches on exposed skin surfaces or the trunk. Any dermatophyte may cause this, but *Trichophyton rubrum* is the most common. Microscopic examination of scrapings or culture confirms the diagnosis.

Tinea cruris manifests as pruritic erythematous lesions in groin area. Microscopic examination or culture confirms the diagnosis.

Tinea pedis starts in interdigital toe infections that progress from dry scaling to maceration, hyperkeratotic skin, and inflammatory vesicular bullous eruptions. Most infections are caused by *Trichophyton* and *Epidermophyton* species. KOH reveals hyphae. Culture is diagnostic.

Tinea versicolor or *pityriasis versicolor* presents as pale macules found on the trunk, arms, or neck. It is caused by a *Microsporum furfur* (now called *Pityrosporum orbiculare*), a yeast. *Pityrosporum* is part of the normal skin flora, but it may overgrow. KOH reveals large, blunt hyphae and spores. Culture is not useful.

Onychomycosis is fungal infection of the nails. It can be caused by dermatophytes, molds, and *Candida*. Mixed in-fections are common. Microscopic examination confirms diagnosis.

DRUG ACTION AND EFFECTS

See Chapter 68.

DRUG TREATMENT PRINCIPLES

Apply by gently massaging into affected skin and surrounding area.

In general, treatment must last long enough for a complete turnover of skin after the symptoms have resolved. If treatment is not carried out long enough, the infection may recur. Some infections require maintenance therapy to prevent recurrence. Several antifungal topical products, such as clotrimazole, are combined with a steroid to relieve itching and inflammation.

Once these symptoms have disappeared, the steroid combination should be discontinued. Continued use of the steroid antifungal combination may allow development of resistant organisms.

Newer antifungals reach high concentrations in the epidermis and appendages that persist over time and have improved effectiveness of treatment of fungal skin diseases, especially of the nails. Ciclopirox is the first topical antifungal to be effective against onychomycosis. However, most antifungals are effective against the common fungal infections. The provider should become familiar with a few agents. Select one of the older agents such as clotrimazole, and select one of the newer more potent agents such as terbinafine. One factor to consider is cost; the older agents are less expensive. Also consider formulation. Decide what formulation would best deliver the medicine to the infection and choose a antifungal to match. Note that the OTC antifungals come in a wider variety of formulations than do the prescription antifungals. Another factor is prior use of antifungals. Ask the patient if he or she has used OTC antifungals before coming to the office. The older antifungals are usually available OTC. If the patient has failed a trial of OTC antifungal, he or she will probably need a more potent, prescription-only antifungal.

HOW TO MONITOR

- Monitor for efficacy and secondary infections.
- Onset of improvement is variable, depending on severity of infection, location of infection, and potency of medication used. Improvement may be seen in 1 day or take as long as 2 weeks or more.

PATIENT VARIABLES

- Older patients are often susceptible to superinfection.
- See Table 14-4 for pediatrics and pregnancy guidelines.

TABLE 14-4 Indications, Patient Variables, and Administration of Antifungals

Medication	Indication	Pediatric	Pregnancy/ Lactation	Administration	Formulation
econazole (Spectazole)	*Tinea pedis* *T. cruris* *T. corporis* *T. versicolor* *Candida*	NI	C/Unknown	qd, 1 mo qd, 2 wk qd, 2 wk qd, 2 wk qd, 2 wk	Rx; 1% cream
clotrimazole (Lotrimin, Mycelex)	*T. pedis* *T. cruris* *T. corporis* *T. versicolor* *Candida*	No: <2 yr; 2-12 yr with supervision	B/Unknown	qd, 4 wk qd, 2 wk qd, 4 wk qd, 4 wk NI	OTC and Rx; 1% cream; topical solution, lotion
ketoconazole (Nizoral)	*T. pedis* *T. cruris* *T. corporis* *T. versicolor* *Candida*	No	C/Unknown	qd, 6 wk qd, 2 wk qd, 2 wk qd, 2 wk qd, 2 wk	Rx; 2% cream, shampoo
miconazole (Monistat, Lotrimin)	*T. pedis* *T. cruris* *T. corporis* *T. versicolor* *Candida*	NI	NI	bid, 1 mo bid, 2 wk bid, 2 wk qd, 2 wk bid, 2 wk	OTC; 2% cream, ointment, powder, spray, spray powder, spray liquid, solution
oxiconazole (Oxistat)	*T. pedis* *T. cruris* *T. corporis* *T. versicolor*	No: <12 yr	NI	1-2/day, 1 mo 1-2/day, 2 wk 1-2/day, 2 wk qd, 2 wk	Rx; 1% cream and lotion
butenafine (Mentax)	*T. pedis* *T. cruris* *T. corporis* *T. versicolor*	No: <12 yr	B/Unknown	bid or qd × 4 wk qd, 2 wk qd, 2 wk qd, 2 wk	Rx; 1% cream
naftifine (Naftin)	*T. pedis* *T. cruris* *T. corporis*	No	B/Unknown in milk	bid, 4 wk bid, 4 wk bid, 4 wk	Rx; 1% cream and gel
terbinafine (Lamisil)	*T. pedis* *T. cruris* *T. corporis*	No: <12 yr	B/Secreted	1-2/day, 1-4 wk 1-2/day, 1-4 wk 1-2/day, 1-4 wk	Rx; 1% cream, 10 mg/g gel
nystatin (Mycostatin)	*Candida*	NI	NI	2-3/day	Rx; 100,000 U/g cream, ointment, powder
haloprogin (Halotex)	*T. pedis* *T. cruris* *T. corporis* *T. manuum* *T. versicolor*	No	B/Unknown	bid, 2-3 wk Intertriginous 4 wk	Rx; 1% cream and solution
tolnaftate (Tinactin)	*T. pedis* *T. cruris* *T. corporis* *T. versicolor*	NI	NI	bid, 2-3 wk bid, 2-3 wk bid, 2-3 wk bid, 2-3 wk	OTC; 1% cream, solution, gel, powder, spray powder, spray liquid
ciclopirox (Penlac)	Onychomycosis	No	B/Unknown	qhs	Rx; 8% topical solution
selenium sulfide (Selsun)	*T. versicolor*	No	C/NI	qd, 1 wk	OTC and Rx; 1%, 2.5% lotion/shampoo, 1% shampoo

NI, Not indicated; *OTC,* over the counter; *Rx,* prescription.

PATIENT EDUCATION

- Before treatment, wash skin with soap and water and dry thoroughly.
- When treating athlete's foot, wear well-fitting, ventilated shoes. Change socks and shoes daily.
- Even though symptoms abate, continue to follow treatment plan for the prescribed amount of time.
- Notify health care provider if symptoms do not improve in 2 weeks (*Tinea cruris* and *corporis*) or 4 weeks (*Tinea pedis*).
- Notify health care provider of any symptoms of irritation at site of application (i.e., redness, itching, burning, blistering, swelling, and oozing). All are possible signs of sensitization.

Specific Drugs

econazole (Spectazole), clotrimazole (Lotrimin, Mycelex), ketoconazole (Nizoral), miconazole (Monistat-Derm, Lotrimin AF), butenafine (Mentax), naftifine (Naftin), terbinafine (Lamisil), nystatin (Nystatin, Mycostatin), haloprogin (Halotex), tolnaftate (Tinactin), ciclopirox (Penlac, Loprox), selenium sulfide lotion 2.5% (Selsun)

See Table 14-4 for specifics regarding antifungal medications.

Contraindications

- Hypersensitivity to any component of the product

Warnings

- Not for ophthalmic use

Precautions

- For external use only. Avoid contact with the eyes.
- If irritation or sensitivity develops, discontinue use and institute appropriate therapy.

Adverse Effects

- Erythema, stinging, blistering, peeling, pruritus, urticaria, burning, and general skin irritation

Topical Antivirals

Specific Drugs

acyclovir (Zovirax), penciclovir (Denavir)

Indications

- Oral antivirals are indicated for herpes zoster infections (see Chapter 70 for further information on antivirals)
- Drug resistance has occurred with topical and oral treatment
- Acyclovir
  - Management of episode(s) of herpes genitalis
  - Limited non–life-threatening monocutaneous herpes simplex infections in immunocompromised patients
  - Active against herpes simplex virus (HSV) types I and II, varicella zoster virus, Epstein Barr virus, and cytomegalovirus
  - Unlabeled use: herpes labialis (cold sores)
- Penciclovir
  - Treatment of recurrent herpes labialis in adults
  - Active against HSVs

Contraindications

- Hypersensitivity or chemical intolerance

Warnings

- For cutaneous use only; do not use in eyes
- Pregnancy *category C*: unknown whether excreted in breast milk
- Safety and efficacy in children not established

Precautions

- Do not exceed the recommended dosage and administration.
- No data demonstrate that acyclovir will either prevent transmission of infection to other people or prevent recurrent infections when applied in the absence of signs and symptoms.
- Do not use to prevent recurrent HSV infections.
- Viral resistance has not been observed, but the possibility exists.

Adverse Effects

- Mild pain with transient burning/stinging (28%), pruritus (4%), edema or pain at application site

Patient Variables

- Pregnancy: *category B*; no information on lactation
- Children: safety and efficacy not established

Patient Education

- For external use only
- Avoid application near eyes
- Ointment must thoroughly cover all lesions
- Use a finger cot or rubber glove to apply ointment to prevent spread of infection
- Start as soon as possible
- Acyclovir ointment is not a cure for herpes simplex infections and is of little benefit in treating recurrent attacks

Dosage and Administration

- Acyclovir: 5% ointment. Apply sufficient amount to cover lesions q3hr six times per day for 7 days.
- Penciclovir: 10 mg cream. Apply every 1 to 2 hours while awake for 4 days. Use on lips and face only.

Scabicides/Pediculicides

General Uses

Indications

- See Table 14-5 for indications.

DISEASE PROCESS

A mite called *Sarcoptes scabiei* causes scabies, a contagious disease. It is frequently found in individuals living in close

TABLE 14-5 Indications for Scabicides and Pediculocides

Medication	*Sarcoptes* (Scabies)	Pediculosis (Lice) Head Lice	Body Lice
crotamiton	X		
lindane*	X	X	X
malathion		X	
permethrin	X	X	X

* Indicated only as a second-line drug.

contact with others and in children. For reasons unknown, blacks rarely acquire scabies.

The mite has a 30-day life cycle. Within 60 minutes after arriving on the skin, the fertilized female burrows into the stratum corneum, where she lays two or three eggs a day. As the female advances, she leaves behind the eggs and fecal matter. The eggs reach the age of maturity in 14 to 17 days. After the mites reach adulthood, they repeat the cycle. The infested person may not experience any symptoms for about 1 month after the initial infestation until the mites increase in number to approximately 20.

Lice cause pediculosis, another contagious disease. They are active and able to move quickly, leading to rapid transmission to others. They are usually found in overcrowded settings or in populations with inadequate hygiene. Elementary school children are at risk. Shared hats or combs can transmit head lice. Blacks rarely get lice.

Three types of lice can affect humans: *Pediculus humanus* var. *capitis* (head lice), *Pediculus humanus* var. *corporis* (body lice), and *Pthirus pubis* (pubic or crab lice). Head and pubic lice nits can be found on hair shafts. Body lice reside on clothing and appear on the skin only to feed.

Lice feed approximately five times a day, using their mouths to pierce the skin, injecting irritating saliva, and sucking blood. After feeding, they develop their characteristic rust coloring. Hypersensitivity is induced by the saliva, which is injected when they pierce the skin, and possibly by fecal matter. The life cycle is about 1 month. Each day the female lays about six eggs, which incubate 8 to 10 days. Lice reach maturity in 18 days.

DRUG TREATMENT PRINCIPLES

Elimination of scabies or pediculosis requires attention to details.

If any step is left out, recontamination is likely. Treat all infected people simultaneously: household members for head lice and sexual partners for body lice.

The instructions specific to the medication selected must be followed completely. Scrupulous cleaning of the environment is vital. All infected persons must be treated simultaneously.

Unless used properly, lindane has a risk of producing neurotoxicity, including seizures. Malathion also has a remote possibility of causing CNS toxicity.

Lindane is absorbed through the skin. Because children have a greater skin surface area relative to body weight, pediatric patients may develop higher blood levels of the drug and are at increased risk for adverse reactions. Because of this risk, new FDA warnings suggest that caution should be used with these products in patients weighing less than 110 lb.

HOW TO MONITOR

- Reevaluate 10 days after treatment. Consider retreatment if the condition is not resolved. Look for sources of reinfection.
- In scabies, pruritus may persist after treatment and does not necessarily indicate need for retreatment.
- In pediculosis, if live lice can be found after 1 week, reapply treatment.

PATIENT VARIABLES

Geriatrics

- In the elderly patient, there may be fewer cutaneous lesions; but the itching is intense.
- The elderly have a decreased immunity, and this may allow greater numbers of mites to survive and multiply.
- In nursing homes, it is possible for all residents to have mites.

Pediatrics

- Epidemics are very common in elementary schools.
- Scabies is not usually suspected in an infant; thus the infant may have a more generalized spread over the body than adults. Regional lymph nodes may swell.

Because lindane is absorbed through the skin and children have more skin surface area relative to body weight, pediatric patients may end up with higher blood levels of the drug.

- Contraindicated in premature infants because their skin may be more permeable than that of a full-term infant and their liver enzymes may not be fully developed.

Pregnancy

- *Category C:* crotamiton, contraindicated topically
- *Category B:* lindane, malathion, and permethrin

Lactation

- Lindane is secreted in low concentrations in breast milk.
- Malathion secretion is unknown, but it is absorbed systemically by the mother.
- The implications of permethrin and crotamiton use during lactation are unknown.

PATIENT EDUCATION

- Shake solution well.
- Apply the drug as directed.
- Treatment of all members of the household may be necessary.
- Wash all clothing and bed linen in soap and hot water.
- Nonwashable clothing should be sealed in plastic bags for 48 to 72 hours and then dry cleaned.
- Reapplication is required in 7 to 10 days only if live lice are present.
- Avoid contact with eyes and mucous membranes. Do not apply to inflamed skin. Flush eyes if exposed.
- Discontinue drug use and notify health care provider if itching or skin irritation persists.
- These drugs are intended for external use only; internal ingestion may produce toxicity.
- Oils may enhance absorption. If using oil-based hair products, wash, rinse, and dry hair before applying.
- Use only one application to avoid overdosing.

Specific Drugs

See Table 14-6 for pharmacokinetics of selected scabicides and pediculicides.

crotamiton (Eurax)

Contraindications

- Known sensitivity to any of the components

Warnings

- For external use only
- Do not apply to acutely inflamed skin, raw weeping surfaces, eyes, or mouth

Adverse Effects

- See Table 14-7 for adverse effects to selected scabicides and pediculicides.

Dosage and Administration

- For scabies, thoroughly massage lotion into the skin of the whole body from the chin down, paying particular attention to all folds and creases.
- A second application is advisable 24 hours later.
- Change clothing and bed linen the next morning.
- Take a cleansing bath 48 hours after the last application.

Overdosage

- Ingestion of crotamiton causes a burning sensation in the mouth; mucosal irritation of mouth, throat, and stomach; nausea and vomiting; and abdominal pain.

TABLE 14-6 Activity and Pharmacokinetics of Pediculicides

	Absorption	Time to Peak	Onset of Action	Kill Time in Pediatrics	Ovicidal Activity in Pediatrics (%)	Residual Activity in Pediatrics	Application Time in Pediatrics	Metabolism	Excretion
malathion	Unknown amount absorbed	12 hr	6 hr	4.4 min	95	Up to 4 wk	8-12 hr		Unknown
permethrin	<2%			10-15 min	75	Up to 10 days	10 min		Urine
lindane	Almost 10%, enhanced by creams and oil	24 hr	6 hr	190 min	45-70	None	4 min	Stored in fatty tissues, including the brain	Urine over 5 days

TABLE 14-7 Common and Serious Adverse Effects of Selected Pediculocides

Drug	Common Side Effects	Serious Adverse Effects
crotamiton	Skin irritation	Allergic sensitivity
malathion	Skin irritation	Remote possibility of systemic toxicity, abdominal cramps, respiratory distress, muscle paralysis, seizures
permethrin	Pruritus; mild transient burning, stinging, itching	Tingling, numbness, rash signify more serious problems
lindane	Skin irritation	In <0.001% of patients, CNS effects, dizziness to convulsions; eczematous eruptions

lindane (Kwell, Scabene)

Contraindications
- Seizure disorders
- Patient weight less than 110 lb

Warnings
- Simultaneous application of creams, ointments, or oils may enhance absorption. Be extremely careful not to overdose, especially in children.
- Although lindane has not shown an increased incidence for liver tumors, in mice, other derivatives of hexachlorocyclohexane have demonstrated carcinogenicity.
- Lindane penetrates the skin and has the potential for CNS toxicity; the young are at a greater risk for toxicity. Contraindicated in neonates.
- Use as second-line drug only.

Drug Interactions
- No drug interactions have been reported.

Overdosage
- Overdose or oral ingestion can cause CNS excitation. Seizures may develop if taken in sufficient quantities.

Dosage and Administration
- For *scabies*, cream and lotion products, apply a thin layer to dry skin and rub in thoroughly. If crusted lesions are present, a tepid bath preceding the medication is helpful. Allow the skin to dry before application. Use of 2 oz is sufficient for an adult. Make a total body application from the neck down. Scabies rarely affects the head of children or adults but may occur in infants. Leave on for 8 to 12 hours; remove by thorough washing. One application is usually curative. Many patients exhibit persistent pruritus after treatment. Do not reapply unless living lice are found after 7 days.
- For *pediculosis pubis*, lotion products, apply sufficient quantity only to thinly cover hair and skin of pubic area and, if infected, thighs and trunk and axillary regions. Rub into skin and hair, leave in place for 12 hours and then wash thoroughly. Reapplication is usually unnecessary unless there are living lice after 7 days. Treat sexual contacts concurrently.
- For *pediculosis capitis*, apply sufficient quantity to cover only affected and adjacent hairy areas. Rub into scalp and hair and leave in place 12 hours; follow by thorough washing. Reapplication is usually not necessary unless there are living lice after 7 days.
- For *pediculosis capitis* and *pubis*, shampoo products, apply a sufficient quantity to dry hair (1 oz for short, 1½ oz for medium, and 2 oz for long hair). Work thoroughly into the hair and allow to remain in place 4 minutes. Add small quantities of water until a good lather forms. Rinse hair thoroughly and towel briskly. Comb with a fine-toothed comb or use tweezers to remove any remaining nits or nit shells. For pediculosis pubis, reapplication is usually not necessary. Reapply if there are demonstrable living lice after 7 days. Treat sexual contacts concurrently. Do not use as a routine shampoo.
- Immediate reapplication of lindane is inappropriate, even if itching continues after the first application. To help prevent overuse, lindane-containing shampoos and lotions are sold only in 1- and 2-oz packages.

malathion (Ovide)

Mechanism of Action
- Malathion has lousicidal and ovicidal properties.
- It is an organophosphate pediculicide liquid for topical application to the hair and scalp and acts via cholinesterase inhibition.
- Malathion binds to the hair shaft, thus giving residual protection against reinfestation.

Precautions
- Malathion topical agents contain flammable alcohol. Avoid exposing lotion and wet hair to open flame or electric heat, including hair dryers. Do not smoke while applying lotion, or while hair is wet.
- Exposure to carbamate- or organophosphate-type insecticides or pesticides of individuals using malathion may increase the possibility of increased systemic absorption of the pesticides or insecticides via the skin or respiratory tract.

Do not use the following:
- Malathion in children less than 2 years of age.
- Permethrin cream in children under 2 months of age, or permethrin liquid in children under 2 years of age.
- Crotamiton in children; safety and effectiveness not established.

Adverse Effects
- Irritation of the scalp can occur.

Drug Interactions
- No drug interactions have been reported with malathion lotion. Malathion inhibits cholinesterase; thus, theoretically, there could be a reaction with some aminoglycosides, anesthetics, antimyasthenics, or cholinesterase inhibitors or succinylcholine.

Overdosage

Malathion is a weaker cholinesterase inhibitor than other organophosphates, but overdose symptoms are the same. The symptoms of toxicity could be delayed up to 12 hours.

The symptoms include abdominal pain, anxiety, unsteadiness, confusion, diarrhea, labored breathing, dizziness, drowsiness, increased sweating, watery eyes, muscle twitching, pinpoint pupils, seizures, and slow heartbeat.

Dosage and Administration
- Sprinkle lotion on dry hair and rub gently until the scalp is thoroughly moistened. Pay special attention to the back of the head and neck.

- Allow the hair to dry naturally; do not use heat, and leave uncovered.
- After 8 to 12 hours, wash the hair with a nonmedicated shampoo. Rinse and use a fine-toothed comb to remove dead lice and eggs.
- If required, repeat with second application in 7 to 9 days. Further treatment is generally not necessary.
- Evaluate other family members to determine if infected; if so, treat.

permethrin (Elimite, Nix)

Mechanism of Action

- Permethrin is a synthetic pyrethroid. It is active against lice, ticks, mites, and fleas.
- It acts on the parasite nerve cell membranes by disrupting the sodium channel current and slowing repolarization, causing paralysis of the pests.

Warnings

- Permethrin is associated with carcinogenesis in mice and an increase in pulmonary adenomas and benign liver adenomas.

Precautions

- Scabies and head lice infestation may be accompanied by erythema, swelling, and itching; permethrin may exacerbate these problems.

Adverse Reactions

Mild, transient symptoms, such as burning, stinging, pruritus, numbness, tingling, erythema, edema, or rash.

Overdosage

- If the drug is swallowed, perform gastric lavage and use general supportive measures.

Dosage and Administration

- For *Sarcoptes scabiei,* thoroughly massage into the skin form the head to the soles of the feet. Treat infants on the hairline, neck, scalp, temple, and forehead. Remove the cream by washing after 8 to 14 hours. Usually 30 g is sufficient for the average adult. One application is curative.
- For *Pediculus capitis*, use after the hair has been washed with shampoo, rinsed with water and towel dried. Apply a sufficient volume to saturate the hair and scalp. Allow to remain on the hair for 10 minutes before rinsing off with water. A single treatment eliminates head lice infestation. Combing of nits is not required for therapeutic efficacy but may be done for cosmetic reasons.

Topical and Oral Acne Preparations

General Uses

- Acne vulgaris

DISEASE PROCESS

Acne is a disease involving the sebaceous glands. Sebaceous glands remain small throughout childhood. At puberty, hormone levels cause increased gland size and sebum secretion. The face, chest, back, and upper arms have the largest and most numerous sebaceous glands.

The sebum is secreted into the follicular canal. Acne begins with the blockage of this canal. Sebum, an irritant fatty acid, causes inflammation and swelling to form a comedone. *Propionibacterium acnes,* an anaerobe, is a normal skin resident and is the primary contaminant of sebum. *P. acnes* modifies the composition of sebum, leading to increased irritation, inflammation, and swelling.

DRUG TREATMENT PRINCIPLES

The effectiveness of treatment depends on the motivation of the patient. If the acne bothers the parent more than the teen patient, then compliance will be low. The face is usually involved and is exposed for all to see. The trunk may also be affected. Acne has a psychological as well as a physical effect on the individual.

Treatment depends on the clinician's assessment of the severity of the acne (Table 14-8). First assess the severity of the acne. Acne is classified as mild (comedonal acne), moderate (papular and pustular acne), and severe (cystic acne).

Start treatment of mild acne with benzoyl peroxide. Add tretinoin or topical antibiotics as needed.

Treatment of moderate acne consists of topical or oral antibiotics. Add benzoyl peroxide or tretinoin as needed.

Treat severe acne with the agents above. If these fail, consider isotretinoin.

Benzoyl Peroxide

The 2.5% concentration of benzoyl peroxide seems to be as effective as higher concentrations but is less irritating. Use water-based, not alcohol-based, preparations to reduce irritation.

Oral and Topical Antibiotics

Many antibiotic topical preparations are used for the treatment of acne. Topical antibiotics used for acne include clindamycin and erythromycin.

The most commonly used oral antibiotics are tetracycline and erythromycin. Tetracycline 500 mg po is commonly used qd.

Topical antibiotics are used for mild papular acne, a patient who refuses or cannot tolerate oral antibiotic, or to wean

TABLE 14-8 Treatment Sequence for Acne

Severity	First-Line Treatment	Second-Line Treatment	Third-Line Treatment
Mild	benzoyl peroxide	tretinoin	Topical antibiotics
Moderate	Topical or oral antibiotics	benzoyl peroxide	tretinoin
Severe	All of the above	isotretinoin	

TABLE 14-9 Dosage and Administration for Common Acne Products

Drug	Dosage	Administration
benzoyl peroxide	Start with lowest dosage. Experiment with various bars, creams, lotions. Increase dosage as tolerated.	Cleansers: wash face once or twice daily. Moisten involved skin areas before application. Rinse well and pat dry. Other dose forms: apply qd, gradually increase to bid-tid. Apply small amount to affected area. Remove with mild soap and water if excessive stinging occurs. Resume treatment the next day.
tretinoin	Start with 0.025% cream, use smallest amount possible to cover area. Use cream for dry skin, gel (90% alcohol) for excessively oily skin. Maintain dosage until response is seen, then gradually decrease.	Start with test area twice a week; gradually increase area of use and frequency. Frequency of three times a week usually adequate; apply before bedtime. Apply when skin is dry, 20 min after washing. After applying, wash hands.

TABLE 14-10 Important Common and Serious Adverse Effects of Acne Preparations

Drug	Common Side Effects	Serious Adverse Effects
benzoyl peroxide	Excessive drying, peeling, inflammation, swelling, allergic contact sensitization/dermatitis	Excessive scaling, erythema, or edema
tretinoin	Skin irritation	Contact allergy is rare; skin may become inflamed, swollen, blistered, or crusted; increased or decreased pigmentation, increased sun sensitivity
isotretinoin	Dried mucous membranes, nosebleeds (up to 80%), cheilitis (>90%), hand and foot epidermis peel, dry eyes; GI effects include dry mouth, nausea, vomiting, abdominal pain, anorexia, weight loss, inflammation of gums	CNS effects include fatigue, headache, visual disturbances; mild to moderate musculoskeletal symptoms

patients under good control from oral to topical preparations (Table 14-9).

Tretinoin (Retin-A), second-line therapy, is a topical vitamin A derivative. It is very effective for the treatment of comedones. Its usefulness is limited by irritation.

Isotretinoin (Accutane), another vitamin A derivative, is an oral third line product for severe acne. It has major medical and legal implications, especially when prescribed to females of childbearing age. Isotretinoin should only be prescribed by a dermatologist. Primary care providers will see patients on isotretinoin for possible follow-up and for other medical problems. The health care provider needs to be aware of and understand the potential drug-related severe health problems and common side effects. Isotretinoin is discussed briefly for this purpose.

Tretinoin and isotretinoin are expensive, and most insurance programs will not reimburse the patient's cost. A letter of medical necessity indicating the product is for acne treatment and not for cosmetic purposes might help the patient obtain reimbursement.

HOW TO MONITOR

- Acne may get worse before it gets better. It may take 4 to 6 weeks to see improvement. Old lesions may take months to fade. Watch for adverse effects (Table 14-10).
- Improvement is judged by the number of new lesions forming after 6 to 8 weeks of therapy.
- Additional time is required to see improvement on the back and chest.

PATIENT VARIABLES

Pediatrics

- Acne usually begins in puberty. It becomes less active in the late teens.
- Safety and efficacy have not been established in children under the age of 12 years.
- Isotretinoin may cause premature closure of the epiphyses.

Pregnancy

- *Category C:* benzoyl peroxide and tretinoin
- *Category X:* isotretinoin is very teratogenic in any amount even for a short period; if pregnancy occurs, abortion must be discussed with the patient

Lactation

- The effects of benzoyl peroxide and tretinoin during lactation are not known.

Race

- Whites are affected more than any other race.

Gender

- Acne affects both males and females. Males frequently have the most severe cases, but the most persistent cases tend to occur in females.

PATIENT EDUCATION

- Current research does not show a link between diet and acne (e.g., that chocolate and French fries increase acne). However, avoid such foods if they are believed to be a trigger to outbreaks.
- Instruct the patient to wash the face two or three times a day with warm water and a mild soap. Do not scrub face, because this may aggravate the condition.
- Use water-based make-up. Avoid oily moisturizers and skin cleansers.
- Avoid digging and squeezing the comedones. This may aggravate the condition and cause scarring.
- Acne may get worse at the beginning of any treatment for acne. Be patient and continue treatment because this is usually only temporary.
- Be consistent and follow all instructions provided by the health care provider. Notify the health care provider of any problems. The health care provider will determine if the treatment should be discontinued.

Specific Drugs

benzoyl peroxide

Mechanism of Action

The primary action of benzoyl peroxide is antibacterial, especially against *P. acnes*. It is believed the bacterial proteins are oxidized by the active or free radical oxygen. As the levels of *P. acnes*, lipids, and free fatty acids drop, resolution of acne is obtained.

Benzoyl peroxide has a drying action and removes excess sebum, which leads to desquamation (drying and peeling) of the skin.

Pharmacokinetics

- Benzoyl peroxide is not absorbed systemically.

Contraindications

- Hypersensitivity. There may be cross-sensitivity with benzoic acid derivatives (cinnamon and certain topical anesthetics).

Warnings

- After reports of tumor development in rodents, benzoyl peroxide was downgraded in 1991 by the Food and Drug Administration from category I (safe and effective) to category III (data insufficient to permit classification).
- There is no evidence benzoyl peroxide is a tumor promoter in humans.

Precautions

- This agent is for external use only. Contact with eyelids, lips, mucous membranes, and highly inflamed or damaged skin should be avoided.
- If accidental contact occurs, rinse with water.
- Discontinue use if severe reaction develops, then institute the appropriate therapy. Product use may be resumed after reaction clears by using less frequent applications.
- The color of hair and fabric may be lightened as a result of the oxidizing effects of benzoyl peroxide.
- Some benzoyl peroxide products contain sulfites. This may cause allergic reactions, including anaphylactic symptoms and asthmatic episodes. In the general population, the prevalence of sulfite sensitivity is unknown. It is most frequently seen in those patients with asthma.

Adverse Effects

- See Table 14-10.

Drug Interactions

- Simultaneous use of benzoyl peroxide with tretinoin may increase skin irritation.
- Transient skin discoloration may occur with the simultaneous use of sunscreens containing *para*-aminobenzoic acid (PABA).

Overdosage

- Excessive scaling, erythema, or edema are effects of overdosage. Treatment involves discontinuing product use and applying cool compresses, emollients, or low-dose topical hydrocortisone.

Patient Education

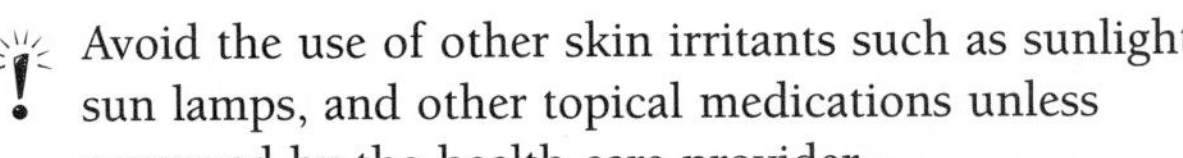

Avoid the use of other skin irritants such as sunlight, sun lamps, and other topical medications unless approved by the health care provider.

- Read patient instructions included with the product.
- Before using, wash the treatment area and allow it to dry.
- Keep product away from eyes, mouth, and mucous membranes. Rinse with water if contact occurs.
- A transitory feeling of warmth or slight stinging may occur. Expect dryness and peeling. Decrease frequency of use or discontinue if excessive redness or discomfort occurs. Discontinue use and contact health care provider if irritation is excessive.
- Water-based cosmetic use is permissible.

Dosage and Administration

- See Table 14-9 for dosage and administration recommendations.

tretinoin (Retin-A Cream, Gel)

- *Unlabeled uses:* topical treatment for different skin cancers and various other dermatologic conditions, to enhance the percutaneous absorption of topical minoxidil and other topical agents, and to improve the appearance of photodamaged skin, especially wrinkling and liver spots.

Mechanism of Action

- Tretinoin promotes and increases cell turnover of both the normal follicle and comedones. Cohesion between keratinized cells is decreased.

- Tretinoin works on the acne precursor lesion, the microcomedone, causing fragmentation and expulsion of the microplug. Closed comedones are converted into open comedones. With continued use, comedone formation is prevented.

Pharmacokinetics

- Tretinoin is metabolized by the skin. Approximately 5% of the compound is excreted in the urine and feces.

Contraindications

- Hypersensitivity to any component of the product

Warnings

Tretinoin is for external use only. Keep it away from the eyes, mouth, angles of the nose, and mucous membranes. Severe local erythema and peeling at application site may be induced.

Use product less frequently or stop use temporarily or completely, if warranted. If applied to reddened skin, a severe local reaction may occur.

Drug Interactions

The stratum corneum becomes thin with the continuous application of tretinoin. This makes the skin more susceptible to irritation from sunburn and sun damage and irritation from wind, cold, or dryness.

- Cosmetics, astringents, alcohol, and acne soaps that have drying properties and strong concentrations of spices or limes may increase the possibility of interaction with tretinoin.
- Use caution when administering tretinoin with sulfur, resorcinol, benzoyl peroxide, or salicylic acid because significant skin irritation may result.

Overdosage

- Topical tretinoin overdose will lead to severe localized skin irritation.

isotretinoin (Accutane)

Indications

- Severe cystic acne not responding to conventional therapy

Mechanism of Action

- The exact mechanism of action is not known. The drug decreases the amount and composition of the sebum lipid. The reduction is maintained while the patient is taking the drug. After the treatment is ended, the composition returns to normal, but the production may not return to pretreatment levels.

Warnings

Isotretinoin must not be used by females who are pregnant. There is an extremely high risk that a deformed infant will result if pregnancy occurs while taking isotretinoin in any amount for even a short period of time.

How to Monitor

The primary health care provider may be asked to monitor the patient while on isotretinoin. Patients must be monitored closely, using the following guidelines:

- Pretreatment: serum pregnancy test, complete blood cell count (CBC), liver function test, triglyceride level
- After 2 to 3 weeks of treatment: triglyceride level, then every 4 weeks; for levels exceeding 350 to 400 mg/dl, repeat in 2 to 3 weeks; for levels exceeding 700 to 800 mg/dl, stop medication because of risk for pancreatitis
- After 4 to 6 weeks of treatment: CBC, liver function
- A monthly pregnancy test should be considered

Precautions

Isotretinoin has the potential for causing many severe health problems. Headaches, which may be indicative of benign intracranial hypertension (especially when combined with minocycline and tetracycline), corneal opacities, decreased night vision, inflammatory bowel disease, hypertriglyceridemia, hepatotoxicity, and musculoskeletal symptoms such as arthralgia may occur. Diabetic patients may demonstrate problems with control of their blood sugar.

- As with the initiation of all acne treatment, the condition may be temporarily exacerbated.

Pharmacokinetics

- Isotretinoin is metabolized in the liver and 99.9% binds to the plasma albumin. It is excreted in urine and bile.

Adverse Effects

- Cheilitis can be easily handled with the use of a petrolatum product such as Aquaphor.
- Dry eyes may make the patient unable to wear contact lenses.

Patient Education

- Roche Laboratories' pregnancy prevention box contains patient qualification checklist, information about treatment, contraception, and serum pregnancy testing information, optional referral form to expert contraception counseling, patient self-evaluation, consent forms, and follow-up survey.

Local Anesthetics

General Uses

Local anesthetics are indicated for a variety of uses, which include minor surgical procedures, suturing, and relief of itching or pain from wounds, burns, and/or hemorrhoids.

Local anesthesia does not depress the patient's level of consciousness, which makes the use much safer than general anesthesia. Local anesthetics may be applied as a powder, gel, lotion, ointment, spray, or injection into a small area. If a larger area is required for anesthesia, a nerve trunk (epidural, spinal) or a single nerve may be injected to provide for regional anesthesia. This discussion is not intended as a complete presentation on local anesthesia but rather to present a brief overview of common local anesthetics used in primary care.

Local anesthetics may be combined with vasoconstrictors (epinephrine) to prolong action by decreasing the systemic absorption. However, at the ends of arteries, such as in the fingers, toes, penis, and nose, vasoconstrictors are not safe for use. In those areas, gangrene may develop because of severe vasoconstriction.

A number of local agents are used safely on mucous membranes, ulcers, or wounds. If agents are applied to the oral cavity, however, the patient may have difficulty swallowing. Therefore food should be withheld for at least 1 hour to prevent aspiration. Use with caution in areas of inflammation.

Do not use if solutions are discolored or contain precipitants. If the solution does not contain a preservative, it must be discarded after opening. Because of some situations of severe anaphylaxis resulting from use of local anesthetics, have resuscitation equipment on hand before use or emergency back-up plans when using any anesthetic. Obtain patient's prior history of local anesthetic use before administration. Patient or guardian should sign a permission form before consenting to any procedure using a local anesthetic.

DRUG ACTION AND EFFECTS

Local anesthesia causes a loss of sensation by first blocking nerve conduction in the smaller unmyelinated fibers that carry pain and then progressing to the larger myelinated fibers for pressure and motor function. The extent of anesthesia depends on a variety of factors: the amount of medication used, body temperature, pH, the amount of protein binding, and dilution by tissue fluids. Local anesthetics work by blocking the flow of sodium ions, thereby preventing depolarization of the nerve fiber and conduction or transmission of the impulse.

Local anesthetics are divided into two groups: esters and amides. Esters are derivatives of *para*-aminobenzoic acid. Hypersensitivity reactions may occur with esters. They are metabolized by hydrolysis. Amides are derivatives of aniline. Allergies to drugs in the amide group are rare. They are metabolized primarily in the liver then excreted primarily in the urine as metabolites. These two groups differ in pharmacokinetics, including protein binding, onset, duration, and allergic potential. The amides are generally more useful clinically.

PHARMACOKINETICS

Absorption is complete, unless epinephrine is added.

Onset depends on the type of block, medication, body fluids, pH, and temperature.

The amides vary in protein binding. Lidocaine and mepivacaine are bound moderately. Etidocaine and bupivacaine are highly bound. The esters are hydrolyzed in the plasma by pseudocholinesterase, and the amides are degraded in the liver by enzymes. Esters are less stable than amides. Esters are metabolized to *para*-aminobenzoic acid, which may cause severe reactions.

Peak concentration of the drug depends on the type but takes from 10 to 30 minutes (Table 14-11).

PATIENT VARIABLES

- Dosage varies according to the weight of the patient as well as the site and type of procedure.
- Children and the elderly are especially prone to aspiration if agents are used in the oral cavity.

Pregnancy

- *Categories B* and *C;* see Table 14-11.

TABLE 14-11 Pharmacokinetics of Local Anesthetics

Drug	Amide or Ester	Onset of Action	Duration of Action	Protein Bound	Pregnancy Category	How Supplied
SHORT ACTING						
procaine	Ester	2-5 min	30-90 min	5.8%	C	1%, 2%, 10%
chloroprocaine	Ester	6-12 min	30-90 min	Unknown	C	1%, 2%, 3%
INTERMEDIATE ACTING						
lidocaine	Amide	<2 min	30-60 min	64.3%	B	0.5%, 1%, 2%, 4%, with and without epinephrine
mepivacaine	Amide	3-5 min	45-90 min	77.5%	C	1%, 1.5%, 2%, 3%
prilocaine	Amide	<2 min	30-120 min	55%	B	4% with and without epinephrine
LONG ACTING						
bupivacaine	Amide	5 min	2-4 hr	95.6%	C	0.25%, 0.5%, 0.75% with and without epinephrine
etidocaine	Amide	3-5 min	5-10 hr	94%	B	1%, 1.5% with and without epinephrine
tetracaine	Ester	15 min	2-3 hr	75.6%	C	1%, 2%, 3%

HOW TO MONITOR

- Monitor for any adverse effects, including cardiac arrhythmias, shock, and/or local reactions.
- Blood pressure, respiratory status, blood flow to the area, ability to swallow, and motor control and sensations should also be monitored.
- Patients may need to be placed on cardiac monitors, depending on the type of procedure and agent used.

PATIENT EDUCATION

- Reactions to local anesthetics range from dermatitis to anaphylactic shock.
- The patient may lose all sensation, including the sensation of temperature, pressure, and touch. Protect area until sensation returns.
- Motor function is lost only if concentrations of the drug are present over time (spinal anesthesia). If regional anesthesia has been achieved, the area of the body needs to be protected from heat, cold, and pressure because those senses will not be intact.
- Local application to the oral cavity results in a decreased ability to swallow and could result in trauma to buccal mucosa or tongue.
- Patients should be advised to use topical anesthetics exactly as prescribed. Aerosols should not be inhaled. Provide instruction for rectal applications. If hemorrhoids are bleeding, systemic absorption will be increased. Suppositories should be refrigerated before use and moistened with water or lubricant before insertion.

Specific Drugs

SHORT-ACTING LOCAL ANESTHETICS

procaine (Novocain)

Indications
- Spinal anesthesia primarily

Contraindications
- Hypersensitivity to procaine.
- Spinal anesthesia is contraindicated in certain CNS diseases and sepsis.

Warnings
- Have resuscitation equipment on hand during use.
- Effect on fetal development not determined.

Precautions
- Use with caution in patients with heart block, rhythm disturbances, or shock.

> Use lowest dose possible for effective anesthesia, especially in children and in elderly or debilitated patients.

- Consult standard references for exact amount of medications for specific procedures and technique.
- If vasopressor is added, use with caution in patients already on any medication likely to raise pressure, for example, monoamine oxidase inhibitors (MAOIs).

Adverse Effects
- May provoke CNS and cardiovascular symptoms

Overdosage
- Hypotension and cardiac arrest are possible
- Other symptoms include nervousness, dizziness, headache, urticaria, and edema

INTERMEDIATE-ACTING LOCAL ANESTHETICS

lidocaine hydrochloride (Xylocaine with and without epinephrine)

Indications
- Lidocaine can be used as a local anesthetic and administered topically in a gel, ointment, spray, lotion, or cream.
- Lidocaine can also be infiltrated into an area for local anesthesia or nerve block.
- Lidocaine has an additional use as an antiarrhythmic and can be administered intravenously by direct injection or continuous infusion.

Contraindications
- Hypersensitivity to lidocaine or to local anesthetics of the amide group

Warnings
- Have emergency resuscitation equipment and drugs on hand.

Precautions
- Safety of use depends on the proper dose and technique and preparedness for emergencies.
- Consult standard textbooks for specifics.

Patient Variables

Pregnancy
- *Category B*

Lactation
- Not known if excreted in human breast milk

Overdosage
- Reactions are similar to other amide anesthetics, which include CNS manifestations of nervousness and euphoria to twitching, convulsions, and unconsciousness.
- Allergic manifestations include urticaria, edema, and anaphylactoid reactions.
- Cardiovascular reactions include bradycardia, hypotension, and shock.
- Neurologic reactions include loss of sensation or motor control and loss of bowel or bladder function.

LONG-ACTING LOCAL ANESTHETICS

bupivacaine hydrochloride (Marcaine with and without epinephrine)

Indications
- Dental and oral surgeries, minor surgical procedures, and therapeutic procedures such as joint injections
- Only the lowest concentration recommended for obstetric procedures
- Chemically, product is related to lidocaine but lasts longer

Contraindications
- Do not give with known sensitivity to bupivacaine or any other local anesthetic.
- Not used for obstetric paracervical blocks.

Warnings
- Do not use 0.075% for obstetric anesthesia.
- Use only if resuscitation equipment and drugs are available.
- Do not use with epinephrine if patient is on MAOIs or antidepressants of the amitriptyline or imipramine types because hypotension may result.
- As results are long lasting, warn patient of inadvertent trauma to lips, buccal mucosa, and tongue.

Patient Variables

Pediatrics
- Not recommended for use in children under 12

Pregnancy
- *Category C*

Overdosage
- Same as other amides: CNS, cardiovascular, and allergic symptoms.

Dosage and Administration
- Dose varies with the procedure, area required, patient's condition, vascularity of tissues, duration of anesthesia desired. Individualize dose.

RESOURCES FOR PATIENTS AND PROVIDERS

CD-ROM

Clinical Dermatology Illustrated: A Regional Approach
Dermatology Procedures, plus VHS tape
Dermatology in Primary Care I and II
Color Atlas and Synopsis of Clinical Dermatology, ed 3
Clinical Dermatology: Diagnosis and Therapy, ed 3
All available from CMEA, Inc. 1(800) 227-CMEA

BIBLIOGRAPHY

Arndt A et al: *Primary care dermatology,* Philadelphia, 1997, WB Saunders.

Bonifaz A et al: Itraconazole in onychomycosis: intermittent dose schedule, *Int J Dermatol* 36:70, 1997.

Cohen BA: *Pediatric dermatology,* ed 2, St Louis, 1999, Mosby.

Cox N, Lawrence C: *Diagnostic problems in dermatology,* St Louis, 1998, Mosby.

Dominguez J et al: Topical isotretinoin vs topical retinoic acid in the treatment of acne vulgaris, *Int J Dermatol* 37:54, 1998.

Edwards F: *Dermatology in emergency care,* Philadelphia, 1997, Churchill Livingstone.

Goldstein BG, Goldstein AO: *Practical dermatology,* ed 2, St Louis, 1997, Mosby.

Van Heerden JS et al: *Tinea corporis/cruris*: new treatment options, *Dermatology* 195(suppl):14, 1997.

CHAPTER 15

Eye, Ear, Throat, and Mouth Agents

Drug Names

Class	Subclass	Generic Name	Trade Name
EYE			
Antiinfectives			
Antibiotics	Quinolones	ciprofloxacin	Ciloxan solution
	Aminoglycosides	gentamicin sulfate	Garamycin ointment and solution
		tobramycin	Tobrex ointment and solution
	Sulfonamides	sulfacetamide sodium	Sodium Sulamyd ointment, solution; Bleph-10
	Macrolides	erythromycin	Ilotycin ointment
	Combination	neomycin, polymyxin B, and bacitracin zinc	Neosporin ointment
		neomycin, polymyxin B, and gramicidin	Neosporin ointment
	Antiviral	trifluridine	Viroptic solution
Nonsteroidal antiinflammatory drugs (NSAIDs)		ketorolac	Acular
Histamine H_2 blocker		levocabastine	Livostin
Mast cell stabilizer		nedocromil	Alocril
Steroid antiinflammatory drugs		dexamethasone	Decadron
Glaucoma Medications			
Sympathomimetics		brimonidine	Alphagan
β-Adrenergic-blocking agents		timolol	Timoptic
Parasympathomimetic (miotics, direct)		pilocarpine	Isopto Carpine, Pilocar, Pilostat
Cholinesterase inhibitors (miotic)		demecarium	Humorsol
Carbonic anhydrase inhibitors		dorzolamide	Trusopt
Other Eye Medications			
Sympathomimetics		phenylephrine hydrochloride	Neo-Synephrine
Vasoconstrictors		naphazoline hydrochloride	Naphcon Forte, Opcon
Lubricant		artificial tears	Lacrisert, generic
Anesthetic		proparacaine hydrochloride	Alcaine, Paracain
Diagnostic		fluorescein sodium, proparacaine	Flucaine, Fluoracaine
EAR		hydrocortisone, neomycin sulfate, polymyxin	Cortisporin otic
		ciprofloxacin and hydrocortisone suspension	Cipro HC otic
NOSE (see Allergic Rhinitis, Chapter 16)			
THROAT/ORAL			
Antifungals		nystatin	Mycostatin
		clotrimazole	Mycelex
OTHER		penciclovir	Denavir
		carbamide peroxide	Gly-Oxide Liquid solution 10%
		chlorhexidine gluconate	Peridex

Eye Agents

General Uses

Indications

- Conjunctivitis

• • •

There are a great many products for the eye. Drugs selected for inclusion are ones seen most commonly, with only one representative drug chosen for many categories. The drugs featured in this chapter have a wide variety of diagnostic and therapeutic uses. The two most common eye diseases seen in primary care that are treated medically are infectious conjunctivitis and seasonal allergic conjunctivitis. Most eye conditions require referral to an ophthalmologist.

DISEASE PROCESS

Anatomy, Physiology, and Pathophysiology

The eye has built-in protective mechanisms. It is lubricated with protective chemicals that are regularly distributed over the lens through the blinking of the eyelid. The lacrimal ducts communicate drain into areas of potential absorption such as nasal and pharyngeal mucosa.

The structures of the eye are recessed within the orbit to further protect the eye from trauma (Figure 15-1). But various processes may penetrate these defenses and produce problems. Conjunctivitis can be caused by bacteria, virus, or allergy. Bacterial conjunctivitis is most often caused by *Streptococcus pneumoniae, Haemophilus influenzae, Staphylococcus aureus, Pseudomonas* species, and *Moraxella* species. Gram-negative infections are less common than gram-positive. *Haemophilus* is common in children. Chlamydial infection is an important cause of blindness.

In glaucoma, the intraocular pressure (IOP) is too high, causing injury and death of nerve cells. Reducing the IOP can arrest the progression of the disease. Open-angle glaucoma has no mechanical obstruction to outflow. In narrow-angle glaucoma, the iris mechanically obstructs outflow (Figure 15-2).

Specific Eye Problems

Bacterial Conjunctivitis

Prolonged use of topical antibiotics may result in overgrowth of nonsusceptible organisms, including fungi. Ophthalmic ointments may retard corneal wound healing.

Topical ocular antiinfectives are used to treat external bacterial infections of the eye and its adnexa, such as conjunctivitis, corneal ulcer, dacryocystitis, and hordeolum. The choice of agent depends on the clinical suspicion of the causative organism. The organisms most commonly associated with different infections are discussed with each individual drug.

Sulfacetamide sodium is usually considered for first line treatment. If the patient is allergic to sulfa, select another medication active against gram-positive bacteria, such as erythromycin. Neosporin is limited by the frequency of allergy to neomycin. Erythromycin prophylaxis is used for ophthalmia neonatorum caused by *Neisseria gonorrhoeae* or *Chlamydia trachomatis.* The usual course of treatment is 3 to 7 days.

Viral Conjunctivitis. Specific viral infections caused by such organisms as herpes simplex are treated with antiviral ophthalmic products.

Trifluridine should be prescribed only for patients who have been clinically diagnosed with herpetic keratitis by an ophthalmologist. Systemic absorption is negligible.

Some practitioners routinely treat viral conjunctivitis caused by an adenovirus with topical antiinfectives to prevent secondary bacterial infections.

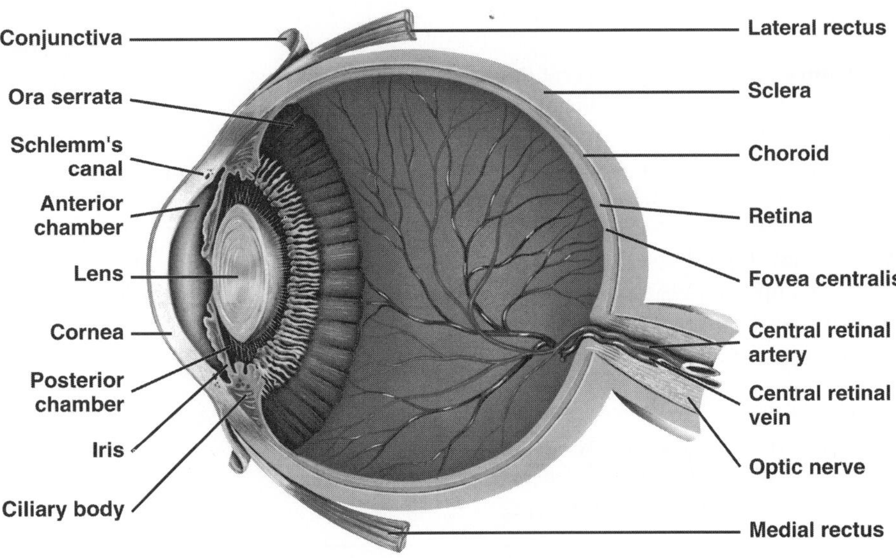

FIGURE 15-1

The globe, looking down on the right eye, showing major anatomic structures. (Courtesy of Glaxo Wellcome.)

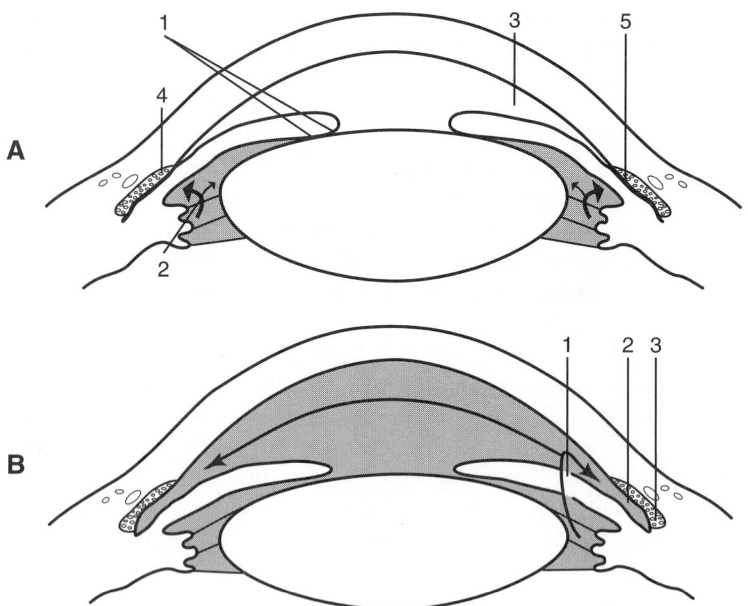

FIGURE 15-2

A, Pupillary block prevents flow of aqueous into the anterior chamber. The iris is pressed firmly against the lens *(1)*, blocking aqueous flow *(2)* into the anterior chamber *(3)*. Instead, the iris is pushed against the trabecular meshwork *(4)*. The peripheral anterior chamber angle is thus closed *(5)*, blocking aqueous outflow and raising IOP. **B,** A small hole in the peripheral iris *(1)* is made with a laser (laser iridectomy), allowing aqueous to enter the anterior chamber of the eye. This opens the anterior chamber angle *(2)* and allows aqueous to drain normally through the trabecular meshwork *(3)*. (From Palay DA, Krachmer JH: *Ophthalmology for the primary care physician,* St Louis, 1998, Mosby.)

Allergic Conjunctivitis. Allergic conjunctivitis is a common problem for patients with allergies. Any allergic rhinitis should be treated appropriately first, unless the ocular symptoms are severe. If ocular symptoms persist after adequate control of the allergies, consider a nonsteroidal antiinflammatory drug, histamine H_2-blocker, or mast cell stabilizer.

 Primary care providers should not prescribe steroid eye drops. Steroids should be ordered only after an ophthalmologist has examined the eye with a slit lamp.

Corticosteroids suppress the body's inflammatory response. They delay healing and allow for serious infections. Steroid eye drops may increase the virulence of a herpes infection and potentiate both fungal and bacterial infections. Chronic use of steroids may lead to glaucoma or cataracts.

Glaucoma. Glaucoma is a condition also managed by the ophthalmologist. It is common for a patient to be on two or more medications for glaucoma. The primary care provider needs to be aware of the possible systemic side effects of the eye drops use or potential drug interactions.

Anesthesia. Topical anesthetics are only used when eye pain makes it impossible for the practitioner to examine the eye. Topical anesthetics retard corneal healing and may allow a corneal abrasion to progress to a corneal ulcer.

 Anesthetics are generally used only by ophthalmologists. If a patient is using them, he or she must use great care not to injure the eye.

Other Eye Problems. Sympathomimetics and vasoconstrictors are common over-the-counter (OTC) agents used for relief of red, irritated eyes. Generally, they are safe and effective. However, chronic use is discouraged because of rebound inflammation.

Ocular lubricants (i.e., artificial tears) are also OTC agents. They are also very safe and effective in the relief of irritated eyes. They are used in elderly patients and in patients who are on medications that cause dry eyes.

Fluorescein is used in the primary care setting when examining the eye for abrasions or foreign bodies. When using the strips, moisten strip with sterile water. Place moistened strip at the fornix in the lower cul-de-sac close to the punctum of the eye. The patient should then blink several times. Allow a few seconds for staining. An injury will show up as an intense green fluorescent color. Rinse out the eye with sterile irrigating solution.

DRUG TREATMENT PRINCIPLES

General Principles

Effective treatment demands accurate diagnosis. Primary care providers collect pertinent information and begin the process of diagnosis. However, many problems require referral to a specialist for care. See Table 15-1 for evaluation and management of potentially serious eye problems.

Ophthalmic solutions are absorbed systemically, and this may pose secondary problems. In general, any adverse reaction that a medication can have when taken orally can occur when the medication is given as an eye drop. Patient factors that increase systemic absorption include lax eyelids and hyperemic or diseased eyes. Absorption is more of a problem in infants and in the elderly. The formulation affects absorption by determining the amount of time the medication stays in contact with the conjunctiva. Ointments are more completely absorbed than suspensions; suspensions are more completely

TABLE 15-1 Evaluation and Management of Potentially Serious Eye Problems

Complaint or Problem	Suggested Treatment
EMERGENCIES	
Chemical burn	Irrigate eye for 15-20 min; send to emergency department
Retinal artery occlusion with sudden, painless loss of vision in one eye	Must be seen by specialist within 90 min to preserve vision
"Something in eye"	Check visual acuity in each eye, document findings; if significant loss of vision or blurring, refer patient to specialist
	Examine eye for foreign body: evert eyelid and if a foreign body is seen, do not irrigate, but flick off with a needle; if fine powder, irrigate
	Stain with fluorescein dye to check integrity of epithelial surface; moisten strip if eye is dry, touch strip to inner conjuctival surface, let patient blink, then shine flashlight (blue filter preferred); epithelial break stains green, refer to specialist
Red eye	Check vision; if vision is decreased, refer to specialist
	Check injection, use finger pressure test to determine if conjuctival or ciliary (Figure 15-3); press lower lid against cornea, draw downward; conjunctiva should blanch; ciliary injection is around the limbus, does not blanch; if ciliary injection, refer to specialist
CONTACT LENSES	
Symptoms: lens wearers are at risk for corneal abrasions and infections and for hypoxic corneal injury	If patient complains of pain, remove contact lens, check for abrasion with fluorescein dye, refer to specialist
CORNEAL ABRASIONS	
Symptoms: pain, foreign body sensation, photophobia, tearing, or blepharospasm immediately after insertion or removal of contact lens or from direct trauma to eye from projected particles	Remove contact lens, stain eye with fluorescein dye, remove foreign body if present; may require topical antibiotic; refer to specialist
Signs: epithelial defect confirms corneal abrasion; may become infected and progress to corneal ulceration	
HYPOXIC CORNEAL INJURY	
Symptoms: during contact lens wear, blurred vision, conunctival hyperemia, pain	Remove contact lens, stain with fluorescein dye, evaluate, and refer to specialist if necessary
Signs: conjuctival hyperemia and ciliary flush, contact lens immobility, diffuse corneal edema; may lead to corneal neovascularization and scarring	
Conjuctivitis	Diagnostic cultures generally not necessary
	Treat with antibiotics: use a broad-spectrum drug or one that covers gram-positive organisms; refer if not resolved in 7 days

absorbed than solutions. Minimize systemic absorption of ophthalmic drops by compressing the lacrimal sac for 3 to 5 minutes after instillation. This retards passage of drops to other areas of absorption.

Eye drops must be properly used to be effective. One drop of medication is all the eye can retain. If more than one drop is used, wait 5 minutes before applying the second drop. Do not use eyecups because of the risk of contamination. See the section on patient education for instructions on how to administer eye medication.

HOW TO MONITOR

Monitor for therapeutic effect and both local and systemic adverse effects.

Antibiotics

Long-term use of topical antibiotic products requires periodic examination for such signs as itching, redness, edema of the conjunctiva and eyelid, or a failure to heal. These could be signs of sensitization. In severe cases of infection, examination of stained conjunctival scrapings and culture studies are recommended.

PATIENT VARIABLES

Geriatrics

- Older patients are susceptible to systemic effects of topical eye drops. For example, β-blocker eye drops used for glaucoma can exacerbate chronic heart failure.
- Use with caution and monitor closely for adverse reactions.
- No change in dosage is required.

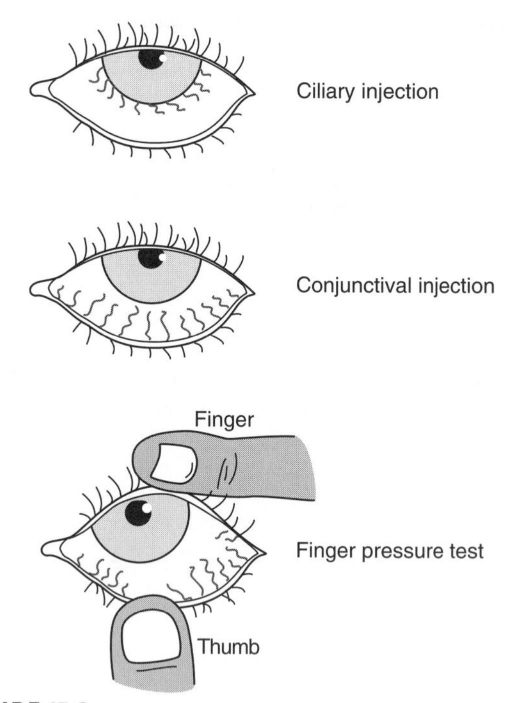

FIGURE 15-3

Diagnostic technique in determining ciliary or conjunctival injection (see Table 15-1).

Pediatrics, Pregnancy, and Lactation

- Table 15-2 lists considerations for ophthalmic drug use in pediatric, pregnant, and lactating patients.

PATIENT EDUCATION

- If the patient experiences any reaction, they should discontinue medication and call the provider.
- Some of the contents of the products may be absorbed by soft contact lenses. Avoid wearing soft lenses while using the medications.
- Store medication as directed on package.

Eye Drops

- Wash hands.
- Tilt head backward or lie down and gaze upward.
- Grasp lower eyelid below eyelashes and pull the eyelid away from the eye to form a pouch.
- Place dropper directly over eye. Avoid contact of the dropper with the eye, finger, or any surface.
- Have patient look upward just before applying a drop.
- After instilling the drop, look downward for several seconds.
- Release the lid slowly and close eyes gently. With eyes closed, apply gentle pressure with fingers to the inside corner of eye for 3 to 5 minutes.
- Do not rub the eye or squeeze the eyelid. Minimize blinking.

Ointments

- Wash hands. Hold ointment in hand for a few minutes to warm ointment and facilitate flow.
- Tilt head backward or lie down and gaze upward.
- Gently pull down the lower eyelid to form a pouch. Place 0.25 to 0.5 inch of ointment with a sweeping motion inside the lower eyelid by squeezing the tube gently and slowly releasing the eyelid.
- Close eye for 1 to 2 minutes, and roll eyeball in all directions. Temporary blurring of vision may occur; use at night.
- Remove excessive ointment around the eye with a tissue.

Antibiotics

- Bacterial conjunctivitis is contagious, usually by direct contact via fingers, towels, handkerchiefs, and similar items moved to the other eye or to other individuals.
- Warm compresses applied to affected eye(s) can aid in the removal of crusting.
- Do not exceed recommended dose or length of treatment; may result in secondary infection.
- Infections can be spread if more than one person uses the medication container.

Specific Drugs

See Table 15-2 for characteristics of eye medications.

ANTIINFECTIVES

See Chapters 58 to 66 for details on particular antiinfective medications.

Antivirals

See Chapter 70 for details on antiviral agents.

NONSTEROIDAL ANTIINFLAMMATORY AGENTS

ketorolac tromethamine (Acular solution)

Indications

- Relief of ocular itching caused by seasonal allergic conjunctivitis.

The drug has no significant effect on IOP and does not appear to potentiate spread of infection.

The mechanism of its action is thought to be due in part to its ability to inhibit prostaglandin biosynthesis. Ocular administration reduces prostaglandin F_2 levels in aqueous humor.

MAST CELL STABILIZERS

nedocromil (Alocril)

Mast cell stabilizers inhibit the Type 1 immediate hypersensitivity reactions. Therefore, they inhibit increased cutaneous vascular permeability that is associated with reagin or IgE and antigen-mediated reactions. This prevents antigen-stimulated release of histamine and other mast cell inflammatory mediators and inhibits eosinophil chemotaxis. The exact mechanism of action is unknown, but the drug has been reported to prevent calcium influx into the mast cell upon antigen stimulation. The drug has no intrinsic vasoconstrictor or other antiinflammatory activity.

ANTIGLAUCOMA MEDICATIONS

See Table 15-2.

TABLE 15-2 Characteristics of Eye Medications

Medication	Indications/ Action	Use in Pediatrics	Use in Pregnancy	Warnings/ Precautions	Common Side Effects	Serious Side Effects
ANTIINFECTIVES					Local discomfort	
Antibiotics	Bacterial conjunctivitis				Local discomfort	Hypersensitivity
ciprofloxacin	Gram positive and negative organisms	>1 yr	C		Local discomfort	Precipitates, hyperemia
gentamicin	Gram positive and negative organisms	>1 yr	C		Local discomfort	Bacterial and fungal corneal ulcers
tobramycin	Gram positive and negative organisms	Safe	B		Local discomfort	
sulfacetamide	Gram positive and negative organisms	>2 mo	C		Local discomfort	Bacterial and fungal corneal ulcers
erythromycin ointment	Gram positive organisms	Neonates	B		Redness	
neosporin ointment	Gram positive organisms	No	C		Redness	Sensitivity to neomycin
neosporin solution	Gram positive organisms	No	C		Redness	Sensitivity to neomycin
Antiviral trifluridine	Herpes simplex virus 1 and 2	>6 yr	C		Mild burning, palpebral edema	Hypersensitivity, viral resistance
NONSTEROIDAL ANTIINFLAMMATORY ketorolac	Allergic conjunctivitis	>3 yr	C	Bleeding tendencies Rheumatoid arthritis, contact lenses	Burning and stinging Superficial keratitis or infections, corneal edema	Hypersensitivity, bleeding Tendency, keratitis, delay wound healing
HISTAMINE H_2 BLOCKER levocabastine	Allergic conjunctivitis	>12 yr	C	Contact lenses	Burning and stinging headache, visual, dry mouth, somnolence	Nausea, rash, dyspnea
MAST CELL STABILIZER nedocromil	Allergic conjunctivitis	>3 yr	B	Contact lenses	Headache, burning irritation, unpleasant taste	Hypersensitivity, asthma
STEROID dexamethasone	Inflammatory conditions	NO	C		Many	Many; see Chapter 52
GLAUCOMA MEDICATIONS						Many systemic
Sympathomimetic brimonidine	Decreased production of aqueous humor Increased outflow of aqueous humor	>NO	B	MAOIs, cardiovascular disease, decreased hepatic or renal	Pruritus, hyperemia, burning, drowsiness, dry mouth	Hypertension, respiratory, muscle pain, systemic sympathomimetic effects, see Chapter 16

MAOI, Monoamine oxidase inhibitor.

Continued

TABLE 15-2 Characteristics of Eye Medications—cont'd

Medication	Indications/ Action	Use in Pediatrics	Use in Pregnancy	Warnings Precautions	Common Side Effects	Serious Side Effects
GLAUCOMA MEDICATIONS—cont'd						
β-Blocker timolol	Decreased production of aqueous humor	NO	C	Atrioventricular block, CHF, bradycardia, bronchospasm, asthma, COPD, diabetes, hyperthyroidism	Discomfort, blurred vision, rash, dizziness, headache, gastrointestinal upset	Cerebrovascular, respiratory, central nervous system and others, see Chapter 21
Parasympathomimetic pilocarpine	Increased outflow of aqueous humor	NO	C	Pupil constriction, retinal detachment, asthma, bradycardia, hypotension	Local irritation, corneal edema, ciliary spasm, miosis, headache, transient night blindness	Systemic beta blocker effects; see Chapter 2
Cholinesterase inhibitor demecarium	Increased outflow of aqueous humor	NO	X	Narrow-angle glaucoma, asthma, PUD, bradycardia, hypotension, recent myocardial infarction epilepsy, parkinsonism	Burning, redness, intense miosis	Iris cysts, systemic anticholinergic
Carbonic Anhydrase Inhibitor dorzolamide	Decreased production of aqueous humor	NO	C	Sulfa allergy, decreased renal or hepatic, respiratory distress, diabetes	Burning, bitter taste, headache, GI distress, paresthesias, tinnitus, myopia	Hypersensitivity, electrolyte imbalance, nephrotoxicity, blood dyscrasias
OTHER						
Sympathomimetics phenylephrine	Minor eye irritation			Headache, dizziness	Excitability, restlessness, palpitations	
Vasoconstrictors naphazoline	Redness	NO	C	Narrow-angle glaucoma, MAOIs, contact lenses, hypertension, cerebrovascular disease, hyperglycemia, hyperthyroidism	Rebound, floaters, congestion, hypersensitivity	Narrow-angle glaucoma, hypersensitivity, systemic adrenergic effects
Lubricant artificial tears	Protection and lubrication	Yes		Reevaluate if irritation increases or persists	Transient stinging	
Anesthetic proparacaine	Diagnostic procedure	NO	C	Cardiac disease hyperthyroidism	Mild local irritation. protect eye from damage, erosions	Hypersensitivity, systemic toxicity, long-term use: corneal opacities, permanent visual loss
Diagnostic fluorescein	Diagnosis of abrasion, foreign bodies	NO	C			Hypersensitivity, stains contact lenses

CHF, Congestive heart failure; *COPD*, chronic obstructive pulmonary disease; *PUD*, peptic ulcer disease.

OTHER OPHTHALMIC MEDICATIONS
Sympathomimetic Agents

phenylephrine hydrochloride (Neo-Synephrine)

- The 0.12% solution is available as an OTC preparation for the relief of minor eye irritation.
- Ophthalmologists use 10% and 12% solutions for vasoconstriction and pupil dilation. These higher percentage solutions can cause significant cardiovascular adverse reactions.
- In the eye, phenylephrine acts locally as a potent vasoconstrictor and mydriatic by constricting ophthalmic blood vessels and the radial muscle of the iris.
- There is little rebound vasodilation, and systemic side effects are uncommon.
- Ophthalmic solutions composed of phenylephrine hydrochlride are contraindicated in persons with narrow-angle glaucoma.

Lubricants

artificial tears (Tears Naturale II, Tears Naturale Free)

- Drugs can be used as often as patient wishes.
- Insert systems are indicated in patients with moderate-to-severe dry eye syndromes such as keratoconjunctivitis sicca, especially in patients who fail a trial of therapy with artificial tear solutions.
- Inserts are also indicated for patients with exposure keratitis, decreased corneal sensitivity, and recurrent corneal erosions.

Anesthetics

proparacaine hydrochloride (Alcaine, Percaine)

- Onset of anesthesia after instillation of one drop occurs in approximately 13 seconds. Duration of action is 15 minutes or longer.

Topical Ear Agents

General Uses

Indications

- Superficial infections of the external auditory canal
- Cerumen removal

There are a large number of otic preparations. Some are prescription only; others are available OTC. The commonly used prescription topical otic preparations are either an antibiotic or an antibiotic plus hydrocortisone. Miscellaneous otic preparations contain a wide variety of combinations of ingredients. Space does not permit a complete listing here, but the components are listed and the most commonly used products are mentioned.

DISEASE PROCESS
Anatomy, Physiology, and Pathophysiology

The pinna is the visible portion of the ear. The outer ear external auditory canal secretes cerumen to move dirt outward through the canal. the external auditory canal is sealed by the tympanic membrane (TM), which mechanically transmits sound to the middle ear. The middle ear is an air-filled cavity, which is connected to the pharynx by the eustachian tube. The eustachian tube opens briefly during swallowing, allowing equalization of the pressures on either side of the TM. The middle ear transmits sound to the inner ear and the inner ear transduces the sound into nerve impulses (Rhoades & Tanner, 1995).

The two most common problems with the outer ear are infection and cerumen impaction. Infections are often caused by swimming, or otherwise getting water in the outer ear. Cerumen impaction is associated with hardening of the cerumen that is associated with old age.

DRUG TREATMENT PRINCIPLES

These medicines act topically, and there is minimal systemic absorption. When treating an ear infection, the other ear may be treated as a preventative measure. A steroid is usually included with the antibiotic to relieve the symptoms of the infection. Use drops for 1 week only.

To prevent infections in patients at risk (swimmers), use a product containing 2% acetic acid, boric acid, isopropyl alcohol, or Burow's solution after exposure. These are available OTC or can be made at home.

To prevent cerumen buildup, use glycerin or an oil such as mineral oil or vegetable oil regularly (usually weekly to monthly). An OTC preparation containing triethanolamine or carbamide may also be used.

To treat impacted cerumen, use OTC ear drops nightly for 4 to 7 days. Avoid ear candles because patients may get burned. Excess cerumen may be removed as an office procedure, if necessary.

For miscellaneous external ear conditions, select an appropriate product from the following list of ingredients:

- Steroids have antiallergic, antipruritic, and antiinflammatory effects.
- Antibiotics have antibacterial activity.
- Phenylephrine is a vasoconstrictor that has a decongestant effect.
- Acetic acid, boric acid, benzalkonium chloride, and aluminum acetate (Burow's solution) have antibacterial and antifungal activity.
- Carbamide peroxide and triethanolamine emulsify and disperse earwax.
- Glycerin is a solvent and vehicle. It has emollient, hygroscopic, and humectant effects.
- Benzocaine is a local anesthetic.
- Antipyrine is an analgesic.

HOW TO MONITOR

Monitor for therapeutic effect and hypersensitivity reactions.

PATIENT EDUCATION

- Use only in the ears. Avoid contact with the eyes.
- Notify health care provider if burning or itching occurs or if the condition persists.
- Use only for a prescribed length of treatment.

- Use ear drops properly:
  1. Wash hands well before instilling eardrops.
  2. Avoid contact of the sterile tip with any part of the ear. For improved accuracy have another individual, if possible, instill drops into the ear canal.
  3. Warm bottle to body temperature by holding in hand for 10 minutes before instillation.
  4. Shake suspension for 10 seconds to mix well.
  5. Patient should lie on side or on back with the affected ear up.
  6. For a child, pull ear down and back.
  7. For an adult, pull ear up and back.
  8. Instill the prescribed number of drops into the ear.
  9. Keep the ear tilted for 2 minutes or insert a cotton plug.
  10. Treat for the recommended amount of time.

Specific Drugs

hydrocortisone 1%, neomycin sulfate 5 mg, polymyxin 10,000 units (Cortisporin otic solution), 2 mg ciprofloxacin and 10 mg hydrocortisone/ml (Cipro HC otic suspension)

Contraindications
- Perforated tympanic membrane
- Hypersensitivity to any component

Precautions
- Prolonged use of antibiotics or steroids may result in the overgrowth of nonsusceptible organisms (e.g., herpes simplex, vaccinia, varicella) and fungus.

Adverse Effects
- Rash, itching, and swelling may be signs of hypersensitivity to components of the product.
- Drainage and pain may signify a middle ear infection, and drops are contraindicated.

Dosage and Administration
- The usual adult dose is four drops instilled three or four times a day. The usual dosage for infants and small children is three drops instilled into the affected ear three or four times a day.
- A wick may be inserted into the canal after the drops have been instilled, and more drops applied to saturate the wick. Instruct the patient to instill a few drops to the wick every 4 hours. Remove wick after 24 hours and continue to instill the appropriate number of drops three to four times a day.

Topical Mouth and Throat Agents

Specific Drugs

ANTIFUNGALS

nystatin (Mycostatin), clotrimazole, other (Mycelex)

Indications
- Oral candidiasis
- Prophylaxis in immunocompromised patients
- Herpes labialis
- Minor sore throat
- Minor irritation of the throat or mouth

See Table 15-3 for characteristics of mouth and throat preparations.

The first group of topical mouth and throat products is antifungals. This section discusses their use only for throat

TABLE 15-3 Characteristics of Mouth and Throat Preparations

Preparation	Contraindications, Warnings, Precautions	Adverse Effects	Pregnancy Class	Formulation	Dosage	Administration
nystatin	Hypersensitivity, not for systemic mycoses	Nausea, vomiting, gastrointestinal distress, diarrhea	C	Oral suspension Troche	Adult and child: 400,000-600,000 U Infants: 200,000 U 200,000 U 1-2 tabs	qid 4-5 times/day
clotrimazole	Hypersensitivity, not for systemic mycoses	Increased AST, nausea vomiting, unpleasant mouth sensations, pruritus	C	Troche	Adult and child >3 yr: 1 troche Prophylaxis: 1 troche during chemotherapy	5 times/day
carbamide peroxide	Irritation	Irritation	NI	Solution, liquid	>2 yr; liquid swish in mouth for 1 min	Up to qid
chlorhexidine	Hypersensitivity, not for necrotizing ulcerative gingivitis, increased calculus deposits	May stain teeth, altered taste perception, minor irritation	B	Oral rinse	>18 yr: 15 ml oral rinse for 30 sec after brushing teeth, expectorate	AM and PM

and mouth fungal infections. These are usually associated with antibiotic treatment and immunocompromised patients.

The antiviral product penciclovir is used (unlabeled) for herpes labialis or cold sores. Carbamide peroxide is indicated for relief of minor oral inflammation such as canker sores, denture irritation, and irritation of inflamed gums.

Pilocarpine taken as a 5-mg tablet is indicated for dry mouth from salivary gland hypofunction caused by radiotherapy or from Sjögren syndrome. Because of the risk of serious parasympathomimetic adverse effects, its use should be reserved for patients with a clear indication and significant consequences from their dry mouth.

There are a wide variety of mouth and throat products with various combinations of ingredients that are used for minor irritation of the throat or mouth. These are generally safe and effective to various degrees. The most frequently used ingredients are the following:

- Carbamide peroxide (urea peroxide) is used to treat minor oral inflammation because it releases oxygen on contact with mouth tissues to provide cleansing.
- Chlorhexidine gluconate is used for gingivitis because it provides microbicidal activity during oral rinsing.
- Antipyrine is an analgesic.
- Benzocaine and cyclonamine are local anesthetics.
- Hydrocortisone and triamcinolone corticosteroids have antiinflammatory activity.
- Cetylpyridinium chloride, eucalyptus oil, thymol, and hexylresorcinol have antiseptic activity.
- Menthol, camphor, capsicum, dyclonine, and phenol have antipruritic, local anesthetic, and counterirritant activity.
- Saliva substitutes are used for relief of dry mouth and throat.
- Tannic acid is used for temporary relief of pain caused by cold sores because it forms a thin, pliable film over sores within 60 seconds of administration.
- Terpin hydrate is an expectorant.

PATIENT EDUCATION

To use the suspension form of the drug:

- Use as directed.
- Divide dose and place half on each side of mouth.
- Retain suspension in mouth for as long as possible before swallowing.
- Continue use for at least 2 days after symptoms disappear.

To use the troche form, patient must be competent enough to allow troches to dissolve slowly:

- Troche should not be chewed or swallowed whole.
- Troche should be dissolved slowly in the mouth.

OTHER MOUTH AND THROAT PREPARATIONS

carbamide peroxide (Gly-Oxide) and chlorhexidine gluconate (Peridex)

- These agents are not appropriate for treatment of severe or persistent sore throat.
- Do not use these products in children under 2 years of age.
- See package labeling for dosage and administration information.

RESOURCES FOR PATIENTS AND PROVIDERS

American Foundation for the Blind, www.afb.org.
Resource for the visually impaired.

National Eye Institute, www.nei.nih.gov.
Information for health professionals.

Self-help for hard-of-hearing people, www.shhh.org.
Enhance quality of life for the hearing impaired.

Supersight, www.supersight.com.
Allows one-stop, direct access to ophthalmology publication websites.

BIBLIOGRAPHY

Eye

Apple DJ, Rabb M: *Ocular pathology,* ed 5, St Louis, 1998, Mosby.

Davey CC: The red eye, *Br J Hosp Med* 33:89-04, 1996.

Ferrell T: *Basic ophthalmology CD-ROM,* St Louis, 1996, Mosby.

Lewis RA, editor: *Glaucoma CD-ROM,* St Louis, 1995, Mosby.

Mauger TF, Craig EL: *Mosby's ocular drug handbook,* St Louis, 1996, Mosby.

Newell FW: *Ophthalmology: principles and concepts,* ed 8, St Louis, 1996, Mosby.

Palay DA, Krachmer JH: *Ophthalmology for the primary care practitioner,* St Louis, 1998, Mosby.

Robert PY, Adenis JP: Comparative review of topical ophthalmic antibacterial preparations, *Drugs* 61:175-185, 2001.

Sassani JW: *Ophthalmic pathology with clinical correlations,* Philadelphia, 1997, Lippincott-Raven.

Shields SR: Managing eye disease in primary care. Part 3. When to refer for ophthalmologic care, *Postgrad Med* 108:99-106, 2000.

Shields SR: Managing eye disease in primary care. Part 2. How to recognize and treat common eye problems, *Postgrad Med* 108:83-86, 91-96, 2000.

Wu T: *Ophthalmology for primary care,* Philadelphia, 1997, WB Saunders.

Ear, Throat, and Mouth

Grossan M: Safe, effective techniques for cerumen removal, *Geriatrics* 55:80, 2000.

McBride DR:Management of aphthous ulcers, *Am Fam Phys* 62:149, 2000.

UNIT 5

Respiratory Agents

Unit 5 discusses drugs that are used to treat diseases of the respiratory system. Respiratory medications represent a very large and quickly changing area of pharmacotherapeutics. Drug formulations and ingredients, particularly for the many medications that have now moved from legend to over-the-counter (OTC) status, vary dramatically from year to year. There is much overlap in the use of these classes of drugs and the conditions they are used to treat. Each drug may be used for many different conditions.

The protocols for drug use in asthma and chronic obstructive pulmonary disease (COPD) have undergone modifications as more drugs become available and more is learned about how to reverse asthmatic changes. Asthma is now viewed as primarily an inflammatory process treated with antiinflammatory medications. Theophylline is no longer a first-line drug. The treatment of COPD and allergic rhinitis involves basically the same medications as those used for asthma, but the medications are used differently.

- **Chapter 16** discusses the many types of medications used to treat upper respiratory infections and allergic rhinitis.
- **Chapter 17** presents a detailed discussion of drugs used in asthma and COPD.

CHAPTER 16

Upper Respiratory Agents

Bonnie R. Bock

Drug Names

Class	Subclass	Generic Name	Trade Name
Decongestants	Oral decongestants	pseudoephedrine HCl	Sudafed (OTC), generic
	Topical nasal decongestants	(P) phenylephrine HCl	Neo-Synephrine (OTC)
		oxymetazoline	Afrin, Neo-Synephrine 12-hour (OTC)
Antihistamines	Sedating antihistamines		
	Ethanolamine	(P) diphenhydramine HCl	Benadryl (OTC), generic
		clemastine fumarate	Tavist (OTC)
	Alkylamine	chlorpheniramine maleate	Chlor-Trimetron (OTC)
	Low-sedating antihistamines		
	Piperadine	(200) cetirizine HCl	Zyrtec (Rx)
	Nonsedating antihistamines	(200) fexofenadine HCl	Allegra (Rx)
	Miscellaneous	(200) loratadine	Claritin (OTC)
		desloratadine	Clarinex (Rx)
	Intranasal miscellaneous	azelastine	Astelin (Rx)
Intranasal steroids		triamcinolone acetonide	Nasacort (Rx)
		beclomethasone dipropionate	Beconase, Vancenase (Rx)
		fluticasone propionate	Flonase (Rx)
Intranasal cromolyn		cromolyn sodium	Nasalcrom (OTC)
Antitussives	Narcotic antitussives	codeine phosphate	Generic (Rx)
	Nonnarcotic antitussives	dextromethorphan HBr	Robitussin DM (OTC)
		benzonatate	Tessalon Perles (Rx)
Expectorants		guaifenesin	Robitussin (OTC), Humibid LA (Rx)

(200), Top 200 drug; (P), prototype drug.

General Uses

Indications

Decongestants

Oral Decongestants

- Nasal congestion caused by the common cold, hay fever, or other upper respiratory allergies
- Nasal congestion associated with sinusitis and eustachian tube congestion
- *Nonlabeled use:* treatment for mild-to-moderate urinary stress incontinence

Topical Nasal Decongestants

- Symptomatic relief of nasal and nasopharyngeal mucosal congestion caused by the common cold, sinusitis, hay fever, or other upper respiratory allergies
- Adjunctive therapy of middle ear infections by decreasing congestion around the eustachian ostia
- Relief of ear block and pressure pain in air travel

Antihistamines

- Symptomatic relief of symptoms associated with perennial and seasonal allergic rhinitis, vasomotor rhinitis, and allergic conjunctivitis; temporary relief of runny nose and sneezing caused by the common cold
- Skin: allergic and nonallergic pruritic symptoms; mild, uncomplicated urticaria and angioedema
- Amelioration of allergic reactions to blood or plasma, dermatographism, and adjunctive therapy in anaphylactic reactions

Intranasal Steroids

- Vasomotor rhinitis and relief of symptoms of seasonal or perennial rhinitis when effectiveness of or tolerance to conventional treatment is unsatisfactory

Intranasal Cromolyn

- Prevention and treatment of allergic rhinitis

Antitussives

Narcotic Antitussives

- Codeine for suppression of cough induced by chemical or mechanical respiratory tract irritation

Nonnarcotic Antitussives

- Dextromethorphan HBr (Robitussin) for control of nonproductive cough
- Benzonatate (Tessalon Perles) for symptomatic relief of cough

Expectorants

Guaifenesin provides symptomatic relief of respiratory conditions characterized by dry, nonproductive cough and in the presence of mucus in the respiratory tract.

• • •

The six classes of drugs discussed in this chapter are used to treat a variety of upper respiratory conditions. The two most common conditions in primary care practice that require these medications are upper respiratory viral infections (URIs or viral rhinitis) and allergic rhinitis (hay fever).

Decongestants and antihistamines are very commonly used both OTC and by prescription for treatment of a variety of conditions. Decongestants are used as first-line drugs for URIs. Antihistamines are first-line treatment for allergic rhinitis. There are too many different antihistamines to include in this text; only those most commonly seen in primary care practice are discussed.

Intranasal steroids and intranasal cromolyn are second-line treatment in upper respiratory conditions. Other formulations of these drugs are used for lower respiratory conditions. These drugs are discussed in detail in Chapter 17; only their intranasal use in upper respiratory conditions is discussed here.

Antitussives and expectorants are also used as adjunct therapy in upper respiratory and lower respiratory conditions and are discussed in this chapter.

Combination drugs containing these categories of medications are available both OTC and by prescription. These combinations can be very confusing. Often OTC combinations contain medications that are not indicated for the condition for which the combination is labeled and can be counterproductive.

Commonly prescribed combination respiratory medications include antihistamine/decongestant combinations (Allegra-D, Claritin-D, Zyrtec-D), decongestant/expectorant combinations (Guaifed PD), antitussive/expectorant combinations (Robitussin AC), which can be useful in treating multisymptom upper and lower respiratory conditions if used appropriately. However, many OTC products are combinations of antihistamines, decongestants, analgesics, and, often, cough suppressants. Many nighttime formulations contain alcohol and acetaminophen, which should not be consumed together. Many consumers use these products erroneously, taking an antihistamine for congestion when actually a decongestant is needed and an analgesic in the absence of pain or fever. Many consumers, particularly the elderly, use these products without considering the ingredients and possible drug interactions with medications they are already taking or preexisting medical conditions that may be adversely affected by certain medications. An example would be patients with hypertension, glaucoma, or urinary retention using pseudoephedrine for congestion. Special formulations are available OTC for patients with hypertension (Coricidin HBP, Coricidin HBP Cough & Cold), and several products are sugar and alcohol free. Despite the multiple-combination preparations available both OTC and by prescription, many authorities recommend prescribing single-ingredient medications to avoid drug errors and over-medicating.

Many patients are self-prescribing OTCs for these diseases. Be sure to ask patients specifically about OTCs they are using. See Chapter 9 for information on OTC use.

DISEASE PROCESS

Anatomy and Physiology

The respiratory system is composed of the upper air passage structure, including the nasal passages, paranasal sinuses, pharynx, and larynx, and the lower air passages, including the trachea, bronchi, and lungs. Air is moved through the upper passages, termed the *conducting portion,* into the lung or respiratory portion, where gas exchange occurs through the alveoli of the lung. The entire airway is lined with epithelial tissue, which contains glands and surface goblet cells that synthesize and secrete thick mucus. Below the larynx to the ends of the bronchi, the airways are lined with columnar epithelial cells that contain hair-like projections or cilia, which continuously beat in an upward motion toward the pharynx. Inhaled irritants stick to the mucus and are moved by the cilia to the pharynx, where they are either swallowed or expectorated.

Pathophysiology

URIs are viral in etiology. Allergic rhinitis is an allergic reaction. A secondary bacterial infection is common in inadequately treated URIs and allergic rhinitis. Acute sinusitis and otitis media are the most common complications, although pneumonia may develop in susceptible patients. Critical decisions revolve around determining whether the problem is viral or bacterial and whether there is an allergic component to the process.

The Disease

Upper Respiratory Infection. URIs are caused by rhinoviruses, adenoviruses, and other viruses. The symptoms are nonspecific and consist of nasal congestion, watery rhinorrhea, headache, sneezing, and scratchy throat along with general malaise. Symptoms are self-limiting, lasting from a few days to a few weeks. On physical examination, the nasal mucosa are reddened and edematous with a watery discharge. Diagnosis is based on clinical observations, after noting absence of signs of bacterial infection–purulent nasal discharge, red tympanic membrane, change in color of discharge, or high fever. URIs should be evaluated by a clinician, particularly if there is any risk of serious disease, including severe acute respiratory syndrome (SARS) is a possible differential.

Allergic Rhinitis. Seasonal allergic rhinitis is usually caused by allergy to pollen: trees in the spring, grasses in the summer, and ragweed in the fall. Perennial allergic rhinitis is usually caused by allergy to dust, molds, or mites. The symptoms are very similar to URI symptoms except that they may be more severe and more persistent, may fluctuate, and often can be related to exposure to allergens. Sneezing, eye irritation, and watery rhinorrhea are often prominent. On physical examination, the turbinates may be pale or violaceous because of venous engorgement rather than red and erythematous as in URIs.

DRUG ACTION AND EFFECTS

Decongestants

Decongestants are sympathomimetic amines that act to stimulate α-adrenergic receptors of vascular smooth muscle, causing vasoconstriction, pressor effects, nasal decongestion, contraction of gastrointestinal and urinary sphincters, pupil dilation, and decreased pancreatic β-cell secretion. Pseudoephedrine also has β-adrenergic properties.

In the sympathetic nervous system, adrenergic effector cells contain two distinct receptors, the α- and β-receptors. Sympathomimetic drugs mimic the action of norepinephrine on sympathetic effector organs, affecting the adrenergic receptors. Important α-adrenergic activities include (1) vasoconstriction of arterioles, leading to increased blood pressure; (2) dilation of the pupils; (3) intestinal relaxation; and (4) bladder sphincter contraction. β-Receptors are divided into β_1- and β_2-receptors because some drugs affect some, but not all, β-receptors. β_1-Adrenergic activity includes (1) cardioacceleration and (2) increased myocardial contractility, whereas β_2 stimulation leads to (1) vasodilation of skeletal muscle, (2) bronchodilation, (3) uterine relaxation, and (4) bladder relaxation.

Pseudoephedrine HCl is an α-adrenergic receptor agonist (sympathomimetic) that produces vasoconstriction by stimulating α-receptors in the mucosa of the respiratory tract and shrinking swollen mucous membranes. It also reduces tissue edema and nasal congestion, increases nasal airway patency, increases drainage of sinus secretions, and opens obstructed eustachian ostia.

Topical application of decongestants to the nasal mucous membranes causes vasoconstriction, resulting in shrinkage, which helps to promote drainage and improve breathing through the nasal passages. Topical agents produce reduced systemic effects compared with oral preparations, achieving decongestion without causing extreme changes in blood pressure, cardiac stimulation, or vascular redistribution.

Oxymetazoline is a direct-acting sympathomimetic amine, which acts on the α-adrenergic receptors of the nasal mucosa, causing vasoconstriction and resulting in decreased blood flow and decreased nasal congestion.

Antihistamines

Antihistamines compete for histamine at the H_1 receptor sites and are used to treat IgE-mediated allergy. Antihistamine therapy is helpful in treating allergic rhinitis and urticaria in most, but not all, patients. They antagonize the pharmacologic effects of histamine. They do not inactivate histamine or block histamine release, antibody production, or antigen-antibody interactions. They also have anticholinergic (drying), antipruritic, and sedative effects to a varying degree. These drugs are classified by the amount of sedation they cause. Azelastine is a topical antihistamine nasal spray with few adverse systemic side effects that is used to treat allergic and vasomotor rhinitis.

Intranasal Steroids

The steroids used in intranasal products have potent glucocorticoid and weak mineralocorticoid activity. Glucocorticoids inhibit cells, including mast cells, eosinophils, neutrophils, macrophages, lymphocytes, and mediators such as histamine, leukotrienes, and cytokines. They exert direct local antiinflammatory effects with minimal systemic effects. Intranasal corticosteroids effectively control the four major symptoms of allergic rhinitis—rhinorrhea, congestion, sneezing, and nasal itch. They are helpful in managing moderate to severe disease and are used in treating both seasonal and perennial allergic rhinitis. These medications must be used consistently on a daily basis for effectiveness, and maximum effects may not be noted for several days to weeks. For details on the immune system, see Chapter 69.

Intranasal Cromolyn

Cromolyn sodium is an OTC intranasal mast cell stabilizer that is used as a preventive agent taken in advance of allergen exposure. It is effective in reducing rhinorrhea, sneezing, and nasal itching, but it has minimal effect on nasal congestion. Cromolyn acts locally on tissue, inhibiting the release of chemical mediators by preventing mast cell degranulation. It has an excellent safety profile, and minimal adverse affects consisting of nasal irritation, stinging, and sneezing. For details, see Chapter 17.

Antitussives

Codeine and dextromethorphan both act centrally by acting on the cough center of the medulla to suppress cough. Dextromethorphan is the *d*-isomer of codeine and lacks the analgesic and addictive properties of codeine. However, it is not as effective as codeine in depressing the cough reflex. Benzonatate anesthetizes stretch receptors in the respiratory passages, reducing the cough reflex at its source.

Expectorants

Guaifenesin increases respiratory tract fluid secretions and helps to loosen bronchial secretions by reducing adhesiveness and tissue surface tension. By reducing the viscosity of secretions, guaifenesin increases the efficacy of the mucociliary mechanism in removing accumulated secretions from the upper and lower airways. As a result, nonproductive coughs become more productive, less frequent, and less irritating to the airways.

DRUG TREATMENT PRINCIPLES

Treatment of Upper Respiratory Infection

Treatment consists basically of symptomatic relief (Figure 16-1). Patient history reveals which symptoms are most troublesome to patients and can be targeted. Decongestants are usually the only medication indicated. Antitussives or expectorants may be helpful. Antihistamines may cause excessive dryness. Because URIs are viral in origin, antibiotics are not indicated. Many patients need this to be explained to them. Nonpharmacologic treatment consists of rest as needed and increased fluids, especially water. Adequate hydration may be more helpful in symptom relief than medication.

Treatment of Allergic Rhinitis

Nonpharmacologic Treatment. Identify environmental precipitants, which may include time of year, work and home

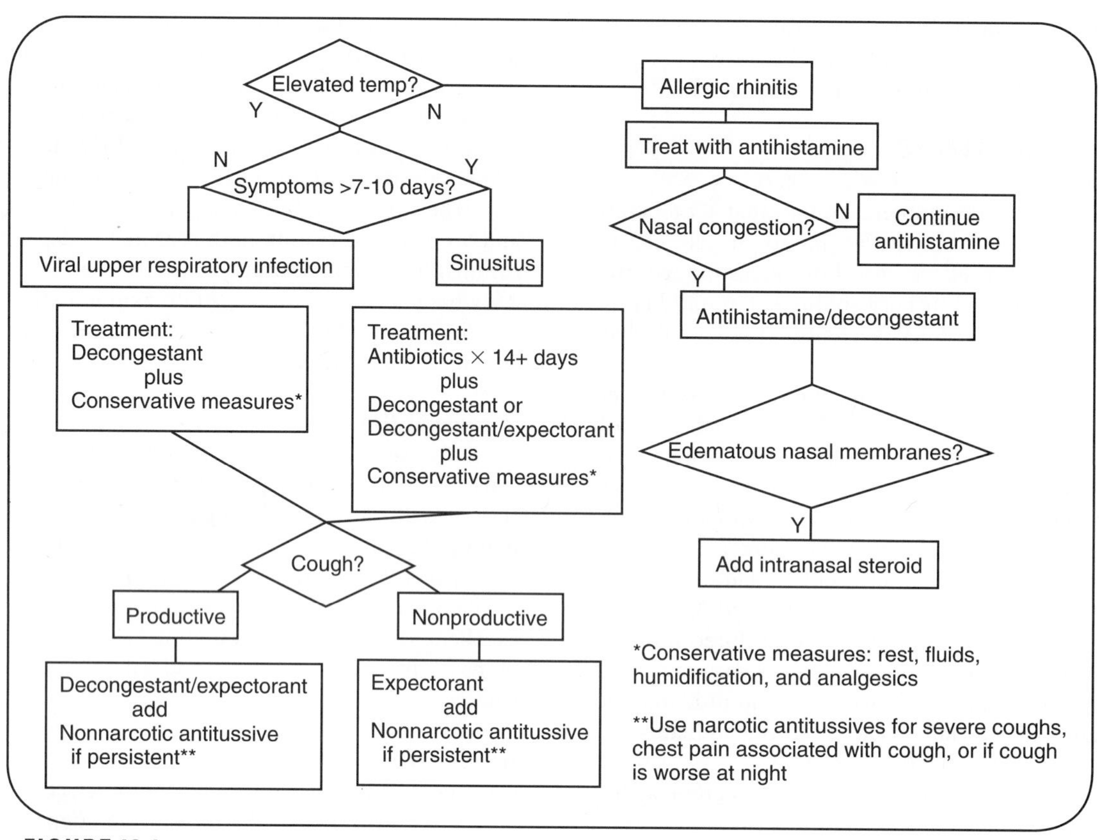

FIGURE 16-1

Treatment plan for URIs and allergies.

environment, and pets. Implement strategies designed to reduce these factors.

Avoid outdoor allergens, use air conditioning in home and car, exercise outdoors in the afternoon when pollen counts are typically low, use HEPA filters in the home, and use a clothes dryer rather than a clothesline, where clothes can collect airborne pollen.

For indoor allergens, use strategies for dust, pet, mold, and cockroach avoidance.

Normal saline nasal sprays or nasal irrigation, twice daily, may help reduce postnasal drip, sneezing, and congestion.

Pharmacologic Treatment. Identify symptoms most problematic to patient for treatment; these may include sneezing, runny nose, itching, and nasal congestion.

Treat mild, intermittent symptoms with a nonsedating oral antihistamine as needed. Add a decongestant if needed.

If the patient is unable to take an oral antihistamine, consider the use of a nasal antihistamine or intranasal cromolyn. Treat moderate, frequent symptoms with a regular- to high-dose intranasal corticosteroid.

Add an oral or a nasal antihistamine and decongestant if necessary.

To treat moderate, persistent symptoms, begin with a combination regimen, consisting of intranasal corticosteroids plus a nonsedating or intranasal antihistamine and decongestant if necessary.

Treat severe symptoms with a combination regimen consisting of a nonsedating antihistamine with or without a decongestant and intranasal corticosteroid. Consider the use of an oral steroid for 5 days, and the use of oxymetazoline as needed for no more than 3 days.

Decongestants

Decongestants are sympathomimetic amines used to relieve nasal congestion caused by colds, allergies, and URIs; they also promote sinus drainage and relieve eustachian tube congestion. Oral forms are often used in combination with antihistamines and expectorants in both OTC and prescription doses (Table 16-1). Topical nasal decongestants provide direct relief to swollen nasal membranes and are sometimes used to decrease congestion of the eustachian tube in middle ear infections and to relieve pressure and blockage of the ear during air travel.

Oral decongestants generally do not cause sedation but may cause systemic effects, including nervousness, dizziness, and difficulty sleeping, particularly in infants and the elderly.

Because of the sympathomimetic effects, decongestants may cause central nervous system (CNS) stimulation, cardiovascular collapse with hypotension, and convulsions. Use them with caution in patients with hypertension, cardiovascular and peripheral vascular disease, hyperthyroidism, diabetes mellitus, prostatic hypertrophy, urinary retention, and increased intraocular pressure.

TABLE 16-1 Commonly Prescribed Respiratory Combination Products

Product Name	Antihistamine	Decongestant	Antitussive	Expectorant
Allegra-D	fexofenadine HCl (60 mg)	pseudoephedrine HCl (120 mg)		
Claritin-D	loratadine (5 mg)	pseudoephedrine sulfate (120 mg)		
Claritin-D 24-hour	loratadine (10 mg)	pseudoephedrine sulfate (240 mg)		
Deconamine SR	chlorpheniramine (8 mg)	pseudoephedrine (120 mg)		
Deconamine CX		pseudoephedrine (30 mg)	hydrocodone (5 mg)	guaifenesin (300 mg)
Entex PSE, Deconsal II, Duratuss		pseudoephedrine HCl (120)		guaifenesin (600 mg)
Guaifed-PD		pseudoephedrine HCl (60 mg)		guaifenesin (300 mg)
Guaifed, extended release		pseudoephedrine HCl (120 mg)		guaifenesin (250 mg)
Phenergan with codeine	promethazine (6.25 mg/5 ml)		codeine (10 mg/5 ml)	
Semprex-D	acrivastine (8 mg)	pseudoephedrine HCl (60 mg)		
Tussi-12	chlorpheniramine (5 mg)		carbetapentane (60 mg)	
Zyrtec D 12-hour	cetirizine (5 mg)	pseudoephedrine (120 mg)		

The clinical problems most often seen with oral decongestants include tachycardia, nervousness, insomnia, palpitations, headache, and irritability, which may be poorly tolerated in the frail elderly, and patients with poorly controlled hypertension may experience an increase in blood pressure. Data suggest that oral decongestants may be used cautiously in patients with controlled hypertension. Sustained-release formulations may have less effect on the cardiovascular system. However, because they may antagonize the effects of hypertensive medications, alternative agents such as topical decongestants should be used for these patients.

Topical decongestants have little systemic effect, but because of rebound congestion (rhinitis medicamentosa), they should only be used in acute conditions for no longer than 3 consecutive days. Rebound congestion is treated by gradual withdrawal, one nares at a time. Saline nasal spray is often helpful.

Overall, topical decongestants are more effective than oral ones, but oral decongestants have longer durations of action and are less irritating.

Antihistamines

Antihistamines are H_1 receptor antagonists often used alone or in combination with decongestants and expectorants to relieve symptoms associated with perennial and seasonal allergies with associated rhinitis, vasomotor rhinitis, allergic conjunctivitis, and cold symptoms such as sneezing and runny nose. They are also used to relieve allergic and nonallergic pruritic symptoms, mild urticaria and angioedema, for prophylaxis against allergic reactions to blood or plasma products, and as adjunctive therapy in anaphylactic reactions.

Antihistamines are often used to treat urticaria. Certain antihistamines also have antiemetic effects and are useful for nausea, vomiting, vertigo, and motion sickness.

Many OTC cold remedies contain antihistamines; however, their use in the treatment of cold symptoms is controversial. Antihistamines are best used to treat allergic symptoms such as rhinorrhea; watery, itchy eyes; postnasal drainage; and sneezing. Decongestants are preferred to treat cold symptoms, such as nasal congestion caused by swollen nasal membranes.

In general, antihistamines are not recommended to treat lower respiratory tract symptoms, including asthma, because anticholinergic effects may cause thickening of respiratory secretions and may impair expectoration. Several reports, however, indicate antihistamines can be safety used in asthmatic patients with severe perennial allergies without exacerbating the asthma.

In general, OTC products are more likely to cause sedation, which may interfere with the patient's activities. Sedating antihistamines are sometimes preferred, particularly to reduce symptoms at night and to induce sleep, and are used in combination with analgesics as a pain reliever and sleep aid. The prescribed antihistamines are less likely to cause sedation and are generally well tolerated. If a particular antihistamine has lost effectiveness or causes untoward side effects, select another antihistamine from a different class. If the patient requires two antihistamines for severe symptoms, drugs from two different classes should be selected.

Intranasal Steroids

Intranasal steroids should be used for at least 1 month before deciding if they are effective. Patients should be warned that improvement usually does not begin until 1 to 2 weeks after starting therapy. Intranasal steroids may help shrink nasal polyps.

Exceeding the recommended dose may result in systemic effects, including suppression of hypothalamic-pituitary-adrenal (HPA) function. Systemic effects are possible with inhaled steroids and less likely with intranasal corticosteroids when used at conventional recommended doses.

Intranasal Cromolyn

For seasonal allergic rhinitis, treatment will be more effective if started before contact with the allergen. Continue treatment throughout exposure. In perennial allergic rhinitis, effects of treatment may require 2 to 4 weeks to become evident when first initiated. The need for the medication may diminish, and it can be discontinued later.

Antitussives

Antitussives are used to control or suppress coughs caused by respiratory tract irritation, colds, or allergies.

It is important to determine the underlying disorder causing the cough, particularly to rule out serious cases of cough, including pneumonia and SARS.

Antitussives should not be given in conditions in which retention of respiratory secretions may be harmful. Antitussives should be used with caution. In general, a cough should not be suppressed. Coughs help bring fluid up from the bronchioles and lungs. However, if a patient is having a nonproductive cough that is causing muscle pain or interfering with sleep, it should be suppressed.

Antitussive preparations come in both liquid and tablet forms. Patients often expect or prefer a cough syrup for cough suppression. Prescribing cough syrups may provide some psychological benefit. A simple cough syrup containing guaifenesin but no other drugs, including alcohol, causes no harm, soothes the throat, and makes the patient feel cared for. A cough syrup with no sugar is made for diabetic patients. These can be used in the patient for whom any other medications are unsafe.

Narcotic Antitussives. Most effective in suppressing coughs are narcotic antitussives. Codeine, as a narcotic antitussive, is used to suppress coughs induced by chemical or mechanical respiratory tract infection. It is also used as a narcotic agonist analgesic for the relief of mild-to-moderate pain (see Chapter 44). The antitussive dose of codeine is lower than the required dose for analgesia, and side effects are less frequent at the antitussive dose. Cough suppression with codeine is therefore beneficial in patients who have cough-related pain or complications such as costochondritis or sleeplessness caused by deep or persistent coughs. Hydrocodone, also a narcotic antitussive and analgesic, has multiple actions similar to those of codeine. Like codeine, it is believed to act directly on the cough center in the brain.

Nausea, vomiting, sedation, dizziness, and constipation are the most common side effects of narcotic antitussives. Allergic reactions to opiates are infrequent and are usually manifested by pruritus and urticaria. Narcotic antitussives should be prescribed in small amounts, and patients should be followed closely to determine effectiveness and to prevent excessive use. They can provide good suppression at doses low enough to provoke few side effects.

Nonnarcotic Antitussives. Nonnarcotic antitussives lack analgesic properties and are not as effective as codeine in suppressing coughs, but they also lack the potential for addiction and other adverse effects of narcotics. Dextromethorphan is a common ingredient in many OTC cold medications and some prescription cough preparations and is frequently used in combination with decongestants, antihistamines, and expectorants (see Table 16-1).

Benzonatate (in the form of capsules that should be swallowed whole) can cause temporary local anesthesia of the oral mucosa if not taken correctly. It also lacks the CNS side effects of codeine or dextromethorphan. However, it is often not as effective. It is often used in patients such as the frail elderly or patients who must continue to perform activities that require maximum mental alertness such as driving who are bothered by their cough but cannot tolerate the CNS side effects of the other cough suppressants.

Expectorants

Guaifenesin (glyceryl guaiacolate) is an expectorant used for the symptomatic relief of a dry, nonproductive cough associated with respiratory tract infections and is used in related conditions such as sinusitis, pharyngitis, bronchitis, and asthma and in the presence of tenacious mucus, mucous plugs, or congestion in the respiratory tract. Guaifenesin is found in many OTC and prescription preparations.

Expectorants are often used in combination with antitussives to provide relief for dry nonproductive coughs and to loosen tenacious mucus or congestion in the respiratory tract. These agents are believed to stimulate the flow of mucus; however, there is no evidence to support this view. Expectorants are often used when the patient insists on a cough remedy when cough suppression is not indicated, or because the patient believes the effect to be beneficial.

Enhancing expectoration by thinning thick secretions helps promote drainage. This can be accomplished through the use of expectorants, by increasing fluid intake, and by increasing air humidification. Fluid intake is probably the most important.

HOW TO MONITOR

Decongestants

- Monitor for symptoms of CNS stimulation in oral use.
- Monitor frequency of use of topical application and monitor for symptoms of rebound congestion (rhinitis medicamentosa).

Antihistamines

- Monitor for relief of targeted symptoms and for excessive drowsiness.

Intranasal Steroids

- Watch closely for development of infections.
- In long-term use, monitor for changes in nasal mucosa.

Antitussives

- Monitor narcotic antitussives for effectiveness and excessive side effects, especially constipation in the elderly.

PATIENT VARIABLES

Decongestants

- Sustained-release products should not be used in nursing mothers or in children under 12 years of age.

Antihistamines

Geriatrics

- Antihistamines are more likely to cause excessive sedation, syncope, dizziness, confusion, and hypotension in elderly patients; a decrease in dosage is usually necessary.

Pediatrics

- Antihistamines may diminish mental alertness.

In young children, antihistamines may produce paradoxical excitation in a syndrome that may include excitement, hallucinations, ataxia, incoordination, muscle twitching, athetosis, hyperthermia, cyanosis, tremor, and hyperreflexia, followed by depression and cardiorespiratory arrest.

Convulsions in children may be preceded by mild depression and indicate a poor prognosis. Dry mouth, fever, fixed dilated pupils, and flushing of the face are common. The convulsant dose of antihistamines is near the lethal dose.

Pregnancy

- *Category B:* diphenhydramine, clemastine, chlorpheniramine, cetirizine, and loratadine
- *Category C:* fexofenadine, desloratadine
- Safety for use in pregnancy has not been established. Several possible associations with malformations have been found, but the significance is unknown. Use only when clearly needed and when the potential benefits outweigh the potential risks to the fetus. Do not use during the third trimester of pregnancy; newborn and premature infants may have severe reactions.
- Because of the higher risk of adverse effects for infants in general, particularly newborns and premature infants, antihistamine therapy is contraindicated in nursing mothers.

Intranasal Steroids

Pediatrics

- Use of intranasal corticosteroids in prepubescent children poses a potential risk of growth suppression. Studies with beclomethasone dipropionate used twice daily have shown a significant decrease in growth velocity. This has not been shown in other intranasal steroids (mometasone furoate monohydrate, budesonide, or fluticasone propionate), and it is possible that growth suppression may be associated with certain agents or may be dose related. Children who are currently taking oral inhaled corticosteroids for asthma are at increased risk. When using intranasal steroids in children, use the lowest dosage for a short period of time, and routinely measure growth.

Pregnancy

- *Category C*

Antitussives: Codeine

Geriatrics

- Administer codeine with caution in elderly and debilitated patients and in those with severe liver impairment of kidney function, hypothyroidism, Addison's disease, urethral stricture, or prostatic hypertrophy.

Pediatrics

- Do not use codeine in premature infants; opiates cross the immature blood-brain barrier to a greater extent, producing significant respiratory depression.
- Give to infants and small children with extreme caution and monitor the dosage carefully.

Pregnancy

- *Category C*

Expectorants

Pediatrics

- Caution is recommended in children up to 12 years of age with a persistent or chronic cough, asthma, or if the cough is accompanied by excessive mucus. A medical evaluation should be conducted before treating with expectorants.

Pregnancy

- *Category C*

PATIENT EDUCATION

Decongestants

- Encourage patients to reduce consumption of caffeine-containing beverages (coffee, tea, and cola) as they may increase the restlessness and insomnia caused by pseudoephedrine in sensitive individuals.

Antihistamines

- Antihistamines are used to treat allergy symptoms and should not be used to treat URIs, including colds and sinusitis.
- Do not use alcohol, sleeping pills, sedatives, or tranquilizers while taking antihistamines.
- Antihistamines may have a sedative effect, causing dizziness in some patients. Patients should avoid driving a car or performing hazardous tasks until the effects of the medication are known.
- Antihistamines should be stored in a tightly closed container in a cool, dry place away from heat, sunlight, and out of the reach of children.
- Some antihistamines may cause stomach upset; they should be taken with food.
- Antihistamines may cause photosensitivity; patient should avoid prolonged sunlight exposure.
- Do not crush or chew sustained-release preparations.

Intranasal Steroids

- Use patient information provided with product.
- Do not exceed recommended dosage.
- Clear secretions from nasal passages before using; use decongestants if necessary.
- Effects are not immediate; results require regular use and usually take a few days.

Intranasal Cromolyn

- Clear the nasal passages before administering the spray and inhale through the nose during administration.
- Do not discontinue therapy abruptly without consulting provider.

Antitussives

- Contact health care provider if cough persists for more than 1 week or is accompanied by a high fever, rash, or persistent headache.

Expectorants

- Instruct patient to drink plenty of water to help loosen mucus in the lungs.
- Contact health care provider if cough persists for more than 1 week or is accompanied by a high fever, rash, or persistent headache.

Specific Drugs

DECONGESTANTS

Oral Decongestants

pseudoephedrine hydrochloride (Sudafed, Entex-PSE [with guaifenesin])

Contraindications

- Hypersensitivity to sympathomimetics, severe hypertension, severe coronary artery disease, or in individuals receiving MAOIs
- Nursing mothers because of the higher than usual risks to infants from sympathomimetic drugs

Precautions

- Diabetes, hypertension, cardiovascular disease, or hyperreactivity to ephedrine

Pharmacokinetics

- See Table 16-2
- Distributed to body tissues and fluids, including fetal tissue, breast milk, and the CNS

Adverse Effects

- See Table 16-3

Drug Interactions

- β-Adrenergic blockers and MAOIs may potentiate the effects of decongestants.
- May reduce the antihypertensive effects of guanethidine, mecamylamine, methyldopa, and reserpine.
- Cocaine use with pseudoephedrine may increase the effects of either one of these medicines on the heart and increase the chance of side effects.
- Caffeine use may increase insomnia and restlessness in sensitive individuals.

Overdosage

- Excessive CNS stimulation, resulting in excitement, tremor, restlessness, insomnia, tachycardia, hypertension, pallor, pupil dilation, hyperglycemia, and urinary retention
- Severe overdose may cause hallucinations, convulsions, CNS depression, cardiovascular collapse, and death

Dosage and Administration

- See Table 16-4

TABLE 16-2 Pharmacokinetics of Common Respiratory Medications

Drug	Absorption	Onset of Action	Half-life	Duration of Action	Metabolism	Excretion
pseudoephedrine	GI; completely absorbed in 30 min	6-8 hr	4-6 hr (30 mg)	8 hr (60 mg) 12 hr (extended release)	Liver	50%-75% in urine
phenylephrine	Nasal mucosa	Immediate		30 min to 4 hr	Liver and intestine, if absorbed	
oxymetazoline	Nasal mucosa	Immediate		5-6 hr with decline over 6 hr		
diphenhydramine	GI	15 min	1-4 hr	4-6 hr	Liver	50%-75% metabolites, 1% unchanged in urine
clemastine	GI	25%-40%	30-60 min	2-6 hr	10-24 hr	Urine
chlorpheniramine	GI	25%-40%	30-60 min	2-6 hr	10-24 hr	Unknown; urine 20%-35%, feces 1%

TABLE 16-2 Pharmacokinetics of Common Respiratory Medications—cont'd

Drug	Absorption	Onset of Action	Half-life	Duration of Action	Metabolism	Excretion
triamcinolone	Nasal mucosa	10-16 hr	4 hr	Varies	Unknown	Unknown
beclomethasone	Nasal mucosa/GI tract	Several days-2 wk	Not determined	Varies	Liver/GI/respiratory tract	Not described
fluticasone	Nasal mucosa	12-48 hr	10 hr	1-2 wk	Liver, if absorbed in GI tract	Unknown in intranasal; fecal (oral dose)
cromolyn	Nasal mucosa	Several days-2 wk	Unknown	Varies	Unknown	Unknown
codeine	GI	30-45 min	2.5-4 hr	4-6 hr	Liver	Urine
dextromethorphan	GI	15-30 min		3-6 hr	Liver; 2D6 substrate, 3A4 substrate (CYP)	Urine
benzonatate	GI	15-20 min		3-8 hr	Unknown	Unknown
guaifenesin	GI		1 hr			Urine

TABLE 16-3 Common and Serious Adverse Effects of Respiratory Medications

Drug	Common Side Effects	Serious Adverse Effects
DECONGESTANTS		
pseudoephedrine	Insomnia, tachycardia, palpitations, headache, dizziness, nausea, nervousness, excitability, agitation, anxiety, weakness, tremor, elevated blood pressure	Arrhythmias, severe hypertension
ANTIHISTAMINES		
diphenhydramine	Somnolence, dry mouth, headache, dizziness, nausea, vomiting, diarrhea, cramps, fever	Dyskinesia, thickening of bronchial secretions
cetirizine	Somnolence, dry mouth, fatigue, pharyngitis, dizziness, abdominal pain, nausea/vomiting, diarrhea	Bronchospasm, hepatitis (rare), hypersensitivity (rare)
loratadine	Headache, somnolence, fatigue, dry mouth, nervousness, abdominal pain	Bronchospasm, hepatitis (rare), hypersensitivity (rare)
azelastine (nasal)	Bitter taste, headache, somnolence, weight increase, myalgia, nasal burning, pharyngitis, dry mouth, paroxysmal sneezing, nausea, rhinitis, fatigue, dizziness	No serious reactions reported
INTRANASAL STEROID		
triamcinolone acetonide	Nasal burning, irritation, dryness, rhinorrhea, sneezing, epistaxis, headache, pharyngitis, dry throat, cough, taste changes, lightheadedness, dyspepsia, nasal ulcer, urticaria, pruritus	Nasal septal perforation, growth suppression (pediatrics), angioedema (rare), bronchospasm (rare), nasopharyngeal candidiasis, increased IOP
INTRANASAL CROMOLYN		
cromolyn sodium	Sneezing, nasal burning, epistaxis, bad taste	Bronchospasm
ANTITUSSIVES		
codeine	Nausea, vomiting, constipation, hypotension, drowsiness, dizziness, rash, pruritus	Respiratory depression (at high doses), abuse potential
dextromethorphan	Nausea, sedation, dizziness, abdominal pain, rash	Serotonin syndrome (rare), abuse potential (rare)
benzonatate	Sedation, headache, dizziness, rash, nausea, dyspepsia, pruritus, confusion, nasal congestion, chest numbness, burning eyes, visual hallucinations	Bronchospasm, laryngospasm, cardiovascular collapse
EXPECTORANT		
guaifenesin	Drowsiness, headache, rash, nausea/vomiting	None noted

TABLE 16-4 Dosage and Administration Recommendations for Common Respiratory Medications

Drug	Dosage/Administration
pseudoephedrine	Adults and children >12 yr: 60 mg PO q4-6hr Sustained release: 120 mg PO q12hr
phenylephrine	Adults and children >12 yr (0.25% and 0.5%): 2-3 drops/sprays per nostril q4hr PRN Children 6-12 yr (0.25% solution): 2-3 drops/sprays per nostril q4hr PRN Children 2-6 yr (0.125% or 0.16% solution): 2-3 drops per nostril q4hr PRN
oxymetazoline	Adults and children >6 yr (0.05% solution): 2-3 drops/sprays bid, both nostrils Children 2-4 yr (0.025% solution): 2-3 drops per nostril bid
diphenhydramine	Adults: 25-50 mg PO tid-qid Sleep aid: 50 mg hs Children (>20 lb): 12.5-25 mg PO tid-qid Maximum dose: 300 mg PO
clemastine	Adults and children >12 yr: 1.34-2.68 mg PO bid-tid PRN; maximum dose: 8.04 mg/day
chlorpheniramine	Adults and children >12 yr: 4 mg PO q4-6hr; maximum dose: 24 mg/24 hr; alternate: 8-12 mg SR q12hr Children 6-12 yr: 2 mg PO q4-6hr; maximum dose: 12 mg/24 hr; alternate: 8 mg SR PO q12hr Children 2-6 yr: 1 mg PO q4-6hr
cetirizine	Adults and children >12 yr: 5-10 mg/day PO; maximum dose: 10 mg/day Children 6-12 yr: 5-10 mg PO qd; maximum dose: 10 mg/day Children 2-6 yr: 2.5 mg PO qd; maximum dose 5 mg/day Children 6 mo-2 yr: see prescribing information
fexofenadine	Adults and children >12 yr: 180 mg PO qd; alternate: 60 mg PO bid; renal dose: 60 mg PO qd Children 6-11 yr: 30 mg PO bid; renal dose: 30 mg PO qd
loratadine	Adults and children >12 yr: 10 mg PO qd; renal dosing (adjust dose frequently), creatinine clearance <30: 10 mg PO qod; hepatic dosing (adjust dose frequently): 10 mg PO qod Children >6 yr: 10 mg PO qd; renal dose, creatinine clearance <30: 10 mg qod; hepatic dose: 10 mg PO qod Children 2-5 yr: 5 mg qd; renal dose, creatinine clearance <30: 5 mg PO qod
desloratadine/loratidine	Adults and children >12 yr: 5 mg qd Renal and hepatic dosing (adjust dose frequently): 5 mg PO qod
azelastine	Adults and children >12 yr: 2 sprays per nostril bid Children 5-11 yr: 1 spray per nostril bid
triamcinolone	Adults and children >12 yr: 1-2 sprays per nostril qd; start 2 sprays per nostril qd Children 6-11 yr: 1-2 sprays per nostril qd; maximum dose: 4 sprays/day Adults: 1-2 sprays per nostril qd; start 2 sprays per nostril qd; maximum dose: 4 sprays/day Children 6-12 yr: 1-2 sprays per nostril qd; start 1 spray per nostril qd; maximum dose: 4 sprays/day
beclomethasone	Adults and children >12 yr: 1 spray per nostril bid-qid; alternate: 2 sprays per nostril bid Children 6-12 yr: 1 spray per nostril tid Adults and children >6 yr: 1-2 sprays per nostril bid Children 6-12 yr: start 1 spray per nostril bid Adults and children >6 yr: 1-2 sprays per nostril qd
fluticasone	Adults: 2 spray per nostril qd; alternate: 1 spray per nostril bid; may decrease to 1 spray per nostril qd Children >4 yr: 1-2 sprays per nostril qd
cromolyn	Adults and children >6 yr: 1 spray per nostril tid-qid; maximum dose: 1 spray per nostril 6×/day
codeine	Adults: 10-20 mg q4-6hr or 10 ml PO q4hr; maximum dose: 60 ml/day Children 6-12 yr: 5-10 mg q4-6hr or 5 ml PO q4hr; maximum dose: 30 ml/day Children 2-6 yr: 2.5-5 mg q4-6hr or 1-1.5 mg/kg/day, codeine divided q4-6h; maximum dose: 30 mg/day

TABLE 16-4 Dosage and Administration Recommendations for Common Respiratory Medications—cont'd

Drug	Dosage/Administration
dextromethorphan	Adults and children >12 yr: 10-20 mg q4hr, do not exceed 120 mg/day; alternate: 30 mg PO q6-8hr Children 6-12 yr: 5-10 mg PO q4hr or 15 mg q6-8hr; maximum dose: 60 mg/day Children 2-6 yr: 2.5-5 mg PO q4hr or 7.5 mg PO q6-8hr; maximum dose: 30 mg/day Adults and children >12 yr: 60 mg (2 tsp) PO q12hr; maximum 120 mg/day (4 tsp), sustained action liquid Children 6-12 yr: 30 mg (1 tsp) PO q12hr; maximum dose 60 mg/day (2 tsp); sustained action liquid Children 2-5 yr: 15 mg (½ tsp) q12hr; maximum 30 mg/day (1 tsp)
benzonatate	Adults and children >10 yr: 1 perle or 1 capsule tid PRN; maximum dose: 500 mg/day
guaifenesin	Adults and children >12 yr: 600-1200 mg PO q12hr; maximum dose: 2400 mg/day or 2-4 tsp PO q4hr; maximum dose: 24 tsp/day Children 6-12 yr: 600 mg SR PO q12hr; maximum dose: 1200 mg/day or 1-2 sp PO q4hr; maximum dose: 12 tsp/day Children 2-6 yr: ½-1 tsp PO q4hr; maximum 6 tsp/day Children <2 yr: 2 mg/kg PO q4hr

Topical Nasal Decongestants

Ⓟ Prototype Drug

phenylephrine hydrochloride (Neo-Synephrine, Sinex)

Contraindications
- MAO inhibitor use within 14 days

Precautions
- Severe hypertension or severe coronary artery disease
- Cautious use in thyroid disease, diabetes mellitus, prostatic hypertrophy
- Topical decongestants should be used in acute states and not longer than 3 to 5 days
- Some products may contain sulfites, which can cause allergic reactions in people with sulfite sensitivities

Drug Interactions
- Anticholinergics, β-blockers, central α_2-agonists, linezolid, MAOIs, sortalol, tricyclic antidepressants

Dosage and Administration
- See Table 16-4

Other Drugs in Class

Other drugs in this class are similar to the prototype except as follows.

oxymetazoline (Afrin)

Warning
- Do not use for longer than indicated or rebound congestion may occur.

ANTIHISTAMINES

Ⓟ Prototype Drug

diphenhydramine hydrochloride (Benadryl)

Contraindications
- Newborn or premature infants, nursing mothers, and patients who have exhibited hypersensitivity to antihistamines

Warnings
- Use with caution in patients with a history of lower respiratory disease, including asthma, because the anticholinergic (drying) effects may thicken secretions and impair expectoration.
- Avoid sedating antihistamines in patients who have a history of sleep apnea.
- Use with caution in patients with increased intraocular pressure, hyperthyroidism, cardiovascular disease, and hypertension.

Precautions
- Use with caution in patients with narrow-angle glaucoma, stenosing peptic ulcer, pyloroduodenal obstruction, symptomatic prostatic hypertrophy, or bladder neck obstruction.

Pharmacokinetics
See Table 16-5.

Adverse Effects
See Table 16-3.

Drug Interactions
- Additive effects with alcohol and other CNS depressants and sedatives.

Overdosage
- CNS depression to stimulation; stimulation is more common in children, whereas in adults, CNS depression, ranging from drowsiness to coma, is more common.
- Coma, cardiovascular collapse, and death may occur.
- Deaths have been reported, particularly in infants and children.

Dosage and Administration
See Table 16-4.

Other Drugs in Class

Other drugs in this class are similar to the prototype except as follows.

clemastine fumarate (Tavist)

Warnings
- Safety and efficacy have not been established in children under the age of 12 and in pregnancy.
- Has an additive effect with alcohol and other CNS depressants and is likely to cause dizziness, sedation, and hypotension in the elderly.

chlorpheniramine maleate (Chlor-Trimeton)

Contraindications
- Narrow-angle glaucoma, prostatic hypertrophy, stenosing peptic ulcer, pyloroduodenal obstruction, bladder neck obstruction
- MAOIs
- Newborn or premature infants

Warnings
- May impair mental alertness; use with caution when performing potentially hazardous tasks or activities.
- Do not administer to infants and children under the age of 6 years.
- May cause inhibition of lactation.

Adverse Effects
- Slight-to-moderate drowsiness is the most common side effect.
- Other possible side effects are similar to those of diphenhydramine; see Table 16-3.

Drug Interactions
- Similar to other antihistamines—MAOIs, alcohol, CNS depressants

cetirizine hydrochloride (Zyrtec)

Contraindications
- Hypersensitivity to hydroxyzine

Precautions
- May produce somnolence in some patients and is considered a low-sedating antihistamine.
- Caution should be exercised when driving or operating dangerous machinery.
- Use caution with concurrent use with alcohol or other CNS depressants.
- Use caution if impaired liver or kidney function present.

Adverse Effects
- Most adverse effects reported with use of cetirizine were mild or moderate.

Drug Interactions
- A small decrease in the clearance of cetirizine was caused by a 400-mg dose of theophylline. Larger doses of theophylline could possibly have a greater effect. No significant interactions were noted with low doses of theophylline, azithromycin, pseudoephedrine, ketoconazole, or erythromycin.
- MAOIs

Overdosage
- Overdosage was reported in one patient taking 150 mg of cetirizine. Somnolence was reported without other abnormal clinical or hematology results.

Dosage and Administration
- Renal dosing: adjust dose amount according to creatinine clearance: <30, give 5 mg PO
- Hepatic dosing: 5 mg PO qd
- See Table 16-4

fexofenadine hydrochloride (Allegra)

- Fexofenadine has a similar clinical profile to other nonsedating antihistamines.
- No significant drug interactions are noted, and serious hypersensitivity reactions are rare.
- Renal dosing should be adjusted frequently.

Miscellaneous Antihistamines

loratadine (Claritin)

- Loratadine is a long-acting tricyclic antihistamine with selective peripheral histamine H_1 receptor antagonistic activity.

Contraindications
- Hypersensitivity to this medication or any of its ingredients

Precautions
- Patients with liver disease should receive a lower dose (10 mg every other day) because of reduced clearance of loratadine
- Impaired renal function
- Use cautiously in nursing mothers
- Safety and effectiveness of use in children under 12 years of age has not been established

Dosage and Administration
- Renal dosing: Adjust dose frequently
- Hepatic dosing: Adjust dose frequently
- See Table 16-4

TABLE 16-5 Pharmacokinetics of Prescribed Antihistamines

Drug	Absorption	Onset of Action	Time to Peak Concentration	Half-Life	Duration of Action	Protein Bound	Metabolism	Excretion
cetirizine (Zyrtec)	20 min-1 hr	1 hr	8.3 hr	24 hr		93%	Liver, partially	Urine, 70%; feces, 80%
fexofenadine HCl (Allegra)	30 min	1-3 hr	1-3 hr	14.4 hr	12 hr	69.4%	Liver, negligible; biliary; renal	Urine, 11%; feces, 80%
loratadine (Claritin)	Enhanced with food	1 hr	1-2 hr	3-20 hr	24+hr	97%	Liver	Urine, 20%; feces, 80%
desloratadine (Clarinex)		1 hr	3 hr	27 hr	24 hr	82%-87%	Liver	Urine and feces
azelastine (Astelin)	40% Systemic absorption	1 hr	2-3 hr	22 hr	4-12 hr	88%	Cytochrome P450	Feces, 75%

desloratadine (Clarinex)

- See Tables 16-4 and 16-5 for specific information regarding dosage and administration recommendations and pharmacokinetics.
- This medication is not recommended for children under 12 years of age.

Intranasal Antihistamines

azelastine (Astelin)

Contraindications
- Known hypersensitivity

Precautions
- Use cautiously if lactating

Dosage and Administration
- Available in 137 μg/spray; see Table 16-4.

Patient Education
- Patients should be instructed to prime the delivery system before initial use and after storage for 3 days or longer.
- Patients should also be instructed to store the bottle upright at room temperature with the pump tightly closed and out of the reach of children.
- Use instructions with package.

INTRANASAL STEROIDS

Ⓟ Prototype Drug

triamcinolone acetonide (Nasacort)

See Chapter 17 for additional details.

Contraindications
- Untreated localized infection
- Hypersensitivity to the drug or a product component
- Ocular HSV infection

Precautions
- Use cautiously in patients with tuberculosis, systemic infection, nasal septal ulcers, or nasal trauma or surgery.
- Localized infections with *Candida albicans* may develop. Treat infection with proper antiinfective therapy.

Dosage and Administration
- Triamcinolone acetonide is supplied as a non-aqueous suspension aerosol nasal inhalation (Nasacort), and aqueous nasal suspension/solution spray (Nasacort AQ)—see Table 16-4 for dosages.
- If the spray pump containing the aqueous suspension or solution is not used for more than 2 weeks, it may need to be partially primed (1 actuation for the suspension and 3 actuations or until a fine mist is observed for the solution).
- The nasal aqueous solution spray pump requires priming—see package insert for instructions.

Other Drugs in Class

Other drugs in this class are similar to the prototype except as follows.

beclomethasone dipropionate (Beconase, Vancenase)

- Has a significant systemic effect, especially on growth in children, as a result of the pharmacokinetics of this older agent.
- Undergoes a low degree of first-pass inactivation (40% to 50%), resulting in a higher posthepatic bioavailability.

fluticasone propionate (Flonase)

- Fluticasone is a very potent nasal corticosteroid. Some studies have compared various intranasal corticosteroids, and results suggest that fluticasone has the potential for more dosage-related systemic effects than other intranasal corticosteroids. It has been shown to suppress systemic markers such as serum and urinary cortisol and serum osteocalcin in adults. Fluticasone suppresses urinary cortisol in children. Compared with triamcinolone, budesonide, and mometasone, fluticasone shows significant adrenal suppression (Lipworth, 2002).

INTRANASAL CROMOLYN

cromolyn sodium (Nasalcrom)

See Chapter 17 for additional information.

Contraindications
- Hypersensitivity to drug or product components

Warnings/Precautions
- Intranasal cromolyn is not to be used for treatment of acute symptoms.

Adverse Effects
- Nasal stinging or sneezing may be experienced. This is rarely a significant problem.
- See Table 16-3.

ANTITUSSIVES

Narcotic Antitussives

codeine phosphate

- Codeine is a narcotic used for suppression of cough caused by chemical or respiratory tract irritation. Codeine acts on the cough center in the medulla to elevate the threshold for cough, and codeine is often combined with other medications (i.e., guaifenesin) in a syrup or elixir.
- See Chapter 44 for details.

Contraindications
- Hypersensitivity
- Use in children under age 2
- Respiratory depression
- Coma

Warnings
- Codeine may be habit forming; psychological and physical dependence and tolerance may occur.
- Codeine may impair the mental and/or physical ability to perform potentially hazardous tasks. Use caution when driving or performing tasks requiring alertness, coordination, or physical dexterity.
- In some ambulatory patients, codeine may produce orthostatic hypotension, dry mouth, and constipation and may cause stomach upset. Take with food or milk.

Precautions
- Use with caution in patients with the following:
  - Head trauma and increased intracranial pressure—the respiratory depressant effects of narcotics and their capacity to elevate cerebrospinal fluid pressure may be exaggerated in these conditions.
  - Patients with seizure disorders
  - Asthma patients
  - Acute abdominal pain
- Use with caution in elderly and debilitated patients and those with severe liver or kidney impairment, hypothyroidism, Addison's disease, and prostatic hypertrophy or urethral stricture.
- Codeine may have a prolonged cumulative effect in patients with liver or kidney dysfunction.

Drug Interactions
- Additive depressant effects occur when used in combination with other narcotic analgesics, phenothiazines, tranquilizers, sedative-hypnotics, antidepressants, alcohol, or other CNS depressants. When used in combination, the dosage of one or both agents should be reduced.
- Caution is advised with using with sedating antihistamines as they may increase the risk of CNS depression and may potentiate opiate analgesic efficacy.

Overdosage
- Serious overdose with codeine is characterized by respiratory depression, extreme somnolence progressing to stupor or coma, skeletal muscle flaccidity, bradycardia, hypotension, and cool, clammy skin. In severe overdoses, apnea, circulatory collapse, cardiac arrest, and death may occur.

Dosage and Administration
- Codeine is combined with guaifenesin as an antitussive syrup, with 10 mg codeine/100 mg guaifenesin/5 ml.
- See Table 16-4.

How to Monitor
- Monitor for effectiveness and excessive side effects, especially constipation in the elderly.

Patient Education
- Narcotic antitussives such as codeine may impair mental and physical abilities. Patients should be cautioned to avoid performing potentially hazardous tasks, such as driving or operating heavy machinery.

Nonnarcotic Antitussives

dextromethorphan hydrobromide (Robitussin DM)

Contraindications
- Hypersensitivity to any component.
- MAOI or MAOI use within 14 days.

Warnings
- Administration of dextromethorphan may be accompanied by histamine release, and the drug should be used cautiously in atopic children.
- According to the World Health Organization (WHO) Expert Committee on Drug Dependence, dextromethorphan can

produce very slight psychic dependence but no physical dependence.
- Do not use for persistent or chronic cough or where cough is accompanied by excessive secretions. Persons with a high fever, rash, persistent headache, nausea, or vomiting should use the drug only under medical supervision.

Precautions
- Use with caution in sedated or debilitated patients and in patients confined to the supine position.
- Lozenges containing dextromethorphan hydrobromide should not be used in children younger than 6 years of age.

Drug Interactions
- The drug may interact with antidepressants—combination may increase risk of serotonin syndrome.
- Avoid use with furazolidone, meperidine, and sibutramine.

Overdosage
- CNS excitement, mental confusion, and respiratory depression (in high doses) are signs of overdosage. Toxic psychosis was reported after ingestion of 20 tablets (300 mg) of dextromethorphan.

Dosage and Administration
- Dextromethorphan 15 to 30 mg is equal to 8 to 15 mg of codeine as an antitussive.

benzonatate (Tessalon Perles)

Contraindications
- Hypersensitivity to benzonatate or related compounds (e.g., tetracaine, procaine)

Warnings
- Do not chew or break capsules, swallow whole.
- Severe hypersensitivity reactions (including bronchospasm, laryngospasm, and cardiovascular collapse) have been reported that are possibly related to local anesthesia effects from chewing or sucking the perle.
- Severe reactions have required intervention with vasopressor agents and supportive measures.

Precautions
- Release of benzonatate in the mouth can produce a temporary local anesthesia of the oral mucosa that could cause choking

Overdosage
- CNS stimulation may cause restlessness and tremors that may proceed to clonic convulsions, followed by profound CNS depression. Overdose may result in death.

Patient Education
- Do not chew or break capsules, swallow whole.

EXPECTORANTS

guaifenesin (Robitussin, Humibid LA)

Contraindications
- Hypersensitivity

Warnings
- Not for use in persistent coughs that occur with smoking, asthma, or emphysema or in coughs with excessive secretions

Drug/Laboratory Test Interactions
- Guaifenesin may increase renal clearance of urate and thereby lower serum uric acid levels.
- Guaifenesin may produce an increase in urinary 5-hydroxyindoleacetic acid and therefore may interfere with the interpretation of this test for the diagnosis of carcinoid syndrome.
- It may falsely elevate the vanillylmandelic acid (VMA) test for catechols.
- Administration of these products should be discontinued 48 hours before collection of urine specimens for such tests.

RESOURCES FOR PATIENTS AND PROVIDERS

American Medical Association, www.ama-assn.org/kidshealth
Provides information on treating kids with asthma.

Managing Your Health, www.hmri.com/
Offers basic patient information on managing your health; has a link to Hoechst Marion Roussel, Inc. AllerDays website, which provides generic allergy information and patient education information available free by calling (800) 824-2896.

Medscape Allergy and Immunology, www.medscape.com/allergy-immunologyhome

University of Utah pathology slides, www-medlib.med.utah.edu/WebPath/ORGAN.html#1info@aafa.org

American Asthma and Allergy Foundation, www.aafa.org, or contact them at AAFA, 1233 20th Street NW, Suite 402, Washington, DC 20036.
They have a nationwide network of chapters and educational support groups. They have Advance, a bimonthly patient newsletter filled with practical tips and the latest news and information. They also have medically reviewed education materials for children, teens, and adults.

BIBLIOGRAPHY

Crisalida T, Kaliner M, Turkeltaub M, editors: *Allergy and asthma pocket guide*, New York, 2002, Adelphi.

Ferguson BJ: Acute and chronic sinusitis: how to ease symptoms and locate the cause, *Postgrad Med* 97:45, 1995.

Goodkin J, editor: Treatment of allergic rhinitis and asthma, *Patient Care Nurse Pract* Fall 2001 (suppl).

Hayden ML, Hendeles L, Ortiz G: *Diagnostic challenges in allergic rhinitis. The changing face of allergic rhinitis: new pieces in the clinical picture*, Monograph 1, Chicago, 2001, Pragmation Office of Medical Education.

Hayden ML, Hendeles L, Ortiz G: *Improving the outcomes of allergic rhinitis treatment. The changing face of allergic rhinitis: new pieces in the clinical picture,* Monograph 2, Chicago, 2001, Pragmation Office of Medical Education.

Kirkpatrick GL: The common cold, *Primary Care* 23:657, 1996.

Lipworth B: Intranasal corticosteroids in allergic rhinitis: safety issues considered, *Respir Dig* 4:13-16, 2002.

Middleton E et al: *Allergy: principles and practice,* ed 5, St Louis, 1998, Mosby.

Pedinoff AJ: Approaches to the treatment of seasonal allergic rhinitis, *Med J* 89:1130, 1996.

Self T, Alloway RR: Treatment of rhinitis, *J Am Acad Nur Pract* 8:135, 1996.

CHAPTER 17

Asthma and COPD Medications

Sandra M. Nettina

Drug Names

Class	Subclass		Generic Name	Trade Name
Short-acting relatively selective β_2-adrenergic agonists		(P) (200)	albuterol (aerosol and tablets)	Proventil, Ventolin, Volmax
			bitolterol mesylate	Tornalate
			levalbuterol	Xopenex
			pirbuterol	Maxair
			terbutaline sulfate	Brethaire, Brethine, Bricanyl
Long-acting relatively selective β_2-adrenergic agonists		(200)	salmeterol xinafoate	Serevent
			formoterol fumarate	Foradil
Methylxanthines		(P)	theophylline	Theo-Dur, Theolair, Slo-bid, Slo-Phyllin
Anticholinergics			ipratropium bromide	Atrovent
Mast cell stabilizers		(P)	cromolyn sodium	Intal
			nedocromil sodium	Tilade
Corticosteroids	Aerosols	(P) (200)	beclomethasone dipropionate	Beclovent, Vanceril, Vancenase
			flunisolide	Aerobid
		(200)	fluticasone	Flovent
			budesonide	Pulmicort
			trimcinolone acetate	Azmacort
	Oral solutions/tablets (see Chapter 52 for details)	(200)	prednisone	Liquid Pred, Deltasone
			prednisolone	Delta-Cortef, Prelone
		(200)	methylprednisolone	Medrol
Leukotriene receptor antagonists		(P) (200)	montelukast	Singulair
			zafirlukast	Accolate
			zileuton	Zyflo
Combination products			albuterol/ipratropium	Combivent
		(200)	fluticasone/salmeterol	Advair

(200), Top 200 drug; (P), prototype drug.

General Uses

Indications

See Table 17-1.

- Asthma
- Chronic obstructive pulmonary disease (COPD)

Unlabeled Uses. Terbutaline, a β_2-adrenergic agonist, is available for emergency management of asthma in subcutaneous form. This is the only form of terbutaline in use, and the drug is not discussed further.

The anticholinergic ipratropium is used as a bronchodilator in patients with asthma who do not tolerate β_2-adrenergic agonists. Inhaled corticosteroids are used as maintenance therapy in patients with COPD, if a trial proves effective. Oral corticosteroids may be used in severe exacerbations of COPD.

• • •

Six classes of medications that work via different mechanisms of action are used in the treatment of asthma and COPD. Each of these six groups is discussed in detail as part of the treatment of asthma or COPD. These drugs are also used in the treatment of a wide variety of other respiratory disorders.

The standards of care for patients with asthma were developed by the National Asthma Education and Prevention Program (NAEPP) Expert Panel Report 2 (ERP2) and NAEPP ERP Update on Selected Topics 2002. Guidelines for standard of care management of COPD can be found in the National Heart, Lung, and Blood Institute–World Health Organization Global Initiative for Chronic Obstructive Lung Disease (GOLD) Executive Summary (2001).

DISEASE PROCESS: ASTHMA

Asthma and COPD are similar in their chronicity and obstructive component. However, asthma differs from COPD in that

TABLE 17-1 Indications for Asthma and COPD Medications

Drug	Indication
Beta agonists	Relief and prevention of bronchospasm in patients with reversible obstructive airway disease in both asthma and COPD
Short-acting:	Acute attacks of bronchospasm
albuterol, salmeterol, and formoterol	Prevention of exercise-induced bronchospasm
Long-acting: β-agonists	Maintenance treatment of asthma
Methylxanthines	Symptomatic relief or prevention of asthma, especially nocturnal symptoms, and reversible bronchospasm associated with COPD
Anticholinergics	Maintenance treatment of bronchospasm associated with COPD
Mast cell stabilizers cromolyn sodium	Prophylaxis of asthma Prevention of exercise-induced bronchospasm
Inhaled corticosteroids	Control of asthma when necessary and moderate COPD
Oral corticosteroids	Short-term management of various inflammatory and allergic disorders such as asthma
Leukotriene antagonists	Prophylaxis and chronic treatment of asthma and allergic rhinitis

TABLE 17-2 Location and Response of Adrenoreceptors

Location	Type	Example of Stimulus Response
Lung (smooth muscle)	α	Mild bronchoconstriction
	β_2	Bronchodilation; dilates arteries; relation of alveolar walls
Mast cells	α	Augments release of histamine and other inflammatory mediators
	β_2	Inhibits release of inflammatory mediators
Heart	β_1	Increases myocardial contraction, force, and volocity; stimulates glycogenolysis
Blood vessels	α	Constriction of most vessels
	β_1, β_2	Dilation of most vessels
Skeletal muscle	β_2	Tremor; stimulates glycogenolysis
Multiple	α	Stimulates glycogenolysis; inhibits norepinephrine and acetylcholine relase
	β_1	Stimulates lipolysis
	β_2	Stimulates norepinephrine release; inhibits acetylcholine release; moves potassium into cells; stimulates insulin release
Eyes (smooth muscle)	α	Mydriasis

Modified from Lees GM: A hitchhiker's guide to the galaxy of adrenoreceptors, *Br Med J* 283:173-178, 1981.

asthma is largely an inflammatory condition with a greater degree of reversibility than COPD. Although the same drugs are used in treatment, asthma and COPD are discussed separately because their responses to pharmacotherapy differ.

Anatomy and Physiology

The respiratory bronchiole is surrounded by smooth muscle and is lined by pseudostratified columnar epithelium containing mucus-secreting goblet cells and cilia. The smooth muscle is innervated by the autonomic nervous system. Parasympathetic stimulation through the vagus nerve and cholinergic receptors in smooth muscle increase bronchial constriction. Sympathetic stimulation through the action of catecholamines such as epinephrine on β_2-adrenergic receptors causes bronchodilation. When there is a need for increased airflow, as in exercise, sympathetic stimulation causes bronchodilation and the bronchoconstrictor tone is inhibited.

The lungs also contain α-adrenergic receptors, and their stimulation results in mild bronchoconstriction. There are no β_1-adrenergic receptors in the lungs. β_1-Adrenergic receptors are the predominant adrenergic receptors of the heart. Their stimulation increases myocardial contractility and conduction, resulting in an increased heart rate (Table 17-2).

Pathophysiology

The key features of asthma are (1) airway hyperresponsiveness, (2) airway inflammation, and (3) airway obstruction that is largely, but not always fully, reversible.

Airway hyperresponsiveness: Triggers include allergens, usually inhaled, aspirin and related nonsteroidal antiinflammatory drugs (NSAIDs), cold air, exercise, airway irritants (i.e., cigarette smoke and air pollution), respiratory infections, and emotional stress. Conditions such as gastroesophageal reflux disease (GERD), chronic sinusitis, and rhinitis exacerbate asthma.

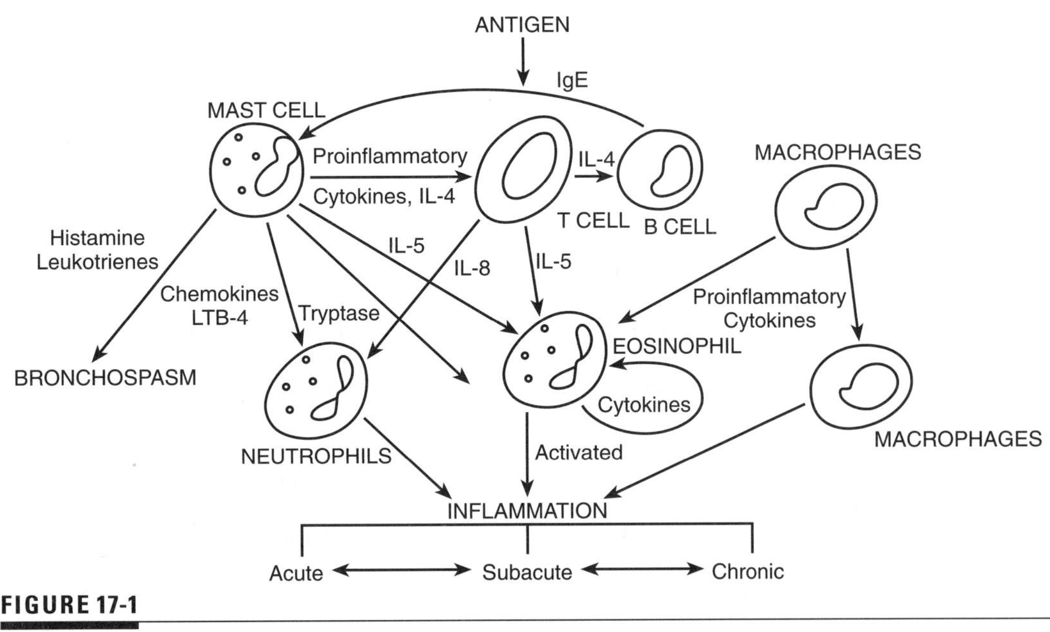

FIGURE 17-1

Cellular mechanisms involved in airway inflammation. (From Expert Panel Report 2: *Guidelines for the diagnosis and management of asthma,* Washington, DC, 1997, US Government Printing Office.)

Airway inflammation: On exposure to an inhaled antigen, mast cells, eosinophils, epithelial cells, macrophages, and activated T cells are released. The chemical mediators they release are cytokines, chemokines, histamine, prostaglandins, and leukotrienes (LTs). Their response in the airways is bronchospasm and inflammation (Figure 17-1); see Chapter 70 on the immune system for more detail.

Airway obstruction: Bronchoconstriction causes the forced expiratory volume in 1 second (FEV_1) to decrease. Inflammatory processes occur within the bronchiole, causing epithelial injury. Chronic inflammation can lead to airway remodeling, thickening of goblet cells and mucus hypersecretion, thickening of the basement membrane by collagen deposition, and hypertrophy of smooth muscle, which all lead to airway obstruction. Thus asthma symptoms may not be reversible.

The Disease

Asthma is the result of complex interactions among inflammatory cells, chemical mediators, and the airways. Asthma is classified based on symptomatology and pulmonary function tests (PFTs); this classification forms a basis for step therapy.

1. *Intermittent:* Less than two daytime symptoms per week, less than two nighttime symptoms per month, peak expiratory flow (PEF) at 80% or more of predicted value, and PEF variability from awakening to before bedtime of less than 20%.
2. *Mild persistent:* More than two daytime symptoms per week but not daily, more than two nighttime symptoms per month, PEF at greater than 80% predicted value, and PEF variability between 20% and 30%.
3. *Moderate persistent:* Daily daytime symptoms, more than one night time symptom per week, PEF between 60% and 80% of predicted, and more than 30% variability in PEF.
4. *Severe persistent:* Continuous daytime symptoms, frequent nighttime symptoms, PEF less than 60% of predicted, and PEF variability more than 30%.

A patient need only have one criterion to move into a new severity rating; thus patients should be reevaluated frequently to determine if the severity has increased or decreased. Signs of worsening asthma may be increased cough, greater degree of breathlessness, the occurrence of wheezing, and increased chest tightness. Use of accessory muscles of respiration and suprasternal retractions indicate severe exacerbation.

Symptoms consist of expiratory wheezing, breathlessness, chest tightness, and nonproductive cough. Patients complain of a feeling of air hunger and breathe more rapidly. The chest should be assessed for deformity, use of accessory muscles, wheezing, and prolonged forced expiration. Wheezing may be absent between episodes of asthma as well as during severe airflow limitation.

Asthma is difficult to diagnose in infants and children younger than 5. Viral respiratory infection is the most common cause of asthma symptoms in this age group.

PFTs, known as spirometry, measure the forced vital capacity (FVC) and the FEV_1 to contribute to the diagnosis and monitoring of asthma. Reduced FVC and FEV_1/FVC values relative to predicted values for the patient's height, age, and sex indicate airflow obstruction. Reversibility can be determined by 12% or greater increase in FEV_1 following inhalation of a short-acting bronchodilator. PEF measurement with an inexpensive handheld meter may be measured twice a day after awakening and then before the midpoint of the day to show variability of 20% or greater with asthma.

DISEASE PROCESS: CHRONIC OBSTRUCTIVE PULMONARY DISEASE

Anatomy and Physiology

Alveoli are thin-walled sacs separated by septa and surrounded by a network of capillaries to facilitate gas exchange. Diffusion of gases across the alveolar capillary membrane can be affected by concentration of oxygen; condition of the lung tissue, which affects the surface area available for diffusion; and thickness of the alveolar capillary membrane.

Pathophysiology

There are several mechanisms involved in the pathogenesis of COPD, including inflammation, edema, fibrosis of the bronchial wall, hypertrophy of submucosal glands and hypersecretion of mucus, loss of elastic lung fibers, and destruction of alveolar tissue. Tobacco smoking or some other noxious stimuli produce an inflammatory response throughout the lungs, including the parenchyma and vasculature. Inflammatory cells invade the area and secrete numerous mediators, including tumor necrosis factor (TNF), interleukin 8, and LTB_4. The larger airways (trachea, bronchi, and bronchioles larger than 2 mm) respond by increasing mucus-secreting glands and reducing mucociliary function. The smaller airways (bronchioles smaller than 2 mm) go through repeated cycles of injury and repair, resulting in remodeling, scaring, thickening, and consolidation. This results in increased airflow resistance as evidenced by FEV_1 and FEV_1/FVC measurements.

As lung parenchyma is destroyed, elastic recoil is lost, reducing the force of expiratory airflow and causing hyperinflation. Hyperinflation leads to lowering and flattening of the diaphragm and barrel chest, which reduce respiratory muscle strength. Loss of alveoli decreases surface area available for gas exchange. Changes in the vasculature of the lungs due to the remodeling process can eventually lead to pulmonary hypertension, cor pulmonale, and severe hypoxia and hypercapnia.

The Disease

COPD has been redefined in the GOLD guidelines (2001) as a disease state characterized by airflow limitation that is not fully reversible, and airflow limitation is usually both progressive and associated with an abnormal inflammatory response of the lungs to noxious particles or gases.

Assessment

Four stages of severity of COPD have been identified:

- Stage 0 (at risk for COPD): Normal spirometry, chronic symptoms may be present
- Stage I (mild COPD): FEV_1/FVC <70%, FEV_1 >80% of predicted, with or without chronic symptoms
- Stage II (moderate COPD): FEV_1/FVC <70%, FEV_1 30% to 80% of predicted, usually symptomatic, often have shortness of breath with exertion
  - Stage IIa: FEV_1 50% to 80% of predicted
  - Stage IIb: FEV_1 30% to 50% of predicted
- Stage III (severe COPD): FEV_1 <30% of predicted, or FEV_1 <50% of predicted plus respiratory failure or right heart failure

Any stage of COPD may be marked by exacerbation of varying severity, but exacerbation is more common in those patients with FEV_1 <50% of predicted value. Many exacerbations are due to respiratory infection or exposure to air pollution, but in about one half of cases, the cause of exacerbation cannot be identified.

The earliest symptom of COPD is often morning cough with sputum that is clear to yellow. Frequent respiratory infections increase the coughing, often turn the sputum yellow or green, and result in periods of wheezing. Later, shortness of breath develops with exertion and becomes progressively more severe. On auscultation, expiration may be prolonged, expiratory wheezing is often present, and crackles may be audible.

Spirometry is the gold standard to make the diagnosis of COPD and determine severity. An FEV_1 measurement and an FEV_1/FVC ratio are determined before and after bronchodilator therapy to make the diagnosis. COPD causes a progressive decline in FEV_1, FVC, and FEV_1/FVC measurements to a greater degree than would be expected with an age-related decline in lung function. Individuals with COPD fail to improve with bronchodilators, unlike asthma patients.

An arterial blood gas measurement is made if the FEV_1 is <50% of the predicted value. Pulse oximetry to measure O_2 saturation in the blood is more easily carried out and can be used for monitoring during rest, activity, and sleep. A chest x-ray film will show hyperinflation of the lungs and flattening of the diaphragm in advanced COPD.

DRUG ACTION AND EFFECTS

β-Adrenergic Agonist Bronchodilators

β-Adrenergic agonists are sympathomimetics. The basic action of the β-agonists is to activate the enzyme adenyl cyclase, which increases the production of cAMP. Intracellular cAMP inhibits phosphorylation of myosin and lowers intracellular concentrations of calcium. The result is smooth muscle relaxation. Bronchodilation reduces airway resistance as shown by increased FEV_1, mid-expiratory flow rate, and vital capacity. Increased cAMP also inhibits the release of mediators from mast cells in the airways.

Nonselective β_2-adrenergic receptor agonists and, to a lesser extent, the relatively selective β_2-adrenergic agonists cause tachycardia by stimulating the β_2-receptors to increase heart rate. Albuterol and the other bronchodilators that are relatively β_2 selective have their greatest effect on β-adrenergic receptors in the bronchial, uterine, and vascular smooth muscles. Bronchodilators developed to date are only relatively selective in stimulating β_2-receptors, and all have the common side effects of increased heart rate and muscle tremor. At higher doses, the selective drugs may lose their receptor selectivity and cause β_1 stimulation. Another problem with β_2-adrenergic agonists is potential tolerance due to downregulation of β-adrenergic receptors with increased use.

Methylxanthines

Methylxanthines cause bronchodilation by competitively inhibiting phosphodiesterase, the enzyme that degrades cAMP, which in turn increases intracellular cAMP. (See β-Adrenergic Agonist Bronchodilators [above] for the action of increased cAMP.) Methylxanthines also act as a direct central nervous system stimulant resulting in vasoconstriction and stimulation of the vagal center, which causes bradycardia. Stimulation of the medulla results in lowering of the respiratory threshold to carbon dioxide, which increases the rate and depth of respiration if respirations are depressed. Cerebral vasoconstriction may decrease cerebral blood flow and increase carbon dioxide tension, which also stimulates respirations in some patients.

Methylxanthines in large doses have a positive inotropic effect on the myocardium and a positive chronotropic effect on the sinoatrial node, causing transient increase in heart rate, force of contraction, cardiac output, and myocardial oxygen demand. At high concentrations, vagal stimulation is masked by increased sinus rate and may result in hypotension, extrasystoles, and arrhythmias. Additional effects of methylxanthines include diuresis through dilation of renal arterioles, increased cardiac output, and inhibition of reabsorption of sodium and potassium in the proximal renal tubules. The gastrointestinal system is affected by relaxation of smooth muscle, causing reduced lower esophageal sphincter pressure and relaxed biliary contraction and the stimulation of gastric secretions.

Anticholinergics

Similar to atropine and other anticholinergics, ipratropium is a nonselective competitive antagonist of muscarinic receptors present in the airways and other organs. The drug blocks acetylcholine-induced stimulation of cyclic guanyl cyclase, thereby reducing production of cyclic guanosine monophosphate (cGMP), a mediator of bronchoconstriction. Airway resistance is reduced, as measured by increases in FEV_1 and the middle half of forced expiratory flow (FEF_{25-75}). Ipratropium may be more effective in COPD because it is believed that cholinergic tone of the airways is increased in COPD.

Ipratropium exhibits greater antimuscarinic effect on bronchial smooth muscle than on secretory glands, especially with oral inhalation of the drug. Additional antimuscarinic effects may include mydriasis, inhibition of salivary and gastric secretions, tachycardia, and spasmolysis; however, clinical trials have shown these effects to be insignificant in healthy individuals and those with COPD.

Mast Cell Stabilizers

Mast cell stabilizers prevent and reduce the inflammatory response in bronchial walls by inhibiting secretion of mediators from mast cells.

The exact mechanism of action of these drugs on mast cells remains to be established. This drug class acts locally to inhibit the release of mediators of type 1 allergic reactions, including histamine and LTs from sensitized mast cells following exposure to an antigen. They also inhibit type III (late) reactions to a lesser extent. These drugs are antiasthmatic and antiallergic, and they may also act as bronchodilators.

Corticosteroids

Corticosteroids are hormonal agents that have a profound anti-inflammatory effect, which acts to reduce airflow obstruction in the bronchioles.

Corticosteroids modify the body's immune responses to diverse stimuli. Corticosteroids suppress cytokine production, airway eosinophil recruitment, and the release of inflammatory mediators. Inhaled corticosteroids provide local therapeutic action with minimal systemic effects. (See Chapter 53 for discussion of mechanism of action in detail.)

Leukotriene Modifiers

Leukotriene (LT) modifiers act on inflammatory mediators of asthma, the LTs (also known as slow-reacting substance of anaphylaxis [SRS-A]), which contribute to airway obstruction.

Cysteinyl LTs (cysLTs) are more potent and longer-acting bronchoconstrictors than histamine. They are produced in a variety of cells (eosinophils, mast cells, basophils, macrophages, and monocytes), from arachidonic acid through several enzyme pathways (Figure 17-2). Arachidonic acid is

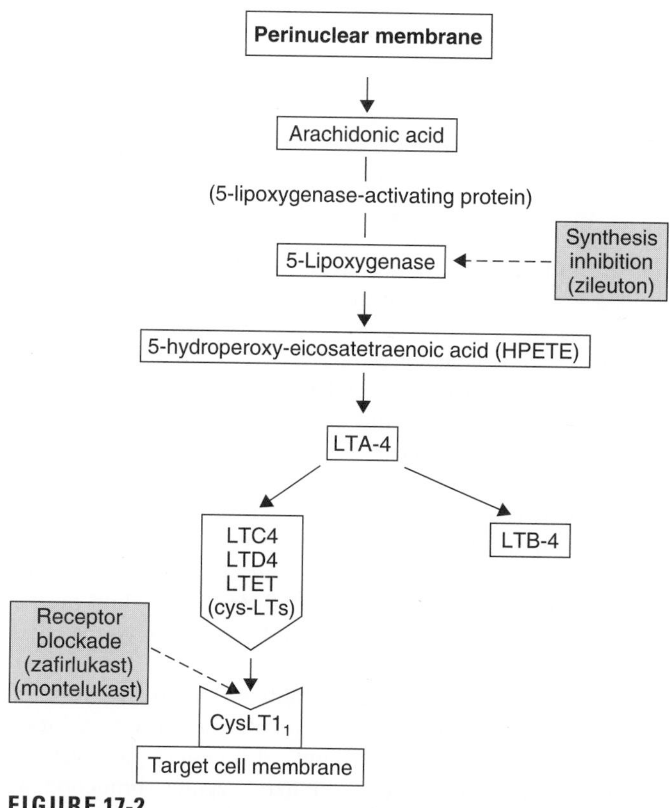

FIGURE 17-2

The action of 5-LO inhibitors and leukotriene receptor antagonists on the production of leukotrienes through the 5-LO pathway. (From Altinger JA: Leukotriene receptor antagonists, *Lippincott's Primary Care Practice* 2(6):634-642, 1998.)

released from cell membranes in response to antigen–antibody reactions, IgE receptor activation, microorganisms, and physical stimuli. LTs enhance responsiveness of the airways to a variety of stimuli and stimulate mucus secretion in the airways. Zafirlukast and montelukast are potent competitive leukotriene receptor antagonists (LTRAs). They block the action of the cysLTs at receptor sites on smooth muscle cells throughout the bronchioles. A single type of receptor is able to mediate profound contraction brought about by the cysLTs. LTRAs prevent the binding of LTs to their receptors in the airways, thereby blocking bronchospasm. Zileuton is a 5-lipoxygenase (5-LO) pathway inhibitor. 5-LO is one of the pathways through which arachidonic acid can be metabolized to form LTs. The effect of both types of drugs is inhibition of the acute bronchoconstriction phase and inhibition of the delayed inflammatory phase of asthma. Bronchodilation with improved FEV_1 and reduced markers of airway inflammation (particularly eosinophils) is the result.

DRUG TREATMENT PRINCIPLES

Asthma Medications

- Long-term control
  - Corticosteroids (inhaled, occasionally systemic)
  - Mast cell stabilizers
  - LTRAs
  - Long-acting β_2-agonists
  - Methylxanthines

- Quick relief
  - Short-acting β_2-agonists
  - Anticholinergics
  - Systemic corticosteroids

The NAEPP EPR guidelines (Tables 17-3 and 17-4) present a stepwise pharmacologic approach that corresponds to the severity of asthma in patients of all ages. The goals of therapy are to gain and maintain long-term control of asthma and to quickly and successfully treat asthma exacerbations. *Control of asthma* is defined as prevention of chronic and troublesome symptoms, maintenance of normal or near-normal pulmonary function, maintenance of normal exercise and activity levels, prevention of recurrent exacerbations, avoidance of adverse effects from drug therapy, and satisfaction of patient and family expectations for asthma care.

Referral to or consultation with an asthma specialist is indicated if there is difficulty maintaining control, if step 4 therapy is needed by the adult or child over 5 years, or if step 3 or 4 therapy is needed by the infant or young child. Referral or consultation may also be considered if the adult or child over 5 years of age requires step 3 therapy or the infant or young child requires step 2 therapy.

Step 1 therapy for adults and children older than 5 years of age with mild intermittent asthma involves a quick relief bronchodilator used intermittently but no long-term medication. Inhaled relatively selective β_2-adrenergic agonist bronchodilators are preferred for all severities of asthma because of their minimal side effect profile; however, oral forms of albuterol, inhaled ipratropium, and oral theophylline may be considered.

Step 2 therapy requires a long-term antiinflammatory medication in addition to a quick relief bronchodilator. Choices of long-term control medication are an inhaled corticosteroid in low dose (preferred), a mast cell stabilizer, an LT modifier, or possibly an oral methylxanthine.

Step 3 therapy uses an inhaled corticosteroid at low-medium dose along with one of the following: an inhaled long-acting β_2-adrenergic agonist, a methylxanthine, or an LT modifier. In some cases, the inhaled corticosteroid dose may need to be increased within the medium range to achieve control. A short-acting β_2-adrenergic agonist is still used for quick relief.

Step 4 therapy uses an inhaled corticosteroid at high dose with a long-acting β_2-adrenergic agonist. An oral corticosteroid may be added, if needed, with frequent attempts to reduce dosage or discontinue. Quick-relief medication continues to be the short-acting β_2-adrenergic agonist. Stepwise therapy for infants and children up to 5 years of age is similar, but preferred choices vary slightly and use of a nebulizer or inhaler with a holding chamber is indicated for delivery of medications.

Education and use of nonpharmacologic management accompany every step of therapy. Nonpharmacologic management involves controlling environmental triggers and using simple breathing techniques to help control airflow. Patients must identify and avoid the factors that trigger their asthma attacks. Allergy skin testing is recommended for indoor perennial allergens. Sinusitis, rhinitis, and GERD should be controlled and influenza should be prevented through the use of yearly influenza immunization.

Early recognition and treatment of exacerbations of asthma are important to reduce the risk of death and help regain control of asthma. Asthma exacerbations are acute or subacute episodes of worsening shortness of breath, cough, wheezing, and chest tightness. Exacerbation can more objectively be determined by decrease in PEF or FEV_1 measurement. Ultimate treatment of exacerbation may involve short-acting β_2-adrenergic agonists, systemic corticosteroids for those with moderate to severe asthma or those who do not respond to inhaled corticosteroids, oxygen to relieve severe hypoxemia, and close monitoring of response through lung function measurements.

Home treatment guidelines are based on comparison of current PEF with personal best or predicted PEF. A PEF value of >50% of personal best value should prompt treatment with two to four puffs of an inhaled short acting β_2-adrenergic agonist every 20 minutes up to three treatments or a single nebulization treatment. Assessment of response 20 to 60 minutes later will determine the next step:

- If symptomatic response is good and PEF is >80% of personal best, short-acting β_2-adrenergic agonist can be continued every 3 to 4 hours for 24 to 48 hours, and patients on inhaled corticosteroids should double their dose for 7 to 10 days. The patient should follow up to ensure resolution of exacerbation and review control measures.
- If symptomatic response is not good and PEF is 50% to 80% of personal best, short-acting β_2-adrenergic agonist should be continued every 3 to 4 hours and an oral corticosteroid should be added. Follow-up should occur as soon as possible.
- If symptomatic response is poor and PEF is <50% of personal best, the short-acting β_2-adrenergic agonist should be repeated immediately, an oral corticosteroid should be started, and the patient should proceed to the emergency department.

Additional treatment may include nebulization therapy, anticholinergics, oxygen, injectable β_2-adrenergic agonists such as epinephrine and terbutaline, and intubation and mechanical ventilation.

Ideally, a written action plan is included in initial education for asthma management. However, it can be designed or redesigned at any time and should definitely be introduced for those patients who have had one or more exacerbation. A system using green, yellow, and red zones is widely used for the PEF categories of >80%, 50% to 80%, and <50%, respectively. Instructions can be individualized based on the guidelines already described. Those patients who are not able to initiate self-management should be instructed to call the clinician, and the same therapy can be initiated over the telephone or in the office.

Chronic Obstructive Pulmonary Disease Medications

- Maintenance
  - Anticholinergics
  - β_2-Adrenergic agonists
  - Methylxanthines
  - Corticosteroids (inhaled, occasionally oral)
  - Expectorants
- Severe exacerbation
  - Anticholinergics
  - β_2-Agonists
  - Methylxanthines
  - Corticosteroids (oral)

TABLE 17-3 Stepwise Approach for Managing Asthma in Adults and Children Older Than 5 Years

	Classify Severity: Clinical Features Before Treatment or Adequate Control		Medications Required To Maintain Long-Term Control
	Symptoms/Day / Symptoms/Night	PEF or FEV_1 / PEF Variability	Daily Medications
Step 4 **Severe Persistent**	Continual / Frequent	≤60% / >30%	• Preferred treatment: —High-dose inhaled corticosteroids AND —Long-acting inhaled β_2-agonists AND, if needed, —Corticosteroid tablets or syrup long term (2 mg/kg/day, generally do not exceed 60 mg/day). (Make repeat attempts to reduce systemic corticosteroids and maintain control with high-dose inhaled corticosteroids.)
Step 3 **Moderate Persistent**	Daily / >1 night/wk	>60% = <80% / >30%	• Preferred treatment: —Low-to-medium–dose inhaled corticosteroids and long-acting inhaled β_2-agonists. • Alternative treatment (listed alphabetically): —Increase inhaled corticosteroids within medium-dose range OR —Low-to-medium–dose inhaled corticosteroids and either leukotriene modifier or theophylline. If needed (particularly in patients with recurring severe exacerbations): • Preferred treatment: —Increase inhaled corticosteroids within medium-dose range and add long-acting inhaled β_2-agonists. • Alternative treatment: —Increase inhaled corticosteroids within medium-dose range and add either leukotriene modifier or theophylline.
Step 2 **Mild Persistent**	>2/wk but <1 ×/day / >2 nights/month	≥80% / 20–30%	• Preferred treatment: —Low-dose inhaled corticosteroids. • Alternative treatment (listed alphabetically): cromolyn, leukotriene modifier, nedocromil, OR sustained release theophylline to serum concentration of 5 = 15 μg/ml.
Step 1 **Mild Intermittent**	≤2 days/wk / ≤2 nights/month	≥80% / <20%	• No daily medication needed. • Severe exacerbations may occur, separated by long periods of normal lung function and no symptoms. A course of systemic corticosteroids is recommended.
Quick Relief **All Patients**	• Short-acting bronchodilator: 2 to 4 puffs short-acting inhaled β_2-agonists as needed for symptoms. • Intensity of treatment will depend on severity of exacerbation; up to 3 treatments at 20-min intervals or a single nebulizer treatment as needed. Course of systemic corticosteroids may be needed. • Use of short-acting β_2-agonists >2 times a week in intermittent asthma (daily, or increasing use in persistent asthma) may indicate the need to initiate (increase) long-term control therapy.		

TABLE 17-4 Stepwise Approach for Managing **Infants** and **Young Children** (5 Years of Age and Younger) with Acute or Chronic Asthma

Classify Severity: Clinical Features Before Treatment or Adequate Control	Symptoms/Day / Symptoms/Night	Medications Required To Maintain Long-Term Control: Daily Medications
Step 4 **Severe Persistent**	Continual / Frequent	• Preferred treatment: —High-dose inhaled corticosteroids AND —Long-acting inhaled β_2-agonists AND, if needed, —Corticosteroid tablets or syrup long term (2 mg/kg/day, generally do not exceed 60 mg/day). (Make repeat attempts to reduce systemic corticosteroids and maintain control with high-dose inhaled corticosteroids.)
Step 3 **Moderate Persistent**	Daily / >1 night/wk	• Preferred treatments: —Low-dose inhaled corticosteroids and long-acting inhaled β_2-agonists OR —Medium-dose inhaled corticosteroids. • Alternative treatment: —Low-dose inhaled corticosteroids and either leukotriene receptor antagonist or theophylline. If needed (particularly in patients with recurring severe exacerbations): • Preferred treatment: —Medium-dose inhaled corticosteroids and long-acting β_2-agonists. • Alternative treatment: —Medium-dose inhaled corticosteroids and either leukotriene receptor antagonist or theophylline.
Step 2 **Mild Persistent**	>2/wk but < 1×/day / > 2 nights/month	• Preferred treatment: —Low-dose inhaled corticosteroid (with nebulizer or MDI with holding chamber with or without face mask or DPI). • Alternative treatment (listed alphabetically): —Cromolyn (nebulizer is preferred or MDI with holding chamber) OR leukotriene receptor antagonist.
Step 1 **Mild Intermittent**	≤2 days/wk / ≤2 nights/month	• No daily medication needed.
Quick Relief **All Patients**		• Bronchodilator as needed for symptoms. Intensity of treatment will depend upon severity of exacerbation. —Preferred treatment: Short-acting inhaled β_2-agonists by nebulizer or face mask and space/holding chamber —Alternative treatment: Oral β_2-agonist • With viral respiratory infection —Bronchodilator q 4–6 hr up to 24 hr (longer with physician consult); in general, repeat no more than once every 6 wk —Consider systemic corticosteroid if exacerbation is severe or patient has history of previous severe exacerbations • Use of short-acting β_2-agonists >2 times a week in intermittent asthma (daily, or increasing use in persistent asthma) may indicate the need to initiate (increase) long-term control therapy.

From National Asthma Education and Prevention Program Expert Panel Report: *Guidelines for the diagnosis and management of asthma—update on selected topics 2002.* NIH Publication No. 02-5075. Washington, DC, US Dept of Health and Human Services. Available at www.nhlbi.nih.gov/guidelines/asthma/index.htm

The GOLD Guidelines treatment of stable COPD is based on severity in a stepwise approach. Treatment with medications alone often does not effectively manage COPD; therefore nonpharmacologic treatment strategies are also important.

The goals of COPD treatment are to alleviate symptoms, increase lung function, improve physical activity, and reduce complications. Pharmacologic treatment does not change the overall long-term decline in lung function; only smoking cessation can slow that progression to the rate of normal age-related decline.

Nonpharmacologic strategies include patient education, nutrition, and exercise. Pulmonary rehabilitation programs are usually multidisciplinary and include individualized, carefully monitored exercise programs as well as patient education and support. Pharmacologic therapy of an adjunct nature includes immunization yearly for influenza and once for pneumococci.

Every effort should be taken to avoid exposing these individuals to upper respiratory infections.

Step 1 therapy for stage I severity COPD begins with a bronchodilator as needed to control symptoms. The choice between an inhaled anticholinergic, inhaled short-acting β_2-adrenergic agonist, inhaled long-acting β_2-adrenergic agonist, and oral methylxanthine should be individualized based on symptomatic response and availability of medication to the patient. In general, short-acting agents have the benefit of being able to reduce acute shortness of breath; however, long-acting agents are more convenient. Inhaled agents are preferred, and combination bronchodilator therapy may produce fewer side effects. Methylxanthines are titrated to therapeutic concentration. All types of bronchodilators have been shown to increase exercise tolerance even without corresponding increase in FEV_1.

Step 2 therapy for stage II severity is the regular use of one or more bronchodilators and an inhaled corticosteroid if a favorable response is shown. A 6- to 12-week trial of inhaled corticosteroid monitored by symptoms and spirometry is recommended for those who have not benefited sufficiently from step 1 therapy. If no appreciable benefit is obtained, the corticosteroid should be discontinued. However, in stage IIb severity, an inhaled corticosteroid is used regardless of the response if there is a history of repeated exacerbations. It has been reported that only 20% of COPD patients will respond to corticosteroid therapy. However, a newer observational study showed an increased 3-year survival rate among COPD patients who were treated with regular dosing of inhaled fluticasone, a corticosteroid, and salmeterol, a long-acting β_2-adrenergic agonists. The use of oral corticosteroids is not included in the GOLD guidelines because there is no evidence that they are beneficial and because potential side effects are great.

Step 3 therapy for stage III severity is the same as step 2 therapy plus the addition of long-term oxygen therapy for those with $PaO_2 \leq 55$ mm Hg or oxygen saturation $\leq 88\%$. Surgical options of bullectomy, lung volume reduction, and lung transplantation may be considered. Another class of drugs that may be tried for moderate to severe COPD but have not been proved is the LT modifiers. It is not recommended by the GOLD guidelines, but if standard therapy is not successful, clinicians may progress to LT modifier therapy. The patient should be evaluated and a beneficial response documented before they are used on a long-term basis, however.

The treatment of acute exacerbations of COPD includes increased bronchodilator dosing and oral corticosteroids. If the patient is not in respiratory acidosis and not in need of ventilatory support, home management with frequent follow-up and monitoring may be appropriate. If not already used for maintenance therapy of stable COPD, an inhaled anticholinergic should be added. The dosage of each particular bronchodilating agent may be increased to the maximum dose range or oral inhaler treatments may be supplemented with nebulization treatments. If improvement is noted on reassessment, this regimen can be continued and stepped down when possible. If improvement does not occur or FEV_1 is <50% of predicted, an oral corticosteroid is added. A course of prednisone 40 mg for 10 days is recommended. Antibiotic therapy is indicated only when worsening shortness of breath and cough are associated with increase in sputum volume and purulence. If hospital management becomes necessary, intravenous methylxanthines and corticosteroids and ventilatory support may be necessary.

HOW TO MONITOR

β-Adenergic Agonist Bronchodilators

- Use of more than one canister of albuterol per month may indicate overreliance on this drug.
- Use of more than two canisters per month poses a risk of increased adverse effects.

Theophylline

- Serum concentration should be measured at peak steady state, which is 8 hours after administration of extended-release formulations and one hour after administration of immediate-release formulations with no dosage change within 3 days.
- Concentration monitoring should take place whenever signs of toxicity are suspected; on initiation of drug and dosage titration until steady state therapeutic concentration is reached; and routinely every 6 months in children and yearly in adults.

Inhaled Corticosteroids

- Monitor the growth of children and adolescents; see Table 17-5 for summary of inhalation systems.

PATIENT VARIABLES

Geriatrics

- Bronchodilators may cause increased adverse reactions. May not tolerate side effects such as tachycardia.
- Theophylline clearance is reduced in the elderly, causing increased risk of drug toxicity and interaction (see Table 17-10, p. 245).
- The total daily dosage should not exceed 400 mg.
- High-dose inhaled corticosteroids and oral corticosteroids that are often used in COPD may cause or worsen osteoporosis in the elderly.
- Nebulization treatment may be useful when elderly patients are unable to use inhalers correctly.

Pediatrics

- Special delivery devices are available for infants and young children. Caregivers must be taught their proper use. Nebulizer treatments are preferred for children aged 2 years and younger. Children aged 3 to 5 years may use either an inhaler with spacer or a nebulizer.
- The rate of theophylline clearance is highly variable in children from infancy to adolescence.
- Ipratropium safety has not been determined in children under 12 years of age.
- NAEPP EPR Update on Selected Topics 2002 states that the use of inhaled corticosteroids in low to medium doses may have the potential for decreasing growth velocity, resulting in differences of up to 1 cm of height in the first year of

TABLE 17-5 Inhalation Delivery Devices

Device/Drugs	Advantages	Disadvantages
Metered-dose inhaler (MDI) β_2-Adrenergic agonists Corticosteroids Mast cell stabilizers Anticholinergic	Small and compact Can be used with open or closed mouth technique; open mouth technique may enhance delivery of drug	Requires slow inhalation Requires coordination of inhalation and actuation Up to 80% of dose deposited in oropharynx
Breath-actuated MDI β_2-Adrenergic agonists	Does not require coordination of inhalation and actuation	Requires slow inhalation for optimal deposition, but not so slow as to prevent actuation
Dry powder inhaler (DPI) β_2-Adrenergic agonists Corticosteroids	Requires rapid, deep inhalation May be easier for children 4 yr old and older	Dose lost if patient exhales through device Delivery may be less than with proper use of MDI
Spacer/holding chamber Can be used with standard inhalers (not breath-actuated and some DPI)	Easier for children 4 yr old and older, or younger than 4 yr with a face mask May perform with tidal breathing rather than slow inhalation followed by breath holding Decreases oropharyngeal deposition and systemic absorption of drug	Simple tube devices still require coordination of inhalation and actuation May be bulky and less convenient to carry Require more extensive cleaning
Nebulizer β_2-Adrenergic agonists Corticosteroids Mast cell stabilizers Anticholinergic	Effective in all age groups and ability Slow tidal breathing with occasional deep breaths most effective	Must have tightly fitting face mask if unable to use mouthpiece Expensive and less portable than other devices

Adapted from National Asthma Education and Prevention Program Expert Panel Report 2: *Guidelines for the diagnosis and management of asthma.* NIH Publication No. 97-4051, Washington, DC, 1997, US Government Printing Office.

treatment. However, this effect is not sustained in subsequent years of treatment, it is not progressive, and it may be reversible.

- Safety and efficacy of montelukast have been established in children 2 to 5 years old at the 4 mg dose.

Pregnancy

- Poorly controlled asthma can result in increased perinatal mortality. In general, there is little evidence to suggest increased risk to the fetus by using the recommended medications to treat asthma.
- *Category C:* β-Adrenergic agonists (except terbutaline), theophylline, corticosteroids, zileuton
- *Category B:* Ipratropium, mast cell stabilizers, montelukast and zafirlukast, and terbutaline.

Lactation

- Most of these medications are excreted in breast milk.
- Theophylline: Breast-feeding may need to be discontinued because the drug can cause serious toxicity in nursing infants.

PATIENT EDUCATION

- Teach basic facts about asthma
- Teach inhaler/spacer/holding chamber technique
- Discuss roles of medications
- Develop self-management plan
- Develop action plan for when and how to take rescue actions, especially for patients with a history of severe exacerbations
- Discuss appropriate environmental control measures to avoid exposure to known allergens and irritants

Proper Use of a Metered Dose Inhaler

1. Remove the cap. (Research studies show 1% of users fail to remove the cap before using the MDI!)
2. Hold the inhaler upright and shake it thoroughly.
3. Tilt head back slightly and breathe out. (Most people take in a large breath before exhaling. This is counterproductive in patients with outflow obstruction and should be specifically noted to patients as a practice to avoid).
4. The MDI may be placed in the mouth with the lips sealed around it, placed 1 to 2 inches away from the opened mouth, or attached to a spacer or holding chamber and the end of the device placed in the mouth and the lips sealed around it. In infants and young children (or anyone unable to self-administer the device), the spacer can be attached to a face mask and the face mask sealed around the patient's face before activating the MDI.
5. Press down on the inhaler to release the medication as you start to breathe in slowly.
6. Breathe in slowly for 3 to 5 seconds.
7. Hold breath for 10 seconds to allow deposition of medication deeply into the lungs.
8. Wait 1 minute and repeat inhalation if additional puffs are prescribed.

For inhaled dry powder medications it is important to close the mouth tightly around the inhaler and breath in rapidly after activating the dose.

Many inhalation aerosol products contain chlorfluorocarbons that may have public health consequences and harm the environment. Alternative products are being created that may require further education and monitoring to ensure the same optimal effect of the drug.

Long-Acting β-Adrenergic Agonist Bronchodilators

- Do not change brands without consulting provider.
- Notify provider if treatment is less effective, symptoms worse, or the need to use this product increases in frequency.
- Usual adverse events include palpitations, chest pain, rapid heart rate, and tremor or nervousness.

Theophylline

- Extended-release capsules should be taken 1 hour before or 2 hours after meals; can take immediate-release forms with food if gastrointestinal upset occurs.
- Do not change brands of theophylline without consulting provider.
- Notify physician if nausea, vomiting, insomnia, jitteriness, headache, rash, severe gastrointestinal pain, restlessness, convulsions or irregular heartbeat occur.
- Avoid caffeine-containing beverages.

Ipratropium

- Avoid contact with eyes, may cause temporary blurring of vision.
- If canister floats in bowl of cold water, it is empty.

Cromolyn

- Do not immerse canister in water.

Corticosteroids

- Rinse mouth after use to reduce systemic absorption and local throat infection.
- Do not abruptly stop medication administration.
- Discard canister when number of doses should be used up; canister cannot be accurately checked.

Leukotriene Receptor Antagonists

- Take regularly, even during symptom-free periods.
- Zafirlukast: Take 1 hour before or 2 hours after meals.
- Zafirlukast and zileuton: Report hepatic dysfunction symptoms (right upper quadrant abdominal pain, nausea, fatigue, lethargy, pruritus, jaundice, flulike symptoms, anorexia).

Specific Drugs

SHORT-ACTING B-ADRENERGIC AGONIST BRONCHODILATORS

(P) Prototype Drug

albuterol (Proventil, Ventolin, Volmax)

Contraindications

Hypersensitivity to albuterol or any component

Warnings

- If paradoxical bronchospasm occurs, it should be discontinued.
- Deterioration of asthma may be signaled by excessive use of inhalations.
- Consider use of an antiinflammatory agent along with albuterol for treatment of asthma.
- May cause adverse cardiovascular effects in some patients, especially those with coronary insufficiency, cardiac arrhythmias, and hypertension.
- Do not exceed recommended dose as it may lead to death.

Precautions

- Administer with caution to patients with cardiovascular disorders, diabetes mellitus, hyperthyroidism, or seizure disorder and the elderly.

Pharmacokinetics

- See Table 17-6.

Adverse Effects

- See Tables 17-7 and 17-8.

Drug Interactions

- Increased sympathomimetic effects with other sympathomimetic agents
- Enhanced toxicity in patients taking methylxanthines
- Decreased bronchodilating effectiveness with patients taking β-adrenergic–blocking agents
- Decreased serum levels and therapeutic effects of digoxin
- Decreased effectiveness of insulin and oral hypoglycemic agents

Overdosage

- Signs and symptoms are those of excessive β-adrenergic stimulation: seizures, hypertension, hypotension, angina, tachycardia, arrhythmias, nervousness, dizziness, etc.
- Cardiac arrest and death may occur.

Dosage and Administration

- See Table 17-9.

Other Drugs in Class

Other drugs in this class are similar to the prototype except as follows.

- Pirbuterol comes in a breath-actuated inhaler that may be easier for some patients to use.
- Terbutaline is no longer widely available in inhaled form. Subcutaneous injection is used in the hospital setting. It should be used cautiously in labor and delivery as it can inhibit labor.
- Less selective β_2-adrenergic agonists such as epinephrine, isoproterenol, and metaproterenol are not recommended due to their potential for cardiac stimulation, especially in high doses.

Text continued on p. 244

TABLE 17-6 Pharmacokinetics of Major Asthma and Chronic Obstructive Pulmonary Disease Medications

Drug	Absorption	Drug Availability (After First Pass)	Onset of Action	Time to Peak Concentration	Half-Life	Duration of Action	Protein Bound	Metabolism	Excretion	Therapeutic Serum Level (ng/ml*)
RELATIVELY SHORT ACTING										
albuterol	Through respiratory and GI tracts	NA	Within 5-15 min	60-90 min (therapeutic effect) 2-4 hr (serum conc.)	3.8 hr	3-4 hr; up to 6 hr in some	NA		Urine	NA
bitolterol	Through respiratory and GI tracts	NA	2-4 min	$^{1}/_{2}$-2 hr (therapeutic effect)	3 hr	5-8 hr	NA		Lungs, urine, feces	NA
levalbuterol	Through respiratory and GI tracts	NA	10-17 min	60-90 min	3.3 hr	5-6 hr	NA		Urine	NA
pirbuterol	Through respiratory and GI tracts	NA	5 min	30-60 min (therapeutic effect)	2 hr	5 hr	NA		Urine	NA
terbutaline										
salmeterol	Through respiratory and GI tracts	NA	10-20 min		5.5 hr	12 hr	96%	Hepatic: hydroxylation	Urine, feces	NA
formoterol	Through respiratory and GI tracts	NA	5 min		10 hr	12 hr	61%-64%	Hepatic: direct glucuronidation	Urine, feces	NA
RELATIVELY LONG ACTING										
theophylline	Rapidly and completely absorbed through GI tract	Nearly 100%		1-2 hr (immediate release) 8 hr (sustained release)	8 hr (varies with age, comorbid illness, and other conditions)	6 hr (immediate release) 8-24 hr (sustained release)	40%	Hepatic: demethylation	Urine	5-15 µg/ml (NAEPP EP2) 10-20 µg/ml (manufacturer information)
ipratropium	Through respiratory tract; swallowed drug is not significantly absorbed	NA	15-30 min	1-2 hr (therapeutic effect)	1.6 hr	4-5 hr	0%-9%	Partially metabolized to inactive ester hydrolysis products		NA

cromolyn sodium	8% Absorbed through respiratory tract; the rest is exhaled or swallowed and excreted	NA		Approximately 2-4 wk for therapeutic effect				Excreted unchanged	Urine, feces	NA
nedocromil	Through respiratory tract	Low systemic absorption		2 wk for therapeutic effect	1.5 hr		89%	Excreted unchanged	Urine	NA
beclomethasone dipropionate	Rapidly absorbed through respiratory and GI tracts	Low systemic absorption; about 20% bioavailability from lungs		Weeks to months for peak therapeutic effect	2.8 hr		87%	Metabolized in the lung and liver (CYP3A)	Feces, urine (small amount)	NA
budesonide	Rapidly absorbed through respiratory and GI tracts	25% Bioavailability from lungs; 5-15% bioavailability from systemic absorption	Improvement in as little as 24 hr	Maximal therapeutic effect in as little as 1-2 wk	2.8 hr		85%-90%	Liver (CYP3A)	Urine, feces	NA
flunisolide	Rapid absorption through respiratory and GI tracts	Low systemic absorption and rapid conversion of systemic drug to inactive metabolite			1.8 hr		NA	Liver	Urine, feces	NA

Continued

TABLE 17-6 Pharmacokinetics of Major Asthma and Chronic Obstructive Pulmonary Disease Medications—cont'd

Drug	Absorption	Drug Availability (After First Pass)	Onset of Action	Time to Peak Concentration	Half-Life	Duration of Action	Protein Bound	Metabolism	Excretion	Therapeutic Serum Level (ng/ml*)
RELATIVELY LONG ACTING—cont'd										
fluticasone proprionate	Majority of the drug is systemically absorbed from the lungs	13%-30%	Improvement in as little as 24 hr	Maximal therapeutic effect in as little as 1-2 wk	3.1 hr		91%	Liver	Feces, urine	NA
triamcinolone acetonide	Rapidly absorbed from the lungs	21.5%			1.5 hr		68%	Liver, kidneys	Feces	NA
montelukast	Rapidly absorbed through the GI tract	64%		2-4 hr	2.7-5.5 hr		99%	Extensively metabolized through the liver (CYP 3A4 and CYP 2C9)	Feces	NA
zafirlukast	Rapidly absorbed through GI tract	Unknown		3 hr	10 hr		99%	Extensively metabolized through the liver (CYP 2C9)	Feces	NA
zileuton	Rapidly absorbed through GI tract	Unknown		1.7 hr	2.5 hr		93%	Metabolized by the liver (CYP 1A2, 2C0, 3A4)	Urine	NA

TABLE 17-7 Common and Serious Adverse Effects by Drug

Drug Class	Drug Name	Common Side Effects	Serious Adverse Effects
Short-acting β-agonists	All	Palpitations, tachycardia, increased BP, cough, dry throat, chest tightness, nausea and vomiting, GI distress, headache, insomnia, tremor, dizziness, vertigo, nervousness, hyperactivity	Arrhythmias, dyspnea
	albuterol	Heartburn, nasal congestion	Angioedema, bronchospasm, hypertension, angina, rash
	bitolterol		Bronchospasm, elevated LFTs
	levalbuterol	Flu-like syndrome, pain, rhinitis, sinusitis, viral infection	
	pirbuterol		Bronchospasm
Long-acting β-agonists	All	Tremor, nervousness, tachycardia	Bronchospasm
	salmeterol	Palpitations, headache, nasal congestion, joint and muscle pain	Immediate hypersensitivity reactions, rash, angioedema
	formoterol	Dizziness, insomnia	Arrhythmias, angina, hypokalemia, metabolic acidosis
theophylline		Tachycardia, palpitations, tachypnea, nausea, vomiting, diarrhea, GI reflux, headache, insomnia, irritability	Arrhythmias, hypotension, seizures, IADH syndrome, hematemesis, proteinuria, circulatory failure, death
ipratropium		Headache, dizziness, fatigue, pain, rash, cough, respiratory infection, palpitations, hypertension, dry mouth, GI distress, constipation, urinary retention, eye pain, alopecia	Anaphylaxis, worsening of narrow-angle glaucoma, bronchospasm, worsening of COPD, tachycardia, urticaria, chest pain
Mast cell stabilizers	All	Headache, nausea, cough, rhinitis	Eosinophilic pneumonitis
	cromolyn	Dizziness, irritation of oropharynx, wheezing, sneezing	Angioedema
	nedocromil	Bad taste, pharyngitis, rash, arthritis, elevated LFTs	Bronchospasm
Inhaled corticosteroids	All	Oral candidiasis; oral, laryngeal, pharyngeal irritation; headache, dyspepsia, cough, respiratory infection	Suppression of HPA axis, cushingoid features, growth velocity reduction, bronchospasm
Leukotriene receptor agonists	All	Headache, fever, rash, dyspepsia, anaphylaxis	
	montelukast	Asthenia, fever	Hepatic eosinophilic inflitrations
	zafirlukast	Dizziness, respiratory infections, elevated LFTs	Systemic eosinophilia, agranulocytosis, bleeding
	zileuton	Dyspepsia, nausea, abdominal pain, asthenia, elevated LFTs, myalgia	Low WBC

IADH, Syndrome of inappropriate ADH secretion; *LFT*, liver function tests.

TABLE 17-8 Adverse Reactions by Body System

Body System	β-Adrenergic Agonists	theophylline	ipatropium	Mast Cell Stabilizers	Leukotriene-Receptor Antagonists
Body, general		Fever, flushing	Fatigue, pain		Fever
Skin		Rash, alopecia	Rash, alopecia		Rash
Hypersensitivity	albuterol and salmeterol: rash, angioedema		Urticaria, angioedema, rash, bronchospasm, pharyngeal edema	Rash, urticaria, angioedama	Anaphylaxis
Respiratory	Cough, bronchospasm, dry throat; dyspnea; albuterol, salmeterol: nasal congestion	Tachypnea, respiratory arrest	Cough, dyspnea, bronchitis, bronchospasm, upper respiratory infection	Bronchospasm, cough, laryngeal edema, nasal congestions, pharyngitis, wheezing, nasal irritation	zafirlukast: infections
Cardiovascular	Palpitations, tachycardia, increased blood pressure, chest tightness, arrhythmias; levalbuterol: hypotension, syncope	Palpitations, tachycardia, hypotension, circulatory failure, life-threatening ventricular arrhythmias	Palpitations, tachycardia, chest pain		
GI	Nausea/vomiting, GI distress	Nausea, vomiting, diarrhea, epigastric pain, hematemesis, GI reflux	Dry mouth, GI distress, nausea, constipation	Nausea	zileuton: abdominal pain, nausea Dyspepsia zafirlukast: nausea, diarrhea
Metabolic and nutritional		Hyperglycemia, inappropriate antidiuretic hormone syndrome			
Musculoskeletal	salmeterol: joint, muscle pain		Back pain	Joint swelling and pain	
Nervous system	Tremor, dizziness/vertigo, nervousness, hyperactivity, headache, insomnia	Headache, insomnia, irritability, seizures, restlessness, reflex hyperexcitability, muscle twitching	Nervousness, headache, insomnia, paresthesia, drowsiness, coordination difficulty, tremor, dizziness	Headache, dizziness	zafirlukast: headache, dizziness zileuton: myalgia
Special senses			Blurred vision		
Hepatic	bitolterol: increased liver function tests				zileuton and zafirlukast: increase LFTs
Genitourinary		Proteinuria, potentiation of diuresis	Urinary retention	Dysuria, urinary frequency	

TABLE 17-9 Dosage and Administration Recommendations for Asthma and COPD Medications

Drug Name	Age Group	Dosage	Administration	Maximum Dose
albuterol (metered-dose aerosol)	Adults and children ≥4 yr	2 inh (100 μg each) *or* 2 inh 15 min before exercise *or* one 200-μg capsule for inh to 2 inh qid	q4-6hr	
albuterol solution for nebulization (0.5% vial for dilution and 0.083% unit dose)	Adults and children >15 kg	2.5 mg (unit dose or dilute 0.5 ml of 0.5% solution with 2.5 ml of sterile saline)	tid-qid	
	Children ≥2 yr; <15 kg	0.1-0.15 mg/kg/dose (for 1.25 mg dilute 0.25 ml of 0.5% solution with 2.75 ml sterile saline)	tid-qid	
albuterol solution for nebulization (0.083% unit dose)	Adults and children 2-12 yr; 15 kg	2.5 mg (3-ml unit dose vial)	tid-qid	
albuterol tablets (extended and immediate release)	Adults and children >12 yr	4-8 mg ER (1-2 tab, 4 or 8 mg each) *or* 2-4 mg IR (1-2 tab, 2 or 4 mg each) Cautiously increase	q12hr tid-qid	32 mg/day
	Children 6-11 yr	4 mg ER (one 4-mg tab) *or* 2 mg IR (one 2-mg tab) Cautiously increase	q12hr tid-qid	24 mg/day
albuterol syrup (2 mg/5 ml)	Adults and children >14 yr	2-4 mg (1-2 tsp) Cautiously increase	tid-qid	32 mg/day
	Children 6-14 yr	4 mg ER (one 4-mg tab) *or* 2 mg IR (one 2-mg tab) Cautiously increase	tid-qid	24 mg/day
	Children 2-6 yr	0.1 mg/kg (should not exceed 2 mg) Cautiously increase to 0.2 mg/kg	tid	4 mg tid
bitolterol (solution for nebulization)	Adults and children >12 yr	2.5 mg 0.2% solution with continuous flow neb; 1 mg with intermittent flow neb	tid-qid with at least 4 hr in between treatments	14 mg (continuous); 8 mg (intermittent)
levalbuterol (solution for nebulization)	Adult and children ≥12 yr	0.63 mg (unit dose 0.63 mg/3 ml) If needed increase to 1.25 mg tid (unit dose 1.25 mg in 3 ml)	tid q6-8hr	
	Children 6-11 yr	0.31 mg (unit dose 0.31 mg/3 ml)	tid	0.63 mg tid
pirbuterol (metered-dose aerosol)	Adults and children ≥12 yr	2 inh (0.2 mg each)	q4-6hr	12 inh daily
salmeterol (metered dose aerosol)	Adults and children ≥12 yr	2 inh (21 μg each) *or* 2 inh 30-60 min before exercise	q12hr	2 doses daily
salmeterol (dry powder for inhalation)	Adults and children ≥4 yr	1 inh (50 μg blister)	q12hr	2 doses daily

inh, Inhalation; *neb*, nebulization; *sol*, solution; *tab*, tablet.

Continued

TABLE 17-9 Dosage and Administration Recommendations for Asthma and COPD Medications—cont'd

Drug Name	Age Group	Dosage	Administration	Maximum Dose
formoterol (dry powder for inhalation)	Adults and children ≥5 yr	1 inh (12-μg capsule)	q12hr	2 doses daily
	Adults and children ≥12 yr	1 inh 15 min before exercise Do not use extra doses if already on regular daily dosing		
theophylline—immediate-release form	Adults and children >45 kg	300 mg/day PO; if tolerated, increase to 400 mg/day after 3 days; if tolerated, increase dose to 600 mg/day after 3 days Dosage based on peak concentration levels	Divided q6-8hr	Concentration not to exceed 20 μg/ml
	Children 1-15 yr	12-14 mg/kg/day; if tolerated, increase to 16 mg/kg/day after 3 days; if tolerated, increase to 20 mg/kg/day after 3 days. Dosage based on peak concentration levels	Divided q6-8hr	Age 6-9 yr: 24 mg/kg/day Age 9-12 yr: 20 mg/kg/day
theophylline—sustained-release form	Adults and children >12 yr	16 mg/kg/day PO or 400 mg/day (whichever is less); may increase by 25% increments every 3 days, if tolerated, and until optimal clinical response is reached	qd or in 2-3 doses spaced 8-12 hr apart	Age 12-16 yr: 18 mg/kg/day Age 16+ yr: 13 mg/kg/day
ipratropium (metered-dose aerosol)	Adults	2 inh (18 μg each)	q6-8 hr	12 inh/24 h
ipratropium (solution for nebulization)	Adults	500 μg (unit dose vial) via neb	q6-8 hr	
cromolyn sodium (metered-dose aerosol)	Adults and children ≥5 yr	2 inh (800 μg each)	qid	
cromolyn sodium (solution for nebulization)	Adults and children ≥2 yr	20 mg (one 2-ml ampule) via neb	qid	
nedocromil (metered-dose aerosol)	Adults and children ≥12 yr	2 inh (1.75 mg each) If good response, can be reduced to tid and then bid	qid	
beclomethasone (metered-dose aerosol) 42 μg and 84 μg	Adults and children ≥12 yr	2 inh (42 μg inhalation) *or* 2 inh double strength (84 μg/inh)	tid-qid bid	20 inh/day 10 inh/day
	Children 6-12 yr	1 or 2 inh (42 μg/inh) *or* 2 inh (84 μg/inh)	tid-qid bid	10 inh/day 5 inh/day
beclomethasone (metered-dose aerosol) 40 μg and 80 μg (CFC free)	Adults	40-80 μg if previously on bronchodilator (1-2 inh 40 μg strength); 40-160 μg if previously on inhaled corticosteroid (1-2 inh 40 μg strength to 1-2 inh 80 μg strength)	bid	640 μg/day
budesonide (inhalation-driven dry powder)	Adults	200-400 μg (200 μg/inh); 400-800 μg if previously on oral corticosteroid	bid	800 μg/day bronchodilator therapy alone; 1600 μg/day if on corticosteroid
	Children ≥6 yr	200 μg (one inh)	bid	800 μg/day

TABLE 17-9 Dosage and Administration Recommendations for Asthma and COPD Medications—cont'd

Drug Name	Age Group	Dosage	Administration	Maximum Dose
budesonide (inhalation suspension for nebulization)	Children 12 mo to 8 yr	0.5-mg respules via neb (0.25 mg/2 ml or 0.5 mg/2 ml); 1 mg if previously on oral corticosteroid	Daily or can be divided into 2 equal doses	0.5 μg/day if on bronchodilator; 1 mg/day if on corticosteroid
flunisolide (metered-dose aerosol)	Adults	2 inh (250 μg/inh)	bid	8 inh (2 mg/day)
	Children 6-15 yr	2 inh	bid	4 inh (1 mg/day)
fluticasone (metered-dose aerosol)	Adults and children ≥12 yr	88 μg (2 inh of 44 μg strength) if previously on bronchodilator; 88-220 μg if previously on inhaled corticosteroid (2 inh of 44 μg strength to 1 or 2 inh of 110 μg strength); 880 μg if previously on oral corticosteroid (4 inh of 220 μg strength)	bid	880 μg/day if on bronchodilator or inhaled corticosteroid; 1760 μg if on oral corticosteroid
fluticasone (dry powder inhalation)	Adults and adolescents	100 μg if previously on bronchodilator (one 100 μg Rotadisk); 100-250 μg if previously on inhaled corticosteroid (one 100 μg or 250 μg Rotadisk); 1 g if previously on oral corticosteroid (four 250 μg Rotadisk)	bid	1 g/day if on bronchodilator or inhaled corticosteroid; 2 g/day if on oral corticosteroid
	Children 4-11 yr	50 μg (one 50-μg Rotadisk)	bid	200 μg/day
triamcinolone (metered dose aerosol)	Adults	2 inh (100 μg each) Alternately 4 inh bid	tid-qid	16 inh/day (1600 μg)
	Children 6-12 yr	1-2 inh (100 μg each) Alternately 2-4 inh bid	tid-qid	12 inh/day (1200 μg)
montelukast (oral tablets)	Adult and adolescents ≥15 yr	10 mg	Daily (evening)	
	Children 6-14 yr	5 mg chewable tab	Daily (evening)	
	Children 2-5 yr	4 mg chewable tab	Daily (evening)	
zafirlukast (oral tablets)	Adults and children ≥12 yr	20 mg	bid	
	Children 7-11 yr	10 mg	bid	
zileuton	Adults and children ≥12 yr	600 mg	qid	
albuterol/ipratropium (metered dose aerosol)	Adults	2 inh (103 μg albuterol and 18 μg ipratropium each inh)	qid	12 inh/day
fluticasone/salmeterol (dry powder inhalation)	Adults and children ≥12 yr	1 inhalation Previously on no corticosteroid therapy, use 100/50 μg strength; previously on inhaled corticosteroid, strength based on dosage of previous corticosteroid	bid	1 inh bid of 500/50 strength

LONG-ACTING RELATIVELY SELECTIVE β_2-ADRENERGIC AGONIST BRONCHODILATORS

salmeterol (Serevent)

Contraindications
- Hypersensitivity to salmeterol or any of its components

Warnings
- Should not be initiated in patients with significant worsening or acutely deteriorating asthma
- Should not be used to treat acute symptoms
- Is not a substitute for inhaled corticosteroids
- Do not exceed recommended dosage.
- May cause paradoxical bronchospasm and immediate hypersensitivity reactions.

Precautions
- Use with caution in patients with coronary insufficiency, hypertension, arrhythmias, thyrotoxicosis, and convulsive disorders.

Drug Interactions
- Action on vascular system may be potentiated by concomitant administration of tricyclic antidepressants or MAOIs
- Decreased effectiveness of bronchodilation with β-adrenergic-blocking agents

Dosage and Administration
- See Table 17-7.
- When using to prevent exercise-induced bronchospasm, use 30 to 60 minutes before exercise.
- Inhalation powder should not be used with a spacer.

Other Drugs in Class

Other drugs in this class are similar to salmeterol except as follows.

formoterol

- Formoterol is administered by capsules inserted into an aerosolize inhaler; store capsules in blister pack until ready for use.

METHYLXANTHINES

Ⓟ **Prototype Drug**

theophylline (Theo-Dur, Theolair, Slo-Bid, Slo-Phyllin, Quibron, Elixophyllin, etc.)

Contraindications
- Hypersensitivity to xanthines, active peptic ulcer disease, and a seizure disorder not controlled by medication

Warnings

! Serious side effects such as ventricular arrhythmias, convulsions, or death may appear as the first signs of toxicity, without warning.

- Theophylline has a very narrow therapeutic window, and toxicity can cause less serious signs of toxicity, including nausea and restlessness.
- Reduced theophylline clearance and increased risk for toxicity have been documented, requiring more intensive monitoring of therapeutic level, in those with the following risk factors: age >60 or <1 year old; comorbid conditions such as impaired liver function, acute pulmonary edema, congestive heart failure, cor pulmonale, hypothyroidism reduced renal function in infants <3 months old, sepsis with multiorgan failure, shock; fever; administration of certain drugs; and cessation of smoking.
- If theophylline toxicity is suspected due to nausea and vomiting, particularly repetitive vomiting, additional doses of theophylline should be withheld and serum concentration of theophylline measure immediately.
- Dosage of theophylline should not be increased in response to acute exacerbation of symptoms.

Precautions
- Use cautiously in patients with seizure disorders and cardiac arrhythmias (not bradyarrhythmias).
- Use cautiously and reduce dosage with hepatic insufficiency.

Drug Interactions
- Many drugs either decrease or increase theophylline levels (see Table 17-10). Theophylline is a cytochrome P450 1A2 substrate. Food-drug interactions include the following:
  - A high-protein/low-carbohydrate diet increases elimination.
  - A high-carbohydrate/low-protein diet decreases elimination.
- Food may alter bioavailability and absorption. Consistent administration while fasting improves consistency of effects.

Overdosage
- Symptoms of overdosage may begin with serum concentrations >20 μg/ml with nausea, tachycardia, vomiting, headache, and insomnia.
- Higher concentrations may cause intractable seizures, hypokalemia, ventricular arrhythmias, and death.

Dosage and Administration
- Theophylline anhydrous and theophylline monohydrate have slightly varying equivalent doses; theophylline anhydrous is 100% theophylline. Dosing intervals vary for immediate-release and extended-release products. Extended-release theophylline products are preferred due to convenience; see Table 17-7, p. 239.
- The dosage should be individualized based on serum concentration measurements to achieve maximal potential benefit with minimal risk of adverse effects (see Table 17-9, pp. 241–243). Therapeutic concentration is 10 to 20 μg/ml; however, the NAEPP recommends 5 to 15 μg/ml for treatment of asthmatic patients. With risk factors for reduced theophylline clearance, give only 16 mg/kg or 400 mg/day.

TABLE 17-10 Theophylline Drug Interactions

Action	Drugs
Agents that increase theophylline concentration	Alcohol, allopurinol, β-blockers (nonselective), calcium channel blockers, cimetidine, corticosteroids, disulfiram, ephedrine, estrogen, influenza virus vaccine, interferon, macrolides, mexiletine, methotrexate, quinolones, tacrine, thiabendazole, thyroid hormones
Agents that decrease theophylline concentration	aminoglutethimide, barbiturates, charcoal, cigarette smoking, ketoconazole, phenytoin, rifampin, sulfinpyrazone, sympathomimetics (β-agonists)
Agents that may increase or decrease theophylline concentration	carbamazepine, isoniazid, loop diuretics, hydantoins
Agents that are affected by theophylline	adenosine, benzodiazepines, erythromycin, halothane, ketamine, lithium pancuronium, phenytoin

ANTICHOLINERGICS

ipratropium bromide (Atrovent)

Contraindications
- Hypersensitivity to ipratropium, atropine, or soya lecithin products such as soybean or peanut (inhalation only)

Warnings
- Do not use as single agent for acute bronchospasm; combine with drug with a faster onset of action.

Precautions
- Immediate hypersensitivity may occur.
- Use with caution in patient with narrow-angle glaucoma, prostatic hypertrophy, or bladder neck obstruction.

Adverse Reactions
- Better tolerated by many than β_2-adrenergic agonist bronchodilators; see Tables 17-7 (p. 239) and 17-8 (p. 240).

tiotropium

- Tiotropium is a longer-acting anticholinergic for inhalation that is used in other countries and is awaiting Food and Drug Administration approval in the United States.
- Twice-daily administration may enhance adherence and thus effectiveness.

MAST CELL STABILIZERS

Ⓟ **Prototype Drug**

cromolyn sodium (Intal)

Contraindications
- Hypersensitivity to cromolyn or to any ingredient in the product being used, such as hypersensitivity to lactose in those using capsules for inhalation

Warnings
- Not for use in the treatment of acute asthma attack
- Dose should be decreased in patients with renal or hepatic impairment.
- Severe anaphylactic reaction may occur.
- Should be discontinued if causes eosinophilic pneumonia.

Precautions
- Use inhalation aerosol cautiously in patient with coronary artery disease because of the propellant.

Drug Interactions
- Animal studies have demonstrated adverse fetal effects at very high parenteral doses in combination with high-dose isoproterenol.

Other Drugs in Class

Other drugs in this class are similar to the prototype except as follows.

cromolyn (Intal)

- Capsules for inhalation are used with a Spinhaler turbo-inhaler for children as young as 2 years and those who have difficulty with the metered dose inhaler.

nedocromil sodium (Tilade)

- Comparable to cromolyn sodium in clinical trials, except that it was slightly less effective in controlling nighttime asthma symptoms.
- For more detailed information, see Chapter 16.

AEROSOL CORTICOSTEROIDS

Ⓟ **Prototype Drug**

beclomethasone dipropionate (Beclovent, Vanceril, Vancenase, QVar)

Contraindications
- Initial treatment of severe, acute asthma attack
- Hypersensitivity to any ingredients

Warnings
- In patients switched from systemic corticosteroids to inhalation, adrenal insufficiency may occur in times of stress; patient may need to resume systemic delivery.
- Severe infection may occur more readily in patients on corticosteroids; therefore immune globulin may be indicated for those people exposed to chickenpox or measles.

- Combined use inhaled corticosteroid and alternate-day systemic therapy leads to HPA axis suppression more readily than either treatment used singly.
- Local fungal infections may occur in the mouth, pharynx, or larynx and may require treatment or discontinuation of the aerosol steroid.
- These products are not indicated for rapid relief of bronchospasm.

Precautions
- Use with caution in patients with active or quiescent tuberculosis; untreated systematic fungal, bacterial, parasiticum or viral infection; or ocular herpes simples.
- Pulmonary infiltrates with eosinophilia may occur.

Other Drugs in Class

Other drugs in this class are similar to the prototype except as follows.

flunisolide (Aerobid)

- Increased levels of orally ingested budesonide in clinical trials
- Absorbed into systemic circulation more readily than other inhaled corticosteroids

fluticasone (Flovent Rotadisk) and budesonide (Pulmicort, Turbuhaler)

- Patient inhalation driven, so may be easier to actuate than most metered dose inhalers
- However, drug delivery may be dependent on force of inhalation.

budesonide (Rhinocort Nasal Inhaler)

- Onset of action of may be faster than with other drugs—within 24 hours.

LEUKOTRIENE RECEPTOR ANTAGONISTS

(P) Prototype Drug

montelukast (Singulair)

Contraindications
- Hypersensitivity to drug or any of its components

Warnings
- Not indicated for acute asthma attacks or as monotherapy in exercise-induced asthma; short-term control medications should be available.

Precautions
- Should not be abruptly substituted for inhaled or oral corticosteroids.
- The 4- and 5-mg chewable tablets of this drug contain phenylalanine.
- Systemic eosinophilia has rarely occurred.

Drug Interactions
- May be decreased effectiveness when CYP P450 inducers such as phenobarbital and rifampin are co-administered.

Other Drugs in Class

Other drugs in this class are similar to the prototype except as follows.

zafirlukast (Accolate)

- Take zafirlukast 1 hour before or 2 hours after meals.
- Zafirlukast inhibits some enzymes of the CYP P450 system; use cautiously with drugs that are metabolized by these enzymes.
- Zafirlukast increases warfarin effect; theophylline and erythromycin decrease levels of zafirlukast; aspirin increases level of zafirlukast.
- Use zafirlukast cautiously in those with liver disease and the elderly; safety in children younger than 5 years has not been established.
- If signs of liver dysfunction develop (right upper quadrant pain, nausea, anorexia, pruritus, jaundice, fatigue), discontinue zafirlukast and measure LFTs and manage accordingly.

zileuton (Zyflo)

- Not indicated for children younger than 12 years.
- May decrease white blood cell count.
- Contraindicated in those with active liver disease; must monitor LFTs and discontinue if enzymes more than three times upper limits of normal.
- Metabolized by certain CYP P450 enzymes, so use cautiously with drugs that inhibit these enzymes; interacts with propranolol, theophylline, and warfarin to increase their effect.

RESOURCES FOR PATIENTS AND PROVIDERS

American Academy of Allergy, Asthma, and Immunology
611 East Wells Street
Milwaukee, WI 53202
(414) 272-6071
www.aaaai.org

American Academy of Pediatrics
How to help your child with asthma
Division of Publications
PO Box 747
Elk Grove Village, IL 60009-0747

Asthma and Allergy Foundation of America
1233 20th Street NW, Suite 402
Washington, DC 20036
(202) 466-7643
www.aafa.org

American Allergy Association
PO Box 7273
Menlo Park, CA 94026
Allergyaid@aol.com

American College of Allergy, Asthma, and Immunology, www.allergy.mcg.edu
Useful information for professionals and the public.

American Lung Association
61 Broadway, 6th Floor
New York, NY 10006
(800) LUNG USA
www.lungusa.org

National Asthma Education and Prevention Program
National Heart, Lung, and Blood Institute Health Information Network
PO Box 30105
Bethesda, MD 20824-0105
(301) 592-8573
www.nhlbi.nih.gov

BIBLIOGRAPHY

Drugs for asthma, *Med Lett* 41:1044, 5-10, Jan 15, 1999.

Finkelstein JA, Fuhlbrigge A, Lozano P: Parent-reported environmental exposures and environmental control measures for children with asthma, *Arch Pediatr Adolesc Med* 156:258-264, 2002.

Gallagher C: Childhood asthma: tools that help parents manage it, *Am J Nursing* 102:71-83, 2002.

Janson S, Lazarus SC: Where do leukotriene modifiers fit in asthma management? *Nurse Practitioner* 27:19-29, 2002.

Lees GM: A hitchhiker's guide to the galaxy of adrenoreceptors, *Br Med J* 283:173-178, 1981.

National Asthma Education and Prevention Program Expert Panel Report 2: *Guidelines for the diagnosis and management of asthma,* NIH Publication No. 97-4051, Washington, DC, 1997, US Government Printing Office.

National Asthma Education and Prevention Program Expert Panel Report: *Guidelines for the Diagnosis and Management of Asthma—Update on Selected Topics 2002,* NIH Publication No. 02-5075, Washington, DC, 2002, US Department of Health and Human Services. Available at www.nhlbi.nih.gov/guidelines/asthma/index.htm

Pauwels RA et al, for GOLD Scientific Committee: Global strategy for the diagnosis, management, and prevention of chronic obstructive pulmonary disease: National Heart. Lung, and Blood Institute and World Health Organization Global Initiative for Chronic Obstructive Lung Disease (GOLD) executive summary, *Respir Care* 46:798-825, 2001. Available at www.goldcopd.com

Quillen DM: COPD: an overview of the gold guidelines, 2001. Medscape Inc. Available at www.medscape.com/viewarticle/4/20891.

UNIT 6

Cardiovascular Agents

There are a wide variety of cardiovascular drugs used for many different diseases. Often the same drug will be used for many different diagnoses. Convention dictates that some cardiovascular drugs be organized by mechanism of action and other cardiovascular drugs be organized by the disease they are used to treat. This large and complex body of knowledge is organized as follows:

- **Chapter 18** focuses on the general guidelines for treatment of hypertension, and on the miscellaneous antihypertensive medications not included in Chapters 21, 22, 23, or 33.
- **Chapter 19** focuses on nitrates. Since nitrates are used predominantly for coronary artery disease, a thorough section on CAD and its treatment is included.
- **Chapter 20** discusses digoxin, used predominantly for chronic heart failure. Use of digoxin in the treatment of arrhythmias is also covered. Other drugs used to treat CHF are discussed in Chapters 21, 22, and 23.
- **Chapter 21** is a general discussion of the many uses of β-blockers.
- **Chapter 22** offers a survey of the numerous uses of calcium channel blockers. The reader is directed also to the chapters on hypertension and coronary artery disease for further discussion of calcium channel blockers.
- **Chapter 23** covers the many uses of ACE inhibitors (ACEIs) and the angiotensin II receptor blockers (ARBs), including their applicability with diabetes mellitus. They are also used to treat hypertension and CHF; discussion of these uses will be found in the respective chapters.
- **Chapter 24** discusses the use of antiarrhythmics in primary care. The class IA drugs, quinidine, procainamide, and disopyramide are covered in detail.
- **Chapter 25** includes an analysis of hyperlipidemias and their treatment.
- **Chapter 26** deals with agents that act on blood. This chapter discusses anticoagulants (emphasizing their use in atrial fibrillation), antithrombolytics, and antiplatelet drugs.

The role of the primary care provider in the treatment of cardiovascular conditions is a complex one that often varies with the comfort level of the provider and the accessibility of specialists. These conditions include some of the most common problems seen in primary care, such as hypertension and coronary artery disease.

CHAPTER 18

Hypertension and Miscellaneous Antihypertensive Medications

Drug Names

Class	Subclass	Generic Name	Trade Name
α_1-Receptor blockers		(P) prazosin terazosin (200) doxazosin	Minipress Hytrin Cardura
Centrally acting α_2-antiadrenergics		(P)(200) clonidine guanabenz guanfacine methyldopa	Catapres Wytensin Tenex Aldomet
Peripherally acting α_2-antiadrenergics		guanadrel reserpine	Hylorel generic
Direct vasodilators		hydralazine minoxidil	Apresoline Loniten

(200), Top 200 drug; (P), prototype drug.

General Uses

Indications

- Hypertension (HTN)

Other Indications and Unlabeled Uses

- α_1-Receptor blockers: either indicated or unlabeled use for the signs and symptoms of benign prostatic hypertrophy (BPH)
- Clonidine: many unlabeled uses, including alcohol and opiate withdrawal, smoking cessation, atrial fibrillation, attention deficit hyperactivity disorder, menopausal flushing, constitution growth delay in children, diabetic diarrhea, pheochromocytoma, restless leg syndrome, ulcerative colitis
- Guanfacine (unlabeled): withdrawal from heroin, migraine
- Methyldopa (unlabeled): hypertension in pregnancy
- Reserpine (indication): for relief of symptoms in agitated psychotic states
- Hydralazine (unlabeled): CHF, aortic insufficiency
- Minoxidil (indication): topical treatment for baldness

See Table 18-1.

The management of hypertension in general will be discussed, with emphasis on the Seventh Report of the Joint National Committee on the Prevention, Detection, Evaluation, and Treatment of High Blood Pressure (JNC 7) guidelines. The drugs most commonly used for hypertension are diuretics, β-blockers, calcium channel blockers, angiotensin-converting enzyme (ACE) inhibitors, and angiotensin II receptor blockers (ARBs). How these drugs are used to treat hypertension is discussed in this chapter. Detailed information on most of these antihypertensives is given in the specific drug chapters. This chapter provides detailed information on several of the other antihypertensives medications.

DISEASE PROCESS

Anatomy and Physiology

Blood pressure (BP) must be kept at a level adequate to maintain tissue perfusion as the blood moves into the capillaries. Peripheral resistance, heart rate, and stroke volume interact to determine the mean arterial pressure and capillary flow. Peripheral resistance is determined by the diameter of the arterioles; constriction of the arterioles raises the BP. Other factors that influence the BP include changes in body position, muscular activity (which causes local warmth, thus dilating vessels), and circulating blood volume. Baroreceptors respond to local changes in BP by constricting or relaxing local smooth muscle to change blood flow. Many hormones also cause contraction or relaxation of arteriolar smooth muscle to bring blood flow to a specific organ. The renin-angiotensin system is also an important regulatory feedback loop component of this system. A drop in the BP to the renal artery stimulates the secretion of renin. The hormone aldosterone, secreted from the adrenal gland, causes reabsorption of sodium in the kidneys, thus leading to water retention, increased blood volume, and increased BP.

Pathophysiology

The cause of primary hypertension (which accounts for as much as 95% of cases of hypertension) remains unknown. Although not completely understood, many factors have been linked to primary hypertension, including some that are

TABLE 18-1 Drugs Commonly Used for Hypertension

Diuretics	
β-Blockers	(BB)
Angiotensin-converting enzyme inhibitors	(ACEI)
Angiotensin II receptor blockers	(ARB)
Calcium channel blockers	(CCB)

genetically determined. Some of the mechanisms involved are elevated peripheral resistance, alteration in the cell membrane related to elevated lipids, endothelial dysfunction, changes in sodium or calcium levels, and hyperinsulinemia. Sympathetic nervous system hyperactivity caused by insensitivity of the baroreflexes may contribute to hypertension accompanied by tachycardia and elevated cardiac output in younger patients.

Dysregulation of the renin-angiotensin system leads to hypertension, although this does not appear to be a major factor in the etiology of hypertension. Black persons with hypertension and older adult patients tend to have lower plasma renin activity. Approximately 10% of hypertensive individuals have high levels, 60% have normal, and 30% have low renin levels.

Some patients have a decreased ability to excrete sodium, which leads to increased blood volume and increased BP. Abnormalities in sodium transport mechanisms lead to an increased level of intracellular sodium in blood cells. This may result in the increased vascular smooth muscle tone characteristic of hypertension.

Environmental, lifestyle, and dietary factors also play important, and modifiable, roles. Obesity leads to increased intravascular volume and increased cardiac output. Alcohol increases BP by increasing plasma catecholamines. Cigarette smoking raises BP by increasing plasma norepinephrine. NSAIDs cause fluid retention, which can lead to hypertension. Excessive intake of sodium (salt) or low levels of potassium can contribute to hypertension by increasing blood volume. Physical inactivity is a recently recognized risk factor.

Hypertension is a powerful risk factor for cardiac disease. The higher the blood pressure, the greater the risk for ischemic heart disease, heart attack, heart failure, stroke, and kidney disease. In adults, each increase of 20 mm Hg in systolic blood pressure (SBP) or 10 mm Hg in diastolic blood pressure (DBP) doubles the risk of cardiovascular disease (CVD). This knowledge has lead to an emphasis on the lower spectrum of blood pressure, resulting in the classification of "prehypertension," which is new to JNC 7.

A metabolic syndrome has recently been identified as a major cardiac risk factor. A patient who has abdominal obesity, hypertension, insulin resistance, and a lipid disorder has a greatly elevated risk of CVD. Instead of being separate risk factors, they work together to increase risk. Table 18-2 lists the major cardiovascular risk factors.

TABLE 18-2 Major Cardiovascular Risk Factors

Metabolic syndrome
- Hypertension
- Dyslipidemia
- Obesity (BMI ≥ 30)*
- Diabetes mellitus

Cigarette smoking
Physical inactivity
Microalbuminuria or estimated GFR < 60 ml/min
Family history of premature cardiovascular disease (men under age 55 or women under age 65)

From Joint National Committee on the Prevention, Detection, Evaluation, and Treatment of High Blood Pressure Education Program: *The seventh report of the Joint National Committee on Prevention, Detection, Evaluation, and Treatment of High Blood Pressure*, National Institutes of Health, National Heart, Lung, and Blood Institute, NIH publication No. 03-5233, May 2003.

*Body mass index is calculated as: $\frac{\text{Weight (in kg)}}{\text{Height (in m}^2)}$.

The Disease

Fifty million Americans have hypertension, with the prevalence increasing with age. Only about 30% of these people are adequately treated. Hypertension is a risk factor for CVD, stroke, CHF, renal failure, and peripheral vascular disease. CVD and stroke are the most common causes of death in the United States. Current levels of cardiovascular morbidity and mortality show that much greater effort needs to be extended to control hypertension.

The pendulum continues to swing regarding which factor is the most important to control: systolic or diastolic BP. The systolic BP was first considered to be most important, then focus shifted to the diastolic BP. Some researchers are exploring the significance of pulse pressure (difference between systolic and diastolic BP). However, ongoing research suggests that both systolic and diastolic BP need to be addressed in management scenarios.

Assessment

The diagnosis of hypertension is based on the average of readings taken at an initial screening and two or more readings taken at each of two or more subsequent visits. The readings on these three separate occasions should not be influenced by any other known mechanism, such as secondary hypertension, recent exercise, anxiety, or an acute illness. Initial evaluation includes a thorough history, physical examination, and laboratory screening (Box 18-1).

Once the diagnosis of hypertension is made, further evaluation of three factors affecting patient's risk is necessary. Determine the severity according to the classification in Table 18-3. Next, evaluate for target organ damage (Table 18-4), the damage the hypertension has all ready caused. Then assess for compelling indications (Table 18-5), which include other conditions managed in parallel with the HTN. These three fators will affect management.

Although primary hypertension is very common, it is essential to rule out secondary causes of hypertension (Table 18-6). Certain laboratory findings are suggestive of secondary causes, and secondary causes should be suspected if the patient's hypertension does not respond to therapy, the hypertension is of sudden onset (especially before age 20 or after age 50), if a patient with well-controlled hypertension has a sudden increase in BP, or if stage 3 hypertension develops.

BOX 18-1

CLINICAL AND DIAGNOSTIC EVALUATION FOR PATIENTS WITH DOCUMENTED HYPERTENSION

THREE MAIN PURPOSES

- Identify known causes of hypertension
- Assess presence/absence of TOD and CVD, extent of disease, and response to therapy
- Identify other cardiovascular risk factors, comorbid conditions; continue/modify treatment as indicated

HISTORY

- BP history, including duration
- Age of onset (<20 or >50 years, think secondary hypertension)
- Levels of hypertension (>180/110 mm Hg, think secondary hypertension)
- Laboratory or diagnostic testing
- All previous treatment and responses to therapy, including adverse events (resistance to therapy, think secondary hypertension)
- Personal or family history or patient symptoms of CHD (especially premature in family), heart failure, cerebrovascular disease, peripheral vascular disease, renal disease, diabetes mellitus, dyslipidemia, or other co-morbidity, such as gout or sexual dysfunction
- Listen for symptoms suggesting causes of hypertension (secondary hypertension), such as headache, daytime somnolence, fatigue, tachycardia, claudication, cold feet, sweating, thinning of skin, flank pain, muscle weakness, tremor
- Lifestyle assessment, including recent weight changes, physical activity profile, cigarette smoking, dietary intake of sodium, alcohol, saturated fat, and caffeine
- Medication history, including over-the-counter drugs, herbal remedies, and illicit drugs
- Psychosocial and environmental factors that may influence hypertension control

Physical Examination

- In particular, look for signs of secondary hypertension, such as variable pressures with tachycardia, sweating or tremors, hyperdynamic apical pulse, murmurs at anterior or posterior thorax, abnormal pulsations in neck, abdominal bruit, abdominal or flank masses, truncal obesity with purple striae, weak femoral pulses, or absent pedal pulses
- Two or more BP measurements, 2 minutes apart, patient either supine or seated and after standing for at least 2 minutes
- Verification in contralateral arm (higher value should be used)
- Height, weight, and waist circumference
- Funduscopic examination
- Examination of neck (assess for carotid bruits, jugular venous distention, or thyroid enlargement)
- Examination of heart (assess for precordial heaves, enlargement, abnormal rate or rhythm, extra sounds, including murmurs, clicks, S3, S4)
- Examination of lungs (assess for evidence of congestion or bronchospasm)
- Examination of abdomen (assess for abnormal aortic pulsations, bruits, enlarged kidneys, masses)
- Examination of extremities (assess for arterial pulses, bruits, or edema)

NEUROLOGIC ASSESSMENT

Initial Diagnostic Screening

- Before initiation of therapy, focus on determining TOD or other risk factors
- Urinalysis
- Complete blood count (CBC)
- Blood chemistries (sodium, potassium, creatinine, fasting glucose, and total and HDL cholesterol)
- Twelve-lead electrocardiogram

Optional Laboratory Tests

- 24-hour urine for microalbuminuria, creatinine clearance, or urinary protein
- Serum calcium
- Uric acid
- Fasting triglycerides and LDL cholesterol
- Glycosylated hemoglobin
- Sensitive TSH
- Limited echocardiography to determine presence of left ventricular hypertrophy (LVH)

From Joint National Committee on the Prevention, Detection, Evaluation, and Treatment of High Blood Pressure Education Program: *The seventh report of the Joint National Committee on Prevention, Detection, Evaluation, and Treatment of High Blood Pressure,* National Institutes of Health, National Heart, Lung, and Blood Institute, NIH Publication No. 03-5233, May 2003.
Material on secondary causes modified from Kaplan NM: *Clinical hypertension,* Baltimore, 1998, Williams & Wilkins.

DRUG ACTION AND EFFECTS

α_1-Receptor blockers

α_1-Receptor blockers act by selectively blocking postsynaptic α_1-adrenergic receptors. This causes dilation of both arterioles and veins and reduces peripheral vascular resistance and supine and standing BP. These drugs tend to affect the diastolic more than the systolic BP. They also relax smooth muscles in the bladder neck and prostate, reducing bladder outlet obstruction without affecting bladder contractility.

Centrally Acting α_2-Antiadrenenrgics

Centrally acting antiadrenergic agents, such as clonidine and methyldopa, act through stimulation of central inhibitory α-adrenergic receptors. They inhibit sympathetic cardioaccelerator and vasoconstrictor centers. Stimulation of α-adrenergic receptors in the brainstem results in reduced sympathetic outflow from the central nervous system (CNS), causing a decrease in peripheral resistance, renal vascular resistance, heart rate, and BP. Renal blood flow and glomerular filtration rate remain essentially unchanged.

TABLE 18-3 New Classification and Management of Blood Pressure for Adults

BP Classification	SBP (mm Hg)	DBP (mm Hg)	Initial Drug Therapy: Without Compelling Indication	Initial Drug Therapy: With Compelling Indication
Normal	<120	and <80	None indicated	Drugs for compelling indications
Prehypertension	120-139	or 80-89		
Stage 1 HTN	140-159	or 90-99	Thiazide-type diuretics for most May consider ACEI, ARB, BB, CCB or combination	Drug(s) for the compelling indications Other antihypertensive drugs (diuretics, ACEI, ARB, BB, CCB) as needed
Stage 2 HTN	≥160	or ≥100	Two-drug combination for most (usually thiazide type diuretic and ACE or ARB or BB or CCB)	

From Joint National Committee on the Prevention, Detection, Evaluation, and Treatment of High Blood Pressure Education Program: *The seventh report of the Joint National Committee on Prevention, Detection, Evaluation, and Treatment of High Blood Pressure,* National Institutes of Health, National Heart, Lung, and Blood Institute, NIH Publication No. 03-5233, May 2003.

DBP, Diastolic blood pressure; *HTN,* hypertension; *SBP,* systolic blood pressure.

TABLE 18-4 Target Organ Damage

- Heart
  - Left ventricular hypertrophy
  - Angina or prior myocardial infarction
  - Prior coronary revascularization
  - Heart failure
- Brain
  - Stroke or transient ischemic attack
- Chronic kidney disease
- Peripheral arterial disease
- Retinopathy

From Joint National Committee on the Prevention, Detection, Evaluation, and Treatment of High Blood Pressure Education Program: *The seventh report of the Joint National Committee on Prevention, Detection, Evaluation, and Treatment of High Blood Pressure,* National Institutes of Health, National Heart, Lung, and Blood Institute, NIH publication No. 03-5233, May 2003.

Peripherally Acting α_2-Antiadrenergics

Peripherally acting antiadrenergic agents inhibit sympathetic vasoconstriction by inhibiting the release of norepinephrine from peripheral nerves. Depletion of norepinephrine causes a relaxation of vascular smooth muscle, which decreases total peripheral resistance and venous return. Guanadrel and guanethidine do not inhibit parasympathetic nerve function nor do they enter the CNS. However, reserpine does enter the CNS, causing side effects.

Direct Vasodilators

Direct vasodilators relax arteriolar smooth muscle and decrease peripheral vascular resistance. This stimulates the carotid sinus baroreceptors, producing reflex increases in heart rate, renin release, and consequently sodium and water retention. Hydralazine and minoxidil result in decreased arterial BP by reducing peripheral vascular resistance. Reflex sympathetic action results in increased heart rate and cardiac output. Neither agent promotes orthostatic hypotension because of the preferential dilation of arterioles as compared with veins. However, reflex renin release leads to production of angiotensin II, which promotes aldosterone release and sodium reabsorption. Hydralazine increases heart rate and sympathetic discharge so it is frequently used in combination with β-blockers, clonidine, or methyldopa. Minoxidil triggers both cardiac and renal homeostatic mechanisms; therefore, it is frequently combined with β-blockers and diuretics.

DRUG TREATMENT PRINCIPLES

Nonpharmacologic Treatment

Lifestyle modification is an important part of treatment for all patients with hypertension (Box 18-2). Those at lower risk may have a longer trial of lifestyle modification only. Individuals at higher risk should have treatment initiated with both lifestyle modification and drug therapy.

The importance of lifestyle modification in the management of hypertension cannot be overstated. Lifestyle modifications

TABLE 18-5 Compelling Indications and Recommended Treatment

Compelling Indication	Diuretic	BB	ACEI	ARB	CCB	Aldosterone Antagonist
Chronic kidney disease			X	X		
Diabetes			X	X	X	
Heart failure	X	X	X	X		X
High-risk for CAD		X	X		X	
Post-MI		X	X	X		
Recurrent stroke prevention	X		X			

From Joint National Committee on the Prevention, Detection, Evaluation, and Treatment of High Blood Pressure Education Program: *The seventh report of the Joint National Committee on Prevention, Detection, Evaluation, and Treatment of High Blood Pressure,* National Institutes of Health, National Heart, Lung, and Blood Institute, NIH Publication No. 03-5233, May 2003.

TABLE 18-6 Secondary Causes of Hypertension

Pathology	Signs and Symptoms	Diagnostic Studies
Coarctation of the aorta	Delayed or absent femoral arterial pulses, decreased BP in lower extremities	ECG, chest x-ray studies, echocardiography, doppler ultrasonography
Cushing syndrome	Chronic steroid use: truncal obesity with purple striae, moon facies	Morning plasma cortisol after 1 mg hs dexamethasone
Pheochromocytoma	Labile HTN tachycardia, headaches, palpitations, pallor, sweating, or tremors	Spot urine for metanephrine
Primary aldosteronism	Muscle weakness, polydipsia, polyuria	Hypokalemia, excessive urinary potassium excretion, suppressed levels of plasma renin activity, elevated sodium level
Chronic kidney disease	Abdominal or flank masses (polycystic kidneys)	Urinalysis, creatinine, renal ultrasound
Renovascular disease	Epigastric or renal artery bruits, atherosclerotic disease of aorta or peripheral arteries	Renal duplex ultrasound, renal arteriography
Sleep apnea	Fatigue, loud cyclic snoring	Polysomnography
Hyperthyroidism	Weight loss, fatigue, tachycardia	TSH, T_4, free T_4, free T_4 index
Hyperparathyroidism	Renal stones, polyuria, constipation	Serum and urine calcium, urine phosphate, serum parathyroid hormone

BOX 18-2

LIFESTYLE MODIFICATIONS

- Lose weight if overweight
- Limit alcohol intake (≤1 oz ethanol/day for men and ≤0.5 oz ethanol/day for women or lighter-weight persons)
- Increase aerobic activity (30 to 45 minutes/day most days of week)
- Reduce sodium intake (≤100 mmol/day 2.4 g sodium or 6 g sodium chloride)
- Maintain adequate intake of dietary potassium (≈ 90 mmol/day)
- Maintain adequate intake of dietary calcium and magnesium
- Stop smoking
- Reduce intake of dietary saturated fat and cholesterol

From Joint National Committee on the Prevention, Detection, Evaluation, and Treatment of High Blood Pressure Education Program: *The seventh report of the Joint National Committee on Prevention, Detection, Evaluation, and Treatment of High Blood Pressure*, National Institutes of Health, National Heart, Lung, and Blood Institute, NIH Publication No. 03-5233, May 2003.

are not easy to adopt or maintain. However, these changes in behavior are inexpensive and have minimal risk. They may prevent hypertension in some individuals, decrease BP or the need for additional therapeutic agents in others, and ultimately reduce other known risk factors for CVD. Health care providers should be prepared to establish long-term therapeutic relationships with patients and to participate as motivators, educators, and role models in community-based programs as an essential part of the team approach needed to sustain these lifestyle changes.

Pharmacologic Treatment

Table 18-3 summarizes hypertension management based on BP stage and compelling indications. Treatment of hypertension is a complex and multifaceted task. Systematic treatment and monitoring such as that illustrated in Figure 18-1 are essential.

The JNC 7 guidelines should be used to determine drug choice.

- Start lifestyle modifications.
- Start drug treatment when indicated in Table 18-3.
- Make the initial drug choice based on stage and compelling indications.
- Titrate dosage. If goal is not achieved, substitute another drug from a different class or add a second agent (usually a diuretic).

The JNC 7 places new emphasis on the use of diuretics as the first choice of drug therapy for uncomplicated hypertension. If there are specific indications for a certain drug, it should be used (see Table 18-5). If there are compelling indications, specific drugs should be used.

Commonly used drugs are diuretics, β-blockers, ACE inhibitors, calcium antagonists, and ARBs. The most commonly used diuretic is hydrochlorothiazide. Loop diuretics are used in patients who have renal insufficiency. Potassium-sparing diuretics such as triamterene are used in combination, usually with hydrochlorothiazide, if the patient has low levels of potassium; they should be administered with caution.

Aldosterone antagonists such as spironolactone, another potassium-sparing diuretic, are often used in patients with congestive heart failure and after MI.

Patients with renal insufficiency and those on ACE inhibitors are at risk for elevated potassium.

ACE inhibitors are very effective and safe for treatment of hypertension. They are cardioprotective. They are useful to preserve renal function but must be used in caution in patients with pre-existing renal failure because of the risk of hyperkalemia. They often are associated with a dry cough. ARBs are as effective as ACE inhibitors but they do not cause cough.

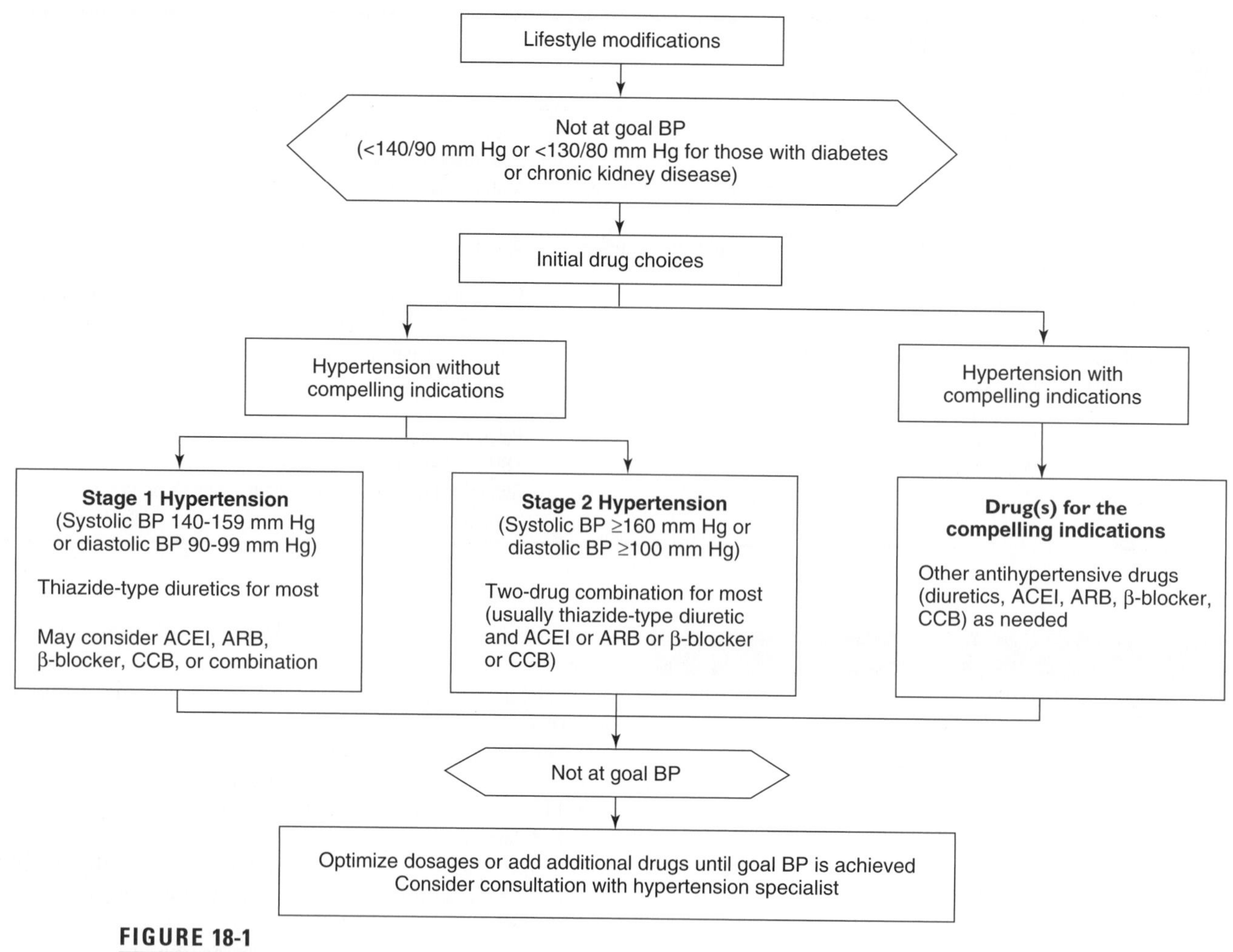

FIGURE 18-1

Hypertension treatment algorithm. (From Joint National Committee on the Prevention, Detection, Evaluation, and Treatment of High Blood Pressure Education Program: *The seventh report of the Joint National Committee on Prevention, Detection, Evaluation, and Treatment of High Blood Pressure,* National Institutes of Health, National Heart, Lung, and Blood Institute, NIH Publication No. 03-5233, May 2003.)

Their effectiveness in providing cardiac and renal protection is less well established.

β-blockers are effective and have well-demonstrated cardioprotective effects. The cardioselective β-blockers have a greater effect on the β_1-cardiac receptors than the β_2-receptors in the bronchi and blood vessels. However, they become less selective as the dosage is increased. Calcium channel blockers do not have the cardioprotective characteristics of ACE inhibitors, ARBs, and β-blockers. Short-acting calcium channel blockers should not be used for treatment of hypertension. Verapamil and diltiazem can affect atrioventricular conduction and should be used with caution in patients on β-blockers.

Cost can be an issue in drug choice. Diuretics, oral clonidine, and some β-blockers (atenolol) are available in generic form and can be inexpensive (less than $10 a month). Other drugs may be very costly, ranging from about $60 to $180 a month. Practitioners should have a good idea of the relative costs of the medications that they prescribe.

Other Antihypertensive Agents

All of the drugs in this chapter can be added when initial monotherapy fails. All of these drugs are in common use.

The α_1-receptor blockers may be used as first-line therapy in patients with benign prostatic hyperplasia (BPH). Prazosin is given less frequently than terazosin or doxazosin because of the increased frequency of first-dose syncope. These cause fewer incidences of reflex tachycardia than the direct vasodilators, but they more frequently cause postural hypotension. They may cause stress incontinence in women and postural hypotension in older adults.

Clonidine is the only antiadrenergic drug in common use. Antiadrenergic agents frequently cause fluid accumulation. Diuretics are usually needed to provide synergistic effects and to prevent fluid accumulation. The centrally acting agents have an increased incidence of adverse CNS effects such as sedation, depression, dry mouth, and impotence. The peripheral adrenergic antagonists are rarely used because of troublesome adverse effects.

Direct vasodilators are usually used in a three-drug regimen. They frequently produce reflex tachycardia but rarely cause orthostatic hypotension. A β-blocker prevents reflex tachycardia caused by decreased peripheral resistance, and a diuretic prevents secondary fluid accumulation. Hydralazine and minoxidil have direct vasodilating actions, but they are reserved for those individuals who do not respond to maximal dosages of other medications. Hydralazine is used more often in patients who have CHF, usually as a fourth-line drug. Minoxidil rarely fails to lower BP, but it should be reserved for patients who have the most severe hypertension refractory to other drugs because it can cause serious adverse reactions such as fluid retention. ACE inhibitors have largely eliminated the need for minoxidil.

HOW TO MONITOR

α_1-Receptor Blockers

- Monitor CBC as indicated. Routine monitoring is not recommended.

Centrally Acting α_2-Antiadrenergics: methyldopa

- Obtain baseline and periodic CBCs.
- Monitor liver function the first 12 weeks of therapy.
- Perform periodic determinations of LFTs, especially during the first 6 to 12 weeks of therapy or when unexplained fevers occur.

Peripherally Acting α_2-Antiadrenergics

- Fluid retention necessitates monitoring serum electrolytes and increases in weight.
- Adjust dosage based on creatinine clearance and renal function studies.

Direct Vasodilators

- Obtain baseline ECG.
- Monitor for blood dyscrasias.
- Monitor renal function studies, weight gain, and signs of edema.
- Obtain baseline ANA before initiation of hydralazine therapy because lupus-type symptoms may occur.

PATIENT VARIABLES

Geriatrics

- Older adults are more likely to have systolic hypertension and more likely to have adverse reactions, such as orthostatic hypotension, which can cause falls
- α_1-Receptor blockers: use is limited because of the side effects of syncope and tachycardia
- Centrally acting α_2-antiadrenergics
  - Clonidine can be useful for isolated systolic hypertension in older adults
  - Be vigilant for orthostatic hypotension, which may cause falls
  - Use with caution in renal failure
  - Clonidine may cause cognitive dysfunction and sedation.
- Direct vasodilators
  - May precipitate angina in patients with coronary artery disease
  - May cause or aggravate pericardial and pleural effusions
  - May increase cerebral and renal blood flow

Pediatrics

None of these drugs are indicated in pediatric patients.

Pregnancy and Lactation

- JNC 7 recommends methyldopa for women whose hypertension is first diagnosed during pregnancy.
- The American Academy of Pediatrics considers methyldopa to be compatible with breastfeeding.

Race

- Incidence of hypertension in whites is 10% to 15%
- Incidence of hypertension in blacks is 20% to 30%; blacks also have higher BP, which is harder to treat
- Black persons respond better than whites to diuretic monotherapy
- ACE inhibitors, ARBs, and β-blockers are less effective unless used with a diuretic
- Calcium channel blockers and ARBs are suitable for use in blacks

Gender

- α_1-Receptor blockers tend to be used in older men because of the positive effect on BPH
- Use minoxidil with caution in women because of hirsutism

PATIENT EDUCATION

All Antihypertensives

- Do not discontinue medication unless directed to do so by the health care provider because rebound hypertension may occur.
- Avoid cough, cold, or allergy medications containing sympathomimetics.
- May cause orthostatic hypotension. If dizziness occurs, avoid sudden changes in position. Use caution when rising from a sitting or lying position. A hot bath or shower may aggravate any dizziness. Dehydration may increase the risk of orthostatic hypotension.

α_1-Receptor Blockers

- Warn of syncope. Make sure the patient takes the first few doses when supine because of the first-dose effect.
- Avoid driving or other hazardous tasks.
- Warn men of the possibility of priapism.

Centrally and Peripherally Acting α_2-Antiadrenergics

- Drowsiness is a common adverse reaction. Take at bedtime.
- Use caution when operating machinery or driving.
- Do not use with alcohol or other CNS depressants; tolerance may be decreased.
- Notify health care provider if severe diarrhea, frequent dizziness, or fainting occurs.
- Use hard candy or frequent mouth care for dry mouth.

TABLE 18-7 Pharmacokinetics of Other Antihypertensive Medications

Drug	Absorption	Drug Availability	Onset of Action	Time to Peak Concentration	Half-Life	Duration of Action	Protein Bound	Metabolism	Excretion
prazosin (Minipress)		48%-68%	2 hr	1-3 hr	2-3 hr	10 hr	92%-97%	Extensive; active metabolites	Bile-feces, 90%; urine, 10%
terazosin (Hytrin)		90%	15 min	1-2 hr	9-12 hr	12-24 hr	90%-94%	70% metabolized	Bile-feces, 60%; urine, 40%
doxazosin (Cardura)		65%			2-3 hr	22 hr	98%	Extensive; several active metabolites	Bile-feces, 63%; urine, 9%
clonidine (Catapres)	GI or transdermal		30-60 min	3-5 hr; 2-3 day transdermal	12-19 hr	12-24 hr		Liver 50%	Kidney, 50%
guanabenz (Wytensin) GI	GI	75%	1 hr	2-4 hr	6 hr	6-12 hr		Rapid	Kidney
guanfacine (Tenex)				1-4 hr	17 hr	24 hr	70%	Liver	Kidney, 40%
methyldopa (Aldomet)	Variable	8%-62%	2 hr	2-4 hr	2 hr	12-24 hr		Complex	Kidney, 70%
guanadrel (Hylorel)			0.5 to 2 hr	1.5-2 hr	10 hr	9-14 hr	<20%	Liver	Kidney, 40%
reserpine			Slow (days)	3.5 hr	33 hr	6-24 hr	96%		
hydralazine (Apresoline)	Rapid	30%-50%	Fast (45 min)	1-2 hr	3-7 hr	6-12 hr	87%	Extensive; liver	Kidney, 12%-14%
minoxidil (Loniten)	Rapid	90%	30 min	2-3 hr	4 hr	24-75 hr	0	90% conjugation	Kidney
guanethidine (Ismelin)	Incomplete	3%-50%	1-3 wk	6-8 hr	2-8 days	24-48 hr		Liver-partial	Kidney, 25%-50%

Direct Vasodilators

- Urine exposed to air may darken.
- Take hydralazine with meals.
- Notify provider if unexplained prolonged fatigue or fever, muscle or joint aches, or chest pain is experienced.

Specific Drugs

α_1-RECEPTOR BLOCKERS

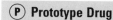

Prototype Drug

prazosin (Minipress)

Contraindications

- Hypersensitivity to prazosin, doxazosin, terazosin, or tamsulosin.

Warnings

Watch for "first-dose" effect. These drugs can cause marked hypotension, especially postural, and syncope. This hypotension with syncope may occur during the first 30 to 90 minutes of the first several doses. Prazosin has a higher incidence of this effect than doxazosin or terazosin.

Priapism occurs rarely.

Administer doxazosin with caution to patients with evidence of hepatic impairment and to patients on other medications metabolized by the liver.

Precautions

- Cardiotoxicity: Rats and mice have had an increased incidence of myocardial necrosis or fibrosis. There is no evidence that this occurs in humans.

Pharmacokinetics

See Table 18-7.

Adverse Effects

See Table 18-8.

Drug Interactions

- Alcohol, β-blockers, cimetidine, and verapamil may increase levels of α-adrenergic blockers.
- Indomethacin may decrease the effect of prazosin.
- α-Adrenergic blockers and prazosin may decrease the effect of clonidine.

Overdosage

- Symptoms involve hypotension.

Dosage and Administration

See Table 18-9.

Other Drugs in Class

Other drugs in this class are similar to the prototype except as follows.

terazosin (Hytrin)

- Hemodilution: small but statistically significant decreases in hematocrit, hemoglobin, white blood cells, total protein, and albumin have been observed with terazosin
- Weight gain with terazosin
- Cholesterol: terazosin and doxazosin have decreased total cholesterol

doxazosin (Cardura)

- Leukopenia/neutropenia with doxazosin
- Mean white blood cell and neutrophil counts were decreased

CENTRALLY ACTING α_2-ANTIADRENERGICS

Clonidine and methyldopa are discussed in detail because they are the only drugs in common use.

Prototype Drug

clonidine (Catapres)

Contraindications

- Hypersensitivity to clonidine or the components of the transdermal system

Warnings

- Use with caution in patients with severe coronary insufficiency, conduction disturbances, recent myocardial infarction (MI), cerebrovascular disease, or chronic renal failure.
- Tolerance may develop.

Precautions

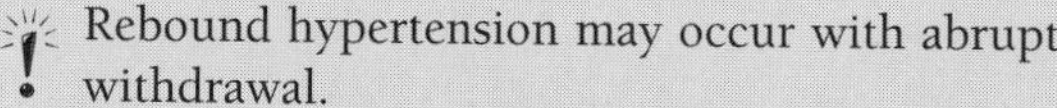

Rebound hypertension may occur with abrupt withdrawal.

- Discontinue the drug gradually.
- Symptoms of rebound hypertension are rapid rise in blood pressure, tachycardia, nervousness, agitation, and headache.
- In addition, tremors and confusion may occur with abrupt withdrawal.
- Sedation or drowsiness is a very common adverse effect.
- With the use of clonidine, retinal degeneration is possible.
- Stop drug within 4 hours of surgery and resume as soon as possible during immediate postoperative course.
- Sensitization to transdermal clonidine may produce a generalized rash.

TABLE 18-8 Common and Serious Adverse Effects of Antihypertensive Medications

Drug	Common Side Effects	Serious Adverse Effects
α_1-Adrenergic blockers	Palpitation, nervousness, asthenia, mild GI distress, urinary frequency, nasal congestion, headache, edema, fatigue	Postural hypotension, syncope, CNS depression, dizziness (10%), dyspnea, blurred vision
clonidine; guanabenz and guanfacine are similar	Dry mouth (40%), drowsiness (33%), dizziness (16%), sedation, constipation (10%), GI distress, headaches, nervousness, impotence	Syncope, CHF, orthostatic hypotension, tachycardia, bradycardia, Raynaud's disease, conduction disturbances; insomnia, hallucinations, thrombocytopenia, weakness, fatigue, MS pain
methyldopa; guanadrel is similar	Headache, asthenia, dizziness, gynecomastia, GI distress	Bradycardia, angina, CHF, orthostatic hypotension, edema. sedation, parkinsonism; toxic epidermal necrolysis, hemolytic anemia, abnormal LFTs, drug fever, arthralgia, myalgia
reserpine	GI distress, impotence, gynecomastia	Arrhythmias, syncope, angina, bradycardia, edema, parkinsonism, dizziness, headache, anxiety, severe depression, nervousness, dyspnea, hypersensitivity
hydralazine	Palpitations, headache, constipation, nausea, vomiting, diarrhea	Tachycardia, angina, paresthesia, dizziness, paralytic ileus, blood dyscrasias, hypersensitivity, edema, dyspnea
minoxidil		Pericardial effusion, angina, cardiac lesions, ECG changes, fluid and electrolyte imbalance, tachycardia, hypersensitivity, hypertrichosis, Stevens-Johnson syndrome

TABLE 18-9 Dosage and Administration Recommendations of Antihypertensive Medications

Drug	Starting Dosage (mg)	Administration	Titration	Maximum Daily Dose
prazosin	1	hs then bid or tid	5-10 mg bid	40 mg
terazosin	1	hs then qd or bid	1-5 mg/day	20 mg
doxazosin	1	hs then qd	2-4 mg/d	8-16 mg
clonidine	0.1 (100 μg topical)	bid qwk	↑ 100 μg weekly ↑ q1-2wk	2400 μg; two 300 μg patches
methyldopa	250	bid or tid	↑ q2days	3 g
hydralazine	10	qid	↑ to 25 mg after 2-4 days, then 50 mg qid	300 mg

mg, Milligrams; *qd*, every day.

Abbreviations used for brevity in this reference table. In clinical practice, we recommend that you follow the communication/abbreviation guidelines of the Joint Commission on Accreditation of Healthcare Organizations (http://www.jcaho.org) and the Institute for Safe Medication Practice (http://www.ismp.org).

- Ophthalmologic effects: perform periodic eye examinations because retinal degeneration has been noted in animal studies.

Drug Interactions

- Clonidine decreases effectiveness of levodopa.
- β-blockers and verapamil increase the effect of clonidine.
- Prazosin and tricyclic antidepressants TCAs decrease the effect of clonidine.

Overdosage

- Symptoms of overdosage include bradycardia, hypotension, CNS depression, respiratory depression, apnea, seizures, and arrhythmias.
- Do not induce emesis; treatment is supportive.

Other Drugs in Class

Other drugs in this class are similar to the prototype except as follows.

methyldopa (Aldomet)

Contraindications

- Active liver disease
- Coadministration with MAOIs and sulfite sensitivity

Warnings/Precautions

- Watch for hemolytic anemia or development of positive Coombs' test.
- Hepatic toxicity has occurred during the first 3 weeks of therapy (elevated liver enzymes, fever, and jaundice); stop drug if this develops.
- Use with caution in patients who have renal insufficiency.
- Transient sedation may occur during initial drug therapy.
- Use lower doses with atherosclerotic vascular disease.

Drug Interactions

- Central effects of levodopa in Parkinson's disease may be potentiated.
- Coadministration of methyldopa and lithium may cause lithium toxicity (i.e., GI distress, tremor, weakness, and lethargy).
- Use of MAOIs leads to excess sympathetic discharge.
- Phenothiazines seriously raise BP.
- Barbiturates may reduce therapeutic response of methyldopa.
- Tricyclic antidepressants blunt the therapeutic effect of methyldopa.

Overdosage

- Sedation, severe hypotension, weakness, nausea, vomiting and CNS and GI alterations are signs of overdosage.
- Gastric emptying should be done if overdosage is caught early.

PERIPHERALLY ACTING α_2-ANTIADRENERGICS

These are not discussed in detail because they are seldom used.

DIRECT VASODILATORS

Only hydralazine is discussed, because minoxidil is seldom used.

hydralazine (Apresoline)

Contraindications

- Hypersensitivity
- CAD, and mitral valve disease

Warnings

- May cause a lupus-type syndrome
- May produce a clinical picture simulating systemic lupus erythematosus (arthralgia, dermatoses, fever, splenomegaly), including glomerulonephritis. Obtain baseline and periodic blood counts and ANA titers
- Renal function impairment: may increase renal blood flow; use with caution
- Bone marrow depression and blood dyscrasias have been reported

Precautions

- Hyperdynamic cardiac status may exaggerate cardiac deficits (pulmonary artery pressure in mitral valve disease; myocardial ischemia or infarction in CAD).
- CAD: myocardial stimulation can cause anginal attacks and ECG changes of ischemia; use with caution in patients with suspected CAD.
- Pulmonary hypertension: use with caution; severe hypotension may result.
- May cause some decrease in total cholesterol.
- Peripheral neuritis as evidenced by paresthesias, numbness, and tingling has been observed.
- Hematologic effects: blood dyscrasias consisting of low CBC, leukopenia, agranulocytosis, and purpura.

Drug Interactions

- β-blockers increase serum levels of hydralazine.
- Indomethacin decreases action of hydralazine.

Overdosage

- Hypotension, tachycardia, headache, and skin flushing to cardiac arrest and shock can occur.

RESOURCES FOR PATIENTS AND PROVIDERS

American Heart Association, www.americanheart.org/, telephone 800-242-8721.

Offers patient teaching information useful for either providers or patients.

American Society of Hypertension, www.ash-us.org.

International Society on Hypertension in blacks, www.ishib.org, telephone 404-875-6263.

Provides information about cardiovascular diseases among various ethnic groups.

Jackson Heart study, www.jsums.edu/jhs/main.html.

Provides information on a study evaluating cardiovascular disease in African Americans.

National Heart, Lung, Blood Institute, www.nhlbi.nih.gov/health or call 301-592-8572.

The latest JNC 7 report is available at this site and may be downloaded. Adobe Acrobat Reader required.

Dash Diet, www.nhlbi.nih.gov/health/public/heart/hbp/dash/index.html, telephone 301-592-8573.

BIBLIOGRAPHY

The ALLHAT Officers and Coordinators for the ALLHAT Collaborative Research Group: Major outcomes in high-risk hypertensive patients randomized to angiotensin converting enzyme inhibitor or calcium channel blocker vs diuretic: The Antihypertensive and Lipid-Lowering Treatment to Prevent Heart Attack Trial (ALLHAT), *JAMA* 288:2981-2997, 2002.

Drugs for hyertension: treatment guidelines, *The Medical Letter* 1(6), 2003.

Goldman G, Braunwald D: *Primary cardiology,* Philadelphia, 1998, Saunders.

Hansson L et al: Effects of intensive blood-pressure lowering and low-dose aspirin in patients with hypertension: principal results of the Hypertension Optimal Treatment (HOT) randomised trial, *Lancet* 351:1755-1762, 1998.

Kaplan NM: *Clinical hypertension,* Baltimore, 1998, Williams & Wilkins. Kasiske BL et al: Effects of antihypertensive therapy on serum lipids, *Ann Intern Med* 122:133, 1995.Labarthe DR: *Epidemiology and prevention of cardiovascular diseases,* Frederick, Md, 1998, Aspen Publishers.

National Heart, Lung, and Blood Institute, National Institutes of Health, National High Blood Pressure Education Program: *The seventh report of the Joint National Committee on Prevention, Detection, Evaluation, and Treatment of High Blood Pressure,* National Institutes of Health, National Heart, Lung, and Blood Institute, NIH Publication No. 03-5233, May 2003.

Sobel BJ, Bakris GL: *Hypertension management,* St Louis, 1995, Mosby.

CHAPTER 19

Coronary Artery Disease and Nitrates

Drug Names

Class	Subclass	Generic Name	Trade Name
Sublingual tablet		(P) (200) nitroglycerin isosorbide dinitrate	Nitrostat Isordil
Translingual spray		nitroglycerin	Nitrolingual
Transdermal patch		nitroglycerin	Nitro-Dur
Topical ointment		nitroglycerin	Nitro-Bid, Minitran
Oral		nitroglycerin isosorbide dinitrate (200) isosorbide mononitrate	Nitrong, Nitro-Bid Isordil ISMO, Monoket, Imdur

(200), Top 200 drug; (P), prototype drug.

General Uses

Indications

Labeled Uses	*Dosage Form*
Acute angina	Sublingual, transmucosal, and translingual spray
Angina prophylaxis	Transdermal, topical, translingual spray, and transmucosal and oral-sustained release forms

Unlabeled Uses	*Dosage Form*
Chronic heart failure (CHF), acute myocardial infarction (MI)	Sublingual, topical, and oral
Raynaud's phenomenon, peripheral vascular disease (PVD)	Ointment

All patients with a history of angina should have sublingual nitroglycerin (NTG) available and they should know how to use it. Medications other than nitrates used to treat coronary artery disease (CAD) include β-blockers (BB), calcium channel blockers (CCB), and angiotensin-converting enzyme (ACEI) and ACE II inhibitors (ARBs). Their use in the treatment of CAD is discussed here. Details on those drugs are discussed in their respective chapters.

Angina persisting longer than 20 minutes or after three doses of NTG 5 minutes apart may indicate progressing infarction, and the patient should go to the nearest emergency department.

The Guidelines for the Management of Patients with Chronic Stable Angina from the American college of Cardiology were released in 2002.

DISEASE PROCESS

Anatomy and Physiology

The myocardium receives its blood supply from the coronary arteries, a system of small arteries that branch from the aorta (Figure 19-1). The right coronary artery lies in a groove between the right atrium and right ventricle and supplies the right ventricle. The left main coronary artery is divided shortly after its origin into two branches—the left anterior descending branch and the circumflex branch. The left anterior descending branch supplies blood to the anterior myocardium, apex, and anterior septum and is located on the surface of the anterior myocardium. The circumflex branch lies in a groove between the left atrium and left ventricle and supplies blood to the left ventricle. Smaller branches arise from the large coronary vessels. In 90% of the population, a posterior descending artery arises from right coronary artery, and in 10%, it arises from the circumflex branch of the left anterior descending artery.

Pathophysiology

Determinants in pathogenesis of myocardial ischemia are the following: atheromatous lesions, increased myocardial oxygen demand, and catecholamine release.

Atheromatous Lesions. The atherosclerotic process is the buildup of plaque in blood vessels. This process occurs throughout the body. The arteries most often affected are coronary arteries (CAD), cerebral vascular arteries (stroke), and the peripheral arteries (PVD). The first step in the process of atherosclerosis is deposition of the fatty streak. Lipid-laden foam cells derived from macrophages or smooth muscle cells accu-

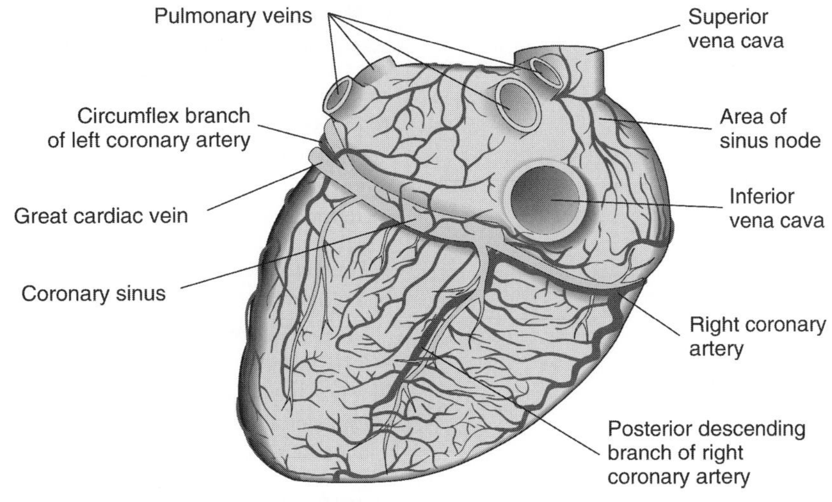

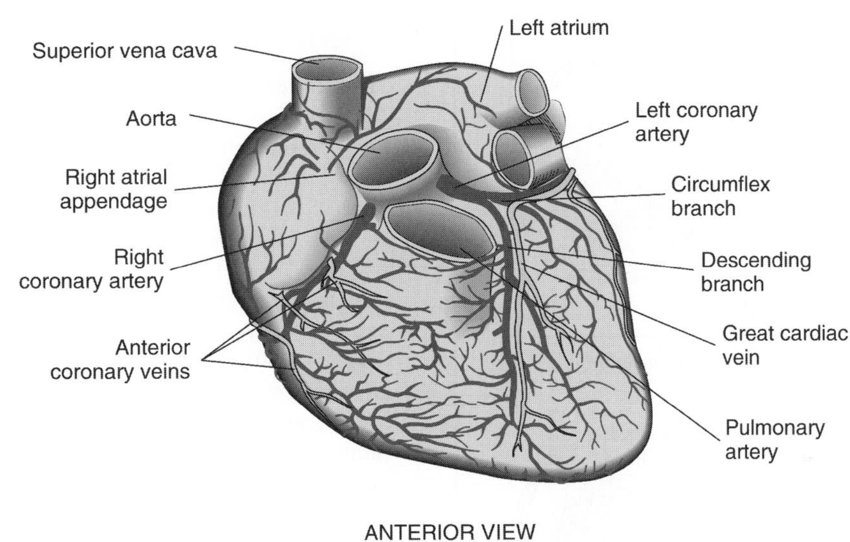

FIGURE 19-1

Anterior and posterior surfaces of the heart, illustrating the location and distribution of the peripheral coronary vessels. (From Berne RM, Levy MW: *Cardiovascular physiology,* ed 7, St Louis, 1997, Mosby.)

mulate on the subendothelial lining. The most important lipids in this step are the low-density lipoproteins (LDLs). Smooth muscle cells migrate into the lesion. At this step, the plaque does not affect circulation. Progression of these fatty streaks leads to the development of a collagen cap. The lesion becomes calcified, and the vessel lumen slowly becomes narrowed.

As the plaque grows, it may develop an internal hemorrhage, which then leaks to the surface. The body reacts by formation of a thrombus. Infarction occurs from total occlusion of the artery by the thrombus (Figure 19-2).

Increased Myocardial Oxygen Demand. Myocardial ischemia can be brought on by increased myocardial oxygen requirements such as exercise, mental stress, or spontaneous fluctuations in heart rate and blood pressure. It can also be caused by decreased oxygen supply such as occurs with vasospasm, platelet plugging, or partial thrombosis. Oxygen supply to the myocardium depends on filling of the coronary arteries during diastole. Filling depends on coronary perfusion pressure and coronary vascular resistance. Coronary vascular resistance depends on the degree of collateralization and the patency of the coronary blood vessels. With exercise, the coronary blood flow may need to increase as much as four to five times above resting level.

Catecholamine Release. Catecholamines release in response to exertional and emotional stress or other activity. Catecholamines cause increased heart rate, blood velocity, and force of myocardial contraction, producing increased oxygen demand and ischemia. Increased heart rate decreases the length

Coronary syndromes: clinicopathological correlates

Syndrome	Coronary pathology
a Stable angina	Stenotic endothelialized atheromatous plaque
b Unstable angina	Ruptured atheromatous plaque with subocclusive thrombus
c Variant angina	Coronary spasm with or without atheromatous plaque
d Myocardial infarction	Ruptured atheromatous plaque with occlusive thrombus

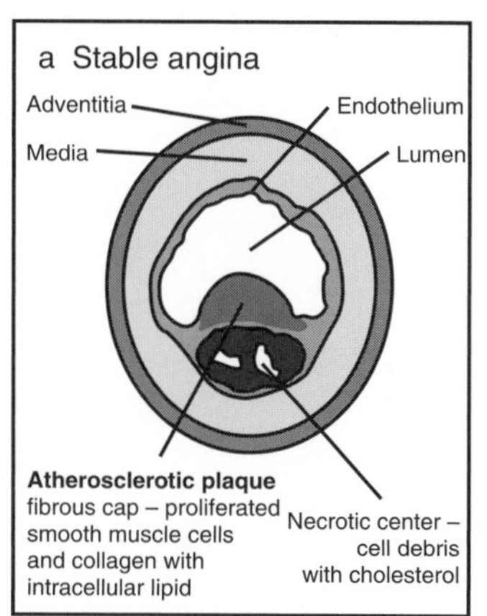

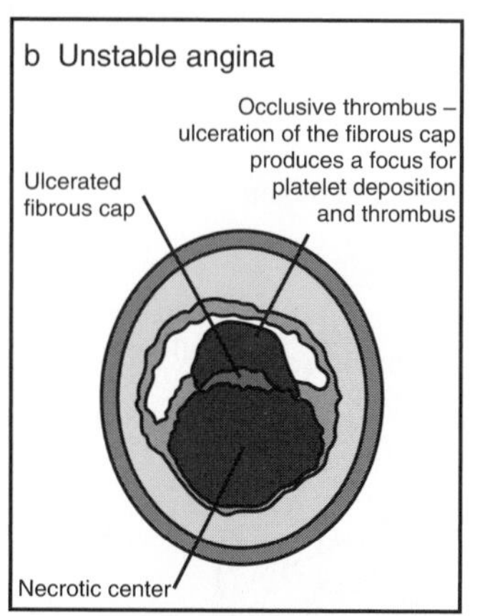

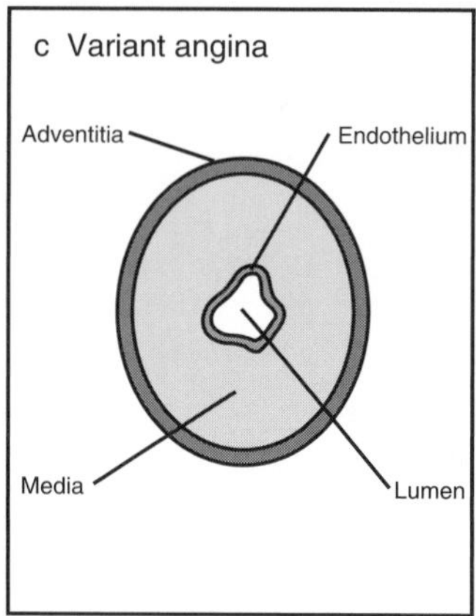

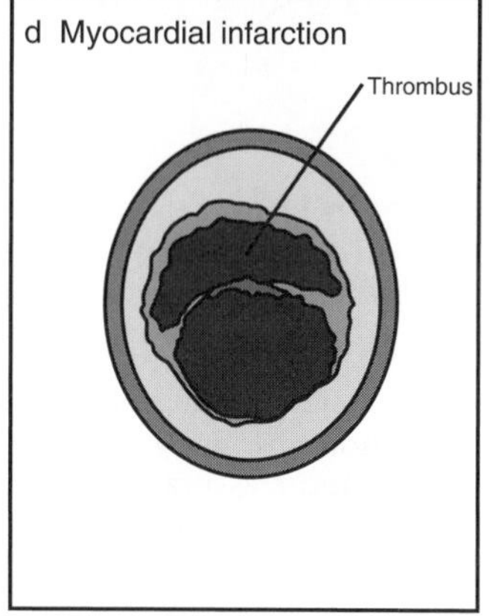

FIGURE 19-2

Plaque formation in coronary syndromes. (From Timmis AD: *Cardiology*, ed 3, London, 1991, Mosby-Wolfe.)

of diastole, which is when the coronary arteries perfuse the myocardium. Ischemia then stimulates further catecholamine release. β-Blockers inhibit this release of catecholamine and help stop the cycle. If the myocardium does not receive enough oxygen, the ischemia may result in pain (angina), arrhythmias, or left ventricular dysfunction (CHF). Ischemia can be either painful or pain free. Silent ischemia is as dangerous as painful ischemia.

BOX 19-1

RISK FACTORS FOR CORONARY ARTERY DISEASE

NONMODIFIABLE OR SLIGHTLY MODIFIABLE
Premature family CAD (before age 50 years)
Age
Male gender

POTENTIALLY MODIFIABLE
Blood lipid abnormalities
Diabetes mellitus
Hypertension
Elevated blood homocysteine levels
Markers of inflammation such as C-reactive protein and hyperfibrinogenemia

MODIFIABLE
Physical inactivity
Cigarette smoking
Obesity

The Disease

Risk Factors. Some large epidemiologic studies have identified certain habits and predisposing conditions that correlate with the development of CAD (Box 19-1). Emerging data suggest that modifying the LDL level to 100 mg/dl or less may slow or possibly reverse the development of atherosclerotic plaque. Elevated levels of serum homocysteine and C-reactive protein (CRP) correlate with the occurrence of CAD. CRP is a marker for underlying systemic inflammation. There is a positive association between homocysteine levels and premature atherosclerotic disease. Serum homocysteine is associated with low dietary folate and deficiencies in vitamins B_6 and B_{12}. Recommendations on the use of tests for homocysteine and CRP are not yet available. Their best use is probably with patients at elevated risk for CAD from other risk factors. Elevations in these tests may indicate a more aggressive approach in prevention.

Angina. There are two major causes of anginal ischemic myocardial pain. By far the most common is arteriosclerotic heart disease described previously. The other cause seen in primary care is coronary vasospasm with or without atherosclerotic CAD.

Definition of Disease. Myocardial ischemia occurs when myocardial oxygen demand exceeds oxygen supply. Increased demand usually occurs from tachyarrhythmias, hypertension, and exercise, all of which increase cardiac workload. Decreased supply usually results from coronary artery stenosis. Angina pectoris is chest pain, pressure, or discomfort caused by myocardial ischemia.

Classification. *Stable angina* is no change in the past 2 months in the frequency, duration (less than 15 minutes), or precipitating causes. There also is a reproducible symptom pattern.

Unstable angina is a change in pattern; increase in frequency, severity, and/or duration of pain and less precipitating factors.

Unstable angina is angina that is new onset, onset with less exertion than the previous pattern, or pain that occurs at rest. Patients with unstable angina should be admitted to a coronary care unit. The treatment of unstable angina is beyond the scope of this text. Immediate care of the patient while awaiting hospitalization is discussed under Drug Treatment Guidelines.

Variant (Prinzmetal's) angina refers to coronary artery spasm. This is very rare. Pain often occurs at rest and develops because of spasm rather than increased myocardial oxygen demand.

Silent ischemia is classified as asymptomatic episodes of myocardial ischemia that can be detected with electrocardiography (ECG) and other diagnostic techniques.

Assessment

The history is crucial to the diagnosis of CAD. Myocardial ischemia causes angina, a symptom of CAD. The sensation of angina is usually described as a heavy substernal pressure or pain, which may radiate to the left arm. It is brought on by exertion and is relieved by rest. The sensation may be described as tightness, squeezing, gas, indigestion, or a vague discomfort instead of a specific description of pain. The pain may be located anywhere from the lower jaw to the epigastrium. It may radiate to the right arm in addition to the left. If the patient identifies the site of pain by pointing to the area of the apical impulse with one finger, angina is unlikely. The episode usually lasts 15 to 30 minutes. Patients are usually most comfortable in a sitting position. They may feel short of breath. Occasionally, a patient may have myocardial ischemia without any symptoms; silent ischemia will show up on ECG.

On physical examination, blood pressure may be elevated or decreased. An occasional extra sound or systolic murmur may be heard. An ECG shows characteristic changes of ischemia in about 75% of the patients with angina. The other 25% have other abnormalities on ECG. The characteristic change is a horizontal or downsloping ST-segment depression that resolves as the angina resolves. T-wave flattening or inversion may also occur. Occasionally ST-segment elevation occurs. Examination of the patient between episodes of angina may be normal, including the ECG.

Basic diagnostic studies include serum lipid levels, CBC, electrolytes, ECG, and exercise testing. Myocardial perfusion scintigraphy uses radionuclide uptake to identify areas of hypoperfusion. An echocardiogram is useful to assess left ventricular function. Coronary angiography is the definitive diagnostic procedure for coronary disease. Newer imaging techniques include computed tomography scanning and magnetic resonance imaging, but their usefulness remains to be determined.

DRUG ACTION AND EFFECTS

Nitrates relax vascular smooth muscle via stimulation of intracellular cyclic guanosine monophosphate production. The major effect of nitrates is to reduce myocardial oxygen demand, primarily by decreasing preload and to a lesser extent by decreasing afterload. Nitrates cause major dilation of the venous bed. Vasodilation results in venous pooling of blood, thereby decreasing venous return. Decreased venous return reduces ventricular end-diastolic volume. This reduction in preload results in reduced filling pressure (decreased pressure of blood against the wall of the heart). Reduced wall tension decreases myocardial oxygen demand.

A relatively minor effect of nitrates is reduction of afterload by arterial relaxation. Reduction of afterload decreases myocardial work, which decreases oxygen consumption.

Another relatively minor effect of nitrates is to improve myocardial oxygen supply by optimizing blood delivery via dilation of coronary arteries. This may be an important mechanism in the prevention and treatment of coronary vasospasm. Nitrates also increase use of coronary collaterals so that there is better perfusion of the inner layers of the myocardium.

DRUG TREATMENT PRINCIPLES

Patients with symptoms suggestive of CAD should be referred to a cardiologist for evaluation and treatment. The primary care provider is usually responsible for follow-up of stable angina.

Risk Reduction

All adults should be educated regarding the efficacy of risk reduction in preventing CAD. Risk reduction is a key component of the treatment of CAD. The three risk factors about which the most effort should be made are hypertension, cigarette smoking, and blood lipid abnormalities. Control of these can significantly reduce a person's risk of CAD. Each of these is important enough to merit a separate chapter in this book. In addition, the control of diabetes mellitus is extremely important. Obesity and physical inactivity should be approached along with lipid reduction. Exercise is important for weight reduction and for regulation of lipids. Bad fats decrease and good fats increase with exercise.

Acute Attack

1. Give NTG sublingually at 3- to 5-minute intervals for 3 doses. If this is not effective, call emergency medical services.
2. Give oxygen, usually at 2 L/min, via nasal cannula.
3. Have the patient chew a regular aspirin (325 mg) while waiting for the ambulance to arrive.
4. Rest and reassurance are helpful.
5. It is important the patient receive thrombolytic therapy as soon as possible, preferably within the first 1 to 3 hours of the MI.

Use of Nitrates in Acute Attack

! Nitrates are taken at the time of an anginal attack. Select a fast-acting nitrate.

The most common form used is a sublingual tablet of NTG. Translingual spray is also acceptable. The usual dose of NTG tablets is 0.4 mg sublingually (SL). Use a smaller dose (0.3 mg) for a small, frail, and/or elderly patient. Increase the dose to 0.4 to 0.6 mg if not completely effective. Sublingual NTG is rapid acting, convenient, relatively safe, and inexpensive. NTG spray is equally as effective as the sublingual tablets but is more expensive. NTG translingual spray may be more convenient for patients who have difficulty handling the small tablets in a stressful situation. It is also more stable and will last longer than the pills. The translingual spray should be sprayed onto or under the tongue, *not inhaled.*

Have the patient take the medicine as soon as pain is experienced. Have the patient lie down and rest. The drug should be effective in 1 to 2 minutes. If the pain is not relieved within 3 to 5 minutes, a second pill may be taken. If the pain is not relieved within another 3 to 5 minutes, a third pill may be taken. If three pills do not relieve the pain, patients should contact their primary care provider or go to an emergency department. If the patient is having an anginal episode at the time of the office visit, an ECG will document the angina. The effectiveness of the nitrate should be evident on a subsequent ECG.

Fast-acting nitrates can also be given before a stressful episode, such as exercise or sex, to prevent angina.

Chronic Stable Angina/Prevention/Post–Myocardial Infarction Management

The following are general steps and cannot include every variable a patient may have. Use these principles with caution (Table 19-1). The previous protocol assumes the patient does not have other concomitant illness. However, angina patients often have other problems, which affect how their angina is treated (Table 19-2).

1. Start with nonpharmacologic lifestyle modifications AFTER the angina is controlled.
2. Manage aggravating factors. Treat other problems and risk factors aggressively:
3. All patients should be given a rapid-acting nitrate and be instructed in its use for treatment of acute angina. See later discussion for specific details.
4. Long-acting nitrates should be considered. The main limitation is tolerance, which can be limited by providing a nitrate-free period of 6 to 10 hours each day. See later discussion for specific details.
5. β-Blocker therapy should be considered in all angina patients. They are the only antianginal agent shown to prevent death in patients with angina. A careful evaluation of the patient's risks and indications for β-blockers should be conducted. Allow 1 to 2 months for a drug trial with β-blockers to adjust dose and monitor for therapeutic response and adverse reactions. See Chapter 21 for more information.
6. Calcium channel blockers are the medications of choice in coronary vasospasm. They may also be useful in stable angina if nitrates and β-blockers have failed. Short-acting nifedipine in moderate to large doses causes an increase in mortality in patients in unstable angina or recently post-MI.
7. Recommend aspirin, unless contraindicated. Every patient with CAD should take aspirin 81 to 325 mg qd.
8. Revascularization procedures include coronary artery bypass grafting, percutaneous transluminal coronary angioplasty, and stenting.

Use of Nitrates in Chronic Stable Angina/Prevention/Post–Myocardial Infarction Management. Nitrates are given on a routine basis to prevent anginal episodes. Angina prophylaxis requires a long-acting transdermal patch, oral sustained release tablet, or topical ointment. A transdermal patch is often used because of its ease of administration. Dosage is measured as release rate in milligrams per hour. The usual starting dosage is 0.2 to 0.4 mg/hr, which is increased or decreased depending on the patient's therapeutic response and the adverse effects. Transdermal patches are more convenient but are more expensive than oral nitrates. Oral nitrates are effective, safe, and economical. The most common oral nitrate used is isosorbide mononitrate. Isosorbide dinitrate is also available. Oral nitrates experience the first-pass phenomenon, in which large amounts of the drug are immediately metabolized by the liver. This means large doses are required to obtain therapeutic effect. Alternative routes of administration, such as transdermal patches and buccal tablets, were developed to avoid this phenomenon.

Tolerance to nitrates is an issue. To prevent tolerance, it is necessary to interrupt therapy for 8 to 12 hours a day. The usual method is to take off the patch or stop the oral medication in the evening and then restart in the morning. The problem with this is that early morning is a dangerous time for ischemia and MI. To avoid this risk, nitrates should be omitted during a quiet period during the day. Another antianginal agent may be necessary during the nitrate-free interval.

HOW TO MONITOR

Patients should be encouraged to keep a record of PRN medication use. This record should be brought to appointments and reviewed by the clinician. Evaluate record for patterns of increased frequency, multiple dosing to eliminate symptoms, or changes in activity that produce angina and point to worsening anginal status. Decreased frequency of anginal episodes will document efficacy of the NTG. If the patient does not have decreased episodes of angina, he or she should notify the provider.

PATIENT VARIABLES

Geriatrics

- Older patients are at increased risk for syncope with administration of NTG.
- Make sure patient is seated or lying down before administering NTG.
- Geriatric patients also usually require a lower dose of nitrates.

Pediatrics

- Safety and efficacy have not been established.

Pregnancy

- *Category C:* safety of use in pregnancy has not been established.

PATIENT EDUCATION

For All Types of Nitroglycerin

NTG is a very unstable medication and great care needs to be taken in handling and storing medication or it will not be effective.

TABLE 19-1 Guide to Comprehensive Risk Reduction for Patients with Coronary and Other Vascular Disease

<table>
<tr><th>Risk Intervention</th><th>Recommendations</th></tr>
<tr><td>Smoking:
Goal
Complete cessation</td><td>Strongly encourage patient and family to stop smoking.
Provide counseling, nicotine replacement, and formal cessation programs as appropriate.</td></tr>
<tr><td>Lipid management:
Primary goal
LDL <100 mg/dl
Secondary goals
HDL >35 mg/dl
TG <200 mg/dl</td><td>Start AHA Step II Diet in all patients: ≤30% fat, <7% saturated cholesterol.
Assess fasting lipid profile. In post-MI patients, lipid profile may take 4 to 6 wk to stabilize.
Add drug therapy according to the following guide:
<table>
<tr><td rowspan="5">LDL <100 mg/dl

No drug therapy</td><td colspan="3">LDL 100-130 mg/dl

Consider adding drug therapy to diet, as follows:</td><td colspan="3">LDL >130 mg/dl

Add drug therapy to diet, as follows:</td><td rowspan="5">HDL <35 mg/dl

Emphasize weight management and physical activity
Advise smoking cessation
If needed to achieve LDL goals, consider niacin, statin, fibrate</td></tr>
<tr><td colspan="6">↘ ↙
Suggested drug therapy</td></tr>
<tr><td colspan="2">TG <200 mg/dl</td><td colspan="2">TG 200-400 mg/dl</td><td colspan="2">TG >400 mg/dl</td></tr>
<tr><td colspan="2">Statin
Resin
Niacin</td><td colspan="2">Statin
Niacin</td><td colspan="2">Consider combined drug therapy (niacin, fibrate, statin)</td></tr>
<tr><td colspan="6">If LDL goal not achieved, consider combination therapy</td></tr>
</table></td></tr>
<tr><td>Physical activity:
Minimum goal
30 min 3-4 times per week</td><td>Assess risk, preferably with exercise test, to guide prescription.
Encourage minimum of 30-60 min of moderate-intensity activity three or four times weekly (walking, jogging, cycling, or other aerobic activity) supplemented by an increase in daily lifestyle activities (e.g., walking breaks at work, using stairs, gardening, household work). Maximum benefit 5-6 hours a week.
Advise medically supervised programs for moderate- to high-risk patients.</td></tr>
<tr><td>Weight management</td><td>Start intensive diet and appropriate physical activity intervention, as outlined previously, in patients >120% of ideal weight for height.
Particularly emphasize need for weight loss in patients with hypertension, elevated triglycerides, or elevated glucose levels.</td></tr>
<tr><td>Antiplatelet agents/ anticoagulants</td><td>Start aspirin 81-325 mg/day if not contraindicated.
Manage warfarin to international normalized ratio = 2-3.5 for post-MI patients not able to take aspirin.</td></tr>
<tr><td>ACE inhibitors post-MI</td><td>Start early post-MI in stable high-risk patients (anterior MI, previous MI, Killip class II [S_3 gallop, rales, radiographic CHF]).
Continue indefinitely for all with LV dysfunction (ejection fraction ≤40%) or symptoms of failure.
Use as needed to manage blood pressure or symptoms in all other patients.</td></tr>
<tr><td>β-Blockers</td><td>Start in high-risk post-MI patients (arrhythmia, LV dysfunction, inducible ischemia) at 5-28 days. Continue 6 months minimum. Observe usual contraindications.
Use as needed to manage angina, rhythm, or blood pressure in all other patients.
Individualize recommendation consistent with other health risks.</td></tr>
<tr><td>Blood pressure control:
Goal
≤140/90 mm Hg</td><td>Initiate lifestyle modification weight control, physical activity, alcohol moderation, and moderate sodium restriction in all patients with blood pressure >140 mm Hg systolic or 90 mm Hg diastolic.
Add blood pressure medication, individualized to other patient requirements and characteristics (i.e., age, race, need for drugs with specific benefits) if blood pressure is not less than 140 mm Hg systolic or 90 mm Hg diastolic in 3 months or if *initial* blood pressure is >160 mm Hg systolic or 100 mm Hg diastolic.</td></tr>
</table>

From American Heart Association Consensus Panel Statement: *Preventing heart attack and death*, Dallas, Tex, 1995, American Heart Association.
ACE, angiotensin-converting enzyme; *MI*, myocardial infarction; *TG*, triglycerides; and *LV*, left ventricular.

- NTG breaks down rapidly and loses its potency. Sunlight speeds up this process.
- Even under the best storage conditions, all types of NTG lose their strength about 3 months after the bottle has been opened. A new prescription should be obtained every 3 months and the old medication discarded. Patients are reluctant to throw away medication they have had to purchase, but most NTG costs only pennies, and patients will eventually learn to discard it.
- Medication should be stored in the original dark glass container. Remove all cotton wadding and keep container tightly capped and out of sunlight. Storage in a plastic or cardboard box allows the nitrate to be absorbed into the container material. If cotton plugs remain in the top of the med-

TABLE 19-2 Treatment of Patients with Comorbid Problems

Clinical Diagnosis	Therapy to Consider
Aortic stenosis	Nitrates (with caution); avoid vasodilators, β-blockers
Asthma, COPD	Avoid β-blockers
Atrial fibrillation	verapamil; if not effective digoxin plus β-blocker
Congestive heart failure	digoxin, ACE inhibitor, nitrates, diuretics
Diabetes mellitus	Use β_1-selective β-blocker or calcium blockers, ACE inhibitor
Hypercholesterolemia	Low-cholesterol diet, exercise, remove stress
Hypertension	Control blood pressure with β-blocker, calcium antagonist, ACEs
Second- or third-degree atrioventricular block	Nitrates; avoid β-blockers, verapamil, and diltiazem
Severe peripheral vascular disease	Avoid β-blockers
Sick sinus syndrome	Nitrates; avoid β-blockers, verapamil, and diltiazem

icine container or other drugs are stored with NTG, the nitrate will be absorbed. Refrigeration helps preserve medication and slow deterioration.

- Natural and predictable side effects of taking NTG include flushing of the face, brief throbbing headache, increased heart rate, dizziness, and lightheadedness when changing position rapidly. Headache usually lasts no longer than 20 minutes and may be relieved by analgesics such as acetaminophen.
- Patients should rest for 10 to 15 minutes after pain is relieved.
- Notify health care provider if blurring of vision, persistent headache, or dry mouth occurs.
- There is no therapeutic value in not taking NTG for anginal pain. It may prevent damage to the myocardium.
- If medication seems not to be as effective after taking it for a while, the patient may be developing a tolerance to the drug. The provider should be notified.
- Patients should keep a record of the frequency of their anginal attacks, the number of pills taken, and any side effects. Bring the record to each appointment.
- Patients should use NTG in anticipation of situations in which they can predict anginal attacks will occur. Taking medication before the activity may prevent or reduce the degree of pain.
- Patients should not change NTG products without notifying the health care provider.
- Alcohol may cause lowered blood pressure with this drug and should be avoided.
- Do not stop taking this medicine abruptly.

Sublingual Tablets

- For acute anginal attacks, take 1 tablet sublingually as soon as pain is experienced. Do not chew or swallow medication; let it dissolve under your tongue. Lie down and rest. If pain is not relieved within 3 to 5 minutes, a second pill may be taken. If pain is not relieved within another 3 to 5 minutes, a third pill may be taken. If pain is not relieved after three tablets, you must go to an emergency department immediately for evaluation.
- Burning under the tongue after sublingual medication is not always a reliable indicator that the drug is still potent. Because some drugs are in a much purer form than others, they do not always produce the characteristic throbbing headache.

Translingual Spray

- Take spray only when lying or sitting down. Because this is a highly flammable product, put out cigarettes and avoid using spray around fire or sparks.
- The spray is more durable than sublingual tablets.

Transdermal Patch

- For transdermal application, select a hairless spot (or clip hair) and apply adhesive pad to skin. Washing, bathing, or swimming does not affect this system. Do not cut or tear patch. If pad should come off, discard it and place a new patch on a different site.
- Discard used NTG patches in a safe place out of reach of children.

Topical Ointment

- For topical ointment, spread thin layer on skin, using applicator and ruler. Do not rub or massage the ointment into the skin. Wash off any medication that may have gotten on hands.
- Keep tube tightly closed.
- Discard used paste in a safe place out of reach of children.

Oral Medication

- Take medication on an empty stomach when possible; follow with a glass of water. Take isosorbide dinitrate 30 minutes to 1 hour before meals; allow 12-hour nitrate-free period to prevent tolerance.
- Take isosorbide mononitrate tablet on awakening and then 7 hours later. For sustained-release products, do not crush or chew; swallow with a half-glassful of water.

Specific Drugs

(P) Prototype Drug

sublingual nitroglycerin (Nitrostat)

Contraindications

- Hypersensitivity or idiosyncrasy to nitrates, severe anemia, closed-angle glaucoma, postural hypotension, early MI, head trauma, and cerebral hemorrhage

Warnings/Precautions

- Use with caution in acute MI, avoid use of long-acting nitrates.

- Postural hypotension may occur accompanied by dizziness, weakness, syncope, or other signs of cerebral ischemia. This is accentuated if patient is standing or has drunk alcohol. Fatalities have occurred.
- Nitrates may aggravate angina caused by idiopathic hypertrophic cardiomyopathy.
- Tolerance to the effects of nitrates frequently occurs. Nitrate-free periods may decrease this tendency. For discussion of tolerance, see *Drug Treatment Principles*.
- Caution is required in administration to patients with open-angle glaucoma because intraocular pressure may be increased.
- Excessive dosage may produce severe headaches. Discontinue the drug if blurred vision or dry mouth occurs.
- Severe hypotension may occur in a patient who is volume depleted or hypotensive for any reason.
- Gradually reduce the dosage to prevent withdrawal reactions.

Pharmacokinetics

- Isosorbide mononitrate is primarily metabolized by the liver but, unlike isosorbide dinitrate, is not subject to the first-pass effect and therefore has nearly 100% bioavailability; see Table 19-3.
- Isosorbide dinitrate is subject to the first-pass effect; therefore there is only 40% to 50% bioavailability after first pass; see Table 19-3.

Adverse Effects

- CNS: headache, dizziness, syncope, anxiety, nervousness, weakness
- GI: nausea, vomiting, diarrhea, dyspepsia, abdominal pain
- Cardiovascular: tachycardia, hypotension, syncope, crescendo angina, rebound hypertension, arrhythmias, premature ventricular contractions, postural hypotension
- Dermatologic: drug rash, exfoliative dermatitis, cutaneous vasodilation with flushing
- Miscellaneous: perspiration, blurred vision, diplopia, edema

Specific dosage formulations cause the following adverse effects:

- Transdermal patch may cause skin irritation. Contact dermatitis may be caused by the transdermal NTG system itself rather than by the NTG molecule.

TABLE 19-3 Pharmacokinetics of Common Nitrates

Drug	Availability (After First Pass)	Onset of Action	Time to Peak Concentration	Half-Life	Duration of Action	Protein Bound	Metabolism
nitroglycerin, sublingual tablet	Poor	1-3 min		1-4 min	30-60 min	60%	Rapidly metabolizes to dinitrates and mononitrates
nitroglycerin, translingual spray		2 min	4 min	5 min	30-60 min		Rapidly metabolizes to dinitrates and mononitrates
nitroglycerin, transdermal patch	NA	2 hr	2 hr to steady state	3 min	Up to 24 hr		Metabolizes to dinitrates, mononitrates, glycerol, and carbon dioxide
nitroglycerin, topical ointment	NA	1 hr	1 hr	3 min	7 hr		Metabolizes to dinitrates, mononitrates, glycerol, and carbon dioxide
nitroglycerin, oral sustained release tablet	20-45 min	3-8 hr					
isosorbide dinitrate, chewable tablet	Highly variable	10%-20%	2.5-3 min	10-15 min	5 hr	2-2.5 hr	
isosorbide dinitrate, sublingual tablet	40%-50%	2-5 min	10-15 min	5 hr	1-3 hr		Metabolizes to mononitrate and sorbitol
isosorbide mononitrate	Not subject to first pass; nearly 100% bioavailability	30-60 min	30-60 min	5 hr	7 hr	<4%	Metabolizes to sorbitol and isosorbide
isosorbide mononitrate, extended release		30-60 min			12 hr after AM dose	5%	Multiple pharmacologically inactive metabolites; metabolized by the liver

- A defibrillator must not be used over an NTG patch; arcing may occur and may burn the patient.
- NTG ointment may cause topical skin reactions and anaphylactoid swelling of oral mucosa and edema of conjunctiva.

Drug Interactions

- Table 19-4 lists common drug interactions of nitrates.

Overdosage

- Signs and symptoms of overdosage result from vasodilation and methehemoglobinemia.
- Methehemoglobinemia is dose related; manifestations include hypotension, headache, tachycardia, flushing, perspiration, palpitations, vertigo, visual disturbances, syncope, nausea, vomiting, possible bloody diarrhea, abdominal cramping, anorexia, slow pulse, initially hyperpnea then dyspnea and slow breathing, heart block,and increased intracranial pressure (indicated by confusion, fever, and paralysis).
- Methehemoglobinemia causes tissue hypoxia that can lead to cyanosis, metabolic acidosis, coma, convulsions, and death.

Treatment of Overdosage

- Induce emesis and perform gastric lavage, followed by charcoal administration only if recently swallowed. NTG is rapidly absorbed.
- Oxygen and intravenous fluids should be administered, and recumbent shock position should be assumed.
- Passive movement of extremities may aid venous return.
- Methehemoglobin should be monitored. Methylene blue should be given slowly to treat methehemoglobinemia at a dose of 1.2 mg/kg.
- An α-antagonist such as phenylephrine or methoxamine may be given to correct hemodynamic effects.
- Epinephrine is ineffective in correcting hypotension and is contraindicated to treat NTG overdose.

Dosage and Administration

Table 19-5 contains a summary of dosage recommendations.

1. NTG sublingual tablets: 0.3 mg (1/200 gr), 0.4 mg (1/150 gr), and 0.6 mg (1/100 gr); 0.4 mg is most commonly used. To administer, dissolve one tablet under tongue. Repeat every 5 minutes until pain is relieved or until three tablets have been taken in 15 minutes.
2. NTG translingual spray: 0.4 mg per metered dose. To use spray, spray onto or under tongue. Use is the same as for sublingual tablets.
3. NTG transdermal patch: 0.1 to 0.8 mg/hr release rates. Generic patches are available in 0.2, 0.4, and 0.6 mg release rates. Tolerance limits efficacy when patches are used for more than 12 hr/day.

TABLE 19-4 Common Drug Interactions with Nitrate Products

Precipitant Drug	Adverse Interaction
Alcohol	Severe hypotension, cardiovascular collapse
aspirin	May increase nitrate serum concentrations or actions
Calcium channel blockers	Marked orthostatic hypotension may occur
dihydroergotamine	Bioavailability of the ergot may increase, causing an increase in mean standing systolic blood pressure or a functional antagonism between the two agents and a decrease in antianginal effects
heparin	May decrease heparin pharmacologic effects
sildenafil (Viagra)	May precipitate severe hypotension and death

TABLE 19-5 Dosage Recommendations for Common Nitrates

Drug			
Generic Name	Trade Name	Initial Dosage	Maintenance Dosage
nitroglycerin sublingual tablet	Nitrostat	0.3 mg	Usual 0.4 to 0.6 mg PRN
nitroglycerin translingual spray	Nitrolingual	0.4 mg/metered dose	
nitroglycerin transdermal patch	Nitro-Dur, Minitran	0.2-0.4 mg/hr for 12 of 24 hr	0.2-0.8 mg/hr for 12 of 24 hr
nitroglycerin topical ointment	Nitro-Bid, Nitrol	½-2 inch on awakening; repeat 6 hr later	½-2 inch on awakening; repeat 6 hr later
isosorbide dinitrate, chewable tablet	Isordil Titradose	5-20 mg q6hr	10-40 mg q6hr
isosorbide dinitrate, sublingual tablet	Isordil SL	2.5-5 mg SL 15 min before activity	Usual 5-20 mg bid-tid; maintenance 10-40 mg bid-tid
isosorbide dinitrate, sustained release	Dilatrate SR	40 mg q8-12hr	40-80 mg q8-12hr
isosorbide mononitrate	ISMO, Monoket, Imdur (extended release)	20 mg on awakening; repeat 7 hr later	20 mg on awakening; repeat 7 hr later
isordil mononitrate, extended release	Imdur	30-60 mg qAM	60-120 mg qd; maximum, 240 mg

4. Topical NTG 2% ointment (15 mg/inch): spread a thin layer on skin using applicator or measuring papers and occlude. Do not use fingers, do not rub or massage ointment into skin. Keep tube tightly closed. The dosage is ½ in to 2 in. Apply first dose upon awakening, give second dose 6 hours later.
5. Isosorbide dinitrate, oral: 5-, 10-, 20-, 30-, and 40-mg scored oral tablets; 40-mg sustained-release tablets.
6. Isosorbide dinitrate, sublingual. For prophylaxis, take 2.5 to 5 mg 2 to 3 hours before anticipated angina. Do not crush chewable tables before administering.
7. Isosorbide dinitrate, extended release; take on empty stomach.
8. Isosorbide mononitrate, oral: 10- and 20-mg tablets; 60-mg extended release tablets. Tablets 20 mg twice daily, given on awakening and 7 hours later. Extended-release tablets, 30 mg (½ tablet) to 60 mg in the morning; may be increased to 120 to 240 mg.
9. Isordil mononitrate, extended release; do not crush or chew. Take with fluid.

evolve For additional information on nitrate product drug formulations, see the supplemental tables on the Evolve Learning Resources website.

RESOURCES FOR PATIENTS AND PROVIDERS

American College of Cardiology, www.acc.org.

American Heart Association. Available at www.americanheart.org

Many provider and patient resources given, including patient education materials. Extensive information about cardiovascular disease with frequent updates and an internal search engine. Topics include research, legislation, politics, publications, nutrition, and heart programs. Comprehensive.

American Society of Hypertension, www.ash-us.org.

Auscultation Assistant. Available at www.wilkes.med.ucla.edu/intro.html

Online teaching tool about heart sounds.

ECG Learning Center. Available at www.medlib.med.utah.edu/kw/ecg/intro.html

University of Utah Medical Library site with information on cardiovascular physiology.

Johns Hopkins Intelihealth. Available at www.intelihealth.com

Provides accurate up-to-date health information on a variety of topics. Click on drugs to learn about nitroglycerin use.

BIBLIOGRAPHY

American Heart Association Consensus Panel statement: *Preventing heart attack and death,* Dallas, 1995, The Association.

Awaty EH et al: Aspirin, *Circulation* 101:1206, 2000.

Antithrombotic Trialists' Collaboration: Collaborative meta-analysis of randomized trials of antiplatelet therapy for prevention of death, myocardial infarction, and stroke in high risk patients, *Br Med J* 324:71, 2002.

Dayspring TD: Coronary artery disease prevention in women, *Female Patient* 26:47-53, 2001.

Fihn SD et al: Guidelines for the management of patient with chronic stable angina: treatment, *Ann Intern Med* 135:616, 2001.

Gibbons RJ et al, American College of Cardiology/American Heart Association Task Force on Practice Guidelines (Committee on the Management of Patients With Chronic Stable Angina): ACC/AHA 2002 guideline update for the management of patients with chronic stable angina—summary article: a report of the American College of Cardiology/American Heart Association Task Force on practice guidelines (Committee on the Management of Patients With Chronic Stable Angina), *J Am Coll Cardiol* 41:159-168, 2003.

Kullo IJ et al: Novel risk factors for atherosclerosis, *Mayo Clin Proc* 75:369, 2000.

Libby P: Current concepts of the pathogenesis of the acute coronary syndromes, *Circulation* 104:365, 2001.

Oberman A: Emerging cardiovascular risk factors, *Clin Rev* 33(Spring):33-38, 2000.

Williams SV et al: Guidelines for the management of patients with chronic stable angina: diagnosis and risk stratification, *Ann Intern Med* 135:530, 2001.

CHAPTER 20

Chronic Heart Failure and Digoxin

Drug Names

Class	Subclass	Generic Name	Trade Name
Glycosides		(200) digoxin	Lanoxin, Digitek

(200), Top 200 drug.

General Uses

Indications

- Chronic heart failure (CHF, formerly called congestive heart failure)
- Atrial fibrillation
- Atrial flutter

• • •

One of the oldest and most widely prescribed primary care medications in the world is the glycoside digoxin. The principal indication for digoxin is CHF. It is also used as an antiarrhythmic to control ventricular response to atrial tachyarrhythmias. Digoxin is one of several cardiac glycosides. It is the most therapeutically important because of its pharmacokinetics, ease of administration, and availability of serum levels. The only glycoside that is discussed in this primary care text is digoxin.

There are many other drugs used to treat CHF, including diuretics and ACE inhibitors, as first-line drugs. Nitrates, hydralazine, β-blockers, ARBs, and CCBs are used as indicated.

! Potential for toxicity is the major disadvantage of digoxin use.

Because of its long half-life and narrow therapeutic window, patients treated with digoxin may easily become toxic. The elderly and the renally impaired are at increased risk for cardiac rhythm disturbances. Digoxin-induced arrhythmias must be differentiated from digoxin-treated ones, and the dose decreased, not increased.

DISEASE PROCESS

Anatomy and Physiology: Important Definitions

- Cardiac output (CO) is the volume of blood ejected from the heart/unit time.
- Stroke volume (SV) is the volume of blood ejected with each beat.
- Heart rate (HR) is the number of beats/minute.
- Calculation of CO: CO = SV × HR
- Left ventricular work and myocardial oxygen consumption depend on HR and blood pressure (HR × BP)
- BP = CO × systemic vascular resistance (SVR) (afterload)
- Afterload is the force against which the ventricle must contract to eject blood, or the arterial pressure, arterial impedance, or resistance.
- Preload refers to the amount of blood going to the heart.
- The Frank-Starling law of the heart: within limits, an increase in the left ventricular filling increases the ventricular force of contraction that increases the SV. After reaching optimal filling, increased volume no longer increases the SV. This is when the heart begins to fail. The Frank-Starling law keeps the output of both ventricles balanced (Figure 20-1)

Pathophysiology

CHF usually originates with left-sided ventricular failure (Figure 20-2). This side is most affected by hypertension, valvular dysfunction, and coronary artery disease. When the ventricle fails to pump enough blood to meet the metabolic needs of the body, baroreceptors in the circulatory system cause reflex sympathetic nervous system activation. Veins and arteries constrict to increase critical organ, especially cardiac, perfusion. The Frank-Starling mechanism increases preload to increase myocardial contractile strength. HR increases, also to ensure perfusion. These changes reduce the blood flow to the kidneys, where receptors act to release renin, starting the angiotensin-aldosterone cascade, leading to further vasoconstriction and sodium and water retention.

As heart failure progresses, the compensatory mechanisms can no longer maintain homeostasis. Rapid heart rhythm reduces the amount of blood pumped and, consequently, oxygen perfusion. Peripheral vasoconstriction forces the heart to pump harder, and the renin-angiotensin-aldosterone mechanism causes overfilling of the heart. The overall result is left-sided ventricular failure. The pulmonary system experiences increasing capillary pressure and fluid leakage into interstitial space, resulting in pulmonary edema. As a further result, blood pools in the right ventricle, causing increased pressure in the systemic circulation (right-sided heart failure). This distends visceral veins, the liver and spleen become engorged, and jugular vein distention (JVD) and tissue edema in the extremities become evident.

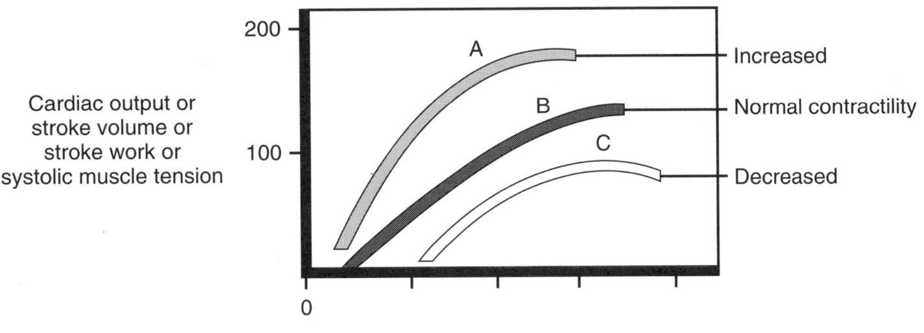

FIGURE 20-1

Frank-Starling's law of the heart, showing the relationship between length and tension in heart. End-diastolic volume determines end-diastolic length of ventricular muscle fibers and is proportional to tension generated during systole as well as to cardiac output, stroke volume, and stroke work. A change in myocardial contractility causes the heart to perform on a different length-tension curve. *A,* Increased contractility. *B,* Normal contractility. *C,* Heart failure or decreased contractility. (From McCance KL, Huether SE: *Pathophysiology,* ed 4, St Louis, 2001, Mosby.)

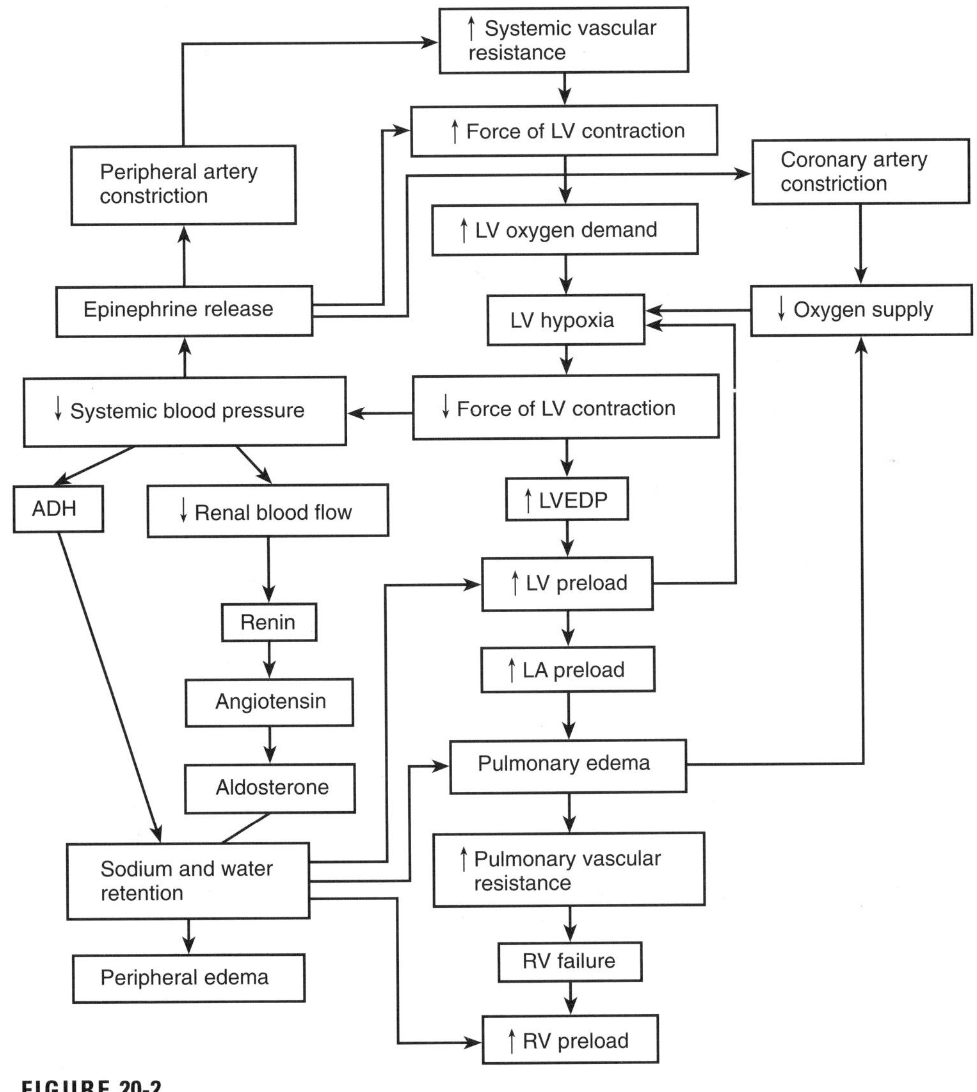

FIGURE 20-2

Left heart failure (chronic heart failure [CHF]) from elevated systemic vascular resistance. Left-sided heart failure leads to right-sided heart failure. Systemic vascular resistance and preload are exacerbated by renal and adrenal mechanisms. *LV,* Left ventricular; *LVEDP,* left ventricular end-diastolic pressure; *LA,* left atrial; *ADH,* antidiuretic hormone; *RV,* right ventricular. (From McCance KL, Huether SE: *Pathophysiology,* ed 4, St Louis, 2001, Mosby.)

TABLE 20-1 Recommended Tests for Patients with Signs and Symptoms of Chronic Heart Failure

Test Recommended	Findings	Suspected Diagnosis
CBC	Anemia	Heart failure caused or aggravated by decreased oxygen-carrying capacity
ECG	Acute ST-T wave changes	Myocardial ischemia
	Atrial fibrillation-tachyarrhythmias	Thyroid disease, rapid ventricular rate
	Bradyarrhythmias	Sick heart
	Left ventricular hypertrophy	Diastolic dysfunction
	Low voltage	Pericardial effusion
	Previous MI	Reduced left ventricular performance
Serum albumin	Decreased	Increased extravascular volume caused by hypoalbuminemia
Serum creatinine	Elevated	Volume overload caused by renal failure
Thyroid studies: T_4 and TSH	Abnormal T_4	Hypothyroidism
	Abnormal TSH	Hyperthyroidism
Urinalysis	Red blood cells and cellular casts	Glomerulonephritis
	Proteinuria	Nephrotic syndrome

Modified from AHCPR: *Quick reference guide for clinicians,* Publication No. 94-0613, Washington DC, 1994, US Government Printing Office.

The Disease

CHF is a clinical syndrome characterized by signs and symptoms of volume overload and inadequate tissue perfusion. Common causes of CHF are ischemic heart disease, systemic hypertension, valve disease, hypertrophic cardiomyopathy from end-stage hypertension, restrictive cardiomyopathies, hypothyroidism and hyperthyroidism, and COPD.

Classification of Severity. Severity of CHF is rated using the New York Heart Association (NYHA) functional classification system:

Class I: Asymptomatic at rest or with ordinary activity; signs or symptoms with severe exercise

Class II: Comfortable at rest; signs or symptoms with ordinary exercise

Class III: Comfortable at rest; signs or symptoms with mild or minimal exercise

Class IV: Signs or symptoms at rest

Assessment

Perform a complete history and physical examination including lying, sitting, and standing BP and pulse. In general, left-sided heart failure manifests itself with pulmonary signs and symptoms; right-sided heart failure causes systemic signs and symptoms. Both left- and right-sided heart failure are present in most patients. The onset is often gradual and subtle. Left-sided symptoms include paroxysmal nocturnal dyspnea (PND), dyspnea on exertion (DOE), S_3 and S_4 heart sounds, arrhythmias, and pulsus alternans. Right-sided symptoms include fatigue, syncope, decreased exercise tolerance, hepatomegaly, peripheral edema, and JVD.

Diagnostic tests (Table 20-1) are performed to rule out other possible causes for the symptoms, determine underlying causes of CHF, and establish a baseline for monitoring the patient. Renal function studies are especially important for dosage determination. Potassium levels are crucial because of the risk for arrhythmia.

Classify CHF according to systolic or diastolic heart failure to determine appropriate treatment.

An ECG should be performed to determine if there are any treatable causes of CHF. Echocardiograms also help assess left ventricular function and measure ejection fraction. In a person with CHF, an ejection fraction less than 40% means left ventricular dysfunction or systolic heart failure; a good ejection fraction means diastolic heart failure. Systolic dysfunction is associated with reduced contractility and increased left ventricular end diastolic volume. Diastolic dysfunction is associated with reduced ventricular filling. Table 20-2 lists factors that may precipitate an episode.

DRUG ACTION AND EFFECTS

Digoxin has an inotropic effect on cardiac cells through enhancement of excitation-contraction coupling triggered by membrane depolarization. It acts at the cellular membrane by inhibiting the sodium-potassium pump, thus causing an increase of intracellular sodium. This causes increased sodium/calcium exchange and subsequent calcium accumulation in the sarcoplasmic reticulum. This results in activation of cardiac contractile proteins, actin, and myosin. The overall result is increased force of contraction of the cardiac muscle.

Cardiac glycosides (1) increase the force of myocardial contraction, (2) depress the sinoatrial node by stimulating vagal activity, (3) prolong conduction to the atrioventricular node via vagal stimulation, (4) increase the refractory period of the atrioventricular node, and (5) increase peripheral resistance. HR is slowed both vagally and extravagally.

In CHF, digoxin increases CO and produces mild diuresis, helping to relieve symptoms. It is most effective in failure caused by decreased left ventricular function and other low-output syndromes. Digoxin is less effective in the high-output syndromes of heart failure such as bronchopulmonary insufficiency, anemia, infection, and hyperthyroidism.

Rapid arrhythmias such as atrial fibrillation, atrial flutter, and paroxysmal atrial tachycardia may provoke pul-

TABLE 20-2 Common Precipitating Factors for Chronic Heart Failure

General Factors	Specific Factors
Patient factors	Alcohol intake Excessive fluid intake Excessive salt intake Increased physical or mental stress Noncompliance with medication regimen Obesity, weight gain
Progression of basic cause	Increasing hypertension, coronary artery disease
Increased cardiac workload	Arrhythmia (possibly caused by digoxin) Electrolyte and acid-base abnormalities Increased or decreased blood volume, anemia Infection (cardiovascular or others such as urinary tract infection) Pulmonary embolism Renal insufficiency
Medications that impair cardiac performance	Cardiovascular drugs Antiarrhythmics β-Blockers Calcium channel blockers Digoxin Corticosteroids Drugs causing fluid retention NSAIDs

monary edema. Oral digoxin maintains tachyarrhythmia suppression.

DRUG TREATMENT PRINCIPLES

The American College of Cardiology/American Heart Association published guidelines for the evaluation and management of heart failure in 1995. These were updated in 2001.

The goals of therapy for the clinician include helping to decrease the signs and symptoms of fluid overload and retention. This will directly help patients maintain their quality of life and their lifestyle as much as possible (Figure 20-3).

Drugs Used to Treat Mild to Moderate Chronic Heart Failure

The following drugs are administered to most patients with heart failure. Figure 20-4 identifies the varying medications and the site of action in treating CHF.

Drug treatment of mild to moderate heart failure proceeds in the following order:

1. *Diuretics in patients with fluid retention:* furosemide is more effective than a thiazide diuretic. Start at 40 mg PO daily, or 20 mg for a small, frail, and/or elderly person. The dosage is then gradually increased until excess fluid retention is relieved. The dosage of furosemide needed to maintain a patient is often less than that needed during an acute exacerbation of CHF; therefore consider decreasing the dosage after the acute episode, and always monitor for dehydration when a patient is on furosemide.
2. *ACE inhibitors or ARBs in all patients unless contraindicated:* add ACE after the diuretic. It is important to make sure the patient is not overdiuresed before starting the ACE inhibitor. If the patient is dehydrated when started on an ACE inhibitor, renal failure may result. The limiting factor for the dose is often hypotension. If patient develops a cough from the ACE inhibitor, change to an ARB. Start with a very low dose and titrate up especially slowly if the patient is elderly, small, or hypotensive.
3. *β-Blockers in all stable (minimal fluid retention) patients unless contraindicated*
4. *Digoxin:* add if needed for treatment of systolic failure. Additional medical conditions that may make digoxin useful include atrial fibrillation and diuretic failure.

If these medications are not sufficient to control heart failure additional drugs may be added.

1. *spironolactone, a potassium-sparing drug, may be added:* spironolactone is an effective diuretic and helps to minimize the risk of hypokalemia from furosemide. Metolazone may be added if the patient is furosemide resistant.
2. *Nitrates and hydralazine:* used only if the patient is unable to tolerate ACE inhibitors.
3. *Calcium channel blockers:* may be useful in diastolic CHF secondary to hypertension but can worsen systolic CHF.

TABLE 20-3 Digoxin Dosing Schedule

Dosing Regimen	To Maintain Therapeutic Level
Loading dose: for adults and children without increased risk for toxicity	0.5 mg, then 0.25 mg q12hr × 2 doses for a total of 1 mg in 24 hr or 0.25 mg bid × 2 days, for a total of 1 mg in 48 hr
Maintenance dose	0.25 mg qd for adults 0.125 mg qd for those at increased risk for toxicity
Maintenance dose for patients with renal insufficiency	0.125 mg qod

digoxin. The administration and dosage of digoxin have changed dramatically over the past few years. In primary care settings, slow digitalization rather than a loading dose is generally recommended because of the risk of toxicity. Digitalization may be achieved within 1 week using small daily maintenance doses. If renal function is poor, modification of dose is required. Digoxin is excreted essentially unchanged, so levels can quickly become toxic.

Start either a loading dose or a maintenance dose, depending on the patient's risk for toxicity and the urgency with which treatment is needed. See Table 20-3 for summary of dosing regimens.

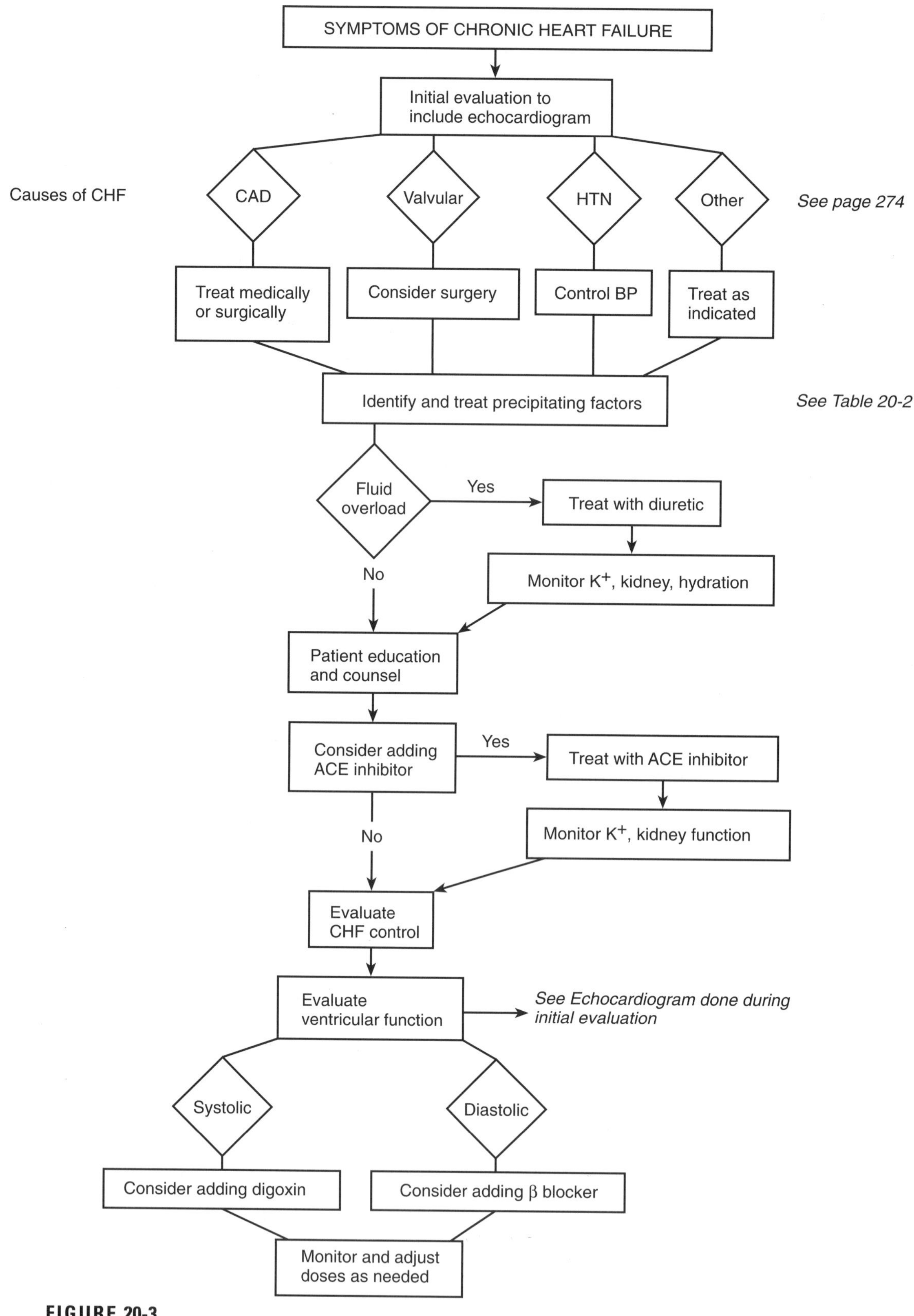

FIGURE 20-3

Treatment algorithm for chronic heart failure. (Modified from AHCPR: *Quick reference guide for clinicians*, Publication No. 94-0613, Washington, DC, 1994, US Government Printing Office.)

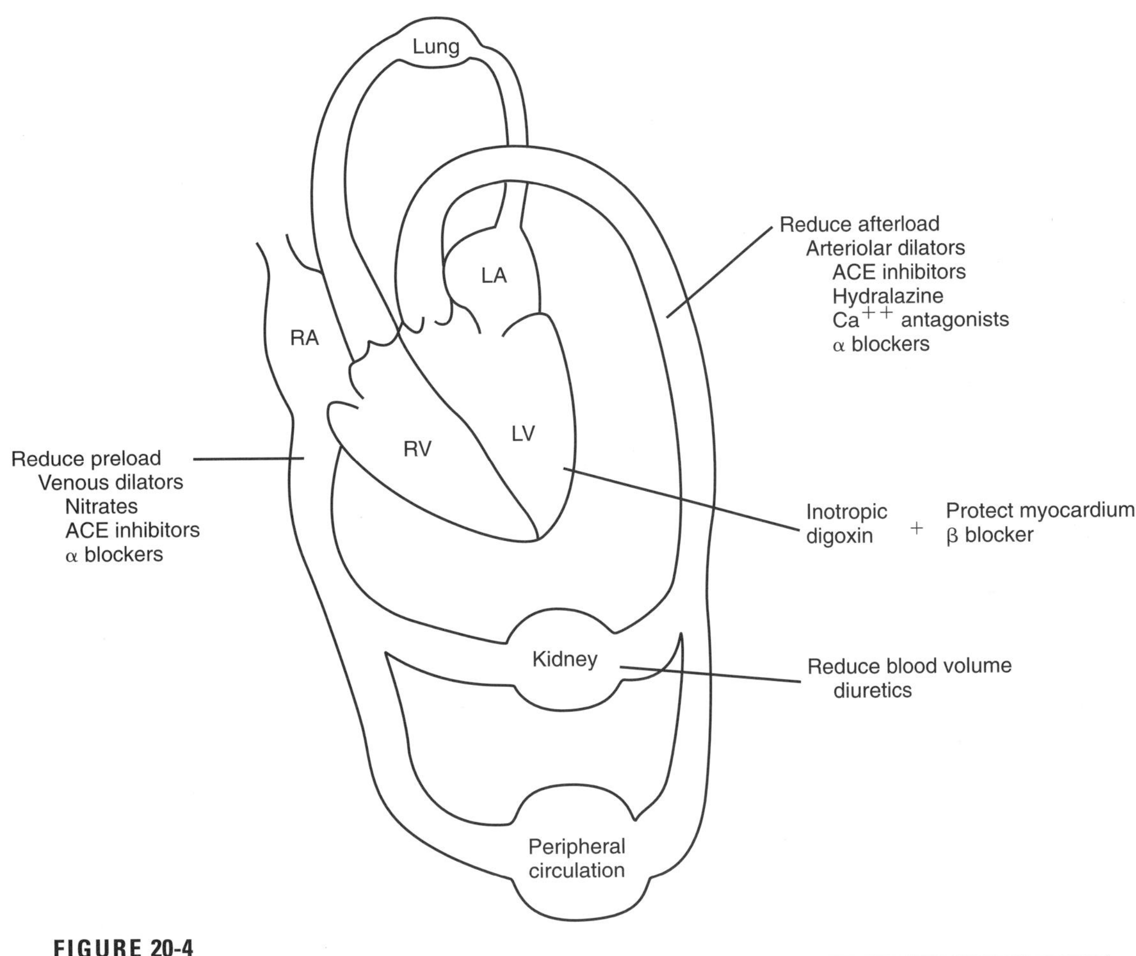

FIGURE 20-4

Sites of action of drugs used in treatment of chronic heart failure. (Data from Hardman J, Limbird L, editors: *Goodman & Gilman's the pharmacologic basis of therapeutics,* ed 10, New York, 2001, McGraw-Hill; Kastrup GK et al, editors: *Facts and comparisons,* St Louis, 1999, JB Lippincott; and Katzung BG: *Basic and clinical pharmacology,* ed 8, Norwalk, Conn, 2000, Appleton & Lange.)

Clinicians should be aware that generic digoxin marketed by different companies may not be bioequivalent to Lanoxin. Write the prescription for the trade or generic medication you desire and then write on the prescription "no substitutions" or "brand medically necessary."

The clinician may need to contact the pharmacy directly to ensure that the medication dispensed each time is the same. Patients should also be instructed to make certain they receive the same product each time the prescription is refilled.

Digoxin has a half-life of 36 hours, so it takes 2 weeks to achieve steady state. Start with a low dose and increase in 2 to 4 weeks if therapeutic effect is not achieved and the patient is not toxic. Perform digoxin levels monthly until stable, then at least every 6 months.

Digoxin, once initiated, is often a lifetime drug. Occasionally a patient with CHF or arrhythmia may stop taking digoxin if the precipitating factors for the heart problem can be eliminated. The drug may be stopped abruptly without adverse effects. The long half-life allows the drug to be excreted over approximately 6 days.

HOW TO MONITOR

Monitor for Therapeutic Effect

- Monitor the patient's clinical response to the digoxin, not just serum drug levels. A therapeutic response may be achieved at a "subtherapeutic" drug level. Use serum levels for monitoring toxicity.
- To monitor for therapeutic effect when digoxin is given for CHF, evaluate both signs and symptoms of heart failure. Patients with CHF should have a gradual disappearance of subjective symptoms. In the physical examination, monitor weight, pulse rate, heart sounds, JVD, breath sounds, and pedal edema.
- To monitor for therapeutic effect when given for arrhythmias, monitor the ventricular rate. The patient may also be aware of rapid or irregular heartbeat, lightheadedness, and dizziness.

Monitor for Toxicity

- To monitor for toxicity, the health care provider must be alert to early signs of toxicity and must obtain a serum level. A digoxin level greater than 2.0 ng/ml indicates toxicity, although some patients become toxic at lower doses. Serum levels should be drawn at least 6 to 8 hours after the last dose and, ideally, just before the next dose.
- The earliest signs of digoxin toxicity are subtle and easy to ignore: increased fatigue, anorexia, weakness, and nausea.
- ECG may show digoxin effect, a nonspecific ST-segment depression, or T-wave flattening.

PATIENT VARIABLES

Geriatrics

- Use caution in the elderly and those with renal impairment. Small body mass requires reduced dosage because of the wide distribution of digoxin in the tissue.

Pediatrics

- Use of digoxin in children requires extra caution, lower doses, and closer monitoring.
- Newborns exhibit a variable tolerance to digoxin.

Pregnancy

- *Category C:* safe use in pregnancy has not been documented.
- Digoxin does appear in breast milk, a possible contraindication to use.

Gender

- Women on digitalis with CHF seem to be at somewhat greater risk of death from all causes.

PATIENT EDUCATION

- Take this drug exactly as directed by the health care provider. If a dose is forgotten, it should be taken as soon as it is remembered. If it is close to the scheduled time for the next dose, do *not* take the missed dose or double the next dose.
- It is important not to switch from trade to different generic products. They may not be the same. Make certain when getting a prescription filled that the same product is received each time.
- For safety, periodic blood tests must be performed to ensure that the drug level is kept within specified limits.
- Because digoxin slows the HR as it strengthens contractions, do not take the medication if HR is very slow. (The health care provider should teach patient and family members how to take a pulse.) Do not take digoxin, without consulting the health care provider, if pulse rate is below 60 beats/minute.
- Do not take OTC medications, especially antacids, cough, cold, allergy, or diet drugs, without first talking with the health care provider.
- Report new or unusual symptoms to the health care provider. Loss of appetite and increased fatigue are two key symptoms that should be reported.
- Digoxin will kill pets and children. Keep it out of the reach of children and others for whom it is not prescribed.
- Patients should carry an identifying bracelet or card stating that they are taking digoxin.
- Reduce overall salt intake. Avoid high-sodium foods, including salted snacks, pork, luncheon meats, and processed cheese. Do not add salt when cooking; do not use extra salt at the table.

Specific Drugs

digoxin (Lanoxin)

Contraindications

- Ventricular fibrillation, ventricular tachycardia, digoxin toxicity, beriberi heart disease, and hypersensitivity to digoxin (allergy is rare)

Warnings

- Sinus node disease and atrioventricular block: because digoxin slows sinoatrial and atrioventricular conduction, the drug commonly prolongs the PR interval and may cause severe sinus bradycardia and sinoatrial block.

! Digoxin toxicity may present with arrhythmias identical to the arrhythmias for which the digoxin is indicated. Make sure the patient is not digoxin toxic before giving the next dose.

- A serum digoxin level may be necessary. An ECG may also be helpful.
- Determine the cause of anorexia, nausea, and vomiting before giving next dose of digoxin because these are frequent symptoms of toxicity.
- Atrial fibrillation may not be controlled with digoxin. Avoid increasing the digoxin dose to toxic levels.
- Acute MI and other severe pulmonary disease or severe cardiac disease may predispose the patient to digoxin toxicity.
- In patients with idiopathic hypertrophic subaortic stenosis (IHSS), use digoxin with extreme caution.
- In Wolff-Parkinson-White syndrome and atrial fibrillation, digoxin may facilitate transmission through accessory pathways, increasing the HR.
- In sick sinus syndrome, digoxin may worsen bradycardia or heart block.
- Amyloid heart disease and constrictive cardiomyopathies do not respond to digoxin.
- Renal function impairment delays excretion of digoxin; adjust dosage. Dialysis has little effect on digoxin.
- Combined renal and hepatic failure may prolong digoxin elimination an additional amount.

Precautions

- Electrolyte imbalances
  - *Potassium:* hypokalemia makes the myocardium more sensitive to digoxin. It may also reduce the positive inotropic effect of digoxin.
  - *Calcium:* hypercalcemia predisposes the patient to digoxin toxicity. Hypocalcemia may make digoxin ineffective.

- *Magnesium:* hypomagnesemia may predispose to digoxin toxicity.
- *Thyroid dysfunction:* hypothyroid patients require less digoxin because of decreased excretion rate. Hyperthyroid patients with heart failure may require larger doses. Arrhythmias caused by hypermetabolic states are particularly resistant to digoxin treatment; it is important to avoid toxicity.
- Digoxin may produce false positive ST-T changes on ECG during exercise testing.

Pharmacokinetics

- *Absorption:* digoxin tablets are 60% to 80% absorbed; the elixir is 70% to 85% absorbed, and the Lanoxi-caps, which are solution-filled capsules, are 90% to 100% absorbed. Because of the variation in bioavailability of some preparations, absorption may vary between different brands of digoxin. Patients who have changed brand names of digoxin have had significantly altered serum levels of digoxin. Unless a meal is very high in fiber, food does not affect the amount of digoxin absorbed.
- *Distribution:* digoxin is widely distributed in the tissues. The highest concentrations are found in myocardium, skeletal muscle, liver, brain, and kidneys. It is not widely distributed in fatty tissue. Digoxin crosses the blood-brain barrier and the placenta. The volume of distribution of digoxin corresponds to the patient's ideal body weight.
- *Metabolism:* most of the digoxin is not metabolized.
- *Excretion:* from 50% to 75% of digoxin is excreted unchanged by the kidneys. In patients with impaired renal function, significant accumulation may occur. This is especially dangerous because of the 36-hour half-life. Approximately 6 days are required to achieve steady state or elimination. Digoxin is not removed by dialysis because it is distributed in tissue, not blood.

Adverse Effects

- Incidence of adverse effects is 5% to 20%; serious effects, 1% to 4%; toxicity, 0.5%; GI disturbances, 0.25%; CNS and other toxicity, 0.25%. The most common adverse effects are as follows:
  - *GI:* anorexia, nausea, vomiting and diarrhea, abdominal discomfort
  - *CNS:* headache, weakness, apathy, drowsiness, visual disturbances (blurred, halo effect and rarely, yellow or green vision), depression, restlessness, seizures, delirium, hallucinations, neuralgia, psychosis
  - *Cardiac:* digoxin toxicity may present as almost any known type of arrhythmia. Ventricular tachycardia and unifocal or multifocal premature ventricular contractions (especially bigeminy or trigeminy) are the most common toxic arrhythmias. Also common are paroxysmal and nonparoxysmal nodal rhythms, atrioventricular dissociation, accelerated junctional (nodal) rhythm, and paroxysmal atrial tachycardia with block. Atrioventricular block, complete heart block, and atrial fibrillation may also occur. The most common cause of death from digoxin toxicity is ventricular fibrillation.

TABLE 20-4 Drug Interactions of Digoxin

Drugs that May Increase Digoxin Levels	Drugs that May Decrease Digoxin Levels
amiodarone	Aminoglycosides
alprazolam, diazepam	Antacids (aluminium and magnesium containing)
bepridil	Antineoplastics (many)
cyclosporine	charcoal, activated
diphenoxylate	cholestyramine
indomethacin	colestipol
itraconazole	kaolin/pectin
clarithromycin, erythromycin	metoclopramide
propafenone	neomycin
propantheline	penicillamine
quinidine	rifampin
spironolactone	St John's wort
tetracycline	sulfasalazine
verapamil	

- Toxicity in children usually presents as an arrhythmia, with fewer GI and neurologic disturbances seen in children than in adults.

Drug Interactions

- Many drugs affect digoxin levels. However, digoxin does not affect the levels of other drugs (Table 20-4). In addition, *β-blockers*, added to digoxin, in patients with atrioventricular conduction abnormalities, can result in complete heart block.

Overdosage

- It is important to monitor closely for digoxin toxicity.

Treatment of Toxicity

- Hold all digoxin until it is certain the patient is not digoxin toxic.
- Treatment of arrhythmias usually requires hospitalization.
- Digitalis immune FAB is a new treatment of digoxin intoxication. Improvement in symptoms usually begins within a half-hour of administration.

Dosage and Administration

- Can be given with or without food; absorption is not affected. Starting dose: 0.125 or 0.25 mg PO daily, depending on size, renal function, and age of patient.
- Adjust dose according to serum digoxin levels.

RESOURCES FOR PATIENTS AND PROVIDERS

Internet

American College of Cardiology, www.acc.org.

American Heart Association. Available at www.americanheart.org

Website has many provider and patient resources, including patient education materials.

American Society of Hypertension, www.ash-us.org.

BIBLIOGRAPHY

Dec GW: Digoxin remains useful in the management of chronic heart failure, *Med Clin North Am* 87:317-337, 2003.

Katz AM: Pathophysiology of heart failure: identifying targets for pharmacotherapy, *Med Clin North Am* 98:303-316, 2003.

Felker FM et al: Inotropic therapy for heart failure: an evidence-based approach, *Am Heart J* 142:393, 2001.

Francis GS: Pathophysiology of chronic heart failure, *Am J Med* 110(Suppl 7A):37S, 2001.

Hunt SA et al: ACC/AHA guidelines for the evaluation and management of chronic heart failure in the adult: executive summary, *Circulation* 104:2996, 2001.

Rathore SS et al: Association of serum digoxin concentration and outcomes in patients with heart failure, *JAMA* 289:871-818, 2003.

Rathore SS et al: Sex-based differences in the effect of digoxin for the treatment of heart failure, *N Engl J Med* 347:1403-1411, 2002.

Stuthers AD: The diagnosis of heart failure, *Heart* 84:334, 2000.

CHAPTER 21

β-Blockers

Drug Names

Class	Subclass	Generic Name	Trade Name
β-Adrenergic blockers	Nonselective	(P) (200) propranolol	Inderal, generic
		carteolol	Cartrol
		nadolol	Corgard
		penbutolol	Levatol
		pindolol	Visken
		sotalol	Betapace, Sotacor
		timolol	Blocadren
	β_1-Selective	(200) atenolol	Tenormin
		(200) metoprolol	Lopressor, Toprol XL
		acebutolol	Sectral
		betaxolol	Kerlone
		bisoprolol	Zebeta
	α-β-Blocker	(200) labetalol	Normodyne, Trandate
		carvedilol	Coreg
		esmolol	Brevibloc

(200), Top 200 drug; (P), prototype drug.

General Uses

Indications

- Hypertension: all except esmolol and sotalol
  - Esmolol and sotalol are used only for arrhythmias and are not discussed further.
- Angina, long-term management: atenolol, metoprolol, nadolol, propranolol
- CHF: metoprolol, carvedilol, bisoprolol
- Selected arrhythmias: acebutolol, esmolol, propranolol, sotalol
- Prophylaxis of migraine: propranolol, timolol
- Propranolol: hypertrophic subaortic stenosis, pheochromocytoma, essential tremor

Unlabeled Uses

- Mitral valve prolapse syndrome
- Alcohol withdrawal

Since the original introduction of propranolol in the early 1960s, β-blockers have proliferated to include a multitude of drugs. Although the drugs have basic similarities, there are important differences. β-blockers are used in a wide variety of cardiac and noncardiac conditions.

DRUG ACTION AND EFFECTS

All β-blockers have a similar mechanism of action. They compete with β-adrenergic receptor–stimulating agents for available β-receptor sites, thereby antagonizing the effects of catecholamines released from the adrenergic nerve endings and the adrenal medulla. β-Blocking agents reduce the metabolic (glycogenolytic, lipolytic), myocardial stimulant, vasodilator, and bronchodilator actions of catecholamines. This represents decreases in chronotropic, inotropic, and vasodilator action. Reduction in heart rate and force of contraction, suppression of renin release, and decrease in outflow of sympathetic vasoconstrictor and cardioaccelerator fibers from the brainstem vasomotor center are produced (Table 21-1).

As a result of β-blockade, cardiac output and heart rate are decreased. Slowing of the atrioventricular conduction system prevents an increase in cardiac automaticity and prolongs the refractory period. Decreased sympathetic peripheral outflow blocks the release of renin (carteolol, labetalol, and pindolol do not consistently inhibit renin release). BP is lowered by the action of β-blockers in decreasing cardiac output, peripheral vascular resistance, venous return, plasma volume, and renin release.

Reducing oxygen demands, decreasing contractility and heart rate, and increasing coronary blood flow as a result of prolonging diastolic ventricular filling time work together to control angina.

CHF is perpetuated by an active renin-angiotensin system coupled with increased tone of the sympathetic nervous system; thus decreasing catecholamine levels reduces cardiac congestion and left ventricular hypertrophy (LVH). β-Blockers may increase β_1-receptor sensitivity and restore inotropic response. β_2-Receptors promote peripheral vasodilation.

β-Blockers prevent arrhythmias by blocking abnormal cardiac pacemaker potentials, decreasing myocardial oxygen

TABLE 21-1 Comparison of Adrenergic Receptors

Receptor	Site	Effect of Stimulation
α_1	Smooth muscle in blood vessels	Vasoconstriction
	Stomach, intestine	Decreased motility and tone
	Kidney	Increased renin secretion
	Liver	Gluconeogenesis
α_2	Smooth muscle in blood vessels	Vasoconstriction
β_1	Cardiac	Increased rate and force of contraction
	Kidney	Increased renin secretion
β_2	Bronchial, vascular, coronary arteriole, uterine smooth muscle, skeletal muscle	Vasoconstriction
	Pancreas	Decreased secretion
	Liver	Gluconeogenesis

TABLE 21-2 Characteristics of Individual Agents

Drug	Selectivity	ISA	MSA	Potency	Lipid Solubility
propranolol	β_1 and β_2	0	+	1.0	High
carteolol	β_1 and β_2	+	0	10.0	Low
nadolol	β_1 and β_2	0	0	1.0	Low
penbutolol	β_1 and β_2	+	0	1.0	High
pindolol	β_1 and β_2	+	+	6.0	Moderate
sotalol	β_1 and β_2	0	0	0.3	Low
timolol	β_1 and β_2	0	0	6.0	Low
atenolol	β_1	0	0	1.0	Low
metoprolol	β_1	0	0	1.0	Moderate
acebutolol	β_1	+	+	0.3	Low
betaxolol	β_1	0	+	1.0	Low-moderate
bisoprolol	β_1	0	0	10.3	Low-moderate
labetalol	α_1, β_1, and β_2	0	0	0.3	Low

ISA, Intrinsic sympathomimetic activity; *MSA,* membrane-stabilizing activity; *+,* present; *0,* absent.

demand, prolonging ventricular filling time, and decreasing microvascular damage of the myocardium.

There are clinically significant differences between β-blockers. They differ in regard to selectivity (β-selectivity, α-blocking receptors), membrane-stabilizing activity (MSA), and intrinsic sympathomimetic activity (ISA), potency, and lipid solubility. See Table 21-2 for characteristics of individual agents.

Selectivity is an important feature of β-blockers. β_1-Selectivity blocks β_1 cardiac receptors with limited influence on β_2 bronchial and vascular receptors, which reduces bronchospasm and peripheral resistance. However, this is dose dependent. Thus the advantage of using β_1-selectivity to reduce bronchospasm and decrease peripheral resistance may be diminished with a high-dose regimen.

ISA, also known as partial agonist activity (PAA), is another property of β-blockers. ISA simultaneously blocks natural catecholamine while only partially activating β-receptors. Thus side effects such as bradycardia, bronchoconstriction, and resting peripheral vascular resistance may be minimized. ISA is not beneficial in alleviating arrhythmias, and may eliminate the effectiveness of the β-blocker in the secondary prevention of MI.

MSA, another feature of this drug class, is described as having a quinidine-like or local anesthetic effect on cardiac action potentials. High concentrations of the β-blocker are needed to reduce arrhythmias, which often produces side effects. Thus the significance of MSA is negligible.

Potency quantifies the amount of drug needed to inhibit catecholamine binding at β-adrenergic sites. The presence of a β-blocker alters the catecholamine response; therefore a higher concentration of catecholamine is required to provoke a response. Esmolol is the least potent β-blocker, and pindolol is the most potent. Potency is relevant when replacing one β-blocker with another.

Lipid solubility denotes the ability of β-blockers to cross the blood-brain barrier. This is important in the management of adverse effects. β-Blockers with high lipid solubility maintain greater volume distribution than those with low lipid solubility. Related side effects involving the CNS, such as lethargy, depression, and sleep disturbances, are more likely to be seen with β-blockers with high lipid solubility. Lipid solubility is an advantage when treating a CNS problem such as migraine or tremor.

DRUG TREATMENT PRINCIPLES

β-Blockers are important drugs known to decrease mortality. However, they must be used with caution because they have many potential problems. They can usually be adequately managed with the proper β-blocker and close monitoring. Selection of agents should be limited to drugs with documented indications and known efficacy. Choose a few β-blockers and become familiar with their use. Propranolol, atenolol, metoprolol, and carvedilol are commonly used.

β-Blockers must be used with caution in certain heart conditions such as heart block, sinus bradycardia, cardiogenic shock, or heart failure.

Bradyarrhythmias, atrioventricular block, heart failure, and exacerbation of peripheral vascular disease (PVD) have occurred. In diabetics, β-blockers may intensify hypoglycemia and prolong gluconeogenesis because of inhibited release of insulin. Clinical signs and symptoms of hypoglycemia may be blocked. Clinical signs and symptoms of thyrotoxicosis may be masked, and abrupt withdrawal may precipitate thyroid storm. Symptoms of depression may be aggravated in individuals with a history of depression. Asthma and COPD may be exacerbated by the use of β-blockers.

Hypertension

β-Blockers are important first-line drugs in the treatment of hypertension. β-Blockers and diuretics remain the two first-choice drugs unless the patient has special circumstances. See Chapter 18 for the management of hypertension.

Angina

β-Blocker withdrawal may exacerbate angina in patients with coronary artery disease (CAD).

β-Blockers are the treatment of choice for chronic long-term stable and unstable angina. Treatment with a β-blocker in variant angina is reserved for patients with significant CAD unresponsive to nitrates and calcium channel blockers. Resting heart rate or drug levels are variable and poor predictors of control. A more precise approach to treatment is drug titration, based on frequency of anginal symptoms and nitrate use (see Chapter 19).

Secondary Prevention Post–Myocardial Infarction

After hospitalization, β-blockers improve survival rates in patients who have had a MI, primarily by reducing the incidence of sudden death in high-risk patients.

Early treatment of MI with β-blockers occurs during the hospital stay. This has shown a small benefit in selected patients.

Chronic Heart Failure

β-Blockers are used in patients with mild to moderate diastolic CHF with stable ejection fractions of greater than 35% to 40%. Benefits are seen in patients with underlying CAD and primary cardiomyopathies. The potential risk of exacerbation of CHF symptoms requires careful monitoring. Carvedilol, metoprolol, and bisoprolol have demonstrated effectiveness in studies. β-Blockers produce increases in ejection fraction and reduction in left ventricular size and mass. Patients have fewer hospitalizations and mortality with a reduction in sudden death and death from CHF.

Arrhythmias

The Cardiac Arrhythmia Suppression Trial in 1994 supported the use of β-blockers in patients with arrhythmias by showing consistent decrease in reoccurrence of arrhythmias. β-Blockers are categorized as class II antiarrhythmic drugs as a result of their reduction in cardiac adrenergic activity. Benefits appear greatest in patients with poor left ventricular function and exercise-induced ventricular tachycardia. Post-MI sudden death most often results from arrhythmias. Ventricular fibrillation is the most common arrhythmia seen in these patients.

Other Uses

Prophylactic treatment of migraine headaches with β-blockers helps reduce the frequency and intensity of headaches. The relative effectiveness is probably influenced by lipid solubility, with more lipid-soluble drugs crossing the blood-brain barrier more easily.

Essential tremor shows marked improvement with propranolol. Atenolol, metoprolol, nadolol, and timolol have been used to treat tremor, but this is a nonlabeled use. Anxiety, with associated tachycardia and tremor, abates with β-blockade of circulating catecholamines. The use of propranolol or timolol in this condition is a nonlabeled use. For performance anxiety, β-blockers have been found to be particularly useful.

Thyrotoxicosis symptoms are surgically or medically managed and respond to propranolol for short-term management.

HOW TO MONITOR

- Blood pressure and pulse should be evaluated weekly until stable and then at least every 3 to 4 months.
- A baseline ECG should be obtained before initiation of drug therapy as needed and on an annual basis thereafter. An ECG provides serial evaluation of electrophysiologic changes during the course of drug therapy and identifies any significant ECG changes such as bradycardia or LVH.
- Based on the specific patient population's appropriate evaluation of blood glucose concentrations, lipid values and renal and hepatic function tests may be warranted.
- Monitor for toxicity manifested by bradycardia and hypotension. In specific patient subsets, observe for progression of cardiac failure and PVD, exacerbation of bronchospasm, hypoglycemia, hyperthyroidism, and depression.

PATIENT VARIABLES

Geriatrics

Recognize the potential for hepatic and renal failure. Drug concentration levels accumulate quickly in the elderly with compromised systems. Thus therapeutic doses need to be small (half normal dosage) and titrated slowly in the elderly.

- Elderly patients have described sedation and sleep disturbances associated with β-blocker use.

Pediatrics

- Safety and effectiveness of β-blockers have not been established in children with the exception of propranolol.

Pregnancy

- The benefits of β-blockers in pregnancy should clearly outweigh any risks. Low birth weight infants have been reported in mothers who used β-blockers during pregnancy.
- *Category B:* acebutolol
- *Category C:* betaxolol, bisoprolol, metoprolol, nadolol, propranolol
- *Category D:* atenolol

Lactation

- β-Blockers appear in breast milk. Either breastfeeding or the drug should be discontinued.

Race

- Effectiveness in hypertensive black persons may be less with β-blockers than with other classes of drugs. This factor most likely is the result of lower plasma renin levels in the black population coupled with greater circulating volume. Diuretics are a better initial choice. β-blockers with ISA may be added later.

PATIENT EDUCATION

- Report shortness of breath, nocturnal cough, or lower extremity edema
- Do not discontinue medication abruptly

- Report use of β-blockers to ophthalmologist
- Monitor pulse and contact health care provider if rate is less than 50
- Diabetic patients: possibility of masked signs of hypoglycemia
- Use caution when performing hazardous tasks

Specific Drugs

NONSELECTIVE β-BLOCKERS

Ⓟ **Prototype Drug**

propranolol (Inderal, Inderal-LA, generic)

Contraindications

- Sinus bradycardia, greater than first-degree heart block, cardiogenic shock, overt cardiac failure, and hypersensitivity

Warnings

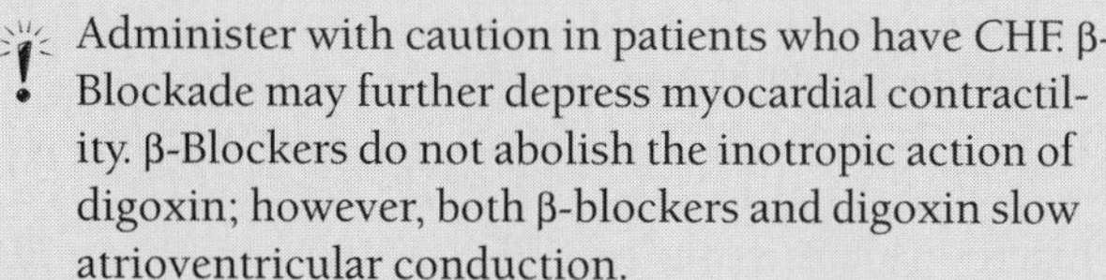
Administer with caution in patients who have CHF. β-Blockade may further depress myocardial contractility. β-Blockers do not abolish the inotropic action of digoxin; however, both β-blockers and digoxin slow atrioventricular conduction.

Abrupt withdrawal may result in withdrawal symptoms (tremulousness, sweating, palpitations, headache, malaise), exacerbation of angina, MI, ventricular arrhythmias, and death.

- In Wolff-Parkinson-White syndrome, the tachycardia may be replaced by a severe bradycardia.
- In patients who have peripheral vascular disease, β-blockers may precipitate or aggravate the symptoms of arterial insufficiency.
- In general, do not administer β-blockers to patients who have bronchospastic disease. β-Blockers with relative β_1-selectivity may be used with caution.
- Bradycardia may be caused by a β-blocker and may be symptomatic.
- Hypotension may occur.
- Anaphylaxis has occurred, with deaths.
- Withdrawal of β-blockers before major surgery and anesthesia is controversial.
- Concomitant use of verapamil or diltiazem may cause heart block
- Use β-blockers with caution in patients with renal or hepatic function impairment.

Precautions

- May mask the signs and symptoms of hypoglycemia
- May mask clinical signs of hyperthyroidism. Abrupt withdrawal may exacerbate symptoms
- May alter serum lipid values, including a nonsignificant increase in triglycerides, total cholesterol, and low- and very low-density lipoprotein cholesterol and a decrease in high-density lipoprotein.
- May potentiate muscle weakness.

Pharmacokinetics

- See Table 21-3.

Adverse Effects

- The most frequent adverse effects are bradycardia, depression, impotence, diarrhea, dizziness, drowsiness, fatigue and weakness, nausea and vomiting, and insomnia. Table 21-4 lists important adverse effects.

Drug Interactions

- Many β-blockers are involved in cytochrome P450 enzyme metabolism; see Table 21-3 for specifics.
- Food may enhance bioavailability.
- See Table 21-5 for drug interactions.

Overdosage

- Symptoms of overdosage are manifested by two features—bradycardia and hypotension.
- Toxicity may also present as cardiac failure, pulmonary edema (particularly with CAD), decreased consciousness, seizures, and bronchospasm.

Dosage and Administration

- See Table 21-6 for dosing information.
- Ethanol: slows the rate of absorption.
- Propranolol and metoprolol: food may enhance bioavailability; take at the same time each day.
- Nadolol, pindolol, acebutolol, atenolol, carteolol, bisoprolol, betaxolol, and penbutolol: take without regard to meals.

Other Drugs in Class

Other drugs in this class are similar to the prototype except as follows.

α-β BLOCKER

labetalol (Normodyne, Trandate)

- Labetalol is a selective α_1- and nonselective β-adrenergic receptor blocker.
- Labetalol produces only minimal reduction in heart rate without reflex tachycardia. Hemodynamically, there is little change in cardiac output and a slight drop in peripheral resistance.

carvedilol (Coreg)

- Nonselective β-blockade and α_1-blockade counteract increased sympathetic activity that causes progressive myocardial damage.
- α_1-Blockade reduces systemic vascular resistance and helps compensate for the initial negative inotropic effects of β-blockade.

TABLE 21-3 Pharmacokinetics of Common β-Blockers

Drug	Absorption	Availability (After First Pass)	Time to Peak Concentration	Half-Life	Duration of Action	Protein Bound	Metabolism	Excretion	Therapeutic Serum Level
propranolol	90%	30%	1-1.5 hr	3-5 hr; 8-11 hr long acting	11 hr	93%	Hepatic 2D6 substrate	Hepatic	50-100 mg/ml
carteolol	90%	90%	1-3 hr	5-6 hr	72 hr	20%-30%	Hepatic, minimal	Renal, 50%-70%	40-160 mg/ml
nadolol	30%	30%	1-4 hr	20-24 hr	21-39 hr	30%	Negligible	Renal	50-100 mg/ml
penbutolol	100%	90%	1.5-3 hr	5 hr	20-24 hr	80%-98%	Hepatic conjugation and oxidation	Renal	
sotalol	70%	90%-100%	2-4 hr	12 hr		0%	Not metabolized	Unchanged in urine	0.5-4.0 mg/ml
timolol	90%	75%		4 hr		10%	Hepatic 2D6 substrate	Renal	0.7-3.0 mg/ml
atenolol	50%	40%-50%	2-4 hr	6-9 hr	24 hr	6%-16%	Hepatic, minimal	Renal, unchanged; feces 50%	0.2-5.0 μg/ml
metoprolol	95%	40%-50%; long acting, 77%	0.5-2.0 hr	3-7 hr	14-24 hr	12%	Hepatic 2D6 substrate	Renal	0.7-3.0 mg/ml; 70-400 long acting
acebutolol	70%-90%	40%	2.5-4 hr	3-4 hr Active metabolite 8-13 hr	24 hr	26%	Hepatic	Bile and intestinal wall Renal, 30%-40%	0.2-2.0 μg/ml
betaxolol	100%	89%	1.5-6 hr	14-22 hr		50%	Hepatic	Hepatic, renal, unchanged	5-20 mg/ml
bisoprolol	>90%	80%	2-4 hr	9-12 hr	24 hr	30%	Hepatic 2D6 substrate	Renal, unchanged, 50%; hepatic, 50%	6-70 mg/ml
labetalol	100%	33%	Oral, 2-4 hr	Oral, 5.5-8 hr		50%	Hepatic, mainly through conjugation to glucuronide metabolites	Renal	0.8-3.0 mg/ml
carvedilol	Rapid	25%-35%	Increased if taken with food	7-10 hr		98%	Hepatic 2D6; 2C9; lesser extent: 3A4; 2C9; 1A2	Unchanged, 2%	

TABLE 21-4 Adverse Reactions to β-Blockers by Body System

Body System	Common Side Effects	Serious Adverse Effects
Body, general	Weight gain, weight loss, decreased exercise tolerance	Lupus-like syndrome, Raynaud's phenomenon, death
Cardiovascular	Bradycardia	Torsades des pointes, cardiac arrest, cardiogenic shock, hypotension, peripheral ischemia, worsening angina, shortness of breath, heart failure, SA block, abnormal ECG, arrhythmias, thrombophlebitis
Circulatory and hematologic		Agranulocytosis, thrombocytopenic purpura, bleeding, thrombocytopenia, eosinophilia, leukopenia, pulmonary emboli, anemia, leukocytosis
Gastrointestinal	Flatulence, gastritis, constipation, nausea, diarrhea, dry mouth, vomiting, heartburn, anorexia, abdominal pain	Ischemia, colitis, dysphagia
Genitourinary	Sexual dysfunction, impotence or decreased libido, dysuria, nocturia, urinary retention or frequency	Renal failure, abnormal renal function
Hepatic		Elevated level of liver enzymes, bilirubin; hepatomegaly, acute hepatitis with jaundice
Hypersensitivity	Pharyngitis, erythematous rash	Photosensitivity, fever with aching and sore throat, laryngospasm, respiratory distress, angioedema, anaphylaxis
Metabolic and nutritional		Hyperglycemia, hypoglycemia, unstable diabetes mellitus
Musculoskeletal	Joint pain, arthralgia, muscle cramps/pain, arthritis	Myalgia, joint disorder, tendinitis, gout
Nervous system	Dizziness, vertigo, tiredness, fatigue, headache, mental depression	Peripheral neuropathy, paralysis, paresthesias, lethargy, somnolence, restlessness, sleep disturbances, nightmares, incoordination, emotional lability, ataxia, seizures, stroke
Respiratory	Cough, nasal stuffiness	Bronchospasm, dyspnea, bronchial obstruction, wheeziness, aryngospasm with respiratory distress, asthma
Skin, appendages	Rash, pruritus, increased pigmentation, sweating, alopecia, dry skin, psoriasis, acne, eczema	Exfoliative dermatitis, peripheral skin necrosis
Special senses	Taste perversion, eye irritation, visual disturbances	Iritis, cataract, diplopia

TABLE 21-5 Drug Interactions of β-Blockers

β-Blocker	Action on Other Drugs	Other Drugs	Action on β-Blockers
β-Blockers	Increased flecainide, clonidine, epinephrine, ergot alkaloids, lidocaine, prazosin	Calcium channel blockers, oral contraceptives, quinidine, diphenhydramine, flecainide, hydroxychloroquine, ciprofloxacin	Increased β-blockers
propranolol	Increased phenothiazines, haloperidol, anticoagulants, gabapentin	aluminum salts, barbiturates, calcium salts, cholestyramine, colestipol, ampicillin, rifampin, nonsteroidal antiinflammatories, salicylates, sulfinpyrazone	Decreased β-blockers
metoprolol, propranolol (lipid soluble)	Increased benzodiazepines, hydralazine		
β-Blockers	Increased and decreased disopyramide	cimetidine, hydralazine, monoamine oxidase inhibitors, propafenone, selective serotonin reuptake inhibitors, thioamines	Increased metoprolol, propranolol
		Thyroid hormones	Decreased metoprolol, propranolol
		haloperidol, loop diuretics, phenothiazines	Increased propranolol

TABLE 21-6 Dosage and Administration Recommendations for β-Blockers

Drug	Indication	Initial Dosage	Titration	Maximum Dosage
propranolol	HTN	40 mg bid SR 80 mg qd	120-240 mg/day bid-tid SR 120-160 mg qd	640 mg
	Angina	80-320 mg bid-qid SR 80 mg qd	SR 160 mg qd	320 mg
	Essential tremor	40 mg bid	120 mg/day	320 mg
carteolol	HTN	5 mg qd		10 mg
nadolol	HTN, angina	40 mg bid	Increase qwk to 80 mg	160-240 mg
penbutolol	HTN	20 mg qd × 2 wk	10 mg q2wk	40-80 mg
pindolol	HTN	5 mg bid × 3-4 wk	Increase 10 mg/day q3-4wk	60 mg
timolol	HTN, migraine CHF	10 mg bid 3.125 mg bid × 2 wk	Increase qwk to 20-40 mg/day Increase to 6.25 mg bid	60 mg Individualize
atenolol	HTN, angina	50 mg qd × 1-2 wk	Increase to 100 mg	100 mg
metoprolol	HTN, angina	100 mg qd or in divided doses	Increase qwk to 450 mg	450 mg
acebutolol	HTN	400 mg qd or 200 mg bid	Increase to 400-800 mg	1200 mg
betaxolol	HTN	10 mg qd × 1-2 wk	Increase to 20 mg	20 mg
bisoprolol	HTN	5 mg qd	Increase to 10 mg	20 mg
labetalol	HTN	100 mg bid	Increase by 100 mg bid q2-3days to 400 mg	2.4 g/day
carvedilol	HTN	6.25 mg bid	Increase to 12.5 mg in 1-2 wk	25-50 mg/day

CHF, Chronic heart failure; *HTN,* hypertension; *qwk,* every week, *SR,* sustained release.

RESOURCES FOR PATIENTS AND PROVIDERS

American College of Cardiology, www.acc.org.
American Heart Association, www.americanheart.org.
American Society of Hypertension, www.ash-us.org.

BIBLIOGRAPHY

Brophy JM et al: Beta-blockers in congestive heart failure, *Ann Intern Med* 134:550, 2001.

CIBIS Investigators and Committees: A randomized trial of β-blockade in heart failure: the cardiac insufficiency bisoprolol study (CIBIS), *Circulation* 90:1765, 1994.

Cruickshank JM: The beta 1 hyperselectivity in β-blocker treatment, *J Cardiovasc Pharmacol* 25(suppl 1):S35, 1995.

Dei Cas L et al: Prevention and management of chronic heart failure in patients at risk, *Am J Cardiol.* 91:10-17, 2003.

Frigerio M et al: Prevention and management of chronic heart failure in management of asymptomatic patients, *Am J Cardiol.* 91:4-9, 2003.

Klein L et al: Pharmacologic therapy for patients with chronic heart failure and reduced systolic function: review of trials and practical considerations, *Am J Cardiol* 91:18-40, 2003.

Miller M, Vogel RA: *The practice of coronary disease prevention,* Baltimore, 1996, Williams and Wilkins.

National Heart, Lung, and Blood Institute, National Institutes of Health, National High Blood Pressure Education Program: *The seventh report of the Joint National Committee on Prevention, Detection, Evaluation, and Treatment of High Blood Pressure,* National Institutes of Health, National Heart, Lung, and Blood Institute, NIH Publication No. 03-5233, May 2003.

Smith AJ et al: Current role of β-blockers in the treatment of chronic congestive heart failure, *Am J Health Syst Pharm* 58:140-145, 2001.

Wink K: Are beta-blockers efficacious as first-line therapy for hypertension in the elderly? *Curr Hypertens Rep* 5:221-224, 2003.

CHAPTER 22

Calcium Channel Blockers

Drug Names

Class	Subclass	Generic Name	Trade Name
Dihydropyridines		(P)(200) nifedipine, nifedipine ER amlodipine felodipine isradipine nicardipine nicardipine SR nisoldipine	Procardia, Adalat Norvasc Plendil DynaCirc Cardene Cardene SR Sular
Phenylalkylamine		(200) verapamil, verapamil SR	Calan, Isoptin, Verelan
Benzothiazepine		(200) diltiazem SR, ER, CD	Cardizem, Tiazac, Cartia-XT
Diarylaminopropylamine		bepridil	Vascor

(200), Top 200 drug; (P), prototype drug.

General Uses

Indications

- Hypertension
- Vasospastic angina
- Arrhythmias (Table 22-1)

Calcium channel blockers are indicated for a variety of cardiovascular conditions. There are four classes of calcium channel blockers. Only one class, the dihydropyridines, includes more than one drug. The main difference between the dihydropyridines and the other classes is that the dihydropyridines do not affect the cardiac conduction system. Diltiazem is generally considered to have effects that are more similar to those of verapamil than those of nifedipine. The new calcium channel blocker bepridil is used only for patients with angina that is not responding to other drugs. About 1% of patients develop a new serious ventricular arrhythmia. Bepridil is not discussed in detail because it is not in common outpatient use.

In 1995, a controversial study reported that persons taking calcium channel blockers to control hypertension were at greater risk of heart attack than were those who were prescribed other types of drugs. The validity of this study has been seriously questioned. Because of this and other studies, the National Heart, Lung, and Blood Institute has issued the following warning.

> ! Short-acting nifedipine should be used very cautiously (if at all), especially at higher doses, in patients with hypertension or unstable angina.

The warning applies *only* to short-acting nifedipine. Further studies are in progress that should help elucidate the role of calcium channel blockers in patients with cardiovascular disease.

DRUG ACTION AND EFFECTS

Although these compounds have diverse chemical structures, they all share a basic electrophysiologic property. They block the inward movement of calcium through the slow channels of the cell membranes of cardiac and smooth muscle cells. The drugs differ in their location of action (Tables 22-2 and 22-3). The three types of tissue cells acted on are as follows:

1. Cardiac muscle (myocardium)
2. Cardiac conduction system: sinoatrial (SA) and atrioventricular (AV) nodes
3. Vascular smooth muscle: coronary arteries and arterioles, peripheral arterioles

Cardiac Muscle

Calcium channel blockers decrease the force of myocardial contraction by blocking the inward flow of calcium ions through the slow channels of the cell membrane during phase 2 (plateau phase) of the action potential. The diminished entry of calcium ions into the cells thereby fails to trigger the release of large amounts of calcium from the sarcoplasmic reticulum within the cell. This free calcium is needed for excitation–contraction coupling, an event that activates contraction by allowing cross-bridges to form between the actin and myosin filaments of muscle. The number of actin and myosin cross-bridges formed within the sarcomere determines the force of the heart's contraction. Decreasing the amount of calcium ions released from the sarcoplasmic reticulum causes fewer actin and myosin cross-bridges to be formed, thus decreasing the

TABLE 22-1 Indications for and Unlabeled Uses of Calcium Channel Blockers

	Indications			Unlabeled Uses			
	Stable Angina	Vasospastic Angina	Hypertension	Migraine	Raynaud's Disease	CHF	Cardiomyopathy
nifedipine		X		X	X	X	X
nifedipine SR		X	X				
amlodipine	X	X	X				
felodipine			X		X	X	
isradipine		X					
nicardipine	X		X			X	
nicardipine SR			X				
nisoldipine			X				
diltiazem	X				X		
diltiazem SR	X	X	X				
verapamil	X	X	X	X			X
verapamil SR			X				

TABLE 22-2 Effects of Selected Calcium Channel Blockers on Cardiac System

Medication	Coronary Vasodilation	Peripheral Vasodilation	Contractility	Automaticity	AV Conduction
verapamil	+++	++	−−−	−−−	−−−
diltiazem	++	++	−−	−−−	−−−
nifedipine	+++	+++	−	−	0

+++, Pronounced increase; ++, moderate increase; *0*, no effect; −, some decrease; −−, moderate decrease; −−−, pronounced decrease.

TABLE 22-3 Effect of Calcium Channel Blockers on Myocardium

Medication Contractility	Myocardial	Cardiac Output	SA Automaticity	AV Refractivity	AV Conduction	Heart Rate	Afterload
nifedipine SR	0	+−	+−	+	+	−	−−−
amlodipine	0	0	0	+−	−	−	−−−
felodipine	0	0	0	−	−	−	−−−
isradipine	0	0	0	+−	+−	0	−−−
nicardipine	+−	+−	0	+	++	0	−−
nicardipine SR	0	0	0	+−	0	0	−−−
nisoldipine	0	0	0	+−	0	0	−−−
verapamil	−−	++	−−−	+−	+−	−−	−−
diltiazem	−	+	−−−	+−	+−	−	−

+++, Pronounced increase; ++, moderate increase; +, some increase; +−, little increase; *0*, no effect; −, some decrease; −−, moderate decrease; −−−, pronounced decrease.

force of contraction and resulting in a negative inotropic effect. This will affect cardiac output.

Cardiac Conduction System (SA and AV nodes)

In these tissues, calcium channel blockers decrease automaticity in the SA node and decrease conduction in the AV node. *Automaticity* means that a cell depolarizes spontaneously and initiates an action potential without an external stimulus. Automaticity is a normal characteristic of the SA nodal cells. *Depolarization* (Phase 0) of the action potential is normally generated by the inward calcium ion current through slow channels. Thus agents that can block the inward calcium ion current across the cell membrane of SA nodal tissue decrease the rate of depolarization and depress automaticity. The result is a variable decrease in heart rate (a negative chronotropic effect) (Figure 22-1). Similarly, an agent that decreases calcium ion influx across the cell membrane of the AV node slows AV nodal conduction (negative chronotropic effect) and prolongs AV refractory time. When AV conduction is prolonged, fewer atrial impulses reach the ventricles, thus slowing the rate of ventricular contractions.

Vascular Smooth Muscle

The smooth muscle of the coronary and peripheral vessels has a significant influence on afterload and the hemodynamics of circulation. The decreased force of smooth muscle contraction results in coronary artery dilation, which lowers coronary resistance and improves blood flow through collateral vessels as well as oxygen delivery to ischemic areas of the heart. Calcium channel blockers dilate the main coronary arteries and arteri-

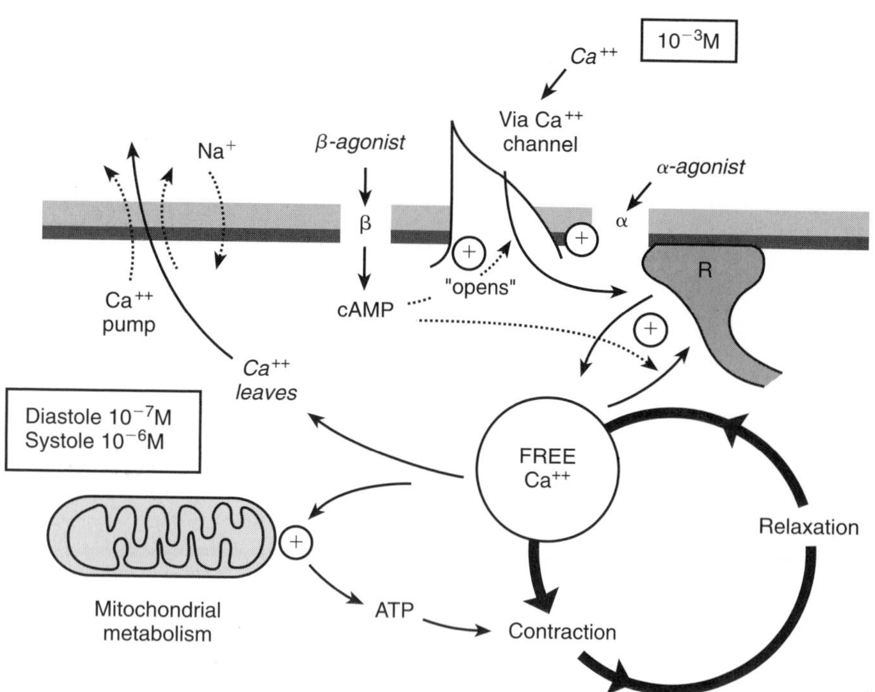

FIGURE 22-1

Physiologic activity of calcium channel blockers. (Data from Hardman J, Limbird L, editors: *Goodman and Gilman's the pharmacological basis of therapeutics*, ed 9, New York, 1996, McGraw-Hill; and National Institutes of Health: *The seventh report of the Joint National Committee on Prevention, Detection, Evaluation and Treatment of High Blood Pressure*, NIH Publication No. 03-5233, Washington, DC, 2003, US Government Printing Office.)

oles, in both normal and ischemic regions. Therefore drugs with these actions are helpful in the treatment of angina pectoris.

Calcium channel blockers reduce arterial pressure at rest and at a given level of exercise by dilating peripheral arterioles and reducing the total peripheral resistance (afterload) against which the heart works. This unloading of the heart reduces myocardial energy consumption and oxygen requirements and probably accounts for the effectiveness of calcium channel blockers in chronic stable angina and causes the decrease in blood pressure.

Calcium channel blockers are a potent inhibitor of coronary artery spasm. The property increases myocardial oxygen delivery in patients with coronary artery spasm and is responsible for the effectiveness of calcium channel blockers in vasospastic angina.

Specific Calcium Channel Blockers

Nifedipine is a potent dilator of vascular smooth muscle causing decreased peripheral vascular resistance in both coronary arteries and peripheral arterioles. Nifedipine has a mild negative inotropic effect, less than that of verapamil. There is usually a small increase in heart rate, a reflex response to vasodilation. Nifedipine has no tendency to prolong AV conduction, prolong SA node recovery time, or slow sinus rate.

Verapamil also dilates vascular smooth muscle, although it is less potent than nifedipine. Verapamil has a significant negative inotropic effect that prevents and blocks reflex tachycardia and relieves coronary artery spasm. This negative inotropic effect decreases myocardial oxygen demand and thus helps to relieve angina-related ischemia and pain. Verapamil also slows conduction in the SA and AV nodes, although it has a greater effect on the AV node.

Diltiazem has a less negative inotropic effect than verapamil and causes less peripheral vasodilation than nifedipine. Diltiazem selectively has more effect on cardiac muscle than on peripheral vascular smooth muscle. It does slow conduction through the SA-AV nodes, but not as much as verapamil.

Bepridil inhibits fast sodium channels in addition to slow calcium channels and has Class I antiarrhythmic properties.

DRUG TREATMENT PRINCIPLES

The dihydropyridines, nifedipine and its relatives, are used differently from verapamil and diltiazem, which are similar to each other.

Nifedipine and *related drugs* cause potent peripheral vasodilation. This often makes them more effective for hypertension than verapamil and diltiazem but more likely to cause peripheral edema. They have no effect on cardiac conduction and will not cause arrhythmias.

Verapamil and *diltiazem* have a significant effect on cardiac conduction and are used to treat arrhythmias in addition to hypertension. They are less likely to cause hypotension than nifedipine and related drugs when used to treat angina in a patient who does not have hypertension. However, they are more likely to cause conduction problems than nifedipine and related drugs when used to treat hypertension. They should be used with β-blockers with much caution, if at all, because β-blockers also affect conduction. Verapamil and diltiazem should be used with caution in patients with CHF because they may have a negative inotropic effect. They may be useful in diastolic dysfunction. evolve For a summary of the major actions and uses of calcium channel blockers, see the supplemental tables on the Evolve Learning Rosources website.

Vasospastic Angina

Calcium channel blockers are the treatment of choice in variant, or Prinzmetal's, angina. The dihydropyridines, verapamil, and diltiazem are all efficacious and are more effective than either nitrates or β-blockers.

Chronic Stable Angina

In chronic stable angina, calcium channel blockers are effective in relieving symptoms of angina and increasing exercise tolerance in formal exercise testing. They also reduce ST-segment changes on ambulatory electrocardiographic monitoring, increase coronary artery blood flow, and improve ventricular dysfunction associated with ischemia. Nitrates and β-blockers remain first-line therapy for angina, with calcium blockers used if symptoms persist or if nitrates and β-blockers are contraindicated or not tolerated.

Hypertension

Diuretics and β-blockers remain first-line therapy for most patients. However, patients unable to tolerate diuretics or β-blockers may tolerate calcium channel blockers. Calcium channel blockers do not have the metabolic adverse effects of diuretics or the central nervous system side effects of β-blockers. Calcium channel blockers are safe and effective for a wide variety of hypertensive patients. They have good patient acceptance because of their low incidence of adverse reactions. They do not affect serum lipid concentrations, and complaints of sexual dysfunction are rare. Black patients, elderly patients, and patients with hyperlipidemia are considered good candidates for calcium channel blockers.

HOW TO MONITOR

- Follow weekly or biweekly while dosages are being titrated upward.
- Once stable, monitor patient periodically, every 3 to 6 months, for adverse responses and control of the disease process.
- Obtain and monitor serum digoxin levels if calcium channel blockers are initiated in patients receiving digoxin.
- Kidney and liver function tests should also be obtained periodically.

PATIENT VARIABLES

Geriatrics

- Lower dosages of calcium channel blockers should be used because older patients are more susceptible to their side effects such as dizziness, weakness, syncopal episodes, and falls. However, calcium channel blockers are generally relatively well tolerated and are often the drug of choice for elderly patients.

Pediatrics

- The safety and effectiveness of calcium channel blockers in children have not been established.

Pregnancy

- *Category C:* teratogenic and embryotoxic effects have been demonstrated in small animals.
- Verapamil, diltiazem, and nifedipine are excreted in breast milk.
- It is not known if the other drugs are excreted in breast milk.

Race and Gender

- No gender differences have been noted.
- Effective in black patients.

PATIENT EDUCATION

- Advise patients they may experience hypotensive effects during titration of dose.
- Urge patients to report signs of CHF (swelling of feet or shortness of breath), irregular heartbeat, nausea, constipation, dizziness, or hypotension.
- Nitrate therapy while patients are on calcium channel blockers may cause some dizziness.
- If taking extended-release tablets, patients may pass inert shell in feces.
- Do not take with grapefruit juice, which is known to affect the liver cytochrome P450 enzyme system and interfere with drug metabolism.

Specific Drugs

DIHYDROPYRIDINES

(P) Prototype Drug

nifedipine (Adalat, Adalat capsules, Procardia, Procardia XL)

Contraindications

- Hypersensitivity
- Nicardipine: advanced aortic stenosis (causes decreased afterload)

Warnings

- Hypotension may occur and may be more common in patients taking concomitant β-blockers. Monitor blood pressure closely.
- CHF may develop rarely when a patient is treated with a calcium channel blocker, usually when used in combination with a β-blocker.
- Antiplatelet effects have caused inhibition of platelet function. Episodes of bruising, petechiae, and bleeding have occurred.

! Withdrawal syndrome: Abrupt withdrawal of calcium channel blockers may cause increased frequency and duration of chest pain. To stop drug, gradually taper dosage.

- Calcium channel blockers do not prevent β-blocker withdrawal symptoms. Be sure to taper any β-blocker, even if starting the patient on a calcium channel blocker.
- Hepatic function impairment causes a longer half-life of nifedipine. Amlodipine, felodipine, nisoldipine, and nimodipine are extensively metabolized by the liver. Half-life is increased, use with caution in patients with impaired liver function.

- Increased angina: rarely, patients, particularly those who have severe obstructive coronary disease, have developed increased frequency, duration, and/or severity of angina or acute myocardial infarction on starting or increasing nifedipine or nicardipine.

Precautions

- Acute hepatic injury with elevations in LFTs has occurred rarely with nifedipine and nimodipine.

- Mild-to-moderate peripheral edema in the lower extremities occurs in about 10% of patients. This is caused by arterial dilation and not left ventricular dysfunction.

Pharmacokinetics

See Table 22-4 for pharmacokinetic information.

Adverse Effects

See Table 22-5 for adverse reactions. evolve For additional information on common side effects of various

TABLE 22-4 Pharmacokinetics of Selected Calcium Channel Blockers

Drug	Onset of Action	Time to Peak Concentration	Half-Life	Therapeutic Serum Level	Duration of Action	Metabolism	Excretion
nifedipine (Procardia)	Oral, 20 min (more rapid when given sublingually)	0.5-1 hr	2-5 hr	22-100 ng/ml	4-8 hr	Liver, 3A4 substrate	Renal, 80%; feces, 20%
amlodipine (Norvasc)	N/A	6-12 hr	30-50 hr	N/A	N/A	Liver, extensive 3A4 substrate	Renal
felodipine (Plendil)	3-5 hr	2.5-5 hr	11-16 hr	N/A	24 hr	Liver, 3A4 substrate	Renal
isradipine (DynaCirc)	2 hr	1.5 hr	8 hr	N/A	12 hr	Liver, 3A4 substrate	Renal
nicardipine (Cardene)	N/A	1 hr	2-4 hr	28-50 ng/ml	8 hr	Liver, 3A4 substrate	Renal
nisoldipine						Liver, extensive	
verapamil (Calan, Isoptin)	Oral, 1-2 hr IV, 1-5 min	1-2 hr	3-7 hr	80-300 ng/ml	Oral: 8-10 hr	Liver, has active metabolite 3A4 substrate Oral, extended release: 24 hr IV, 2 hr	Renal and feces
diltiazem (Cardizem)	30 min	2-3 hr		50-200 ng/ml	48 hr	Liver, has active metabolite 3A4 substrate	Renal and bile
diltiazem SR (Cardizem SR)	30-60 min	6-11 hr	3.5-7 hr	50-200 ng/ml	12 hr	Liver, has active metabolite 3A4 substrate	Renal and bile

TABLE 22-5 Adverse Reactions to Calcium Channel Blockers

Body System	diltiazem	nifedipine	verapamil
Skin, appendages	Rash, erythema multiforme, Stevens-Johnson syndrome	Edema, flushing	Rash, Steven-Johnson syndrome, erythema multiforme
Respiratory	Dyspnea	Cough, dyspnea	Dyspnea
Cardiovascular	Angina, hypertension, hypotension, AV block, bradycardia, angina, atrial fibrillation, MI, palpitations, syncope	Palpitations, angina, bradycardia, hypotension, syncope, tachycardia	ECG, abnormal bradycardia, AV block, CHF, hypotension, angina, syncope, palpitations, MI, tachycardia
GI	Constipation, diarrhea, nausea	Constipation, nausea	Constipation, diarrhea, nausea
Circulatory and lymphatic	Ecchymosis	Leukopenia, thrombocytopenia	Ecchymosis
Musculoskeletal	Arthralgia, muscle cramps	Arthralgia, muscle cramps	Muscle cramps, myalgia
Nervous system	Headache, paresthesia, insomnia	Headache, tremor, weakness, fatigue, asthenia, dizziness, anxiety, ataxia, confusion, depression	Headache, dizziness, fatigue, ataxia, paresthesia, confusion
Genitourinary	Impotence	Impotence	Impotence

calcium channel blockers, see the supplemental tables on the Evolve Learning Resources website.

Table 22-6 compares the adverse reactions among different types of dihydropyridines.

Drug Interactions

- The combination of dihydropropyridine and β-blockers is usually well tolerated but may increase the likelihood of CHF, severe hypotension, or exacerbation of angina.
- Many calcium channel blockers are cytochrome P450 3A4 substrates.
- Drug interactions vary by individual drug (see Table 22-7).

Dosage and Administration

- Nifedipine: avoid administration with grapefruit.
- Nisoldipine: avoid administration with a high-fat meal. Available as extended-release tablet.
- Nicardipine: immediate release has prominent peak effects, which increases risk of adverse reactions. See Table 22-8 for specific dosage and administration information.

TABLE 22-6 Comparison of Adverse Effects (in Percentages) Among Dihydropyridines

Drug	Edema	Flushing	SOB	Dizziness	Headache
nifedipine	20	25	6	10	15
amlodipine	8	2	1	3	7
felodipine	8	5	2	3	12
isradipine	4-30	3	3	5	15
nisoldipine	12	0	1	6	22

SOB, Shortness of breath.

TABLE 22-7 Drug Interactions of Calcium Channel Blockers

Calcium Channel Blocker	Action on Other Drugs	Drug	Action on Calcium Channel Blockers
DIHYDROPYRIDINES		cimetidine, ranitidine, β-blockers	Increased dihydropyridine
Dihydropyridines	Increased anesthetics	cisapride, diltiazem, quinidine	Increased nifedipine
nifedipine	Increased digoxin, quinidine, tacrolimus, vincristine	melatonin, nafcillin, St John's wort	Decreased nifedipine
		erythromycin	Increased felodipine
nifedipine, isradipine, nicardipine	Increased β-blockers	carbamazepine, oxcarbazepine	Decreased felodipine
		Azole antifungals	Increased nisoldipine
felodipine, nicardipine	Increased cyclosporine	itraconazole, rifampin	Increased felodipine, isradipine, nifedipine
isradipine	Decreased lovastatin		
		cyclosporine	Increased nifedipine, felodipine
VERAPAMIL AND DILTIAZEM			
verapamil and diltiazem	Increased midazolam, triazolam, buspirone, carbamazepine, digoxin, statins, imipramine, quinidine, sirolimus, tacrolimus, theophylline, β-blockers, anesthetics	barbiturates	Decreased nifedipine, felodipine
		phenytoin	Decreased felodipine, nisoldipine
		valproic acid	Increased nimodipine
verapamil	Increased disopyramide, flecainide, doxorubicin, ethanol, nondepolarizing muscle relaxants, prazosin, cyclosporine	amiodarone, cimetidine, ranitidine, β-blockers	Increased verapamil and diltiazem
		rifampin	Decreased verapamil and diltiazem
diltiazem	Increased nifedipine, methylprednisolone, moricizine	Barbiturates, calcium salts, phenytoin, antineoplastics	Decreased verapamil
		nifedipine	Increased diltiazem
		moricizine	Decreased diltiazem

TABLE 22-8 Dosage and Administration Recommendations for Calcium Channel Blockers

Drug	Dosage Form	Initial Dosage	Titration	Maximum Dose
nifedipine	Capsules	10 mg tid	Increase q1-2wk: 10-20 tid to 20-30 qid	120 mg/day
	Tablets, ER	30 mg qd	Increase to 60 mg in 1-2 wk	120 mg
amlodipine	Tablets	5 mg qd	Increase to 10 mg qd	10 mg
felodipine	Tablets, ER	5 mg qd	Increase to 10 mg in 2 wk	10 mg
isradipine	Capsules	2.4 mg bid	Increase by 5 mg/day q2-4wk	20 mg/day
	Tablets, CR	5 mg qd	Increase by 5 mg q2-4wk	20 mg/day
nicardipine	Capsules	20 mg tid	Increase to 40 mg tid q3days	
	Capsules, SR	30 mg bid	Increase to 60 mg bid	
nisoldipine	Tablets, ER	20 mg qd	Increase by 10 mg/wk to 20-40 mg	60 mg
verapamil	Tablets and capsules, ER	120 mg qd	Increase to 180-240 mg qd	480 mg
diltiazem	Tablets	30 mg qid	Increase to q1-2 mg/day to 180 mg/day	360 mg/day
	Capsules, ER	20-120 mg qd	Increase to 180-240-360 mg q2wk	480 mg

PHENYLALKYLAMINE

verapamil hydrochloride (Calan, Calan SR, Isoptin, Isoptin SR, Verelan)

Contraindications

- Hypersensitivity
- Sick sinus syndrome or second- or third-degree block except in patients with functioning artificial pacemaker
- Hypotension less than 90 mm Hg
- Patients with atrial flutter/fibrillation and an accessory AV pathway may develop rapid ventricular response or ventricular fibrillation

Warnings

- Hypotension may occur during initial dosing or dosage increases and may be more common in patients taking concomitant beta blockers. Monitor blood pressure.
- Use with caution in patients with heart failure because the negative inotropic effect may precipitate CHF.
- Cardiac conduction: may cause first-degree AV block and transient bradycardia.
- Elevated liver enzymes, including elevated transaminases, alkaline phosphatase, and bilirubin, have been reported. Periodic monitoring is prudent. Verapamil is highly metabolized by the liver and should be administered with caution to patients with hepatic insufficiency.
- Renal function impairment: 70% is excreted as metabolites in the urine. Administer with caution to patients with impaired renal function.
- Antiplatelet effects: bruising, petechiae, and bleeding have occurred.
- Patients with idiopathic hypertrophic cardiomyopathy (IHSS) may experience a variety of serious side effects, including pulmonary edema and severe hypotension, with verapamil.
- Abrupt withdrawal may cause increased frequency and duration of chest pain.

Pharmacokinetics. See Table 22-4.

Adverse Effects. See Table 22-5.

Drug Interactions

- Verapamil is a cytochrome P450 3A4 substrate (see Table 22-7 for drug interactions).

RESOURCE FOR PATIENTS AND PROVIDERS

American Heart Association. Available at www.amhrt.org/Heart-StrokeAtoZGuide/calccb.html

Internet site discussing calcium channel blockers.

BIBLIOGRAPHY

Black HR et al: Principal results of the Controlled Onset Verapamil Investigation of Cardiovascular End Points (CONVINCE) trial, *JAMA* 289:2073-2082, 2003.

Cheng JW, Behar L: Calcium channel blockers: association with myocardial infarction, mortality, and cancer, *Clin Ther* 19:1255, 1997.

Epstein M: *Calcium antagonists in clinical medicine,* ed 2, St Louis, 1997, Hanley & Belfus.

Flack JM, Mensah GA, Ferrario CM: Using angiotensin converting enzyme inhibitors in African-American hypertensives: a new approach to treating hypertension and preventing target-organ damage, *Curr Med Res Opin* 16:66-79, 2000.

Joint National Committee on the Prevention, Detection, Evaluation, and Treatment of High Blood Pressure Education Program: *The seventh report of the Joint National Committee on Prevention, Detection, Evaluation, and Treatment of High Blood Pressure,* National Institutes of Health, National Heart, Lung, and Blood Institute, NIH Publication No. 03-5233, May 2003.

Kirpichnikov D, Sowers JR: Role of ACE inhibitors in treating hypertensive diabetic patients, *Curr Diab Rep* 2:251-257, 2002.

Saseen JJ, MacLaughlin EJ, Westfall JM: Treatment of uncomplicated hypertension: are ACE inhibitors and calcium channel blockers as effective as diuretics and beta-blockers? *J Am Board Fam Pract* 16:156-164, 2003.

Summaries for patients. Effects of blood pressure drugs in patients with diabetes and kidney disease, *Ann Intern Med* 138:542-549, 2003.

Where do calcium antagonists fit in the management of hypertension? *Drug Ther Perspect* 15:10-11, 2000.

CHAPTER 23

ACE Inhibitors and Angiotensin Receptor Blockers

Drug Names

Class	Subclass	Generic Name	Trade Name
Angiotensin-converting enzyme inhibitors (ACEIs)	Sulfhydryl-containing	(200) captopril	Captoten
	Dicarboxyl-containing	(P) (200) lisinopril hydrochloride	Prinivil, Zestril, Zestoretic
		(200) benazepril hydrochloride	Lotensin
		(200) enalapril maleate	Vasotec
		(200) quinapril hydrochloride	Accupril
		moexipril hydrochloride	Univasc
		(200) ramipril	Altace
		trandolapril	Mavik
	Phosphorus-containing	fosinopril sodium	Monopril
Angiotensin II receptor blockers (ARBs)		(P) (200) losartan	Cozaar, Hyzaar
		candesartan	Atacand
		eprosartan	Reveten
		(200) irbesartan	Avapro
		telmisartan	Micardis
		valsartan	Diovan

(200), Top 200 drug; (P), prototype drug.

General Uses

Indications

Angiotensin-converting enzyme inhibitors

- Hypertension
- CHF
- MI
- Left ventricular dysfunction
- Diabetic nephropathy

Unlabeled Uses

- Captopril: hypertensive crises
- Angiotensin II receptor antagonists: hypertension
- CHF
- Diabetic nephropathy

This chapter discusses the angiotensin-converting enzyme inhibitors (ACEIs) and angiotensin II receptor antagonists (blockers) (ARBs) as a unit because these drugs are quite similar; exceptions are noted.

An advantage of ACEIs and ARBs is their freedom from serious adverse reactions. Abrupt withdrawal of these agents has not resulted in rebound hypertension. ACEI-induced cough is the most commonly recognized class adverse reaction, whereas hyperkalemia, hypotension, and acute renal failure are potentially serious problems. This cough does not occur with ARBs.

DRUG ACTION AND EFFECTS

ACEIs suppress the renin-angiotensin-aldosterone system. They block the conversion of angiotensin I to the active angiotensin II, a potent endogenous vasoconstrictor, by inhibiting the converting enzyme (Figure 23-1). ACEIs reduce local angiotensin II at vascular and renal sites and may attenuate the release of catecholamines from adrenergic nerve endings. The reduction of plasma angiotensin II causes a subsequent increase in plasma renin activity and reduced aldosterone secretion (loss of the negative feedback because of decreased angiotensin II). Reduction in aldosterone secretion results in less sodium–potassium exchange in the distal renal tubule, causing a slight increase in serum potassium.

ACEIs block the action of ACE in other reactions beside angiotensin II. ACE blocks the degradation of bradykinin, a potent, naturally occurring vasodilator. This is thought to be the cause of the cough commonly experienced by patients taking this drug.

There are two types of angiotensin receptors, called AT_1 and AT_2. Most of the biological effects of angiotensin II are mediated by the AT_1 receptor. AT_2 receptors may exert antiproliferative and vasodilatory effects.

Captopril is the only ACE inhibitor that contains a sulfhydryl group. It has been speculated that this is a factor in the development of rash, taste disturbances, and neutropenia.

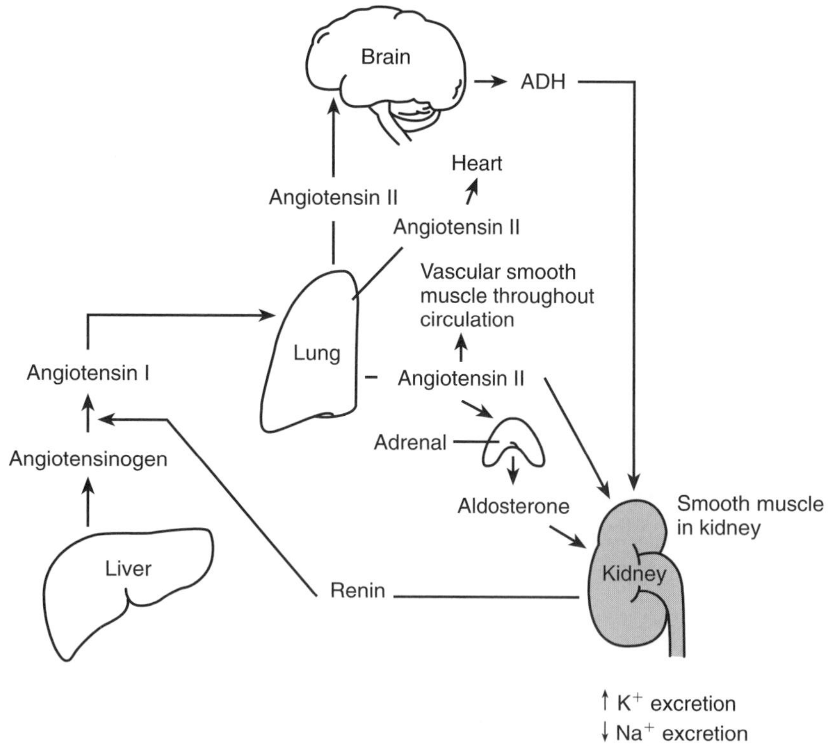

FIGURE 23-1

Schematic representation of the essential components of the renin-angiotensin-aldosterone system. (Modified from Berne RM, Levy MN: *Physiology*, ed 4, St Louis, 1998, Mosby.)

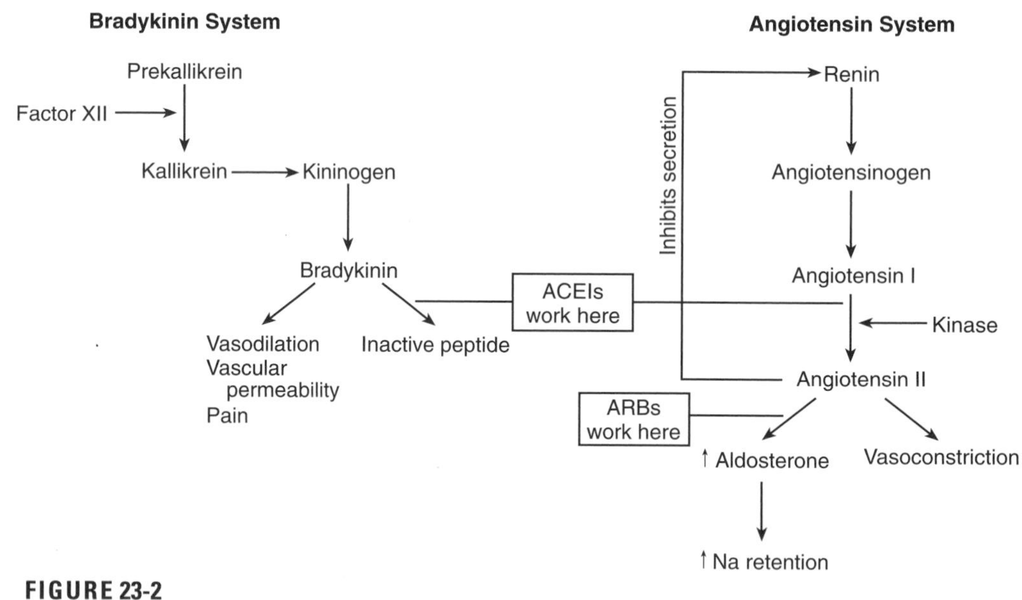

FIGURE 23-2

Sites of action of the ACE inhibitors and the receptor antagonists. (Modified from McCance KL, Huether SE: *Pathophysiology*, ed 4, St Louis, 2001, Mosby.)

ARBs block the effects of angiotensin II by blocking the binding of angiotensin II to its receptors. They do not affect bradykinin (Figure 23-2). The receptor affinity is highest by candesartan > irbesartan > eprosartan > telmisartan > valsartan > losartan.

ARBs differ from ACEIs in the following four respects:

1. ARBs are more active against AT_1 receptors than are ACEIs.
2. ACE inhibition is not associated with increased levels of angiotensin II, as are ARBs.
3. ACEIs may increase angiotensin levels more than do ARBs.
4. ACEIs increase levels of bradykinin, unlike ARBs.

Whether these differences cause significant clinical outcomes is unknown.

The pharmacologic effects of ACE inhibition result in a reduction in systemic vascular resistance, with either no effect or a moderate increase in cardiac output. Blood pressure is lowered through decreased systemic vascular resistance. Blood pressure reduction is not accompanied by changes in heart rate. Renal perfusion is increased and renal vascular resistance is decreased, but the glomerular filtration rate is usually unchanged. In patients with CHF, ACEIs significantly decrease preload and afterload. This causes a modest increase in ejection fraction and a decrease in ventricular end-diastolic pressure and volume. These in turn improve myocardial energy metabolism. ACEIs act on the renal vasculature to reduce arteriolar resistance. which improves renal hemodynamics. This may improve the course of patients with diabetic nephropathy and other renal diseases with glomerular hypertension.

DRUG TREATMENT PRINCIPLES

ACEIs and ARBs have an extremely low incidence of adverse reactions compared with other drugs for hypertension and angina. ACEIs have similar therapeutic and adverse reactions. They differ basically in pharmacokinetics (Table 23-1). Some come as prodrugs that must be metabolized by liver into the active compound. The duration of hypotensive effects is critical. Many products claim that they provide 24-hour protection, but their effect may wear off before 24 hours. Blood pressures should be checked shortly before the time of administration to ensure 24-hour control of blood pressure. They differ in tissue distribution, which may cause differences in the renin-angiotensin systems affected. Except for fosinopril, they are cleared predominantly by the kidney. ACEIs are generally considered safe and effective in patients with mild to moderate renal impairment; however, dosage reduction is required in patients whose renal clearance is diminished. Fosinopril, lisinopril, and ramipril are eliminated by both hepatic and renal mechanisms, having the ability to compensate for renal dysfunction by shifting to hepatic elimination. Dehydration and renal insufficiency increase the risk of elevated K^+ when an ACE is started.

ARBs are very similar to ACEIs. Their advantages are that they do not cause the dry cough characteristic of ACEIs and that the incidence of angioneurotic edema is less. However, because of their cost, ARBs are usually reserved for patients unable to tolerate the cough from ACEIs.

Hypertension

ACEIs are of particular value for treatment of hypertensive patients who have concomitant illnesses such as diabetes mellitus, renal insufficiency, left ventricular dysfunction, and CHF. ACEIs cause regression of left ventricular hypertrophy in hypertensive patients. It is possible that ACEIs reduce the incidence of heart disease in hypertensive patients more than do other antihypertensive medications, including diuretics and β-blockers. Studies are ongoing. Blood pressure reduction may be progressive with maximal effects achieved in 2 to 4 weeks. Combination therapy with thiazide diuretics provides an additive effect. Orthostatic effects are more commonly seen in volume- or salt-depleted patients. Abrupt withdrawal of ACEIs has not been associated with rebound hypertension.

Post–Myocardial Infarction/High Risk of Cardiovascular Events

ACEIs prevent ventricular remodeling after myocardial infarction. They improve endothelial function. They decrease the action of fibrin, reducing clotting. In one study, they decreased the rate of MI, stroke, and death in a variety of patients who did not have CHF but had vascular disease, diabetes, and one other risk factor for cardiovascular disease. This study suggests ACEIs may be beneficial for a large number of patients.

Chronic Heart Failure

ACEIs should be given to all patients with impaired left ventricular systolic function regardless of whether they are experiencing symptoms of heart failure, because they have been shown to prevent or delay the progression of heart failure. They reduce ventricular dilation, restore the heart to its normal elliptical shape, and reverse ventricular remodeling. They induce a more favorable hemodynamic state, including reduced afterload, increased cardiac output, decreased heart rate, decreased systemic blood pressure, renovascular resistance decreases, and renal blood flow increases, which causes natriuresis. The patient should not be dehydrated before starting therapy or the drug may precipitate renal failure.

Prevention of Renal Failure in Diabetes

ACEIs prevent or delay the progression of renal disease due to diabetes and many other diseases. They are used in mild to moderate renal insufficiency; but they must be used with increased caution as the renal insufficiency progresses. They are effective in both type I and type 2 diabetes regardless of baseline renal function or blood pressure. They may also decrease retinopathy in type 1 diabetics.

HOW TO MONITOR

- All patients should have a baseline and a periodic electrolyte panel (serum Na^+, K^+, total CO_2), serum blood urea nitrogen and creatinine, and urinalysis. Once dosage is stable, serum creatinine and potassium should be checked in 2 and 4 weeks. Patients without risk factors for renal deterioration should have these parameters checked every 3 to 6 months during stable maintenance therapy.
- Monitor WBCs for leukopenia periodically.
- Monitor supine blood pressure weekly while titrating dose. Patients with severe hypertension should be monitored more frequently during initial titration.

PATIENT VARIABLES

Geriatrics

- Useful in the elderly
- A lower dose may be needed in patients with renal or hepatic insufficiency

Pediatrics

- Safety and effectiveness of ACEIs in children have not been established.
- Irbesartan is indicated in children over 6 years old.

TABLE 23-1 Pharmacokinetic Properties of ACE Inhibitor Agents

Drug (Active Metabolite)	Potency	Effect of Food on Absorption	Availability (After First Pass)	Onset of Action	Duration of Action	Time to Peak Concentration	Half-Life	Protein Bound	Metabolism	Excreted Unchanged
captopril		Reduced absorption	60%-75%	0.25 hr	6 hr	1 hr	1.5-2 hr	25%-30%	50%	Urine, 40%-50%
lisinopril		None	25%-50%	1 hr	24 hr	6 hr	12 hr	NA		Urine, 100%
benazepril	High	None	37%	1%	24 hr	2-4 hr	10-11 hr	>95%	Prodrug to active in the liver	Urine and bile, metabolites <1%
enalapril (enalaprilat)		None	36%-44%	1 hr	24 hr	4-6 hr	11 hr	NA	Prodrug to active in the liver	Urine, 90% active metabolite
quinapril (quinaprilat)		Reduced	60%	1 hr	24 hr	2-4 hr	2 hr	90%	Prodrug in the liver	Active metabolites
moexipril (moexiprilat)		Reduced	13%	1.5 hr	24 hr	3-6 hr	2-10 hr	50%	Prodrug in the liver	Active and inactive metabolites predominantly in urine
ramipril (ramiprilat)		Reduced	56%	1-2 hr	24 hr	1.1-4.5 hr	13-17 hr	56%	Prodrug in liver	Active and inactive metabolites excreted by kidney
trandolapril (trandolquilat)		Reduced		4 hr	24 hr		5 hr	80%	Liver, 14%	Urine, 33%; feces, 56%
fosinopril (fosinoprilat)	High	None	36%	1 hr	24 hr	2 hr	4 hr	95%	Prodrug to active in the liver	Metabolites in urine and bile
losartan (Cozaar)		Well absorbed	33%	1 hr		3-4 hr	6-9 hr	99%	CYP 450 2C9 substrate and 3A4 substrate active metabolites	Urine, 35%; feces, 60%
candesartan			15%				9 hr	99%	Liver	Urine, 33%; feces, 67%
eprosartan		Reduced absorption	13%				5-9 hr	98%	Liver	Urine, 7%; feces, 90%
irbesartan (Avapro)		Rapidly absorbed	60%-80%			1.5-2 hr	11-15 hr	90%	CYP 2C9	Urine and bile, 20%
telmisartan		Reduced	50%				24 hr	99.5%	11% converted to metabolites	Feces, 97%
valsartan (Diovan)		Reduced	25%		24 hr	2-4 hr	6 hr	95%	Liver, 20%; not CYP 450	Urine, 13%; feces, 83%

Pregnancy

- *Category C:* first trimester
- *Category D:* second and third trimesters

These drugs can cause fetal and neonatal morbidity and death. Discontinue as soon as possible after patient becomes pregnant. Several ACEIs have been found in breast milk.

Race

- Less effective in blacks than in nonblacks when used as monotherapy
- Use of ACEIs in combination with diuretics has been successful in blood pressure reduction in blacks at comparable rates as in nonblacks

PATIENT EDUCATION

- Take a missed dose as soon as possible. Skip the missed dose if it is almost time for the next dose. Do not take two doses at the same time.
- Common side effects include nonproductive cough, dizziness or lightheadedness.
- *The patient should call the practitioner immediately if any of these serious adverse effects occur:*
  - Swelling (face, mouth, hands, tongue, or feet), difficulty breathing or swallowing, hives, severe itching, fainting, cloudy urine, sore throat, fever
  - Signs of excess potassium in the body: irregular heartbeat, leg weakness, numbness or tingling of hands or feet, extreme nervousness
- Avoid the use of potassium-containing medicines or salt substitutes while receiving this drug.

Specific Drugs

Ⓟ Prototype Drug

lisinopril (Prinivil, Zestril, Zestoretic)

Contraindications

- Hypersensitivity with angioedema with any ACEI

Warnings

- Neutropenia and agranulocytosis have occurred with captopril and occasionally with enalapril, lisinopril, and quinapril. Data are lacking to document whether other ACEIs cause agranulocytosis. Monitor WBCs.
- Anaphylactoid reactions, including angioedema of face, extremities, lips, mucous membranes, tongue, glottis, or larynx, have occurred.
- Proteinuria or nephrotic syndrome has occurred with captopril.

Watch for first-dose effect. Initial dose of ACEI may cause a precipitous, symptomatic fall in blood pressure, particularly in patients receiving diuretics, on sodium-restricted diets, or on dialysis.

- Drug may be associated with oliguria, progressive azotemia, or, rarely, acute renal failure and death. If possible, withhold diuretic for 24 to 72 hours before starting ACEI
- Renal impairment dose reductions are indicated. There is a potential for exacerbation of renal insufficiency and hyperkalemia.
- Volume-depleted patients (i.e., patients using diuretics or dialysis, or with vomiting or diarrhea, salt depletion) are at increased risk for symptomatic hypotension.
- Ramipril and fosinopril are primarily metabolized to active drug; increased inactive drug levels may occur with hepatic failure. In severe hepatic dysfunction, dose adjustments may be needed.
- In renal artery stenosis, a potential for increases in serum creatinine exists.
- Hypertensive patients with CHF have increased risk of symptomatic hypotension.

Precautions

- Hyperkalemia or use of potassium-sparing diuretics or salt substitutes can induce hyperkalemia.
- Valvular stenosis: Patients with aortic stenosis are theoretically at risk of decreased coronary perfusion.
- Cough has occurred with the use of all ACEIs. The cough is nonproductive and persistent and resolves within 1 to 4 days after therapy is discontinued. It has a higher incidence in women. Incidence ranges from 5% to 25% and can be as high as 39%.
- Photosensitivity may occur.

Pharmacokinetics

- See Table 23-1.

Adverse Effects

- See Table 23-2.

Drug Interactions

- See Table 23-3.

Dosage and Administration

- See Table 23-4 for dosage and administration directions for all ACEIs and ARBs.
- In general, it takes about 2 weeks for blood pressure reduction to be seen and 4 weeks to see the full effect.
- Food affects the rate but not the extent of absorption of fosinopril.
- Take captopril and moexipril 1 hour before meals.
- Ramipril capsules can be opened and mixed with food or water.
- The rate and absorption of quinapril are reduced approximately 25% when taken with a high-fat meal.
- Lisinopril, captopril, enalapril, ramipril: Decrease dose in renal insufficiency.

TABLE 23-2 Adverse Reactions to ACEIs and ARBs by Body System

Body System	ACEIs and ARBs
Skin, appendages	Rare: rash, diaphoresis, erythema multiforme, exfoliative dermatitis, flushing, photosensitivity, pruritus
Hypersensitivity	Angioedema (0.1%-0.5%)
Respiratory	Common: cough (ACEIs only); rare: asthma, bronchospasm
Cardiovascular	Orthostatic hypotension; rare: angina, CVA, MI
GI	Rare: abdominal pain, nausea, diarrhea, constipation
Hemic and lymphatic	Leukopenia, agranulocytosis
Musculoskeletal	Myalgia, arthralgia
Nervous system	Headache (<5%), dizziness (3%), fatigue (2%); ataxia, confusion, asthenia
Hepatic	Hepatitis
Genitourinary	Renal insufficiency, hyperkalemia, impotence

*Rare (>1%) unless noted.

TABLE 23-3 Drug Interactions of ACEIs and ARBs

ACEI/ARB	Action on Other Drugs	Drug	Action on ACEIs and ARBs
ACEIs	Increased digoxin, lithium, potassium preparations/potassium-sparing diuretics	Phenothiazines	Increased ACEIs
		capsaicin	Increased ACEIs (cough)
captopril	Increased allopurinol	Antacids, indomethacin	Decreased ACEIs
quinalapril	Decreased tetracycline	probenecid	Increased captopril
telmisartan	Increased digoxin	rifampin	Decreased enalapril
telmisartan	Increased and decreased warfarin	cimetidine, fluconazole	Increased losartan
		indomethacin, phenobarbital, rifampin	Decreased losartan

ACEI, angiotensin-converting enzyme inhibitor.

TABLE 23-4 Dosage and Administration Recommendations for ACEIs and ARBs

Drug	Indication*	Starting Dose	Usual Dosage	Maximum Daily Dosage
captopril	HTN	25 mg bid or tid	50 mg tid	450 mg
	CHF	25 mg tid	50-100 mg tid	450 mg
	Diabetic neuropathy	25 mg tid		
lisinopril	HTN	10 mg qd	20-40 mg	80 mg
	CHF	5 mg qd	5-20 mg	
benazepril	HTN	10 mg qd	20-40 mg	80 mg
enalapril	HTN	5 mg qd	10-40 mg qd or divided doses	40 mg
	CHF	2.5 mg bid	2.5-20 mg/day	40 mg
quinapril	HTN	10-20 mg	20-60 mg qd or divided doses	
moexipril	HTN	7.5 mg	7.5-3.0 qd or divided doses	60 mg
ramipril	HTN	2.5 mg qd	2.5-20 qd or divided doses	
	CHF	1.25-2.5 mg bid for 1 wk	Increase q3wk to 5 mg bid as tolerated	
	Cerebrovascular risk reduction	2.5 mg qd for 1 wk	5 mg qd for 3 wk; then 10 mg	
fosinopril	HTN	10 mg qd	20-40 mg qd or divided doses	80 mg
ANGIOTENSIN II RECEPTOR BLOCKERS				
losartan	HTN	80-160 mg qd	Increased q2-4wk	320 mg
	CHF	40 bid	80-160 mg bid	320 mg
candesartan	HTN	16 mg qd	8-32 mg qd or divided doses	
eprosartan	HTN	600 mg qd	400-800 mg qd or divided doses	800 mg
irbesartan	HTN	150 mg qd	300 mg qd	300 mg
	Nephropathy in type 2 diabetes		Target dose 300 mg qd	
telmisartan	HTN	40 mg qd	20-80 mg	80 mg
valsartan	HTN	80-160 mg qd	80-320 mg qd	320 mg
	CHF	40 mg bid	80-160 mg bid	320 mg

CHF, Chronic heart failure; *HTN,* hypertension.
*HTN dose is when patient IS NOT on a diuretic; CHF dose is when patient IS on a diuretic and digitalis.

RESOURCES FOR PATIENTS AND PROVIDERS

Internet

American Heart Association, www.americanheart.org

This site has many provider and patient resources, including patient education materials.

Heartpoint, www.heartpoint.com

A source of high-quality patient information on heart disease.

Video and Books

Goldman GW, Braunwald R, Zorab R: *Primary cardiology,* Philadelphia, 1998, WB Saunders.

Kahn mg: *Cardiac drug therapy,* ed 6, St Louis, 2003, WB Saunders.

Labarthe DR: *Epidemiology and prevention of cardiovascular diseases,* Frederick, MD, 1998, Aspen Publishers.

BIBLIOGRAPHY

Andersson PE et al: Regression of left ventricular wall thickness during ACE-inhibitor treatment of essential hypertension is associated with an increase in insulin-mediated skeletal muscle blood flow, *Blood Press* 7:118, 1998.

Anker SD: Catecholamine levels and treatment in chronic heart failure, *Eur Heart J* 19(Suppl F):F56, 1998.

Antonelli Incalzi R et al: Trends in prescribing ACE-inhibitors for congestive heart failure in elderly people, *Aging Clin Exp Res* 14:516-521, 2002.

Burnier M et al: Angiotensin II type 1 receptor blockers, *Circulation* 103:904, 2001.

Cheng A et al: Use of angiotensin-converting enzyme inhibitors as monotherapy and in combination with diuretics and calcium channel blockers, *J Clin Pharmacol* 38:477, 1998.

Franz IW et al: Time course of complete normalization of left ventricular hypertrophy during long-term antihypertensive therapy with angiotensin-converting enzyme inhibitors, *Am J Hypertens* 11(6 Pt 1): 631, 1998.

Gabbay E et al: Angiotensin-converting enzyme inhibitor cough: lessons from heart-lung transplantation, *Respirology* 3:39, 1998.

Gattis WA et al: Is optimal angiotensin-converting enzyme inhibitor dosing neglected in elderly patients with heart failure? *Am Heart J* 136:43, 1998.

Hamlin R et al: Plasma ACE inhibition by five different ACE Inhibitors, *Vet Q* 20(Suppl 1):S109, 1998.

Moore MA: Drugs that interrupt the renin-angiotensin system should be among the preferred initial drugs to treat hypertension, *J Clin Hypertens* 5:137-144, 2003.

Moser M et al: The role of combination therapy in the treatment of hypertension, *Am J Hypertens* 11(6 Pt 2):73S, 1998.

Rahman M: Initial findings of the AASK: African Americans with hypertensive kidney disease benefit from an ACE inhibitor, *Cleve Clin J Med* 70:304-305, 309-310, 312, 2003.

Remme WJ: The sympathetic nervous system and ischaemic heart disease, *Eur Heart J* 19(Suppl F):F62, 1998.

CHAPTER 24

Antiarrhythmic Agents

Elizabeth Monsen and Maren Stewart Mayhew

Drug Names

Class	Subclass	Generic Name	Trade Name
I	IA	quinidine	Quinidex Extentabs, Quinaglute Duratabs
		procainamide	
	IB	lidocaine	Xylocaine
		mexiletine	Mexitil
		tocainide	Tonocard
	IC	flecainide	Tambocor
		propafenone	Rythmol
II	β-Adrenergic blockers	propranolol	Inderal
		metoprolol	Tenormin
III		amiodarone	Cordarone
		sotalol	Betapace
IV	Calcium channel blockers	verapamil	Calan
		diltiazem	Cardizem
Other		digoxin	Lanoxin
		adenosine	Adenocard

General Uses

Indications

- Paroxysmal supraventricular tachycardia
- Atrial fibrillation
- Premature ventricular contractions (see Table 24-1 for indications for each medication)

• • •

Antiarrhythmics are used for the treatment of fast, slow, or irregular heartbeats. The antiarrhythmics most likely to be seen in an outpatient setting are class IA drugs, quinidine; class II, propranolol; class III, amiodarone; class IV, verapamil; and other, digoxin. Class II, class IV, and digoxin are discussed in detail in separate chapters. Quinidine and amiodarone are discussed in this chapter. The primary care provider who has a patient taking an antiarrhythmic should consult the most recent sources for complete, updated information on the drug and should work closely with a cardiologist or experienced physician.

All antiarrhythmic medications have potentially serious side effects including the induction of other serious and even fatal arrhythmias.

National guidelines for management of atrial fibrillation were published in 2003.

DISEASE PROCESS

Only the three arrhythmias most commonly managed in the outpatient setting are discussed in detail: paroxysmal supraventricular tachycardia (PSVT), atrial fibrillation (AF), and premature ventricular contractions (PVCs).

Anatomy and Physiology

The heart is composed of specialized myocardial muscle cells that have the capacity to generate an electrical potential (automaticity) and spread the electrical current from cell to cell (conductivity) (Figure 24-1). Many cells within the myocardium can serve as a pacemaker of the heart. The primary pacemaker is found in the sinoatrial node. Electrical waves of depolarization spread through the atrium, the atrial-ventricular junction, and down the left- and right-bundle branches, producing synchronized atrial and ventricular muscular contraction. When the dominant pacemaker slows, or does not fire, other cells take over and continue the heartbeat, although at a slower rate. Sometimes aberrant cells take over the pacemaker role, creating irregular rhythms and/or tachyarrhythmias.

Action potential (Figure 24-2) refers to the difference in electrical charge across the myocardial cell membrane, resulting in polarization and depolarization. *Depolarization* is the electrical impulse that results in the contraction of muscle. *Repolarization* is the recovery stage after muscle contraction.

Pathophysiology

The mechanism of an arrhythmia is theoretically important in determining which drug will be effective. The two basic tachy-

TABLE 24-1 Antiarrhythmic Medication Indications

Class	Drug	Indications
IA	quinidine	Atrial flutter Paroxysmal and chronic atrial fibrillation Paroxysmal ventricular tachycardia without complete heart block
II	propranolol	Paroxysmal atrial tachycardias, especially induced by catecholamines, digitalis, or Wolff-Parkinson-White syndrome Persistent sinus tachycardia Tachycardias and arrhythmias caused by thyrotoxicosis Persistent atrial extrasystoles Atrial flutter and fibrillation when rate cannot be controlled by digitalis
III	amiodarone	Documented life-threatening recurrent ventricular arrhythmias not controlled by antiarrhythmic drugs Recurrent ventricular fibrillation Recurrent hemodynamically unstable ventricular tachycardia
VI	verapamil	Atrial fibrillation, to control ventricular rate, with digoxin Repetitive paroxysmal supraventricular tachycardia
Other	digoxin	Atrial fibrillation, to control ventricular rate Atrial flutter

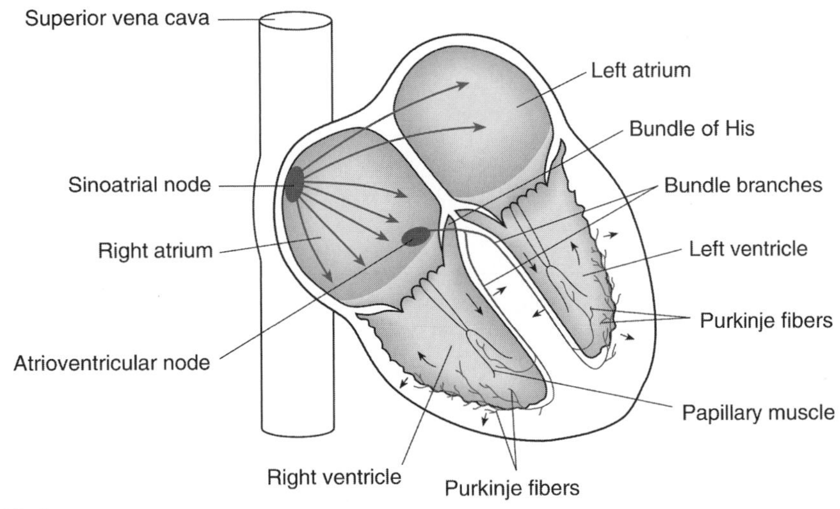

FIGURE 24-1

Conduction system of the heart. (From Berne RM, Levy MN: *Cardiovascular physiology*, ed 7, St Louis, 1997, Mosby.)

arrhythmic mechanisms within the heart are (1) increased automaticity resulting in an ectopic focus and (2) reentry through abnormal conduction pathways. However, it is often clinically impossible to determine the mechanism. Arrhythmias that are caused by irritability or increased automaticity are treated with drugs that prolong the action potential, thus decreasing the rate at which impulses can be generated (Figure 24-3). Sustained ventricular tachycardia is usually reentry, and it is treated with a drug that prolongs the effective refractory period.

The Disease

PSVTs are a group of tachyarrhythmias. The most common mechanism is reentry within the atrioventricular (AV) node, but it can also be caused by increased automaticity within the atria or AV node. It is characterized by an atrial and ventricular rate of 130 to 250, 1:1 conduction, and a narrow QRS complex. PSVTs are often seen in patients with no underlying heart disease. The therapy depends on the patient's ability to tolerate the tachycardia, mechanism of the arrhythmia, and how frequently the arrhythmia presents.

AF occurs due to a total lack of organized activation in the atria. Attempts to convert the patient to normal sinus rhythm are not usually successful over time. Sustained AF is associated with two problems. The first is rapid ventricular response. The ventricular response is usually 150 to 220 beats/min. This rapid rate may be poorly tolerated, precipitating CHF. The second issue with AF is the risk of thromboembolism. Clots may form in the atria and be released into systemic circulation, causing arterial occlusions and strokes.

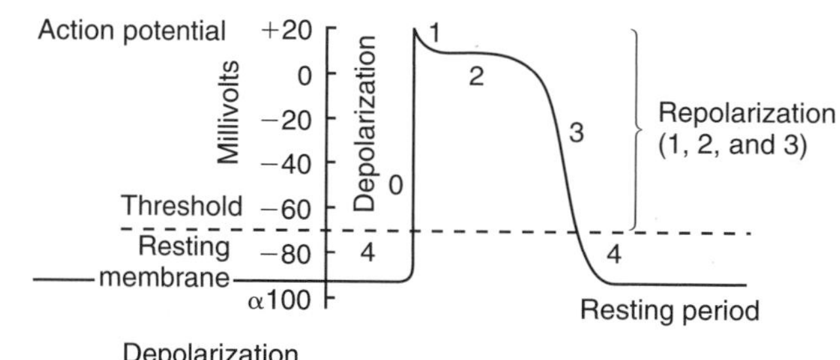

A

Depolarization
Phase 0—membrane becomes permeable to Na^+ which rapidly flows into the cell

Repolarization
Phase 1—membrane potential becomes slightly positive because of the rapid influx of Na^+
Phase 2—slow inward flow of Ca^{++} and outward flow of K^+
Phase 3—rapid outward flow of K^+

Resting period
Phase 4—cell membrane actively transports Na^+ outside and K^+ inside, returning cell membrane to state of polarization

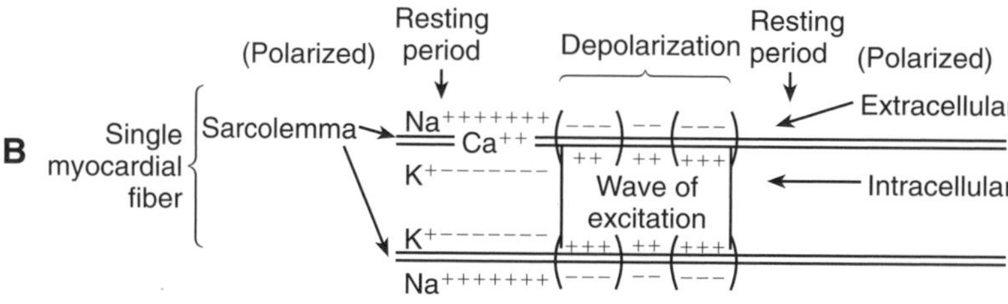

FIGURE 24-2

A, Action potential of a single myocardial fiber (cell). **B**, Ionic exchanges that occur across the cell membrane of a single myocardial fiber during an action potential. (From McKenry LM, Salerno E: *Mosby's pharmacology in nursing*, ed 22, St Louis, 2002, Mosby.)

PVCs are caused by increased automaticity. They are classified according to both prevalence and morphologic characteristics. The most important factor in determining whether to treat PVCs is the presence of underlying heart disease. Underlying heart disease (especially myocardial ischemia or recent MI) greatly increases the risk associated with even simple PVCs. Additional factors that place the patient at increased risk are the presence of cardiac scarring, hypertrophy, and/or left ventricular dysfunction. PVCs that are frequent, paired, or sustained are particularly dangerous. PVCs that occur during the QT interval are also a risk for starting ventricular fibrillation. Because of the risks inherent in antiarrhythmic therapy, patients should not be treated unless clearly indicated. Torsades de pointes is a life-threatening ventricular tachycardia associated with prolongation of the QT interval. It is most often seen as a drug reaction.

Assessment

Take a thorough health history, including history of hypersensitivity, drug history of other medications that may cause drug interactions, other medical problems, and other antiarrhythmic agents that could cause an additive cardiac depressant effect. The patient with an arrhythmia may have no complaints or may complain of palpitations, dizziness, weakness, or syncope. The palpitations may be described as fluttering, pounding, skipped beats, or "heart jumping out of the chest." They are often noticed when the patient is sitting quietly or lying in bed.

Auscultation often gives clues as to the type of arrhythmia. AF is irregularly irregular. PSVT is regular tachycardia. PVCs are a regular rhythm interrupted by premature beats, with a compensatory pause. Premature atrial contractions (PACs) are a regular rhythm with an occasional skip, but no compensatory pause.

Obtain relevant laboratory studies, such as a chest radiograph, graded exercise test, ECG, echocardiogram, and 24-hour Holter monitor result. Obtain baseline laboratory such as CBC, electrolytes, thyroid panel, and renal and hepatic function tests.

Identify and remove, or correct, any precipitating factors. Treat any underlying factors that may cause arrhythmias, such as hypoxia, acid-base imbalance, increased or decreased potassium, thyroid dysfunction, excessive catecholamines, or drug toxicity. Anxiety, caffeine, cigarettes, or stimulants

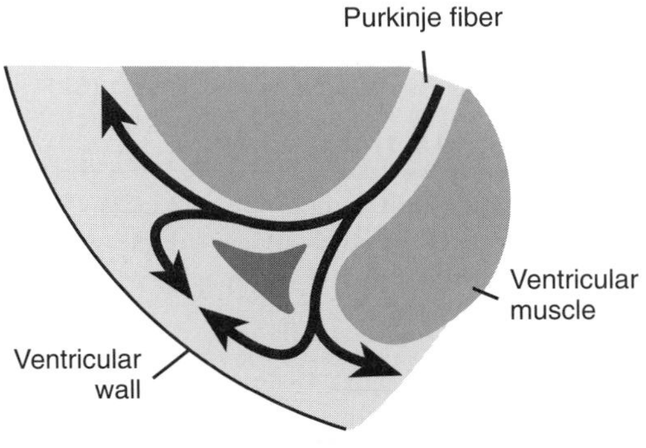

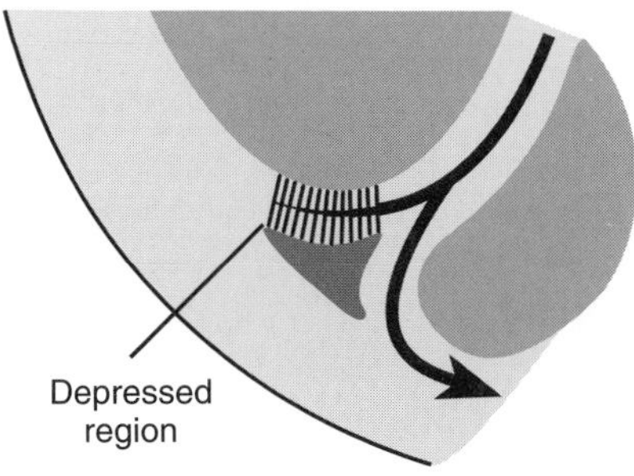

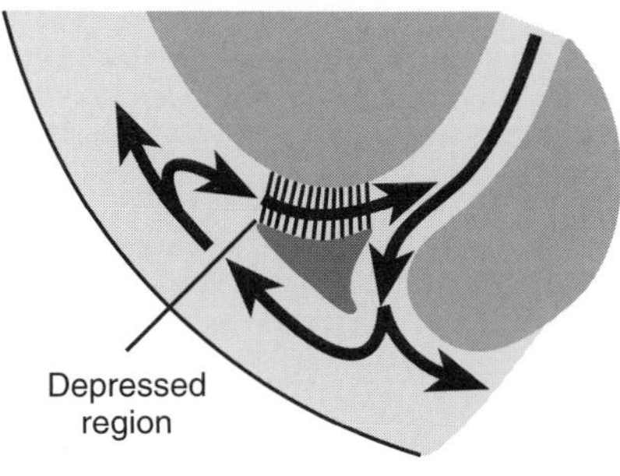

FIGURE 24-3

Mechanisms of arrhythmias.

such as decongestants, diet pills, amphetamines, theophylline, nicotinic acid, or alcohol may also precipitate arrhythmias.

DRUG ACTION AND EFFECTS

Antiarrhythmics act to reduce electrical irregularity of the heart. They do this by acting on the action potential of cardiac cells (Figure 24-4, Table 24-2). All antiarrhythmics have the potential to cause arrhythmias. The 1995 CAST Study revealed the dangers of aggressive medical treatment of arrhythmias.

Class IA drugs (quinidine, procainamide) depress phase 0 depolarization, lengthening the effective refractory period of atrial and ventricular myocardium by depressing the inward sodium current and decreasing the automaticity and excitability of ectopic foci of cardiac muscle. Class IB drugs depress phase 0 slightly. Class IC depress phase 0 markedly and profoundly slow conduction.

β-Blockers compete with β-adrenergic receptor–stimulating agents for available β-receptor sites, thereby antagonizing the effect of catecholamines released from the adrenergic nerve endings and the adrenal medulla. β-Blocking agents reduce the metabolic (glycogenolytic, lipolytic) actions of catecholamines. This decreases chronotropic, inotropic, and vasodilator action. Reduction in heart rate and force of contraction, suppression of renin release, and decreased outflow of sympathetic vasoconstrictor and cardioaccelerator fibers from brainstem vasomotor center are produced.

Amiodarone lengthens the cardiac action potential, prolonging phase 3 repolarization. It blocks sodium and potassium channels, which contribute to slowing of conduction, and prolongs refractoriness in the AV node. Its vasodilatory action decreases cardiac workload and therefore decreases myocardial oxygen consumption.

Class IV drug verapamil inhibits calcium ion influx through slow channels into conductile and contractile myocardial cells and vascular smooth muscle cells, slows AV conduction, and prolongs the effective refractory period within the AV node.

Digoxin decreases action potential duration.

DRUG TREATMENT PRINCIPLES

The primary care provider must work in collaboration with the cardiologist. The cardiologist determines the appropriate medication and begins treatment. The patient, once stable, may be turned over to the primary care provider for long-term monitoring. Table 24-3 outlines specific treatment principles for each type of arrhythmia.

Paroxysmal Supraventricular Tachycardia

Prophylaxis of PSVT usually involves digoxin. Verapamil or β-blockers are a second choice. These may also be used in combination. It must be remembered that verapamil increases digoxin serum levels. If the patient has significant heart disease, he or she may require a class IA, IC, or III drug. Radiofrequency ablation is frequently used to eliminate the accessory pathway. This avoids the problems with the safety of the antiarrhythmic drugs.

Atrial Fibrillation

The treatment of chronic AF is twofold. Control of rapid ventricular response is accomplished with digoxin, a β-blocker, or a calcium channel blocker. Prevention of thromboembolic events is accomplished by anticoagulation. Warfarin is the treatment of choice. If the patient is unable to be safely anticoagulated with warfarin, aspirin may be given at 325 mg/day (see Chapter 26).

Premature Ventricular Contractions

In general, PVCs are treated if *any* of the following apply:

- Complex PVCs are present
- The patient is 1 year or less post-MI
- The patient has underlying heart disease
- The patient has angina

PVCs are not treated if *all* of the following apply:

- The patient is asymptomatic
- The patient has a normal heart
- The PVCs are simple
- The PVCs disappear with exercise on a graded exercise test

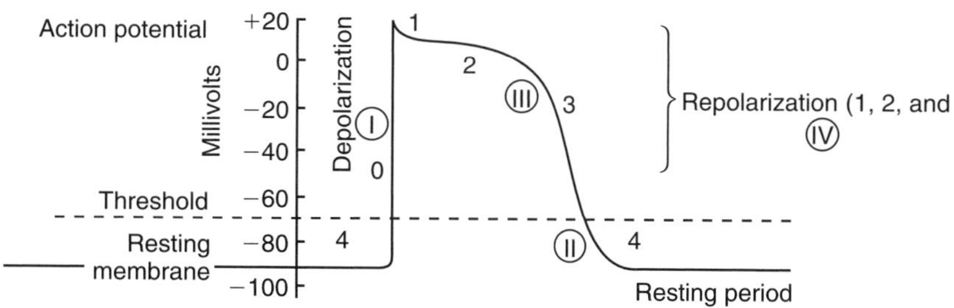

FIGURE 24-4

Phases of the action potential and location of action of the classes of antiarrhythmics. Circled Roman numerals indicate the major site of action of that category of antiarrhythmic.

TABLE 24-2 Mechanism of Action of Antiarrhythmic Medications

Drug	Heart Rate	Automaticity of Ectopic Foci	Conduction Velocity: AV Node	Conduction Velocity: Ventricle	Refractory Period: Atrium	Refractory Period: Ventricle	Accessory Pathway	ECG Changes: PR Interval	ECG Changes: QRS	ECG Changes: QT Interval
IA										
quinidine	±	↓	±	↓	↑↑	↑	↑	±	↑	↑
procainamide	±	↓	±	↓	↑	↑	↑↑	±	↑	↑
IB										
lidocaine	0	↓	0	0	0	±	↑↓	0	0	↓
mexiletine	0	↓	0	0	0	↑	↑	0	0	0
tocainide	0	↓	0	0	↓	↓	↑	0	0	↓
IC										
flecainide	0	↓	↓	↓↓	0	↑	↑↑	↑	↑↑	↑
propafenone	0	↓	↓	↓	0	↑	↑	↑	↑	↑
II (β-ADRENERGIC BLOCKERS)										
propranolol	↓	↓	↓	↓	±	0	↑	↑	0	↓
metoprolol	↓	↓	↓	0	±	0	↑	↑	0	↓
tenormin	↓	↓	↓	0	±	0	↑	↑	0	↓
III										
amiodarone	↓	↓	↓	↓	↑	↑	↑	↑	↑	↑↑
sotalol	↓	↓	↓	0	↑↑	↑↑	↑	↑	0	↑↑
IV (CALCIUM CHANNEL BLOCKERS)										
verapamil	↓	↓	↓	0	0	0	0	↑	0	0
OTHER										
digoxin	↓	↑	↓	↓	±	↓	↑↓	↑	0	↓
adenosine	↑	↓	↓	0	0	0	0	↑	0	0

TABLE 24-3 Suggested Treatment of Common Arrhythmias

Arrhythmia	Treatment Indicated for Acute Problem	Treatment Indicated for Chronic Prophylaxis
Paroxysmal supraventricular tachycardia	IV adenosine Verapamil	digoxin propranolol verapamil
Premature ventricular contractions	Lidocaine IV Procainamide	quinidine or procainamide amiodarone
Atrial flutter/atrial fibrillation	IV β-Blocker IV calcium channel blocker IV digoxin Cardioversion	digoxin propranolol verapamil Anticoagulants

Chronic treatment to suppress ventricular tachycardia is usually determined by provocative testing in an acute care setting. Drugs that may be effective include the class IA drugs and amiodarone. All of the drugs that may be effective are known to cause the arrhythmia that is being treated. Patients for whom medications are not effective or tolerated may be considered for implantable cardiac defibrillators.

HOW TO MONITOR

Monitor for Therapeutic Effect

A treatment goal specific to the patient is necessary. Total elimination of all irregular beats is not an appropriate goal. The goal is usually to prevent a potentially fatal arrhythmia or prevent certain targeted symptoms.

Monitor for Toxicity

An antiarrhythmic may cause the arrhythmia one is trying to suppress. A worsening of an arrhythmia after starting the drug may be an adverse reaction to the drug. At each visit ask about specific adverse effects. Monitor drug levels and electrocardiograms as needed. These drugs have significant adverse effects that require close monitoring. See the specific drug section for adverse effects.

quinidine. Therapeutic plasma level is around 3 to 6 μg/ml in most laboratories.

Perform periodic CBC and hepatic and renal function tests.

amiodarone. Plasma concentrations may be helpful in evaluating nonresponsiveness or unexpectedly severe toxicity.

Perform baseline chest radiographs and pulmonary function tests, including diffusion capacity, before initiation of therapy. Patient history, physical examination, and chest radiograph should be done every 3 to 6 months.

Thyroid function is needed at baseline and periodically during therapy.

Assess liver enzymes on a regular basis.

Perform regular ophthalmic examination, including funduscopy and slit-lamp examination.

PATIENT VARIABLES

Geriatrics

- A normal change of aging is loss of conduction fibers in the heart predisposing them to benign arrhythmias. If treated, the elderly are at increased risk for adverse reactions to the medications they may require a decreased dosage due to possible impaired renal or hepatic function.
- Amiodarone: Healthy subjects older than 65 years show lower clearances of amiodarone than younger subjects and an increased half-life (20 to 47 days).

Pediatrics

- Safety and efficacy of these drugs have not been established.

Pregnancy

- *Category B:* lidocaine
- *Category C:* quinidine, procainamide, mexiletine, tocainide, flecainide, propafenone, propranolol, verapamil, digoxin, and adenosine
- *Category D:* amiodarone

Lactation

- Drugs are excreted in breast milk.

PATIENT EDUCATION

- Wear a medical alert bracelet and carry a medical identification card specifying that you are taking this drug.
- Report any new or uncomfortable symptoms to your health care provider.

quinidine

- Take quinidine with food to decrease chances of having an upset stomach.
- Notify the provider of signs of cinchonism: ringing in the ears, hearing loss, headache, nausea, dizziness, vertigo, lightheadedness, and disturbed vision.

amiodarone

- Photosensitivity occurs in about 10% of those on amiodarone. Advise patients to use sunscreen and protective clothing.
- Advise to call for breakthrough arrhythmia, dyspnea, or cough.
- Advise patients of need to monitor for toxic effects.

Specific Drugs

CLASS I DRUGS

Subclass IA Drugs

quinidine (Quinidex Extentabs, Quinaglute Dura-Tabs)

Contraindications. Do not use in the presence of hypersensitivity to quinidine, or in patients with second- or third-degree AV block, intrav-entricular conduction defects, structural heart disease, renal failure with significant azotemia, severe CHF, severe ventricular conduction defects, and abnormal rhythms caused by escape mechanisms.

Warnings/Precautions

Treat AF and atrial flutter with digoxin before adding quinidine, or an extremely rapid ventricular rate may result.

Use with caution in patients with severe heart disease (because the drug depresses myocardial contractility), renal disease (because of potential accumulation of quinidine in plasma), hypotension (because it may further reduce blood pressure), digitalis intoxication, electrolyte abnormalities (increases the risk of torsades de pointes), or myasthenia gravis (because of anticholinergic effects). Give a test dose for hypersensitivity with a short-acting quinidine sulfate.

Preexisting asthma, muscle weakness, and infection with fever may mask quinidine hypersensitivity.

Pharmacokinetics

- See Table 24-4 for a comparison of the pharmacokinetics of major antiarrhythmic medications.

Adverse Effects. See Table 24-5.

TABLE 24-4 Pharmacokinetics of Common Antiarrhythmic Medications

Drug	Absorption	Drug Availability (After First Pass)	Onset of Action	Time to Peak Concentration	Half-Life	Duration of Action	Protein Bound	Metabolism	Excretion	Therapeutic Serum Level
IA										
quinidine	70%	—	30 min	6 hr	6-8 hr	6-8 hr	80%-88%	Hepatic	Hepatic	2-6 mg/L
procainamide	85%	—	30 min	—	3 hr	3+ hr	20%		Renal	3-10 mg/ml
IB										
lidocaine	—	—	—	—	1-2 hr	15 min	40%-80%	Hepatic	Renal	1.5-6 mg/ml
mexiletine	90%	—	—	2-3 hr	10-12 hr	24 hr	50%-60%	Hepatic	Hepatic	0.5-2 mg/ml
tocainide	100%	100%	—	0.5-2 hr	15 hr	—	10%	—	Renal	4-10 mg/ml
IC										
flecainide	100%	100%	—	3 hr	12-27 hr	—	40%	Hepatic	Renal	0.2-1 mg/ml
propafenone	100%	3%-10%	—	3.4 hr	2-10 hr	—	97	Hepatic	Hepatic	0.06-1 mg/ml
II										
propranolol	100%	—	30 min	—	2-3 hr	—	90%-95%	Hepatic	Hepatic	0.05-1 mg/ml
metoprolol	100%	50%		—	3-7 hr	—	12%	Hepatic	Hepatic	—
tenormin	50%	—	—	2-4 hr	6-7 hr	24 hr	16%	—	Renal	—
III										
amiodarone	35%-65%	—	2 days- 2wk	3-7 hr	15-142 days	Weeks-months	96%	Hepatic	Hepatic	1-2.5 mg/L
sotalol	90%-100%	—	—	2.5-4 hr	12 hr	—	0%	—	Renal	—
IV										
verapamil		13%-65%	30 min		3-7 hr		88%-92%	Hepatic		0.08-0.3 mg/ml
OTHER										
digoxin	60%-80%	—	0.5-2 hr	—	30-40 hr	24 hr	20%-25%	—	Renal	0.5-2 ng/ml
adenosine	—	—	—	—	<10 sec	1-2 min	—	—	—	—

TABLE 24-5 Common and Serious Adverse Effects of Antiarrhythmic Agents

Drug	Common Minor Effects	Serious Adverse Effects
IA		
quinidine	Lightheadedness, diarrhea, nausea, vomiting, heartburn, esophagitis, fatigue, palpitations, weakness, rash, visual problems, tremor	Cinchonism, hepatotoxicity, bronchospasm, lupus erythematosus–like syndrome, convulsions, ventricular tachycardia, ventricular fibrillation, torsades de pointes
procainamide	Myalgias, anorexia, nausea, vomiting, diarrhea, rash	Positive ANA titer, lupus erythematosus–like syndrome, blood dyscrasia, agranulocytosis, neutropenia, hypoplastic anemia, thrombocytopenia, CHF, asystole, ventricular fibrillation, hypotension, hepatic dysfunction
IB		
lidocaine	Lightheadedness, nausea, blurred vision, paresthesias, tremors	Respiratory depression/arrest, bradycardia, hypotension, cardiac arrest, allergic reactions
mexiletine	Palpitations, increased PVCs, nausea, vomiting, diarrhea, heartburn, constipation, dizziness, tremor, fatigue, weakness, blurred vision, paresthesias	Hepatic dysfunction, blood dyscrasias, ventricular tachycardia, ventricular fibrillation, angina, hypotension, bradycardia, second- or third-degree heart block, supraventricular arrhythmias, cardiogenic shock
tocainide	Fatigue, palpitations, chest pain, nausea, vomiting, anorexia, diarrhea, dizziness, paresthesias, tremor, headache, anxiety, blurred vision, diaphoresis, increased PVCs	Blood dyscrasias, agranulocytosis, leukopenia, neutropenia, aplastic/hypoplastic anemia, thrombocytopenia, pulmonary fibrosis/edema, interstitial pneumonitis, CHF, hypotension, bradycardia, ventricular tachycardia, ventricular fibrillation
IC		
flecainide	Dizziness, visual disturbances, dyspnea, headache, nausea, fatigue, palpitations, chest pain, asthenia, tremor, constipation, edema	CHF, bradycardia, second- or third-degree block, ventricular tachycardia, ventricular fibrillation, supraventricular arrhythmias, hepatic dysfunction, blood dyscrasias, death
propafenone	Unusual taste, nausea, vomiting, headache, fatigue, weakness, palpitations, diarrhea, anorexia, anxiety blurred vision	CHF, bradycardia, second- or third-degree heart block, ventricular tachycardia, ventricular fibrillation, torsades de pointes, bronchospasm
II		
propranolol	Fatigue, lightheadedness, depression, short-term memory loss, nausea, vomiting, diarrhea	Bronchospasm, bradycardia, CHF, hypotension, second- or third-degree heart block
metoprolol	Fatigue, dizziness, depression, headache, nightmares, insomnia, peripheral edema, nausea, diarrhea, pruritus, rash	Bronchospasm, bradycardia, CHF, hypotension, second- or third-degree heart block
tenormin	Fatigue, lightheadedness, lethargy, depression, nausea, diarrhea, dyspnea	Bronchospasm, bradycardia, second- or third-degree heart block, hypotension, CHF
III		
amiodarone	Photosensitivity, hyperthyroidism, hypothyroidism, malaise, fatigue, tremor, poor coordination, nausea, vomiting, constipation, anorexia	Pulmonary toxicity, hepatic failure, second- or third-degree heart block, blue-gray skin discoloration, bradycardia, ventricular tachycardia, ventricular fibrillation, torsades de pointes, optic neuropathy/neuritis, vision loss, peripheral neuropathy, CHF
sotalol	Elevated blood glucose levels, elevated liver enzymes, fatigue, dyspnea, asthenia, dizziness, infection, chest pain, palpitations, edema, headache, insomnia, depression, anxiety, mood change, nausea, vomiting, diarrhea, dyspepsia, abdominal pain, asthma, sexual dysfunction, back pain, rash, visual problems	Torsades de points, ventricular tachycardia, ventricular fibrillation, bradycardia, syncope, CHF, AICD discharge, hypotension, second- or third-degree heart block, bronchospasm, asystole
IV		
verapamil	Constipation, headache, rash, bleeding, visual problems, upper respiratory infection, dizziness, fatigue, edema, nausea, flushing	Second- or third-degree heart block, bradycardia, CHF, hypotension
OTHER		
digoxin	Palpitation, ventricular extrasystoles, tachycardia, anorexia, nausea, vomiting, diarrhea, headache, dizziness, mental disturbances, rash	Cardiac arrest, second- or third-degree heart block, ventricular tachycardia, ventricular fibrillation
adenosine	Facial flushing, headache, dyspnea, chest pressure, hyperventilation, lightheadedness, paresthesias, blurred vision, heaviness in arms, neck/back pain, nausea, metallic taste tightness in throat	Prolonged asystole, ventricular tachycardia, ventricular fibrillation, bradycardia, atrial fibrillation, bronchospasm

CHF, Chronic heart failure.

TABLE 24-6 Dosage and Administration Recommendations for Antiarrhythmic Agents

Drug	Age Group	Starting Dosage	Maintenance Dosage	Administration	Maximum Dose
IA					
quinidine	Pediatric and adult	300 mg q12hr	300 mg q8hr	PO q8-12hr	Variable, dependent on serum therapeutic range and presence of ECG changes
procainamide	Adult	500 mg bid	Dependent on body weight, see prescribing information	PO q12hr	5000 mg/day
IB					
lidocaine	Pediatric and adult	400 mg q8hr	Individualize	IV or injection	Dependent of weight
mexiletine	Adult	200 mg q8hr	200-300 mg q8hr	PO q8-12hr	1200 mg/day
tocainide	Adult	400 mg q8hr	400-600 mg q8hr	PO q8-12hr	2400 mg/qd
IC					
flecainide	Adult	100 mg bid	150 mg bid	PO q8-12hr	400 mg/day
propafenone	Adult	150 mg q8hr	225 mg q8hr	PO q6-8hr	900 mg/day
II					
propranolol	Pediatric and adult	10-40 mg bid	80-160 mg bid	PO q8-12hr	640 mg/day
metoprolol	Adult	25 mg bid (Lopressor) 25 mg qd (Toprol XL)	50 mg bid (Lopressor) 100 mg qd (Toprol XL)	PO q12-24hr	200 mg/day
tenormin	Adult	25 mg qd	50-100 mg/day	PO qd	200 mg/day
III					
amiodarone	Adult	800-1600 mg/day (loading dose for 1-3 wk) Requires baseline and periodic PFTs, laboratory tests, ophthalmology examination	200-400 mg/day	PO qd (loading doses may require bid scheduling)	600 mg/day
sotalol	Adult	80 mg bid Monitor ECG closely for prolonged QT interval with initiation or increase in therapy	240-320 mg/day	PO q8-12hr Reduced creatinine clearance requires longer dosing intervals	640 mg/day
IV					
verapamil	Adult	80 mg q8hr 120 mg SR qd	120-480 mg/day PO qd (SR)	PO q6-8hr	480 mg/day
OTHER					
digoxin	Pediatric and adult	0.125 mg (adult)	0.125-0.25 mg qd	PO qd	0.5 mg/day
adenosine	Pediatric and adult	6 mg (adult)	None	6 mg rapid IV bolus through peripheral line, may repeat with 12 mg if no conversion after 1-2 min	May repeat 12 mg IV

Drug Interactions

> ! Quinidine increases digoxin plasma levels. Concurrent administration requires a decrease in digoxin dosage. Quinidine reduces prothrombin levels and causes bleeding in patients on warfarin anticoagulants.

Thiazide diuretics prolong quinidine half-life. The anticholinergic effect of quinidine is additive with other anticholinergic drugs and antagonistic with cholinergic drugs. Other antiarrhythmic agents exert an additive cardiac depressant effect. Phenobarbital and phenytoin may reduce plasma half-life of quinidine by 50%.

Dosage and Administration. Give a test dose of quinidine and monitor for adverse reactions in a controlled setting before sending the patient home.

Dosage may vary considerably. Decreasing ectopic activity at the lowest dosage is the therapeutic goal (see Table 24-6).

CLASS III DRUGS

amiodarone (Cordarone)

Only the oral form of amiodarone will be discussed here. Parenteral form is used only in acute care settings. Sotalol is initiated in acute care settings.

Contraindications

- Hypersensitivity to the drug or its components
- Severe sinus node dysfunction, marked sinus bradycardia, second- and third-degree AV block, syncope caused by bradycardia

Warnings/Precautions. Amiodarone can exacerbate arrhythmias. Significant heart block or sinus bradycardia has occurred.

 Hypersensitivity pneumonitis or interstitial/alveolar pneumonitis has occurred in as many as 10% to 17% of patients at doses of 400 mg/day.

A higher percentage of patients have abnormal diffusion capacity without symptoms. Any new respiratory symptoms may represent pulmonary toxicity and should be evaluated with a complete history, physical examination, chest radiograph, and pulmonary function tests with diffusion capacity. A gallium scan should also be considered. Pre-existing pulmonary disease does not seem to increase the risk of developing pulmonary toxicity, but such patients have a poorer prognosis if pulmonary toxicity occurs.

Liver injury is common but usually mild and manifested only by abnormal liver enzymes. If the increase is greater than three times normal or doubles in a patient with elevated baseline enzymes, consider discontinuing or decreasing the dose. Overt liver disease has occurred and has been fatal in a few cases.

Optic neuropathy or optic neuritis resulting in visual impairment has occurred. Some cases have progressed to permanent blindness. Optic neuropathy or neuritis may occur at any time during treatment.

Amiodarone inhibits peripheral conversion of thyroxine (T_4) to triiodothyronine (T_3). It is also a potential source of large amounts of inorganic iodine; therefore, amiodarone can cause hypothyroidism or hyperthyroidism. Thyroid function should be monitored at baseline and periodically during therapy, especially in the elderly and in any patient with a history of thyroid nodules, goiter, or other thyroid dysfunction. Altered thyroid function and abnormal thyroid function tests may persist for several weeks or months following discontinuation of amiodarone. Hypothyroidism is managed with dose reduction or a thyroid hormone supplement. Hyperthyroidism may be a greater threat to the patient because of the possibility of aggravation of the arrhythmia. Aggressive medical treatment is needed, including dose reduction or discontinuation of the amiodarone. Antithyroid drugs, β-adrenergic blockers, or temporary corticosteroid therapy may be necessary. The action of antithyroid drugs may be delayed in amiodarone-induced thyrotoxicosis because of substantial quantities of preformed thyroid hormones stored in the gland.

Adverse Effects. See Table 24-5.

Drug Interactions. The potential for drug interactions exists during use of the drug. Interactions may occur with drugs administered after amiodarone is discontinued, secondary to the long and variable half-life of 3 to 107 days.

Anticoagulants: Potentiation of anticoagulation response can occur, which can result in serious or fatal bleeding. A 30% to 50% reduction in anticoagulant dose reduction is usually required. Onset is 3 to 4 days and may persist for months after amiodarone is discontinued.

Antiarrhythmics: Effects of β-blockers, calcium channel blockers, digoxin, flecainide, lidocaine, procainamide, and quinidine are increased in the presence of amiodarone. Concomitant use of antiarrhythmics can increase risk of hypotension, bradycardia, and potentially fatal arrhythmias.

Dosage and Administration. See Table 24-6 for loading and maintenance dosages.

RESOURCES FOR PATIENTS AND PROVIDERS

American Heart Association. Available at www.americanheart.org

Has many provider and patient resources including patient education materials.

ECG Home Page. Available at www.homepages.enterprise.net/djenkins/ecghome.html

This is a 12-lead ECG library.

Heartpoint. Available at www.heartpoint.com

A source of high-quality patient information on heart disease.

BIBLIOGRAPHY

Ferry DR, O'Rourke RA: *Basic electrocardiography in ten days,* New York, 2000, McGraw-Hill Professional.

Kowey PR et al: Pharmacologic and nonpharmacologic options to maintain sinus rhythm: guideline-based and new approaches, *Am J Cardiol* 91:33-39, 2003

Laiken RJ, Laiken JK, Karliner KJ: *Interpretation of electrocardiograms: a self-instructional approach,* ed 2, Philadelphia, 1998, Lippincott-Raven.

Mandel M: *Cardiac arrhythmias,* ed 3, Baltimore, 1995, Williams & Wilkins.

Naccarelli GV et al: Old and new antiarrhythmic drugs for converting and maintaining sinus rhythm in atrial fibrillation: comparative efficacy and results of trials, *Am J Cardiol* 91:15-26, 2003.

Nul DR et al: Heart rate is marker of amiodarone mortality reduction in severe heart failure, *J Am Coll Cardiol* 29:1199-1205, 1997.

Phillips RE, Feeney MK: *The cardiac rhythms: a systematic approach to interpretation,* ed 3, Philadelphia, 1997, WB Saunders.

Saoudi N, Hoels W, El-Sherif N: *Atrial fibrillation and atrial flutter: from basic to clinical applications,* Philadelphia, 1998, Futura.

Snow V et al: Management of newly detected atrial fibrillation: a clinical practice guideline from the American Academy of Family Physicians and the American College of Physicians, *Ann Int Med* 139(12): 1009-1017, 2003.

Wagner GS, Marriott HJL: *Marriott's practical electrocardiography,* ed 10, Philadelphia, 2001, Lippincott, Williams & Wilkins.

CHAPTER 25

Antihyperlipidemic Agents

James D. Hoehns and Courtney D. Eckhoff

Drug Names

Class	Subclass	Generic Name	Trade Name
HMG-CoA reductase inhibitors		(P)(200) atorvastatin	Lipitor
		lovastatin	Mevacor
		(200) fluvastatin	Lescol
		(200) pravastatin	Pravachol
		(200) simvastatin	Zocor
		rosuvastatin	Crestor
Fibric acid derivatives		(P)(200) gemfibrozil	Lopid
		fenofibrate	Tricor
Bile acid sequestrants		(P) cholestyramine	Questran, Questran Light
		colestipol	Colestid
		colesevelam	Welchol
Selective cholesterol absorption inhibitors		ezetimibe	Zetia
Other agents		nicotinic acid (niacin)	Niaspan, generic
Combination products		lovastatin/niacin	Avicor

(200), Top 200 drug; (P), prototype drug.

General Uses

Indications

- Hyperlipidemia

Currently there are five classes of antihyperlipidemic drugs, and each class has its own mechanism for lowering lipid levels and somewhat unique indications. The 3-hydroxy-3-methylglutaryl coenzyme A (HMG-CoA) reductase inhibitors are indicated for patients with primary hypercholesterolemia; that is, low-density lipoprotein (LDL) is the primary lipid elevation with minor elevations in triglycerides. Fibric acid derivatives are indicated for reducing the risk of developing cardiovascular heart disease (CHD) in patients without a history of CHD and who have low high-density lipoprotein (HDL) cholesterol levels in addition to elevated LDL cholesterol and triglyceride levels. They are also indicated for adults with marked hypertriglyceridemia who are at risk of pancreatitis and who have not responded adequately to dietary therapy. Bile acid sequestrants are indicated as adjunctive therapy to diet for reducing LDL cholesterol in patients with primary hypercholesterolemia. Niacin is indicated for patients with hyperlipidemia (all forms of elevated total cholesterol or triglycerides) who respond inadequately to dietary therapy. Selective cholesterol absorption inhibitors are used as adjunctive therapy to diet for the reduction of elevated total cholesterol, LDL cholesterol, and apolipoprotein B in patients with primary hypercholesterolemia.

This chapter incorporates the guidelines for the treatment of hyperlipidemia from the National Cholesterol Education Program (NCEP), 2001.

DISEASE PROCESS

Anatomy and Physiology: Lipids and Lipoproteins

Cholesterol and triglycerides are classified as lipids, and both are normal and vital constituents of plasma. Because they are hydrophobic and insoluble, they are transported in the plasma by lipoproteins. There are four classes of lipoproteins: chylomicrons, very low-density lipoproteins (VLDL), LDL, and HDL. Chylomicrons and VLDL are considered triglyceride-rich lipoproteins, whereas LDL and HDL are considered cholesterol-rich lipoproteins. Of the lipoproteins, evaluation of LDL and HDL levels is of primary importance. These two lipoproteins differ in several respects, including their cholesterol transport activities. Simply stated, LDL transport cholesterol from the liver to peripheral tissues and, conversely, HDL remove cholesterol from the periphery and transport it to the liver. Chylomicrons are the largest and least dense of the lipoproteins, followed in order of increasing density and decreasing size by VLDL (or pre-β), intermediate low-density lipoproteins (ILDL or broad β), LDL (or β) and HDL (or α).

Pathophysiology: Lipoprotein Abnormalities

There are a variety of different lipid disorders that can occur as either a primary event or secondary to some underlying disease.

TABLE 25-1 Primary Dyslipidemia and Associated Abnormalities

Dyslipidemia	Primary Abnormality	Frequency*
Familial hypercholesterolemias	Defective or absent LDL receptors (increased LDL)	0.2%
Familial defective apo-B	LDL receptor binding decreased because of abnormal apo-B (increased LDL)	0.2%
Familial combined hyperlipidemia	Apo-B and VLDL overproduction	0.5%
Familial hypertriglycerideemia	Decreased lipoprotein lipase activity, high VLDL production	1%
Familial hypoalphalipoproteinemia	Decreased apo-A-1 production, increased HDL catabolism	1%

apo, Apolipoprotein; *HDL,* high-density lipoprotein; *LDL,* low-density lipoprotein; *VLDL,* very low-density lipoprotein.
*Percent of general population.

Dyslipidemia can result from genetic disorders, concomitant disease states, or environmental factors. Alterations in lipoprotein metabolism are complex and often multifactorial. The primary dyslipidemias are associated with overproduction or impaired removal of lipoproteins. Primary dyslipidemias and their associated abnormalities are listed in Table 25-1. Often the cause of primary dyslipidemia is not identified and plays little or no role in the diagnosis and treatment of most patients.

Table 25-2 provides a list of causes that contribute to secondary hyperlipidemia. If the clinician determines a patient's hyperlipidemia may be secondary to another process, correction or modification of this process should be sought before pharmacologic treatment of the hyperlipidemia is pursued. Not mentioned in Table 25-2 is obesity, which may also produce lipoprotein alterations. In diabetes, triglyceride levels are related to the degree of diabetic control. In hypothyroidism, lipid abnormalities are corrected with thyroxine replacement. In uremia, a low HDL level is observed. Elevated lipids in nephrotic syndrome are related to urinary loss of albumin and protein. In drug-induced hyperlipidemias, estrogens may increase HDL, whereas β-blockers, progestins, and anabolic steroids may decrease HDL. evolve For additional information on the classification of hyperlipidemias, see the supplemental tables on the Evolve Learning Resources website.

The Disease

Overwhelming scientific evidence supports a causal relationship between hyperlipidemia and CHD. Premature coronary atherosclerosis, leading to manifestations of CHD, is the most common and important consequence of hyperlipidemia. Elevated LDL cholesterol is a significant and positive predictor of CHD. Although cholesterol likely contributes to CHD in multiple ways, a major mechanism is LDL oxidation. The oxidation causes the lipoproteins to be "sticky" and facilitates its adhesion to the endothelium of blood vessels causing atherosclerosis. There is an inverse correlation between HDL and CHD risk so that elevated HDL cholesterol is considered protective against the development of CHD. Roughly 50% of Americans have cholesterol levels that place them at an increased risk of CHD.

Elevated triglycerides are now known to be an independent risk factor for CHD. Obesity, inactivity, cigarette smoking, excess alcohol, high carbohydrate intake, diseases (type 2 diabetes, renal failure, nephrotic syndrome), and drugs (corticosteroids, estrogens, retinoids) are known to be risk factors for elevated triglycerides.

TABLE 25-2 Disorders Associated with Secondary Hyperlipoproteinemia

Underlying Disorder	LDL/ Cholesterol	VLDL/ Triglycerides
ENDOCRINE/METABOLIC		
Diabetes mellitus		↑↑↑
Cushing syndrome	↑↑	↑
Hypothyroidism	↑↑↑	
Anorexia nervosa	↑↑	
RENAL		
Uremia		↑↑↑
Nephrotic syndrome	↑↑↑	↑↑
HEPATIC		
Primary biliary cirrhosis	↑	
Acute hepatitis		↑↑↑
IMMUNOLOGIC		
Systemic lupus erythematosus		↑↑
Monoclonal gammopathies		↑↑
STRESS INDUCED		
Acute myocardial infarction		↑↑
Sepsis, excessive burns		↑↑
DRUG INDUCED		
Alcohol		↑↑
Thiazide diuretics	↑	↑↑
β-Blockers		↑↑
Glucocorticoids		↑
Estrogens	↓	↑↑↑
Progestins	↑↑	
Anabolic steroids	↑↑	
Retinoids	↑	↑↑↑

LDL, Low-density lipoprotein; *VLDL,* very low-density lipoprotein.

Assessment

As a screening measure, a fasting lipoprotein profile should be obtained every 5 years in adults, beginning at the age of 20 years. Serum cholesterol should be assessed more frequently in patients who have risk factors for CHD. Lipid profiles should be obtained in the fasting state (>12 hours since last meal) for an accurate measurement of triglycerides and LDL. Patients should be evaluated for common secondary causes of hyperlipidemia (diseases and drugs). Assessment of the patient's lifestyle including diet and exercise is crucial.

DRUG ACTION AND EFFECTS

HMG-CoA Reductase Inhibitors

These drugs (commonly called "statins") are reversible, competitive inhibitors of HMG-CoA reductase, which is the rate-limiting enzyme in cholesterol biosynthesis. HMG-CoA reductase catalyzes the conversion of HMG-CoA to mevalonate, a cholesterol precursor, in the liver. Inhibition of this enzyme decreases cholesterol synthesis, particularly causing a decrease in the serum LDL level. Although the mechanism of action appears straightforward, most LDL lowering observed with these drugs results from secondary, compensatory changes resulting from enzyme inhibition. Inhibition of HMG-CoA reductase reduces intracellular cholesterol concentrations, leading to an increased synthesis and expression of LDL receptors in the liver. This up-regulation of LDL receptors is a compensatory response to restore intracellular cholesterol homeostasis. As the concentration of LDL receptors increases, there is a resulting rise in the catabolic clearance of LDL from the plasma.

In addition to their impressive LDL-lowering effect, HMG-CoA reductase inhibitors increase HDL and decrease triglycerides modestly. New research suggests these drugs may also decrease levels of C-reactive protein, decreasing inflammatory processes that may be associated with atherosclerosis.

Fluvastatin is the first entirely synthetic HMG-CoA reductase inhibitor and has a chemical structure unrelated to the others in this class.

Fibric Acid Derivatives

Despite our lengthy experience with gemfibrozil, several uncertainties surround its precise mechanism of action. Its primary lipoprotein effect is to decrease plasma VLDL and triglyceride concentrations. The ability of gemfibrozil to lower triglycerides is attributed to an increase in lipoprotein lipase activity, which results in an increased catabolism of VLDL. Gemfibrozil may also suppress lipolysis in adipose tissue, decrease free fatty acid flux, and lower the rate of triglyceride synthesis. The increase in HDL observed with gemfibrozil may be the result of an increased synthesis of apolipoprotein A-1 or may be indirectly related to the drug's ability to lower VLDL. Gemfibrozil exerts a variable and minor effect on LDL levels.

Fenofibrate is a prodrug that is converted to its active metabolite, fenofibric acid. Fenofibric acid inhibits triglyceride synthesis and accelerates the removal of lipoproteins.

Bile Acid Sequestrants

Bile acid sequestrants are unique among the antihyperlipidemics because they are not absorbed systemically and are the safest drugs available for treatment of hypercholesterolemia. Although they differ in their chemical structure, all are large copolymers that function as anion-exchange resins in the intestinal lumen. Here they bind to bile acids, forming an insoluble complex, and result in a large increase in the fecal excretion of bile acids. The pathways involved in cholesterol and bile acid metabolism are intertwined and closely related. Although the resin agents are sequestering bile acids and interrupting their enterohepatic recirculation, there is a threefold to tenfold increase in the diversion of cholesterol into bile acid synthesis. This resultant decline in intracellular cholesterol concentrations leads to two compensatory changes: an acceleration of HMG-CoA reductase activity and an up-regulation of LDL cell-surface receptors. The two homeostatic changes increase intracellular cholesterol concentrations for conversion to bile acids, either by increased cholesterol synthesis or by increased uptake and removal of LDL from plasma. Therefore bile acid sequestrants increase the diversion of cholesterol to bile acid synthesis, lower intracellular stores of cholesterol, and result in an increased catabolism of LDL by the liver.

nicotinic acid (niacin) (Niaspan)

Niacin is believed to act on a hormone-sensitive lipase that leads to inhibition of release of free fatty acids from adipose tissue (lipolysis). The inhibition of lipolysis leads to reduced free fatty acid transport to the liver and therefore decreased synthesis of VLDL. This decrease in VLDL in turn causes a reduction in LDL. An increase in lipoprotein lipase activity by nicotinic acid is believed to increase the rate of chylomicron triglyceride removal from the plasma. The mechanism underlying the increase in HDL remains uncertain.

Selective Cholesterol Absorption Inhibitors

Ezetimibe is the first agent in a new class of drugs referred to as selective cholesterol absorption inhibitors. Ezetimibe is known to localize in the intestinal wall, where it is converted to its active glucuronide metabolite. It appears to act on the brush border of intestinal epithelial cells, where it selectively inhibits the absorption of cholesterol from dietary and biliary sources. The reduced cholesterol absorption results in a decrease in the delivery of cholesterol to the liver. Less cholesterol is thus available in hepatic stores, allowing more cholesterol to be cleared from the blood. Ezetimibe does not affect the absorption of fat-soluble vitamins or triglycerides, a benefit over bile acid sequestrants. Ezetimibe and/or its glucuronide conjugate circulates enterohepatically, repeatedly delivering the agent back to the intestine and reducing systemic exposure.

DRUG TREATMENT PRINCIPLES

The most widely recognized treatment guidelines for hyperlipidemia are those of the National Cholesterol Education Program (NCEP), most recently updated in 2001. An important tenet to these guidelines is that the intensity of evaluation and treatment depends on the patient's overall risk status for CHD (Box 25-1). That is, those patients with preexisting CHD or with CHD risk equivalents or those who are at high risk (more than two risk factors) of CHD in the near future are treated more aggressively. Next, patients with two or more risk factors should be further classified into 10-year risk groups based on their Framingham point scores. (See Framingham tables at www.nhlbi.nih.gov/guidelines/cholesterol/risk. Framingham scores are based on age, total cholesterol level, smoking status, HDL cholesterol, and systolic blood pressure. They are used to assess the individual's 10-year risk of developing CHD. Three levels of 10-year risk are identified greater than 20%, 10% to 20%, and less than 10%. Those found to have

TABLE 25-3 Treatment Decisions Based on LDL Cholesterol Levels

Risk Category	Initiate Lifestyle Change (mg/dl)	Initiate Drug Therapy (mg/dl)	LDL Goal (mg/dl)
CHD or risk equivalent (10-yr risk >20%)	≥100	≥130	<100
2+ Risk factors (10-yr risk ≤20%)	≥130	10-yr risk 10-20% ≥130 10-yr risk <10% ≥160	<130
No CHD and <2 risk factors	≥160	≥190	<160

CHD, Coronary heart disease; *LDL*, low-density lipoprotein.

BOX 25-1

NCEP CHD RISK EQUIVALENTS

Noncoronary vascular disease
Type 2 diabetes
10-Year CHD risk >20% (based on Framingham tables)

NCEP RISK FACTORS FOR CORONARY HEART DISEASE OTHER THAN LDL CHOLESTEROL

Positive Risk Factors

Age
- Male >45 years
- Female >55 years

Family history of premature CHD
- CHD in male first-degree relative <55 years or female first-degree relative <65 years

Current cigarette smoking
Hypertension
- Blood pressure >140/90 mm Hg or presently taking antihypertensive medication

Low HDL cholesterol (<40 mg/dl)

Negative Risk Factor

High HDL cholesterol (>60 mg/dl)

a risk greater than 20% are categorized as if they had a CHD risk equivalent (for further information see NCEP guidelines).

A second important feature of the NCEP guidelines is that both dietary and drug treatment decisions are based on LDL cholesterol levels (Table 25-3). For example, an individual whose blood pressure is 150/95 mm Hg who currently smokes and has a 10-year risk of 8% would have lifestyle changes initiated at an LDL level of 130 mg/dl or greater. According to the recommendations this individual would initiate drug therapy with an LDL level of 160 mg/dl or greater. In contrast, an individual with the risk factors listed earlier and a 10-year risk of 12% would initiate therapeutic lifestyle changes and drug therapy at an LDL of 130 mg/dl or greater.

Nonpharmacologic Treatment

The importance of dietary therapy and exercise should not be overlooked. Readers are advised to review the NCEP guidelines for further discussion of dietary strategies. Consider referring the patient to a dietitian for further instruction on low saturated fat and low cholesterol diets. Try to improve CHD risk factors that can be modified: smoking, hypertension, diabetes, inactivity, and obesity.

TABLE 25-4 Comparative Percentage Changes in Lipoprotein Concentrations Observed with the Antihyperlipidemic Medications

Drug	LDL (%)	HDL (%)	TG (%)
Bile acid sequestrants	↓15-30	↑3-5	↑5-30
niacin	↓10-25	↑15-35	↓20-50
HMG-CoA inhibitors	↓20-50	↑5-15	↓10-25
gemfibrozil	↓0-15	↑10-15	↓20-50
fenofibrate	↓20-25	↑10-15	↓30-50
ezetimibe	↓15-18	↑2-4	↓4-6

HDL, High-density lipoprotein; *LDL*, low-density lipoprotein.

Pharmacologic Treatment

The treatment of elevated LDL cholesterol in patients with no prior history of CHD is considered *primary prevention*. Treatment of patients with prior CHD is termed *secondary prevention*. Although therapeutic lifestyle changes are the mainstay of primary prevention, recent evidence shows that lipid-lowering drugs reduce the risk for developing CHD. In the case of secondary prevention, it is clear that antihyperlipidemic drugs reduce major coronary artery events, coronary artery procedures, stroke, as well as coronary and total mortality.

Although the focus of the NCEP guidelines is on LDL, consideration of the triglycerides and HDL should be included in drug selection (Table 25-4). If triglycerides are greater than 200 mg/dl after the LDL goal is reached, NCEP recommends setting a goal for non-HDL cholesterol (total cholesterol minus HDL cholesterol) 30 mg/dl higher than LDL goal. Once the LDL goal has been reached and triglycerides are less than 200 mg/dl, the focus should turn to the patient's HDL. The first step in treatment is to increase physical activity and lose weight if overweight. Drug therapy, nicotinic acid or fibric acid derivatives, may be used if the patient's HDL level remains below 40 mg/dl.

HMG-CoA Reductase Inhibitors. These are the most expensive drugs for treating hyperlipidemia, but they are also the best tolerated by patients and are highly efficacious at lowering LDL. Adverse effects are similar for all six of these agents. However, a switch from one drug to another may be advisable if adverse reactions occur. Their onset of activity is evident within 2 weeks, with maximal lipoprotein changes occurring 4 to 6 weeks after initiation. Serum lipoprotein concentrations typically return to baseline values within a similar period after drug discontinuation. These drugs generally work well at the lower dosages; seldom does increasing the dosage confer

TABLE 25-5 Comparative Efficacy of Currently Available Statins

HMG-CoA Reductase Inhibitor (mg)						Change in Lipid and Lipoprotein Levels (%)			
atorvastatin	lovastatin	fluvastatin	pravastatin	simvastatin	rosuvastatin	Total	LDL	HDL	Triglycerides
—	20	40	20	10	—	−22	−27	4-8	−10 to 15
10	40	80	40	20	—	−27	−34	4-8	−10 to 20
20	80	—	—	40	—	−32	−41	4-8	−15 to 25
40	—	—	—	80	10	−37	−48	4-8	−20 to 30
80	—	—	—	—	40	−42	−55	4-8	−25 to 35

HDL, High-density lipoprotein; *LDL*, low-density lipoprotein.
Data from Maron DJ, Fazio S, Linton MF: Current perspectives on statins, *Circulation* 101:207-213, 2000.

additional benefit. Because of this and the cost of the increasing dosages, lower dosages are generally used.

At clinically relevant dosages, the LDL-lowering potential of the six drugs in this class can be roughly ranked in the following order: atorvastatin > simvastatin > pravastatin = lovastatin > rosuvastatin > fluvastatin. The comparative potency and efficacy of the HMG-CoA reductase inhibitors are summarized in Table 25-5.

Fibric Acid Derivatives. Both are highly effective at decreasing triglycerides and increasing HDL but are less effective than the HMG-CoA reductase inhibitors at lowering LDL levels, which may actually increase in some patients. Gemfibrozil and fenofibrate are well tolerated but can cause hepatotoxicity and cholelithiasis. Gemfibrozil's maximal effect observed within 4 to 5 weeks. Generic gemfibrozil is available and costs less than the HMG-CoA reductase inhibitors.

Fenofibrate results in a decrease in cholesterol and triglyceride levels and an elevation of HDL. Uric acid levels may also be decreased in some patients receiving fenofibrate because of uricosuric activity observed with the drug.

Bile Acid Sequestrants. The three bile acid sequestrants are equally efficacious. Patient acceptance is a primary concern because of gastrointestinal adverse effects such as constipation, bloating, and nausea. Selection between agents should be based on cost and palatability. Questran Light (aspartame used for flavoring) should be used before Questran, which contains sucrose and provides unneeded calories for many patients (diabetics, obese). Colesevelam and colestipol are available in tablet form and may be preferred by patients who dislike the inconvenience and taste associated with the powder resin.

LDL concentrations begin to decline within a few days with a maximal effect observed within 1 month. Triglycerides and VLDL concentrations rise initially in treatment and tend to return to baseline levels after 1 month. Patients who have preexisting elevations in triglycerides may experience a greater and more sustained increase in triglyceride levels. HDL levels are not predictably altered with bile acid sequestrants.

Niacin. Niacin is one of the most effective antihyperlipidemics at lowering triglycerides and increasing HDL and is similar to the bile acid sequestrants in lowering LDL. The main limitation to niacin use is the adverse effect of flushing, although tolerance to this phenomenon generally occurs with continued use. Flushing occurs shortly after ingestion and can be blunted with aspirin (30 minutes before) and a slow escalation in niacin dosage over 3 to 4 weeks to 500 to 100 mg three times a day. Sustained-release niacin products cause less flushing than immediate- release tablets but may cause more serious liver toxicity; hence the immediate- release tablets are usually recommended first. Niacin impairs glucose tolerance and may cause hyperuricemia. It should be used with caution in patients with diabetes or gout. Niacin remains the least expensive antihyperlipidemic available and is probably underused in practice.

Selective Cholesterol Absorption Inhibitors. Ezetimibe is the only available agent in this novel drug class. When compared with placebo, ezetimibe has been shown to decrease intestinal cholesterol absorption by 50%. As monotherapy, ezetimibe can decrease LDL, increase HDL, and decrease triglycerides. When used in combination with a low-dose statin, an additional 18% reduction in LDL cholesterol has been seen compared with statin monotherapy. The reduction in LDL cholesterol may be seen as early as 2 weeks following initiation of ezetimibe.

Combination Therapy. Treatment with several drugs may be required to keep blood levels within the appropriate range, but combination treatment also contributes to the increased risk of adverse effects. Combining statins with a fibric acid derivative increases the risk of rhabdomyolysis. Statins, fibric acid derivatives, and niacin are known to cause hepatotoxicity. Ezetimibe may also cause hepatotoxicity. This adverse effect is multiplied when the drugs are used together.

HOW TO MONITOR

All Medications

Lipid profiles should be performed to obtain a baseline level and repeated at 4 to 6 weeks, and perhaps again at 3 months, after initiation of therapy to assess response. For long-term monitoring, total cholesterol can be obtained at most follow-up visits, with a lipoprotein profile (and LDL estimation) performed annually.

Liver function tests (LFTs [AST/ALT]) should be performed at baseline, at 6 and 12 weeks after initiation of therapy or dose escalation, every 3 months for a year, and periodically thereafter (e.g., annually or semiannually).

Statins, fibric acid, and nicotinic acid

Ask the patient about myalgias and check CPK if present. Otherwise routine monitoring of CPK is probably not necessary.

If statins, niacin, or fibric acid derivatives are used in any combination, monitor LFTs and CPK more frequently (e.g., every 4 weeks initially, then every 2 months). This is because of concerns of additive risk of hepatotoxicity and myopathy.

HMG-CoA Reductase Inhibitors

Pravastatin may require less frequent monitoring of LFTs (i.e., at baseline and 3 months only). If AST or ALT is three times the upper limit of normal or greater, a dosage reduction or discontinuation of therapy is recommended. Some clinicians advocate even less frequent monitoring of LFTs due to the statin's low risk of toxicity. Less than 1% of patients typically develop LFT results greater than three times the upper limit of normal during therapy.

Fibric Acid Derivatives

For gemfibrozil, monitor complete blood cell count every 3 months for the first 12 months of administration.

Bile Acid Sequestrants

No routine laboratory monitoring for adverse effects is necessary.

For patients receiving other drugs, monitor for a decreased pharmacologic response and/or drug level of these medications when bile acid resins are initiated. This is especially necessary for patients receiving digoxin, warfarin, levothyroxin, or thiazide diuretics.

nicotinic acid (niacin) (Niaspan)

Repeat lipid profile 4 to 6 weeks after reaching dosage of 500 mg three times daily, and perhaps again at 3 months, to assess response. For long-term monitoring, total cholesterol can be obtained at most follow-up visits, with a lipoprotein profile (and LDL estimation) performed annually.

ezetimibe

When used in combination with a statin, LFTs (AST/ALT) should be performed at baseline and as indicated for the statin.

When used as immunotherapy, LFTs are not routinely necessary.

PATIENT VARIABLES

Geriatrics

In general, the antihyperlipidemics may achieve maximal cholesterol reductions in the elderly at somewhat smaller dosages than those required in younger patients. Significant pharmacokinetic alterations in the elderly do not appear to be a major concern with the available antihyperlipidemics.

A common dilemma is deciding how aggressively to treat hyperlipidemia in the elderly. Statin therapy does not pose an increased safety risk for older patients with hypercholesterolemia or established cardiovascular disease. Drug therapy is warranted for patients 65 to 75 years of age due to the association between hypercholesterolemia and CHD. Those without CHD but who have several risk factors and a markedly elevated LDL should also be strongly considered for drug therapy. No data on patients over the age of 75 is available and lipid-lowering therapy is controversial. For patients who are currently on therapy it should be continued. Before initiating therapy in individuals over 75 a number of factors other than chronologic age need to be considered: quality of life, life-span limitations, comorbid conditions, and physiologic age. Although benefits of lipid-lowering therapy in the middle aged are well accepted, the CHD risk reduction associated with treatment in the elderly (>70 years old) is less certain. Taking these factors into consideration, elderly patients with established CHD and elevated LDL cholesterol should ordinarily be treated.

Pediatrics

Managing hypercholesterolemia in children primarily involves dietary and lifestyle changes. Cholestyramine and colestipol are the only Food and Drug Administration–approved drugs for managing hypercholesterolemia in children, yet they are rarely used. If pharmacotherapy is recommended, cholestyramine is presently the drug of choice because it is not absorbed systemically and is considered quite safe. Scientific evidence shows a 15% to 20% LDL cholesterol reduction with bile acid sequestrants in pediatrics. It is advised that antihyperlipidemics be prescribed to children only under the supervision of a lipid specialist.

Pregnancy

Triglyceride and cholesterol levels increase during pregnancy, but the increases are not usually considered clinically significant. Drug therapy for hyperlipidemia should be discontinued during pregnancy. The safety of lipid-lowering drugs in pregnant women has not been established. Therapy with HMG-CoA reductase inhibitors is contraindicated during pregnancy and lactation. For patients with severe forms of hyperlipidemia, consultation with a lipid specialist should be considered.

- *Category B:* colesevelam
- *Category C:* fenofibrate, clofibrate, gemfibrozil, niacin, cholestyramine, and ezetimbe
- *Category X:* ezetimibe, fluvastatin, lovastatin, pravastatin, simvastatin, and rosuvastatin
- No fetal harm is expected when cholestyramine and colestipol are given in recommended dosages although they may interfere with absorption of fat-soluble vitamins

PATIENT EDUCATION

All Medications

Patients should report any signs and symptoms of liver dysfunction.

Statins, fibric acid, and nicotinic acid

Promptly report any muscle pain, tenderness, or weakness that is unexplained, particularly if malaise or fever is also present.

HMG-CoA Reductase Inhibitors

May cause photosensitivity. Advise to use sunscreens, limit prolonged sun exposure, or wear protective clothing until tolerance is ascertained.

Bile Acid Sequestrants

The powders can be blended and stored with any consumable liquid. Mixing the powders with fruit juice tends to be more palatable than mixing them with water. They can be mixed with hot food but should not be cooked.

The resins often interfere with absorption of other drugs. Other medications should be taken 1 hour before, or 3 to 4 hours after, taking cholestyramine, colestipol, or colesevelam.

nicotinic acid (niacin) (Niaspan)

Facial and upper extremity flushing commonly occurs with niacin use. Pruritus, warm sensations, and tingling also may occur. These adverse effects tend to diminish in severity with continued use. Avoid taking niacin with hot fluids because these may worsen flushing episodes. If very bothersome, aspirin (325 mg) may blunt this effect if given 30 minutes before niacin ingestion.

Specific Drugs

HMG-CoA REDUCTASE INHIBITORS

Ⓟ **Prototype Drug**

atorvastatin (Lipitor)

Contraindications

- Active liver disease or unexplained persistent elevation in transaminases
- Pregnancy and lactation

Warnings

! Liver dysfunction: HMG-CoA reductase inhibitors have been associated with biochemical abnormalities of liver function. Liver function tests should be monitored. With an increase in transaminase level of three times the upper limit of normal a dose reduction or withdrawal from the medication is recommended. Patients reporting myalgias should receive prompt evaluation. With dose reduction, interruption, or discontinuation, transaminase levels usually return to baseline without sequelae.

! Skeletal muscle: rare cases of rhabdomyolysis with acute renal failure secondary to myoglobinuria have been reported. Patients should be instructed to report immediately unexplained muscle pain, tenderness, or weakness. Therapy should be discontinued if markedly elevated creatinine phosphokinase levels occur.

Pharmacokinetics

See Table 25-6.

Adverse Effects

Statins are generally well tolerated (see Table 25-7).

Drug Interactions

Administration of atorvastatin with either cholestyramine or colestipol decreases atorvastatin AUC by 25%. However, LDL reduction was greater with the combination than with either drug alone (see Table 25-8).

Dosage and Administration

In general, take in the evening (see Table 25-9).

Other Drugs in Class

Other drugs in this class are similar to the prototype except as follows.

lovastatin (Mevacor)

Lovastatin should be taken with meals.

- Altocor, extended-release lovastatin, provides a slower, prolonged exposure to lovastatin compared with immediate release.
- Lovastatin is the only HMG-CoA reductase inhibitor available in generic form at this time.
- A combination product, Advicor, combines extended-release niacin and lovastatin. The rationale for this combination is a result of the potent LDL-lowering effects of lovastatin and the effects of niacin on HDL and triglycerides.

fluvastatin (Lescol)

If patient requires an 80 mg total daily dose, it should be divided into 40 mg twice daily. Fluvastatin 80 mg is available in an extended-release form so that it may be administered once daily.

pravastatin (Pravachol)

The most hydrophilic statin on the market, it enjoys favorable data from many of the large outcome-based clinical trials.

simvastatin (Zocor)

After 1 year of therapy, LFTs are not required with simvastatin use. However, LFTs should be monitored at baseline and every 6 months for the first year.

rosuvastatin (Crestor)

Elevated levels have been found in Asian populations; use lower dosage with caution.

TABLE 25-6 Pharmacokinetics of Antihyperlipidemic Agents

Drug	Absorption	Drug Availability (After First) Pass)	Time to Peak Concentration	Half-Life	Protein Bound	Metabolism	Excretion
atorvastatin		14%	1-2 hr	14 hr	≥98%	Hepatic CYP 3A4	Feces, >90%; urine, <5%
lovastatin (prodrug)		30%	2 hr	3 hr	>95%	Hepatic CYP 3A4	Feces, 83%; urine, 10%
fluvastatin		24%	<1 hr	2.5 hr	98%	Hepatic CYP 2C9 (75%) 2C8 (5%) 3A4 (20%)	Feces, >90%; urine, <10% Urine, 70%;
pravastatin	34%	17%	1-1.5 hr	2 hr	50%	Hepatic CYP 3A4	Feces, 60%; urine, 20%
simvastatin (prodrug)		5%	<2 hr		95%	Hepatic	Feces, 60%; urine, 16%
rosuvastatin		20%	3-5 hr		90%	CYP 2C9 (10%)	Feces, 90%; urine (unchanged), 10%
gemfibrozil			1-2 hr	1.5 hr	98%	Hepatic	Feces, 6%
fenofibrate			6-8 hr	20 hr	99%	Plasma esterases; hepatic conjugation	Urine, 60%; feces, 25%
cholestyramine	NA	NA	NA	NA	NA	NA	Feces, 100%
colestipol	NA	NA	NA	NA	NA	NA	Feces, 100%
colesevelam	NA	NA	NA	NA	NA	NA	Feces, 100%
ezetimibe (prodrug)			4-12 hr	22 hr	>90	Glucuronidation (hepatic and small intestine)	Feces, 78%; urine, 11%
niacin				0.75 hr		Hepatic	Urine, 88%

NA, Not applicable.

FIBRIC ACID DERIVATIVES

Ⓟ **Prototype Drug**

gemfibrozil (Lopid, various generics)

Contraindications

Hepatic dysfunction, primary biliary cirrhosis, severe renal dysfunction, preexisting gallbladder disease, or hypersensitivity to gemfibrozil

Warnings

Some earlier clinical trials with patients receiving gemfibrozil (or chemically similar clofibrate) demonstrated increases (or no change) in all-cause mortality compared with groups receiving placebo. This increase in noncardiovascular mortality has been related to increases in cancer and other unknown etiologies (e.g., accidental and violent deaths). More recent large-scale clinical trials have shown significant decreases in CHD events with gemfibrozil use.

When gemfibrozil is administered concomitantly with HMG-CoA reductase inhibitors, patients may be at an increased risk of myositis or rhabdomyolysis. Gemfibrozil monotherapy may also be associated with the development of these conditions. Persistent increases in serum transaminases (e.g., AST or ALT) may be observed; thus LFTs should be monitored periodically (e.g., at baseline, 6 and 12 weeks, and twice yearly thereafter). Any elevations in serum transaminases are usually reversible with drug discontinuation. Gemfibrozil may increase cholesterol excretion into bile, leading to an increased risk of cholelithiasis. If a patient develops cholelithiasis while receiving gemfibrozil, the drug should be discontinued.

Dosage and Administration

Gemfibrozil should be taken twice daily 30 minutes before meals. Fenofibrate can be taken once daily (see Table 25-9).

Text continued on p. 323

TABLE 25-7 Common and Serious Adverse Effects of Antihyperlipidenic Agents by Body System

Body System	Statins	Fibric Acid Derivatives—gemfibrozil	Fenofibrate	Bile Acid Sequestrants	Selective Cholesterol Absorption Inhibitor	niacin
Body, general	Fatigue	Fatigue		Fatigue, weight loss/gain, swollen glands, edema, weakness	Fatigue	Flushing
Skin, appendages	Rash, pruritus	Eczema, rash	Rash, pruritus, eczema			Rash, pruritus
Hypersensitivity			Skin rash, Stevens-Johnson syndrome, urticaria, rash	Urticaria, dermatitis, asthma, wheezing, rash		
Respiratory	Cough		Cough, asthma	Shortness of breath	Cough	
Cardiovascular	Chest pain, syncope	Atrial fibrillation	Angina, hypertension, abnormal ECG, peripheral vascular disorder, hypotension, tachycardia, atrial fibrillation	Chest pain, angina, tachycardia (infrequent)		Atrial fibrillation and other cardiac arrhythmias, orthostasis GI
GI	Nausea, vomiting, diarrhea, abdominal pain, constipation, flatulence, dyspepsia, dysgeusia, cholestasis	Dyspepsia, abdominal pain, diarrhea, nausea, vomiting, constipation, acute appendicitis, cholelithiasis	Pancreatitis, cholelithiasis, dyspepsia, flatulence, constipation, diarrhea, nausea, vomiting, increased appetite, rectal disorder, esophagitis, gastritis, colitis, vomiting, anorexia	Common: constipation Lees frequent: abdominal pain, distention, cramping, GI bleed, nausea, vomiting, diarrhea, indigestion, flatulence, perianal irritation anorexia, steatorrhea, dental bleeding, sour taste Less common: pancreatitis, diverticulitis, cholecystitis, cholelithiasis, impaction	Diarrhea, abdominal pain	GI upset, activation of peptic ulcer, nausea, vomiting, abdominal pain, diarrhea, dyspepsia, cholestasis

Hemic and lymphatic	Ecchymosis, anemia, lymphadenopathy, thrombocytopenia, petechiae	Anemia, leukopenia, bone marrow hypoplasia, eosinophilia, thrombocytopenia	Anemia, leukopenia, thrombocytopenia, bone marrow hypoplasia	Increased prothrombin time, ecchymosis, anemia		
Metabolic and nutritional		Increased glucose		Malabsorption		Decreased glucose tolerance, hyperglycemia
Musculoskeletal	Rhabdomyolysis, arthralgia, myalgia	Rhabdomyolysis, myopathy, myositis	Rhabdomyolysis, myositis, myalgia, arthritis	Backache, muscle/joint pains, arthritis	Back pain, arthralgia, no rhabdomyolysis seen	Rhabdomyolysis
Nervous system	Headache, dizziness, asthenia, insomnia, paresthesia	Vertigo, headache, paresthesia	Headache, dizziness, insomnia, depression, vertigo, anxiety	Headache, anxiety, vertigo, dizziness, insomnia, fatigue, tinnitus, syncope, drowsiness, femoral nerve pain, paresthesia	Dizziness	Headache
Special senses	Ophthalmoplegia, progression of cataracts	Taste perversion	Conjunctivitis	Uveitis		Toxic amblyopia, vision disturbances
Hepatic	Increased LFTs, hepatitis, jaundice	Hepatotoxicity, increased LFTs	Increased LFTs, hepatitis		Unknown	Increased LFTs, severe hepatic toxicity
Genitourinary	Gynecomastia, loss of libido, erectile dysfunction	Decreased renal function	Decreased renal function	Hematuria, dysuria, burnt odor to urine, diuresis, increased libido		Hyperuricemia

TABLE 25-8 Potential Drug–Drug Interactions

Lipid-Lowering Agent	Interaction	Result
atorvastatin	digoxin	Increased digoxin concentrations 20%
	cyclosporine	Increased risk of rhabdomyolysis
	gemfibrozil/fenofibrate	
	niacin	
	erythromycin	
	itraconazole/ketoconazole	
	Bile acid sequestrants	Decreased atorvastatin AUC 25%
lovastatin	warfarin	Increased anticoagulation response
	ketoconazole/itraconazole/fluconazole	Increased risk of rhabdomyolysis
	cyclosporine	
	gemfibrozil	
	niacin	
	erythromycin	
	danazol	
fluvastatin	cyclosporine	Increased risk of rhabdomyolysis
	gemfibrozil	
	niacin	
	erythromycin	
	Bile acid sequestrants	Decreased fluvastatin AUC 50%
	ranitidine/cimetidine/omeprazole	Increased fluvastatin AUC
	rifampin	Decreased fluvastatin AUC
pravastatin	cyclosporine	Increased risk of rhabdomyolysis
	gemfibrozil	
	niacin	
	erythromycin	
	warfarin	Increased anticoagulation response
simvastatin	ketoconazole/itraconazole/fluconazole	Increased risk of rhabdomyolysis
	cyclosporine	
	gemfibrozil	
	niacin	
	erythromycin	
	digoxin	Increased digoxin level (minor)
	warfarin	Increased anticoagulation response
rosuvastatin	cyclosporine	Increased risk of rhabdomyolysis
	warfarin	Increased INR
	gemfibrozil, fenofibrate	Increased risk of rhabdomyolysis
	Antacids	Decreased rosuvastatin levels
	Oral contraceptives	Increased hormone levels
Fibric acid derivatives	HMG-CoA reductase inhibitors	Increased risk of rhabdomyolysis
	warfarin	Increased hepatotoxicity
	Bile acid sequestrants	Increased anticoagulation response
		Decreased gemfibrozil absorption
Bile acid sequestrants	warfarin	Decreased absorption; take all medications 1 hr before or 4 hr after ingesting the resin agent
	levothyroxine	
	digoxin	
	thiazides	
	phenobarbital	
	Tricyclic antidepressants	
niacin	HMG-CoA reductase inhibitors	Increased risk of rhabdomyolysis
	gemfibrozil	
ezetimibe	fibric acid derivatives	Increased bioavailability of ezetimibe
	Bile acid sequestrants	Decreased ezetimibe levels
	cyclosporine	Increased ezetimibe levels

TABLE 25-9 Dosage and Administration

Drug	Age Group	Starting Dosage	Maintenance Dosage	Administration	Maximum Dosage
atorvastatin	Adults	10 mg	Increase q4 wk 10-80 mg	qd	80 mg/day
lovastatin	Adults	20 mg	10-80 mg	Once daily with evening meal	80 mg/day
fluvastatin	Adults	20-40 mg	20-80 mg	qHS	80 mg/day
pravastatin	Adults	10-20 mg	10-40 mg	qHS	40 mg/day
simvastatin	Adults	5-10 mg	5-40 mg	qHS	40 mg/day
rosuvastatin	Adults	5-20 mg	10 mg	qd	40 mg/day
gemfibrozil	Adults	600 mg	600 mg	q12 hr	1200 mg/day
fenofibrate	Adults	67 mg	67-201 mg	qd	201 mg/day
cholestyramine	Children Adults	240 mg/kg/day 4 g/day	 4-24 g/day	3 Divided doses 1-6 Divided doses	 24 g/day
colestipol	Adults	Granules 5 g Tablets 2 g	5-30 g increase q4 wk 2-16 g	qd or in divided doses	30 g 16 g
colesevelam	Adults	1.875 g	1.875 g	bid (or 3.75 g once daily)	4.375 g/day
ezetimibe	Adults	10 mg	10 mg	qd	10 mg/day
niacin	Adults	100 mg	500-1000 mg	tid	3-4 g/day
niacin (extended release)	Adults	250 mg	250 mg-2 g	qd	2 g/day
niacin/lovastatin	Adults	500 mg/20 mg	500/20-2000/40 mg	qHS	2000 mg/40 mg

BILE ACID SEQUESTRANTS

Ⓟ Prototype Drug

cholestyramine (Questran, Questran Light, generic)

Contraindications

- Complete biliary obstruction
- Hypersensitivity either to cholestyramine or colestipol

Warnings

Patients with phenylketonuria (an inborn error of phenylalanine metabolism) should avoid Questran Light (or its generic equivalent), which contains aspartame for flavoring and contains 16.8 mg phenylalanine per 5-g dose.

Precautions

Both agents may interfere with normal fat and fat-soluble vitamin (vitamins A, D, E, and K) absorption and thus chronic use may be associated with an increased bleeding potential caused by hypoprothrombinemia associated with vitamin K deficiency. Worsening of constipation, fecal impaction, and aggravation of hemorrhoids have been associated with their use. Earlier animal studies suggested cholestyramine may be associated with increased gastrointestinal cancers, although this has not been substantiated in humans.

Pharmacokinetics

Because these drugs are not absorbed systemically, they are not metabolized and are entirely eliminated by fecal excretion (Table 25-6).

Adverse Effects

Severe adverse effects are very uncommon with these drugs because they are not systemically absorbed (see Table 25-7).

Drug Interactions

Bile acid sequestrants are notorious for binding within the gastrointestinal tract to coadministered drugs and substantially decreasing their absorption. If patients are taking any other medications they should be advised to take them either 1 hour before or 4 hours after ingesting the resin agent, to minimize this effect (see Table 25-8).

Dosage and Administration

Bile acid sequestrants are commonly titrated upward slowly (over several weeks) to minimize gastrointestinal-related adverse effects. They are usually taken before meals. Cholestyramine administration at mealtime is recommended to decrease gastrointestinal-related adverse effects (see Table 25-9).

It is important to explain to patients that they should not ingest the dry resin powders but must first mix each scoopful or packet with 2 to 6 oz of water or another beverage. Mixing the resins with fruit juice is one vehicle that has shown improved palatability in comparison with water.

Colestipol and colesevelam tablets should be swallowed whole. They should not be chewed, cut, or crushed.

OTHER AGENTS

nicotinic acid (Niaspan, various generics)

Contraindications. Hypersensitivity to niacin, active liver disease, active peptic ulcer, pregnancy, or lactation

Warnings. Niacin may lead to persistent increases in serum transaminases, and its use has been associated with jaundice and chronic hepatic toxicity. LFTs should be assessed at baseline, at 6 and 12 weeks after beginning therapy, and periodically thereafter (e.g., twice yearly). If used in conjunction either with HMG-CoA reductase inhibitors or gemfibrozil, LFTs should be monitored more frequently (e.g., every 2 months), and periodic creatinine kinase levels should be considered. This is because of a concern regarding an increased risk of hepatotoxicity or myopathy with these combinations. Myopathy and elevations of creatine kinase have been observed in patients receiving niacin alone or with other antihyperlipidemics. Patients with a history of liver or gallbladder disease should use niacin with caution.

Niacin typically worsens glycemic control in diabetic patients and has been shown to increase plasma glucose concentrations by 16% (niacin dosage was 1.5 g three times daily. Close monitoring of blood glucose is recommended if niacin is used in patients with diabetes. Niacin may also worsen peptic ulcer disease and can cause hyperuricemia. Patients with a history of gout or peptic ulcer disease should use niacin with caution.

Dosage and Administration. Acute adverse effects (flushing, nausea) are lessened with use of the sustained-release products, but they may cause somewhat increased hepatotoxicity compared to immediate-release formulations (see Table 25-9).

Niacin should be taken with meals because it may cause nausea and dyspepsia.

Patients should not be directly switched from immediate-release to sustained-release preparations at the same dosage per day. A lower dosage (approximately half of the previous immediate-release dosage) of the sustained-release product should be prescribed.

The majority of adverse effects associated with niacin are dose related, which is the rationale for titrating dosages slowly.

SELECTIVE CHOLESTEROL ABSORPTION INHIBITORS

ezetimibe (Zetia)

Contraindications

- Hypersensitivity
- The combination of ezetimibe and HMG-CoA reductase inhibitors is contraindicated in patients with active liver disease or unexplained persistent elevations in serum transaminase

Precautions

- When administered with HMG-CoA reductase inhibitors it should be in accordance with product labeling for that HMG-CoA reductase inhibitor.
- Use is not recommended in hepatic insufficiency.

Adverse Reactions. Most adverse reactions appear with the same frequency with ezetimibe as with placebo. However, the drug is very new and rare adverse effects may not have been seen (see Table 25-7). No LFT elevation or rhabdomyolysis has been found in monotherapy.

Drug Interactions. The combination of gemfibrozil, fenofibrate, or cholestyramine with ezetimibe is not recommended at this time (see Table 25-8).

Dosage and Administration. Ezetimibe may be administered with HMG-CoA reductase inhibitors for incremental effect and for convenience the two drugs may be administered together (see Table 25-9).

Ezetimibe may be taken once daily without regard to meals.

RESOURCES FOR PATIENTS AND PROVIDERS

American Heart Association, www.americanheart.org
Provides many provider and patient resources, including patient education materials, recipes, risk assessment, and treatment options.

Lipids Online, www.lipidsonline.org
Provider information on preventing and managing cardiovascular disease.

NCEP guidelines, www.nhlbi.nih.gov/guidelines/cholesterol
Includes 10-year risk calculator, executive summary of guidelines, and patient information.

University of Iowa Virtual Hospital, www.vh.org
Provider and patient information on diet strategies and smoking cessation.

BIBLIOGRAPHY

American Association of Clinical Endocrinologists: AACE lipid guidelines, *Endocr Pract* 6:162, 2000.

Betteridge JD, editor: *Lipids: current perspectives,* St Louis, 2000, Martin Dunitz.

Elliott HL: *Current issues in cardiovascular therapy,* St Louis, 1997, Martin Dunitz.

Expert Panel on Detection, Evaluation, and Treatment of High Blood Cholesterol in Adults: Executive summary of the Third Report of the National Cholesterol Education Program (NCEP) Expert Panel on Detection, Evaluation, and Treatment of High Blood Cholesterol in Adults (Adult Treatment Panel III), *JAMA* 285:2486, 2001.

Farnier M. Ezetimibe in hypercholesterolemia, *IJCP* 56:611, 2002.

Feher MD, Richmond W: *Pocket picture guide to lipids and lipid disorders,* ed 2, St Louis, 1997, Mosby.

Gotto AM: *Contemporary diagnosis and management of lipid disorders*, ed 2, Newton, PA, 2001, Handbooks in Health Care.

Kashyap ML, et al: Long-term safety and efficacy of a once-daily niacin/lovastatin formulation for patients with dyslipidemia, *Am J Cardiol* 89:672, 2002.

Keenan JM: Treatment of patients with lipid disorders in primary care: treatment guidelines and their implications. *South Med J* 97:266-276, 2003.

Malloy MJ, Kane JP: Agents used in hyperlipidemia. In *Basic and clinical pharmacology,* ed 8, New York, 2001, McGraw-Hill.

Maron DJ, Fazio S, Linton MF: Current perspectives on statins, *Circulation* 101:207-213, 2000.

McGowan MP: Lipid-lowering therapy in women: new treatment options. *Prev Cardiol Clin* 2002.

McEvoy GK, editor: *American hospital formulary service: drug information,* Bethesda, MD, 2001, American Society of Health-System Pharmacists.

McKenney JM: New guidelines for managing hypercholesterolemia, *J Am Pharm Assoc* 41:596, 2001.

Robins SJ, Collins D, et al: VA-HIT Study Group. Veterans Affairs High-Density Lipoprotein Intervention Trial. Relation of gemfibrozil treatment and lipid levels with major coronary events: VA-HIT: a randomized controlled trial, *JAMA* 285:1585, 2001.

Stevermer JJ, Meadows SE: What is the target for low-density lipoprotein cholesterol in patients with heart disease? *J Fam Pract* 51:893, 2002.

Shepherd J, Gaw A, Packard C: *Statins: HMG-CoA reductase inhibitors in perspective,* St Louis, 1998, Martin Dunitz.

Steinmetz KL: Colesevelam hydrochloride, *Am J Health Syst Pharm* 59:932, 2002.

Teo KK, Burton JR: Who should receive HMG CoA reductase inhibitors? *Drugs* 62:1707, 2002.

CHAPTER 26

Agents that Act on Blood

Theresa Pluth Yeo

Drug Names

Class	Subclass	Generic Name	Trade Name
Heparin group	Heparin	(P) heparin sodium	Generic
	Low molecular weight heparin (LMWH)	enoxaparin sodium	Lovenox
		ardeparin sodium	Normiflo
		dalteparin	Fragmin
	Heparinoid	danaparoid	Orgaran
		fondaparinux	Arixtra
Oral anticoagulants		(P) warfarin	Coumadin and generics
		dicumarol	Dicumarol
		anisindione	Miradon
Antiplatelet agents		(P) acetylsalicylic acid (ASA)	aspirin, Ecotrin, Halfprin, generic
		dipyridamole	Persantine
	Platelet glycoprotein IIb/IIIa inhibitors	clopidogrel	Plavix
		ticlopidine	Ticlid
		tirofiban	Aggrastat
		eptifibatide	Integrilin
		anagrelide	Agrylin
		abciximab	ReoPro
Thrombolytic agents		(P) alteplase (tPA)	Activase
		reteplase	Eliminase
		streptokinase	Streptase
		reteplase	Retavase recombinant
		urokinase	Abbokinase
Peripheral vascular dilators (hemorheologics)		pentoxifylline	Trental, Pentoxifylline ER

(P), Prototype drug.

General Uses

Indications

- Prevention and treatment of thromboembolic events such as stroke, MI, deep vein thrombosis (DVT), and pulmonary emboli (PE)

Drugs that act directly on blood include the antithrombotic agents (heparins, anticoagulants, and antiplatelet agents or platelet-active drugs), thrombolytics, and peripheral vasodilators.

The following drugs are not discussed because their use is seldom or never seen in primary care. Anisindione is not commonly used. The antiplatelet agents dipyridamole, tirofiban, epifibatide, anagrelide, and abciximab are also not seen in primary care. Dipyridamole is an old drug that is seldom used because aspirin is more effective. Thrombolytic agents are used for acute treatment of myocardial infarction (MI), pulmonary embolism (PE), systemic embolism, ischemic cerebrovascular events, and chronic heart failure (CHF) in acute care settings (Table 26-1). The glycoprotein IIb/IIa inhibitors are used as second-line therapy in stroke prevention. Pentoxifylline is limited to use in patients who have peripheral arterial disease. Drugs recommended here follow the sixth ACCP Consensus Guidelines on Antithrombic Treatment and the Stroke Council of the American Heart Association statement on primary prevention of stroke.

DISEASE PROCESS

Anatomy and Physiology

There is a delicate balance between the fluidity of the bloodstream and the ability of blood to clot quickly to prevent hemorrhage. In the coagulation system, there are two pathways necessary for clotting. The *intrinsic clotting pathway* refers to coagulation that occurs without the addition of any chemical agents; that is, the clotting factors needed for coagulation are intrinsic to the blood. The *extrinsic clotting pathway* is triggered by the addition of thromboplastin. The intrinsic and extrinsic pathways merge in what is referred to as the *final common pathway* (Figure 26-1).

TABLE 26-1 Indications for Drugs that Act on Blood

Category	Drug	Indications
Heparin group	heparin and low molecular weight heparin (LMWH)	Acute treatment of thromboembolic event (DVT, PE, stroke, ACS); early treatment of acute MI, cardiac surgery, vascular surgery, during and after coronary angioplasty, coronary stents, selected patients with acute stroke, unstable angina, atrial fibrillation, precardioversion of atrial fibrillation; prophylaxis of DVT and PE in postoperative and high-risk patients
Oral anticoagulants	warfarin	Venous thromboembolism, high-risk surgery, prophylaxis (abdominal and orthopedic surgery); short-term treatment of single episode of DVT or PE (3-6 mo); prevention of thromboembolic events (DVT and PE); indefinite treatment of recurrent DVT or PE, prevention of systemic embolism, postmechanical prosthetic heart valve replacement, cardiomyopathy, acute MI (3 mo); AC cardioversion in atrial fibrillation, tissue cardiac valve replacement (3 mo), atrial fibrillation, valvular heart disease, mechanical prosthetic heart valves
Antiplatelet agents	aspirin	Prophylaxis against thromboembolic complications in cardiovascular disease, recurrent MI or unstable angina, acute ischemic stroke, suspected acute MI, men with TIAs
	clopidogrel	Recent MI, stroke, established peripheral arterial disease: reduce risk of new stroke, MI
	ticlopidine	Prevention of thrombotic stroke in patients who cannot take aspirin; second-line choice in ischemic stroke
	dipyridamole	Adjunctive therapy with warfarin in prevention of postoperative thromboembolic complications in cardiac valve replacement; plays no helpful role in ischemic stroke or TIA
	abciximab	Adjunct therapy in percutaneous transluminal coronary angioplasty procedure to prevent acute cardiac ischemic complications; systemic embolism, heart failure
Peripheral vasodilators	pentoxifylline	Intermittent claudication caused by chronic occlusive arterial disease of the limbs

ACS, Acute coronary syndrome; *DVT*, deep vein thrombosis; *MI*, myocardial infarction; *PE*, pulmonary embolism; *TIA*, transient ischemic attack.

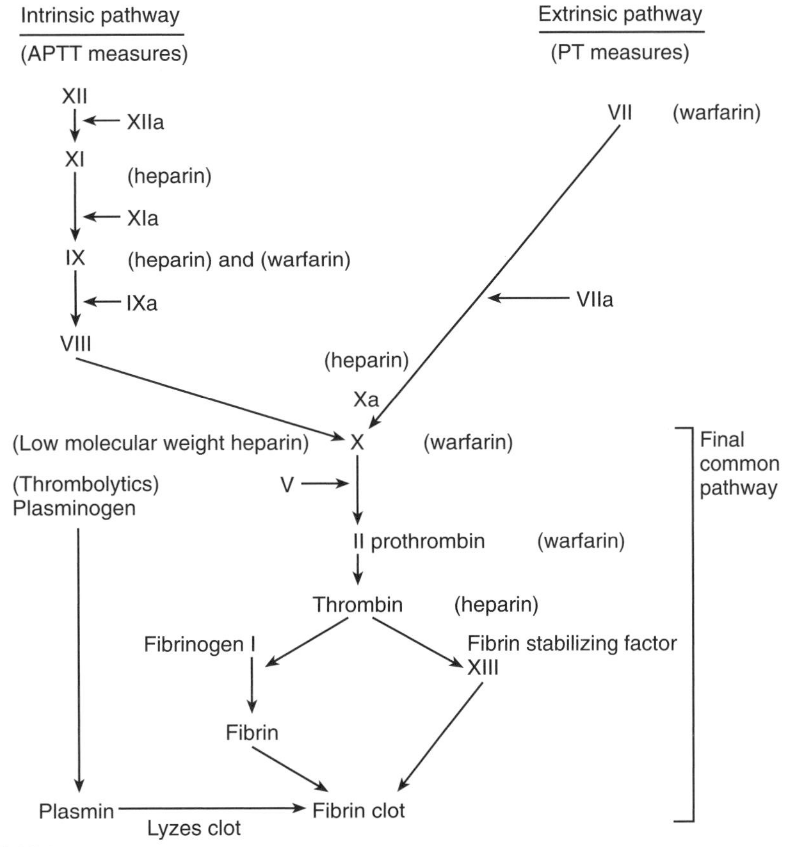

FIGURE 26-1

Coagulation and fibrinogen systems. Site of action of antithrombotic and thrombolytic drugs.

The intrinsic pathway is triggered when blood comes into contact with damaged endothelium or collagen. The intrinsic pathway is much slower than the extrinsic pathway in producing thrombin. Substances that are released by damaged tissues trigger the extrinsic pathway. The ultimate outcome of the extrinsic pathway is the conversion of prothrombin to thrombin. In the final common pathway, thrombin enzymatically converts fibrinogen to fibrin to form a fibrin-bound clot.

When there is direct tissue injury in the body, thrombin is released, thus initiating the fibrinogen system. Activated by thrombin, adenosine diphosphate (ADP), serotonin, and epinephrine, the platelets adhere to the damaged cell wall and trigger formation of the active clotting factors VII and X. Factors VII and X facilitate conversion of prothrombin to thrombin, which in turn converts fibrinogen to fibrin. The fibrin-bound clot framework itself further stimulates activation of more platelets. The platelets release thromboxane A_2, serotonin, and ADP, which enhance platelet aggregation and reinforce the formed clot.

Pathophysiology

The normally protective mechanism can become destructive to the body and the source of further pathology when clots form in areas that prevent tissues from receiving blood. Tissue ischemia and necrosis occur distal to the thrombosis. The thrombosis of MI, venous thromboembolism, PE, stroke, and chronic peripheral arterial occlusive disease are examples of this destructive process.

There are a number of factors associated with increased risk for a thromboembolic event (Box 26-1). Most of these factors are linked to decreased circulation, reduced mobility, or obstruction of blood flow. Many of these factors are the result of other diseases or disability. One of the critical decisions a clinician needs to make is whether it is possible to reduce or control risk factors in order to minimize the chance of thromboembolic events.

The Disease

Most of these drugs are used to prevent or treat blood clots that cause thromboembolic events such as stroke, MI, deep vein thrombosis (DVT), and PE. The most important pathogenic mechanism in angina and MI is an intracoronary platelet-rich thrombus on a disrupted, ulcerated, or eroded atherosclerotic plaque leading to partial or complete coronary artery occlusion. The same process occurs in the blood vessels of the brain causing strokes. DVTs and PEs are generally caused by clots that form in the atria of the heart, becoming lodged in arterioles.

The majority of cases of chronic peripheral arterial occlusive disease are caused by atherosclerosis. The femoropopliteal, tibioperoneal, aortoiliac, carotid, vertebral, splanchnic, renal, and brachiocephalic arteries are those most commonly involved. In chronic arterial occlusive disease, the goal of antithrombotic drug therapy is to relieve symptoms of pain and claudication and to prevent progression of disease leading to loss of the limb.

BOX 26-1

RISK FACTORS FOR THROMBOEMBOLIC EVENTS

- Age >40 years
- General anesthesia >30 minutes
- Cancer
- Oral contraceptive pills
- Prior oral contraceptive therapy
- Polycythemia
- Varicose veins
- Obesity
- Trauma
- Venous stasis
- Bed rest
- Chronic heart failure
- Immobility

Assessment

Assess personal and family history of bleeding and vascular disorders.

Check platelets, prothrombin time/international normalized ratio (PT/INR), activated partial prothrombin time (aPTT), complete blood cell count (CBC) with platelets, stool hemoccult, creatinine/blood urea nitrogen, and liver function tests.

DRUG ACTION AND EFFECTS

Heparin

Heparin has no effect on existing clots; it prevents or retards formation of new thrombi. Heparin blocks antithrombin III. Antithrombin III neutralizes activated factor X. Factor X is responsible for initiating the final common pathway in the clotting cascade (see Figure 26-1), which ends in clot formation. Antithrombin III inhibits the conversion of prothrombin to thrombin and prevents the activation of fibrin stabilizing factor, which converts fibrinogen to fibrin.

Low molecular weight heparin has several advantages over unfractionated heparin. It has a more predictable anticoagulant effect with a higher ratio of anti–factor Xa to anti–factor IIa, thus inhibiting the generation of thrombi higher in the clotting cascade.

Oral Anticoagulants

Warfarin competitively blocks vitamin K–binding sites, as well as inhibiting the synthesis of vitamin K–dependent coagulation factors VII, IX, X, and II (prothrombin) and anticoagulant proteins C and S. The degree of suppression is dose dependent. At therapeutic levels, warfarin decreases liver synthesis of vitamin K–dependent cofactors by 30% to 50%, exerting its therapeutic anticoagulation effects. Oral anticoagulants do not reverse ischemic damage or lyse an established thrombus but rather prevent extension of the existing thrombus and the formation of new thrombi.

Antiplatelet Agents

Aspirin (ASA) prevents platelet aggregation by inhibiting cyclooxygenase in platelets and endothelial cells, thereby preventing the synthesis of thromboxane A_2 and prostacyclin, both of which are potent platelet aggregators and vasoconstrictors.

Clopidogrel inhibits platelet aggregation by inhibiting the binding of ADP to its platelet receptor and the subsequent ADP mediated activation of the glycoprotein IIb/IIIa complex.

The effect is irreversible; platelets exposed to clopidogrel are affected for the remainder of their life span.

Ticlopidine inhibits platelet aggregation by altering the function of the platelet membrane and prolonging the bleeding time.

Dipyridamole increases the body's adenosine levels, producing vasodilation, particularly of the coronary arteries, which improves blood flow. It also inhibits phosphodiesterase, the enzyme responsible for elevating levels of cyclic adenosine monophosphate (cAMP). Low levels of cAMP are associated with reduced platelet adhesiveness.

The glycoprotein IIb/IIIa inhibitors are the newest group of antiplatelet drugs available for use. The glycoprotein IIb/IIIa receptor sites bind fibrinogen and von Willebrand factor to platelets, leading to normal aggregation. The glycoprotein IIb/IIIa inhibitor drugs reversibly block the binding sites, inhibiting platelet aggregation. The different drugs vary in their ability to bind with plasma protein; tirofiban is 65% protein bound, whereas eptifibatide is only 25% bound.

The mechanism of action of anagrelide, which reduces platelet counts, is unknown at this time.

Thrombolytic Agents

The thrombolytic drugs dissolve blood clots at sites of intravascular injury. They activate tissue plasminogen, which hastens the conversion of plasminogen to plasmin. Enhanced levels of plasmin (a proteolytic enzyme) digests fibrin-bound clots and coagulation factors.

Peripheral Vascular Agents

Pentoxifylline decreases blood viscosity, improves erythrocyte flexibility, increases leukocyte deformability, and inhibits neutrophil adhesion and activation. Although the precise mechanism of action is unknown, these actions improve blood flow through microcirculation and increase tissue oxygenation to the affected area.

DRUG TREATMENT PRINCIPLES

heparin

Low-dose heparin prophylaxis is recommended preoperatively and postoperatively in patients undergoing selected general surgical procedures and major orthopedic procedures to prevent venous thromboembolism. Standard heparin, LMWH, or heparinoid may be used. Typically the first dose is given 1 to 2 hours preoperatively and then every 8 or 12 hours postoperatively.

Begin standard heparin load with a 5000-unit bolus, then give 20,000 to 40,000 units every 24 hours or give as 15 to 25 U/kg/hr. Begin monitoring blood work as soon as medication is started so that any necessary adjustment to the dosage may be made. LMWH dosing depends on the product used (e.g., enoxaparin [Lovenox], 30 mg bid).

Generally, treatment is discontinued when the patient is past the risk of thromboembolic complications, which varies with the specific indication. Heparin is most often administered intravenously for 5 to 10 days. Oral anticoagulation with warfarin is usually required after heparin treatment to completely interrupt the thrombotic process and is begun concurrently with heparin at day 3 of therapy (Figure 26-2).

Heparin resistance is seen in febrile patients and those with active thrombosis, phlebitis, infections, MI, cancer, and heparin-induced thrombocytopenia (HIT). There is concern about increasing the risk of osteoporosis with prolonged standard heparin administration (>3 months, at an accumulated dose of 20,000 U). Another advantage of the LMWHs is that they produce less HIT and osteoporosis.

The rate of cross-reactivity between standard heparin and LMWH is 80% to 100%; therefore if there is need for continued anticoagulation in a situation in which standard heparin has been used, LMWH cannot be used. The heparinoid danaparoid or warfarin may be used as alternative therapies.

Oral Anticoagulants

The goals of oral anticoagulant therapy are to stop expansion of an established clot, prevent thromboembolic complications, and prevent formation of new thrombi. Warfarin therapy is often started concurrently with inpatient heparinization. Warfarin therapy is then continued as short-term adjunct therapy in DVT, post-MI, PE, and after total joint replacement for up to 3 months. It is used indefinitely in recurrent DVT, PE, chronic atrial fibrillation (AF), post–embolic stroke, cardiomyopathy, left ventricular aneurysm, valvular heart disease, and mechanical cardiac valve replacement. There is no con-

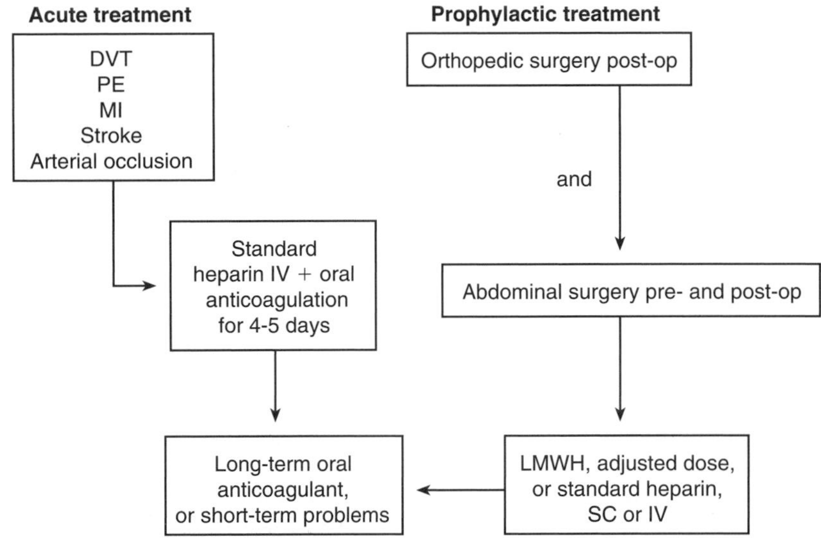

FIGURE 26-2

Algorithm for heparin administration decisions.

sensus with regard to perioperative management of patients on warfarin. According to the American Heart Association, the INR must be 1.5 or less before surgery can be safely performed.

Recommendations for how much medication to start with have grown more conservative over time. Usually begin with 2.5 or 5 mg and then adjust according to INR.

Use the generic warfarin (5 mg tablets) with caution because higher doses may be required to achieve INR goals. Patients taking Coumadin brand warfarin should not use generic warfarin interchangeably because of differing bioavailability factors. Difficulty maintaining a steady state may be encountered.

Stop warfarin temporarily when INR is greater than 6.0 and hemoglobin is stable but the patient has evidence of minor bleeding (ecchymoses, petechiae, gum bleeding, prolonged oozing from superficial trauma). Warfarin may be restarted when the INR is less than 4.0. The INR should be monitored every 3 days until INR and dose are again stable. Determine the source of overanticoagulation; possibilities include medication administration error, dietary indiscretion, alcohol overuse, acute febrile illness, diarrhea, new prescription or over-the-counter (OTC) medications, new herbal remedies, or vitamin supplements.

Factors that increase sensitivity to warfarin include travel, diet, environment, physical state, prolonged hot weather, increased age, poor nutritional status, vitamin K deficiency, malabsorption, CHF, vascular damage, hepatitis, obstructive jaundice, biliary fistula, febrile states, hyperthyroidism, bowel sterilization for surgery, and recent surgery.

Factors that decrease the response to warfarin include diabetes mellitus, hyperlipidemia, hypothyroidism, edema, hypercholesterolemia, and hereditary or acquired resistance to warfarin.

Antiplatelet Agents

ASA is the antiplatelet agent of choice for reducing thromboembolic events in patients with atherosclerosis (as evidenced by recent stroke, MI, or peripheral arterial disease). It decreases the incidence of MI and/or death in men over 50 years of age and patients with unstable angina, non–Q-wave infarction, acute MI, or cerebrovascular disease.

The effectiveness of ASA in preventing *arterial* thrombosis is well documented; however, its effectiveness in postoperative prevention of *venous* thromboembolism is controversial. LMWH and warfarin are more effective in decreasing the incidence of venous thromboembolism than is ASA.

Clopidogrel, a platelet glycoprotein IIb/IIIa inhibitor, inhibits platelet aggregation and is useful when a rapid antiplatelet effect is required. It is more effective than ASA in reducing stroke in patients who have had a TIA or minor stroke. Its effectiveness has been demonstrated primarily in preventing acute and intermediate complications in high-risk coronary angioplasty patients.

Ticlopidine is closely related to clopidogrel. However, it has more side effects (diarrhea, neutropenia, thrombocytopenia) than ASA or clopidogrel and is seldom used.

Thrombolytic Agents

The eligibility criteria for thrombolytic therapy include absence of brain injury or hemorrhage on computed tomography scan and initiation of intervention within 3 to 6 hours from onset of stroke symptoms. Intracerebral hemorrhage is the major complication, and its incidence increases when thrombolytic treatment has been delayed and when the duration of cerebral injury is longer than 3 to 6 hours.

Peripheral Vascular Agents

Treatment of occlusive arterial disease includes a regular walking program, control of serum cholesterol, smoking cessation, surgical consideration, and adjunct medical therapy.

Pentoxifylline is used in patients with chronic occlusive arterial disease to treat intermittent claudication. It is generally considered to be useful only if the disease is of moderate severity. In the treatment of peripheral vascular disease (PVD), pentoxifylline helps relieve symptoms and increase patient functioning. Improvement may be seen in about 2 to 4 weeks. If improvement is not seen by 8 weeks of therapy, discontinue the medication. If the patient takes the medication and exercises regularly, the arterial disease may improve to the extent that the drug is no longer needed. A trial off medication is recommended after 6 months of therapy to assess benefits.

HOW TO MONITOR

Standard heparin

Monitor patient for adverse effects, particularly bruising and bleeding.

Obtain regular laboratory studies to keep medication within therapeutic range (Table 26-2). Coagulation parameters useful in monitoring the effect of the anticoagulant ~~and thrombolytic~~ agents include the following

- aPTT, which reflects the intrinsic pathway, particularly thrombin, factor Xa, and factor IXa
- PT, which measures the extrinsic pathway and reflects depression of vitamin K–dependent factors VII, X, and II
- INR; the validity of PT determinations depends on the thromboplastin reagent used to perform the test (laboratories report both determinations [PT/INR] when a PT is ordered).

The goal of prolonging the PT 1.5 to 2.5 times normal has been replaced by a specific INR goal recommendation for each individual clinical indication. The typical INR goal is 2.0 to 3.0, except in mechanical cardiac valve replacement, where a higher INR is necessary to prevent clot formation.

low molecular weight heparin

The purification process used to develop LMWH renders it incapable of being monitored by the aPTT or PT/INR. The patient should be observed for clinical signs of bleeding, and a CBC with a platelet count should be obtained if side effects are suspected.

Oral Anticoagulants

Monitor INR every 3 days until goal is reached, then weekly, decreasing to every 2 weeks, and finally monthly when stable dose and INR are demonstrated.

Obtain regular CBC with platelets, liver function tests, stool for occult blood, and urinalysis for albumin and hemoglobin.

TABLE 26-2 Parameters to Monitor in Heparin Therapy

Type of Heparin	Parameters to Monitor
Parenteral heparin	Laboratory indexes Monitor aPTT q6hr Daily platelets for HIT Daily hemoglobin for hemorrhage
Subcutaneous heparin	
Standard heparin: fixed or low dose	Prolong aPTT 1.1-2× normal; often not necessary to closely monitor aPTT unless there is associated hepatic failure or heart failure
LMWH	No need to monitor aPTT Observe for signs/symptoms of bleeding: ecchymoses, purpura, hematuria, CNS changes, headache
Intravenous heparin	Check stool frequently for occult blood; aPTT q6hr, platelets and hemoglobin daily
Subcutaneous low dose standard heparin or LMWH	Usually no need to monitor coagulation parameters Suspected HIT: serotonin-release test, heparin-induced antibodies Stool for occult blood

aPTT, Activated partial thromboplastin time; *HIT,* heparin-induced thrombocytopenia.

Selected patients manage their warfarin using a home coagulation monitor. The Boehringer-Mannheim CoaguCheck Plus Coagulation Monitor is approved by the Food and Drug Administration and expensive ($2000) and the level of decision-making ability required renders home coagulation monitoring impractical for most patients.

Query patient at each visit regarding signs and symptoms of bleeding, drug side effects, dietary vitamin K intake/changes, missed doses, alcohol intake, recent illness, new prescription medications, use of OTC medications, vitamin supplements, and herbal remedies. Gingko has been linked to prolonged clotting times.

Antiplatelet Agents

- Monitor for GI upset and hypersensitivity reactions
- Routine monitoring of coagulation parameters is not necessary
- Monitor CBC with platelets, urinalysis, and stool hemoccult periodically based on coexistent medical conditions

Peripheral Vascular Dilators

Obtain an objective measure of the patient's exercise tolerance, such as the number of blocks the patient can walk before beginning treatment. Monitor ability to walk as a measure of the drug's effectiveness.

Assess patient's subjective and objective improvement in pain-free walking distance at 4-week intervals.

Monitor patients for bleeding, including hematocrit or hemoglobin if the patient has any increased risk for bleeding.

PATIENT VARIABLES

Geriatrics

- *Heparin:* elderly patients may have low levels of antithrombin III and therefore have increased thrombotic potential. It may be difficult to achieve therapeutic aPTT levels.
- *Warfarin:* liver function declines with aging, resulting in slower metabolism of warfarin; therefore a decreased dose is warranted. The elderly exhibit a greater tendency to bleed into the skin while on warfarin because of thinning of the epithelial layer.
- *Thrombolytics:* use with caution in adults older than 75 years due to increased risk of CNS bleeding.
- *Clopidogrel:* no dosage adjustment is needed.
- *Pentoxifylline:* older patients may have renal insufficiency with a decreased ability to excrete this drug. Thus the geriatric patient may be at higher risk of toxicity.

Pediatrics

- Use of oral anticoagulants in children is not well documented.
- *Heparin, thrombolytics, clopidogrel,* and *pentofylline:* safety in children has not been established.
- Children and teenagers should not take ASA without consulting their provider regarding Reye's syndrome. Safety has not been established in children younger than 18 years.

Pregnancy

- Heparin *(Category C):* does not cross the placental barrier. Carcinogenic potential and reproductive effects have not been evaluated. If anticoagulation is necessary, heparin is the drug of choice, despite category C classification.
- Warfarin *(Category X):* do not use warfarin in pregnancy because it crosses the placental barrier. Low birth weight, growth retardation, spontaneous abortion, and stillbirth have been seen when given to pregnant women. Carcinogenicity and mutagenicity have not been determined. If patient becomes pregnant while on warfarin, she may need to consider termination of pregnancy. Refer patient to high-risk pregnancy obstetric/gynecology specialist.
- Thrombolytics *(Category C):* it is not known whether drugs cause fetal harm.
- Clopidogrel *(Category B):* there are no adequate studies.
- ASA *(Category C):* ASA should not be taken in the last 3 months of pregnancy.
- Pentoxifylline *(Category C)*

Lactation

- Heparin: not excreted in human milk.
- Warfarin: can be taken by nursing mothers because it does not appear to have an anticoagulant effect on breast-fed infants.
- Thrombolytics and clopidogrel: not known if these are excreted in human milk.
- Pentoxifylline and its metabolites: excreted in breast milk.

Gender

- Research has confirmed effectiveness of ASA in men for prevention of venous thrombosis and TIA; research is on-going to determine effectiveness in women.

PATIENT EDUCATION

For All Products

Emphasize the seriousness of any signs or symptoms of bleeding, what the patient should look for, and when to return to or call the health care provider.

Encourage patients to practice to use safety measures and fall prevention in the home to decrease risk of injury and bleeding and bruising.

heparin

Report any hypersensitivity reactions, such as skin rashes, hives, swelling, itching.

Oral Anticoagulants

Consistency is the key to successful warfarin treatment. Remind patient to take medication at the same time every day.

For missed doses, caution patient not to "double-up" the next day. Take warfarin as soon as possible on the same day or not at all that day.

Inform patient of increased risk of bleeding, and signs and symptoms that indicate major or minor bleeding.

Review relevant safety issues with the patient. Caution in particular about prolonged bleeding associated with falls, abrasions, or cuts.

Emphasize the importance of laboratory monitoring to keep clotting parameters within the therapeutic range.

Have patient inform other health care providers, particularly dentists, about anticoagulation medications.

Diet to include a low-fat, high-fiber diet with consistent vitamin K intake (Box 26-2).

The effect of alcohol on warfarin can be unpredictable, increasing or decreasing the INR.

Patient should be aware that many nonprescription multivitamin supplements contain vitamin K. Have patient bring in all OTC preparations, herbs, and vitamins to check labels for hidden sources of vitamin K.

Vitamin C, vitamin E, selenium, and many herbal remedies can interact with warfarin. Patient should inform provider of all preparations taken.

Patient should not start new OTC medications or alternative therapies, such as acupuncture or massage without discussing or informing provider.

Address the following safety issues with the patient:

- Fall-proof home with nonslip rugs, nightlights, and handrails to decrease risk of falls with potential for serious injury and hemorrhage.
- Obtain medical alert identification (wear bracelet/necklace and carry identification in wallet/purse).

Instruct patient regarding the signs and symptoms of bleeding. Request that patient promptly report any unusual symptoms or unexplained bruising and bleeding.

Patient should document any missed warfarin doses and any variations in diet or alcohol consumption. These should be brought to office appointments and included in patient's record.

Provider should stress importance of regular laboratory monitoring of PT/INR to maintain therapeutic clotting levels and avoid complications of warfarin therapy.

BOX 26-2

VITAMIN K CONTENT OF COMMON FOODS (PER SERVING)

HIGH VITAMIN K CONTENT (>150 μg)
Broccoli, cucumber with peel, endive, kale, red lettuce, raw mint, raw parsley, spinach, Swiss chard, green tea, raw turnip, watercress, brussels sprouts

MODERATE VITAMIN K CONTENT (<150 μg)
Green beans, raw cabbage, canola oil, coleslaw, green lettuce, salad oil, mayonnaise

LOW VITAMIN K CONTENT (<30 μg)
Apple, artichoke, dried beans, butter, cauliflower, celery, coffee, cereal, dairy products, eggs, fish, flour, fruit, tomato juice, green pepper, meat, peanut butter, root vegetables, onion, tomato

Antiplatelet Agents

- Caution patients that they may bleed longer than usual if they sustain minor cuts.
- Caution about easy bruisability.
- Report bleeding, bruises, and injuries to provider.
- Inform dentist and surgeons of drug use before invasive procedures.

Peripheral Vascular Dilators

- Take this drug with meals to minimize possible GI discomfort.
- Regular leg exercise is important. Daily walking is usually recommended. Patients are to walk until claudication begins, immediately stop and rest for 3 min, then resume walking. This should be done at least eight times a day.
- Cessation of smoking is an extremely important component of treatment.

Specific Drugs

HEPARIN GROUP

(P) Prototype Drug

heparin sodium

Contraindications

- Hypersensitivity to heparin
- Thrombocytopenia or previous HIT

- Uncontrolled active bleeding
- Inability to complete coagulation tests

Warnings
Hemorrhage can occur at any site. Signs and symptoms will vary with the location and extent of bleeding. Adrenal, ovarian, and retroperitoneal hemorrhage has occurred.

Patients who have had large embolic strokes or uncontrolled hypertension should not receive anticoagulation for 5 to 14 days after the event because of predisposition for hemorrhagic transformation.

Thrombocytopenia has occurred in up to 30% of patients. There are two forms:

- Type I: Early, benign, reversible nonimmune thrombocytopenia
- Type II: A more serious IgG-mediated platelet aggregation form.

There is an increased incidence of thromboembolic events associated with HIT. Monitor daily platelet count and immediately refer patient to specialist if platelet count is declining from preheparin baseline.

Advanced age, high body mass index, low preoperative hemoglobin, obesity, and CHF contribute to failure rates for low dose heparin prophylaxis.

Do not give heparin intramuscularly; it can cause hematoma formation.

Heparin may increase serum triglyceride levels.

Administer heparin with caution if there is a previous history of allergy. If necessary to use heparin, a test dose may be given with epinephrine 1:1000 subcutaneous injection available, in conjunction with hematologic consultation.

Thrombi can form because of heparin-induced platelet aggregation, called "white clot syndrome." This can lead to skin necrosis, gangrene, MI, PE, stroke, and death.

Precautions
Use with caution in patients with liver disease, jaundice, malnutrition, subacute bacterial endocarditis, brain tumors, hypotension, and continuous tube drainage from stomach or small intestine.

Elevated liver function tests are sometimes seen.

Pharmacokinetics
See Table 26-3 for pharmacokinetics.

Adverse Effects
See Table 26-4 for important adverse reactions to heparin.

Drug Interactions
Platelet inhibitors, ASA, dextran, ibuprofen, indomethacin, or dipyridamole given with heparin can result in bleeding.

Streptokinase and warfarin can potentiate heparin activity; administer heparin cautiously in conjunction with these agents.

Digoxin, tetracycline, nicotine, and antihistamines inhibit the anticoagulation action of heparin. See Box 26-3 for a list of the most common drug interactions.

Dosage and Administration
See Table 26-5 for heparin dosing schedule, Table 26-6 for administration recommendations, and Table 26-7 for weight-based intravenous heparin dose nomogram.

Overdosage
Signs of overdosage include the following

- Minor bleeding: hematoma, ecchymosis, oozing from superficial skin breaks and catheter placement sites, hematuria, mucous membrane bleeding
- Major bleeding: intracranial hemorrhage, sudden unexplained drop in hematocrit, sudden hypotension

Protamine sulfate (1%) up to 50 mg is given by slow infusion over at least 10 minutes for reversal of heparinization. Dose of 1 mg protamine neutralizes 100 U heparin. Side effects of protamine include hypotension and anaphylactic reactions.

low molecular weight heparin and heparinoid

LMWH has at least equivalent antithrombotic effects to standard heparin in most circumstances. In DVT, it has become the preferred therapy. It has a longer half-life because of reduced binding to plasma proteins and endothelial cells. The reported incidence of minor bleeding is less, but no difference has been found in the incidence of major bleeding.

The heparinoid danaparoid (Orgaran), which is a mixture of heparin sulfate, dermatan, and chondroitin sulfate, is similar to standard heparin both pharmacologically and in clinical properties. It has much less cross-reactivity with standard heparin than LMWH and can be used to treat patients with HIT in whom continued anticoagulation is needed. Danaparoid, however, cannot be used interchangeably with standard heparin. Danaparoid is approved for postoperative use to prevent DVT.

ORAL ANTICOAGULANTS

(P) Prototype Drug

warfarin (Coumadin)

Contraindications
Active bleeding in GI, genitourinary, and respiratory tracts; known blood dyscrasias; hemorrhagic tendencies or hemophilia; polycythemia vera; purpura; leukemia; bleeding diathesis history; cerebral hemorrhage; peptic ulcer disease; ulcerative colitis; recent surgery or surgical wounds; pending brain, eye, spinal cord surgery, or prostatectomy; patients undergoing regional or lumbar block anesthesia; polyarthritis; diverticulitis; cerebral or dissecting aortic aneurysm; eclampsia, preeclampsia, therapeutic abortion, or threatened abortion; malignant hypertension; pericarditis; subacute bacterial endocarditis; known vitamin C or K deficiency; laboratory monitoring is unavailable; lack of patient cooperation, or if unsupervised senility, psychosis, or alcoholism is present.

TABLE 26-3 Pharmacokinetics of Heparin, Oral Anticoagulants, Thrombolytic Agents, and Antiplatelet Agents

Drug	Absorption	Drug Availability (After First Pass)	Onset of Action	Time to Peak Concentration	Half-Life	Duration of Action	Protein Bound	Metabolism	Excretion	Therapeutic Serum Level
heparin sodium	Not absorbed through GI mucosa	Reduced with SC route	Immediate, IV; 1-2 hr, SC	3 hr, SC	Dependent on dose; 1, 2.5, 5 hr	Effect gone within hours of discontinuation	Yes	Hepatic and partly renal	Primarily through the reticuloendothelial system; small amount in urine	Monitor aPTT, 1.5-2.5 × normal; narrow therapeutic index; check platelets daily with IV infusion
warfarin	Rapid from GI tract, within 1 hr		1 hr	2-8 hr	25-60 hr, mean 40 hr	2-5 days	99%	Liver and kidneys R-1A2 substrate R-3A4 substrate S-2C9 substrate	Urine and feces	Monitor PT/INR according to specific indications
aspirin (ASA)	80%-100%	50%-70% decreased by first-pass effect	5-30 min	0.25-2 hr	15-20 min	Depends on form given	Poorly bound	Liver	Urine	NA
dipyridamole (Persantine)	Incomplete absorption		24 min	75 min	10 hr	3 hr	Tightly bound	Liver	Feces and urine	NA
clopidogrel (Plavix)	Rapid		30 min	1 hr	8 hr	2 hr	98%	Liver	Urine, 50%; feces, 40%	NA
ticlopidine (Ticlid)	Rapid, 80%			2 hr	12.6 hr		98%	Liver	Urine and feces	NA
abciximab (ReoPro)			10 min	2 hr	30 min	6 hr	Bound to platelet receptor			Check PT, aPTT, platelets before administration and after infusion
alteplase	Not absorbed after oral administration	80% cleared in 10 min	Immediate	30-90 min	5 min	7 hr	Yes	Liver	Urine	NA
streptokinase	Not absorbed when given orally	Rapidly cleared	Immediate	Varies, 2-4 hr	Initial 18-23 min, then 83 min	12 hr	Yes	Liver	Urine	NA

aPTT, Activated partial thromboplastin time; *PT*, prothrombin time.

TABLE 26-4 Adverse Effects of Drugs Affecting Blood

Drug	Major Adverse Effects
heparin sodium	Bleeding: nosebleeds, hematuria, tarry stools, easy bruising and petechiae formation
	Hypersensitivity reactions may include urticaria, rhinitis, asthma, cyanosis, tachypnea, tachycardia, hypertension, fever, and chills
	There is an association between long-term heparin therapy and osteoporosis, occurring when the total heparin dose has exceeded 20,000 U/day for longer than 3 months
	Heparin can inhibit aldosterone synthesis, which is usually of no clinical importance
	Hyperkalemia and other metabolic derangements have been reported
warfarin (Coumadin)	Minor bleeding and hemorrhage is reported in 2%-20% of patients. GI hemorrhage is responsible for 25% of all deaths caused by oral anticoagulant toxicity
	Reported skin and joint manifestations include rash, gangrene, leg and foot pain, skin ulcers, and mylagias
Thrombolytic agents	
alteplase (tPA)	Allergic reactions, arrhythmias, nausea, vomiting, fever, hypotension, thrombocytopenia
streptokinase	Bleeding, strongly antigenic, allergic reactions, anaphylaxis, fever, hypotension, arrhythmias
urokinase	Bleeding, fever, mild allergic reactions, bleeding—20% of patients
pentoxifylline (Trental)	Nausea, vomiting, dyspepsia, belching, bloating, and flatulence (cause 5% of patients to discontinue therapy
	Dizziness, headache tremor, nervousness, or agitation
	Angina edema, hypotension, dyspnea, flushing, and palpitations
	Other adverse effects are cholecystitis, constipation, dry mouth, depression, seizures, epistaxis, laryngitis, nasal congestion, brittle fingernails, pruritus, rash urticaria, angioedema, blurred vision, conjunctivitis, earache, scotoma, bad taste, excessive salivation, leukopenia, and weight change

BOX 26-3

DRUG INTERACTIONS WITH ANTICOAGULANTS (BOTH HEPARIN AND WARFARIN)*

MEDICATIONS ASSOCIATED WITH AN INCREASE IN INR RESPONSE

acetaminophen
alcohol
allopurinol
aminosalicylic acid
amiodarone
Anabolic steroids
aspirin
Biaxin
Bromelains
chenodiol
chloral hydrate
chlorpropamide
cholestyramine
chymotrypsin
cimetidine
ciprofloxacin
clofibrate
cotrimoxazole
danazol
dextran
dextropropoxyphene
dextrothyroxin
diazoxide
diflunisal
disopyramide
disulfiram
fenoprofen
fluconazole
5-fluorouracil
fluoxetine
fluvoxamine
glucagon
halothane
heparin
ibuprofen
ifosfamide
indomethacin
influenza virus vaccine
isoniazid
itraconazole
keterdac
ketoprofen
levamisole
levothyroxin
liothyronine
lovastatin
mefenamic acid
methyldopa
methylphenidate
metolazone
metronidazole
miconazole
Monoamine oxidase inhibitors
moricizine
nalidixic acid
naproxen
Nonsteroidal antiinflammatory drugs
ofloxacin
omeprazole
pentoxifylline
phenylbutazone
phenytoin
piroxicam
propafenone
propranolol
Pyrazolones
quinidine
quinine
ranitidine
Salicylates
simvastatin
sulfinpyrazone
Sulfonamides
sulindac
tamoxifen
tetracycline
Thyroid drugs
tolbutamide
tolectin
trimethoprim/sulfamethoxazole

MEDICATIONS THAT DECREASE INR RESPONSE

Adrenocortical steroids
alcohol
aminoglutethimide
Antacids
Antihistamines
azathioprine
Barbiturates
carbamazepine
chloral hydrate
chlordiazepoxide
cholestyramine
Cyclosporins
dicloxacillin
Diuretics
ethchlorvynol
etrelinate
glutethimide
griseofulvin
haloperidol
meprobamate
moricizine hydrochloride
nafcillin
Oral contraceptives
paraldehyde
primidone
ranitidine
rifampin
sucralfate
trazodone
vitamin C

*No known effect: atenolol, bumetanide, diflunisal, and enoxacin.

TABLE 26-5 Heparin Dosing Schedule

Type of Heparin	Dosage Schedule Recommendation
Standard unfractionated heparin IV	5000 U bolus followed by 800-1000 U/hr infusion
Weight-based IV heparin	Initial dose: 80 U/kg bolus followed by 18 U/kg/hr infusion, then follow Table 26-5
Adjusted-dose IV heparin	Give only amount needed to raise aPTT 2-5 sec above the control level
Prophylactic SC heparin	
Unfractionated standard heparin	5000 U SC bid or tid
enoxaparin (LMWH)	30 mg SC bid
dalteparin (LMWH)	40-60 mg SC bid
danaparoid (heparinoid)	Therapeutic anticoagulation: 2500 U bolus, followed by 400 U/hr for 4 hr, then 300 U/hr for 4 hr, then 150-200 U/hr Prophylactic anticoagulation: 750 U q12hr for 7-10 days

aPTT, Activated partial thromboplastin time; *LMWH,* low molecular weight heparin.

TABLE 26-6 Dosage and Administration Recommendations

Medication	Dosage	Administration
heparin sodium	5000 U	SC
	Low-dose prophylaxis preoperative	5000 U SC, 2 hr before surgery
	For age >40 yr	5000 U SC, q12hr postoperatively for 7 days
enoxaparin (Lovenox)	30 mg bid	SC, postoperatively for 7-10 days in total hip replacement
dalteparin (Fragmin)	2500 U qd	SC, 1-2 hr after abdominal surgery for 5-10 days
danaparoid (Orgaran)	Postoperatively for prevention of DVT; useful in HIT	SC, IV
aspirin (ASA)	MI: 160 mg-325 mg	PO
	TIA and stroke: 650 mg qd or 325 mg qid	PO
dipyridamole (Persantine)	75-100 mg	PO qid
clopidogrel (Plavix)	75 mg	PO bid, take with or without food
ticlopidine (Ticlid)	250 mg	PO bid, take with food

DVT, deep vein thrombosis; *HIT,* heparin-induced thrombocytopenia; *PTCA,* percutaneous transluminal coronary angioplasty.

TABLE 26-7 Weight-Based IV Heparin Dose Nomogram

aPTT	Dosage
Initial dose	80 U/kg bolus, then 18 U/kg/hr
aPTT <35 sec	80 U/kg/bolus, then 4 U/kg/hr
aPTT 36-45 sec	40 U/kg/bolus, then 2 U/kg/hr
aPTT 46-70 sec	Therapeutic range, no change
aPTT 71-90 sec	Decrease rate by 2 U/kg/hr
aPTT >90 sec	Hold infusion 1 hr, then decrease rate by 3 U/kg/hr

aPTT, Activated partial thromboplastin time.
Modified from Hirsh J, Raschke R, et al: Heparin: mechanism of action, pharmacokinetics, dosing, considerations, monitoring, efficacy, and safety, *Chest* 108 (Suppl 4):258S, 1995.

Warnings/Precautions

- Look for unsuspected source of bleeding; peptic ulcer disease, or neoplasm when bleeding occurs with therapeutic PT/INR.
- Risk of complications increases in patients with protein C deficiency. Suspect if there is family history of recurrent thromboembolic disorders.
- Abrupt cessation of therapy is not recommended; taper dose over 3 to 4 weeks to prevent rebound hypercoagulable state.
- Use with caution in severe-to-moderate hypertension, severe renal disease, and hepatic dysfunction.
- Administer cautiously to patients with indwelling catheters.
- Trauma or surgery may cause internal bleeding when patient is anticoagulated.
- Necrosis and/or gangrene of skin related to local thrombosis usually occurs within days of start of therapy. Concurrent use of heparin may minimize tissue necrosis.
- Warfarin may enhance release of atheromatous plaque emboli and systemic cholesterol microembolization. "Purple-toe" syndrome develops between 3 and 10 weeks of initiation of warfarin.

Adverse Effects

The risk of hemorrhage in warfarin therapy is related to the intensity and duration of treatment (see Table 26-4).

Acetaminophen is an unrecognized source of overanticoagulation in warfarin therapy. Daily use of 4 regular-strength acetaminophen tablets, or 28 tablets per week, greatly increases the risk of a prolonged INR of greater than 6.0.

Many patients anecdotally report a sensation of feeling cold that is subjectively attributed to "thin blood." No controlled studies have evaluated this common complaint.

Drug Interactions
Warfarin reacts with many other drugs. Some of these drug interactions are unpredictable, increasing or decreasing warfarin responsiveness in different patients (Box 26-3).

Overdosage
Excessive overanticoagulation with or without bleeding can be reversed in many instances by discontinuing the drug on a temporary basis. If minor bleeding progresses to major bleeding, parenteral vitamin K may be needed. See Table 26-8 for management of prolonged INR. Vitamin K should not be given indiscriminately because its use reduces future response to warfarin. In emergency situations of hemorrhage, 200 to 500 ml fresh frozen plasma or whole blood can restore clotting factors to normal.

Signs and symptoms of over anticoagulation include the following:

- Minor bleeding (drop in hemoglobin of 3%): ecchymoses and easy bruisability, excessive bleeding from superficial cuts, (e.g., shaving), bleeding from oral mucous membranes, nosebleeds, heavy menstrual bleeding, vaginal bleeding, hematuria, hematemesis, joint swelling, and pain
- Major bleeding (drop in hemoglobin >5%): headache, blurred vision, dysarthria, stroke symptoms, weakness, extreme fatigue, and melena

Dosage and Administration
Daily maintenance dose of warfarin is between 2 and 12 mg. The dose is titrated to achieve the INR goal for the specific anticoagulation indication (see Table 26-8).

Other Drugs in Class

Other drugs in this class are similar to the prototype except as follows.

anisindione (Miradon)

Anisindione (Miradon) is a synthetic coagulant indanedione derivative. Its pharmacokinetic properties are similar to those of warfarin. It is reserved for use in cases of warfarin allergy or sensitivity. Managing anisindione and achieving stable, therapeutic PT/INR values is more difficult than with warfarin. It can itself cause a severe hypersensitivity reaction and should be monitored carefully. Do not use in acute stroke patients. See Box 26-3 for drug interaction information.

ANTIPLATELET AGENTS

aspirin (ASA)

The optimal dose of ASA needed for prevention of stroke remains controversial. Presently a wide dosing range is used from 325 to 1300 mg/day.

Routine monitoring of coagulation parameters is not necessary.

Assess sodium content of ASA preparation in patients with heart failure or edema.

Individuals with delayed gastric emptying may retain enteric-coated aspirin products. Use with caution in patients with increased risk of bleeding from trauma or surgery.

Use with caution in patients with hepatic impairment.

clopidogrel (Plavix)

Contraindications

- Hypersensitivity
- Active pathologic bleeding

Warnings

- Thrombotic thrombocytopenia purpura has been reported rarely and requires prompt treatment.
- Hepatic function impairment: use with caution

Precautions

- Bleeding risk: use with caution in patients who may be at risk of increased bleeding. Discontinue clopidogrel 5 days before surgery.
- GI bleeding: use with caution in patients with conditions at risk for bleed as in ulcers.

Adverse Effects. See Table 26-4.

Drug Interactions

- Clopidogrel inhibits CYP 450 2C9.
- Coadministration with nonsteroidal antiinflammatory drugs is associated with increased GI bleed.
- Safety of coadministration with warfarin has not been established.

Dosage and Administration. No dose adjustments are needed in elderly patients or those with renal disease.

TABLE 26-8 Management of Prolonged INR from Warfarin

INR Value	Signs and Symptoms of Bleeding	Treatment
4.0-6.0	None	Omit dose for 3 days. Resume at lower dosage or determine transient source of elevation.
6-10	None	Give 0.5-1.0 mg vitamin K; if INR not <6.0 in 24 hr, may repeat dose. Determine source of elevation. Resume usual dosage or lower by 10%.
10-20	None	Give 3 mg vitamin K; repeat INR q6-12hr. Repeat vitamin K if necessary
>20	Serious bleeding	Give 10 mg vitamin K; monitor INR q6hr, may repeat vitamin K q12hr. supplement with fresh frozen plasma or whole blood.
	Life-threatening hemorrhage	Give 10 mg vitamin K, fresh frozen plasma or whole blood to restore clotting factors.

Overdosage. Reported intentional overdose (1050 mg) of clopidogrel did not result in adverse events or sequelae.

ticlopidine (Ticlid)

Ticlopidine can cause life-threatening hematologic adverse reactions including neutropenia/agranulocytosis and thrombotic thrombocytopenia purpura.

PERIPHERAL VASCULAR DILATORS

pentoxifylline (Trental)

Contraindications

- Recent cerebral, retinal hemorrhage and sensitivity to pentoxifylline or methylxanthines, such as caffeine, theophylline, and theobromine
- The drug is not to be used in patients with severe hepatic disease because it is metabolized by the liver

Warnings/Precautions. Caution should be exhibited when prescribing pentoxifylline in patients who have increased risk for hemorrhage, such as recent surgery, peptic ulceration, and current warfarin use. These patients need to be monitored closely for bleeding with frequent checks of prothrombin times and hematocrit/hemoglobin.

Renal function impairment may necessitate lower dosage.

Patients with chronic occlusive arterial disease of the limbs often have other manifestations of arteriosclerotic disease such as angina, hypotension, and arrhythmia. Monitor the patient for other signs and symptoms of arteriosclerotic disease.

Adverse Effects. See Table 26-4.

Drug Interactions. Concomitant use with theophylline may lead to increased theophylline levels and theophylline toxicity.

Concomitant use with warfarin may cause bleeding and prolonged PT. Frequently monitor PT in patients taking warfarin.

Dosage and Administration. Usual dose is 400 mg three times daily with meals. If patient develops adverse digestive or central nervous system side effects, the dose can be lowered to 400 mg twice daily. An extended-release product is also now available.

RESOURCES FOR PATIENTS AND PROVIDERS

Internet

American Heart Association. Available at www.amhrt.org
Dupont-Merck. Available at www.dupontmerck.com
Medical Consult. Available at www.mediconsult.com
Pharmacology Information Database. Available at www.pharminfo.com
Risk Management Foundation, Harvard Medical Institutions. Available at www.rmf.harvard.edu/default.asp?v=flash

Educational Materials

Dupont Pharma CoumaCare Program
Call (800) 4Pharma for outpatient management and educational materials on Coumadin, including audiocassettes, videos, and brochures for patients.

BIBLIOGRAPHY

Aschenbrenner D, Cleveland L, Venable S: *Drug therapy in nursing*, Philadelphia, 2002, Lippincott, Williams & Wilkins.
Ansell J, Oertel L, Wittowsky A: *Managing oral anticoagulation therapy: clinical and operational guidelines*, Frederick, MD, 1997, Aspen Publishers.
Cushinotto N: Clinical considerations of heparization, *J Am Acad Nurse Pract* 9:6, 1997.
Goldstein L, et al: Primary prevention of stroke: a statement for healthcare professionals from the Stroke Council of the American Heart Association, *Circulation*, 103:1, 2001.
Self T: Warfarin interactions: update on the most common and clinically significant, *Consultant*, March 2002
Sixth ACCP Consensus Conference on Antithrombotic Therapy, *Chest* 119(1 suppl):1S-370S, 2001.
The National Institute of Neurological Disorders and Stroke (NINDS) rt-PA Stroke Study Group: Tissue plasminogen activator for acute stroke, *N Engl J Med* 333:24, 1995.

UNIT 7

Gastrointestinal Agents

Unit 7 discusses drugs that are used to treat a wide variety of gastrointestinal (GI) conditions. Some GI drugs are grouped by mechanism of action and others by condition treated. Unfortunately categorization of GI drugs inevitably produces a large miscellaneous section. We have attempted to cover the drugs and the conditions commonly seen in primary care.

- **Chapter 27** discusses antacids and the management of gastroesophageal reflux disease (GERD).
- **Chapter 28** discusses medications that decrease acidity, including H_2 antagonists and proton pump inhibitors used to treat peptic ulcer disease (PUD).
- **Chapter 29** focuses on the use of laxatives to treat constipation.
- **Chapter 30** discusses antidiarrheals and their use to manage diarrhea.
- **Chapter 31** discusses antiemetics to manage nausea and vomiting.
- **Chapter 32** deals with other GI medications. It discusses medications used to treat irritable bowel syndrome. Other drugs discussed are gallstone solubilizers, GI stimulants/prokinetic agents, prostaglandins, ulcerative colitis medication, and locally acting agents.

CHAPTER 27

Antacids

Drug Names

Class	Subclass	Generic Name	Trade Name
Calcium salts		(P) calcium carbonate	Tums, Rolaids
Sodium bicarbonate			Alka-Seltzer
Aluminum salts		aluminum hydroxide aluminum carbonate	Amphojel Basaljel
Magnesium salts		magnesium hydroxide	Milk of Magnesia
Combination products		aluminum hydroxide and magnesium hydroxide; alginic acid, magnesium trisilicate, calcium stearate	Maalox, Mylanta, Gelusil Gaviscon

(P), Prototype drug.

General Uses

Indications

- Hyperacidity: heartburn, GI reflux, and acid indigestion
- Hyperacidity associated with peptic ulcer, gastric hyperacidity, and sour stomach
- Aluminum carbonate: hyperphosphatemia; low-phosphate diet to prevent formation of phosphate urinary stones
- Magnesium oxide: magnesium deficiencies; magnesium depletion from malnutrition, restricted diet, alcoholism, or magnesium-depleting drugs

Unlabeled Uses

- Gastroesophageal reflux disease (GERD)
- Antacids with aluminum and magnesium or aluminum hydroxide: prevent stress ulcer bleeding; duodenal ulcer, may be gastric ulcer
- Calcium carbonate: prevent and manage osteoporosis

• • •

These medications are used commonly for gastroenterologic diseases such as reflux esophagitis and peptic ulcers. The most common antacids prescribed have at least one of the following elements as their main ingredient: calcium carbonate, aluminum salts, or magnesium. The ingredient alginate may provide barrier protection.

The prototype antacid will be considered to be calcium carbonate because of its widespread popularity. However, combination antacids—in particular, combinations of aluminum hydroxide and magnesium hydroxide—are probably the most commonly used antacids. Antacids vary in sodium content, in magnesium content (a problem in kidney failure), and in the tendency to cause diarrhea or constipation.

DISEASE PROCESS

Anatomy and Physiology

Saliva is basic, causing the contents of the esophagus to be neutral to basic. Esophageal peristalsis and salivary bicarbonate serve to protect the esophageal mucosa. The stomach contents are highly acidic, which helps digest food.

Pathophysiology

When food moves from the stomach back into the esophagus, highly acid material moves into a basic area. The acid causes ulceration of the mucosal lining.

Many factors may lead to GERD. A very important factor that contributes to GERD is an incompetent lower esophageal sphincter (LES). Reflux occurs during spontaneous relaxation of the LES. A decrease in the LES pressure allows acidic gastric contents to enter the lower portion of the esophagus. This happens at rest but increases with stress such as abdominal straining, lifting, or bending. The highly acidic gastric contents are damaging to the esophageal mucosa.

Delayed gastric emptying may be caused by gastroparesis or partial gastric outlet obstruction. This can increase GERD because the food stays in the stomach longer. During sleep, peristalsis is decreased, causing an increase in symptoms. Saliva is basic and helps neutralize the stomach contents. Anything that decreases salivation such as anticholinergic medications can exacerbate GERD. Hiatal hernias are common and are not a cause of GERD. If the patient with a hiatal hernia has GERD, more reflux will occur.

The Disease

GERD is a very common condition, consisting of stomach contents moving back into the esophagus. Most patients have a very mild disease, although it is possible for the patient to develop complications such as active erosive esophagitis, esophageal adenocarcinoma, and esophageal stricture.

The main symptom of GERD is heartburn occurring 30 to 60 minutes after meals and when the patient bends over or lies down. Relief is usually reported after taking antacids. Other symptoms may include nonspecific GI symptoms such as regurgitation of sour or bitter gastric contents, belching, and fullness of the stomach. Atypical symptoms include chronic cough, chronic laryngitis, asthma, sore throat, and noncardiac chest pain. Erosive esophagitis may have more severe symptoms such as pain and dysphagia but also may be relatively asymptomatic. Esophagitis is divided into four grades, which are determined endoscopically. Grade 1 is defined by erythema of the distal esophagus. Grade 2 consists of scattered erosions. Grade 3 is confluence of erosions involving less than 50% of the diameter of the esophagus, whereas grade 4 involves greater than 50% of the diameter.

Providers must ask specifically about antacids and other OTC remedies when taking a medication history. Many patients will have tried OTC remedies before going to their primary care provider. Most will have tried antacids and OTC histamine blockers (see Chapter 28). Many patients do not consider antacids to be a medication and will not mention taking them when asked about medication use.

An upper endoscopy with biopsy is the standard diagnostic procedure. It confirms the diagnosis and documents the type and extent of tissue damage. Uncomplicated GERD responsive to first-line therapy does not require an endoscopy. For most patients, empiric treatment is initiated based on history and physical examination. Patients who do not respond or those with suspected complications should have an endoscopic examination.

The differential diagnosis includes peptic ulcer, cholelithiasis, nonulcer dyspepsia, and angina pectoris.

DRUG ACTION AND EFFECTS

Antacids are weak bases that neutralize gastric hydrochloric acid by combining with it to form salt and water. This decreases the amount of gastric acid in the stomach, raising the pH. Antacids decrease pepsin activity because pepsin is rendered inactive in alkaline conditions. Antacids also increase LES tone, reducing reflux. Aluminum ions inhibit smooth muscle contraction, inhibiting gastric emptying. This is counterproductive, because in GERD, prompt gastric emptying is beneficial.

Antacids do not protect the stomach by coating the mucosal lining. Alginic acid is not an antacid. In the presence of saliva, it reacts with sodium bicarbonate to form sodium alginate and protect the mucosa with its foaming, viscous, and floating properties.

The ability of antacids to neutralize gastric acid has been labeled the *acid-neutralizing capacity* (ANC). This ANC is the quantity of 1 M HCl (expressed in milliequivalents) that can be brought to pH 3.5 in 15 minutes (expressed as mEq/ml). Antacids with high ANC are usually more effective.

DRUG TREATMENT PRINCIPLES

The goal of treatment is symptomatic relief and prevention of complications. GERD is a lifelong disease that requires lifestyle modifications and medications as indicated.

Nonpharmacologic Treatment

Lifestyle modifications are the foundation of treatment. Many patients can resolve their symptoms by lifestyle changes without taking medications. Lifestyle modifications include diet, weight loss if overweight, activity, cessation of smoking and alcohol use, and avoidance of drugs that decrease LES pressure (Table 27-1).

Pharmacologic Treatment

Medical treatment depends on the symptoms.

Mild, Intermittent Symptoms. Antacids are used for immediate relief of intermittent heartburn. Because their duration of action is only 2 hours, H_2-blockers can be used if the symptoms last longer than 2 hours or occur at night. OTC doses are usually sufficient. These drugs take at least 30 minutes to take effect; they can also be taken before a meal expected to cause heartburn.

Moderate Symptoms. Patients who experience symptoms several times a week or daily should be treated with a prescription strength H_2-blocker. Twice-a-day dosing will provide 24-hour reduction in acidity. Proton pump inhibitors are seen being used for moderate symptoms. Their advantage is once-a-day dosing, but they are much more expensive and do not come in an OTC form. Treatment should continue for 8 to 12 weeks. Intermittent treatment (treatment when symptoms recur) is the usual plan of treatment for mild to moderate disease.

Severe Symptoms and Erosive Disease. If the patient has severe symptoms, has failed the treatment for milder symp-

TABLE 27-1 Lifestyle Modification Treatment for GERD

Lifestyle Area	Modification
Activity	Sit up for at least 1 hr after eating Elevate head of bed 6-8 in, using blocks Pillows are less effective and can be countereffective if they caused bending at the waist Avoid straining, lifting, and bending over, specially on a full stomach
Avoidance of causative drugs	Avoid drugs that decrease lower esophageal sphincter pressure, such as theophylline, nitrates, calcium channel blockers, and benzodiazepines Avoid anticholinergics and other drugs that decrease salivation; avoid drugs that decrease peristalsis
Diet	Avoid foods that decrease lower esophageal sphincter pressure Avoid foods that are irritants, such as citrus and coffee
Smoking and alcohol intake	Cease smoking and alcohol to decrease GI irritation
Weight loss	Strive for a gradual, sustained loss of 2 lb per month

toms, or has erosion documented by endoscopy, he or she should be started on proton pump inhibitor. Initial dosing is the usual starting dose once a day. If this is not effective, increase the dose to twice a day. The usual course of therapy is 8 to 12 weeks, to allow for healing of the erosions. Repeat endoscopy is not required if the patient responds to treatment. Most patients should be allowed a trial off medication, although relapse is frequent, with a rate of about 80%. If relapse occurs (usually within the first 3 months), the patient will require maintenance therapy. The dose for maintenance therapy may not need to be a high as it was for initial treatment. If patients do not respond to therapy, refer for consideration of surgery.

Promotility drugs such as metoclopramide or bethanechol reduce reflux by increasing LES tone and increasing peristalsis and gastric emptying. Because of their potential for serious adverse effects, they are not recommended for GERD unless nonresponsive to other therapy.

Additional Considerations. Antacids with the highest ANC are sodium bicarbonate and calcium carbonate. Sodium bicarbonate is not suitable for long-term use because of side effects. Calcium carbonate requires monitoring for long-term effects.

One critical decision for the clinician to consider is drug formulation, which affects efficacy. Suspension and gel formulations have higher ANC than powders or tablets. Tablets must be chewed thoroughly to be effective and work best if taken with a full glass of water. Tablets may be more convenient for occasional indigestion.

Timing of antacids is important; for the greatest effectiveness, take 1 hour after meals. This increases the amount of time the antacid is in the stomach and functioning as an antacid. Taking antacids on an empty stomach is not as effective because of the short transit time through the stomach. Taken properly, their duration of action is 2 hours. To avoid drug interactions, it is important to take antacids either 1 hour before or 2 hours after taking other medications.

Antacids with calcium may cause constipation. Aluminum may cause constipation; magnesium may cause diarrhea. These second two ingredients are usually given together to balance the effect on the bowels. Antacids with sodium bicarbonate have sufficient sodium to cause problems in patients with hypertension CHF. Other antacids vary by brand name in their sodium content. If the patient is on a low-salt diet, the sodium content of the antacid should be checked before prescribing. If the patient has any renal insufficiency, magnesium intake should be limited, and, if given, magnesium levels should be checked periodically. Antacids with calcium may precipitate kidney stones in the predisposed patient.

HOW TO MONITOR

- Monitor electrolytes (magnesium, sodium, or calcium levels as indicated) with long-term use of antacids.
- Evaluate therapeutic effect by following symptom resolution.
- Assess GI and renal status.
- Monitor for adverse effects.

PATIENT VARIABLES

Geriatrics

- Avoid using antacids containing magnesium in elderly patients with renal failure because they may develop hypermagnesemia.
- Avoid sodium-containing antacids because of fluid retention.

Pediatrics

- Safety is not established in children.

Pregnancy

- No Food and Drug Administration (FDA) category has been established, although antacids are generally considered safe for use in pregnancy.

PATIENT EDUCATION

- The patient should notify the health care provider if taking any other medications. Antacids may interact so they should be taken either 2 hours before or after taking other medications.
- If a chewable antacid is prescribed, chew tablet completely and follow this with at least an 8-oz glass of water.
- Shake liquid preparations thoroughly before taking to ensure accurate dosage.
- Store liquid formulations in a cool place but do not freeze. Refrigeration may make them taste better.
- Antacids may cause constipation or diarrhea. Either should be reported to the health care provider.
- Notify provider if you see symptoms of bleeding, such as black tarry stools or "coffee ground" vomitus.
- The effectiveness of antacids decreases with the age of the medication. Be sure to discard out-of-date antacids.

Specific Drugs

CALCIUM SALTS

Ⓟ **Prototype Drug**

calcium carbonate (Tums, Rolaids)

- Tums produce a rapid, prolonged, and powerful neutralizing effect.

Warnings

- Sodium content of antacids can be important in patients with hypertension, CHF, or renal failure or on a low-salt diet.

Acid Rebound

Antacids may cause dose related rebound hyperacidity. The stomach responds to the higher pH by producing more gastric acid. This is compensated for by the antacids.

It is not clear whether acid rebound is clinically important, except when antacids are discontinued. Monitor for increased symptoms when routinely administered antacids are discontinued.

TABLE 27-2 Common and Serious Adverse Effects of Antacids

Drug	Common Minor Effects	Serious Adverse Effects
All antacids		Acid rebound Milk alkali syndrome (dose dependent)
calcium	Constipation	Milk alkali syndrome
sodium		Sodium retention Milk alkali syndrome
aluminum	Constipation	Hypophosphatemia; aluminum intoxication; accumulation in serum, bone, CNS, encephalopathy Osteomalacia in patients who have renal failure
magnesium	Diarrhea	Hypermagnesemia in patients who have renal failure

- Milk-alkali syndrome: this is an acute illness with the symptoms of headache, nausea, irritability, and weakness) or a chronic illness with alkalosis, hypercalcemia, and possibly renal impairment. This can occur with high doses of calcium carbonate or sodium bicarbonate.
- Hypophosphatemia: prolonged use of aluminum-containing antacids may result in hypophosphatemia if phosphate intake is not adequate. Hypophosphatemia can cause anorexia, malaise, muscle weakness, and osteomalacia.
- Use with caution in patient with renal function impairment. Hypermagnesemia and toxicity may occur in patient with impaired renal function because of decreased clearance of the magnesium ion. Osteomalacia: prolonged use of aluminum containing antacids in patient with renal failure my cause or worsen osteomalacia. Aluminum is deposited in bone. Calcium is relatively safe.

Precautions

- GI hemorrhage: use aluminum hydroxide with care in patients with recent massive upper GI hemorrhage.
- Lipid effects: antacids may have an effect on lipid levels but this effect is not well studied.
- Aspirin: do not use in combination in chronic pain syndromes. Alkalinization of the urine accelerates aspirin excretion and systemic alkalosis of increased sodium load may occur.

Adverse Effects

- Adverse effects depend on the major ingredient(s). Most adverse effects are self-limiting and mild, especially for short-term use (Table 27-2). In long-term use, significant adverse effects can occur.

Pharmacokinetics

- Antacids vary in the amount they are absorbed. Sodium bicarbonate is most extensively absorbed. About 15% of the calcium is absorbed. Small amounts of aluminum are absorbed systemically.

Approximately 5% to 20% of the magnesium can be systemically absorbed. It is the systemic absorption that is responsible for many of the adverse reactions.

- The antacids that are not absorbed pass through the intestines and are eliminated in the feces. Aluminum-containing antacids bind with phosphate ions in the intestine to form insoluble aluminum phosphate that is excreted in the feces.
- If ingested 1 hour after meals, antacids reduce gastric acidity for about 2 to 3 hours. However, when ingested when fasting, antacids reduce acidity for only 20 to 40 minutes because of rapid gastric emptying.

Drug Interactions

- Antacids inhibit the absorption of many drugs. Take drugs 2 hours before or after an antacid to avoid drug interactions.
- Drug interactions are an important consideration (Table 27-3). There are three different mechanisms for drug interactions. The first is by increasing the gastric pH alters the disintegration, dissolution, solubility, ionization, and gastric emptying time. This decreases the absorption of weakly acidic drugs (digoxin, phenytoin, chlorpromazine, isoniazid). Weakly basic drugs absorption is increased possibly resulting in toxicity or adverse reactions (pseudoephedrine, levodopa).
- The second mechanism of drug interaction is by adsorbing or binding drugs to the antacid surface, resulting in decreased bioavailability (tetracycline). Magnesium antacids have the greatest adsorption; calcium and aluminum have an intermediate ability to adsorb medications.
- The third mechanism of drug interaction is by increasing urinary pH. This affects the rate of drug elimination. This inhibits the excretion of basic drugs (quinidine, amphetamines) and enhances excretion of acidic drugs (salicylates). The sodium antacids have the greatest effect on urinary pH. Have the patient take the antacid 2 hours before or after taking other medications to reduce the likelihood of adverse actions.

Dosage and Administration

- See Table 27-4.

TABLE 27-3 Drug Interactions with Antacids

Antacid	Effect
Calcium	Decreased action of fluoroquinolones, hydantoins, iron salts
Sodium	Increased action of amphetamines, flecainide
	Decreased action of benzodiazepines, iron salts, ketoconazole, lithium, methotrexate
Aluminum	Increased action of benzodiazepines
	Decreased action of allopurinol, chloroquine, corticosteroids, diflunisal, digoxin, ethambutol, histamine H_2 antagonists, iron salts, isoniazid
Magnesium	Increased action of dicumarol
	Decreased action of benzodiazepines, chloroquine, corticosteroids, digoxin, histamine H_2 antagonists, hydantoins, iron salts, nitrofurantoin

TABLE 27-4 Dosage and Administration Recommendations for Antacids

Drug	Dosage	Administration
calcium salts		
Tums	0.5-1.5 g	As needed
Rolaids chewable	0.5-1.5 g	As needed
sodium bicarbonate	Two tablets dissolved in 6 oz of water	q4hr; maximum eight tablets per day
aluminum hydroxide (Amphojel)	500-1800 mg	Three to six times daily, between meals and qHS
aluminum carbonate (Basaljel)	One or two capsules or tablets or 10 ml of suspension in water or fruit juice	q2hr; may use up to 12 times per day
magnesium salts		
magnesium hydroxide (Milk of Magnesia)	>12 yr: 5-15 ml liquid or 650 mg-1.3 g tablets	qid
magnesium oxide	140-400 mg tablet	tid-qid
combination products		
alginic acid, sodium bicarbonate, magnesium trisilicate, calcium stearate (Gaviscon)	Two to four tablets or 15-30 ml	qid (after meals and at bedtime)
aluminum hydroxide and magnesium hydroxide (Maalox)	Two to four tablets; suspension 10-20 ml	qid (after meals and at bedtime)
aluminum hydroxide and magnesium hydroxide (Mylanta, Mylanta double strength)	10-12 ml	Between meals and at bedtime, as needed

Other Drugs

Other antacids are similar to the prototype except as follows.

SODIUM SALTS

sodium bicarbonate (Alka-Seltzer)

- Sodium bicarbonate is a well-known antacid often used OTC by patients that has more adverse effects than other antacids and is not recommended for use. It is usually found in combination with other medications such as aspirin.

ALUMINUM SALTS

aluminum hydroxide (Amphojel)

- These drugs have relatively high risk of significant adverse reactions when used on a long-term basis.

MAGNESIUM SALTS

magnesium hydroxide (Milk of Magnesia)

- Adverse reactions occur primarily in patients with renal failure.
- Avoid in geriatric patients.
- Do not use in children younger than 12 years.

RESOURCES FOR PATIENTS AND PROVIDERS

Educational Materials

CD-ROMs available from CMEA, Inc at (800) 227-CMEA: *Gastroenterology: Electronic Reference and Review.*

BIBLIOGRAPHY

Bytzer P: Goals of therapy and guidelines for treatment success in symptomatic gastroesophageal reflux disease patients, *Am J Gastroenterol* 98(suppl): S31-S39, 2003.

Erstad BL: Dyspepsia: initial evaluation and treatment, *J Am Pharm Assoc* 42:460-468, 2002.

Gremse DA: Gastroesophageal reflux disease in children: an overview of pathophysiology, diagnosis, and treatment, *Am J Gastroenterol* 98(3 suppl):S24-S30, 2003.

Quigley EM: Factors that influence therapeutic outcomes in symptomatic gastroesophageal reflux disease, *J Pediatr Gastroenterol Nutr* 35(suppl 4):S297-S299, 2002.

Ramakrishnan A, Katz PO: Pharmacologic management of gastroesophageal reflux disease, *Curr Gastroenterol Rep* 4:218-224, 2002.

Richter JE: Gastroesophageal reflux disease during pregnancy, *Gastroenterol Clin North Am* 32:235-261, 2003.

CHAPTER 28

Histamine-2 Blockers and Proton Pump Inhibitors

Drug Names

Class	Subclass	Generic Name	Trade Name
H_2-Receptor antagonists		(P)(200) ranitidine	Zantac
		(200) cimetidine	Tagamet
		famotidine	Pepcid
		nizatidine	Axid
Proton pump inhibitors		(P)(200) omeprazole	Prilosec
		(200) lansoprazole	Prevacid
		(200) rabeprazole	Aciphex
		(200) esomeprazole	Nexium
		(200) pantoprazole	Protonix

(200), Top 200 drug; (P), prototype drug.

General Uses

Indications

- H_2-blockers
  - Duodenal ulcer treatment and maintenance
  - Gastric ulcer treatment
  - Gastroesophageal reflux disease (GERD)
  - Pathologic hypersecretory conditions
- Proton pump inhibitors (PPIs)
  - Gastric and duodenal ulcers
  - GERD
  - Pathologic hypersecretory conditions
  - *Helicobacter pylori*

Both histamine H_2-blockers (antagonists) and PPIs are acid antisecretory agents. They decrease the amount of acid the stomach produces. The two categories do this via different mechanisms of action. The indications and unlabeled uses for the different H_2-blockers are inconsistent and confusing (see Table 28-1 for a list). They are based on what indication the drug company applied for rather than any difference between the drugs. These distinctions are not always observed in practice. All H_2-blocker drugs, except for cimetidine, have the same mechanism of action and have similar effectiveness and side effect profiles.

PPIs are generally considered to be more powerful in action than the histamine H_2-blockers as they decrease stomach acidity to a greater extent. There are five PPIs, with little difference between them except for duration of action.

DISEASE PROCESS

Anatomy and Physiology

Several protective factors work together to protect the stomach mucosa from injury. The gastric mucosal barrier resists backward diffusion of hydrogen and thus has the ability to contain a high concentration of hydrochloric acid (HCl) within the gastric lumen unless an injurious agent breaks the barrier.

Endogenous prostaglandins are thought to provide cytoprotection against injurious agents and are synthesized abundantly in the mucosa of the stomach and duodenum. They are known to stimulate secretion of both mucus and bicarbonate and to maintain mucosal blood flow.

Mucus also mediates mucosal protection. It is secreted by surface epithelial cells and forms a gel that covers the mucosal surface and physically protects the mucosa from abrasion. It also resists the passage of large molecules such as pepsin. Bicarbonate is produced in small amounts by surface epithelial cells and diffuses up from the mucosa to create a thin layer of alkalinity between the mucus and the epithelial surface. Other protective factors include mucosal blood flow, epithelial renewal, and epidermal growth factor that is secreted in saliva and by the duodenal mucosa.

The mucosal surface of the stomach is divided according to the type of glands, namely, the oxyntic (parietal) gland area, which secretes acid, and the pyloric gland area, which does not. The most important cell types in these glandular areas are mucous and peptic cells, which are found in both glandular areas; oxyntic cells, which occur only in the oxyntic gland area;

TABLE 28-1 Indications and Unlabeled Uses for Histamine H_2 Blockers

	cimetidine	famotidine	nizatidine	ranitidine
Duodenal ulcer treatment and maintenance	•	•	•	•
GERD	•	•	•	•
Gastric ulcer treatment maintenance	•	•	•	•
Peptic ulcer	X	X	X	X
Prophylaxis of stress ulcers	X	X		X
Pathologic hypersecretory conditions	•	•		•
Heartburn/indigestion, sour stomach	•	•		•
Erosive esophagitis, maintenance				•
Prevent upper GI bleeding	•	X		X
Prevention of gastric NSAID damage				X

•, Indication; X, unlabeled use.

and endocrine cells, which are scattered throughout both glandular areas. The oxyntic gland area occupies most of the mucosal surface of the stomach. The oxyntic cells secrete hydrochloric acid (HCl) using an energy-dependent active transport mechanism and intrinsic factor (IF), a protein required for the absorption of vitamin B_{12}.

The stomach has three naturally occurring secretagogues, which are stimulants to secretion. The three major secretagogues are acetylcholine (a neurotransmitter), gastrin (a hormone), and histamine (a paracrine substance). Receptor activation by these secretagogues initiates biochemical steps leading to active transport of hydrogen by the oxyntic cell. Histamine, released by mast cells, binds to the histamine H_2-receptor that activates intracellular stimulatory protein G and eventually activates the membrane-bound ATPase. This proton pump provides the energy to extrude hydrogen from the oxyntic cell in exchange for potassium. In this manner histamine initiates a train of intracellular events that stimulates the continuous secretion of acid.

The rate of secretion varies greatly, depending on the time of day or night and the proximity to eating a meal. When the stomach is at rest, the rate of secretion is quite low. This basal rate is in great contrast to the high rate of secretion found at mealtime. Basal secretion in the human stomach exhibits a circadian rhythm, characterized by a maximal rate in the evening and a minimal rate in the morning.

The high rates of acid secretion surrounding mealtimes are reduced to the basal rate of secretion through inhibitory processes that begin to occur during a meal. Abatement of hunger suppresses the cephalic phase of gastric secretion. Secretion of HCl by oxyntic cells causes antral mucosal surface pH to fall below 3.0, prompting the release of the paracrine substance, somatostatin. Somatostatin decreases gastrin release from the G cells and directly inhibits oxyntic cell secretion of acid.

Pathophysiology

Drugs that decrease acid production, or antisecretory agents, are used to prevent the autodigestion of the upper gastrointestinal (GI) tract by the acid–pepsin complex. Drugs or foods that increase acid production may provoke autodigestion. This is often the pathogenesis of peptic ulcer disease. These agents not only cause injury themselves but also augment the injury initiated by other agents.

The mucosa of the upper GI tract is susceptible to injury from a variety of conditions and agents. Endogenous agents include acid, pepsin, bile acids, and other small intestine contents. Exogenous agents include ethanol, aspirin, and NSAIDs.

Acid is essential for the occurrence of peptic injury. A pH of 1 to 2 maximizes the activity of pepsin. In addition, mucosal injury from aspirin, other NSAIDs, and bile acids is augmented in the presence of acid. On the other hand, ethanol causes mucosal injury with or without acid. Corticosteroids, smoking, and physiologic and psychologic stress predispose some people to mucosal injury via mechanisms that are not completely understood. When negative feedback is overwhelmed or ineffective, an erosion (<5-mm lesion) or an ulcer (≥5 mm in diameter) may result. Ulcers represent a loss of the enteric surface epithelium that extends deeply enough to reach or penetrate the muscularis mucosa. Because pepsin is active only at a pH of 1 to 4, neutralization of acid or inhibition of acid production eliminates the harmful effects of pepsin.

The Disease

Peptic ulcer is defined as a break in the gastric or duodenal mucosa that arises when the normal mucosal defensive factors are impaired or overwhelmed. Duodenal ulcers are more common between the ages of 30 and 55 years; gastric ulcers are more common between the ages of 55 and 70 years. Ulcers are five times more common in the duodenum than the stomach. Duodenal ulcers are almost never malignant, whereas 3% to 5% of gastric ulcers are malignant.

A peptic ulcer results from damage to the gastric or duodenal mucosa. An ulcer occurs when the normal mucosal defenses are weakened, or aggressive factors such as acid and pepsin are increased. There are three important causes of peptic ulcer disease: NSAIDs, *H. pylori,* and acid hypersecretory states such as Zöllinger-Ellison syndrome.

DRUG ACTION AND EFFECTS

Medications that inhibit acid secretion can act in several ways at several locations on or in the oxyntic cell. Histamine H_2-receptor antagonist drugs can bind to the H_2-receptor, thereby displacing histamine from receptor binding sites and preventing stimulation of the oxyntic cell by the secretagogue. The four H_2-receptor antagonists have similar chemical structures. They reversibly inhibit basal or histamine-, pentagastrin-, or meal-stimulated acid secretion in a linear, dose-dependent manner by interfering with histamine at the H_2-receptors on the gastric parietal cells. As much as 90% inhibition of vagal and gastrin-stimulated acid secretion occurs with these agents, reflecting the importance of histamine in the mediation of cholinergic and gastrin-stimulated acid secretion. Near-complete inhibition of nocturnal acid secretion may be achieved as well.

The PPIs irreversibly inhibit the acid secretory pump embedded within the parietal cell membrane by altering the activity of H^+,K^+-ATPase. This enzyme affects the secretory pump in the gastric parietal cell by inhibiting hydrogen ion transport into gastric lumen and by decreasing stimulated acid secretion. It decreases the volume of gastric fluid. There is an increase in the serum gastrin concentrations. Because PPIs act on the basolateral membrane of the parietal cell, they do not affect gastric emptying, basal or stimulated pepsin output, or secretion of intrinsic factor. This type of drug does not seem to affect ATPase of other organ systems.

TABLE 28-2 Usual Length of Treatment

Type of Medication	Indication	Length of Time
H_2 blockers	Duodenal ulcer	8 wk
	Eradication of *H. pylori*	Short tem
	Erosive esophagitis	Long term
	Gastric ulcer	12 wk
	GERD	12 wk
	Heartburn	Short term
	Hypersecretory conditions	Long term
	Prevention of gastric NSAID damage	Long term
	Upper GI bleeding	Short term
Proton pump inhibitors	Active duodenal ulcer	4-8 wk
	GERD	4-8 wk
	Hypersecretory conditions	Long term

DRUG TREATMENT PRINCIPLES

Nonpharmacologic Treatment

Lifestyle modifications for peptic ulcer therapy (PUD) are integral to treatment. Recommendations no longer include bland or restrictive diets. Patients should eat balanced meals at regular times. Patients should avoid foods that exacerbate symptoms. High fiber is encouraged. Caffeine causes increased acid secretion and should be avoided. Alcohol can aggravate an ulcer but usually does not appear to be harmful in moderation. Smoking should be strongly discouraged.

Pharmacologic Treatment

The goal is relief of symptoms and healing of ulcer. Treatment consists of a course of either a histamine H_2-blocker or a PPI. H_2-blockers are generally considered the first-line treatment of mild to moderate PUD. PPIs should be used for severe PUD. They may also be used for the more mild to moderate cases. If the patient does not start to see improvement within a few days, increase the dose of medication or change from an H_2-blocker to a PPI. See Table 28-2 for recommendations on usual length of therapy.

***H. pylori* Ulcer.** The *H. pylori* organism must be eradicated to prevent recurrences; there are several treatment regimens. In general, an acid suppressant (H_2-blocker or PPI) is combined with an antibiotic or antibiotics. Occasionally this regimen includes bismuth. After this treatment is completed, continue treatment of the ulcer with an acid suppressant. See Table 28-3 for dosing regimens for *H. pylori* treatment.

TABLE 28-3 Regimen for *H. pylori* Eradication

Drug	Dosage Schedule
TRIPLE THERAPY	
tetracycline or amoxicillin	500 mg qid for 2 wk
metronidazole	250 mg tid for 2 wk
Pepto-Bismol	Two tablets qid for 2 wk
H_2-BLOCKER DOUBLE THERAPY	
Prilosec	20 mg bid for 2 wk, then 20 mg qd
Biaxin	500 mg tid for 2 wk
COMBINATION PRODUCTS	
Helidac (bismuth subsalicylate, metronidazole, and tetracycline)	In addition to an H_2 antagonist: chew and swallow 525 mg bismuth subsalicylate (two tablets), and swallow 250 mg metronidazole, and 500 mg capsule tetracycline with glass of water qid (at meals and bedtime) for 2 wk
Tritec (ranitidine and bismuth citrate)	Take 400 mg ranitidine and bismuth bid for 4 wk along with clarithromycin 500 mg tid for first 2 wk; can take with or without food

NSAID-Induced Ulcer. Discontinue the NSAID if possible and use a standard dosing regimen of an acid suppressant. Prevention of ulcers in patients on NSAIDs is used for high-risk patients such as those with history of ulcer disease, concurrent therapy with corticosteroids or anticoagulants, serious illness, or advanced age. Options include using a cyclooxygenase-2–selective agent, misoprostol, or a PPI.

Refractory Ulcers. Refractory ulcers are uncommon with PPIs. Consider pathologic hypersecretory conditions and refer the patient to a gastroenterologist. Patients with a nonhealing gastric ulcer should be evaluated for cancer by repeating the endoscopy after 3 to 4 months. Symptomatic response does not preclude the presence of a gastric malignancy.

Histamine H_2-Blockers. All H_2-receptor blockers are capable of healing duodenal ulcers, relieving symptoms, and preventing complications. They are well tolerated and have a remarkably low incidence of side effects, less than 3%.

Single dosing at bedtime of H_2-receptor antagonists is approved for the treatment of acute peptic ulcers. Evening dosing appears to provide optimal 24-hour inhibition. Early evening is the optimal time for once-daily dosing. Because all H_2-blockers have basically the same efficacy, there is no reason to switch from one to another if there is no symptomatic response. Cimetidine is sold over the counter, but it is often involved in drug interactions.

Proton Pump Inhibitors. One advantage of PPIs is their once-a-day dosing, which improves patient compliance. Because PPIs affect the actively secreting parietal cells, they should be given at mealtime. H_2-receptor antagonists should not be used concurrently with PPIs.

HOW TO MONITOR

- Check stools and emesis for blood. It takes 72 hours to clear stool from the GI tract from a former bleed. Once the stool is negative for blood, no further hemoccult test is necessary unless symptoms return or worsen.
- Assess for confusion, especially in elderly or debilitated patients and those with renal or hepatic dysfunction.
- Unusual weakness or tiredness may suggest blood dyscrasias.

H_2-Blockers

- Monitor liver enzymes.
- Consider monitoring renal function, especially in the elderly.

PATIENT VARIABLES

Geriatrics

- Decreased liver and renal function may decrease elimination of the drugs; reduce dose by one half.
- No adjustment of dosage is necessary with PPIs.

Pediatrics

- Clinical experience in children is limited. Safety and efficacy have not been established. Cimetidine is not recommended for children under 16 years of age.

Pregnancy

- All H_2-receptor antagonists cross the placenta and, although believed safe, are not recommended in the first trimester of pregnancy or for nursing mothers.
- *Category B:* H_2-blockers, lansoprazole, rabeprazole, pantoprazole
- *Category C:* omeprazole

Lactation

- H_2-blockers and PPIs are secreted in the milk.

Race

- Higher levels of omeprazole with equivalent doses have been noted in Japanese and Asian subjects. Consider lowering dose.

PATIENT EDUCATION

H_2-Blockers

- Do not take within 2 hours of antacid ingestion.
- H_2-receptor antagonists should be given after meals and at bedtime. If using once-a-day dosing, give medication before bedtime.
- Report any blood in vomitus or stool or any dark tarry stools, any unusual weakness or tiredness (may suggest blood dyscrasias) or confusion, especially in the elderly.
- Oral suspensions should be shaken vigorously for 5 to 10 seconds before each use.
- Unused constituted oral suspensions should be discarded after 30 days.

Proton Pump Inhibitors

- The capsule should be swallowed whole; instruct patients not to crush or chew capsules.
- PPIs should be taken before meals.
- PPIs and H_2-blockers should not be used concurrently. H_2 blockers are sold OTC.

Specific Drugs

H_2-RECEPTOR ANTAGONISTS

(P) Prototype Drug

ranitidine (Zantac)

Contraindications

- Hypersensitivity

Warnings

- Hypersensitivity reactions: rare cases of anaphylaxis
- Reversible hepatitis and blood dyscrasias occur rarely.
- Because H_2-blockers are excreted by the kidney, dosage should be adjusted in patients with impaired renal function.
- Use with caution in patients with hepatic dysfunction.

Precautions

Symptomatic response to these agents does not preclude gastric malignancy.

TABLE 28-4 Pharmacokinetics for Medications that Reduce Acidity

Drug	Availability (After First Pass)	Time to Peak Concentration	Half-Life	Duration of Action	Protein Bound	Metabolism	Urinary Excretion of Oral Dose
ranitidine	50%-60%	1-3 hr	2-3 hr	—	15%	CYP 2D6 substrate; liver	30%-35%, unchanged
cimetidine	60%-70%	1-2 hr	1.5-2 hr	—	13%-25%	CYP 1A2, 2C9, and 3A4 inhibitor	Unchanged
famotidine	40%-45%	1-3 hr	2.5-3.5 hr	—	15%-20%	Liver	30%, unchanged
nizatidine	>90%	1-2 hr	1.1-1.6 hr	—	35%	Liver	>90%, unchanged
omeprazole	30%-40%	0.5-3.5 hr	0.5-1 hr	>2 hr	95%	Liver; CYP 1A2, 2C9, and 10; CYP 3A4 inhibitor	77%, metabolites
lansoprazole	>80%	1.7 hr	1.5 hr	24 hr	97%	CYP 2C substrate; liver	33%, metabolites
rabeprazole	52%	2.5 hr	1-2 hr	24 hr	96.3%	Liver	90%, metabolites
esoprazole	90%	1.5 hr	1.5 hr	—	97%	CYP 2C19 and 3A4	80%, metabolites
pantozol	77%	2.4 hr	1 hr	>24 hr	98%	Liver	71%, metabolites

TABLE 28-5 Common and Serious Adverse Effects of Cimetidine

Drug	Common Minor Effects	Serious Adverse Effects
H_2-blockers	Very low incidence of side effects, most 1%	Very rare; skin reactions, blood dyscrasias, elevated
ranitidine	Vertigo	Blurred vision, malaise, reversible leukopenia, anaphylaxis
cimetidine	Diarrhea, arthralgias, myalgia	CNS effects: confusion, dizziness, somnolence, headache, hallucination; peripheral neuropathy, galactorrhea, epidermal necrolysis
famotidine	Headache, anorexia, dry mouth	Musculoskeletal pain
nizatidine	Fatigue, sweating	Tachycardia, hyperuricemia
Proton pump inhibitiors	Well tolerated, headache, diarrhea with increased doses	Hypertension, tachycardia
omeprazole	Headache, diarrhea, nausea, flatulence, abdominal pain, constipation, dry mouth	Bradycardia, peripheral edema, high blood pressure, severe skin reactions, pancreatitis, interstitial nephritis
lansoprazole	Constipation	Gallbladder disease, esophagitis
rabeprazole		Migraine, bradycardia, tachycardia
esomeprazole	Headache, diarrhea, nausea, flatulence, abdominal pain, constipation, druy mouth	Bradycardia, peripheral edema, high blood pressure, severe skin reactions, pancreatitis, interstitial nephritis
pantoprazole		Insomnia, dizziness, somnolence, convulsions, rash, pancreatitis

- Reversible central nervous system effects have occurred with cimetidine: disorientation, mental confusion, agitation, psychosis, depression anxiety, hallucinations.
- Use of cimetidine in the elderly is not recommended.
- Hepatocellular injury with nizatidine and ranitidine as evidence by elevated liver enzymes (AST, ALT, or alkaline phosphatase). All abnormalities reversed on discontinuation of the drug.

Pharmacokinetics

- See Table 28-4 for pharmacokinetics of all acid antisecretory drugs.
- All H_2-receptor antagonists are rapidly absorbed from the small intestine but not the stomach. Absorption is unaffected by food but may be decreased by 30% or more by antacids and/or sucralfate. H_2-receptor antagonists are mostly metabolized by the liver except for nizatidine, which is largely excreted by the kidneys.

Adverse Effects

- H_2-blockers, except for cimetidine, have a very low rate of side effects and are very safe. Because of drug interactions and increased incidence of side effects, cimetidine is not as safe (see Table 28-5 for adverse effects).

Drug Interactions

- See Table 28-6 for a summary of the drug interactions of H_2-blockers.

TABLE 28-6 Drug Interactions

Acid Antisecretory Drug	Effect on Other Drug	Other Drugs	Effect on Antisecretory Drugs
H_2-blockers	Increased action of ethanol	Antacids, anticholinergics, metoclopramide	Decreased action of H_2-blockers
ranitidine	Increased action of procainamide, salicylates, sulfonylurea, warfarin	clarithromycin, sucralfate	Decreased action of omeprazole
cimetidine	Increased action of flecainide, fluorouracil, procainamide, succinylcholine, narcotic analgesics Decreased action of iron salts, indomethacin, ketoconazole, tetracyclines, digoxin, fluconazole, tocainide	sucralfate	Decreased action of lansoprazole
famotidine	None listed		
nizatidine	Increased action of salicylates		
Proton pump inhibitors			
omeprazole	Increased action of benzodiazepines, phenytoin, clarithromycin		
lansoprazole			

Other Drugs in Class

Other drugs in this class are similar to the prototype except as follows.

nizatidine (Axid)

- Nizatidine does not inhibit the cytochrome P-450 (CYP)–linked drug-metabolizing enzyme system; therefore drug interactions mediated by inhibition of hepatic metabolism are not expected to occur.

cimetidine (Tagamet)

- Cimetidine has extensive drug interactions, many related to its metabolism by the CYP 1A2, 2C9, 2D6, and especially 3D4 enzymes.
- Cimetidine interacts with over 100 medications. Consult a reference for a complete listing.
- Toxic doses may be associated with respiratory failure and tachycardia that may be controlled by assisted respiration and β-blockers. Severe central nervous system symptoms such as unresponsiveness have been reported with doses between 20 and 40 g.

PROTON PUMP INHIBITORS

Ⓟ Prototype Drug

omeprazole (Prilosec)

Contraindications

- Hypersensitivity

Warnings/Precautions

- Omeprazole should be prescribed only for the conditions, dosages, and duration described.
- It is unknown whether the drug crosses the placenta or is distributed in breast milk.
- Patients should be cautioned that capsules should not be opened, chewed, or crushed and should be swallowed whole.
- Safety and effectiveness in children have not been established.

Pharmacokinetics

- Because the absorption of PPIs is enhanced in an alkaline medium, more is absorbed as they inhibit the secretion of gastric acid.
- The half-life of the drugs is about 60 minutes; however, they have a very long duration of action of at least 72 hours. It takes about 3 to 5 days for gastric acid secretion to return to normal after the discontinuation of these drugs because H^+, K^+-ATPase enzyme needs to be synthesized again.
- Tolerance and rebound hypersecretion after discontinuation do not appear to be issues.
- Protein binding is 95% to 97%. The drugs are metabolized extensively in the liver and then excreted in urine.

Adverse Effects

- PPIs have an even lower incidence of adverse reactions than do H_2-blockers.

Drug Interactions

- See Table 28-6 for specific interactions. Omeprazole inhibits CYP 1A2, 2C, and 3A4 isoenzyme systems and may interfere with the metabolism of other drugs using these systems. Lansoprazol uses the CYP 350 3A and 2C19 enzymes, without clinically significant drug interactions. Pantoprazole uses the C19 and 3A4 without significant interactions.
- Because these drugs decrease gastric acid, they may interfere with the absorption of drugs that need an acid stomach to be absorbed; these include ketoconazole, ampicillin, iron salts, digoxin, and cyanocobalamin.

Other Drugs in Class

Other drugs in this class are similar to the prototype except as follows.

rabeprazole (Aciphex)

- Only pantoprazole is less expensive.
- This drug comes in a small pill and is easy to swallow.

esomeprazole (Nexium)

- Essentially identical to omeprazole, except it has a longer duration or action, needing only once-a-day dosing.

pantoprazole (Protonix)

- The least expensive of the PPIs.
- This drug comes as a small pill and is easy to swallow.

RESOURCES FOR PATIENTS AND PROVIDERS

Inside tract of GI treatment: do you have H. pylori? Patient education information available free by calling (800) 824-2896 for AMA booklet on GERD (also in Spanish).

BIBLIOGRAPHY

Cappell MS: Gastric and duodenal ulcers during pregnancy, *Gastroenterol Clin North Am* 32:263, 2003.

Friedman SL, et al: *Current diagnosis and treatment in gastroenterology*, ed 2, New York, 2002, McGraw-Hill/Appleton & Lange.

Graham D: Therapy of *Helicobacter pylori:* current status and issues, *Gastroenterology* 118:S2, 2000.

Wolfe MM, et al. Acid suppression: optimizing therapy for gastroduodenal ulcer healing, gastroesophageal reflux disease, and stress-related mucosal disease, *Gastroenterology* 118:S9, 2000.

Yamada T, et al: *Handbook of gastroenterology*, Philadelphia, 1998, Lippincott, Williams & Wilkins.

Zulloa A, et al: A new highly effective short-term therapy schedule for *Helicobacter pylori* eradication, *Aliment Pharmacol Ther* 14:715, 2000.

CHAPTER 29

Laxatives

Drug Names

Class	Subclass	Generic Name	Trade Name
Bulk laxatives		(P) psyllium methylcellulose calcium polycarbophil Bran	Metamucil, Fiberall Citrucel FiberCon, Fiberall Chewable
Emollients/fecal softeners		(P) docusate sodium docusate calcium	Colace Surfak
Osmotic laxatives		lactulose sorbitol polyethylene glycol glycerol (glycerin)	Chronulac, Cephulac MiraLax, GoLYTELY Generic suppositories
Stimulants	diphenylmethane derivatives anthraquinone derivatives	(P) bisacodyl cascara sagrada senna casanthranol	Dulcolax Milk of Magnesia Senokot, X-Prep
Saline laxatives		(P) magnesium hydroxide magnesium sulfate magnesium citrate	Milk of Magnesia Epsom salts Generic
Enemas		sodium phosphate Soap suds Tap water Oil retention–mineral oil	Fleet enema

(P), Prototype drug.

General Uses

Indications

- All
  - Constipation
  - Prophylaxis of constipation
  - Surgical or procedural preparation: polyethylene glycol (GoLYTELY), sodium phosphate enema, magnesium citrate
  - Expedite cleansing of the body of toxins or parasites
- Psyllium: irritable bowel syndrome and diverticular disease
- Polycarbophil: irritable bowel syndrome, diverticulosis, acute nonspecific diarrhea
- Mineral oil enema: relief of fecal impaction
- Lactulose: hepatic encephalopathy

• • •

Laxatives are divided into six primary categories, which vary in mechanism of action, potency, effect, indication, and cost. The six categories are bulk, stool softeners, osmotic, stimulants, saline, and enemas.

DISEASE PROCESS

Anatomy and Physiology

The large intestine contains a mixture of the remnants of several meals ingested over 3 to 4 days. The ascending colon holds the contents of the stomach for about an hour. The transverse colon is the primary site for processing feces. The descending colon is a holding tank and conduit for feces for about 24 hours. The sigmoid colon and rectum also act as reservoirs. The nerves responsible for the activation of mass movements are located in the descending colon. Skeletal muscles that maintain continence are located in the surrounding pelvic floor. The integrity of the nervous system is necessary for coordination of the defecation process.

Contractions occur almost continuously in the large intestine. There are two basic types of contractions. The segmental pattern of motility occurs in the transverse colon, where most of the removal of water and electrolytes occurs and feces are moved forward very slowly. The circular muscles are responsible for segmental contractions. Ring-like contractions divide the colon into chambers called *haustra*. Haustrations mix and compress the feces, facilitating absorption of water while moving the feces backward and slowly forward. The second type of contraction, the mass movement (power propulsion) is a different process that occurs in the transverse and descending colon to promote bowel movements. Evacuation is also aided by (1) voluntary muscles of the abdomen that contract to promote propulsion, (2) relaxation of the circular muscles, with disappearance of haustral contractions, and (3) distention of the gut caused by increased contents of the bowel. The increase in mass movements after a meal is called the *gastrocolic reflex*.

Pathophysiology

An abnormality anywhere in the evacuation system can cause constipation. Without enough mass, the contractions are not stimulated. Disruption of the nerves controlling the process prevents proper stimulation of the muscles. Weakness of the muscles of the abdominal wall, the circular muscles (segmental contractions), or the muscles controlling mass movement will inhibit a bowel movement. Pain with stretching of the gut inhibits contractions. Any structural defect will form a physical barrier to proper transit.

The Disease

Constipation is a very common complaint in all ages. Constipation means very different things to different patients. Often it is perceived as infrequent or difficult defecation. Some of these changes normally occur if a patient becomes less active or eats less food. The frequency of bowel movements in normal patients ranges from 3 to 12 a week. Changes in consistency are generally due to changes in the amount of fiber eaten. The objective definition of constipation is 2 or fewer bowel movements per week, or excessive difficulty and straining at defecation. True clinical constipation includes the diagnostic findings of a large amount of feces in the rectal ampulla on digital examination and/or excessive fecal loading of the colon, rectum, or both on abdominal radiograph.

There are many causes of constipation, ranging from inadequate fiber to colon cancer. Medications are an important cause (Table 29-1). Systemic disease may cause constipation through neurologic gut dysfunction, myopathies, and electrolyte imbalances. Diabetic patients may have autonomic nerve dysfunction. Structural causes can be the result of a congenital defect or the structural obstruction of a mass, which may be cancerous. Any sudden change in bowel habits warrants a thorough investigation.

Practitioners should ask specifically about any OTC laxatives that the patient has taken. Evaluate for laxative abuse. Prolonged and habitual use of laxatives can cause cathartic colon, thereby causing reliance on laxatives for a regular bowel movement. Laxative abuse syndrome (LAS) is difficult to diagnose; it is often seen in women with depression, personality disorders, or anorexia nervosa. Clinical features of laxative abuse include factitious diarrhea, electrolyte imbalance, osteomalacia, protein-energy malnutrition, cathartic colon, liver disease, and steatorrhea. Many agents can be detected in urine or stool samples.

TABLE 29-1 Medications and Other Agents that Contribute to Constipation

Agents	Example
Analgesics	codeine morphine Prostaglandin inhibitors
Antacids	aluminum hydroxide calcium carbonate
Anticholinergics	Antidepressants Antihistamines Antiparkinson drugs Antipsychotics Antispasmodics Anxiolytics
Other	Anticonvulsants Antihypertensives barium sulfate Iron Lead MAO inhibitors Polystyrene resins verapamil

DRUG ACTION AND EFFECTS

All laxatives work by either increasing fluid retention in the colon, resulting in bulkier and softer stools; by decreasing absorption of luminal water through actions on the colonic mucosa; or by increasing intestinal motility. Expected results vary from 5 minutes to several days.

Bulk Laxatives

Bulk laxatives are nondigestible and nonabsorbable. They swell in water to form a viscous solution or gel that absorbs water and expands, increasing both bulk and moisture content of the stool. The increased bulk stimulates peristalsis and the absorbed water softens the stool. They also stimulate colonic bacterial growth that increases the weight of the stool and stretches the intestinal wall, further stimulating peristalsis.

Stool Softeners

Stool softeners act to soften stool by lowering surface tension, allowing the fecal mass to be penetrated by intestinal fluids. They also inhibit fluid and electrolyte reabsorption by the intestine.

Docusate sodium is an anionic surfactant that lowers the surface tension of stool to allow mixing of aqueous and fatty substances, which softens the stool and permits easier defecation. It stimulates cyclic adenosine monophosphate (cAMP) to increase secretion of water, sodium, and chloride into the gut.

Osmotic Laxatives

Osmotic laxatives are largely nonabsorbable sugars, although small amounts may be absorbed. Bacteria metabolize them into lactic acid, formic acid, acetic acid, and carbon dioxide. These act via osmosis. This means they are in solution in higher concentration in the bowel, causing water to move from the tissue into the bowel to equalize the osmotic pressure. The increased bulk increases colonic peristalsis. Most are disaccharides. Lactulose is a semisynthetic disaccharide of fructose and galactose. Sorbitol is a nonabsorbable sugar. However, glycerin is a naturally occurring trivalent alcohol suppository that acts via hyperosmotic action and local irritation and lubrication.

Stimulants

Stimulant or irritant laxatives increase peristalsis via several mechanisms, depending on the subclass. Stimulants have a direct action on intestinal mucosa or nerve plexus. Diphenylmethanes (bisacodyl) stimulate sensory nerves in the intestinal mucosa and increase intestinal chloride secretion. Anthraquinonenone derivatives (i.e., cascara sagrada, senna, casanthranol) primarily stimulate colonic intramural nerve plexuses.

Senna is protected from small intestinal absorption by their glucose molecules. Colonic bacteria cleave the glucose molecules, releasing active rheinanthrones and producing an action that is specific to the colon.

Saline Laxatives

Saline laxatives attract and retain water in the bowel, increasing intraluminal pressure. Saline laxatives produce an osmotic effect, drawing water into the intestinal lumen of the small intestine and the colon and inducing contractions. Magnesium hydroxide also stimulates the release of cholecystokinin, which increases intestinal secretion and stimulates peristalsis and transit.

Enemas

Enemas work primarily by inducing evacuation as a response to colonic distention and by lavage. They create a barrier between the feces and the colon wall that prevents colonic reabsorption of fecal fluid, thus softening the stool. The lubricant effect also eases the passage of feces through the intestine. Mineral oil retention enemas also work by lubricating the rectum and colon. Soap suds enemas provide an irritant action.

DRUG TREATMENT PRINCIPLES

Treat the underlying cause of constipation first if possible. Start treatment for constipation immediately if it is causing significant discomfort. Understanding the underlying cause of the constipation will help determine which class of laxative is most likely to be successful. For example, constipation caused by diseases such as hypothyroidism should resolve with treatment of the hypothyroidism.

Nonpharmacologic Treatment

Nonpharmacologic measures are cost effective and do not have the complications associated with laxative use. These measures should be used in all patients with constipation regardless of whether a medication is prescribed. No medication is an adequate replacement for these measures. Nonpharmacologic management of chronic constipation is encouraged for all ages, especially the young and old. In the absence of disease, adequate colonic movements can be accomplished by a regimen based on four basic components:

- First, adequate fluids are crucial both for laxatives to work and to prevent constipation, with 1500 ml/day minimum essential for maintaining normal bowel activity. Adequate fluids act by keeping fluid in the feces as it passes through the colon. This maintains the bulk of the feces and allows for normal transit. Fluids that are diuretics, such as those containing caffeine, do not work as well to keep water in the feces. Flavored waters are often an acceptable substitute for plain water.
- Second, a high-fiber diet is important. An adult should have a daily intake of 15 to 30 g of fiber; a child should receive 1 g per year of age plus 5 g/day after 2 years of age. This fiber is best obtained from high-roughage foods like bran or vegetables and fruits. See Table 29-2 for a list of foods high in fiber. Bran is the outer coating of various grains. The two most commonly found are wheat bran and oat bran, which have large amounts of fiber. Other whole grain, unpolished grains, and rice have the outer coating still on, have good amounts of fiber, and may be easier to tolerate than concentrated bran. Sudden increases in fiber in the diet can cause bloating and gas. A high-fiber diet is better tolerated if the change is made gradually. Another method of getting enough fiber is the regular use of a bran slurry (see Box 29-1 for ingredients). Start with 1 tablespoon a day and work up to 3 tablespoons twice a day as needed. It can be mixed in with cereal or other foods. Make sure the patient continues to drink enough fluids.
- Third, patients should establish and maintain a regular exercise schedule. Any type of activity is helpful. Simply walking briskly every day helps facilitate digestion and keeps muscles of the body better toned.

TABLE 29-2 Foods High in Fiber

Type of Food	Examples
Fruits (most fruits contain fiber, especially those listed)	Apples Blackberries Peaches Pears Raspberries Strawberries
Grains	Bran cereals Brown rice Popcorn Rye bread Whole wheat bread
Vegetables (most vegetables have fiber; the ones listed are especially high in fiber content)	Beans Broccoli Cabbage Carrots Cauliflower Celery Corn Peas Potatoes Squash

BOX 29-1

BRAN SLURRY RECIPE

3 cups applesauce (low sugar)
2 cups wheat or oat bran
1½ cups unsweetened prune juice

TABLE 29-3 Drugs of Choice in Treatment of Constipation

	Short Term	Long Term
First line	Mild: bulk, stool softeners	Bulk, stool softeners
Second line	Severe: enema	Osmotics
Third line	Stimulants, saline	Stimulants, saline

- Fourth, a regular toileting schedule should be established. This includes going to the toilet at the same time each day, 15 to 45 minutes after a meal. Patient should allow for 10 to 15 minutes on the toilet without interruption, stress, or need to hurry. Patients should not ignore or postpone the urge to defecate.

Pharmacologic Treatment

Pharmacologic treatment may be added if nonpharmacologic treatment is not sufficient or when immediate or thorough cleansing is indicated. Selection is based on matching the patient characteristics to the effects of the different categories of laxatives. Important factors to consider include cause of constipation, long- or short-term use, severity, age of patient, oral food and fluid intake, and prior laxative use (Table 29-3).

One important decision is the medication formulation. Remedies are available as oral, rectal suppositories, and enemas. Oral formulations can come in tablet, capsule, syrup, powder, or liquid forms. Some are dissolved in water. Oral treatment is used for long-term use; it is essential to find a formulation that the patient is willing and able to tolerate on a long-term basis. Oral medications can also be used on a short-term for severe constipation. Rectal suppositories and enemas should be used only for short-term management because irritation of the rectum can occur with chronic use.

Management

Short Term

- Short-term relief of constipation, whether occasional or caused by external factors, is treated by a short-acting laxative. Another short-term use is preparation for a surgery or procedure.
- Mild short-term constipation can be treated with bulk laxatives or stool softeners.
- If the patient is severely constipated, he or she might need an enema or one of the more potent laxatives. Laxative categories used for severe short-term treatment include stimulants, saline, and enemas. Enemas are useful when the patient has stool in the rectum but is unable to push it out. If the patient is impacted, they must be manually disimpacted before any laxative is used. Stimulants and saline laxatives are used for constipation higher in the colon.
- If the patient has chronic constipation with a short-term exacerbation, long-term management will be necessary.

Long Term

- Choose a laxative based on the patient's characteristics and initiate treatment. Table 29-3 provides drug choices.
- If the patient has mild constipation, simple long-term treatment is adequate.
- If the patient has severe constipation, short-term treatment should be instituted while the long-term program is being started. The patient must continue a regimen for at least a week before evaluating the effectiveness. Increase dose as necessary.
- If first-line treatment is not effective, consider changing laxatives or adding a second laxative. Change to a more potent category. Use caution if adding a second laxative. Do not use two laxatives from the same category. Bulk and stool softeners can be combined safely with other laxatives. However, they will not be needed if the patient is placed on osmotic laxatives, because these also soften stools. Stimulants, saline, and enemas may be given as needed for a short-term problem. Monitor the frequency of their use; if needed often, this means the long-term plan needs adjustment. Stimulant, saline, and osmotic laxatives should not be combined with each other because of increased risk of adverse reactions.

Chronic Laxative Abuse

- Many patients have all ready used pharmacologic treatment and have developed cathartic colon from LAS. These patients should be weaned from their stimulant and saline laxatives and placed on safer long-term laxatives. Long-term management should be initiated with a bulk or stool softener for milder constipation.
- Usually, however, these patients will need a stronger laxative such as an osmotic. Then start gradually decreasing their use of the stimulant or saline laxative as tolerated. Patient education is crucial to success.

Bulk Laxatives. Bulk laxatives are the most commonly used first-line laxative to treat or prevent mild short-term constipation. They are especially helpful for long-term use because of a good safety profile. A patient with severe constipation may need a more potent laxative, especially at first. These products come as powder that is mixed with water. Some form a gritty residue that is unpalatable. Some also come as wafers or tablets.

Patients likely to benefit from bulk-forming laxatives include postpartum, elderly, and debilitated patients. Patients who eat a small quantity of food or have a low level of mobility are also likely to benefit. However, they can be dangerous in patients with poor fluid intake. They can be used to wean patients from long-term stimulant laxatives. Bulk laxatives may reduce the risk of colon cancer. Psyllium lowers serum cholesterol by binding bile salts in the intestine.

Stool Softeners. Fecal softeners are mild acting and frequently used in long-term treatment and prevention of constipation produced by a delay in rectal emptying. They are also useful when it is important to reduce straining at stool, as in patients with hernia or cardiovascular disease, during postpartum, or after rectal surgery. Fecal softeners can be helpful in elderly patients unable to drink adequate fluids for bulk laxatives to be effective.

Mineral oil is now regarded as not safe for oral ingestion and its use is not recommended. Lipid pneumonitis may result from oral ingestion and aspiration of mineral oil, especially when the patient reclines.

Osmotic Laxatives. Use of osmotic laxatives has greatly increased in recent years. They are used for short- and long-term constipation and bowel cleansing. They are especially useful for moderate to severe chronic constipation. They are preferred over stimulant and saline laxatives because of a better safety profile but are not as potent. One drawback is their cost, and unlike most other laxatives, they require a prescription.

Sorbitol is used in the short-term treatment of constipation. It is also mixed with activated charcoal in the management of poisonings or drug overdoses.

Lactulose is used to treat constipation and also is useful for reducing urea production in the colon, thus lowering blood ammonia levels in patients with portal systemic encephalopathy. It comes as a thick syrup that many patients find unpalatable.

Polyethylene glycol comes in two forms: MiraLax powder for chronic constipation and GoLYTELY for bowel cleansing before a procedure. MiraLax comes as a powder that dissolves in water and is tasteless and nongritty. Because polyethylene glycol is an isotonic solution, dehydration does not occur.

Glycerin suppositories aid rectal evacuation and are useful in bowel retraining programs and in reestablishing normal function in those who are laxative dependent. It may be used on an occasional basis in the management of chronic constipation. They do not have a powerful osmotic effect.

Stimulants. Stimulants are the most potent class of laxatives. These are recommended for use in short-term treatment but may also be used on an occasional basis in a patient with chronic constipation. They should be used after other methods have failed. They are also used to cleanse the bowel in preparation for endoscopic examination, x-ray studies, or surgery. Bisacodyl suppositories are used to cleanse the colon in pregnant women before delivery.

Saline Laxatives. Saline laxatives are also potent laxatives. Saline laxatives are used to cleanse the bowel in preparation for endoscopic examination, x-ray studies, or surgery. They are used to hasten evacuation of worms after administration of anthelmintics and after the ingestion of poisons to hasten elimination of toxic material. They are the laxative of choice for securing a stool specimen.

Milk of Magnesia (MOM) may also be used on an occasional basis in a patient with chronic constipation. If MOM alone is ineffective, MOM with Cascara may be given. MOM is a very popular OTC laxative and a cause of LAS. The magnesium laxatives have a significant risk for adverse reactions with long-term use; they may cause an accumulation of magnesium, which may be a problem in patients with renal insufficiency.

Enemas. Enemas are used for short-term constipation while the patient is being started on a bowel regimen. They are also used to prevent discomfort and tearing or laceration of hemorrhoids or fissures. An enema may be necessary to soften stool after abdominal or rectal surgery. Repeated enemas can cause rectal irritation. Fleet enemas contain only a small amount of liquid to fill the rectum. Oil enemas are very helpful for softening hard stool. Enemas using soap suds or tap water use more liquid and go farther up the colon; this may be effective for a high impaction but puts the patient at risk for electrolyte imbalance.

Pulsed irrigation enhanced evacuation in children and adults is used to treat fecal impaction that otherwise may require operative disimpaction.

Normal saline or air enemas are used under ultrasound guidance in nonoperative management of ileocolic intussusception. They may be used for treatment of acute fecal impaction if phosphate-containing enemas are contraindicated.

HOW TO MONITOR

Short-Term Use

- Monitor for effectiveness.

Long-Term Use

- All laxatives promote fluid loss; monitor fluid and electrolytes.

PATIENT VARIABLES

Geriatrics

- Constipation increases with age, with as many as 30% of healthy older persons regularly using laxatives. Laxatives are second only to analgesics as the most commonly used OTC drugs by the elderly.
- Older adults are more susceptible to dehydration and electrolyte imbalance from laxatives than are younger patients.

Pediatrics

- Constipation in children may have many causes; contributing factors include emotional, dietary, and environmental changes.
- Dosage adjustments are indicated under specific drugs.
- Magnesium salts and phosphate enemas can cause serious metabolic disturbances in infants and young children. Administer with caution. Do not administer enemas to children younger than 2 years. Infants receiving lactulose may develop hyponatremia and dehydration.

Pregnancy

Constipation is common during pregnancy and is thought to be due to an increase in circulatory progesterone. This is compounded by the fact that vitamins, iron, and calcium taken during pregnancy tend to be constipating as well.

- *Category B:* lactulose, magnesium sulfate
- *Category C:* casanthranol, cascara sagrada, docusate sodium, docusate calcium, mineral oil, senna
- *Contraindicated*
    - Castor oil during pregnancy, as its irritant effect may induce premature labor
    - Improper use of saline cathartics can lead to dangerous electrolyte imbalance; bulk-forming or stool softeners are preferred

Lactation

- Although their absorption is limited, laxatives may be excreted in breast milk

Race and Gender

- Constipation is more frequent in women and in nonwhites than in men and whites.

Sociocultural

- Individuals with a low income and less education are at increased risk for constipation.

PATIENT EDUCATION

- Patients and/or parents may need to be educated about what constitutes a normal bowel movement.
- Nonpharmacologic measures should be reviewed; specific instructions should be written on a prescription pad.
- Handouts on high-fiber foods should also be provided to the patient.

ORAL LAXATIVES

The following is applicable to all categories of oral laxatives.

Contraindications

- Hypersensitivity, symptoms of appendicitis, fecal impaction, intestinal obstruction, undiagnosed abdominal pain, perforation, or toxic megacolon

Warnings

- Constipation: before using laxatives, consider living habits affecting bowel function, including disease state and drug history. Implement nonpharmacologic treatment. Restrict self-medication to short-term therapy of constipation. Chronic use of laxatives (particularly stimulants) may lead to dependence.
- Fluid and electrolyte balance: excessive laxative use may lead to significant fluid and electrolyte imbalance. Monitor patients periodically.
- Abuse/dependency: chronic use of laxatives may result in fluid and electrolyte imbalances, steatorrhea, osteomalacia, diarrhea, cathartic colon, and liver disease (LAS or cathartic colon).

Precautions

- Rectal bleeding or failure to respond may indicate a serious condition, which may require further medical attention.
- Some of these products contain tartrazine, to which patients may be allergic.

Adverse Effects

- Diarrhea, nausea, vomiting, perianal irritation, fainting, bloating, flatulence, cramps.

Pharmacokinetics

Only lactulose and magnesium are absorbed in appreciable amounts (Table 29-4).

Drug Interactions

Laxatives can affect the absorption of drugs absorbed in the intestine by decreasing transit time, giving the bowel less time to absorb the medication. Important medications here are oral anticoagulants, digoxin, and aspirin. They should be taken 2 hours apart to avoid drug interactions (Table 29-5).

Dosage and Administration

See Table 29-6.

Overdosage

- Diarrhea; discontinue the laxative, and monitor fluids.

TABLE 29-4 Pharmacokinetics

Drug	Onset of Action	Site of Action
BULK LAXATIVES		
psyllium	24-72 hr	Small and large intestines
methylcellulose	24-72 hr	Small and large intestines
calcium polycarbophil	12-24 hr	Small and large intestines
Bran powder	Days	Colon
STOOL SOFTENERS		
docusate sodium	12-72 hr	Small and large intestines
docusate calcium	12-72 hr	Small and large intestines
OSMOTIC LAXATIVES		
lactulose	24-48 hr	Colon
sorbitol	24-48 hr	Colon
polyethylene glycol	3-24 hr	Colon
glycerol (glycerin)	0.25-1 hr	Colon
STIMULANT LAXATIVES		
bisacodyl	6-8 hr	Colon
	1 hr	Rectum
cascara	6-8 hr	Colon
senna	6-12 hr	Colon
casanthranol	6-12 hr	Colon
SALINE LAXATIVES		
magnesium hydroxide	3-12 hr	Small and large intestines
magnesium sulfate	3-12 hr	Small and large intestines
magnesium citrate	3-6 hr	Small and large intestines
sodium phosphate	1-6 hr	Small and large intestines
ENEMAS		
sodium phosphate	5-15 min	Rectum
Soap suds	5-15 min	Rectum
Tap water	5-15 min	Rectum
Mineral oil		Rectum

Specific Drugs

BULK LAXATIVES

Ⓟ Prototype Drug

psyllium (Metamucil, Sugar-Free Metamucil, Fiberall)

Contraindications

- Swallowing disorders, intestinal stricture

Precautions

- Always give with one or more full glasses of water.
- Psyllium products with dextrose should be used cautiously in patients with diabetes.
- Bulk-forming agents may cause impaction, particularly if feces is temporarily arrested in their passage through the alimentary canal (e.g., patients with esophageal stricture). Administer bulk-forming agents with plenty of fluid (240 dl/dose), especially in elderly or immobile patients.

Adverse Effects

- Abdominal distention and borborygmi are common symptoms, particularly when bulk laxatives are first initiated.
- Bloating appears to be more of a problem with bran.

TABLE 29-5 Drug Interactions

Laxative	Action on Drugs	Drugs	Effect on Laxative
Surfactants	Increased effect of mineral oil	Milk, antacids, H_2 blockers, PPI	Increased effect of bisacodyl
Mineral oil	Decreased action of lipid-soluble vitamins	Antacids	Decreased action of lactulose
Bulk laxatives	Decreased action of digitalis, salicylates, coumadin	neomycin and other antiinfectives	lactulose (conflicting reports)
Saline and magnesium	Decreased action of tetracycline		
Magnesium salts	Decreased action of digoxin, chlordiazepoxide, chlorpromazine, dicumarol, isoniazid		

PPI, Proton pump inhibitor.

TABLE 29-6 Dosage and Administration Recommendations

Drug	Age Group	Dosage	Administration	Maximum Daily Dose
BULK LAXATIVES				
psyllium	Adult	Half adult dosage	In water; bid	
	Child	1 tsp-1 tbsp	In water; up to tid	
methylcellulose	Adult >12 yr	1 tbsp powder	In water	
	Child 6-12 yr	Half adult dosage	In water	
calcium polycarbophil	Adult >12 yr	625 mg tablet	qd-qid	4 g
	Child 6-12 yr	500 mg	qd-qid	2 g
Bran powder	Adult	6-20 g	qd	
	Child	5 g	qd	
STOOL SOFTENERS				
docusate sodium	Adult >12 yr	100 mg capsule	qd-tid	
	Child 6-12 yr	100 mg	qd	
docusate calcium	Adult >12 yr	240 mg capsule	qd	
OSMOTIC LAXATIVES				
lactulose	Adult	15-30 ml syrup	qd; may be mixed with other liquids	60 mg
sorbitol				
polyethylene glycol (MiraLax)		17 g powder	In 8 oz liquid, qd	
GoLYTELY	Adult	4 L	Before GI examination; 240 ml q10 min	
glycerol (glycerin)		One suppository in rectum, retain 15-30 min	qd	
STIMULANT LAXATIVES				
bisacodyl	Adults >12 yr	10-15 mg	Swallow whole, qd	
	Child 6-12 yr	5 mg	qd	
senna	Adult >12 yr	8.6 mg; two tablets	qd	Four tablets
	Child 6-12 yr	One tablet	qd	Two tablets
	Child 2-6 yr	Half tablet	qd	One tablet
casanthranol	Adult >12 yr	One tablet	qd	
cascara	Adult >12 yr	One tablet	qd	
SALINE LAXATIVES				
magnesium hydroxide	Adult >12 yr	30-60 ml granules	Take with liquid	
magnesium sulfate	Adult >12 yr	5-10 ml suspension	In 4 oz of water	
	Child 6-12 yr	2.5-5 ml	In 4 oz of water	
	Children 2-5 yr	5-15 ml	In 4 oz of water	
magnesium citrate				
ENEMAS				
sodium phosphate	Adult >12 yr	118 ml liquid	PRN	
	Child 2-12 yr	59 ml liquid	PRN	
Mineral oil			Insert into rectum	

Other Drugs in Class

Other drugs in this class are similar to the prototype except as follows.

methylcellulose (Citrucel) and calcium polycarbophil (FiberCon, Fiberall Chewable)

- Contraindicated inpatients for whom extra calcium is dangerous and in children under 3 years of age.
- Calcium levels may be monitored in those on calcium polycarbophil.
- Calcium polycarbophil releases calcium following ingestion that may impair absorption of tetracycline. This is avoided by spacing the dose of these 2 or more hours apart.

Bran

- See instructions on high-fiber diet and slurry (Box 29-1).

FECAL SOFTENERS

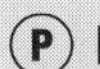 **Prototype Drug**

docusate sodium (Colace)

Warnings
- Docusate sodium should be avoided in patients with edema or heart failure and those on sodium-restricted diets.

Adverse Effects
- Docusate: throat irritation, and a bitter taste have been associated with docusate; rash is uncommon but may occur.

OSMOTIC LAXATIVES

lactulose (Chronulac, Cephulac)

Contraindications
- Patients who require a low galactose diet

Warnings
- To avoid inadequate acidification of stool in treating encephalopathy, other laxatives should not be used concurrently with lactulose.
- Electrocautery procedures: a theoretical hazard may exist for patients being treated with lactulose.

Precautions
- Diabetics: lactulose syrup contains galactose and lactose; use with caution.

Adverse Effects
- Lactulose can cause abdominal distention, epigastric pain, anorexia, hypernatremia, and lactic acidosis.
- Cramping can be as frequent as a 20% incidence; to avoid, start with a low dose.

Overdosage
- Hypernatremia and lactic acidosis have been seen with high doses of lactulose.

Other Drugs in Class

Drugs that are from the same category or subcategory are similar to lactulose except in the following ways.

sorbitol

- Sorbitol may cause hypernatremia and abdominal bloating.

polyethylene glycol (MiraLax and GoLYTELY)

- MiraLax powder dissolves in water, where it is undetectable.

STIMULANTS

Ⓟ **Prototype Drug**

bisacodyl (Dulcolax)

Warnings
- Stimulants have high risk for electrolyte abnormalities and fluid imbalance.
- Daily use of bisacodyl suppositories can cause rectal burning, proctitis, or sloughing of the epithelium.

Precautions
- All stimulant laxatives have a high abuse potential and can cause cathartic bowel with prolonged use. These laxatives should not be used longer than 1 week.

Adverse Effects
- Cramping and nausea and vomiting are more frequent with stimulants.

Drug Interactions
- Bisacodyl should not be ingested within 1 hour of antacids or foods because the tablets have an enteric that interacts with food and can cause severe cramping in the stomach or duodenum. Stimulant laxatives should not be taken within 2 hours of other oral medications.

Overdosage
- Large doses can cause nephritis. Hepatotoxicity may result from tannic acids absorbed from excess bisacodyl tannex laxatives.

Other Drugs in Class

Other drugs in this class are similar to the prototype except as follows.

Anthraquinone Derivatives

cascara sagrada

- Usually in MOM with cascara for added stimulant effect
- Both cascara sagrada and senna may discolor acidic urine to yellow-brown or black; and alkaline urine to pink-red, red-violet, or red-brown

Melanosis coli
- A darkened pigmentation of the colonic mucosa resulting from chronic use of anthraquinone derivatives (casanthranol, cascara sagrada, senna)

senna

- Has been associated with finger clubbing
- Considered to be herbal and hence safe by many patients, but should not be used on a chronic basis
- X-Prep (a powdered concentrate of senna) must be used cautiously in diabetic patients because it contains 50 g of glucose per bottle

SALINE LAXATIVES

Ⓟ Prototype Drug

magnesium hydroxide (Milk of Magnesia)

Contraindications

- Laxatives containing magnesium are contraindicated in patients with impaired renal function.
- Saline laxatives containing magnesium are contraindicated in children under 6 years of age.

Warnings

- In pregnancy, sodium salts may promote sodium retention and result in edema.
- Individuals on a sodium-restricted diet, and in the presence of edema, CHF, renal failure, or borderline hypertension, should use preparations containing sodium cautiously.
- Megacolon, bowel obstruction, imperforate anus, or CHF: Do not use sodium phosphate and sodium biphosphate in these patients; hypernatremic dehydration may occur.
- Renal function impairment: up to 20% of the magnesium in magnesium salts may be absorbed. Use caution with products containing phosphate, sodium, magnesium, or potassium salts in the presence of renal dysfunction. Use sodium phosphate and sodium biphosphate with caution in these patients; hyperphosphatemia, hypernatremia, acidosis, and hypocalcemia may occur.

Precautions

- Saline cathartics can produce dehydration if used without adequate fluid replacement.
- Phosphate salts can result in hypocalcemia in children less than 2 years of age.
- Magnesium levels may need to be monitored.

Adverse Effects

- Dizziness, palpitations, weakness, and dehydration have been reported with saline laxatives.
- Excessive bowel activity and cramping may occur.

Overdosage

- Large doses of magnesium can cause respiratory depression and alterations in neuromuscular activity from hypermagnesemia.
- Other symptoms of hypermagnesemia include muscle weakness, electrocardiographic changes, sedation, and confusion.

Other Drugs in Class

Other drugs in this class are similar to the prototype except as follows.

magnesium sulfate (Epsom Salts) and magnesium citrate

- Same characteristics as the prototype drug.
- Magnesium citrate cherry flavor may produce a red color in the urine.
- Use for bowel preparation before surgery or procedures. Refrigerate to improve taste. Take with a full glass of water.
- Sulfate salts are considered to be the most potent saline laxative.

ENEMAS

sodium phosphate (Fleet Enema)

Contraindications

- Enemas should not be given before manual removal of fecal impaction because of the potential for rectal wall perforation.
- Phosphate enemas are contraindicated in children under 2 years of age, in patients with inflammatory disease with a high risk of mucosal laceration or bowel perforation, and in those with impaired renal function.

Warnings

- Phosphate that is absorbed systemically can cause fluid retention and hyperphosphatemia and should be used cautiously in children 2 to 5 years of age, especially in those with underlying bowel disease or renal dysfunction.

Precautions

- Mechanical trauma can occur when sensitive rectal tissues are probed. The lubricated tip should be inserted gently in the adult (3 to 4 inches), child (2 to 3 inches), and infant (1½ inches). Use no more than 200 ml of fluid in those with impaired renal function or who cannot tolerate a large volume of fluid.
- Enemas should not be relied on to maintain bowel regularity because they disrupt normal defecation reflexes and may result in dependence. Monitor electrolyte losses.

Adverse Effects

- Cramping, distention, and mucorrhea may result.

Overdosage

- Hypovolemia and potassium depletion may occur when excessive lavage is used. Fatal hyperphosphatemia and hypocalcemia have been associated with excess phosphate doses.

Other Drugs in Class

Soap Suds, Tap Water, Oil Retention, Saline Enemas

- Soap suds enemas are irritating and can cause proctitis and should be avoided in the elderly.
- Hyperkalemia may result when potassium-based soaps are used.

- Hot water use in enemas can cause acute proctitis.
- Cold water administration can cause extreme cramping.
- Repeated tap water enemas can result in water toxicity and/or circulatory overload.

BIBLIOGRAPHY

Friedman SL et al: *Current diagnosis and treatment in gastroenterology*, ed 2, New York, 2002, McGraw-Hill/Appleton & Lange.

Jacobs TQ, Pamies RJ: Adult constipation: a review and clinical guide, *J Natl Med Assoc* 93:22-30, 2001.

Motola G et al: Self-prescribed laxative use: a drug-utilization review, *Adv Ther* 19:203-208, 2002.

Morgan C: Constipation during pregnancy. Fiber and fluid are keys to self-management, *Adv Nurse Pract* 9:57-58, 2001.

Smith C et al: Patient and physician evaluation of a new bulk fiber laxative tablet, *Gastroenterol Nurs* 26:31-37, 2003.

Suarez F: Intestinal gas, *Clin Perspect Gastroenterol* July/August:209, 2000.

Wanitschke R et al: Differential therapy of constipation—a review, *Int J Clin Pharmacol Ther* 41:14-21, 2003.

Yamada T et al: *Handbook of gastroenterology*, Philadelphia, 1998, Lippincott, Williams & Wilkins.

CHAPTER 30

Antidiarrheals

Drug Names

Class	Subclass	Generic Name	Trade Name
Opiate and opioid derivatives		(P) diphenoxylate hydrochloride and atropine sulfate	Lomotil, Lofene, Lomanate, Lomodix
		loperamide hydrochloride	Imodium, Imodium A-D, Kaopectate II, Pepto Diarrhea Control
		tincture of opium	Paregoric
Adsorbents		bismuth subsalicylate	Pepto-Bismol, Bismatrol, Pink Bismuth
		attapulgite	Kaopectate Advanced Formula, Children's Kaopectate, Diasorb, Kaopectate Maximum Strength Caplets, Rheaban

(P), Prototype drug.

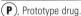

General Uses

Indications

- Acute nonspecific diarrhea
- Functional chronic diarrhea
- Loperamide (unlabeled use): for treatment of traveler's diarrhea in combination with trimethoprim-sulfamethoxazole
- Attapulgite: mild-to-moderate diarrhea
- Bismuth: indigestion, nausea, control of traveler's diarrhea, and as an adjunct to treatment of *Helicobacter pylori* peptic ulcer disease.

Antidiarrheal agents are used as temporary adjunctive therapy in the management of acute nonspecific diarrhea and functional chronic diarrhea. Acute episodes of diarrhea are usually benign and self-limiting, by definition lasting less than 1 week and usually lasting only 1 to 2 days.

If diarrhea persists for longer than 72 hours, or if there is gross blood in the stool, the patient should be evaluated further.

Diarrhea should always be evaluated before pharmacologic treatment is begun. Diarrhea is a symptom, so therapy should aim at treatment of the underlying cause.

Many antidiarrheal agents are now available over the counter (OTC) and therefore may be overused. Opioid agents may prolong acute infectious diarrhea, leading to potentially serious consequences. Antidiarrheals should never be used for more than 48 hours without supervision by a health care provider. Short-term use is generally considered safe but should not be a substitute for determining the cause of the diarrhea. The American Gastroenterological Association 1999 guidelines are the basis for the recommendations for this chapter.

DISEASE PROCESS

Anatomy and Physiology

See Chapter 29 for anatomy and physiology of the bowel.

Pathophysiology

Large-volume diarrhea is caused by excessive amounts of water or secretions in the intestines. Small-volume diarrhea is caused by excessive intestinal motility.

Large-volume diarrhea can be caused by osmosis. A nonabsorbable substance (such as lactose and nonabsorbable sugar) in the gut causes fluids to be drawn into the lumen by osmosis. This condition may also be caused by excessive mucosal secretions. Bacterial toxins and neoplasms producing hormones also stimulate secretions.

Large-volume diarrhea can also be caused by excessive motility of the intestine. Conditions affecting the autonomic nervous system control of digestion (e.g., diabetic neuropathy) increase transit time, preventing adequate absorption of water and electrolytes from the feces.

Small-volume diarrhea is usually caused by an inflammatory condition affecting gut mucosa.

The Disease

Medically it is considered diarrhea if the patient has increased frequency, which is usually more than two or three bowel movements per day, or the stools are liquid, not just "soft."

Diarrhea is divided into acute and chronic. By definition acute diarrhea persists for less than 3 weeks, usually a few days to 1 week. It is subdivided into either noninflammatory or inflammatory diarrhea. Noninflammatory diarrhea is watery, nonbloody, and is usually caused by a bacterium or virus that is self-limiting. Inflammatory diarrhea has white blood cells (WBCs) in the stool, reflecting invasion of the organism or toxin into the wall of the intestine (Table 30-1).

TABLE 30-1 Causes of Acute Infectious Diarrhea

Cause	Noninflammatory	Inflammatory
Viral	Norwalk, rotavirus	Cytomegalovirus
Protozoal	*Giardia, Cryptosporidium*	
Bacterial		
Preformed toxin	*Staphylococcus aureus, Bacillus cereus*	*Escherichia coli, Vibrio parahaemolyticus, Clostridium difficile C. perfringens*
Enterotoxin production	*E. coli, Vibrio cholerae*	
Mucosal innervation		*Shigella, Campylobacter jejuni, Salmonella,* enteroinvasive *E. coli, Chlamydia, Neisseria, Listeria*

TABLE 30-2 Causes of Chronic Diarrhea

- Lactose intolerance
- Irritable bowel disease
- Fecal impaction
- Inflammatory bowel disease
  - Ulcerative colitis
  - Crohn's disease
- Microscopic colitis
- Malignancy
- Radiation
- Malabsorption
  - Celiac sprue
  - Pancreatic disease
- Neuropathy
- Chronic infections
  - *C. difficile*
  - Parasites
  - HIV related

Chronic diarrhea has an extensive number of etiologies. Evaluate the patient carefully for the cause of the diarrhea and treat the disease, not the symptom. Medications that can cause diarrhea include laxatives, antacids, magnesium-containing products, and antibiotics (Table 30-2).

Assessment

The American Gastroenterological Association guidelines emphasize comprehensive evaluation of a patient before treatment. The history is important to diagnosis. Similar illness in contacts points to an infection. Ingestion of improperly prepared or stored food suggests infection or bacterial toxins. Exposure to impure water suggests parasites. Travel abroad exposes patients to infections characteristic of the local area. Antibiotic use points to *Clostridium difficile*.

DRUG ACTION AND EFFECTS

Opioids

Opioid antidiarrheal agents act on the smooth muscle of the intestinal tract to slow gastrointestinal (GI) motility and propulsion. Slowed transit time of intestinal contents allows more fluid to be absorbed from the stool, decreasing fecal volume, and decreasing fluid and electrolyte loss. There is little or no analgesic activity.

The opioids (except loperamide hydrochloride) may be habit forming. Atropine sulfate is added to some formulations to discourage deliberate overdose.

Adsorbents

Adsorbents act by reducing intestinal motility and by adsorbing fluid. In infectious diarrhea they bind bacteria and toxins in the GI tract.

DRUG TREATMENT PRINCIPLES

This section discusses the empirical treatment of diarrhea appropriate in the following conditions: initial treatment before diagnostic testing is completed, diarrhea without diagnosis, and diarrhea with diagnosis but no cure. The American Gastroenterological Association guidelines address empirical therapy.

Acute Diarrhea

Acute diarrhea is usually mild and self-limited. Nonpharmacologic measures, especially a liquid diet, provide bowel rest and adequate hydration. Rest, reassurance, and fluid and electrolyte replacement are also helpful. Oral hydration with electrolyte solution (Gatorade or Pedialyte) is recommended in moderate to severe cases; cola or ginger ale may be sufficient in milder cases. The patient should then be progressed to the BRAT format (banana, rice, applesauce, toast) as tolerated. If the patient is not able to replace liquids as fast as he/she is losing them, further treatment is needed to prevent dehydration. Children and frail patients with severe diarrhea may need antidiarrheals or IV rehydration (which can be accomplished in the emergency department [ED] without hospitalization).

Treatment of acute diarrhea with antidiarrheals can prolong the infection and should be avoided if possible. If patients find the diarrhea significantly inconvenient, they may be given antidiarrheals on a limited basis. Antidiarrheals may be used safely in patients with acute mild to moderate diarrhea. Their main use is for patient comfort. Do not use in patients with bloody diarrhea, high fever, or systemic toxicity because they may worsen the disease. Discontinue if not effective and pursue the etiology of the diarrhea. Used short term, they are safe and effective for patient relief, allowing patients to function in their usual activities and avoiding distressing episodes of incontinence. Patients with acute inflammatory diarrhea that does not improve within a few days may require antibiotic therapy.

Chronic Diarrhea

Once the etiology of the chronic diarrhea has been optimally treated, antidiarrheals may be used as needed to control symptoms and prevent dehydration. Opioids are generally safe and effective if used as directed.

Opiates and Opioid Derivatives

Opiates decrease the stool number and liquidity and reduce fecal urgency. They are best used for chronic diarrhea.

Adsorbents

Bismuth reduces symptoms through its antiinflammatory and antibacterial properties and decreases nausea and vomiting, and is best used for acute diarrhea.

HOW TO MONITOR

- Monitor number and character of stools and have the patient keep a record as needed.
- Monitor hydration status, fluid and electrolyte loss, hypotension, and signs of dehydration.
- Observe for signs of toxicity (see specific drug).
- Acute diarrhea should improve within 48 hours of treatment initiation.
- Chronic diarrhea should improve within 10 days.

PATIENT VARIABLES

Geriatrics

- Fecal impaction associated with use of adsorbents is more common in debilitated geriatric patients.
- Diarrhea can be caused by liquid stool leaking around an impaction.

Pediatrics

- Antidiarrheals are not recommended in young children.
- Opioids are contraindicated in children younger than 2.
- Bismuth and attapulgite are not recommended for children younger than 3 years of age.

Pregnancy

- *Category B:* loperamide
- *Category C (D* in third trimester*):* bismuth
- Diphenoxylate and atropine are excreted in breast milk

PATIENT EDUCATION

- Supportive therapy including rest, hydration, and appropriate diet is the recommended first-line treatment for acute diarrhea.
- Use safety precautions in driving or operating machinery requiring alertness because the drug may produce drowsiness or dizziness.
- When using opioid agents, avoid alcohol or other CNS depressants; do not exceed the prescribed dose.
- Antidiarrheal agents should not be used for self-medication for more than 48 hours. If diarrhea is not controlled within 48 hours or if fever develops, the patient should consult a health care provider.

Specific Drugs

OPIATES AND OPIOID DERIVATIVES

(P) Prototype Drug

diphenoxylate (2.5 mg) and atropine sulfate (0.025 mg) (Lomotil)

Contraindications

- Known enterotoxin-producing bacterium, pseudomembranous enterocolitis, obstructive jaundice, advanced liver disease, known hypersensitivity to diphenoxylate or atropine

Warnings

- Diarrhea: may aggravate diarrhea associated with organisms that penetrate intestinal mucosa.
- Fluid and electrolyte balance: must also treat fluid replacement. Dehydration increases adverse effects.
- Advise safety precautions related to possible drowsiness and dizziness.
- May prolong the half-life of drugs metabolized in the liver.
- Ulcerative colitis: may induce toxic megacolon.
- Renal and liver disease: use with extreme caution in patients with advanced hepato-renal disease and in all patients with abnormal liver function tests because hepatic coma may be precipitated.
- Atropine: may cause anticholinergic side effects. Avoid in patients in whom anticholinergic drugs are contraindicated. Although the dose of atropine is subtherapeutic, take precautions related to the use of atropine. Signs of atropinism may occur even in recommended doses, especially in children and patients who have Down's syndrome.

Precautions

Schedule V drugs may be habit forming.

Safety is not established in children younger than 12 years of age. In treatment of acute enteritis, diphenoxylate (Lomotil) may cause fluid retention in the intestines great enough to mask depletion of extracellular fluid and electrolytes, especially in younger children.

Pharmacokinetics

See Table 30-3 for pharmacokinetic information. Diphenoxylate is rapidly metabolized by ester hydrolysis to diphenoxylic acid (diphenoxylate HCl), which is biologically active.

Adverse Effects

- Mild: drowsiness, dizziness, nervousness, restlessness, headache, depression, dry mouth, difficult urination, blurred vision
- Severe: paralytic ileus, urinary retention, respiratory depression

Drug Interactions

Concurrent administration with monoamine oxidase (MAO) inhibitors may lead to hypertensive crisis.

Effects of barbiturates, tranquilizers, and alcohol are increased with coadministration of these products.

Dosage and Administration

See Table 30-4.

Overdosage

Symptoms of overdosage include drowsiness, hypotension, blurred vision, dry mouth, and meiosis. Overdosage may lead to severe respiratory depression and coma, possibly leading to brain damage or death, especially in children.

Other Drugs in Class

Other drugs in this class are similar to the prototype except as follows.

loperamide hydrochloride (Imodium)

It is more specific, longer acting, and two to three times more potent on weight basis than diphenoxylate. Loperamide has no analgesic activity.

Overdosage may be produced at doses around 60 mg. Symptoms of overdosage include CNS and respiratory depression, GI cramping and irritation, nausea, vomiting, and constipation.

camphorated tincture of opium (Paregoric)

Hypersensitivity to opium or its other components is also a contraindication.

TABLE 30-3 Pharmacokinetics of Selected Antidiarrheal Agents

Drug	Absorption	Onset of Action	Time to Peak Concentration	Half-Life	Duration of Action	Metabolism	Excretion
diphenoxylate hydrochloride and atropine sulfate	Well absorbed via oral route; bioavailability 90%	45-60 min	2 hr	12-14 hr	Varies	Liver: diphenoxylic acid is active metabolite	Feces, 50%; urine, 14%; excreted unchanged in urine, 1%
loperamide hydrochloride	Oral route: <40%; very low levels in breast milk; <50% available after first pass	0.5-1 hr	2.5 hr (soln) 4-5 hr (caps)	11 hr	Depends on many factors	Liver	Unchanged in feces, 25%; urine, 1%
camphorated tincture of opium (Paregoric)			No information			Liver	Urine
bismuth subsalicylate	Bismuth minimally absorbed across GI tract; salicylate readily absorbed		No information			Chemical dissociation to bismuth salts in GI tract	Urine, 90%
attapulgite	Not absorbed after oral administration		No information			Liver	NA

TABLE 30-4 Dosage and Administration for Antidiarrheal Agents

Drug	Administration and Dosage
diphenoxylate hydrochloride and atropine sulfate	Tablets: two tablets (5 mg) qid Liquid: 10 ml (5 mg) qid; maximum dose 20 mg/day
loperamide hydrochloride	4 mg initially, then 2 mg after each diarrheal stool; maximum dose 8 mg/day
camphorated tincture of opium (Paregoric)	Adults: 5-10 ml, qd-qid Children: 0.25-0.5 ml/kg qd-qid
bismuth subsalicylate	Take recommended dose every 30 min to 1 hr as needed; chew or dissolve tablets in mouth before swallowing; Adult: 524 mg, maximum eight doses/24 hr (30 ml, two tablets, or two caplets) Child 9 to12 yr: 262 mg, maximum eight doses/24 hr (15 ml, one tablet, or one caplet) 6 to 9 yr: 2 tsp (10 ml), 2/3 caplet, or 2/3 tablet 3 to 6 yr: 1 tsp (5 ml), 1/3 caplet, or 1/3 tablet
attapulgite	Liquid: take recommended dose after each loose bowel movement Adult, child >12 yr: 2 tbsp up to six times per day (maximum 9000 mg/24 hr) Child 3-6 yr: 1/2 tbsp; 6 to 12 yr: 1 tbsp Caplets: swallow whole caplets; one dose after each loose bowel movement Adult: 2 caplets (maximum 12 caplets/24 hr) Child 3 to 6 yr: 1 caplet (maximum 6 cap/24 hr)

It is a schedule III drug; may be habit forming.

Use with caution in patients who have respiratory, hepatic, renal dysfunction, or a history of narcotic abuse.

ADSORBENTS

bismuth subsalicylate (Pepto-Bismol)

Contraindications

- In patient with influenza or chickenpox it could mask symptoms of Reye syndrome.
- Known hypersensitivity to salicylates
- History of severe GI bleeding
- History of coagulopathy
- Known allergy to aspirin or nonaspirin salicylates

Precautions. Use with caution in patients taking medication for anticoagulation, diabetes, and gout.

Adverse Effects. These products may cause darkening of stool and tongue discoloration.

Drug Interactions. There is increased risk of toxicity with concurrent use of aspirin, warfarin, and hypoglycemics. Decreased effect is often seen with concurrent use of tetracyclines and uricosurics.

Overdosage. Salicylate toxicity symptoms include tinnitus and fever.

attapulgite (Kaopectate)

Do not use this drug if there is hypersensitivity to any component.

This agent may impair absorption of oral clindamycin, tetracyclines, penicillamines, and digoxin.

BIBLIOGRAPHY

American Gastroenterological Association medical position statement: Guidelines for the evaluation and management of chronic diarrhea, *Gastroenterology* 116:1461, 1999.

Chassany O et al: Drug-induced diarrhoea, *Drug Saf* 22:53, 2000.

Misiewicz JJ et al: *Mosby CD atlas of clinical gastroenterology,* St Louis, 1996, Mosby.

CHAPTER 31

Antiemetics

Drug Names

Class	Subclass	Generic Name	Trade Name
Antidopaminergics	Phenothiazines	(P) chlorpromazine	Thorazine
		prochlorperazine	Compazine
		promethazine	Phenergan
	Prokinetic	metoclopramide	Reglan
Anticholinergics	Antihistamines	(P) meclizine	Antivert
		dimenhydrinate	Dramamine
	Other	trimethobenzamide HCl	Tigan
		scopolamine	Transderm-Scop
Serotonin 5-HT_3 receptor antagonists		(P) ondansetron HCl	Zofran
		granisetron HCl	Kytril

(P), Prototype drug.

General Uses

Indications

- Nausea and vomiting
- Motion sickness
- Vertigo

The mechanisms of action will not be discussed in detail because drugs with similar mechanisms of action can be found in other chapters. The use of these drugs as antiemetics will be discussed in this chapter (Table 31-1).

The phenothiazine subclass of the antidopaminergic antipsychotics includes the drugs prochlorperazine and promethazine, which are used for nausea and vomiting. See Chapter 50 for a detailed discussion of the phenothiazine antipsychotics.

The anticholinergics are divided into two subclasses. The antihistamines commonly used as antiemetics are meclizine and dimenhydrinate. See Chapter 16 for a detailed discussion of antihistamines. The other subclass of anticholinergics include trimethobenzamide and scopolamine. These are similar to other anticholinergics which are discussed in detail in Chapter 32.

The serotonin 5-HT_3 receptor antagonists ondansetron and granisetron have a similar mechanism of action to tegaserod which is discussed in Chapter 32.

The prokinetic agent, metoclopramide, is also discussed in Chapter 32.

In all cases of nausea and vomiting or vertigo, the underlying cause should be established. Nausea and vomiting are symptoms. Severe nausea and vomiting may be the presenting symptoms of underlying conditions such as brain tumors, intestinal obstruction, or appendicitis, and the use of antiemetic medication may slow the diagnosis.

DISEASE PROCESS

Anatomy and Physiology

A "vomiting center" (VC) in the medulla coordinates the respiratory and vasomotor centers and the vagus nerve innervation of the GI tract. This may have four different sources of stimuli. The chemoreceptor trigger zone (CTZ) is located outside the blood-brain barrier near the vomiting center in the medulla (Table 31-2).

Pathophysiology

Normal peristalsis moves the contents of the gut forward. If the forward passage is impeded, reverse peristalsis (retroperistalsis) propels the bolus away from the obstructed segment. During the act of vomiting, retroperistalsis begins in the small intestine. The gastroduodenal junction, stomach wall, and gastroesophageal junction relax to permit passage of the bolus.

Vertigo is caused by inflammation of semicircular canals of the inner ear. Motion sickness is caused by repetitive motion, such as angular, linear, or vertical motion.

The Disease

Nausea is a vague but intensely unpleasant sensation of feeling "sick to the stomach," "queasy," or "about to vomit." This is different than the feelings of discomfort associated with anorexia. Vomiting must be distinguished from the effortless regurgitation that may accompany gastroesophageal reflux disease (GERD).

Nausea and vomiting can be caused by a wide variety of different factors. These range from benign fleeting stimuli, such as emotion, to extremely serious diseases, such as a brain tumor. Sometimes the cause is obvious, as in motion sickness or reaction to chemotherapy. On other occasions, the diagnosis may be elusive. Accurate diagnosis of the cause also determines which class of antiemetic will probably be most effective.

TABLE 31-1 Specific Indications for Antiemetics

Drug	Nausea and Vomiting from Many Causes	Nausea and Vomiting from Drugs	Motion Sickness	Vertigo
Phenothiazines		X		
meclizine			X	X
dimenhydrinate			X	
trimethobenzamide	X		X	
scopolamine			X	X
Serotonin 5-HT_3 receptor antagonists		X		

TABLE 31-2 Sources of Stimuli to the Vomiting Center

Source of Stimuli	Type of Stimulus	Receptors Involved
GI tract: afferent vagal and splanchnic fibers	Distention, irritiation, infections, obstruction, dysmotility	Vagal: serotonin 5-HT_3
Vestibular system	Motion, infections	Histamine H_1 and muscarinic cholinergic
Higher CNS centers	Increased intracranial pressure, infections, tumors, hemorrhage Psychogenic: sights, smells, emotions	Various
Chemoreceptor trigger zone (located outside the blood-brain barrier near the medulla)	Drugs such as opioids, chemotherapy, toxins, hypoxia, uremia, acidosis, and radiation therapy	Serotonin 5-HT_3 and dopamine D_2

Motion sickness causes intense nausea and mild vomiting. Patients with vertigo experience whirling or a feeling of the room spinning around. In true vertigo the patient can identify the direction the room is circling. These patients respond to the sensation with swaying, weakness, and lightheadedness. With either of these conditions the patient may experience sweating, pallor, rapid breathing, and nausea and vomiting.

DRUG ACTION AND EFFECTS

Antiemetics act on the VC in the medulla through the four different sources of stimuli input. See Table 31-2.

Antidopaminergics

Phenothiazines block dopamine receptors in the CTZ as well as other areas of the brain.

metoclopramide. Metoclopramide antagonizes the central and peripheral dopamine recptors, preventing stimulaton of CTZ.

Anticholinergics

Anticholinergics have antiemetic, anticholinergic, and antihistaminic properties. These antihistamines reduce the sensitivity of the labyrinthine apparatus. This may be mediated through nerve pathways to the VC from the CTZ, peripheral nerve pathways, or other CNS centers. These drugs have a suppressant action on hyperstimulated labyrinthine function. The precise mode of action is not known.

trimethobenzamide. The precise mechanism of action of trimethobenzamide is unknown, but it is thought to be mediated through the CTZ. However, direct impulses to the VC are not inhibited.

scopolamine. Scopolamine causes inhibition of vestibular input to the central nervous system (CNS), which results in inhibition of the vomiting reflex. Scopolamine may also have a direct action on the VC within the reticular formation of the brainstem.

Serotonin 5-HT_3 Receptor Antagonists

These are selective inhibitors of type 3 serotonin (5-HT_3) receptors that exhibit antiemetic activity. It is uncertain whether the antiemetic activity of the drug is mediated peripherally, centrally, or both; however, current data suggest that serotonin receptors play a major role in acute emesis but only a minor role in delayed nausea and vomiting.

DRUG TREATMENT PRINCIPLES

Types of vomiting can be divided into two categories: acute vomiting and anticipated vomiting precipitated by a predicted cause such as motion sickness or chemotherapy.

Acute Vomiting

Nonpharmacologic Treatment. Most causes of acute vomiting are self-limiting and require no specific treatment. The focus of treatment of acute nausea and vomiting is to replace fluids and electrolytes to prevent dehydration. General supportive treatment for nausea and vomiting consists of a diet of clear liquids and small amounts of dry foods as tolerated.

Pharmacologic Treatment. If the patient is unable to keep intake up with the fluid loss, antiemetics should be given.

Antiemetics may also be given for comfort measures if the patient is uncomfortable. If the patient is experiencing predominantly nausea, an oral antiemetic may be effective. If the patient is unable to keep down a pill, a rectal suppository may be given. Rectal suppositories are effective for short-term use for acute nausea and vomiting but will cause rectal irritation with regular use. Once the vomiting is under control, the patient may be switched to oral antiemetics to prevent recurrence of vomiting until the cause of the vomiting is resolved.

If the vomiting is not controlled, dehydration may occur with associated hypokalemia and metabolic alkalosis. These patients will need to be treated with IV medications and fluid replacement in a hospital or emergency department setting.

Anticipated Vomiting

In many situations, nausea and vomiting may be anticipated. These include motion sickness and chemotherapy. The choice of drug depends on the cause of the vomiting. In these cases, antiemetics are most effective if they are given before the emetogenic stimulus. Some chemotherapeutic agents are so emetogenic that patients may refuse further chemotherapy. Premedicating the patient may be necessary in order for the patient to receive the full therapy.

Antidopaminergics. In general, the antidopaminergic medications work most effectively in drug-induced emesis. Commonly used agents include prochlorperazine, promethazine, and metoclopramide. These agents have wide dosing ranges and may be started at the lowest dosage and increased as needed for symptom control. Metoclopramide is given IV for anticipated vomiting from chemotherapy.

Anticholinergics. Anticholinergic agents seem to be more effective in motion sickness or vertigo. Like the antidopaminergic drugs, these have wide dosing ranges allowing for dose modification for symptom control. Scopolamine is best used as the transdermal patch for motion sickness.

Serotonin 5-HT$_3$ Receptor Antagonists. For nausea and vomiting related to chemotherapy, 5-HT$_3$ serotonin receptor antagonists alone or in combination with other agents are the drugs of choice to bring about relief.

HOW TO MONITOR

Monitor for effectiveness and adverse effects.

PATIENT VARIABLES

Geriatrics

- The elderly may require dose reduction and close monitoring because of the increase in adverse effects in this population.

Pediatrics

- The use of antiemetics is discouraged in uncomplicated vomiting.
- Anticholinergics/antihistamines: can cause hallucinations, convulsions, or death; mental alertness may be diminished; can produce excitation.
- In combination with viral illnesses, there may be an increase in the risk of developing Reye syndrome.
- The dopaminergics raise the risk of extrapyramidal symptoms occurring secondary to the drugs. Children with acute illnesses such as chickenpox, influenza, and so on, are more susceptible to the neuromuscular adverse effects of these drugs than are adults.
- Do not give any antiemetic drugs to children younger than 12 years except:

  promethazine, dimenhydrinate: do not use in children younger than 2 years of age.

  ondansetron: little is known about use in children younger than 3 years of age.

Pregnancy

- None of the antiemetic drugs should be used for nausea and vomiting during pregnancy. Nursing mothers also should not use these products.

PATIENT EDUCATION

- These drugs may have sedative effects.
- Patients should not drive or operate dangerous equipment and should use caution while driving or performing other tasks that require concentration.
- Alcohol and other CNS depressants should be avoided.
- Adequate dosing before riding in a vehicle must be ensured for the prevention of motion sickness.
- The antidopaminergics may exacerbate preexisting psychiatric conditions.

Specific Drugs

ANTIDOPAMINERGICS

Phenothiazines

Ⓟ Prototype Drug

chlorpromazine hydrochloride (Thorazine)

Indications

Control of nausea and vomiting; relief of intractable hiccoughs.

Mechanism of Action

Phenothiazines block dopamine receptors in the chemoreceptor trigger zone as well as other areas of the brain.

Warnings/Precautions

Extrapyramidal reactions, such as tardive dyskinesia, may occur.

Use with caution in patients with hepatic or renal disease, glaucoma, or prostatic hypertrophy.

Adverse Effects

Sedation, dry mouth, blurred vision, mydriasis, constipation, obstipation, atonic colon, urinary retention, decreased sweating, impotence, hyperthermia, hypothermia, hypotension, tachycardia, increased pulse, syncope, dizziness, urticaria, erythema, eczema, photosensitivity.

Overdosage
Symptoms involve extrapyramidal reactions, hypotension, and sedation. CNS depression and coma with areflexia may occur. Early signs of overdose may include restlessness, confusion, and excitement. Treatment generally involves symptomatic with supportive care.

Other Drugs in Class

Other drugs in this class are similar to the prototype except as follows.

Prokinetic

metoclopramide (Reglan)

Indications. Given parenterally, prevents nausea and vomiting associated with cancer chemotherapy. Also has potential value in controlling nausea and vomiting from a variety of causes.

Mechanism of Action. Metoclopramide, like the phenothiazines, is an antidopaminergic agent that blocks the dopamine receptors in the chemoreceptor trigger zone of the brain. It is especially effective in preventing nausea and vomiting associated with cancer chemotherapy.

Warnings. May cause somnolence, nervousness, dystonic reactions, Parkinsonism, and tardive dyskinesias. May also cause increased pituitary prolactin release, galactorrhea, and menstrual disorders.

ANTICHOLINERGICS

Ⓟ Prototype Drug

meclizine (Antivert)

Meclizine has an onset of action of 30 to 60 minutes, depending on dosage. Duration of action is 4 to 6 hours to 12 to 24 hours, also depending on dosage.

Adverse Effects
See Table 31-3.

Dosage and Administration
See Table 31-4.

TABLE 31-3 Adverse Effects by Body System

Body System	Antidopaminergics	Anticholinergics: Antihistamines	Anticholinergics: tigan	Anticholinergics: scopolamine	$5\text{-}HT_3$ Receptor Antagonists
Skin, appendages		Rash, urticaria		Allergic skin reactions	Pruritus
Hypersensitivity	Hypersensitivity	Hypersensitivity	Hypersensitivity	Hypersensitivity	Hypersensitivity
Respiratory					Hypoxia, bronchospasm
Cardiovascular		Hypotension, palpitations, tachycardia	Hypotension		Hypertension, tachycardia
GI		Dry mouth, anorexia, nausea, vomiting, diarrhea, constipation	Diarrhea		Abdominal pain, constipation, diarrhea, nausea, vomiting
Hemic and lymphatic			Blood dyscrasias		Blood dyscrasias
Musculoskeletal		Muscle cramps			Musculoskeletal pain
Nervous system		Drowsiness, restlessness, excitation, nervousness, insomnia, euphoria, auditory and visual hallucinations	Parkinson-like symptoms, coma, convulsions, depression, disorientation, dizziness, drowsiness, headache	Drowsiness (15%), restlessness, disorientation, memory disturbances, dizziness, restlessness, hallucinations, confusion	Anxiety, dizziness, drowsiness, headache, malaise, fatigue, chills/shivering
Special senses		Blurred vision, diplopia, vertigo, tinnitus	Blurred vision	Blurred vision, dilation of pupils	
Hepatic			Jaundice		↑ ALT, AST
Genitourinary		Urinary frequency, difficult urination, urinary retention			Urinary retention
Other		Dry nose and throat		Dry mouth (67%)	Fever

TABLE 31-4 Dosage and Administration Recommendations for Antiemetics

Drug	Age Group	Dosage	Administration	Maximum Daily Dose
chlorpromazine	Adult	10-25 mg PO 50-100 mg PR	q4-6 hr q6-8 hr	
	Child	0.55 mg/kg PO 1.1 mg/kg PR	q4-6 hr q6-8 hr	
prochlorperazine	Adult	5 mg PO	q6 hr	15 mg
promethazine	Adult	25 mg PO	bid take 30 min before travel	
	Child	0.25-0.5 mg/kg	q4-6 hr	
dimenhydrinate	Adult	50-100 mg	q4-6 hr	400 mg
	Child 6-12 yr	25-50 mg	q6-8 hr	150 mg
	Child 2-6 yr	12.5-25 mg	q6-8 hr	75 mg
trimethobenzamide	Adult	250 mg PO 200 mg PR	tid-qid tid-qid	
	Child (30-90 lb)	100-200 PO mg 100-200 PR mg	tid-qid tid-qid	
scopolamine	Adult	1.5 mg/patch	Apply patch behind ear, change q3d	
ondansetron	Adult >12 yr	8 mg PO	bid, 1 hr before chemotherapy	
	Child 4-11 yr	4 mg PO	q4 hr × 3, 30 min before chemotherapy	
granisetron	Adult	2 mg PO	qd or 1 mg q12 hr, 1 hr before chemotherapy	

Other Drugs in Class

Other drugs in this class are similar to the prototype except as follows.

scopolamine (Transderm-Scop)

The transdermal system allows for reaching steady state plasma levels rapidly and maintains steady state for 3 days. Onset of action is approximately 4 hours.

SEROTONIN 5-HT$_3$ RECEPTOR ANTAGONISTS

(P) Prototype Drug

ondansetron hydrochloride (Zofran)

Contraindications

- Hypersensitivity to the drug (rare but sometimes severe with IV use)

Warnings

- Does not stimulate intestinal or gastric peristalsis. Not to be used instead of nasogastric suction.
- Patients should be informed to stop drug if rash develops.
- Use may mask progressive ileus and/or gastric distention in patients undergoing abdominal surgery.
- In patients with severe hepatic impairment, dosage should be reduced and used with caution. The manufacturer recommends that the total daily dose not exceed 8 mg in patients with severe hepatic impairment.

Pharmacokinetics

Half-life is 1.5 hours.

Adverse Effects

See Table 31-3.

Drug Interactions

Rifampin will decrease the levels of ondansetron.

Overdosage

Hypotension, faintness, and short episodes of blindness have been seen.

BIBLIOGRAPHY

American Gastroenterological Association Medical Position Statement: Nausea and vomiting, *Gastroenterology* 120:261, 2001.

Chen JJ et al: Efficacy of ondansetron and prochlorperazine for the prevention of postoperative nausea and vomiting after total hip replacement or total knee replacement procedures: a randomized, double-blind comparative trial, *Arch Intern Med* 158(9):2124, 1998.

Feyer P et al: Radiotherapy-induced emesis: an overview, *Strahlenther Onkol* 174 (suppl 3):56, 1998.

CHAPTER 32

Other Gastrointestinal Agents

Drug Names

Class	Subclass	Generic Name	Trade Name
IBS treatment	Antispasmodics/anticholinergics	(P) dicyclomine hydrochloride	Bentyl
		hyoscyamine sulfate	Levsin, NuLev
	5-HT_4 Receptor agonist	tegaserod maleate	Zelnorm
GI stimulants/prokinetic agents		metoclopramide	Reglan
Prostaglandin		misoprostol	Cytotec
Ulcerative colitis treatment		mesalamine	Asacol
		sulfasalazine	Azulfidine
Locally acting agent		simethicone	Phazyme, Gas-X
Gallstone-solubilizing agent		ursodiol	Actigall

(P), Prototype drug.

General Uses

Indications

See Table 32-1.

This chapter discusses many diverse classes of medications; the only thing they have in common is that they are used for GI conditions. Each class is discussed separately. The disease that is discussed in this chapter is irritable bowel syndrome (IBS).

Irritable Bowel Syndrome

Antispasmodic agents (e.g., dicyclomine hydrochloride [Bentyl], hyoscyamine sulfate [Levsin]) are used primarily to treat IBS and other functional GI disorders. There are a large number of antispasmodics on the market, but they are not often used. Only the two most common antispasmodic drugs will be discussed in this chapter. Dicyclomine will be used as the prototype.

Tegaserod maleate (Zelnorm), a new drug in the 5-HT_4 receptor agonist subclass, is used exclusively to treat IBS in women.

DISEASE PROCESS

Pathophysiology

Pathophysiology of IBS is not fully understood, but bowel motility is affected. Normal bowel motility has segmenting contractions to slow the transit through the bowel. If these are increased, constipation results. If they are decreased, frequent loose stools result. External factors include stress, psychologic factors, abuse, food intolerance, and menstruation.

The Disease

IBS is a common chronic functional bowel disorder. Other names for IBS are spastic colitis, mucous colitis, nervous colitis, spastic colon, nervous colon, irritated colon, or unstable colon. Functional bowel disorders are composed of combinations of chronic or recurrent GI symptoms not explained by structural or biochemical abnormalities. Generally the diagnosis is a clinical one based on a cluster of symptoms with the exclusion of a specific organic cause. Diagnostic criteria have been developed to make the diagnosis of IBS more consistent. The history of the patient is critical for diagnosis of IBS. Common symptoms are abdominal pain, altered bowel frequency and stool consistency (often alternating diarrhea and constipation), abdominal distention or bloating, and varying degrees of anxiety or depression. The pain is described as sharp, burning, or cramping. The location is usually diffuse. A careful history is necessary to determine what the patient means by such words as “diarrhea,” “constipation,” and “regular.” Nocturnal diarrhea may indicate a more serious problem.

DRUG ACTION AND EFFECTS

Antispasmodic/anticholinergic agents are also known as antimuscarinic drugs. The muscarinic nervous system is a subcategory of the anticholinergic nervous system. The other subcategory, the nicotinic nervous system is seldom involved in pharmacology. Anticholinergic agents decrease motility, relax smooth muscle tone in the GI tract, and decrease secretions.

Antispasmodics decrease GI motility by relaxing smooth muscle tone. These medications have anticholinergic properties, thus they compete with acetylcholine for receptors at postganglionic fibers of the parasympathetic nervous system.

Dicyclomine has indirect and direct effects on the smooth muscle of the GI tract. It indirectly blocks the acetylcholine-

TABLE 32-1 Indications for Use of Miscellaneous GI Drugs

Drug Category	Individual Drugs	Indications
Antispasmodics/anticholinergics	dicyclomine, hyoscyamine	IBS, PUD, hypermotility disorders, ulcerative colitis, diverticulitis
IBS management	tegaserod	IBS with constipation
GI stimulants/prokinetic agents	metoclopramide	Diabetic gastroparesis, severe GERD
Prostaglandins	misoprostol	Reduce risk of NSAID PUD
Ulcerative colitis treatment	mesalamine	Ulcerative colitis
	sulfasalazine	Ulcerative colitis, RA, JRA
Locally acting agents	simethicone	Flatulence
Gallstone-solubilizing agents	ursodiol	Gallstones

GERD, Gastroesophageal reflux disease; *IBS,* irritable bowel syndrome; *JRA,* juvenile rheumatoid arthritis; *PUD,* peptic ulcer disease; *RA,* rheumatoid arthritis.

receptor sites and directly antagonizes bradykinin and histamine in GI tract smooth muscle. Both of these actions help relieve smooth muscle spasm.

Hyoscyamine, a belladonna alkaloid, inhibits the muscarinic actions of acetylcholine at postganglionic parasympathetic neuroeffector sites, including smooth muscle, secretory glands, and CNS sites. Thus this drug has an effect on peripheral cholinergic receptors present in the smooth muscle of the GI tract. Specific anticholinergic responses are dose related. Low doses inhibit salivary and bronchial secretions and sweating. Next, pupil dilation and accommodation are affected, and heart rate is increased. Higher doses decrease motility of GI and urinary tracts, and then inhibit gastric acid.

Tegaserod is a 5-HT_4 receptor partial agonist. It stimulates the peristaltic reflex and intestinal secretion and inhibits visceral sensitivity to normalize impaired motility in the GI tract.

DRUG TREATMENT PRINCIPLES

Nonpharmacologic Treatment

Treatment of IBS begins with patient education. The patient must be reassured there is no organic cause for the symptoms. Teach that this is a chronic condition that will not lead to an organic problem.

Diet is the cornerstone of treatment. The amounts of fiber and fluid usually need to be increased. Fiber should be increased gradually to avoid bloating. (See Chapter 29 for a list of high-fiber foods.) The patient should drink six to eight glasses of water a day. The patient should identify and eliminate foods that cause symptoms. Foods that commonly cause problems include brown beans, brussels sprouts, cabbage, cauliflower, raw onions, grapes, plums, raisins, coffee, red wine, beer, and caffeine. Exclude lactose intolerance.

Other important lifestyle changes include good bowel habits and exercise. See Chapter 29 for a discussion of bowel training. The best exercise is usually regular walking.

Pharmacologic Treatment

The first medications used are usually bulk-forming laxatives. Given with adequate fluid, these regulate the bowels and decrease both the diarrhea and constipation of IBS. If a patient's problem is not controlled by the preceding measures, specific drugs to treat the condition may be required. (See Chapters 29 and 30 for additional treatment options.)

If the patient has problems with gas, including explosive bowel movements, belching, or flatus, simethicone may be used.

If the preceding treatment is not effective, antispasmodics may be added to the regimen. These are often helpful for the cramping abdominal pain. They are particularly useful for short-term treatment of exacerbations of IBS caused by external stress.

Tegaserod is used for short-term treatment of women with IBS whose primary symptom is constipation.

HOW TO MONITOR

Monitor for therapeutic response: The patient should be able to report fewer episodes of abdominal cramping and less diarrhea and constipation.

Monitor for anticholinergic effects: Evaluate for increased heart rate and blood pressure, dry mouth, constipation, blurred vision, or urinary retention.

PATIENT VARIABLES

Geriatrics

Lower doses of antispasmodics should be prescribed to geriatric patients because this population may react with increased adverse effects such as agitation or excitement.

Pediatrics

Safety and efficacy are not established. Hyoscyamine has been used in infant colic. Dicyclomine is contraindicated in infants younger than 6 months of age.

Pregnancy

- *Category B:* dicyclomine, tegaserod
- *Category C:* hyoscyamine
- It is not known whether tegaserod is excreted in milk.

Gender

The safety and efficacy of tegaserod has not been established in men.

PATIENT EDUCATION

Antispasmodics

- Refrain from activities that require mental alertness while taking these medications.
- Stay out of hot and humid environments while taking these medications.
- Take 30 to 60 minutes before a meal.
- Notify physician of side effects, especially eye pain, rash, or flushing.
- Gum or sugarless hard candy may relieve dry mouth.

Specific Drugs

ANTISPASMODICS/ANTICHOLINERGICS

(P) Prototype Drug

dicyclomine hydrochloride (Bentyl)

Contraindications

- Hypersensitivity
- Glaucoma
- Cardiovascular: tachycardia, unstable cardiovascular status in hemorrhage, myocardial infarction (MI)
- GI tract obstructive disease (pyloroduodenal stenosis, etc.), paralytic ileus, severe ulcerative colitis, and hepatic disease
- Myasthenia gravis
- Genitourinary (GU): obstructive uropathy, caused by prostate hypertrophy; renal disease

Warnings

! Heat prostration potential with extremely high temperatures. These drugs can cause a reduction in sweating, which can predispose a patient to heatstroke and fever.

Use with caution when patients have diarrhea. Diarrhea may be an early sign of incomplete bowel obstruction. Patients who are sensitive to anticholinergic drugs may exhibit signs of psychosis.

Precautions

Use with caution in the following:

- Cardiovascular: CAD, CHF, arrhythmias, tachycardia, HTN
- GI: hepatic disease; early evidence of ileus, hiatal hernia associated with reflux esophagitis (may aggravate)
- GU: renal disease; prostatic hypertrophy.
- Ocular; glaucoma
- Pulmonary: COPD reduces bronchial secretions; asthma, allergies
- May contain tartrazine, sulfites

Pharmacokinetics

Compared with the belladonna alkaloids (hyoscyamine) dicyclomine is poorly and unreliably absorbed orally. It does not cross the blood-brain barrier; therefore CNS and ophthalmic effects are less likely. The duration of action is more prolonged than the belladonna alkaloids.

Adverse Effects

Dry mouth, dizziness, blurred vision, nausea, lightheadedness, drowsiness, weakness, nervousness, urinary hesitancy and retention, tachycardia, palpitations, mydriasis, cycloplegia, increased ocular pressure, loss of taste, headache, insomnia, nausea, vomiting, impotence, constipation, and bloated feeling.

Drug Interactions

The anticholinergics increase the pharmacologic effects of digoxin and atenolol and decrease the effects of phenothiazine. Amantidine, phenothiazines, and TCAs increase the side effects of the anticholinergics.

They may decrease or antagonize effects of medications used to treat glaucoma. Antacids may decrease absorption of anticholinergics.

Dosage and Administration

- Adult: 20 to 40 mg qid ac and qhs
- Geriatric: start with 10 mg bid to qid; increase slowly as tolerated

Other Drugs in Class

Other drugs in this class are similar to the prototype except as follows.

hyoscyamine sulfate (Levsin)

Hyoscyamine is a belladonna alkaloid, unlike dicyclomine. It is rapidly absorbed. It readily crosses the blood-brain barrier and affects CNS. Thus is has a greater risk of CNS adverse effects than dicyclomine.

Dosages: *adult* 0.125 to 0.25 mg tid to qid; *geriatric* 0.125 mg ½ tablet bid to qid

tegaserod maleate (Zelnorm)

Mechanism of Action. Tegaserod is a 5-HT_4 receptor partial agonist. It has a high affinity for 5-HT_4, with little affinity for 5-HT_1, 5-HT_3 or dopamine receptors. As an agonist, it triggers further release of neurotransmitters such as calcitonin. 5-HT_4 receptors in the GI tract stimulate the peristaltic reflex and intestinal secretion and inhibit visceral sensitivity. It normalizes impaired motility and moderates visceral sensitivity.

Contraindications

- Hypersensitivity
- Severe renal impairment
- Moderate or severe hepatic impairment
- History of bowel obstruction
- Symptomatic gallbladder disease
- Suspected sphincter of Oddi dysfunction
- Abdominal adhesions

Warnings

- Carcinogenesis: produces hyperplasia in mice
- Pregnancy: *Category B*

- Lactation: not known if it is secreted in breast milk
- Children: safety and efficacy have not been established in children younger than 18 years of age

Precautions

- Diarrhea: do not start treatment in patients who are currently experiencing or frequently experience diarrhea.
- Increased abdominal surgeries have been noted, but a causal relationship has not been established.

Pharmacokinetics. Bioavailability is 10%. Peak plasma concentrations are reached 1 hour after dosing. It is 98% protein bound. Metabolized by hydrolysis in the stomach and conjugation to a metabolite. Half-life 11 hours after IV dosing Most is excreted unchanged in the urine; the rest is excreted in urine as metabolites.

Adverse Effects

- Nausea, abdominal pain, diarrhea, nausea, and headache

Drug Interactions

- Tegaserod decreased effectiveness of digoxin and oral contraceptives
- Bioavailability is decreased with food

Dosage and Administration. Give 6 mg bid 30 min before meals for 4 to 6 weeks. If effective, an additional 3- to 6-week course may be considered. Has not been studied beyond 12 weeks.

GI STIMULANTS/PROKINETIC AGENTS

metoclopramide (Reglan)

Cisapride (Propulsid), a related drug, has been removed from primary care because of the risk for serious adverse reactions and potentially fatal drug interactions.

Indications

- Diabetic gastroparesis; severe GERD unresponsive to standard therapy

! Although very effective, this drug has the potential for very serious adverse reactions.

Drug Action and Effects. Metoclopramide stimulates the upper GI tract. Although the exact mode of action is unclear, it appears to increase the responsiveness of the tissues in the GI tract to acetylcholine. Metoclopramide increases the tone and amplitude of gastric contractions and relaxes the pyloric sphincter and duodenal bulb. This drug has also been shown to accelerate gastric emptying by increasing peristalsis of the duodenum and jejunum. Increased resting tone of the lower esophageal sphincter has also been shown to be an action of metoclopramide. Its antiemetic properties are related to metoclopramide's antagonism of the central and peripheral dopamine receptors.

How to Monitor. The patient should be monitored during the first 24 to 48 hours for any adverse reactions. Should extrapyramidal symptoms (EPS) occur, treat with diphenhydramine (Benadryl IM) or benztropine (Cogentin IM). Should parkinsonian symptoms occur (usually within the first 6 months), discontinue use of metoclopramide. Stop the medication if the patient develops tardive dyskinesia.

Patient Variables

Geriatrics

- Older patients may have a slight decrease in elimination of these drugs.

Patients are at increased risk for adverse effects such as confusion and extrapyramidal symptoms. Use with caution.

Pediatrics. Safety and effectiveness of these drugs are not established, and thus use of them is not recommended. Metoclopramide has been used in infants and children for symptomatic GERD. Methemoglobinemia has occurred. Infants and children ages 21 days to 3.3 years with GERD have been treated with metoclopromide at dosage of 0.5 mg/kg/day; symptoms improved.

Pregnancy

- *Category B:* no adequate studies; metoclopramide crosses the placenta and is excreted into breast milk.

Patient Education

- Do not drink alcohol while taking this drug.
- Do not operate heavy equipment or drive a vehicle for at least 2 hours after taking this medication because of the risk of sedation and drowsiness.
- Inform health care provider of the occurrence of any involuntary movements or twitching.

Contraindications

- Hypersensitivity to the drug or to sulfonamides
- When stimulation of GI motility might be dangerous such as GI hemorrhage, obstruction, or perforation
- Pheochromocytoma: may cause a hypertensive crisis
- Epilepsy: people receiving drugs are likely to experience extrapyramidal reactions

Warnings

- Depression: with suicidal ideation, has occurred in patients with and without prior history of depression

! EPS manifested as acute dystonic reactions may occur, usually within the first 24 to 48 hours; seen more frequently in children and young adults, and in geriatric patients.

- Parkinson-like symptoms occur with in the first 6 months of treatment; use with caution in patients with Parkinson's disease

- Tardive dyskinesia, a syndrome of potentially irreversible, involuntary, dyskinetic movements, may develop. Highest likelihood is among the elderly.
- Hypertension has occurred in patients.
- Anastomosis or closure of the gut. Metoclopramide theoretically increases pressure on suture lines.
- Elevated prolactin levels persist during chronic administration.

Precautions
- Hypoglycemia in diabetics
- Use caution in hazardous tasks

Adverse Effects. Common mild side effects in 20% to 30% of patients include restlessness, anxiety, drowsiness, fatigue, lassitude, insomnia, headache, dizziness, sedation, nausea, diarrhea, rash, decreased libido, bowel disturbances, and fever.

Potentially serious adverse reactions include EPS, tardive dyskinesia, dystonic reactions, akathisia, prolactin secretion, hypo-/hypertension, depression with suicidal ideation, seizures, and hallucinations.

Drug Interactions. Drug interactions are a common problem. Metoclopramide may decrease the levels of digoxin and cimetidine. It may increase the levels of alcohol, cyclosporine, monoamine oxidase inhibitors (MAOIs), succinylcholine, and levodopa. Levodopa, anticholinergics, and narcotic analgesics decrease the effect of metoclopramide. There may be an increased risk of extrapyramidal reactions when phenothiazine and butyrophenone antipsychotics are given with metoclopramide.

There may be increased CNS depression when metoclopramide is given concurrently with antihypertensives, alcohol, sedatives, and tricyclic antidepressants.

Dosage and Administration
- For gastroesophageal reflux: 10 to 15 ml po qid, 30 minutes before each meal and at bedtime
- For diabetic gastroparesis: 10 mg qid, 30 minutes before meals and at bedtime

Overdosage. Symptoms of metoclopramide overdose include drowsiness, disorientation, and extrapyramidal reaction and are usually self-limiting (disappear after about 24 hours).

PROSTAGLANDINS

misoprostol (Cytotec)

General Uses. Misoprostol is used with an NSAID to decrease incidence of gastric side effects.

Drug Action and Effects. Misoprostol is a synthetic prostaglandin, similar in action to natural substances produced by the body. Unlike H_2 blockers and acid pump inhibitors, this protective agent does not inhibit the release of acid. Misoprostol shields the stomach's mucous lining from the damage of acid by increasing mucus and bicarbonate production and by enhancing blood flow to the stomach. NSAIDs cause ulceration by blocking prostaglandin synthesis that, in turn, decreases bicarbonate and mucus production. Misoprostol binds with prostaglandin receptor sites, thus causing the increased production of bicarbonate and mucus. Prostaglandin receptor sites are saturable, reversible, and stereospecific. These sites have a high affinity for misoprostol.

How to Monitor
- Ask patient specifically about diarrhea at follow-up visits.
- Check stool for occult blood.
- If patient is of childbearing age, administer pregnancy test before starting drug.

Patient Education
- Do not take if pregnant or planning to become pregnant. Make it clear to female patients who are in their child-bearing years that pregnant women taking misoprostol may experience a miscarriage. They also may experience life-threatening bleeding as a result of the miscarriage.
- Emphasize the importance of not giving this drug to anyone else.
- Take drug with food to minimize risk of GI side effects.

Contraindications

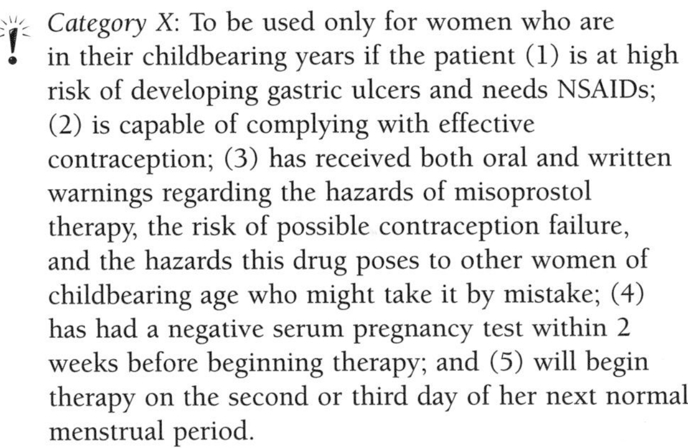

Category X: To be used only for women who are in their childbearing years if the patient (1) is at high risk of developing gastric ulcers and needs NSAIDs; (2) is capable of complying with effective contraception; (3) has received both oral and written warnings regarding the hazards of misoprostol therapy, the risk of possible contraception failure, and the hazards this drug poses to other women of childbearing age who might take it by mistake; (4) has had a negative serum pregnancy test within 2 weeks before beginning therapy; and (5) will begin therapy on the second or third day of her next normal menstrual period.

- Avoid if patient has allergy to any prostaglandins.

Warnings/Precautions. The safety and efficacy in children has not been established.

Adverse Effects. The most common adverse effects are diarrhea, abdominal pain, nausea, flatulence, headache, dyspepsia, vomiting, constipation, vaginal spotting, uterine cramps, hypermenorrhea, and dysmenorrhea.

Drug Interactions. Concomitant use with antacids may decrease plasma concentration levels of misoprostol.

Dosage and Administration. Usual recommended dose 200 µg qid. It is often necessary to start at 100 µg bid and slowly increase dose to avoid excessive diarrhea.

ULCERATIVE COLITIS DRUGS

sulfasalazine and mesalamine

Mechanism of Action. Sulfasalazine is split into sulfapyridine and mesalamine (5-ASA) by bacteria in the colon. Mesalamine is thought to be the active component. Mesalamine is an aminosalicylate. The mechanism of action of sulfasalazine and mesalamine is unknown. It is thought to be topical rather than systemic. They act by blocking cyclooxygenase and inhibiting prostaglandin production in the colon.

Contraindications
- Hypersensitivity to mesalamine, salicylates, or any component of the formulation

Warnings
- Intolerance/colitis exacerbation: acute intolerance syndrome may occur with cramping, acute abdominal pain, and bloody diarrhea.
- Pancolitis: some patients have developed pancolitis although it occurred less often with mesalamine then with placebo.
- Renal function impairment: has occurred. Use caution with patients with renal impairment.
- Pregnancy: *Category B*; no adequate studies.
- Lactation: low concentrations of mesalamine have been detected.
- Safety and efficacy for use in children have not been established.

Precautions
- Pericarditis has occurred rarely with sulfasalazine; investigate chest pain
- Sulfite sensitivity

Pharmacokinetics
- Sulfasalazine is not absorbed; it acts locally. Mesalamine is absorbed.

Adverse Effects. Well tolerated. Most effects are mild and transient. Most common are headache, abdominal pain/cramps/discomfort, eructation, diarrhea, constipation, and nausea. Rare are chest pain, anxiety, confusion, and agranulocytosis. Capsules have fewer adverse reactions than tablets. Elevated levels of AST<ALT, alk phos creatinine, BUN, amylase, lipase, GGTP, and LDH. Hepatitis rarely occurs.

Drug Interactions. There are no known drug interactions.

Dosage and Administration
- 1 g capsules qid for a total dose of 4 g for up to 8 weeks
- Tablets 800 tid for a total dose of 2 to 4 g/day for 6 weeks
- Suppositories and suspension for rectal instillation are also available
- Swallow tablets whole
- Shake suspension well before inserting into rectum

Overdosage. Symptoms of salicylate toxicity may be possible, such as tinnitus, vertigo, headache, confusion, drowsiness, sweating, hyperventilation, vomiting, and diarrhea.

LOCALLY ACTING AGENTS

simethicone (Phazyme, Gas-X)

The antiflatulent agent simethicone is used to help relieve painful symptoms of trapped air and gas in the GI tract. An overproduction of gas may occur when eating certain foods or swallowing air in the process of eating or chewing. This medication is OTC.

Mechanism of Action. Simethicone is a defoaming agent and thus acts by altering the surface tension of gas bubbles trapped in the GI tract. This action causes the gas bubbles to coalesce and the trapped gas to be expelled through belching or rectal flatus.

Contraindications
- Hypersensitivity to simethicone

Adverse Effects
- Excessive episodes of belching and rectal flatus

Patient Education
- Do not take this medication indiscriminately.
- Patients should report any symptoms that persist to the health care provider.

Dosage and Administration
- Ages 12 years and up: 40 to 125 mg after each meal and qhs
- Children (ages 2 to 12 years): 0.6 ml qid after meals and qhs
- Infants (younger than age 2 years): 0.3 ml qid after meals and qhs

GALLSTONE-SOLUBILIZING AGENTS

ursodiol (Ursodeoxycholic Acid) (Actigall)

General Uses. Ursodiol is used to dissolve radiolucent non-calcified gallstones in those patients who either refuse surgery or are poor surgical risks. Ursodiol is also used to prevent stone formation in those undergoing rapid weight loss after gastric bypass surgery or from low-calorie diets. A functional gallbladder is needed for the drug to be used.

Drug Action and Effects. Ursodiol is a naturally occurring bile acid that suppresses hepatic synthesis and cholesterol secretion and inhibits intestinal absorption of cholesterol. This increases the concentration level at which saturation of cholesterol occurs. The bile changes from cholesterol precipitating to cholesterol solubilizing.

How to Monitor
- Monitor for fever, pain, and jaundice.
- Monitor for an acute condition in the abdomen that can occur if stones move and block the common bile duct.
- In weight-loss patients, monitor for nausea.
- Check baseline LFTs and monitor periodically.

Patient Variables

Pediatrics
- Safety and usage in children have not been established.

Pregnancy
- *Category B:* it is not known if ursodiol is excreted in breast milk; use with caution if administered to a nursing mother.

Patient Education
- Therapy is continued for at least 3 months after apparent dissolution.
- If there is no dissolution after 12 months, surgery may be necessary. As long as there is progress toward dissolution, the drug may be continued.

Contraindications. Patients with stones larger than 20 mm, acute condition in the abdomen, known sensitivity to the drug, acute pancreatic gallstones, or acute cholecystitis are not candidates for the drug.

Warnings. Bile-sequestering agents and aluminum-based antacids may reduce absorption. Oral contraceptives, estrogens, and clofibrate increase cholesterol secretion in the liver and may counteract the effectiveness of ursodiol.

Adverse Effects. Diarrhea, pruritus, rash, dry skin, stomatitis, flatulence, headache, fatigue, myalgia, and rhinitis are reported adverse effects.

Dosage and Administration. Dosage is 8 to 10 mg/kg/day twice a day; in rapid weight loss, 300 mg twice a day. Some health care providers recommend 300 mg at bedtime.

BIBLIOGRAPHY

Barkin JS, Rogers AI: *Difficult decisions in digestive diseases,* ed 2, St Louis, 1994, Mosby.

Drossman DA, Rome II: *The functional gastrointestinal disorders,* ed 2, New York, 2002, Degnon.

Hann LR, Sorrells SC, Harding JP, et al: Additional investigations fail to alter the diagnosis of IBS in subjects fulfilling the Rome criteria, *Am J Gastroenterol,* 94:1279-1282, 1999.

Kantsevoy S, Margolois S: *The Johns Hopkins white papers: digestive disorders,* Baltimore, 2002, Rebus.

Kowdley KV: Update on therapy for hepatobiliary diseases, *Nurse Pract* 21(7):78-88, 1996.

UNIT 8

Renal/Genitourinary Agents

The renal system plays a major role in the excretion of drugs and in the maintenance of body health and integrity. Attention to the use of diuretics in the treatment of hypertension dwindled in past years as new products entered the market. The last few years have seen a resurgence of interest in diuretics, which remain the mainstay of hypertensive treatment.

Other new products for the treatment of a variety of GU problems have entered the market and are discussed in detail.

- **Chapter 33** discusses the physiology behind why diuretics may be effective in reducing hypertension, CHF, and renal failure. The physiology comprises a foundational understanding of the actions of different diuretics. Both the advantages and disadvantages of diuretic use are described and represent mandatory information for clinicians.
- **Chapter 34** covers male genitourinary agents. This is a small but important group of medications, representing drugs for benign prostatic hypertrophy and new drugs for erectile dysfunction.
- **Chapter 35** outlines other renal/genitourinary agents, focusing on the management of urinary incontinence and other urinary problems.

CHAPTER 33

Diuretics

Sandra L. Cotton and Karen MacKay

Drug Names

Class	Subclass		Generic Name	Trade Name
Diuretics	Carbonic anhydrase inhibitors		acetazolamide	Diamox, Diamox Sequels
	Loop (Na-K-2Cl inhibitors)	(P)(200)	furosemide	Lasix
			bumetanide	Bumex
			ethacrynic acid	Edecrin
			torsemide	Demadex
	Thiazides and thiazide-like (NaCl inhibitors)	(P)(200)	hydrochlorothiazide	HydroDIURIL, Esidrix, Oretic
			chlorothiazide	Diuril
			chlorthalidone	Hygroton
			indapamide	Lozol
			metolazone	Zaroxolyn
Potassium-sparing diuretics	Na channel blockers	(P)(200)	triamterene	Dyrenium
			amiloride	Midamor
	Aldosterone antagonists		spironolactone	Aldactone
Fixed-dose combination therapies			hydrochlorothiazide/amiloride	Moduretic
		(200)	hydrochlorothiazide/spironolactone	Aldactazide, Spirozide, spironolactone
			hydrochlorothiazide/triamterene	Dyazide, Maxzide
Potassium supplements			potassium chloride	Kaon-Cl, K-Dur, K-Lor, K-Tab, Micro-K, Slow K

(200), Top 200 drug; (P), prototype drug.

Diuretics, Potassium-Sparing Diuretics, and Combination Therapies

General Uses

Indications

- Hypertension
- Chronic heart failure
- Renal failure
- Cirrhosis

The four major classes of diuretics (Table 33-1) act by decreasing sodium (Na) reabsorption at different sites along the nephron. The four classes differ by the specific site of action in the nephron. The ability to augment urinary losses of Na and water is useful in a variety of clinical situations, including hypertension, congestive heart failure, renal failure, and cirrhosis. There are a large number of thiazide diuretics; only the five most commonly used are discussed. The use of potassium supplementation is discussed separately at the end of the chapter.

DRUG ACTION AND EFFECTS

Sodium (Na), chloride (Cl), and water are freely filtered across the glomerulus. Under normal circumstances more than 99% of these substances are reabsorbed along the renal tubule. This requires the renal tubules to reclaim nearly 3 lb of sodium chloride each day. The reabsorption of Na is, in general, an active transcellular process. By contrast, chloride reabsorption may be passive or active, but is most commonly coupled to Na reabsorption, which explains the parallel reabsorption of these two ions. Water reabsorption occurs by diffusion, which is driven by solute, particularly Na, reabsorption.

The first step of Na and water reabsorption at each site involves the transport of Na from the tubular lumen into tubular epithelial cells. It is this first step that is inhibited by diuretics. Each segment of the nephron contains different luminal transport proteins or channels that facilitate the entry of filtered Na into the cell. These transport systems are predominantly inhibited by only certain types of diuretics. It is this specificity that determines the diuretic's site of action. Once Na has entered the tubular cells it is pumped out of the other side of the cell by a sodium-potassium exchanger into the interstitial fluid, from where it may be returned to the circulation.

The sites of action of the different types of diuretics are outlined in Figure 33-1 and Table 33-1. The ability of each type of diuretic to increase urinary Na excretion depends on two factors: the amount of Na reabsorbed at its site of action and the ability of more distal sites to reclaim that Na. The carbonic anhydrase inhibitors act on the proximal tubule. These drugs have limited clinical utility as diuretics because Na lost at this site is effectively reclaimed at more distal sites along the nephron. Loop diuretics are the most potent diuretics. They act in the ascending limb of

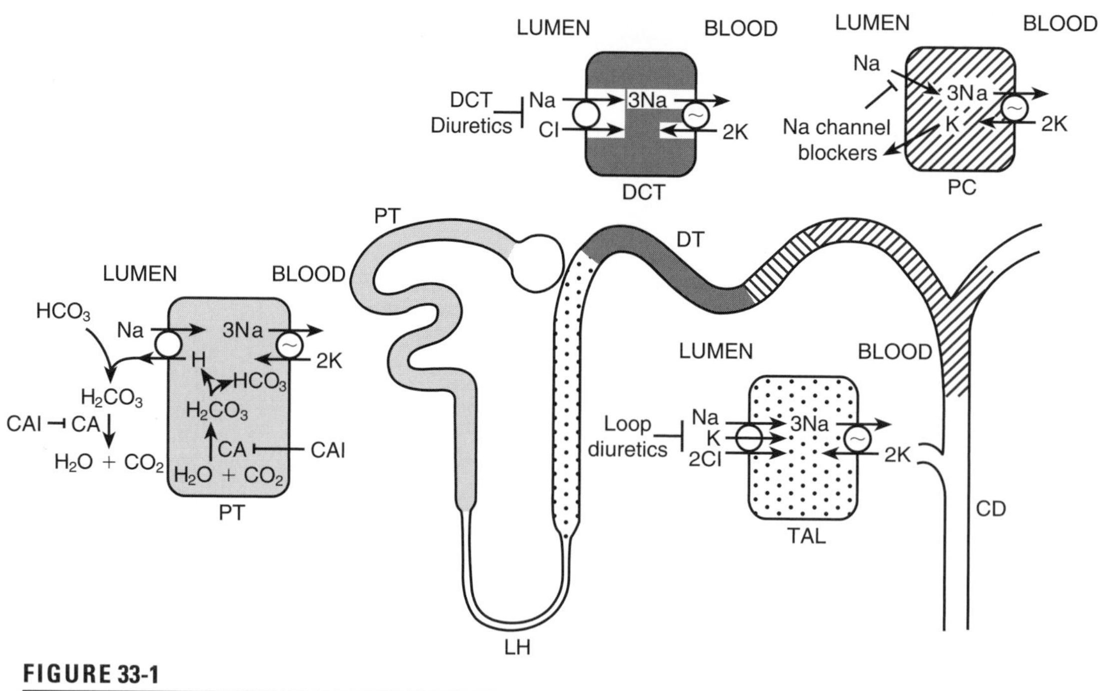

FIGURE 33-1

Sites and mechanisms of diuretic drugs. *PT,* Proximal tubule; *LH,* loop of Henle; *TAL,* thick ascending limb; *DT,* distal tubule; *DCT,* distal convoluted tubule; *CD,* collecting duct; *PC,* principal cell; *CA,* carbonic anhydrase; *CAI,* carbonic anhydrase inhibitor; ~, indicates primary active transport. Spironolactone (not shown) is a competitive aldosterone antagonist and acts primarily in the collecting duct. (From Ellison DH: The physiologic basis of diuretic synergism: its role in treating diuretic resistance, *Ann Intern Med* 114(10):887, 1991.)

TABLE 33-1 Classification of Diuretics

Proximal Tubule *Carbonic Anhydrase Inhibitors*	Loop of Henle *Na-K-2Cl Inhibitors*	Distal Convoluted Tubule *NaCl Inhibitors*	Collecting Tubule *Na Channel Blockers* and Aldosterone Antagonists
acetazolamide (Diamox)	furosemide (Lasix) bumetanide (Bumex) ethacrynic acid (Edecrin) torsemide (Demadex)	hydrochlorothiazide (HCTZ) metolazone (Zaroxolyn) chlorthalidone (Hygroton) indapamide (Lozol)	triamterene (Dyrenium) amiloride (Midamor) spironolactone (Aldactone)

Modified from Ellison DH: In-depth review: diuretic drugs and the treatment of edema: from clinic to bench and back again, *Am J Kidney Dis* 23(5):627, 1994.

the loop of Henle, where 25% of Na is normally reclaimed. The thiazide diuretics act on the distal tubule, where 5% to 10% of Na is normally reclaimed. The collecting duct is the site of action of the potassium-sparing diuretics. Normally only 3% to 5% of Na is reabsorbed at this site. These drugs, as their group name implies, limit the urinary losses of potassium.

Carbonic Anhydrase Inhibitors

Approximately 50% to 75% of filtered Na is reabsorbed in the proximal tubule. An important Na transport pathway at this site is the sodium/hydrogen (Na/H) exchanger that is located in the luminal membrane of proximal tubular cells (see Figure 33-1). An important factor in maintaining Na/H exchange is the removal of hydrogen ions from the tubular lumen. If hydrogen ions accumulate, then the activity of the Na/H exchanger is slowed. Carbonic anhydrase facilitates the removal of luminal hydrogen ions by promoting the dissociation of carbonic acid, H_2CO_3, (formed by the association of filtered bicarbonate with the hydrogen ions secreted into the tubular lumen by the Na/H exchanger) to yield carbon dioxide and water. This process of carbonic acid formation and dissociation maintains low luminal hydrogen ion levels and thus allows the Na/H exchanger to continue to reabsorb Na. If carbonic anhydrase is inhibited, luminal hydrogen ion concentrations rise and the activity of the Na/H exchanger is inhibited. The carbonic anhydrase inhibitors are relatively weak diuretics because of the ability of more distal sites to increase their reabsorption of Na.

An important consequence of carbonic anhydrase inhibition is its interference with bicarbonate reabsorption (see Figure 33-1). The distal nephron sites are not able to reclaim all of this additional bicarbonate and, as a result, bicarbonate is lost into the urine. This loss of bicarbonate can be an advantage in the treatment of individuals with severe metabolic alkalosis where this bicarbonate loss can limit alkalemia. However, loss of urinary bicarbonate can also lead to severe metabolic acidosis.

Loop Diuretics

Twenty-five percent of filtered Na is reclaimed in the loop of Henle. A cotransporter in the ascending limb moves one molecule of Na and potassium and two molecules of chloride (Na-K-2Cl) from the tubular lumen into the tubular epithelial cells (see Figure 33-1). The majority of reabsorbed potassium then moves back out of the cell into the tubular lumen via potassium channels. This Na-K-2Cl cotransporter is inhibited by the loop diuretics. Diuretics that act at this site are very potent because of the large amount of Na usually reabsorbed at this site and the relatively limited ability of more distal sites to increase Na reabsorption.

Inhibition of the Na-K-2Cl cotransporter also decreases absorption of calcium and magnesium and leads to increased urinary losses of these cations.

Thiazide Diuretics

Five to ten percent of filtered NaCl is reabsorbed in the distal tubule. This resorption occurs via an NaCl cotransporter that is inhibited by thiazide diuretics. The mechanisms that underlie the efficacy of thiazides in the treatment of hypertension are not completely known. Volume loss likely plays an important role. However, during chronic therapy these drugs may also act to decrease peripheral vascular resistance.

Potassium-Sparing Diuretics

Na Channel Blockers. The collecting duct plays a major role in the day-to-day regulation of NaCl and potassium excretion. Na resorption along this segment, which reabsorbs only 3% to 5% of filtered Na, occurs via a luminal Na channel. The reabsorption of Na generates a voltage gradient that drives potassium from the tubular cell into the tubular lumen and hence into the urine. If Na resorption at this site is blocked, this slows potassium excretion and leads to the potassium retention for which diuretics acting on this segment are named.

Aldosterone Antagonists. Tubular epithelial cells in the collecting duct possess high-affinity receptors for the hormone aldosterone. Occupancy of these receptors by aldosterone initiates a number of events, including the activation of previously inactive luminal Na channels, transport of more Na channels from the cytosol to the luminal cell membrane, and stimulation of the production of more Na channels. Spironolactone competes with aldosterone for binding to high-affinity aldosterone receptors and thereby blocks the physiologic actions of aldosterone. Spironolactone is most efficacious in situations in which the body is producing high amounts of aldosterone.

DRUG TREATMENT PRINCIPLES

An important factor in diuretic efficacy is the patient's ability to adhere to a low-sodium diet. As drug concentration falls, a period of positive Na balance, the period of postdiuretic Na retention, may follow. If dietary salt intake is high, then the amount of Na lost in response to diuretic may be partially or completely offset by postdiuretic Na retention.

Renal function is another important variable in determining diuretic response. Patients become less responsive to diuretics as renal function declines. Loop diuretics typically retain efficacy even in the face of moderately severe renal insufficiency; however, patients require higher diuretic doses to achieve an effect. Most of the thiazides are relatively inef-fective in individuals with glomerular filtration rates of less than 30 to 40 ml/min. The exceptions to this are metolazone and indapamide. Potassium-sparing diuretics should be used with great caution or avoided in patients with renal insufficiency because of their potential to induce life-threatening hyperkalemia.

In addition, length of time on therapy may contribute significantly to the responsiveness of the kidneys to diuretics. The ability of the diuretic to increase renal NaCl excretion declines over time. This phenomenon, termed "diuretic resistance" is thought to occur in one out of three patients with chronic heart failure (CHF). The addition of a second drug may act synergistically to mitigate this adaptive process.

For diuretic resistance, evaluate and treat these factors: patient noncompliance (either not taking drug or high NaCl intake), CHF, renal failure, nephrotic syndrome, and cirrhosis. Drugs that can cause diuretic resistance include NSAIDs, captopril, cimetidine, and antihypertensives (Boxes 33-1 and 33-2).

BOX 33-1

CAUSES OF DIURETIC RESISTANCE

Patient Noncompliance
Not taking drug
High NaCl intake

Impaired Bioavailability
Chronic heart failure*
Idiopathic edema

Impaired Diuretic Secretion by Proximal Tubule
Renal failure
Old age
Renal transplantation
Chronic heart failure*
Drugs
NSAIDs (loop and DCT diuretics), furosemide (Captopril), amiloride and triamterene (Cimetadine)

Protein Binding in Tubule Lumen
Nephrotic syndrome

Hemodynamic (Reduced Glomerular Filtration Rate [GFR])
Drugs
Antihypertensives
NSAIDs
Hypoxemia
Reduced "fullness" of arterial vascular system

Enhanced NaCl Reabsorption
Primary
Chronic heart failure*
Nephrotic syndrome
Cirrhosis
Secondary to drugs
NSAIDs
Adaptation to chronic diuretic therapy

*Chronic heart failure alters primarily the time course of diuretic absorption rather than the percentage of administered dose that is absorbed.
From Ellison DH: The physiologic basis of diuretic synergism: its role in treating diuretic resistance, *Ann Intern Med* 114(10):889, 1991. Used by permission of The American College of Physicians.

BOX 33-2

APPROACH TO DIURETIC RESISTANCE IN PATIENTS

Assess Compliance with Medical Regimen (Diet and Drugs)
Measure daily Na excretion
If >100 mmol/day, reduce intake
If <100 mmol/day, proceed as below

Assess Status of Underlying Disease
Does patient really need further reduction of extracellular fluid volume?
Can treatment of underlying disease be improved?

Discontinue NSAIDs and Consider Reducing Vasodilators (especially if blood pressure is low)

Change to a Loop Diuretic and Increase Dosage until Diuretic Threshold or Maximum Safe Dose is Attained
Consider constant diuretic infusion
May block postdiuretic NaCl retention and be useful for hospitalized patients

Consider Diuretic Combinations
Add DCT diuretic (usually the best choice is metolazone or hydrochlorothiazide)
Add distal diuretic (amiloride, triamterene, and spironolactone are primarily effective in cirrhotic edema)
Add proximal diuretic (carbonic anhydrase inhibitors)

From Ellison DH: The physiologic basis of diuretic synergism: its role in treating diuretic resistance, *Ann Intern Med* 114(10):889, 1991. Used by permission of The American College of Physicians.

As with any medication it is important to determine the patient's previous response to treatment and history of any adverse events. Additional considerations include cost, mobility, or toileting concerns that may affect a patient's adherence to the prescribed diuretic therapy.

Osmotic Diuretics

Osmotic diuretics, such as mannitol, act by inhibiting Na absorption in the proximal tubule and loop of Henle. Their clinical use is limited primarily to inpatient settings in which they may be used to reduce intracranial pressure or to reduce intraocular pressure in glaucoma. Osmotic diuretics are not used in edematous states or in outpatients because of their potential to induce intravascular volume expansion and pulmonary edema in susceptible patients. These drugs will not be considered further.

Carbonic Anhydrase Inhibitors

Carbonic anhydrase inhibitors are relatively weak diuretics. Their primary use is in the treatment of open-angle glaucoma and the prophylaxis and treatment of acute mountain sickness. The risk of mountain sickness is directly related to the rate of ascent. Acetazolamide is efficacious above 4000 meters when ascent rates are higher than 500 meters per day. Acetazolamide may also be used, usually in combination with other diuretics, to treat edema associated with CHF. The ability of carbonic anhydrase inhibitors to increase urinary losses of bicarbonate may be useful in treating individuals with severe metabolic alkalosis.

Loop Diuretics

The major use of loop diuretics involves the treatment of states of volume excess that include CHF, nephrotic syndrome, acute and chronic renal insufficiency, and cirrhosis. They may also be used to treat hypertension in patients with diminished renal function. Because all loop diuretics are similar in their mechanism of action, if a patient fails to respond to one loop, another should not be tried. Instead, a combination of diuretics that are pharmacologically different should be prescribed.

The major toxicities related to these potent diuretics lie in their ability to induce fluid and electrolyte imbalances. Na and water losses may lead to volume depletion and hypotension. Hypokalemia, hypomagnesemia, metabolic alkalosis, and hypocalcemia may also result.

The amount given as a once-a-day dosage is more effective than the same amount given in divided doses. Dosage adjustment is usually required before achieving the expected outcome or deeming the drug ineffective.

Thiazides

Thiazides are used most frequently to treat hypertension. Thiazide diuretics may also be useful in the treatment of edematous states such as CHF, cirrhosis, nephrotic syndrome, and chronic renal insufficiency. Because the thiazide diuretics do act distally, they are a particularly useful strategy in combination with loop diuretics for patients who have developed diuretic resistance.

Thiazides are useful in the treatment of hypocalciuric stone disease because of their ability to decrease renal calcium excretion; however, this may contribute to osteoporosis. They may also be used to decrease urine volume in patients with nephrogenic diabetes insipidus. Thiazide diuretics in combination with a low-salt diet in the management of Ménière's disease may decrease the natural progression of sensorineural hearing loss and treat vertigo through prevention of flare-ups.

As is the case with most diuretics, the major complications of thiazide therapy include fluid and electrolyte abnormalities. Of concern is the increased incidence of sudden death seen in patients whose hypertension was treated with thiazides. This is thought, although not proven, to be a consequence of diuretic-induced hypokalemia.

As a general recommendation, thiazides should be started at the lowest dosage, given once or twice daily for those with shorter half-lives. The smallest effective dose should be used for the treatment of hypertension because the adverse effects of hypokalemia, increased cholesterol, and possibly the increase in sudden death seen in thiazide-treated patients appear to be dose related.

Patients whose edematous state is not sufficiently improved with maximum-dose thiazides should be evaluated for causes of diuretic resistance or renal or hepatic insufficiency and changed to a loop diuretic if no remediable cause is identified.

Potassium-Sparing Diuretics

The major use of potassium-sparing diuretics is in combination with other diuretics. Concomitant use of potassium-sparing diuretics augments urinary Na losses and blunts the hypokalemia typically produced by the use of thiazide and loop diuretics as single agents. See later discussion on combination diuretics.

Spironolactone is particularly useful in physiologic states associated with high levels of aldosterone production. These states include primary aldosteronism and secondary hyperaldosteronism associated with cirrhosis, nephrotic syndrome, and CHF. Recent studies have underscored the benefit select patients with CHF may receive through the careful addition of spironolactone to standard therapy. Spironolactone has also been used in the treatment of hirsutism.

Amiloride is also useful in treating the polyuria associated with lithium use.

Combination Diuretics

Diuretic combinations are used for two general purposes. The first is as a second diuretic to remedy an electrolyte abnormality induced by another. The most common example of this is the use of a potassium-sparing diuretic to blunt the hypokalemia induced by a thiazide diuretic. The other rationale for combination diuretics is to increase urinary Na losses by blocking Na reabsorption at two sites along the nephron. An example of this is the use of a loop diuretic and a thiazide to effect diuresis in individuals with resistance to the effects of loop diuretics used alone. Simultaneous use of two diuretics of the same class (i.e., two loop diuretics or two thiazides) has no therapeutic benefit that could not be achieved by maximizing the dose of a single agent. Four combinations of diuretics—thiazide and potassium-sparing, loop and thiazide, loop and potassium-sparing, and loop and carbonic anhydrase inhibitors—may be prescribed. Only thiazide and potassium-sparing agents are available as a fixed dosage. All four combinations of diuretic agents are discussed below.

Thiazide and Potassium-Sparing Combinations. Fixed-dose combinations of thiazide and potassium-sparing diuretics are convenient and may enhance patient compliance. Their disadvantage is that they limit flexibility in dose titration. Ideally, the correct dose of individual agents should be determined first, and then the patient changed to a fixed-dose product if one exists that matches his or her needs. Unfortunately, differences in bioavailability require caution when changing from one product to another. Cautions and adverse effects are similar to those for the individual agents.

Loop and Thiazide Diuretics. Patients may become resistant to the effects of diuretics during treatment. Patients may tolerate these regimens better if the thiazide is administered every other day or only two or three times a week.

The combination of loop and potassium-sparing diuretics is frequently used to treat patients with decompensated liver disease and ascites. These individuals typically have high aldosterone levels and, as a result, maximally conserve Na in the collecting duct. Adding spironolactone is more efficacious than either agent used independently. A typical starting combination of these drugs is 40 mg of furosemide with 100 mg of spironolactone. Amiloride, which also acts in the collecting duct, may be used in lieu of spironolactone. Its onset of action is faster and it does not have the complication of gynecomastia that may be associated with spironolactone.

Loop and Carbonic Anhydrase Inhibitors. Two factors occur during loop diuretic therapy that may make the addition of a carbonic anhydrase inhibitor useful. The first is that loop diuretic–induced volume loss stimulates an increased absorption of Na in the proximal tubule. This increased proximal reabsorption of Na may blunt the efficacy of the loop diuretic. Second, loop diuretics increase urinary losses of hydrogen ions and, as a consequence, may contribute to the development of a metabolic alkalosis. The addition of a carbonic anhydrase inhibitor may enhance urinary Na losses and prevent or minimize the development of a metabolic alkalosis.

The combination of a loop diuretic and a carbonic anhydrase inhibitor should be given with caution. Hypovolemia, hypokalemia, and metabolic acidosis are potential complications of this therapy. The health care provider should have a clear understanding of the patient's acid-base status before using a carbonic anhydrase inhibitor. For example, if the patient's serum bicarbonate is elevated as an appropriate response to acute or chronic respiratory acidosis, then the addition of a carbonic anhydrase inhibitor could lead to severe acidemia. A full discussion of acid-base balance is beyond the scope of this chapter.

HOW TO MONITOR

Fluid and electrolyte abnormalities are the most common adverse effects of diuretic use. Up to 50% of patients receiving diuretic therapy experience potassium levels below 3.5 mEq/L. The "renaissance" of spironolactone highlights that the losses of potassium and/or magnesium through administration of thiazides in CHF and in hypertension are not without consequences. Volume status should be assessed initially and periodically during therapy. Patients can be instructed to record their weight and amount of edema on a daily basis at home. Major changes in electrolytes generally occur within the first few weeks of therapy, and, contrary to popular belief, potassium depletion is not progressive with continued treatment. Serum electrolytes should be checked before diuretic therapy is initiated, after 1 to 2 weeks of therapy, and at intervals warranted by changes in therapy or in the patient's clinical condition thereafter. To prevent significant cardiovascular events such as fatal dysrhythmias, in some patients, supplementation with magnesium as well as potassium may need to be considered. See the discussion on monitoring under "Potassium Supplementation in Diuretic-Treated Patients" later in this chapter.

PATIENT VARIABLES

Geriatrics

Older patients are at an increased risk for diuretic-induced electrolyte disturbances and renal insufficiency. Because diuretic response decreases with declining renal function, the fall in glomerular filtration rate seen with aging may decrease diuretic response. Orthostatic hypotension causes the elderly to be at an increased risk of falls. In many elders, diastolic or isolated systolic hypertension may be successfully treated with low-dose diuretic monotherapy.

Pediatrics

There are limited data regarding the safety and efficacy of diuretic therapy in pediatric patients. The following therapies are used in a variety of clinical situations, including edema, glaucoma, and epilepsy. Acetazolamide is used for glaucoma and epilepsy only. Bumetanide and ethacrynic acid are not recommended in children younger than 18 years of age. Furosemide should be avoided in the premature infant with respiratory distress syndrome because it may increase the risk of persistent patent ductus arteriosus. Chlorothiazide, hydrochlorothiazide, spironolactone, and hydrochlorothiazide and spironolactone have been safely used in pediatric patients for the treatment of edema and hypertension. Careful monitoring is essential because pediatric patients may be less tolerant of small shifts in fluid and electrolytes.

Subtle changes related to diuretic or potassium replacement therapies may not manifest themselves in pediatric as in adult patients. Infants especially cannot report symptoms related to weakness, confusion, paresthesias, or muscle cramps. Changes in personality, eating or sleeping patterns, and restlessness should be reported and investigated promptly.

Pregnancy

Category C

Race and Gender

Gender has not been identified as a consideration in diuretic therapy.

Race can be a factor. In treatment of hypertension (HTN), African-Americans often respond better to diuretics than other hypertensive medications.

PATIENT EDUCATION

- Importance of dietary Na restriction in determining diuretic efficacy.
- Symptoms of hypovolemia, including weakness and orthostatic dizziness, which might indicate a need for diuretic dose adjustment.
- Signs and symptoms of hypokalemia or hyperkalemia, including profound weakness. Patients should report these symptoms promptly so that electrolytes may be checked.
- Adherence with intermittent dosing schedules, such as alternate day or weekly dosing, may improve if patients use a calendar to record medication use.
- Patients may wish to avoid taking their diuretics late in the day to minimize disturbance of sleep patterns.
- Urinary volume is expected to increase. Therefore easy access to a bathroom is essential, especially with initiation of drug therapy. For some patients, this effect does not improve over time.
- May need to monitor daily weights; to rapid weight loss (more than 1 to 2 lb/day) might be harmful.

Specific Drugs

DIURETICS

Carbonic Anhydrase Inhibitors

acetazolamide (Dazamide, Diamox, Diamox Sequels)

Contraindications

- Hepatic cirrhosis because the impaired renal excretion of ammonia caused by the drugs can precipitate hepatic encephalopathy
- Advanced renal insufficiency, respiratory acidosis, or metabolic acidosis: the loss of bicarbonate in the urine induced by these drugs may cause severe acidemia in these patients
- Hyponatremia or hypokalemia may be substantially worsened by the use of carbonic anhydrase inhibitors
- Sulfa allergy

Precautions. Because these drugs may cause hypokalemia and metabolic acidosis, patients should be monitored with serum electrolyte values before and at regular intervals during treatment. A complete blood count before treatment and periodically thereafter will detect hematolytic toxicity, which can occur with sulfonamides such as acetazolamide.

Drug Interactions

- Salicylates and diflunisal may increase the activity of carbonic anhydrase inhibitors.
- Acetazolamide can increase cyclosporine levels and decrease levels of primidone.

Dosage and Administration. See Table 33-2 for all dosages and administration.

LOOP DIURETICS

(P) Prototype Drug

furosemide (Lasix)

Contraindications

- Volume-depleted patients: these drugs can induce substantial losses of Na and water.
- Sulfa allergy

Warnings

Diuretic-induced hypokalemia is a very common consequence of loop diuretic therapy. The potency of loop diuretics requires careful patient monitoring to assess volume status and to monitor for deficiencies in potassium. Careful monitoring of daily weights at home can help identify patients with too rapid volume loss (more than 1 to 2 lb/day).

Precautions

Loop diuretic–induced hypercalciuria could increase the frequency of stone formation in susceptible individuals. Laboratory abnormalities associated with loop diuretic use include hyperuricemia, which may lead to clinical episodes of gout, impaired glucose tolerance, and increases in low-density lipoprotein (LDL) cholesterol. The adverse effects on lipid levels may dissipate during chronic therapy.

Pharmacokinetics

See Table 33-3. These drugs are highly protein bound and thus are not filtered into the tubular lumen through the glomerulus. Instead they gain access to the tubular lumen via an organic ion transporter in the proximal tubule.

Adverse Effects

See Table 33-4. The most common adverse effects are related to fluid and electrolyte abnormalities.

TABLE 33-2 Dosage and Administration Recommendations for Diuretics

Drug	Diagnosis	Dosage	Administration	Maximum Daily Dose
acetazolamide	Glaucoma Mountain sickness prevention CHF	250-1000 mg 750-100 mg 250-375 mg	qd Divided doses, start 24-48 hr prior to ascent qd, best qod or qd × 2 then 1 day off	1000 mg
furosemide		20-80 mg	qAM	200 mg tid
bumetanide		0.5-2 mg	qd, may be repeated q2-5hr	10 mg
ethacrynic acid		50-100 mg qd		200 mg bid
torsemide	CHF, renal failure HTN	10-20 mg 5-10 mg	qd qd	200 mg/dose 200 mg/dose
hydrochlorothiazide	HTN Edema	12.5-50 mg 25-100 mg	qd qd	>50 mg, lose K^+
chlorothiazide	HTN, edema	0.5-100 mg	qd-bid	1 g
chlorthalidone	HTN Edema	25-50 mg 50-100 mg	qd qd	100 mg 200 mg
indapamide	Edema due to CHF	2.5 mg	qAM	5 mg
metolazone	HTN, CHF	0.5-1 mg	qd	20 mg
triamterene		50-100 mg	qd	300 mg
amiloride		5-10 mg		20 mg
spironolactone		25-100 mg	qd or divided doses	100 mg

hr, Hour; *mg,* milligram; *ml,* milliliter; >, greater than; <, less than; *q,* every.

TABLE 33-3 Pharmacokinetics of Diuretics

Drug	Oral Absorption	Onset of Action	Half-Life	Duration of Action	Elimination
acetazolamide	NC	Tabs, 1-1.5 hr Caps, 2 hr	6-9 hr	Tabs, 8-12 hr Caps, 18-24 hr	Renal
furosemide	10%-90%	0.3-1 hr	0.5-1 hr	6-8 hr	Renal, 60%; liver, 40%
bumetanide	72%-95%	0.5-1 hr	1-1.5 hr	4-6 hr	Renal, 65%; liver, 35%
ethacrynic acid	NC	<0.5 hr	0.5-1 hr	6-8 hr	Renal, 65%; liver, 35%
torsemide	79%-91%	1 hr	0.8-6 hr	6-8 hr	Renal, 30%; liver, 70%
hydrochlorothiazide	65%-75%	2 hr	15 hr	6-12 hr	Liver, 70%; renal
chlorothiazide	10%-21%	2 hr	0.75-2 hr	6-12 hr	Renal; liver, 20%-60%
chlorthalidone	60%-70%	2 hr	35-50 hr	24-72 hr	Renal, 65%; liver, 10%; unknown, 25%
indapamide	NC	1-2 hr	10-22 hr	36 hr	Liver
metolazone	65%	1 hr	8 hr	12-24 hr	Renal, 80%; liver, 20%
triamterene	30%-70%	2-4 hr	1.6-2.5 hr	12-16 hr	Liver
amiloride	50%	2 hr	6-9 hr	24 hr	Renal
spironolactone	90%	24-72 hr	1.3-2 hr	48-72 hr	Liver

ID, Insufficient data; *NC,* nearly complete.

TABLE 33-4 Adverse Effects of Diuretics

Drug	Common	Serious
CARBONIC ANHYDRASE INHIBITORS	Metabolic acidosis, hemolytic anemia, erythema multiforme, bone marrow depression	
acetazolamide	Drowsiness, paresthesias, confusion, tinnitus, transient myopia, anorexia, altered taste, nausea, vomiting, diarrhea, polyuria, and mild electrolyte imbalances	Severe electrolyte imbalances GI bleeding, aplastic anemia, and sulfonamide-type reactions, including toxic epidermal necrolysis and Stevens-Johnson syndrome
LOOP DIURETICS	Orthostatic hypotension, excessive diuresis, leading to dehydration/hypovolemia and hemoconcentration, with subsequent hypotension and severe electrolyte imbalances of potassium, chloride, magnesium, and Na; ototoxicity Tinnitus Vertigo Hyperuricemia	Cardiovascular collapse Encephalopathy with preexisting liver disease Severe electrolyte imbalances (Ca, Cl, K, Mg, Na)
furosemide	Photosensitivity	Anemia, neutropenia, and agranulocytosis Hyperglycemia
bumetanide	Mild electrolyte imbalances	Reversible azotemia, metabolic alkalosis
ethacrynic acid	Anorexia Diarrhea	Neutropenia Agranulocytosis
torsemide	Hyperglycemia	ECG changes
THIAZIDE DIURETICS	Orthostatic hypotension, dizziness, drowsiness, syncope, weakness, nausea, GI irritation, hypermotility, electrolyte imbalances, hemoconcentration, transient elevation in BUN, hypovolemia, depressed respirations and lethargy leading to coma, and elevated glucose levels	
hydrochlorothiazide	Anorexia, nausea, vomiting Abdominal pain, cramping Rash, urticaria	Leukopenia, thrombocytopenia Agranulocytosis
chlorothiazide	Paresthesias, weakness Photosensitivity	Pancreatitis Leukopenia, agranulocytosis, aplastic anemia, anaphylactic reactions
chlorthalidone	Vertigo Rash Urticaria Hyperuricemia	Jaundice, pancreatitis Leukopenia, thrombocytopenia
indapamide	Headache Fatigue Muscle cramps/spasms Hyperglycemia Hyperuricemia	Necrotizing angiitis Vasculitis Cutaneous vasculitis Pruritus
metolazone	Headache	Lassitude, muscle cramps Joint pain/swelling, chest pain
POTASSIUM-SPARING DIURETICS	Dehydration Hypotension Hyperkalemia Nausea Vomiting GI disturbances Weakness	
triamterene	Nephrolithiasis Headache Weakness Fatigue	Acute renal failure and megaloblastic anemia Electrolyte imbalances of hyper- or hypokalemia Anaphylactic reactions

TABLE 33-4 Adverse Effects of Diuretics—cont'd

Drug	Common	Serious
POTASSIUM-SPARING DIURETICS—cont'd		
amiloride	Headache	Severe hyperkalemia Encephalopathy
spironolactone	Headache, lethargy, GI irritation Deepening of the voice	Severe hyperkalemia Dehydration and hyponatremia Agranulocytosis, mental confusion Endocrine and androgenic effects with high doses Gynecomastia, irregular menses or amenorrhea Postmenopausal bleeding, hirsutism

Drug Interactions

Concomitant use of loop diuretics and aminoglycosides or cisplatin can increase ototoxicity. Diuretic-induced volume depletion increases the risk of aminoglycoside-induced acute renal failure. Loop diuretics can increase the activity of anticoagulants and salicylates and increase blood levels of β-blockers and lithium. Probenecid decreases the efficacy of loop diuretics.

Other Drugs in Class

Other drugs in this class are similar to the prototype except as follows.

bumetanide (Bumex), torsemide (Demadex), ethacrynic acid (Edecrin)

Bumetanide and torsemide are metabolized in the liver. They are better absorbed, more bioavailable, and have a longer duration of action than furosemide. For patients with CHF in whom variation of furosemide absorption may be clinically significant, treatment with more completely absorbed loop diuretics may be indicated. Thrombocytopenia is a rarely reported complication of bumetanide use. Ethacrynic acid is a phenoxyacetic acid derivative; severe diarrhea has been reported.

Thiazides and Thiazide-like Diuretics

Ⓟ Prototype Drug

hydrochlorothiazide (HCTZ) (HydroDIURIL, Esidrix, Microzide, Oretic)

Contraindications

- Hypersensitivity to sulfonamides
- Glomerular filtration rates of 30 ml/min or less

Warnings

Use with caution in patients with moderate chronic renal insufficiency or hepatic dysfunction because of the potential of both these conditions to deteriorate with volume depletion or electrolyte imbalances.

Precautions

- Serum electrolytes should be checked before treatment is initiated and periodically thereafter. Hypokalemia is a common complication of thiazide use (Box 33-3).
- Women may have a greater decrease in serum potassium concentration than men.
- The glucose intolerance seen with thiazide use appears to be a consequence of diuretic-induced hypokalemia.
- Because thiazides interfere with the kidney's ability to completely dilute the urine, patients may retain free water with resultant hyponatremia.
- Thiazides decrease uric acid excretion and may predispose susceptible individuals to episodes of gout.
- The decrease in renal calcium excretion, which may be advantageous in patients with calcium-containing stone disease, may lead to hypercalcemia, particularly in those with hyperparathyroidism.
- Dose-related increases in LDL are seen early in therapy. These increases tend to return to baseline with chronic therapy.
- Thiazide diuretics have been reported to worsen disease in individuals with systemic lupus erythematosus.

Potassium supplementation is often required (Box 33-4).

Pharmacokinetics

A variety of preparations exist that differ primarily in their duration of action; see Table 33-3.

BOX 33-3

SIGNS AND SYMPTOMS OF HYPOKALEMIA

Arrhythmias, weak irregular pulse, flattened T waves, U waves
Potentiation of digitalis toxicity
Fatigue
Muscle weakness, cramps
Soft and flabby muscles
Decreased reflexes
Postural hypotension
Rhabdomyolysis
Confusion
Glucose intolerance
Polyuria
Metabolic alkalosis
Nausea and vomiting
Decreased GI motility, ileus

BOX 33-4

FOOD SOURCES RICH IN POTASSIUM

HIGH: 5-10 mEq/SERVING (195-390 mg)

Dairy
Milk, 1%

Meats, Dry Beans, Eggs, and Nuts
Almonds
Beef, lean, ground, broiled/fried
Black bean soup
Chicken, ½ breast
Mussels, cooked
Pork, center loin, broiled
Tuna, canned in water
Turkey, without skin, roasted
Swordfish

Vegetables
Broccoli, boiled
Carrot, raw
Tomato, raw

Fruits
Apple juice
Grapefruit juice
Peaches, canned in water
Pear, raw
Strawberries, raw

VERY HIGH: >10 mEq/SERVING (>390 mg)

Dairy
Milk, skim
Yogurt, plain, fat free

Meats, Dry Beans, Eggs, and Nuts
Baked beans, vegetarian or pork, or refried beans
Kidney beans, boiled
Lima beans, boiled

Vegetables
Marinara sauce
Potato, baked with skin
Spinach, boiled

Fruits
Banana
Cantaloupe, raw
Orange juice, canned
Raisins

Condiments
Salt substitutes (1 mEq = 30 mg potassium)

Adverse Reactions
A variety of uncommon adverse effects have been described with the different thiazides (see Table 33-4).

Drug Interactions
Thiazides may increase the effects of anesthetics, prolong chemotherapy-induced leukopenia, increase the toxicity of digitalis and lithium, and increase calcium levels in patients also treated with calcium and/or vitamin D supplementation. Decreases in efficacy of anticoagulants, antigout agents, oral hypoglycemics, and insulin may be seen with concomitant thiazide use. Anticholinergics may increase thiazide absorption, whereas bile acid sequestrants decrease it. Methenamines and NSAIDs may decrease the efficacy of thiazide diuretics.

Other Drugs in Class

Other drugs in this class are similar to the prototype except as follows.

chlorothiazide (Diuril), chlorthalidone (Hygroton), indapamide (Lozol), metolazone (Mykrox, Zaroxolyn)

Exceptions to avoiding thiazides in patients with glomerular filtration rates of 30 ml/min or less are metolazone and indapamide. These two thiazides are effective in patients with diminished glomerular filtration rates. In addition, increased cholesterol does not occur during treatment with indapamide.

POTASSIUM-SPARING DIURETICS

(P) Prototype Drug

triamterene (Dyrenium, Maxzide)

Contraindications
- Life-threatening hyperkalemia can result if triamterene is used in patients with elevated pretreatment serum potassium, patients receiving concomitant potassium supplementation, or patients with moderate or severe renal insufficiency.
- Do not use with other potassium-sparing diuretics.
- Hypersensitivity

Warnings
Potassium-sparing diuretics can cause life-threatening hyperkalemia. Clinical manifestations of hyperkalemia include profound weakness, paresthesias, flaccid paralysis, bradycardia, hypotension, and ECG abnormalities, including peaked T waves and prolongation of the P-R, QRS, and Q-T intervals. Patients should be advised to avoid large amounts of high-potassium foods, particularly if they were encouraged to eat such foods before therapy with a potassium-sparing diuretic was initiated. Salt substitutes that contain potassium chloride and potassium supplements should be avoided. Electrolytes should be monitored before initiation of therapy and frequently thereafter.

Patients with diabetes-related renal insufficiency are at higher risk of hyperkalemia, and these drugs should be used in these patients only with considerable caution and careful monitoring of electrolytes.

Precautions
Hyponatremia may occur with these drugs, particularly when used in combination with other diuretics

that predispose to the development of hyponatremia. Drugs in this group can also cause a metabolic acidosis.

- Triamterene has been found as a component of renal stones; use with caution in patients with a history of renal stones
- Triamterene is a weak folic acid antagonist and can contribute to folate deficiency states
- Triamterene photosensitivity
- Glucose intolerance

Drug Interactions

Angiotensin-converting enzyme inhibitors commonly raise serum potassium levels and should be used with great caution in combination with potassium-sparing diuretics. Spironolactone may decrease the effectiveness of anticoagulants and mitotane. Triamterene increases amantadine levels. Cimetidine appears to increase the effects of triamterene by increasing its bioavailability and decreasing its clearance.

Other Drugs in Class

Other drugs in this class are similar to the prototype except as follows.

amiloride (Midamor), spironolactone (Aldactone)

Spironolactone may cause gynecomastia, decreased libido, hirsutism, and menstrual irregularities. Spironolactone was also found to be tumorigenic in rats. Amiloride and spironolactone have complex effects on the elimination of digitalis and may blunt its inotropic activity. NSAIDs lower the therapeutic effect of amiloride and spironolactone and may increase the risk of hyperkalemia.

Potassium Supplements

General Uses

Most potassium supplements consist of the chloride salt of potassium (KCl). A smaller number are provided as potassium salts of bicarbonate, acetate, citrate, or *l*-lysine. Potassium chloride is the preferred replacement for most patients with diuretic-induced hypokalemia because diuretics induce losses of both potassium and chloride. For this reason only potassium chloride replacement agents are reviewed. When metabolic acidosis is present, the use of bicarbonate, citrate, acetate, or gluconate potassium salts may be indicated.

Volume loss associated with diuretic use can stimulate aldosterone production that further increases urinary potassium losses. New guidelines on potassium replacement from the National Council on Potassium in Clinical Practice were released in 2000. These new guidelines underscore the importance of preventing potassium loss as well as replacement in patients with hypertension, CHF, patients with cardiac arrhythmias, stroke, diabetes, and those patients with renal impairment. It is recommended that increasing potassium intake should be considered when serum potassium levels are between 3.5 and 4 mmol/L. A target goal of at least 4 mmol/L is suggested for patients with asymptomatic hypertension, CHF, and patients with cardiac arrhythmias.

Approaches to avoiding hypokalemia in patients treated with diuretics include using the lowest effective diuretic dose, restricting dietary Na intake to 75 to 100 mEq/day, increasing dietary potassium intake (see Box 33-4), or making concomitant use of potassium-sparing agents (see earlier discussion). Patients who require a second agent to control hypertension or who have specific types of cardiac disease could be considered for treatment with medications that tend to increase serum potassium concentrations (e.g., ACE inhibitors).

DRUG ACTION AND EFFECTS

Potassium is the major intracellular cation, and it has major regulatory roles in cell metabolism. Many cellular functions may be adversely affected by hypokalemia. For example, hypokalemia may decrease the kidney's ability to respond to antidiuretic hormone, leading to polyuria. Hypokalemia may also impair insulin secretion and lead to worsened glucose control in diabetic patients. Of major importance is the role of potassium in defining resting membrane potential. Because of this role, hypokalemia may predispose to the development of arrhythmias and smooth and skeletal muscle dysfunction. Patients taking digitalis are particularly prone to the arrhythmic potential of hypokalemia. The signs and symptoms associated with hypokalemia are listed in Box 33-3.

HOW TO MONITOR

Serum electrolytes should be monitored before diuretic treatment is initiated. Because patients typically become hypokalemic within the first weeks of therapy, their electrolytes should be checked after 1 to 2 weeks of therapy. Hypokalemic patients can increase their potassium intake by augmenting their dietary intake of potassium (see Box 33-4) and/or by using potassium supplements (Table 33-5). Potassium levels should be rechecked approximately 2 weeks after changes are made to assess the effect of these changes. At that time a new steady state exists, and potassium levels may then be checked based on clinical concerns or additional changes in therapy.

The amount of potassium replacement required to normalize serum potassium must be determined individually. Relatively low doses (10 to 30 mEq) may be required in the patient on a low-dose thiazide who is compliant with a higher potassium and sodium-restricted diet, whereas much higher doses are required in the patient on higher doses of a loop diuretic who is unable to maintain a low Na and high-potassium diet.

PATIENT VARIABLES

Common Considerations

A normal diet contains approximately 50 to 100 mEq of potassium each day. Individuals whose diet is low in potassium-containing food and those with poor general dietary intake are

TABLE 33-5 Potassium Chloride Preparations

Form	Form and Concentration	
	Brand Name	Concentration (%)*
Liquid	Cena-K	10
		20
	Generic KCl	10
	Kaochlor	10
	Kaon-Cl	20
	Kay Ciel	10
	Klorvess	10
	Kolyum	10
	Potasalan	10
	Rum-K	15 (30 mEq/15 ml)
Powder	Generic	10
	Gen-K	20, 25
	Kato	20
	Kay Ciel	20
	K+Care	15, 20, 25
	K-ide	20
	K-Lor	15, 20, 25
	Klor-Con	20, 25
	Klorvess	20
	K-Lyte/Cl	25
	K-sol	20
Suspension	Micro-K LS	20
Effervescent tablets	Gen-K/Cl	20
	Klorvess	20
Tablets/capsules	Generic	8, 10
	Kaon-Cl	6.7, 10
	K-Dur	10, 20
	K-Lease	10
	K-8	8
	K+10	10
	K-Norm	10
	Klor-Con	8, 10
	Klotrix	10
	K-Tab	10
	Micro-K	8, 10
	Slow-K	8
	Ten-K	10

*10%: 20 mEq/15 ml; 15%: 30 mEq/15 ml; 20%: 40 mEq/15 ml.

particularly vulnerable to the development of diuretic-induced hypokalemia.

As indicated above, individuals with underlying cardiac disease and those treated with digitalis are more vulnerable to hypokalemia-induced arrhythmias. Also, patients with preexisting difficulties with any of the symptoms listed in Box 33-3 may be more likely to experience an exacerbation of these symptoms should hypokalemia be allowed to develop.

Geriatrics

Because many elders are on concomitant digitalis therapy, patients should be carefully monitored for previously described concerns regarding hypokalemic-related arrhythmias. Because elders are more susceptible to the development of potassium chloride–induced GI lesions, careful monitoring for GI side effects in this population is an additional concern. Because renal function declines with age, monitoring for hyperkalemia secondary to impaired potassium excretion gains increased importance.

Pediatrics

The safety and efficacy of the use of potassium replacement therapy in children have not been established.

Pregnancy

Category C

Race and Gender

Race and gender have not been identified as considerations in potassium replacement therapy.

PATIENT EDUCATION

In general, GI upset is a frequent concern regarding adherence to the prescribed potassium replacement therapy. This side effect may be prevented or decreased if the potassium is taken with meals and a full glass of water or other liquid. Because electrolyte imbalances may have severe consequences, educating patients to seek medical care if they develop symptoms of hyperkalemia or hypokalemia (described later) is of top priority.

The following should be discussed with patients before they begin oral potassium replacement therapy and periodically reinforced as needed:

- Taking potassium with food and a full glass of water or other liquid may prevent nausea or GI upset.
- Do not chew or crush tablets or capsules.
- Mix or dissolve oral liquids, soluble powders, or effervescent tablets completely in 3 to 8 ounces of water, juice, or other liquid.
- Take as prescribed (i.e., frequency and amount), especially if on diuretic or digitalis preparation.
- Report difficulties with swallowing tablets or capsules.
- Because the wax matrix of capsules from which the body has extracted the potassium is not absorbed in the GI tract, patients may observe this in their stool.
- Extended-release liquid suspension contains docusate sodium, a stool softener, as a dispersing agent. Therefore character or consistency of stool may change.
- Notify primary care provider if tarry stools or other signs of GI bleeding develop.
- Do not use potassium-containing salt substitutes while taking potassium supplements.
- Report for potassium monitoring as directed.
- Because potential drug interactions with ACE inhibitors exist, patients may need closer monitoring of potassium levels to check for hyperkalemia.
- Report the following signs and symptoms of hyperkalemia or hypokalemia to primary care provider: tingling in hands or feet; unusual tiredness or weakness; leg cramps or muscle weakness; feeling of heaviness in legs; nausea/vomiting; abdominal pain; black or tarry stools; weak, slowed, or irregular pulse; or low blood pressure.

Specific Drugs

potassium chloride (Kaon-Cl, K-Dur)

Pharmacokinetics. Absorption of orally administered potassium is nearly complete. In terms of distribution, the majority of potassium is located intracellularly where potassium concentration is 150 mEq/L. Extracellular potassium concentrations normally range from 3.5 to 5 mEq/L. Biotransformation of potassium does not occur, and the kidney represents the dominant site of excretion with only very small amounts of potassium lost in the stool (5 to 10 mEq/day) or sweat (0 to 10 mEq/day). Potassium is freely filtered through the glomerulus, and then almost completely reabsorbed in the proximal tubule. Excretion of potassium into the urine occurs as a function of potassium secretion in the collecting tubule. Plasma potassium concentration and aldosterone normally determine the amount of potassium lost in the urine. The normal kidney is capable of regulating potassium excretion to markedly increase excretion in situations of increased potassium intake or to markedly decrease potassium excretion in times of low potassium intake.

Contraindications. Sensitivity to tartrazine (found in some potassium preparations, e.g., Kaon-Cl or Kaochlor) may produce some allergic-type reactions. This same sensitivity is frequently seen in patients who are also sensitive to aspirin. The combined use of potassium supplements and potassium-sparing diuretics can lead to life-threatening hyperkalemia. The administration of potassium to patients with chronic renal insufficiency may overwhelm the kidneys' limited ability to excrete potassium and may also lead to severe hyperkalemia.

Tablets or capsules can cause GI ulceration in patients with impaired GI transport. Liquid forms of potassium replacement should be used in these patients.

Warnings. Life-threatening hyperkalemia may occur in patients whose ability to excrete potassium is impaired by either renal insufficiency or the concomitant use of potassium-sparing diuretics. Potassium chloride tablets may cause GI ulceration, bleeding, or strictures, particularly if the tablets are rapidly dissolving.

Adverse Effects. It is important to recognize that hyperkalemia may be entirely asymptomatic, manifesting itself only by an elevated serum potassium level (6.5 to 8 mEq/L) and by characteristic ECG changes. The elevated serum potassium level predisposes the patient to arrhythmias. Late manifestations include muscle paralysis and subsequent cardiovascular collapse (9 to 12 mEq/L). Unpleasant taste and GI irritation with abdominal discomfort, nausea, vomiting, and diarrhea are the most common adverse effects. More serious complications include hyperkalemia, GI ulceration, bleeding, and, rarely, perforation.

Drug Interactions. The combination of potassium supplements with medications that tend to raise serum potassium levels can cause life-threatening hyperkalemia. The concomitant use of potassium supplementation and potassium-sparing diuretics should be completely avoided or used only under extreme circumstances with vigilant monitoring. The combination of ACE inhibitors and potassium replacement may also induce hyperkalemia. However, this drug combination may be necessary in patients also treated with diuretics. These patients obviously require very careful monitoring.

Dosage and Administration. Dosage must be individualized based on periodic monitoring of serum potassium levels. Approximately 20 mEq/day is typically required to prevent and 40 to 100 mEq/day to treat patients with hypokalemia. The National Council on Potassium in Clinical Practice recommends administering supplements orally in moderate dosages over a period of several days to weeks to achieve full potassium repletion.

How Supplied. Potassium preparations are available in a number of forms, including liquid, powder, effervescent tablets, capsules, and controlled or extended-release tablets. The potassium concentration of the liquid preparations varies from 20 to 45 mEq/15 ml, powders from 15 to 25 mEq per packet, effervescent tablets 20 to 50 mEq, and capsules or tablets 6.7 to 20 mEq. The liquids, effervescent tablets, and powders may be less likely to cause GI ulceration but are frequently poorly tolerated because of their unpleasant taste (see Table 33-5).

BIBLIOGRAPHY

Appel, LJ: The verdict from ALLHAT—thiazide diuretics are the preferred initial therapy for hypertension, *JAMA* 288(23):3039-3042, 2002.

Brater DC: Diuretic therapy, *N Engl J Med* 339(6):387-395, 1998.

Brater DC: Pharmacology of diuretics, *Am J Med Sci* 319(1):38-50, 2000.

Cohn JN, Kowey PR, Whelton PK, Prisant LM: New guidelines for potassium replacement in clinical practice: a contemporary review by the National Council on Potassium in Clinical Practice, *Arch Intern Med* 160(16):2429-2436, 2000.

Doggrell SA, Brown H: The spironolactone renaissance, *Expert Opin Investig Drugs* 10(5):943-954, 2001.

Dumont L, Mardirosoff C, Tramer MR: Efficacy and harm of pharmacological prevention of acute mountain sickness: quantitative systemic review, *BMJ* 321:267-272, 2000.

Ellison DH: Diuretic resistance: physiology and therapeutics, *Semin Nephrol* 19(6):581-597, 1999.

Kelly J, Chambers J: Inappropriate use of loop diuretics in elderly patients, *Age Aging* 29:489-493, 2000.

Laragh JH, Sealey JE: K+ depletion and the progression of hypertensive disease or heart failure: the pathogenic role of diuretic-induced aldosterone secretion, *Hypertension* 37(part 2):806-810, 2001.

Pennington JAT, editor: *Bowes and Church's food values of portions commonly used*, ed 16, Philadelphia, 1994, JB Lippincott.

Sica DA et al: Importance of potassium in cardiovascular disease, *J Clin Hypertens* 4(3):198-206, 2002.

The ALLHAT Officers and Coordinators for the ALLHAT Collaborative Research Group: major outcomes in high-risk hypertensive patients randomized to angiotensin-converting enzyme inhibitor or calcium channel blocker vs diuretic, *JAMA* 288(23):2981-2997, 2002.

CHAPTER 34

Male Genitourinary Agents

Drug Names

Class	Subclass	Generic Name	Trade Name
Drugs for benign prostatic hypertrophy	α-Adrenergic agonist	(P) tamsulosin	Flomax
		alfuzosin	Uroxatral
		doxazosin	Cardura
		terazosin	Hytrin
	Androgen hormone inhibitor	finasteride	Proscar
Drugs for erectile dysfunction (ED)	PDE5 inhibitor	(P) sildenafil	Viagra
		tadalafil	Cialis
		vardenafil	Levitra
	Other	alprostadil	Caverject
		yohimbine	Yocon

(P), Prototype drug.

The drugs used for BPH and those for ED are discussed in separate sections of this chapter.

Drugs for Benign Prostatic Hypertrophy

General Uses

Indications

- Benign prostatic hypertrophy (BPH)

The drugs commonly used in the management of BPH are the α_1-adrenergic receptor blockers such as doxazosin and terazosin. Tamsulosin (Flomax) is an α-adrenergic receptor blocker that is specific to the prostate and is indicated only for treatment of symptoms of BPH. Also used is finasteride, an androgen hormone inhibitor.

DISEASE PROCESS

BPH is a benign neoplasm of the prostate gland, which if large enough, causes voiding dysfunction. Prostatism has three components: histologic prostatic hyperplasia, an increase in outflow resistance, and the response of the bladder (detrusor) muscle to obstruction. The prostate depends on the androgen 5 α-dihydrotestosterone (DHT) for growth. The enzyme 5 α-reductase metabolizes testosterone to DHT in the prostate gland, liver, and skin. DHT induces androgenic effects by binding to androgen receptors in the cell nuclei of these organs. BPH is extremely common in the aging male. By age 85, prevalence is approximately 90%. Prostate cancer is also common and must be considered in the diagnostic evaluation.

The Agency for Health Care Policy and Research (AHCPR) *Guideline on Benign Prostatic Hyperplasia: Diagnosis and Treatment* is an essential guide for providers dealing with this condition, although there are new medications available since these guidelines were released. Their suggested medical history focuses on the urinary tract and overall health problems that could affect the urinary system such as diabetes, Parkinson's disease, or stroke. Medications that can affect bladder function are anticholinergics and sympathomimetics. Symptom evaluation is best done using a standard scale for rating and classifying symptoms. The American Urological Association symptom index for benign prostatic hyperplasia is the scale commonly used.

The physical examination emphasizes the digital rectal examination (DRE) and the neurologic system. The DRE is used to estimate the size of the prostate gland, evaluate anal sphincter tone, and to raise suspicion of prostate or rectal malignancy.

Required laboratory tests to assess renal function include urinalysis and serum creatinine and BUN. The prostate-specific antigen (PSA) is considered optional in the AHCPR report. Other tests that may be performed are uroflowmetry, postvoid residual, and pressure flow studies. Tests that are not recommended by the AHCPR guidelines are filling cystometry, urethrocystoscopy, or imaging of the urinary tract unless indicated by prostatism complicated by additional disease or symptoms.

DRUG ACTION AND EFFECTS

The α-adrenergic receptor inhibitors antagonize contractions in the prostate and bladder neck. Tamsulosin is an α_{1A}-adrenoceptor antagonist. Because α_{1A}-receptors predominate in the prostate, tamsulosin and alfuzosin are more selective antagonists and may cause fever but few other systemic side effects.

Finasteride is a competitive and specific inhibitor of DHT, the potent androgen upon which the development of the prostate gland is dependent. It is a 5 α-reductase inhibitor that blocks the conversion of testosterone to dihydrotestosterone.

It reduces the size of the gland but may often take 6 months for maximum effect.

DRUG TREATMENT PRINCIPLES

The goals of treatment are to alleviate symptoms and to maintain the function of the kidneys.

Surgery is the primary treatment of BPH. Treatment of BPH depends on the severity of symptoms and the patient's surgical risk. Surgery is indicated if the patient has refractory retention, recurrent urinary tract infections (UTIs), hematuria, bladder stones, or renal insufficiency. Medical treatment is used when the patient is reluctant or unable to have surgery or the symptoms are mild enough that surgery is not warranted. The decision is generally made with the patient discussing his options with a urologist. See algorithm for decision making in the treatment of BPH.

All of the α-blockers indicated for hypertension are effective in treatment of BPH and should be considered in patients with concomitant BPH and hypertension. If the patient does not have hypertension, tamsulosin is probably the first choice. These drugs have a relatively quick onset of action.

Although the α-blockers are best for quick symptom relief, finasteride can prevent growth of the prostate in the long term. Finasteride therapy may also decrease the incidence of urinary retention and the need for operative treatment. Thus each medication serves a different purpose, and they can be used together.

Herbal treatment of BPH is popular. Saw palmetto, echinacea, and pollen extract are used. Their safety and efficacy are unknown.

HOW TO MONITOR

- Monitor for symptom relief utilizing the American Urological Association (AUA) Symptom Index.
- Monitor closely for complications of BPH, such as obstructive uropathy.

PATIENT VARIABLES

Geriatrics

- BPH is very commong in elderly men

Pediatrics

- Not indicated for use in children

Pregnancy

- *Category C:* other α_1-adrenergic blockers
- *Category X:* finasteride

> ! Finasteride is teratogenic. Finasteride tablets must not be touched by a woman who may potentially be pregnant because the product may be absorbed through the skin. A pregnant woman should not come in contact with the semen of a man who is taking tamsulosin.

Gender

- Tamsulosin is not indicated for females

PATIENT EDUCATION

- Report immediately any signs and symptoms of obstructive uropathy.

Specific Drugs

α-ADRENERGIC ANTAGONISTS

(P) Prototype Drug

tamsulosin (Flomax)

Contraindications

- Hypersensitivity
- Female sex

Warnings/Precautions

- Priapism is rare
- Reduced male fertility with tamsulosin is reversible

Pharmacokinetics

See Table 34-1.

Adverse Effects

See Table 34-2.

Drug Interactions

- Potentiates other α-adrenergic blocking agents.
- Alcohol, β-blockers, and cimetidine increase the risk of hypotension.

Dosage and Administration

Give 0.4 mg po qd. It should be administered approximately 30 minutes following the same meal each day. If patient fails to respond after 2 to 4 weeks, increase to 0.8 mg. If therapy is interrupted, restart at 0.4 mg dose.

Other Drugs in Class

Drugs that are from the same category or subcategory are similar to the prototype except in the following ways.

alfuzosin (Uroxatral)

Contraindications

- Moderate to severe hepatic impairment
- Concomitant use with potent 3A4 inhibitors
- Concomitant use with ED drugs

Drug Interactions. Inhibitors of CYP 3A4; can increase serum levels.

Dosage and Administration. 10-mg extended release tablet is given with a meal every day. No dosage change is required in elderly or with renal impairment.

finasteride (Proscar)

Contraindications

- Hypersensitivity
- Pregnancy

TABLE 34-1 Pharmacokinetics of Male Genitourinary Agents

Drug	Absorption and Availability	Onset of Action	Half-life	Duration of Action	Protein Bound	Metabolism	Excretion
tamsulosin (Flomax)	Decreased with food; 90% available after first pass				94%-99%	Hepatic PCY 450 pathway not known	Urine, 60% metabolized; urine, 10% unchanged; feces, 20%
alfuzosin (Uroxatial)			10 hr			CYP 3A4	Metabolites in feces, urine
finasteride (Proscar)	63% available after first pass	1-2 hr to peak	6 hr		90%	Hepatic 2D6 3A4	Urine, 40% as metabolites; feces, 60%
sildenafil (Viagra)	Rapid, 40% ↓ with high-fat meal	Onset 30-60 min 27 min	Peak 2 hr	4 hr	96%	3A4 2C9	Metabolites in feces
tadalafil (Cialis)		45 min	17.5 hr	3-6 hr		CYP 3A4	Metabolites in feces, urine
vardenafil (Levitra)	15% bioavailable ↓ with high-fat meal	26 min	4-5 hr	4 hr		CYP 3A4	Feces
alprostadil injection	Absorbed from urethra	30 sec	10 min	1 hr	81%		Metbolized in lungs 90% kidney as metabolites

TABLE 34-2 Adverse Effects of Drugs Affecting the Urinary Tract

Drug	Adverse Effects
tamsulosin	Orthostasis, dizziness, somnolence, rhinitis, diarrhea, abnormal ejaculation, fatigue, headache
alfuzosin	Dizziness (5%), syncope (rare), hypotension (rare) Abnormal ejaculation has not occurred QT interval increase (dose higher than 40 mg)
finasteride	Impotence; decreased libido; decreased volume of ejaculate; breast tenderness and enlargement; hypersensitivity reactions, including lip swelling and skin rash, testicular pain
sildenafil, vardenafil	Headaches, flushing, dyspepsia, rhinitis, urinary tract infection, abnormal vision, diarrhea, dizziness, rash, hypotension
alprostadil injection	Priapism, penile fibrosis, penile pain, hematoma, decreased blood pressure, increased heart rate, headache, respiratory tract infection, hypertension

Warnings

- A woman who may become pregnant should not handle crushed tablets or come in contact with semen of men taking drug because birth defects may occur.
- Treatment with drug will decrease serum levels of PSA.

Precautions

- Obstructive uropathy: not all patients have a response to finasteride; monitor carefully for obstructive uropathy.

Drug Interactions. None noted at this time.

Dosage and Administration

- Take 5 mg once a day. May be taken without respect to meals. Early improvement may be seen. At least 6 to 12 months of therapy may be necessary to assess full response.
- This product is marketed as Propecia to treat male pattern hair loss: 1 mg qd.

Drugs for Erectile Dysfunction

General Uses

Indications

- Erectile dysfunction (ED)
- vardenafil (Levitra) is about ten times as potent as sildenafil.
- tadalafil (Cialis) has a different chemical structure than sildenafil and vardenafil. It has less affinity for PDE6 (retina), but more affinity for PDE11. PDE11 is found in skeletal muscle, testes, heart, prostate, kidney, liver, and pituitary, but its function is unknown.

- alprostadil (Caverject): treatment of ED resulting from neurogenic, vasculogenic, or psychogenic causes, or that of mixed etiology
- yohimbine (Yocon): there are no Food and Drug Administration (FDA)-sanctioned indications.
- Unlabeled uses include treatment of ED resulting from vascular or diabetic origins, or caused by the use of serotonin reuptake inhibitors; it is also used for orthostatic hypotension and as an aphrodisiac.

DISEASE PROCESS

ED is defined as the consistent inability to maintain an erect penis with sufficient rigidity to allow sexual intercourse. It is common and increases with age.

Erection and ejaculation involve complex interactions with psychologic, hormonal, neural, and vascular functions. Both sympathetic and parasympathetic pathways are used. Parasympathetic (cholinergic) stimulation controls erection of the penis. Sympathetic (adrenergic) pathways produce ejaculation by causing contraction of the prostate and seminal vesicles along with effects on the bulbocavernous and ischiocavernous muscles.

ED may result from malfunction in one or more areas. Causes are categorized into psychologic or organic. Psychologic causes are usually abrupt in onset, and incidence varies with partner, position, or situation. This etiology occurs more commonly in younger men. Organic causes usually have a gradual onset and are more consistent.

Workup for ED should include a complete history, including information about sexual history, emotional upheavals, and any drug use. Testing may include measurement of nocturnal penile tumescence with mechanical and elective devices. Injections of papaverine have also been used as a screening measure. If the patient fails to have an erection after injection, he may have vasculogenic impotency, and further workup may be necessary. Vascular angiography and hormone levels (e.g., testosterone and prolactin levels) may also be obtained to assist with evaluation.

Neurologic causes for ED include diabetes, multiple sclerosis, spinal cord damage, nerve damage after a prostatectomy, decreased blood flow to penis because of atherosclerosis, or vascular damage resulting from injury, for example, renal transplant, bypass procedures, hyperprolactinemia, and structural abnormalities. Numerous drugs may also be responsible (e.g., antihypertensives, opioids, antidepressants, antianxiety agents, antipsychotic agents, ethyl alcohol, chemotherapeutic agents, cimetidine, estrogenic agents).

ED in men with diabetes often is associated with diabetic neuropathy and peripheral vascular disease. It occurs at an earlier age in men with diabetes than in men in the general population, and several studies have demonstrated that ED affects 35% to 75% of men with diabetes.

DRUG ACTION AND EFFECTS

PDE5 inhibitors have a very specific mechanism of action. Erection involves release of nitric oxide (NO) in the corpus cavernosum in response to stimulation. NO increases levels of cyclic guanosine monophosphate (cGMP), producing smooth muscle relaxation in the corpus cavernosum and allowing inflow of blood. Phosphodiesterase type 5 (PDE5) degrades cGMP in the corpus cavernosum, causing the blood flow to decrease. These drugs work by inhibiting PDE5.

The PDE5 enzyme is very specific to receptors in the corpus cavernosum's smooth muscle. It is also found in much lower concentrations in platelets, vascular and visceral smooth muscle, and skeletal muscle. PDE3 is found in cardiac contractility; therefore, these drugs are not active there. It is closely related to PDE6, which may explain the abnormalities in color vision seen with PDE5 inhibitors.

Alprostadil has many actions. Vasodilation and inhibition of platelet aggregation are the most important. It induces erection by relaxation of trabecular smooth muscle and by dilation of cavernosal arteries. This causes expansion of lacunar spaces and entrapment of blood by compressing the venules against the tunica albuginea. This is called the corporal veno-occlusive mechanism.

Yohimbine is an alkaloid derived naturally from the West African tree *Corynanthe yohimbine*. Yohimbine is an alkaloid similar to reserpine with both sympatholytic and mydriatic properties. It is an α_2-adrenergic antagonist affecting erectile function by stimulating presynaptic norepinephrine release in the lower nerve centers. Antidiuresis also occurs from the release of antidiuretic hormone.

DRUG TREATMENT PRINCIPLES

Nonpharmacologic Treatment

There are many nonpharmacologic treatments for erectile dysfunction. Vascular reconstruction may be appropriate in patients with decreased blood flow. Vacuum constriction devices are safe and effective. There is a wide variety of implanted penile prostheses.

Pharmacologic Treatment

Hormonal replacement with testosterone injections or topical patches can be used for men with documented androgen deficiency and no contraindications. This requires a thorough endocrine evaluation.

PDE5 inhibitors have been shown to be very safe and effective drugs if used properly. The major risk with its use is in patients with cardiac conditions. Treatment with these drugs in controlled studies has suggested that erectile function improved regardless of patient age, the duration of ED, or the duration of diabetes. PDE5 inhibitors are effective 50% to 80% of the time.

Injection of a vasoactive prostaglandin such as alprostadil is acceptable for most men.

Yohimbine has not demonstrated effectiveness in trials, but patients are still interested in its use. There are no data that show how yohimbine should be used.

HOW TO MONITOR

- Monitor for effectiveness.
- Monitor for adverse reactions, especially priapism.

PATIENT VARIABLES

Geriatrics

- sildenafil: reduce dose
- vardenafil, tadalafil: no adjustment necessary
- alprostadil, yohimbine not indicated

Pediatrics

- PDE5 inhibitors, yohimbine: not indicated
- alprostadil: generally not indicated; however, may be used in newborns with congenital heart defects

Pregnancy

- sildenafil: *Category B:* safety has not been established
- alprostadil: do not use for sexual intercourse with a pregnant woman unless a condom is used
- yohimbine: do not use

Gender

- PDE5 inhibitors, alprostadil, yohimbine: not indicated for use in women

PATIENT EDUCATION

See individual drug.

Specific Drugs

PDE5 INHIBITORS

Ⓟ **Prototype Drug**

sildenafil (Viagra)

Contraindications

- Hypersensitivity
- Coadminister very carefully in patients taking nitrates or a patient who has taken nitrates, even intermittently

Warnings

- Renal and hepatic function impairment: clearance is reduced, consider lower dose.
- Do not use in patients who have severe hepatic impairment.

Precautions

- Cardiovascular status: there is a potential for cardiac risk associated with sexual activity. Treatments for ED, including sildenafil, generally should not be used in men for whom sexual activity is inadvisable because of their underlying cardiovascular status.

> ! Serious cardiovascular events, including MI, sudden cardiac death, ventricular arrhythmia, cerebrovascular hemorrhage, transient ischemic attack, and hypertension have been reported in temporal association with sildenafil.

- It is not possible to determine whether these events are related directly to sildenafil, to sexual activity, to the patient's underlying cardiovascular disease, to a combination of these factors, or to other factors.
- Deformation of penis/priapism: use with caution in patients with anatomic deformation or the penis or with risk factors for priapism.
- Bleeding disorders: sildenafil has an effect on platelets but has shown no effect on bleeding time when taken alone or with aspirin. Administer with caution in patients with bleeding disorders or active peptic ulceration.
- Visual disturbances: mild, transient, dose-related impairment of blue/green color discrimination has been noted.
- May be associated with retinitis pigmentosa.

Pharmacokinetics

See Table 34-1. Sildenafil absorption is slowed by a high-fat meal.

Drug Interactions

Sildenafil is a 3A4 and 2C9 substrate; inhibitors of these enzymes may reduce sildenafil clearance, causing an increase in plasma concentrations. Inducers will decrease sildenafil concentration.

- Use lower dose of sildenafil when used with ritonavir, ketoconazole, itraconazole, erythromycin. Do not use with nitrates or α-blockers.
- May add to hypotensive effect of other antihypertensive drugs.

Patient Education

- Discuss with patients the potential cardiac risk of sexual activity in patients with preexisting cardiovascular disease
- Advise patients who experience symptoms (e.g., angina pectoris, dizziness, nausea) upon initiation of sexual activity to refrain from further activity and discuss the episode with their provider.
- Priapism is an emergency. For any erections that last longer than 4 hours, seek immediate medical assistance
- Take 1 hour before expected use, lasts for 4 hours, take only one a day.
- May alter color vision temporarily, producing blue-green hazy vision.

Dosage and Administration

ED: 50 mg before sexual activity; may be taken anywhere from 4 hours to 30 minutes before. Use once a day with maximum dose of 100 mg; 25 mg recommended in geriatric patients or those with hepatic impairment, severe renal impairment, and concomitant use of potent P450 3A4 inhibitors.

Other Drugs in Class

Drugs that are from the same category or subcategory are similar to the prototype except in the following ways.

vardenafil (Levitra)

Manufacturer states that it has a shorter onset of action than sildenafil, but studies have not substantiated this claim.

Warning. Vardenafil can cause a slight prolongation of the QT interval. Do not use with antiarrhythmic drugs or in patients with hepatic insufficiency.

Adverse Reactions. Headache, facial flushing, dyspepsia, rhinitis, back pain, myalgia, and hypotension.

Drug Interactions

- Concomitant use with potent 3A4 inhibitors could increase serum levels of vardenafil.
- May potentiate the hypotensive effects of nitrates; do not use concomitantly because it might cause myocardial ischemia.
- May increase hypotensive effect of α-blockers, concomitant use is contraindicated.

Dosage and Administration. May only be taken once daily. Recommended starting dose is 10 mg with or without food, about 60 minutes before sexual activity. Lower dose in elderly with moderate hepatic impairment. Dosage can be increased to 20 mg or lowered to 5 mg depending upon effects.

tadalafil (Cialis)

- Tadalafil has a longer duration of action than sildenafil or vardenafil; it may last up to 36 hours.
- Does not produce visual changes.

Drug Interactions

- Do not use with nitrates or any α-blocker except tamsulosin.
- Does not interact with hypertensive drugs.
- Potent CYP 3A4 inhibitors increase serum level of tadalafil.

Dosage and Administration. Take ½ hour before intercourse. Initial dose is 10 mg without regard to meals. Dosage is 5 mg with mild hepatic impairment. May increase to 20 mg.

OTHER ED DRUGS

alprostadil (Caverject)

Contraindications

- Hypersensitivity
- Conditions that might dispose the patient to priapism
- Anatomic deformation of the penis
- Patients with penile implants
- Men in whom sexual activity is inadvisable or contraindicated

Warnings

- Priapism has occurred; to avoid, use lowest dose possible
- Penile fibrosis may occur
- Penile pain after intracavernosal administration is reported in up to 37% of patients; administer slowly
- Hematoma/ecchymosis may occur due to faulty injection technique
- Hemodynamic changes such as decreased blood pressure and increased rate have been observed

Drug Interactions. Alprostadil increases the effect of anticoagulants and decreases cyclosporine blood concentration. Use with vasoactive agents is not recommended.

Overdosage. Systemic effects may occur.

Dosage and Administration. First dose must be given in office. Use a tuberculin syringe.

Patient Education

- The patient requires an explanation on how to use that is beyond the scope of this text
- Instructions for injection are included in the package
- Do not change dose
- Use condom if partner is pregnant

yohimbine (Yocon)

Contraindications

- Hypersensitivity
- Renal disease

Warnings

- Special risk patients: do not use in patients with cardiorenal problems or psychiatric disorders with a history of gastric or duodenal ulcer

Pharmacokinetics. Information is not available.

Adverse Effects. Yohimbine penetrates the CNS to cause central excitation, including elevated blood pressure and heart rate, increased motor activity, nervousness, irritability, and tremor. Dizziness, headache, and skin flushing have also occurred.

Drug Interactions. Do not use with antidepressants.

Overdosage. Symptoms include increased heart rate and blood pressure, piloerection, and rhinorrhea. Other symptoms include paresthesias, incoordination, tremulousness, and a dissociative state. Death can occur via respiratory paralysis.

Dosage and Administration. One 5.4 mg tablet three times a day. If side effects occur, may cut the dose in half.

BIBLIOGRAPHY

Benign Prostatic Hypertrophy

Barry MJ et al: The American Urological Association symptoms index for benign prostatic hyperplasia, *J Urol* 148:1549, 1992.

Kreder KJ: Combination drug therapy for benign prostatic hyperplasia, *JAMA* 274:359, 1995.

Medina JJ et al: Benign prostatic hyperplasia (the aging prostate), *Med Clin North Am* 83:1213, 1999.

USDHHS, PHS, AHCPR: *Guidelines on benign prostatic hyperplasia: diagnosis and treatment,* Clinical Practice Guideline No. 8. AHCPR Publication No, 94-0582, February 1994.

Erectile Dysfunction

Burnett AL: New options for erectile dysfunction, *Therapeutic Spotlight—Supplement to Clinician Reviews,* 3-7, June, 1998.

Goldstein I et al: Oral sildenafil in the treatment of erectile dysfunction: sildenafil study group, *N Engl J Med* 338:1397, 1998.

Padma-Nathan H, Forrest C: Diagnosis and treatment of erectile dysfunction: the process of care model, *Nurse Practitioner* (suppl 25) (5): 4-10, 2000.

Sterling L: Pharmacologic options for erectile dysfunction, *Therapeutic Spotlight—Supplement to Clinician Reviews,* 8-10, June, 1998.

CHAPTER 35

Other Renal/Genitourinary Agents

Drug Names

Class	Subclass	Generic Name	Trade Name
Anticholinergics/antispasmodics		(P) oxybutynin chloride tolterodine propantheline flavoxate	Ditropan XL Detrol LA Pro-Banthine Urispas
Cholinergic agonist		bethanechol chloride	Urecholine
Posterior pituitary hormone		desmopressin	DDAVP
Urinary tract analgesia		phenazopyridine	Pyridium

(P), Prototype drug.

Urinary Tract Medications

General Uses

Indications

Urinary incontinence (UI)

- Oxybutynin XL: treatment of overactive bladder with symptoms of urge urinary incontinence, urgency, and frequency
- Tolterodine LA: treatment of patients with an overactive bladder with symptoms of urinary frequency, urgency, or urge incontinence
- Propantheline: indicated for adjunctive therapy in the treatment of peptic ulcer
  Unlabeled uses of propantheline:
  Treatment of urinary incontinence due to involuntary ureteral and bladder contractions for its antisecretory and antispasmodic effects; it is similar to dicyclomine (Bentyl) (discussed in Chapter 32).
- Flavoxate for the symptomatic relief of dysuria, urgency, nocturia, suprapubic pain, frequency, and incontinence as may occur in cystitis, prostatitis, urethritis, and urethrocystitis/urethrotrigonitis
- Bethanechol chloride: urinary retention: acute postoperative and postpartum nonobstructive (functional) urinary retention and neurogenic atony of the urinary bladder with retention
- Desmopressin (DDAVP): indicated for primary nocturnal enuresis (intranasal)
  Unlabeled use of desmopressin:
  Treatment of overactive bladder in adults
- Phenazopyridine (Pyridium): symtomatic relief of pain, burning, urgency, frequency, and other discomforts arising from irritation of the lower urinary tract mucosa caused by infection, trauma, surgery, or endoscopic procedures
  Unlabeled use of phenazopyridine:
  Interstitial cystitis

• • •

This chapter contains two categories of drugs used for UI, a drug for treating nocturnal enuresis in children, and a urinary tract analgesic drug. The disease discussed is UI, primarily in women. Many of the drugs commonly used to treat symptoms of urinary incontinence do not have FDA approval for the indication of urinary incontinence. The anticholinergics/antispasmodics and a cholinergic agonist, which are FDA approved for this condition, are discussed in detail in this chapter. α-Adrenergic agonists, α-adrenergic antagonists, tricyclic antidepressants, sympathomimetics, and estrogens are also used, and information about those drugs may be found in the relevant chapters. The Agency for Health Care Policy and Research (AHCPR) *Clinical Practice Guideline for Urinary Incontinence in Adults* is a vital, but dated resource for any provider caring for these patients.

Desmopressin is a new medication used in children with primary nocturnal enuresis. Phenazopyridine is used short term for urinary analgesia, usually from an acute urinary tract infection (UTI).

DISEASE PROCESS

Urinary incontinence is involuntary leakage of urine.

There are four categories of incontinence: stress, urge, overflow, and functional. Stress incontinence is loss of urine associated with increased intraabdominal pressure such as coughing, sneezing, lifting, or exercise. It is usually associated with laxity of the pelvic floor musculature in multiparous menopausal women, especially those who are obese. The sphincter function is insufficient to prevent loss of urine.

Urge incontinence is the loss of urine preceded by a strong urge to void. It is seen with inflammatory or neurogenic disorders of the bladder and common in elderly women. It is caused by detrusor hyperreflexia or sphincter dysfunction.

Overflow incontinence results from chronic urinary retention with distended bladder. It is seen in neurologic conditions such as multiple sclerosis and with benign prostatic hyperplasia (BPH). When a full bladder receives more urine, the pressure in the bladder exceeds the sphincter outlet resistance and a small amount of urine dribbles out.

Functional incontinence occurs when the patient is unable to get to the toilet. This usually occurs in elderly demented patients who no longer recognize the need to void or in patients who are physically unable to get to the toilet. There is no neurologic dysfunction; the cause is physical deconditioning or cognitive deficit.

Mixed types of incontinence are not uncommon. Patients frequently have a combination of stress and urge incontinence.

Assessment

Any new onset of UI should be evaluated for transient incontinence. Table 35-1 lists common causes of transient urinary incontinence.

The history will provide the most useful information to diagnose the type of incontinence. A voiding diary may help provide clues to the type of incontinence and is useful in documenting whether the treatment is effective. The physical examination should focus on abdomen, rectum, and genitalia in men, and rectum and pelvis in women.

A urinalysis and postvoid residual are required laboratory tests. Other tests that may be indicated are urine culture, provocative stress testing and observation of voiding, urine cytology, and blood tests. Further evaluation by qualified specialists may include urodynamic, endoscopic, and imaging tests.

DRUG ACTION AND EFFECTS

Anticholinergics/Antispasmodics

Anticholinergic agents have many actions. They block muscarinic actions (a subset of the parasympathetic nervous system). The primary effects are blurred vision, urinary retention, constipation, dry mouth, tachycardia, and confusion.

Anticholinergic medications used for urge incontinence include those in this chapter, tricyclic antidepressants (TCAs), and dicyclomine (discussed in Chapter 48).

The anticholinergic agents inhibit the action of acetylcholine on bladder smooth muscle. This blocks contraction of

TABLE 35-1 Common Causes of Transient Urinary Incontinence

Cause	Comment
Delirium	In the elderly, incontinence is an associated symptom that abates with treatment of the underlying cause.
Urinary tract infection (UTI)	Dysuria and urgency may cause an elderly patient to be unable to reach the toilet in time. Asymptomatic bacteriuria is rarely a cause of incontinence. A UTI can cause both transient incontinence and delirium in an elderly patient.
Atrophic urethritis or vaginitis	May present as dysuria, dyspareunia, burning on urination, urgency, agitation (in demented patients), and occasionally as incontinence. Both disorders are treated with estrogen.
Medications	
Sedative hypnotics, opiates	Benzodiazepines may accumulate in elderly patients and cause confusion and secondary incontinence. Alcohol, used as a sedative, can cloud the sensorium, impair mobility, and induce a diuresis, resulting in incontinence; opiates can cause sedation and confusion.
Diuretics	Diuresis can overwhelm bladder capacity and lead to polyuria, frequency, and urgency, thereby precipitating incontinence in frail elderly.
Anticholinergics, antihistamines, antidepressants, antispasmodics	Anticholinergic effects include urinary retention with associated urinary frequency and overflow incontinence. Also can cause decreased sphincter tone.
Antipsychotics	May cause sedation, rigidity, and immobility.
α-Adrenergics (decongestants, alpha-$_1$ adrenergic blockers)	Sphincter tone in the proximal urethra can be increased. This can cause stress incontinence in women. An older man with BPH may develop acute urinary retention and overflow incontinence.
Calcium channel blockers	Reduce smooth muscle contractility in the bladder and occasionally can cause urinary retention and overflow incontinence.
Psychologic factors	Severe vegetative depression may lead to functional incontinence.
Excessive urine production	Excess intake, endocrine conditions that induce diuresis (e.g., hypercalcemia, hyperglycemia, and diabetes insipidus), and expanded volume states (e.g., CHF), lower extremity venous insufficiency, drug-induced ankle edema, and low albumin states cause polyuria and can lead to incontinence.
Restricted mobility	Arthritis, poor eyesight, Parkinson's, orthostatic hypotension, etc. may prevent the patient from getting to the toilet in time.
Stool impaction	May present with either urge or overflow incontinence and may have fecal incontinence as well.

the bladder. This is used to decrease the urodynamic response of detrusor overactivity, the problem in urge incontinence. These actions result in increased bladder capacity, delayed desire to void, and diminished frequency of involuntary bladder contractions.

Oxybutynin has both anticholinergic and direct smooth-muscle relaxant properties, a direct antispasmodic effect. This is not antimuscarinic. It is a direct relaxant effect on smooth muscle by way of phosphodiesterase inhibition.

Tolterodine is a muscarinic receptor antagonist that is selectively more active on the bladder than on the salivary glands. It was originally marketed to be as effective as oxybutynin with decreased incidence of adverse effects such as dry mouth, but research has not confirmed those claims.

Propantheline's effectiveness in UI is based on its anticholinergic properties.

Flavoxate acts as a direct smooth-muscle relaxant. This effect causes a relief of bladder spasticity and thereby produces an increased bladder capacity. It also has a local anesthetic and analgesic action.

Cholinergic Agonist

Bethanechol has the opposite effect of the anticholinergics. It stimulates the parasympathetic nervous system, causing a release of acetylcholine at parasympathetic nerve endings. This increases detrusor muscle tone. This increased tone causes a contraction that initiates voiding and bladder emptying, useful in some cases of overflow incontinence.

desmopressin (DDAVP)

Desmopressin is a synthetic analog of vasopressin and acts as an antidiuretic. Vasopressin is a naturally occurring antidiuretic hormone (ADH). Desmopressin's action is stronger as an antidiuretic than as a vasopressor and smooth muscle. It decreases urine output for approximately 6 hours.

Urinary Tract Analgesia

Phenazopyridine is an azo dye that is excreted in the urine, where it exerts a topical analgesic effect on urinary tract mucosa. It is useful only for the relief of symptoms. Phenazopyridine is compatible with antibacterial therapy.

DRUG TREATMENT PRINCIPLES

The mainstay of treatment of most UI is nonpharmacologic. Treatment of UI includes behavioral, pharmacologic, and surgical options. There are also many devices used to manage incontinence.

Nonpharmacologic Treatment

Consider referral to a specialist if the patient is motivated to try nonpharmacologic treatments. Behavioral techniques can be very effective for stress, urge, and mixed incontinence. These methods are not indicated and should not be used in overflow incontinence. Some of these techniques can be adapted to manage functional incontinence. They include bladder retraining (resisting urge), habit training (timed voiding), prompted voiding, and pelvic muscle exercises. Biofeedback, vaginal cone retention, and electrical stimulation can also be used.

Treatment of UI depends on the type of incontinence. Four algorithms heavily focusing on diagnosis are described in the AHCPR guidelines. They describe decision-making steps in dealing with stress incontinence, urge incontinence, incontinence in males, and functional incontinence. However, over time new advances in medications have changed the pharmacologic choices described in these guidelines.

Pharmacologic Treatment

In female stress incontinence, α-adrenergic agonists and estrogens are used, alone or together. Estrogen (topically) may be considered first-line therapy in elderly women with atrophic vaginitis that contributes to the incontinence. Pseudoephedrine 30 to 60 mg orally up to four times a day can also be used, although high blood pressure is a risk for some individuals. TCAs increase bladder outlet resistance, which allows for better storage of urine. Imipramine is the most commonly used (25 mg orally at bedtime). Onset of effect may take several weeks.

In urge incontinence, first-line pharmacotherapy is oxybutynin or tolterodine. Second-line medications are estrogen or the TCAs. These drugs are additive to the anticholinergic agents and are often used in combination. Propantheline has strong anticholinergic side effects and is now considered a low-priority second-line choice. The theoretic advantage of flavoxate with its direct action on smooth muscle has not been effective in trials. Hyoscyamine or dicyclomine can also be considered.

Bethanechol, a urinary cholinergic, is used for the short-term treatment of urinary retention. The cause of the retention must be diagnosed and treated.

Phenazopyridine is used in interstital cystitis.

HOW TO MONITOR

- Clinical effectiveness may be monitored by the use of a bladder diary, including voiding pattern, incontinent episodes, urge symptoms, and urine volumes.
- Monitor for anticholinergic side effects.
- Monitor cardiovascular status in patients with cardiac disease.
- Intake and output should be monitored with bethanechol.

PATIENT VARIABLES

Geriatrics

- All types of UI are very common.
- Elderly patients are extremely sensitive to the anticholinergic effects, and both confusion and extreme cardiac effects are commonly seen.

Pediatrics

- Anticholinergics: oxybutynin is not indicated in children younger than 5 years of age; tolterodine: safety and efficacy in children younger than 12 years have not been not established
- Cholinergics are not indicated in children
- Primary nocturnal enuresis is common in children; desmopressin may be used in children 6 years of age or older

Pregnancy and Lactation

- *Category B:* anticholinergics: not established; lactation: not known

- *Category C:* bethanechol in lactation is unknown
- *Category B:* desmopressin

Gender

- Causes of incontinence vary by gender.

PATIENT EDUCATION

- Careful patient teaching concerning response and side effects is necessary.
- Avoid driving or participating in other hazardous activities until the reaction to the drug is known.
- A dry mouth may be relieved by sugar-free gum or hard candy. Patients need to be cautioned to maintain adequate fluid and fiber intake to prevent constipation.
- Avoid hot environments due to suppression of sweat gland activity and an increased risk for heatstroke. This is a particular problem for the elderly due to age-related reduction in sweat gland activity.
- Alcoholic beverages should be avoided.
- Elderly or debilitated patients should be warned that it is possible that they may experience agitation, confusion, excitement, or drowsiness with a usual dose. If this happens, they should stop taking the drug and notify the practitioner.
- Postural hypotension and tachycardia may occur during early therapy.
- Bethanechol: Take on an empty stomach in order to avoid the side effects of nausea and vomiting.
- Because orthostatic hypotension may occur, patients need to be taught how to change positions slowly.

Specific Drugs

ANTICHOLINERGICS/ANTISPASMODICS

(P) Prototype Drug

oxybutynin chloride (Ditropan, Ditropan XL)

Contraindications

- Hypersensitivity to oxybutynin or to any other anticholinergic agent
- Untreated narrow-angle glaucoma, partial or complete GI obstruction, paralytic ileus, intestinal atony in the elderly or debilitated, megacolon, ulcerative colitis, and obstructive uropathy, myasthenia gravis, unstable cardiovascular status, and in acute hemorrhage

Warnings

When taken by patients living in areas of high environmental temperature, there is an increased risk for heatstroke due to suppression of sweat gland activity.

- Diarrhea may be an early sign of intestinal obstruction in patients with a colostomy or ileostomy. In this situation, the use of oxybutynin chloride would be harmful.
- Use with caution in patients who have gastroesophageal reflux disease (GERD) or are taking drugs (such as bisphosphonates) that may cause or exacerbate esophagitis.
- May induce drowsiness or blurred vision. The concomitant use of alcohol or other sedating drugs may enhance the drowsiness caused by oxybutynin.
- Use with caution in patients with clinically significant bladder outflow obstruction because of the risk of urinary retention.
- Renal/hepatic function impairment: use with caution in patients with hepatic or renal impairment.

Precautions

All drugs that have anticholinergic and smooth-muscle relaxant properties have troublesome systemic anticholinergic side effects. The elderly are particularly sensitive to these effects. Careful dosing and the close monitoring of clinical response and tolerance of side effects are essential. The medication may aggravate the symptoms of heart disease (including angina, CHF, arrhythmias, tachycardia, hypertension), hyperthyroidism, reflux esophagitis, hiatal hernia, and prostatic hypertrophy.

Pharmacoknetics

See Table 35-2.

Adverse Reactions

See Table 35-3.

Drug Interactions

Concurrent use of other anticholinergics or drugs with an anticholinergic activity may enhance the anticholinergic effects of oxybutynin chloride.

Oxybutynin may increase serum concentrations of digoxin, decrease serum concentrations of haloperidol, and enhance the development of tardive dyskinesia.

Dosage and Administration

The usual dosage for adults is 5 mg two or three times a day. This may be increased to 5 mg four times a day. The recommended geriatric dosage is 2.5 to 5 mg twice daily. This may be increased by 2.5 mg increments every 1 or 2 days. The dosage for the XL formulation is 5 mg once daily; increase gradually to 30 mg as needed.

The usual pediatric dosage for children 5 years of age and older is 5 mg twice a day. This may be increased to 5 mg three times a day.

Other Drugs in Class

Other drugs in this class are similar to the prototype except as follows.

tolterodine LA (Detrol)

Theoretically, tolterodine produces a lower incidence of dry mouth than oxybutynin. Both now have long-acting formulations, which have fewer side effects than the short-acting formulations. Perhaps oxybutynin is more potent whereas tolterodine may cause fewer dry mouth symptoms.

TABLE 35-2 Pharmacokinetics of Medications Used in Treating Urinary Tract Conditions

Drug	Absorption	Onset of Action	Half-Life	Duration of Action	Protein Bound	Metabolism	Excretion
oxybutynin XL	6%-10%	Onset 30-60 min	6-10 hr		Protein-bound 0	Hepatic	Renal, 1%
tolterodine	50%	Onset 30-60 min	9 hr			Hepatic	Renal, 1% 2D6
propantheline	NI	Onset 30-45 min	1.6 hr	Duration NI	Protein-bound NI	Hepatic, GI tract	Renal, 70% as metabolites
flavoxate	NI	60 min; 112 min to peak concentration	NI	Duration NI	Protein-bound NI	Metabolism NI	Renal, 10%-30%
bethanechol	NI	Onset 30-90 min	1-6 hr	1 hr	Protein-bound NI	Metabolism unknown	Unknown
desmopressin	Intranasal, 3.3%-4.1%	Onset of action 40-45 min to peak	3.5 hr	Duration 6 hr	Protein-bound NI	Metabolism NI	Unknown
phenazopyridine	3%	Onset 1 hr	2-4 hr	Duration 4 hr	Protein-bound NI	Metabolism 2D6 and 3A4	Excretion urine, 65% unchanged

NI, No information.

TABLE 35-3 Common and Serious Adverse Effects of Medications Used in Treating Urinary Tract Conditions

Drug	Common Side Effects	Serious Adverse Effects
Anticholinergics	Dry mouth, constipation, diarrhea, ↓ sweating, headache, dizziness, anxiety, vision changes, fatigue, sinusitis, dysuria, somnolence	Urinary retention, ↑ IOP, drowsiness, confusion and delirium in elderly
oxybutynin	60% dry mouth	
tolterodine	Possibly lower incidence of dry mouth	
propantheline	High incidence of adverse effects	
flavoxate	Decreased anticholinergic effects. Antispasmodic effects: nausea, vomiting, nervousness, vertigo	Tachycardia
bethanechol	Flushing, sweating, abdominal cramps, colicky pain, nausea, belching, diarrhea, borborygmi, salivation, lacrimation, malaise, urinary urgency, headache	Bronchial constriction, asthma, miosis, orthostatic hypotension, fecal incontinence
desmopressin	Nasal irritation, nosebleed when given intranasally	Severe fluid overload and hyponatremia
phenazopyridine	Headaches, rash, vertigo, GI disturbances, staining of contact lenses	Anaphylactoid-like reaction, renal and hepatic toxicity

IOP, Intraocular pressure.

Dosage and Administration. Give 2 mg bid with or without food. Give 1 mg bid if frail, hepatic insufficiency, or taking other drugs that inhibit the CYP 3A4 enzyme system. With extended-release formulation, give 4 mg once daily.

propantheline (Pro-Banthine)

Drug Interactions. An increased effect will occur with narcotic analgesics, type I antiarrhythmics, antihistamines, phenothiazine, TCAs, corticosteroids, CNS depressants, amiodarone, β-blockers, and amoxapine.

Dosage and Administration. The usual adult dosage is 15 mg three times a day 30 minutes before meals and 30 mg at bedtime. The dosage will need to be adjusted as needed and tolerated with a maximum dose not to exceed 120 mg daily. The recommended geriatric dosage is 7.5 mg two or three times a day. The dosage may require adjustment as needed and tolerated with a maximum dosage not to exceed 30 mg three times a day. The usual pediatric dose is 0.375 mg/kg of body weight four times a day with adjustment as needed and tolerated (pediatric administration is limited due to available dosage form).

If the patient is also receiving antacids, propantheline should be taken at least 1 hour before or after the other drug.

flavoxate (Urispas)

Dosage and Administration. The usual dosage for adults and for children older than 12 years of age is 100 to 200 mg three times a day. A reduction of dosage may be considered with improvement of symptoms.

CHOLINERGIC AGONISTS

bethanechol chloride (Urecholine)

Contraindications. Hypersensitivity, hyperthyroidism, asthma, peptic ulcer disease (PUD), bradycardia, AV conduction defects, recent urinary or GI surgery, CAD, hypotension, hypertension, parkinsonism, epilepsy, and vasomotor instability.

Warnings/Precautions
- Reflux infection: in urinary retention, if the sphincter fails to relax as bethanechol contracts the bladder, urine may be forced up the ureter into the kidney pelvis. If there is bacteriuria, this may cause reflux infection.
- Some products containing tartrazine may cause allergies.

Drug Interactions
- When bethanechol chloride is given concomitantly with other cholinergics, additive cholinergic effects and toxicity may occur.
- Ganglionic-blocking compounds may raise the level of bethanechol, causing severe abdominal symptoms and a critical fall in blood pressure.
- Quinidine and procainamide can raise the level of bethanechol and antagonize the cholinergic effects of bethanechol.

Dosage and Administration. The dosage is highly individualized. The minimally effective dosage should be determined by beginning the adult patient on 5 to 10 mg, then repeating hourly to a maximum of 50 mg until there is a satisfactory response. Take medication on an empty stomach.

POSTERIOR PITUITARY HORMONE

desmopressin

Primary nocturnal enuresis should be used as an adjunctive to behavioral conditioning or other nonpharmacologic intervention. Desmopressin is effective in some cases that are refractory to conventional therapies. Desmopressin rapidly reduces the number of wet nights per week. However this tends to not be maintained after cessation of therapy. Desmopressin is more expensive than TCAs but is safer. Alarm interventions are intermediate in cost and are more disruptive, but do not have the potential for adverse effects.

Contraindications
- Hypersensitivity: severe allergic reactions. Anaphylaxis has not been reported with intranasal administration.
- Intranasal delivery may be inappropriate when there is an impaired level of consciousness.

Warnings
- Water intoxication: fluid overload and hyponatremia may result from excessive fluid intake. Severe hyponatremia may induce seizures and coma. Serum electrolyte monitoring is a reasonable precaution with initiation of the medication. Patients with electrolyte or fluid balance abnormalities, such as CHF and cystic fibrosis, should be monitored carefully. Pay particular attention to the possibility of the rare occurrence of an extreme decrease in plasma osmolality that may result in seizures, leading to coma. Very young or elderly patients should be cautioned to drink only enough fluid to satisfy thirst in order to decrease the potential for water intoxication and hyponatremia.
- Desmopressin: children and infants require careful fluid intake restriction to prevent possible hyponatremia and water intoxication.

Precautions
- Cardiovascular effects: high intranasal dosage has infrequently produced a slight elevation of blood pressure that disappears with dosage reduction. Use with caution in coronary artery insufficiency or hypertensive cardiovascular disease.
- Nasal mucosa changes (e.g., scarring, edema, discharge, blockage, congestion, severe atrophic rhinitis)
- Decreased response with time (longer than 6 months) has been reported.

Drug Interactions
- Desmopressin may increase the effect of pressor agents.
- Carbamazepine and chlorpropamide may potentiate the effects of desmopressin.

Administration and Dosage. Individualize dosage. Initial dose 20 μg intranasally at bedtime. It may be increased up to 40 μg or decreased to 10 μg depending on the response. Give one-half dose in each nostril. Duration of treatment is usually 4 to 8 weeks. The bottle accurately delivers 25 or 50 doses. Discard any solution remaining after 25 or 50 doses because the amount delivered may be less than that prescribed.

Urinary Tract Analgesia

phenazopyridine (Pyridium)

Contraindications

- Hypersensitivity, renal insufficiency, glomerulonephritis, or severe hepatitis

Precautions

- Use with caution in GI disturbances, glucose-6-phosphate dehydrogenase deficiency.
- Do not delay definitive diagnosis and treatment of the etiologic condition.
- Discontinue when symptoms of infection are controlled, usually within 2 days.

Adverse Effects. Stains urine (and underwear) orange.

Dosage and Administration. The usual dosage for adults is 200 mg three times a day after meals. Continued use after 2 days when used with an antibiotic for the treatment of a urinary tract infection is not recommended. It is available over the counter (OTC) at 100 mg and by prescription at 200 mg.

Patient Education

- Stains the urine orange or red and may stain fabrics.
- Notify provider if patient develops a yellowish tinge to the skin and/or sclera.
- Do not use long term.

RESOURCES FOR PATIENTS AND PROVIDERS

USDHSS, PHS, Agency for Health Care Policy and Research: Urinary Incontinence in Adults, Rockville, Maryland, Department of Health and Human Services, Rep No. AHCPR92-0038, 1992.

Patient education pamphlets on urinary incontinence available from the American College of Obstetricians and Gynecologists, 409 12th Street, SW, Washington, DC 20024-2188.

BIBLIOGRAPHY

Fantyl JA et al: *Urinary incontinence in adults: acute and chronic management: clinical practice guideline,* No. 2, 1996 Update. Rockville, MD, US Department of Health and Human Services, Public Health Service, Agency for Health Care Policy and Research; March 1996, AHCPR Publications Nl. 96-0682. Available at www.ahrq.gov.

Franks M, Chartier-Kastler E, Chancellor MB: New pharmacologic and minimally invasive therapies for the overactive bladder, *Drug Benefit Trends* 12(5):49-57, 2000.

Frenchman IB: Cost of urinary incontinence in two skilled nursing facilities: a prospective study, *Clin Geriatr* 9(1):1-4, 2001.

Glazener CMA, Evans JHC: Desmopressin for nocturnal enuresis in children (Cochrane Review). In *The Cochrane Library,* Issue 2, Oxford, 2002, Update Software.

Newman DK: New technology for women for stress incontinence, *Contemp OB/GYN* 15:69-70,74-75, 79-83, 2000.

Sampselle CM et al: Continence for women: a test of AWHONN's evidence-based protocol in clinical practice, *J Obstet Gynecol Neonatal Nurs* 29:18-26, 2000.

Sussman D, Garely A: Treatment of overactive bladder with once-daily extended-release tolterodine or oxybutynin: the antimuscarinic clinical effectiveness trial (ACET), *Current Medical Research Opinions* 18(4):177-184, 2002.

UNIT 9

Musculoskeletal Agents

Unit 9 focuses on drugs used in the treatment of common musculoskeletal conditions in primary care.

- **Chapter 36** discusses acetaminophen, an important medication used for many different conditions, particularly in the treatment of mild pain and fever. Acetaminophen (available OTC) is closely related to the drugs in Chapter 37, but it lacks the antiinflammatory action that the nonsteroidal antiinflammatory drugs (NSAIDs) possess.
- **Chapter 37** contains a discussion of aspirin and NSAIDs. Their use to treat acute muscle strain and osteoarthritis is explored.
- **Chapter 38** discusses disease modifying antirheumatic drugs (DMARDs) that are used to treat rheumatoid arthritis. These drugs are seldom ordered in primary care and are only discussed briefly. Immune modulators are also discussed briefly. These drugs should be prescribed and monitored by a specialist.
- **Chapter 39** discusses the different classes of medications used to treat gout.
- **Chapter 40** explores the use of bone metabolism regulators and selective estrogen receptor modulators used to prevent and treat osteoporosis in postmenopausal women and elderly men.
- **Chapter 41** discusses muscle relaxants, drugs usually used as adjunctive treatment in the management of acute muscle strain.

CHAPTER 36

Acetaminophen

Drug Names

Class	Subclass	Generic Name	Trade Name
		(200) acetaminophen	Tylenol

(200), Top 200 drug.

General Uses

Indications

- Antipyretic
- Analgesic: acute mild to moderate pain and chronic pain
- Weak antiinflammatory effects

Unlabeled use

To decrease fever and pain in children receiving diphtheria, pertussis, and tetanus (DPT) vaccination

• • •

Acetaminophen (APAP) is an over-the-counter (OTC) medication commonly used to alleviate fever and mild pain. It can be used in patients who have experienced gastric irritation with aspirin (ASA) or nonsteroidal antiinflammatory drugs (NSAIDs). Acetaminophen is similar to aspirin in its effectiveness in decreasing fever and pain. It is the drug of choice for relief of minor pain in children, adults, and the elderly. APAP is different from aspirin in that it has a weak antiinflammatory effect and no impact on platelet aggregation. Usually well tolerated at recommended dosage of 4 g/day.

Acetaminophen is a metabolite of phenacetin. Phenacetin was introduced in 1887, used extensively for many years, then taken off the market because it led to nephropathy. APAP has been in use since 1893 but has become very popular since 1949. APAP has the effectiveness of phenacetin without the adverse reactions.

The use of acetaminophen in the management of fever is discussed in this chapter. For additional information on the use of APAP in the treatment of pain, see Chapter 42.

DISEASE PROCESS

Pathophysiology

Fever is an elevation of the setpoint of body temperature. The hypothalamus is the site of the heat-regulating center. The setpoint is elevated by several mechanisms. The most common is through the monocyte-macrophages, that, when stimulated, release pyrogenic cytokines, including interleukin-1. These stimulate the heat-regulating center to raise the setpoint. This prompts increased heat production via shivering or decreased heat loss through peripheral vasoconstriction.

The Disease

It is essential to determine and treat the cause of the fever and not just the symptoms. Fever is a symptom with many causes, the most common being infection. The danger in treating a fever is the risk of masking symptoms of a worsening infection. A fever may be an important indication of antibiotic resistance. Fever of unknown origin is defined as unexplained cases of fever exceeding 38.3°C on several occasions for at least 3 weeks in patients without neutropenia or immunosuppression. Causes of fever and hyperthermia are listed in Table 36-1.

DRUG ACTION AND EFFECTS

Acetaminophen reduces fever by direct action on the hypothalamic heat-regulating center, lowering the setpoint to normal. It does this by inhibiting the action of pyrogenic cytokines on the heat-regulating centers. This action increases dissipation of body heat via vasodilation and sweating.

Acetaminophen is a centrally acting analgesic. The site and mechanism of analgesic action are not clear. It may be the result of inhibition of prostaglandin synthetase in the CNS. APAP differs from ASA in that it does not inhibit peripheral prostaglandin synthesis. This may account for the absence of antiinflammatory and platelet-inhibiting effects.

DRUG TREATMENT PRINCIPLES

Acetaminophen is an OTC medication, and many patients self-administer this product. Ask specifically about acetaminophen when taking a medication history. Generic acetaminophen is equally effective as and less expensive than brand-name products.

APAP use is straightforward in adults. However, in children it becomes more complicated with many opportunities for error. There are different dosages for different age groups and many formulations with different strengths. See Table 36-2 for a list of formulations and strengths. Note the confusing array of products with different strengths. Failure to give the proper concentration and dosage may lead to serious acetaminophen toxicity. Drops are three times more concentrated than the elixir. Two teaspoonfuls of the elixir are approximately equal to one adult dose of 325 mg.

Fever

Acetaminophen is the drug of choice for reduction of fever. Treatment of minor fever is not generally indicated. Symptomatic relief of a fever greater than 40°C is usually required. Treatment of a temperature greater than 41°C is a medical emergency.

TABLE 36-1 Causes of Fever and Hyperthermia

Common Causes of Fever	Less Common Causes of Fever	Causes of Hyperthermia
Infections: bacteria, virus, rickettsia, fungus, parasites	Cardiovascular disease: myocardial infarction, thrombophlebitis, pulmonary embolism	Heatstroke
Autoimmune diseases	GI disease: inflammatory bowel disease, alcoholic hepatitis, granulomatous hepatitis	Malignant hyperthermia of anesthesia
CNS disease, including head trauma and mass lesions	Medication: drug fever	Malignant neuroleptic syndrome
Malignant disease especially renal cell, liver, leukemia, and lymphoma	Other: sarcoidosis, tissue injury, hematoma, and factitious	

TABLE 36-2 Strengths (in mg) of Various Formulations

Formulation	80	100	120	125	160	300	325	500	650
Drops	0.8 ml								
Elixir	2.5 ml 5 ml		5 ml		5 ml				
Liquid					5 ml			15 ml	
Solution with dropper	1.66 ml								
Solution		1 ml							
Capsules, sprinkle	X	X							
Caplets					X			X	X
Capsule							X	X	
Gelcap								X	
Tablet, chewable	X				X				
Tablet					X		X	X	X
Suppository	X		X	X		X	X		X

These vary in flavors and ingredients—saccharin, alcohol, phenylalanine, aspartame, sucrose, corn syrup, etc.

The decision to treat a fever depends on the circumstances. All fevers do not need to be treated with an antipyretic. Fever may be a protective physiologic mechanism. Treating the fever may prolong the course of the infection, obscure symptoms, or make it is difficult to assess the patient's response to the infection.

Fever should be treated if it is deleterious to the patient, or the patient is in significant discomfort from the fever. For example, the elderly can have tachycardia from fever that may decompensate their CHF. Children may have seizures if their temperature is high. The patient may experience fluid and electrolyte imbalance from the perspiration.

Nonpharmacologic treatment of fever consists of heat removal measures such as alcohol or cold sponge baths or ice bags. An untreated fever may cause fluid and electrolyte losses through perspiration; these fluid and electrolyte losses must be replaced.

Pharmacologic treatment of fever may be with aspirin, NSAIDs, or APAP. APAP is generally preferred in children. Some adults may find aspirin or ibuprofen more effective. Acetaminophen is given every 4 hours. If the patient has an illness causing a fever, it is often advisable to give the medication routinely rather than as needed to prevent uncomfortable swings in temperature.

Acute Mild to Moderate Pain

Acetaminophen is useful in the treatment of mild to moderate noninflammatory acute pain such as headaches, muscle aches, and the malaise accompanying minor viral infections. It is commonly used to relieve the pain of teething in children. It is not effective in the treatment of acute inflammation. The effectiveness of pain relief is better if APAP is given on a routine basis and not on a prn basis.

Chronic Pain

Acetaminophen is a very effective pain medication for chronic pain of both malignant and nonmalignant origin. It is useful for the pain of osteoarthritis in the elderly who often cannot tolerate NSAIDs. It is often used in combination with other medications to enhance their effectiveness. It is frequently combined with codeine and similar opioids as an adjunct medication and to prevent drug abuse by injection of the codeine. See Chapter 44 for discussion of analgesics.

When given in combination products, such as acetaminophen with codeine, it is important to monitor the daily intake of acetaminophen to avoid an overdose.

DPT Vaccination Use

A dose of acetaminophen should be given immediately following vaccination and every 4 to 6 hours for 48 to 72 hours. This will decrease the incidence of fever and injection site pain.

PATIENT VARIABLES

Geriatrics

Geriatric patients often have subclinical hepatic insufficiency and are at risk for APAP toxicity. Use APAP with caution in geriatric patients, especially in combination with alcohol or in a patient with known impaired hepatic function. Use lower doses and increased dosage intervals. It is safer than other drugs for treatment of chronic pain.

Pediatrics

Acetaminophen is commonly used for pain and fever in children and is generally well tolerated. Use caution to avoid overdosage. Unlike aspirin, acetaminophen may be given to children with viral infections because it is not associated with Reye syndrome. Children should *never* receive aspirin because of concern about Reye syndrome.

Pregnancy and Lactation

Acetaminophen crosses the placenta. It is routinely used in pregnancy and appears safe for short-term use. There is no evidence of a relationship between APAP ingestion and congenital malformations.

Acetaminophen is excreted in breast milk. No adverse effects in nursing infants have been reported.

PATIENT EDUCATION

- Keep medication away from children.
- Severe pain or high fever may indicate serious illness. If symptoms persist, consult a health care provider.
- Avoid large amounts of alcohol consumption while taking acetaminophen because of the increased risk of liver damage.

Specific Drugs

acetaminophen (Tylenol)

Contraindications

- Hypersensitivity to acetaminophen, known G6PD problems, or liver disease

Warnings/Precautions

- Do not exceed recommended dosage.
- Use with caution in patients with hepatic function impairment.
- Use with caution in patients with chronic alcoholism.

Pharmacokinetics. Acetaminophen is rapidly and almost completely absorbed from the GI tract. Peak plasma concentration occurs in 30 minutes to 2 hours. Liquid preparations are absorbed faster than tablets. The rate and amount of absorption from rectal suppositories are variable. The half-life is 1 to 3 hours. It is metabolized in the liver. About 4% is metabolized via cytochrome P450 oxidase system, and the toxic metabolite is detoxified with hepatic glutathione. Hepatic necrosis can occur if the glutathione stores have been depleted by chronic or toxic doses of acetaminophen. Approximately 95% of this drug is metabolized and excreted in the urine.

Adverse Effects. Used as directed, adverse effects are rare. Hypersensitivity presents as skin eruptions, urticarial and erythematous skin reactions, and fever. Extremely rare hematologic reactions include hemolytic anemia, leukopenia, neutropenia, and pancytopenia. Other reactions are hypoglycemia and jaundice. Adverse effects are usually dose-dependent. Hepatic toxicity may occur following greater than 7.5 g within 8 hours or less. Alcoholics are more susceptible to hepatic toxicity.

Drug Interactions. Concurrent use with the following drugs may increase the risk of hepatotoxicity: barbiturates, hydantoins, carbamazepine, rifampin, sulfinpyrazone, and ethanol.

Overdosage. Call a poison control center if a patient takes more than 50 mg/kg in a single dose. Acute overdosage of acetaminophen can result in hepatotoxicity and is life threatening. APAP is metabolized to a highly toxic intermediate, which is normally immediately detoxified by glutathione. When the glutathione is depleted, the toxic intermediate attacks other cells, causing necrosis. Symptoms are nausea, vomiting, drowsiness, confusion, liver tenderness, low blood pressure, cardiac arrhythmias, jaundice, and acute hepatic and renal failure. The patient should immediately receive activated charcoal. Further treatment should take place in a hospital setting with the patient receiving acetylcysteine, the specific antidote for acetaminophen poisoning. The proper amount is based on serum level of APAP.

Chronic overdosage of 5 to 8 g/day for several weeks or 3 to 4 g/day for 1 year can cause liver damage, renal tubular necrosis, and myocardial damage.

TABLE 36-3 Dosage of acetaminophen by Age

Age Group	Dosage (mg)
0-3 mo	40
4-11 mo	80
1 to <2 yr	120
2-3 yr	160
4-5 yr	240
6-8 yr	320
9-10 yr	400
11 yr	480
12-14 yr	640
>14 yr	650
Adult	1000

Dosage and Administration. See Table 36-3. Dosage for adults is simple. Give 325 to 650 mg for fever and 325 to 1000 mg for pain. Administer every 4 hours. It can be given either prn or routinely. Maximum dose is 1000 mg every 4 hours or five times per 24 hours. One dose per day should be skipped to minimize the chance of overdosage. Elderly patients frequently do well on 1000 mg every 6 hours because they metabolize it more slowly.

Dosage for children is based on the formula 10 to 15 mg/kg. Administer every 4 to 6 hours for neonates. For children older than 2 months of age, administer every 4 hours. Skip one dose per day to minimize the chance of overdosage. By 8 years of age, most children can take one adult 325-mg tablet. Teenagers who weigh more than 100 lb can take the adult dose. See Table 36-3 for a list of dose by age.

Formulation is an issue for children. (There are many confusing, different formulations.)

The infant formulations may be less concentrated than the child formulations. Chewable tablets come in two strengths and are easily confused. Suppositories are needed if the child is vomiting or refuses the medication. Give specific instructions on the type of formulation recommended. Instruct the parent to read the label carefully to avoid overdosage.

BIBLIOGRAPHY

Bryant S, Bellamy L, Paloucek F, Wahl M: Acute acetaminophen poisoning in children: kids aren't just little adults, *J Emerg Med* 24(4):472-473, 2003.

Canoso B: *Rheumatology in primary care,* Philadelphia, 1997, WB Saunders.

Clark EA, Plint A, Correl R, Gaboury I, Passi B: Analgesia for musculoskeletal injuries in children: a randomized, blinded, controlled trial comparing acetaminophen, ibuprofen, and codeine, *Acad Emerg Med* 10(5):469, 2003.

Evered LM: Does acetaminophen treat fever in children? *Ann Emerg Med* 41(5):741-743, 2003.

Harris NS, Wenzel RP, Thomas SH: High altitude headache: efficacy of acetaminophen vs ibuprofen in a randomized, controlled trial, *J Emerg Med* 24(4):383-387, 2003.

Mackowiak PA: Concepts of fever, *Arch Intern Med* 158:1871, 1998.

CHAPTER 37

Aspirin and Nonsteroidal Antiinflammatory Drugs

Drug Names

Class	Subclass	Generic Name	Trade Name
Salicylate		(P) acetylsalicylic acid	Aspirin
NSAIDs	Propionic acids	(P) (200) ibuprofen	Motrin, OTC brands
		fenoprofen	Nalfon
		flurbiprofen	Ansaid
		ketoprofen	Orudis, Oruvail
		(200) naproxen	Naprosyn, Anaprox
		oxaprozin	Daypro
	Acetic acids		
	Indole and indene acetic acids	indomethacin	Indocin
		etodolac	Lodine
		sulindac	Clinoril
	Heteroaryl acetic acids	diclofenac	Voltaren, Cataflam
		ketorolac	Toradol
		tolmetin sodium	Tolectin
	Alkanones	(200) nabumetone	Relafen
	Fenamates (anthranilic acids)	meclofenamate	Meclomen
		mefenamic acid	Ponstel
	Oxicams	piroxicam	Feldene
		meloxicam	Mobic
	COX-2 inhibitors	(200) celecoxib	Celebrex
		valdecoxib	Bextra

(200), Top 200 drug; (P), prototype drug.

General Uses

Indications

Aspirin

- Acute or long-term symptomatic treatment of mild to moderate pain, rheumatoid arthritis, and osteoarthritis
- Reduces risk of recurrent transient ischemic attacks (TIAs) or stroke in patients who have had TIAs due to fibrin platelet emboli
- Reduces the risk of death or nonfatal myocardial infarction (MI) in men with previous infarction or unstable angina pectoris

Unlabeled Uses

- Prevention of cataracts, toxemia in pregnancy
- Reduction of risks for colorectal adenomas

Most NSAIDs

- Osteoarthritis (OA)
- Rheumatoid arthritis (RA)
- Mild to moderate pain: dental extractions, minor surgery, soft tissue athletic injury
- Primary dysmenorrhea

Unlabeled Uses

- Tendinitis, bursitis, migraine

This chapter discusses the use of salicylates and NSAIDs in the treatment of osteoarthritis and acute inflammatory/pain conditions. Salicylates and NSAIDs are closely related. They have antiinflammatory, analgesic, and antipyretic effects. Aspirin (ASA) is the only salicylate discussed because it is the only salicylate in common use.

All of these drugs can cause GI irritation and bleeding, which can be fatal. GI bleeding may occur without any prodromal symptoms.

NSAIDs are a large group of drugs used to treat a large variety of conditions. The official FDA indications vary among the NSAIDs and do not correlate well with their common usage. Table 37-1 lists some indications for use of aspirin and individual NSAIDs. Recent research suggests that long-term NSAID use may decrease the incidence of Alzheimer's disease. However, these neurologic effects are negated if the individual has been taking ASA for its cardioprotective effects. The different classes are chemically unrelated but share the same therapeutic actions and adverse effects. For the purpose of this chapter, they will be divided into seven classes: propionic acids, indole and indene acetic acids, heteroaryl acetic acids, alkanones, fenamates, oxicams, and COX-2 inhibitors. There are significant differ-

TABLE 37-1 Indications for Specific Drugs

	OA	RA	Mild to Moderate Pain	Primary Dysmenorrhea	Juvenile RA	Acute Gout	Acute Tendinitis/ Acute Bursitis
Aspirin	X	X	X				
ibuprofen	X	X	X	X			
fenoprofen	X	X	X		Y		
flurbiprofen	X	X		Y		Y	
ketoprofen	X	X		X	Y		
naproxen	X	X		X	X	X	X
oxaprozin	X	X					
indomethacin	X	X				X	X
etodolac	X	X	X			Y	Y
sulindac	X	X			Y	X	X
diclofenac	X	X		X	Y		
ketorolac			X				X
tolmetin	X	X			X		
nabumetone	X	X					
meclofenamate	X	X	X	X			
mefenamic acid			X	X			
piroxicam	X	X		Y	Y		
meloxicam	X						
celecoxib	X	X		X			
valdecoxib	X	X		X			

X, Indication; *Y,* unlabeled use.

ences among the drugs. Ibuprofen is considered the prototype NSAID. It was the first one on the market and remains widely used. Although COX-2 inhibitors may decrease the risk of GI side effects, they are much more expensive.

DISEASE PROCESS

Anatomy and Physiology

In joints, the ends of the bones are capped by cartilage, and the joint structure is held together by a very tight capsule. Lining that capsule is a very fine membrane, the synovium. The synovium normally stops at the point where the cartilage begins. The synovium does not extend across the whole joint; otherwise there would be trauma to the synovium every time the joint was flexed (Figure 37-1). The tendons attach to the bones, and, when the muscle contracts, the joint opens or closes.

Inflammation. The inflammatory response is necessary for the body's survival when faced with stressors from the environment. A number of stimuli can trigger the inflammatory response. These include infectious agents, ischemia, antigen-antibody interactions, and thermal or other injury. In many of the conditions the cause of the inflammation is not known. The inflammatory response has three phases: (1) acute, transient, local vasodilation and increased capillary permeability; (2) delayed, subacute infiltration of leukocytes and phagocytic cells; and (3) chronic proliferative tissue degeneration and fibrosis.

Polymorphonuclear (PMN) leukocytes or granulocytes are composed of neutrophils, eosinophils, basophils, and mast cells. Other white blood cells (WBCs) include monocytes/macrophages. When the monocytes are released into the bloodstream, they migrate to various tissue sites where they differentiate (mature) and become macrophages. The third type of WBCs are the lymphocytes, the B and T cells. These do not participate in nonspecific inflammatory response.

The inflammatory response begins when circulating proteins and blood cells come into contact with a stimulus. Neutrophils arrive at the site first and phagocytose (ingest the particles causing the inflammation). The mast cells are already present in the loose connective tissues close to blood vessels. Monocytes and macrophages arrive and begin phagocytosis. Mast cells, monocytes, and macrophages release many substances called collectively mediators or facilitators of inflammation. The mast cell is the most important activator of the inflammatory response.

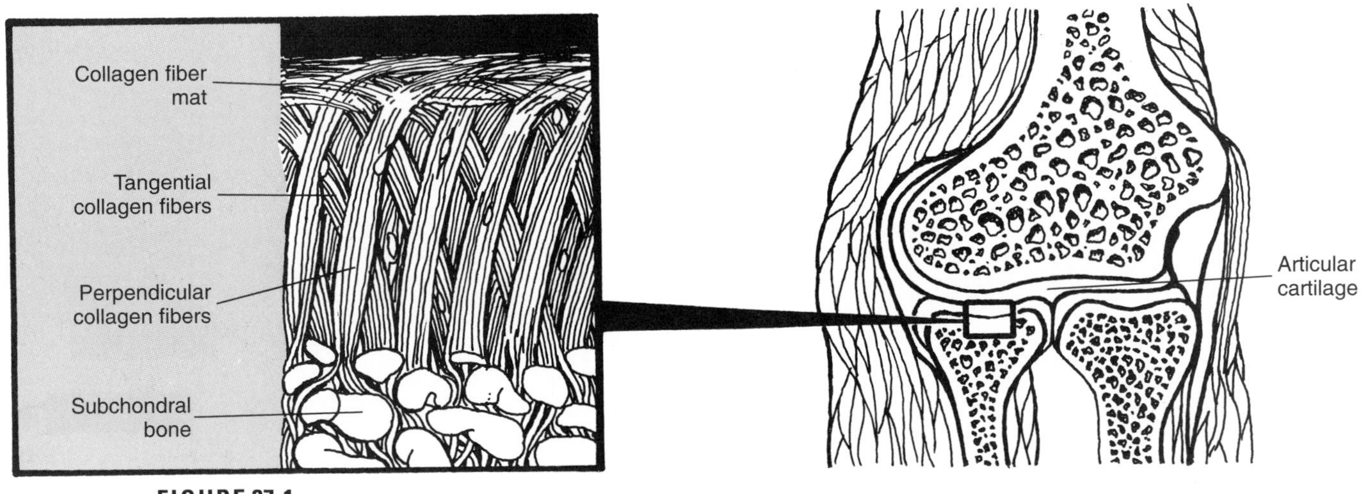

FIGURE 37-1

Organization of collagen fibers in articular cartilage. (From McCance KL, Huether SE: *Pathophysiology,* ed 4, St Louis, 2001, Mosby.)

The mast cell immediately releases substances from their granules, which cause immediate inflammation. These substances include histamine, neutrophil chemotactic factor, and eosinophil chemotactic factor. The mast cell also synthesizes then releases leukotrienes and prostaglandins, which cause long-term inflammation (Figure 37-2). These facilitators start a chain of reactions, producing exudate that defends against infection and facilitates tissue repair and healing. Whereas there are many mediators of inflammation, this discussion focuses on the prostaglandins, which are affected by aspirin and NSAIDs.

Prostaglandins cause increased vascular permeability and neutrophil chemotaxis (movement), and induce pain. Increased vascular permeability allows diffusion of the large molecule inflammatory substances across cell walls into the site of inflammation. Prostaglandins are made in the mast cell from arachidonic acid by the action of the enzyme cyclooxygenase (COX) and are classified into groups according to their structure. Prostaglandins E_1 and E_2 are active in the inflammatory response. Aspirin and NSAIDs act to block the enzyme cyclooxygenase from producing prostaglandins, thereby inhibiting inflammation (see Figure 37-2).

There are two types of cyclooxygenase: COX-1 and COX-2. COX-1 is found in the blood vessels, stomach, and kidneys; COX-2 is found in the brain and kidneys. The inhibition of COX-2 is necessary to prevent inflammatory action.

COX-1 prostaglandins protect the gastric mucosa. Prostaglandins encourage mucosal blood flow and elaboration of bicarbonate to produce a more neutral or less acid layer next to the gastric mucosa. Prostaglandins also produce a significant layer of mucus that serves as a barrier to the acid. They also maintain normal renal function, mental function, and temperature. It is through COX-1 inhibition that salicylates and NSAIDs are thought to have their direct detrimental effect on gastric mucosa. The selective COX-2 inhibitor drugs are designed to primarily inhibit COX-2 while sparing COX-1. Because this selectivity is not perfect, these drugs may still exert some detrimental effect on gastric mucosa.

When there is an inflammatory process, the synovium becomes lumpy. The synovium also starts to grow into and across the cartilaginous area, producing pits in the cartilage. At the same time, the tendon sheath that surrounds the tendon becomes inflamed so that motion of the joint is painful. If this process is not checked, ultimately the ends of the bones are denuded and bone grates upon bone, with eventual destruction of the joint (Figure 37-3). The inflammatory response is accompanied by symptoms of erythema, edema, tenderness, and pain. Inflammation protects the body from attack from foreign substances. However, some inflammatory responses are detrimental to the body. This is generally when the body reacts to itself.

Pathophysiology: Osteoarthritis

In OA, the articular cartilage degenerates, is roughened, and then worn away. The body attempts to repair the lost cartilage, but the integrity of the new cartilage is inferior to the original and the integrity of the surface of the cartilage is lost. The bone compensates by hypertrophy at the articular margins, forming spurs and lipping at the edge of the joint surface. The synovial membrane thickens, but the synovial membrane does not form adhesions. There usually is a low level of inflammation (see Figure 37-3).

The Disease

There are more than 100 types of arthritis. The one thread common to all arthritic conditions is inflammation. Treating the inflammation is only one component of treating arthritis, but it is extremely important.

Characteristic symptoms of OA are pain with movement and weight bearing that is relieved by rest. The patient often has brief morning stiffness (less than 15 minutes) with minimal articular inflammation and no systemic manifestations. Joints commonly affected are terminal joints of the fingers, thumb, hip, knee, and spine. There are no signs of acute inflammation and the erythrocyte sedimentation rate (ESR) is normal.

DRUG ACTION AND EFFECTS

Acetaminophen (APAP) is different from salicylates and NSAIDs in that it does not have significant antiinflammatory

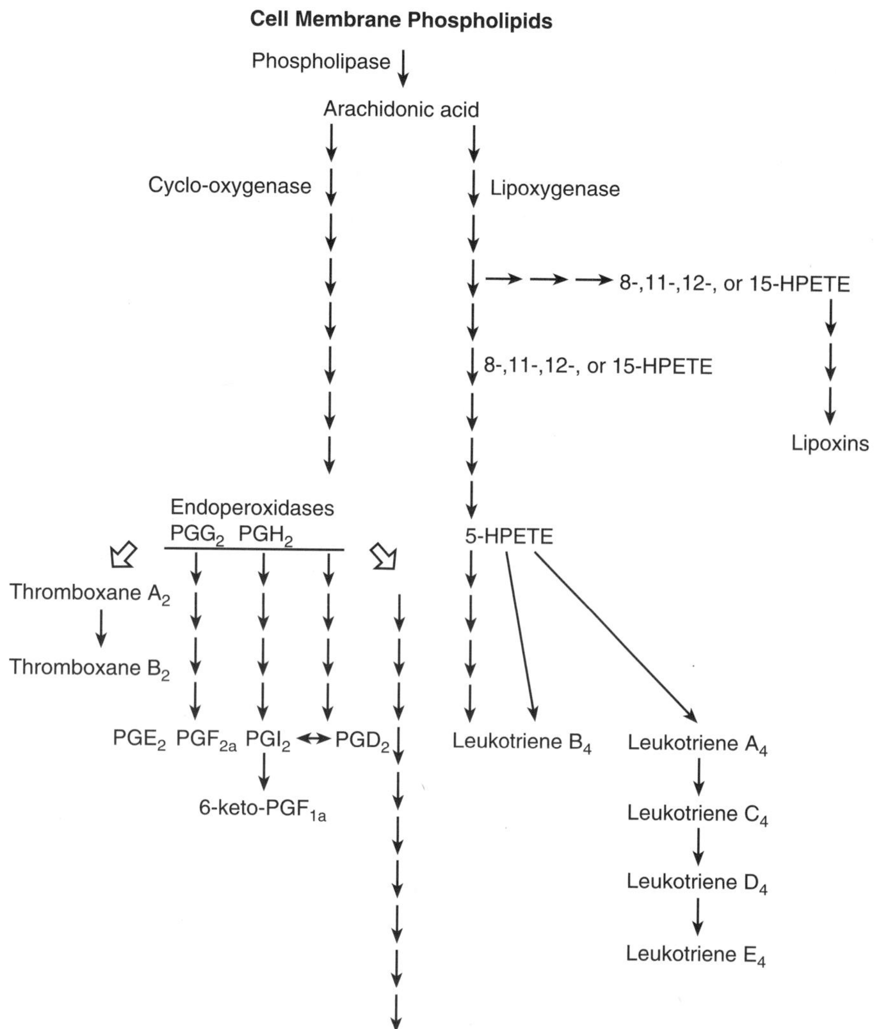

FIGURE 37-2

Arachidonic acid synthesis to prostaglandins. (Modified from Melmon K, Morrelli-Howard F: *Clinical pharmacology: basic principles in therapeutics,* ed 3, New York, 1992, McGraw-Hill.)

action. This is because APAP affects cyclooxygenase in the brain but not in peripheral tissue.

Salicylates and NSAIDs reduce inflammation by inhibiting the production of prostaglandins in both central nervous system (CNS) and peripheral tissue. They do this by blocking the production of cyclooxygenase, an enzyme that is necessary for the biosynthesis of prostaglandins. This is the major mechanism involved for most of the effects achieved by salicylates and NSAIDs (see Figure 37-2). The incidence of colon cancer has been found to be lower in patients who take ASA on a regular basis.

Pain

The mechanism for decreasing pain is through the anti-inflammatory process. Pain is relieved when inflammation is decreased and when prostaglandins are reduced. Salicylates may cause some pain reduction centrally at subcortical sites.

Antipyretic Effects

ASA also blocks the effect of interleukin-1 on the hypothalamus, which is responsible for temperature control. Peripherally salicylates also reduce fever by causing vasodilation of superficial blood vessels. This effect results in dissipation of heat.

Platelet Effects

Prostaglandins have an important effect on platelet aggregation. Prostaglandins produce thromboxane, which prevents platelet aggregation from occurring. Any drug that decreases prostaglandins will reduce the production of thromboxane. This effect is used in treating cardiovascular disease. Aspirin causes an irreversible inactivation of cyclooxygenase, allowing decreased production of prostaglandins for the life of the platelet. Thus the platelet is unable to produce prostaglandin to produce platelet aggregation during its life span of 8 to 10 days. NSAIDs, however, have a reversible inactivation of cyclooxygenase, lasting only the duration of the drug activity so continuous platelet aggregation is not found. This is why aspirin but not NSAIDs are used for prevention of stroke and MI.

In fact, regular NSAID use may block the cardioprotective effect of ASA.

Ongoing research is examining the use of NSAIDs in treatment of a variety of problems:

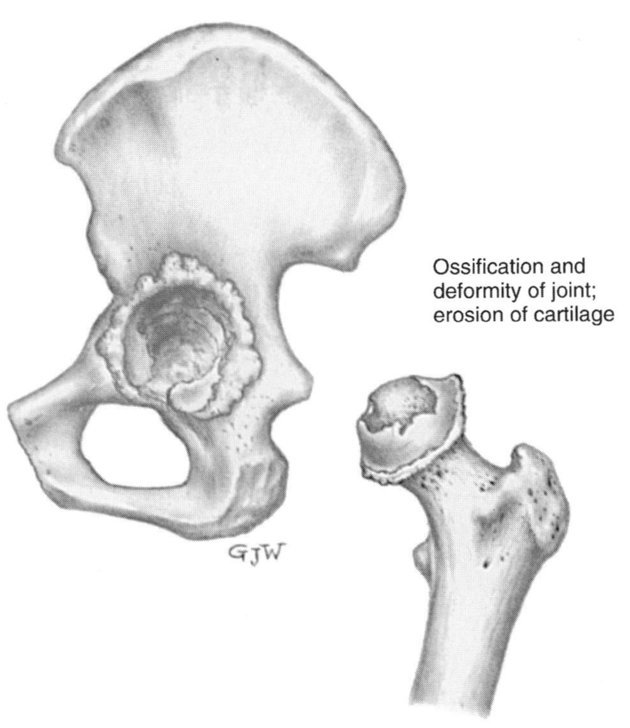

FIGURE 37-3

Osteoarthritis (OA). Cartilage and degeneration of the hip joint from osteoarthritis. (From Mourad L: *Orthopedic disorders*, St Louis, 1991, Mosby.)

1. The use of NSAIDs to reduce the risk of Alzheimer's is under study at the NIH.
2. There seems to be a strong inverse link between breast cancer and NSAID use.
3. NSAIDs may protect against Parkinson's disease.

Adverse Effects

When prostaglandins are inhibited, more gastric acid is produced. So ASA and NSAIDs, by inhibiting prostaglandins, increase gastric acid production at the same time they decrease the defense to that acid. This is the basis for the adverse GI effects of these medications.

Kidneys that are impaired also rely on prostaglandins to cause vasodilation. When prostaglandins are inhibited, there is less vasodilation and decreased blood flow to the kidneys.

DRUG TREATMENT PRINCIPLES

The underlying goals of treatment are to limit the inflammatory process, protect the joint, and relieve pain.

Nonpharmacologic methods are important in all of the uses of NSAIDs. If a patient has moderate pain, consider starting NSAIDs at the same time as nonpharmacologic treatment.

Drug Choice

Each of the NSAID drugs differs in a number of drug properties. Evaluation of these properties in relationship to the patient and his/her condition will aid drug choice. There is wide variation in how patients will respond to a particular medication. As always, when there are many drugs in the same class, select a few and become familiar with them. Clinically there are no clear guidelines, no evidence-based decision making, to assist the provider in selecting the most appropriate NSAID for a particular patient.

Aspirin can be effective and inexpensive. It requires up to 12 tablets a day, so compliance can be difficult. Salicylates are generally less expensive than NSAIDs. Because salicylates almost always cause GI distress or ulceration, there is significant limitation on their use.

The following drug characteristics must be considered:

- Degree of COX-1 versus COX-2 inhibition. There are varying degrees of COX-1 inhibition. Even the COX-2 inhibitors have a small amount of COX-1 inhibition. These differences cause differences in the frequency of adverse GI effects.
- Potency of the different therapeutic effects. For example, one drug may be a relatively weak antiinflammatory but a potent analgesic. This is used for pain rather than for inflammation.
- Pharmacokinetics to consider include duration of action (frequency of dosing), protein binding (drug interactions), and renal excretion (renal function).
- Relative frequency of adverse effects, especially GI, renal, hepatic, cardiovascular.
- The specific use that is intended and the specific indications for each drug.
- Whether the drug is over the counter (OTC) or prescription only.

Patient variables to consider include the following:

- Medical condition, especially renal and hepatic function, cardiovascular status
- Age
- Ability to comply with dosing schedules
- Reliability of the patient in promptly reporting adverse effects
- Cost

See Table 37-2 for other unique properties of antiinflammatory drugs.

Initiate treatment with starting dose. The analgesic effect should be noticed within 1 to 4 hours of administration. However the full antiinflammatory effect will not be noted until a few weeks. Increase the dose until therapeutic effects are seen or patient experiences adverse effects. Patient response to one NSAID does not predict what the response will be to any other one, even within the same drug class. If pain cannot be adequately managed with NSAIDs, see Chapter 44 for analgesia.

If the patient experiences GI distress or is at high risk for GI bleed, coadministration of misoprostol may be considered. H_2-blockers, and proton pump inhibitors may have some benefit, but only misoprostol is acceptable as a means of preventing both gastric and duodenal ulcers. Misoprostol may be started at a much lower dose than recommended (100 mg bid, not 200 qid) and slowly increased, to avoid the severe diarrhea it often produces.

! Women who are of childbearing age should not take misoprostol unless appropriate contraception is being used, as it is an abortifacient.

TABLE 37-2 Individual Characteristics of Aspirin and NSAIDs

	Inflammation	Pain	COX-1*	COX-2	Renal AR	Hepatic AR	Comments
Aspirin			↑				High risk AR; cardioprotective
ibuprofen	↑		↑				Prototype
fenoprofen		↑					AR: headache
flurbiprofen		↑					
naproxen			↑			2C9, ↑	
oxaprozin						2C9	
indomethacin	↑		↑	↑	↑	↑	High risk AR, esp CNS, headache, hyperkalemia; aggravates epilepsy and parkinsonism; short-term use only
etodolac			↓	↑		↓ 2C9	
sulindac					↓	↑	AR: pancreatitis; prodrug, bypasses kidney hepatic risk
diclofenac		↑	↑			↑	
ketorolac	↓	↑↑	↑↑			2C9	↑ AR: headache, black box warning; short-term use, not primary care
tolmetin		↑					
nabumetone			↓	↓	↓	2C9	Prodrug
meclofenamate			↑				Toxicity manifests as diarrhea
mefenamic acid			↑			2C9	Toxicity manifests as diarrhea, ↑ AR
piroxicam			↑		↑	↓	High risk of AR; qd dosing, largely replaced by COX-2 inhibitors
meloxicam			↓	↑		2C9	↑ GI in dose >30 mg
celecoxib			↓↓	↑			AR: headache, sulfa allergy, qd dosing
valdecoxib			↓↓	↑	↑	↑3A4 2D9	Sulfa allergy, qd dosing

Blank, Average; *0,* none; *AR,* adverse reaction; ↑, increased; ↓, decreased.
*COX action correlates to GI AR.

Aspirin products have largely been replaced by the use of NSAIDs. There is a trend toward increasing use of COX-2 inhibitors because they have a reduced risk of GI distress. This has allowed for NSAID treatment for many patients formerly unable to use them. However they still have adverse renal, hepatic, and cardiovascular effects. Cost is the major limitation. Insurance companies often limit reimbursement or require preauthorization unless patient has had an adverse reaction to NSAIDs.

Osteoarthritis Treatment

Nonpharmacologic treatment includes proper exercise with rest periods. A supervised walking program can improve functional status. Recommend weight loss to over-weight patients to reduce strain on joints. The patient must be realistic about the limitations of the medications and their prognosis.

Acetaminophen may be effective in the treatment of the pain of osteoarthritis because many patients have minimal inflammation. Patients with mild OA should be started on acetaminophen. If this is not effective, NSAIDs can be used. NSAIDs are more effective than acetaminophen for OA of the knee or hip. They are also more effective in moderate to severe disease. Some patients can be managed on chronic acetaminophen therapy with short-term use of NSAIDs for flareups. Because of the decreased risk of GI toxicity, COX-2 inhibitors are useful for long-term management of OA in elderly patients.

Intraarticular injection of steroids can be used on a limited basis. Topical creams such as capsaicin may also help with the pain. Surgical measures such as hip or knee replacement may be necessary in joints that are seriously affected.

Rheumatoid Arthritis

NSAIDs are frequently prescribed in RA and other rheumatologic diseases. See Chapter 38.

Acute Mild to Moderate Pain

Nonpharmacologic treatment includes rest, ice, compression, and elevation (RICE) for the first 24 to 48 hours, as indicated. These actions are the cornerstones of therapy.

For minor problems, start the patient on NSAIDs immediately. In large muscle injury with the possibility of continued bleeding into the tissue, wait 24 hours because of the NSAID effect on platelets. Usually short-acting products are used, such as ibuprofen. These are given for a limited amount of time, usually 1 to 2 weeks.

In addition to these indications, NSAIDs are used for a large variety of minor musculoskeletal problems such as low back pain, bursitis, and tendinitis. NSAIDs are also frequently used for chronic pain. See Chapter 44 for more information.

Primary Dysmenorrhea

NSAIDs should be started when the patient starts menstrual bleeding. The medication should be taken on a routine basis for 2 to 3 days. It is important that NSAIDs are not used during pregnancy.

Reduction of Cardiovascular Risk

Aspirin at the dosage of 325 mg taken every other day or 81 mg daily is effective in reducing the incidence of MI. A higher dose appears necessary for stroke prevention, such as 325 mg daily. An 81 mg enteric-coated aspirin is commonly used because of the decreased risk of GI toxicity.

HOW TO MONITOR

All Drugs

- Adverse reactions, especially GI distress
- Monitor renal and hepatic function
- Subjective report of relief of pain

Salicylates

- Monitor for vertigo, tinnitus, or impaired hearing.
- Serum concentration can be measured.

NSAIDs

- Short-term: acute, minor pain should be relieved within 1 hour.
- Long-term: get a baseline complete blood count (CBC) and differential, creatinine, U/A, K^+, liver function tests (LFTs). Check when product is started and then every 3 months until the patient is stable, then every 3 to 6 months.
- Follow patients weekly after initial prescription to determine pain relief and/or early side effects.
- Relief of pain such as in rheumatoid arthritis may take up to 2 weeks.
- GI bleeding can occur at any time during therapy. Assess for bleeding tendencies by monitoring CBC, prothrombin time (PT), U/A and stool for occult bleeding.

PATIENT VARIABLES

Geriatrics

Elderly patients are more susceptible to the adverse effects, especially the GI, CNS, and renal effects. NSAIDs can cause confusion in the elderly patient. Renal clearance may be decreased. Rarely observed increases in serum potassium can occur in the elderly, those with renal disease, or those on potassium-sparing diuretics. Use with antihypertensive agents requires monitoring for increasing hypertension (especially with diclofenac), edema, or other signs of CHF.

Pediatrics

There is a possible association between the development of Reye syndrome and the use of salicylates as an antipyretic in children and teenagers who have varicella or an influenza virus infection. Dehydrated children have increased susceptibility to salicylate toxicity.

The use of NSAIDs in the pediatric population is not common, except in children with a diagnosis of juvenile arthritis. Ibuprofen, naproxen, and indomethacin are available in liquid form. Naproxen may be useful because it does not have to be given as often as ibuprofen and is safer than indomethacin. The elixir or suspension dosage should be watched carefully because the drug concentration may vary. It is very easy to give a small child an overdose if the correct product and dosage are not followed.

Pregnancy

- The use in pregnant women generally is not recommended; NSAIDs must be discontinued prior to the expected due date to prevent excess bleeding
- *Category B:* NSAIDs (e.g., naproxen, ibuprofen)
- *Category C:* NSAIDs (e.g., COX-2 inhibitors)
- *Category D:* salicylates (aspirin); may be teratogenic or produce hemorrhage; avoid use during pregnancy, especially in the third trimester
- *Category D:* NSAIDs are not recommended in third trimester or near delivery

Lactation

Salicylates and NSAIDs (e.g., naproxen, ibuprofen, COX-2 inhibitors) are excreted in milk.

PATIENT EDUCATION

All Drugs

These drugs can cause serious GI bleeding. Report immediately signs of GI irritation, pain, emesis, diarrhea, presence of blood; stop taking the drug.

- Take with meals or with food or milk to avoid GI distress. A full glass of water is also recommended.
- May take with antacids.
- Refrain from drinking alcohol.
- Take medication around the clock (e.g., every 6 hours, not just qid) for best serum concentration.
- Do not take more than one drug from these two classes of drugs concurrently.

Salicylates

- Discard aspirin if tablets exude a strong vinegar-like odor.
- Stop taking aspirin 2 weeks before surgery to avoid any problem with platelets.

NSAIDs

- Patients should notify health care provider if they become aware of shortness of breath (SOB), wheezing, dizziness, GI distress, pruritus, or skin rash.

- Stop medication 1 week before surgery to avoid any problem with platelets.

Specific Drugs

SALICYLATES

Ⓟ **Prototype Drug**

Aspirin

Contraindications

- Suspected hypersensitivity to salicylates or NSAIDs because anaphylaxis is not uncommon

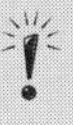

Cross-sensitivity may occur between aspirin and other NSAIDs that inhibit prostaglandin synthesis and between aspirin and tartrazine. Aspirin hypersensitivity is more prevalent in patients with asthma, nasal polyps, and chronic urticaria.

- Hemophilia, bleeding ulcers, and hemorrhagic states

Warnings

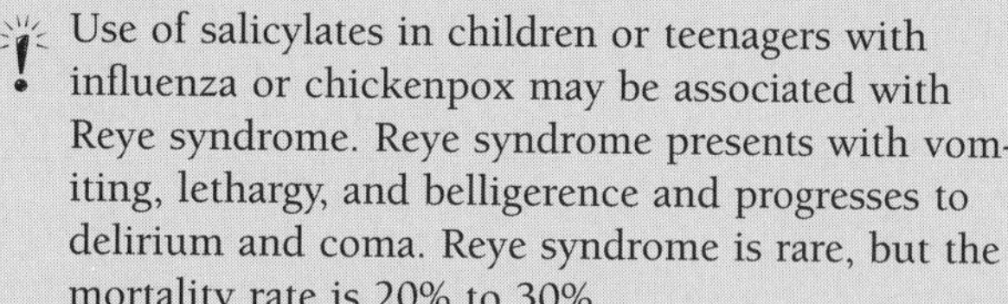

Use of salicylates in children or teenagers with influenza or chickenpox may be associated with Reye syndrome. Reye syndrome presents with vomiting, lethargy, and belligerence and progresses to delirium and coma. Reye syndrome is rare, but the mortality rate is 20% to 30%.

- Hypersensitivity may be exhibited by acute bronchospasm, generalized urticaria and angioedema, severe rhinitis, and shock within 3 hours of ingestion. Foods containing salicylates may contribute to a reaction. These include curry powder, paprika, licorice, Benedictine liqueur, prunes, raisins, tea, and gherkins.
- Tinnitus, dizziness, or impaired hearing probably represents high blood salicylic acid levels and can be helpful in dosage titration. Temporary hearing loss disappears gradually when the drug is discontinued.
- Hepatic function impairment, hypothrombinemia, and vitamin K deficiencies: ASA may cause hepatotoxicity and bleeding.
- Administration of aspirin to patients should be avoided for 1 to 2 weeks before any surgical procedure because of bleeding tendency.

Precautions

- Chronic renal insufficiency: ASA can impair renal function.
- Gastric ulcer, peptic ulcer, mild diabetes, gout, erosive gastritis, or bleeding tendencies because of GI irritation and bleeding.
- Severe anemia, history of coagulation defects, or patients on anticoagulants because aspirin interferes with hemostasis.
- Patients taking long-term therapy should not take other salicylates such as nonprescription analgesics.
- Controlled-release aspirin has a long onset of action and is not recommended for fever or short-term pain control or for children younger than 12 years of age. It is also contraindicated in children with fever and dehydration.

Pharmacokinetics

Rapid and complete absorption of aspirin occurs after oral administration (Table 37-3). The bioavailability of aspirin depends on the dosage formulation, particle size, presence of food, gastric emptying time, gastric pH, and antacids or buffering agents in the stomach. Food slows the absorption of salicylates. Bioavailability of enteric-coated products may be erratic. Absorption from rectal suppositories is slow with lower salicylate levels. They are partially hydrolyzed to salicylic acid during absorption. Salicylic acid is distributed to all body tissues and fluids, including the CNS.

Adverse Effects

See Table 37-4.

Drug Interactions

See Table 37-5.

Overdosage

An overdosage of salicylates is life threatening and requires intensive supportive treatment in a hospital. Initial symptoms are respiratory alkalosis with hyperpnea and tachypnea, nausea, vomiting, hypokalemia, tinnitus, neurologic abnormalities, dehydration, hyperthermia, hyperactivity, and hematologic abnormalities, progressing to coma and respiratory collapse.

Dosage and Administration

See Table 37-6.

NSAIDS

Ⓟ **Prototype Drug**

ibuprofen (Motrin, etc.)

Contraindications

- Hypersensitivity
- NSAID: potential of cross-sensitivity to other NSAIDs or salicylates. If patient has had asthma, rhinitis, urticaria, nasal polyps, angioedema, bronchospasm, or other symptoms of allergic or anaphylactoid reactions, he or she should never receive another NSAID
- Ketorolac: contraindicated in patients with previously documented peptic ulcers and GI bleeding
- Indomethacin: do not give in patients with active GI lesions or a history of recurrent GI lesions unless the high risk is warranted and the patients can be monitored closely

TABLE 37-3 Pharmacokinetics of Aspirin and NSAIDs

Drug	Drug Availability, After First Pass	Time to Peak Concen-tration	Half-Life	Protein Bound	Metabolism	Excretion
Aspirin	Variable	NI	15-20 min	76%-90%	Oxidation conjunction	Renal, depends on urinary pH
ibuprofen	80%	1-2 hr	1.8-2 hr	99%		45%-79%, renal
fenoprofen	NI	2 hr	3 hr	99%		90%
flurbiprofen	NI	1.5 hr	5.7 hr	99%		70%
ketoprofen	90%	0.5-2 hr	2.1 hr	99%		80%
naproxen	95%	2-4 hr	12-17 hr	99%		95%
oxaprozin	95%	3-5 hr	42-50 hr	99%	2C9	65%; fecal, 35%
indomethacin	98%	21.5 hr	4.5 hr	90%		60%; fecal, 33%
etodolac	80%	1.5 hr	7.3 hr	99%	2C9	72%; fecal, 16%
sulindac	90%	2-4 hr	7.8 hr	93%		50%; fecal, 25%
diclofenac	50%-60%	2 hr	2 hr	99%		65%
ketorolac	100%	2-3 hr	5-6 hr	99%	2C9	91%
tolmetin	NI	0.5-1 hr	2-7 hr	NI		100%
nabumetone	80%	9-12 hr	22.5 hr	99%	2C9	80%; fecal, 9%
meclofenamate	100%	0.5-2 hr	1.3 hr	99%		70%; fecal, 30%
mefenamic acid	NI	2-4 hr	2 hr	90%	2C9	52%; fecal, 20%
piroxicam	NI	3-5 hr	50 hr	99%	2C9	NI
meloxicam	89%	4-5 hr	15-20 hr	99%		50%; fecal, 50%
celecoxib	NI	3 hr	11 hr	97%	2C9	27%; fecal, 57%
valdecoxib	83%	3 hr	8-11 hr	98%	3A4/2C9	90%

NI, No information.

TABLE 37-4 Common and Serious Adverse Effects of Salicylate and NSAIDs (by Body System)

Body System	Common Side Effects	Serious Adverse Effects
Body, general	Headache, dizziness	
Skin, appendages	Increased sweating, photosensitivity	Rash, pruritus
Hypersensitivity	Rash, pruritus, fever	Urticaria, Stevens-Johnson syndrome, toxic epidermal necrolysis, anaphylaxis, pulmonary infiltrates, asthma
Respiratory		Asthma, acute bronchospasm
Cardiovascular	Palpitations, tachycardia	Hypertension, MI, CHF, arrhythmia, PE
GI	Diarrhea, nausea, constipation, flatulence, dyspepsia	GI bleeding
Hemic and lymphatic		Blood dyscrasias
Nervous system		CVA, sedation, confusion
Special senses	Taste disturbances	Blurred vision
Hepatic	↑ LFTs	Hepatic failure, tinnitus, hearing loss, vertigo*
Genitourinary	↑ Creatinine	Fluid and electrolyte changes, sodium and water retention, hyperkalemia, acute renal failure

*Salicylates only.

TABLE 37-5 Drug Interactions of Salicylates and NSAIDs

Salicylate/NSAID	Action on These Drugs
ASA	↑ Anticoagulants, heparin, carbonic anhydrase inhibitors nitroglycerin, valproic acid, methotrexate, sulfonylureas, insulin
ASA	↓ NSAIDs, angiotensin-converting enzyme (ACE) inhibitors, β-blockers, loop diuretics, probenecid, sulfinpyrazone, spironolactone
NSAIDs	↑Aminoglycosides, anticoagulants, cyclosporine, hydantoin, lithium, methotrexate, penicillamine, ASA
NSAIDs	↓ ACE inhibitors, β-blockers, loop diuretics, lithium
ibuprofen, indomethacin	↑ Digoxin
indomethacin	↑ Dapiprazole
indomethacin, naproxen, sulindac	↓ Thiazides
indomethacin, diclofenac	↓ Potassium-sparing diuretics
valdecoxib	↑ Dextromethorphan

Drugs	Action on Salicylate/NSAID
Oral anticoagulants, alcohol, ammonium chloride, ascorbic acid, methionine, carbonic anhydrase inhibitors, nizatidine	↑ ASA
Antacids, urinary alkalinizers, charcoal, corticosteroids	↓ ASA
cyclosporine, bisphosphonates, probenecid	↑ NSAIDs
cholestyramine, colestipol, sucralfate	↓ NSAIDs
diflunisal	↑ Indomethacin
fluconazole	↑ Celecoxib, valdecoxib
cimetidine	↑↓ NSAIDs
ketoconazole	↑ Valdecoxib
phenobarbital	↓ Fenoprofen
Salicylates	↓ NSAIDs, except ↑ ketorolac

TABLE 37-6 Dosage and Administration of Salicylates and NSAIDs

Medication	Formulation	Acute	Chronic	Administration	Maximum Dose
Aspirin	Many	325-650 mg q4hr	3.2-6 g/day	dd	500 mg q3hr
ibuprofen	Liquid, tablet	200 mg q4-6hr	300 mg	qid	3.2 g
fenoprofen	Caplet	200 mg q4-6hr	300-600 mg	tid-qid	2400 mg
flurbiprofen	Tablet	NI	200-300 mg/day	dd	300 mg
ketoprofen	Caplet	25-50 mg q6-8hr	75 mg	tid	300 mg/day
naproxen	Liquid, tablet	500 mg q12hr	25-500 mg	bid	1500 mg/day short term
oxaprozin	Tablet	NI	600-1200 mg	qd	1800 mg
indomethacin	Liquid, tablet	75-150 mg/day	25 mg	bid-tid	150-200 mg
etodolac	Tablet	200-400 mg q6-8hr	300 mg	bid-tid	1000 mg
sulindac	Tablet	200 mg bid	150 mg	bid	400 mg
diclofenac	Tablet	50 mg tid	100-150 mg/day	dd	200 mg
ketorolac	Tablet, injection	20 mg	NI		40 mg/day, 5 days
tolmetin	Tablet	NI	400 mg	tid	1800 mg
nabumetone	Tablet	NI	1000 mg	qd	1500-2000 mg
meclofenamate	Caplet	50 mg q4-6hr	200-400 mg/day	dd	400 mg
mefenamic acid	Caplet	500 mg, then 250 mg q6hr	NI		1 week
piroxicam	Caplet	NI	10-20 mg	qd	20 mg
meloxicam	Tablet	NI	7.5 mg	qd	15 mg
celecoxib	Caplet	400 mg, then 200 mg bid	200	qd	400 mg
valdecoxib	Tablet	20 mg bid	10 mg	qd	40 mg

dd, Divided doses; *NI,* no information.

Warnings

- GI effects: serious toxicity such as inflammation, bleeding, ulceration, and perforation of the stomach and small or large intestine, can occur at any time, with or without warning symptoms, in patients treated chronically with NSAID therapy. Although minor upper GI problems (e.g., dyspepsia) are common, usually developing early in therapy, remain alert for ulceration and bleeding even in the absence of previous GI tract symptoms
- CNS effects: depression, drowsiness, headache, and dizziness, especially in the elderly
- Renal function impairment: NSAID metabolites are eliminated primarily by kidneys; use with caution in those with renal function impairment. Reduce dosage.
- Hepatic function impairment may occur.

Precautions

! A patient with a prior history of GI disease should exercise extreme caution. The risk for GI bleeding increases with age.

- The risk of GI bleeding for a person between the ages of 25 and 49 is almost zero; the risk increases steeply from 60 to 69 years; and from 70 to 80 years of age, the risk almost doubles.
- Corticosteroids: NSAIDs are not a substitute for corticosteroids. Do not discontinue corticosteroids abruptly. Corticosteroid should not be given concurrently with NSAIDs.
- NSAIDs reversibly inhibit platelet aggregation.
- Cardiovascular effects: may cause fluid retention and peripheral edema. Use caution in compromised cardiac function, hypertension, in patients on chronic diuretic therapy, or other conditions predisposing to fluid retention. Agents may be associated with significant deterioration of circulatory hemodynamics in severe heart failure and hyponatremia presumably because of inhibition of prostaglandin-dependent compensatory mechanisms.
- Ophthalmic effects: perform ophthalmologic studies in patients who develop eye complaints during therapy. Effects include blurred or diminished vision, scotomata, changes in color vision, corneal deposits, and retinal disturbances. Discontinue therapy if ocular changes are noted.
- Infection: NSAIDs may mask the signs of infection.
- Renal effects: acute renal insufficiency, interstitial nephritis with hematuria, nephrotic syndrome, proteinuria, hyperkalemia, hyponatremia, renal papillary necrosis, and other renal medullary changes may occur. Administer with caution in dehydrated patients. Hyperkalemia is a potentially serious NSAID-induced renal electrolyte abnormality.
- Hepatic effects: borderline liver function test elevations may occur in about 15% of patients and may progress, remain essentially unchanged, or become transient with continued therapy. The ALT test is probably the most sensitive indicator of liver dysfunction.
- Alcoholics are at risk for adverse effects because of the toxic effect of alcohol on the gastric mucosa and liver. Remember that patients underreport their drinking, so all patients should be warned about the risk of bleeding from concurrent use of alcohol and NSAIDs.
- Photosensitivity may occur.

Pharmacokinetics

See Table 37-3. Analgesic effect onset is generally 30 to 60 minutes and lasts 4 to 6 hours. Antiinflammatory response onset may take 1 to 3 weeks. Indomethacin has a faster onset of antiinflammatory effect than other NSAIDs.

Adverse Effects

The most important adverse effects have been discussed in the warnings and precautions. These drugs have a large number of possible side effects. *Drug Facts*, a well-known drug compendium, lists 175. The frequency of the various adverse reactions vary by drug. The most common ones are listed in Table 37-4.

Drug Interactions

See Table 37-5.

Dosage and Administration

See Table 37-6.

Other Drugs in Class

Other drugs in this class are similar to the prototype except as follows.

fenoprofen (Fenoprofen): used for pain.

flurbiprofen (Ansaid): used for acute pain secondary to musculoskeletal injuries; relative high risk of GI adverse reactions.

ketoprofen (Orudis): used in osteoarthritis.

naproxen: now over the counter. Has longer half-life than ibuprofen. Can be used bid instead of qid ibuprofen. Excellent for both musculoskeletal pain and arthritis.

indomethacin (see Chapter 39): very good with acute inflammation, but very high adverse reaction risk.

etodolac (Lodine): lower risk of GI adverse reactions than most.

sulindac (Clinoril): lower risk of renal adverse reactions.

diclofenac (Voltaren): good for pain; relatively high risk of GI adverse reactions.

ketorolac (Toradol): acute to severe pain only; increased adverse reactions.

tolmetin (Tolectin): once more popular drug used in arthritis treatment; used as alternative drug now.

nabumetone (Relafen): relative low risk of GI and renal adverse reactions. Commonly used for acute musculoskeletal injuries.

meclofenamate (Meclomen): high incidence of adverse reactions. Used in patients with chronic arthritis who need alternative medications.

mefenamic (Ponstel): increased adverse reactions.

piroxicam (Feldene): long half-life with qd dosing, but high GI and renal adverse reactions. Not used much anymore.

meloxicam (Mobic): very low risk of GI AR and increase COX-2 but not quite as low on GI adverse reactions as the COX-2 inhibitors. Is a very good drug.

celecoxib (Celebrex): COX-2 with probably the least amount of adverse reactions seen, especially GI and renal. Maybe used qd with chronic pain of arthritis. Cannot be used by people who are allergic to sulfa.

valdecoxib (Bextra): COX-2 good for acute flares of arthritis or acute soft tissue injuries.

RESOURCES FOR PATIENTS AND PROVIDERS

Arthritis Foundation, ftp.netcom.com/pub/ar/arthritis/arthritis. html. *Information about arthritis.*

Borenstein BM, Wiesel W, Boden RJ: *Low back pain: medical diagnosis and comprehensive management,* ed 2, Philadelphia, 1995, WB Saunders.

REFERENCES

Cherkin DC et al: Medication use for low back pain in primary care, *Spine* 23(5):607, 1998.

Dionne R: Relative efficacy of selective COX-2 inhibitors compared with over-the-counter ibuprofen, *Int J Clin Pract* Suppl (135):18-22, 2003.

Gabriel SE et al: Costs and effectiveness of nonsteroidal anti-inflammatory drugs: the importance of reducing side effects, *Arthritis Care Res* 10(1):56, 1997.

Geba GP et al: Efficacy of rofecoxib, celecoxib, and acetaminophen in osteoarthritis of the knee. A randomized trial, *JAMA* 287:64, 2002.

Henry D, McGettigan P: Epidemiology overview of gastrointestinal and renal toxicity of NSAIDs, *Int J Clin Pract* Suppl (135):43-49, 2003.

Hochberg MC: COX-2: where are we in 2003? Be strong and resolute: continue to use COX-2 selective inhibitors at recommended dosages in appropriate patients, *Arthritis Res Ther* 5(1):28-30, 2003.

Ibuprofen interferes with aspirin's benefits, *Health News* 9(4):6, 2003.

Pincus T et al: A randomized, double-blind, crossover clinical trial of diclofenac plus misoprostol versus acetaminophen in patients with osteoarthritis of the hip or knee, *Arthritis Rheum* 44:1587, 2001.

Simon R, Namazy J: Adverse reactions to aspirin and nonsteroidal antiinflammatory drugs (NSAIDs), *Clin Rev Allergy Immunol* 24(3):239-252, 2003.

Wolfe MM: Risk factors associated with the development of gastroduodenal ulcers due to the use of NSAIDs, *Int J Clin Pract* Suppl (135):32-37, 2003.

CHAPTER 38

Disease-Modifying Antirheumatic Drugs and Immune Modulators

Drug Names

Class	Subclass	Generic Name	Trade Name
Gold salts		gold sodium thiomalate aurothioglucose auranofin	Myochrysine Solganal Ridaura
Antimalarials		hydroxychloroquine sulfate	Plaquenil
Sulfonamides		sulfasalazine	Azulfidine
Antineoplastics		methotrexate sodium penicillamine	Rheumatrex, Folex Cuprimine
Immunosuppressants		azathioprine cyclosporine tacrolimus	Imuran Sandimmune Prograf
Immunomodulators	Cytokine blockers	etanercept infliximab anakinra leflunomide	Enbrel Remicade Kineret Arava
Corticosteroids		prednisone	generic

General Uses

Indications

See Table 38-1.

The drugs in this section are generally prescribed by a rheumatologist but are seen by the primary care provider. All patients with suspected rheumatoid arthritis (RA) should be referred to a specialist for evaluation and initiation of medication. Primary care providers should work with the specialist in monitoring the course of the disease and identifying possible adverse reactions. Therefore this chapter emphasizes the principles of drug use and how to monitor. Methotrexate is discussed in detail because it is by far the most commonly used drug-modifying antirheumatic drug (DMARD). The drugs in this chapter include old DMARDs now seldom used and very recently introduced medications whose place in management has not yet been determined. Practitioners should refer to the latest information on RA therapy because it is a rapidly changing field.

DISEASE PROCESS

Anatomy and Physiology of Inflammation

See immunization and NSAID chapters for additional discussion of inflammation and how the body recognizes a foreign substance and attacks with two nonspecific white blood cells (WBCs)—polymorphonuclear leukocytes (neutrophils, eosinophils, basophils, and mast cells) and monocytes/macrophages. The lymphocytes (B and T cells) respond to specific antigens. There are two basic antiinflammatory actions: phagocytosis (ingestion of unwanted material) and secretion of substances that mediate the inflammatory response. There is an almost bewildering array of these substances with overlapping sources and functions.

Reduced to its most basic elements, the granulocytes (neutrophils, eosinophils, and basophils) are the leukocytes minus the mast cells. They are phagocytes. Neutrophils provide immediate phagocytosis of foreign and dead material, and then die. Eosinophils help to control the inflammatory response and act directly against parasites. The monocytes/macrophages provide more prolonged phagocytosis than the neutrophils.

Mast cells respond with immediate degranulation (release) of histamine, neutrophil chemotactic (movement) factor, and eosinophil chemotactic factor. Then they synthesize and release leukotrienes and prostaglandins. The mast cell production of prostaglandins is the site of action of the NSAIDs. Basophils function similar to mast cells.

Macrophages, mast cells, T-helper cells, natural killer cells, and others secrete many cytokines, including colony-stimulating factor interleukins, tissue necrosis factor, and interferon.

T-cell lymphocytes produce lymphokines, many of which are interleukins or interferons. Interferons are active against viruses.

TABLE 38-1 Important Characteristics of DMARDs

	Indication	Formulation	Onset of Action	% Who Respond
gold salts	RA	po or injection	3-6 mo	60
hydroxychloroquine	SLE, RA, malaria	Tablets, take with food	2-4 mo	25-50
sulfasalazine	RA, ulcerative colitis, JRA	Tablets	1-2 mo	60
methotrexate	Severe RA	Tablets, SC qwk	1-2 mo, some relief in 2-6 wk	50
penicillamine	RA, Wilson's disease	Tablets, on empty stomach	2-3 mo	
azathioprine	RA, transplant	Tablets, injection	1-2 mo	
cyclosporine	RA, transplant	po, bid, on empty stomach	1-2 mo	
tacrolimus	Transplant, unlabeled: RA	Capsules, injection		
etanercept	RA	25 mg SC twice a week		70
infliximab	RA	IV		42
anakinra	RA	SC qd		38
leflunomide	RA	po qd		50

SLE, Systemic lupus erythematosus.

Platelets stop bleeding and release serotonin, which has vascular effects similar to histamine.

There are three plasma protein systems located in the plasma of blood, not inside a cell. These include the complement, clotting, and kinin systems. Each initiates a cascade of reactions, ending with potent biochemical mediators of the inflammatory response. The complement system is a nonspecific mediator of inflammation that is potent against bacterial infection. IgG or IgM usually initiates the cascade by forming an immune complex. The kinin system begins with bradykinin, which causes dilation of vessels, acts with prostaglandins to induce pain and increase vascular permeability and is important in the prolonged phase of inflammation. The clotting system is discussed in Chapter 26.

Pathophysiology

The pathophysiology of RA is much the same as for any autoimmune disease. For some reason the body fails to distinguish between self- and non–self-protein found in the body, and proteins carried by foreign invaders. In all individuals it is not uncommon for a T– or B–immune cell lymphocyte to react to a self-protein during its development in the thymus or bone marrow. Normally these self-reactive immune cells are destroyed, but occasionally they escape destruction. Years later they are activated to trigger an immune response. Activation is thought to occur after infection with a common bacterium or virus that contains a protein with a stretch of amino acids that match a stretch of amino acids on a tissue protein. The most common organisms implicated in this activation include *Streptococcus, Mycoplasma,* and *Borrelia* (the agent of Lyme disease), although retroviruses may also be responsible.

In RA the causative agents first gain access to the joint and cause an inflammatory response. This causes damage to small blood vessels and leads to the accumulation of inflammatory cells (macrophages and lymphocytes). Macrophages process the pathogenic material and transfer the antigen to lymphocytes. Among the lymphocytes, the B cells produce antibodies, and the T cells produce cytokines that activate B cells and cytotoxins that attack tissues directly inside the joint capsule, causing synovitis. As the disease progresses, the inflammatory process spreads from the synovium into the cartilage and bone, with collagen-destroying enzymes causing destruction of the joint. These changes begin within the first 2 years of the disease, making early diagnosis and aggressive treatment very important.

The Disease

The clinical presentation of RA is extremely variable. Articular signs and symptoms include symmetric joint swelling with stiffness, warmth, tenderness, and pain. Stiffness is usually worse in the morning. Duration of stiffness is a method of evaluating disease activity. Although any joint may be affected, the joints most often affected are the proximal interphalangeal (PIP) and metacarpophalangeal (MCP) and the wrists, knees, ankles, and toes. Systemic symptoms include a prodrome of malaise, fatigue, fever, and weight loss.

Physical examination shows acute inflammation of the joint: heat, tenderness, and swelling. Anemia, high-spiking fevers, rash, and other extraarticular features occur in onset systemic juvenile arthritis. Later in the disease the examination becomes specific for RA. X-rays of the wrists or feet are usually the earliest to show changes but are not diagnostic in the early phase of RA. The erythrocyte sedimentation rate (ESR) is a very nonspecific but sensitive indication of inflammation. It will be elevated in active disease and is usually monitored as an indicator of the effectiveness of therapy. RA factor (an IgM antibody) is positive in 75% to 85% of patients with RA. Antinuclear antibodies (ANA) are elevated in approximately 20% of patients with RA.

Over time, the disease involves skin and blood vessels, lymph tissues, eyes, chest cavity, lungs, nerves, and blood. Patients with classic RA and a need for aggressive treatment have joint symptoms that persist beyond 2 years, positive rheumatoid factor, poor functional status, a large number of inflamed joints, and extraarticular manifestations of disease.

DRUG ACTION AND EFFECTS

DMARDs

DMARDs have antiinflammatory effects that may slow the progress of the disease. The exact mechanism of how they work in RA is unclear.

gold salts

Gold salts can prevent or suppress but not cure arthritis and synovitis. Macrophage phagocytosis is inhibited and prostaglandin synthesis and lysosomal enzyme release are decreased. In addition, gold salt compounds interfere with antibody production and lymphocyte, neutrophil, and monocyte function.

hydroxycholoroquine

It has been suggested that hydroxychloroquine sulfate acts by mimicking the action of its parent compound, chloroquine. The antimalarials possess antiinflammatory properties, possibly through inhibiting the conversion of arachidonic acid to prostaglandin F_2. In vitro, these agents also interfere with the chemotaxis of polymorphonuclear leukocytes, macrophages, and eosinophils.

Sulfonamides

Sulfasalazine's mechanism of action remains unknown. It has antiinflammatory action and reaches high concentrations in serous fluids in connective tissue.

Antineoplastics

Methotrexate is used because it possesses both antiinflammatory and immunosuppressive properties. This agent acts by inhibiting dihydrofolate reductase and 5-amino-imidazole-4-carboxamide ribonucleotide transferamylase, resulting in impaired DNA synthesis. Furthermore it exhibits inhibitory effects on cytokines, especially interleukin-1, and may alter arachidonic acid metabolism. Methotrexate also exerts an antiproliferative effect on synovial cells.

Penicillamine's mechanism of action is unknown. It may inhibit T-lymphocyte function. It may also protect lymphocytes against the harmful effects of H_2O_2 produced in inflammation.

Immunosuppressants

Although the immune response is generally beneficial, it is advantageous to reduce its effectiveness in autoimmune disease and organ transplantation.

Azathioprine is an immunosuppressive, with the greatest effects on delayed hypersensitivity. It suppresses cell-mediated hypersensitivity, antibody production, and T-cell effects. It inhibits the lymph node hyperplasia that precedes the onset of the signs of the disease.

Cyclosporine is an immunosuppressant that suppresses some humoral immunity and cell-mediated immune reactions. It inhibits the immunocompetent lymphocytes, mainly the T lymphocytes but also interleukin-2 or T-cell growth factor. Lymphokine production is inhibited. Cyclosporine does not cause bone marrow suppression.

Tacrolimus is a new, macrolide immunosuppressant. It inhibits T-lymphocyte activation. The T lymphocytes produce interleukin-2 and gamma interferon.

Immunomodulators

Agents that regulate the extent and duration of the immune response are known as immunomodulators. Interferons and interleukins are some of the many substances the body releases during the inflammatory response. Through genetic research, these agents have been cloned so that they can be produced outside the body and given to patients who are immunodeficient. Some are indicated for multiple sclerosis. They show promise in RA but specific usage is still unclear.

Cytokines are cellular hormones that seem to stimulate target cells and recruit new cells into the inflammatory milieu.

Cytokines are cellular messengers that initiate and perpetuate the inflammatory response by stimulating the production of cartilage-degrading enzymes and allowing pannus, an inflammatory exudate, to attach to cartilage and bone. The two cytokines targeted by the new immune modulators are tumor necrosis factor (TNF) and interleukin (IL)-I.

Although each cytokine blocker has its own benefits, they share common untoward effects. Serious infections, sepsis, and fatalities have been observed in treated patients, many of whom were receiving other immunosuppressive agents concomitantly. There have been rare cases of TB. All candidates for cytokine-blocker therapy should be assessed for TB risk; anti-TB therapy should be considered before starting the cytokine blocker with those deemed to be at risk. People with serious chronic infections or those who require live-virus vaccinations should not be given a cytokine blocker.

Etanercept and infliximab bind to tumor necrosis factor and block its interaction with cell surface receptors. Tumor necrosis factor is a cytokine that is involved in the inflammatory response.

Anakinra is an interleukin-1 receptor antagonist. It blocks the activity of interleukin-1, which mediates inflammatory and immunologic responses in a wide range of activities.

Leflunomide blocks the synthesis of pyrimidine, which is required for proliferation of T cells.

Corticosteroids

Corticosteroids inhibit the production of interleukins. This inhibition decreases the immune response through the diminished activity of the T cells. Corticosteroids also affect both the type and number of leukocytes and monocytes in the serum. Corticosteroids' antiinflammatory effects overlap with their immunosuppressive actions. They also affect carbohydrate, protein, and lipid metabolism and increase hepatic gluconeogenesis. Detailed information regarding corticosteroids can be found in Chapter 52.

DRUG TREATMENT PRINCIPLES

Treatment of RA must include nonpharmacologic measures. These include patient education, addressing the emotional impact of RA, physical and occupational therapy, systemic rest, articular rest, exercise, use of heat and cold applications, assistive devices, splints, and weight loss if overweight.

The management of RA has changed considerably with the advent of new classes of drugs and new uses for older agents. First-line therapy for this disease has been NSAIDs and glucocorticoids that were given to reduce pain and inflammation. A DMARD was added if these medications were not adequate. As a diverse group of drugs, what the DMARDs have in common is their use in slowing the disease process in RA. On the negative side, DMARDs have a high incidence of adverse effects and drug interactions, some of which can lead to death.

New trends focus on early aggressive disease-modifying treatment. Use the DMARD as the first-line drug as soon as the disease is diagnosed to prevent joint destruction and deformity. Methotrexate and leflunomide are considered first-line choices in patients with more aggressive rheumatic disease (synovitis plus extraarticular manifestations). If the disease is mild, gold salts, hydroxychloroquine, and sulfasalazine may be used because they are considered to be lower in serious adverse effects than the other DMARDs.

Because gold is a heavy metal, it is very slow to be removed. Thus adverse effects may be prolonged. Use extreme caution in patients with a history of blood dyscrasias, allergy to medications, skin rash, previous kidney or liver disease, hypertension, or compromised cerebral or cardiovascular circulation.

Use hydroxycholorquine with caution in patients with renal/hepatic function impairment or history of alcohol use. It can cause irreversible retinal damage. Patients should wear sunglasses in bright sunlight because the eyes may become photosensitive.

Cyclosporine is considered the most effective immunosuppressant agent on the market today. Cyclosporine uses the CYP450 3A4 enzyme system and will interact with other drugs using the same system.

Combination therapy is increasingly used because it is safe, more effective, and provides a more sustained response. Immune modulators have changed treatment but their place in the therapeutic regimen has not been well elucidated. This is a very new, rapidly developing area and these drugs are just starting to be seen in primary care.

HOW TO MONITOR

- The rheumatologist should follow the patient closely.
- Indicators of reduced disease activity are decreased ESR and C-reactive protein. The ESR is used over time to monitor disease activity.
- Patients should be monitored closely for adverse effects. The usual parameters to monitor include the following:
    - CBC with differential and platelets for blood dyscrasias, hepatic and renal function, and urinalysis.
    - Gold salts: before instituting treatment, rule out pregnancy, perform a CBC with differential, platelet, hemoglobin, WBC and erythrocyte counts, urinalysis, and renal and liver function tests. Perform urinalysis for protein and sediment changes prior to each injection. Perform CBC including platelets, before every second injection (every 2 weeks) throughout treatment. Purpura and ecchymoses always require a platelet count. Inquire regarding pruritus, rash, sore mouth, metallic taste, and indigestion before each injection. Observe the patient at least 15 minutes after injections. For oral gold, monitor CBC with differential, platelet count, and urinalysis at least monthly.
    - Hydroxychloroquine: periodic blood cell counts during prolonged therapy. Refer to ophthalmologist for baseline and every-3-month examination. Assess patient for muscle strength and knee and ankle reflexes.
    - Sulfasalazine: perform CBC, including differential WBC, and liver function tests before starting, and every second week during the first 3 months of therapy. During the second 3 months, perform the same tests once monthly and thereafter once every 3 months and as clinically indicated. Also perform urinalysis and an assessment of renal function periodically during treatment.
    - Methotrexate: CBC, albumin, creatinine, and LFT baseline and then monthly for 6 months and every 1 to 2 months thereafter. Baseline alkaline phosphatase, chest radiograph, and hepatitis B and C serology in high-risk patients.
    - Penicillamine: urine for proteinuria and hematuria, LFTs every 6 months, CBC with differential and platelets every 2 weeks for the first 6 months then monthly.
    - Azathioprine: CBC with platelets weekly during the first month, twice monthly for the second and third months of treatment, then monthly or more frequently as dosage is altered.
    - Cyclosporine: monitor renal and hepatic function. Hepatotoxicity usually occurs in the first month of therapy. Blood levels of cyclosporine may be useful.
    - Tacrolimus and infliximab: test for tuberculosis before beginning treatment. Monitor renal function and CBC. Watch for infection. No specific guidelines.
    - Etanercept: update vaccines before initiating therapy; assess for infections or risk factors for infections.
    - Infliximab: tuberculin (TB) test before initiation of therapy; assess for infections or risk factors for infections.
    - Anakinra: neutrophil counts at baseline and then monthly for 3 months and every 3 months thereafter. Assess for infections of risk factors for infections.
    - Leflunomide: CBC, LFTs; at minimum perform ALT at baseline and monthly.

PATIENT VARIABLES

Use with caution in patients with hepatic or renal insufficiency because the drug may accumulate and cause toxicity.

Geriatrics

Geriatric patients are more susceptible to adverse effects. The frail elderly do not usually tolerate this very aggressive category of drugs. Use methotrexate with caution; decrease the dose, due to diminished hepatic and renal function in this population.

Pediatrics

Use extreme caution when administering these drugs to children. These agents have caused deaths.

Pregnancy

These agents are class C, D, or X and should be used with great caution if the patient is of childbearing age. Metho-

TABLE 38-2 Common and Serious Adverse Effects of DMARDs and Immune Modulators

Drug	Adverse Reactions
gold salts	Blood dyscrasias, thrombocytopenia (1%-3%), proteinuria, rash, anaphylaxis, syncope, bradycardia, diarrhea, infection, bruising, bleeding, swelling
hydroxychloroquine	Irreversible retinal damage, agranulocytosis, skin reaction, GI distress, muscular weakness, CNS toxicity (irritability, psychosis, dizziness, convulsions), alopecia
sulfasalazine	GI intolerance; deaths from hypersensitivity, agranulocytosis, aplastic anemia, or other dyscrasias; renal and liver damage; irreversible neuromuscular and CNS changes; fibrosing alveolitis; anorexia; headache; reversible oligospermia (33%); infection; bruising; bleeding; swelling
methotrexate	Hepatotoxicity, lung disease, bone marrow depression, GI distress, thrombocytopenia, hypertension, rash/pruritus, diarrhea, alopecia, dizziness, headache, infection, fetal death
penicillamine	Rash, agranulocytosis, thrombocytopenia (4%), Goodpasture syndrome and myasthenia gravis, hepatotoxicity, autoimmune syndromes, pemphigus vulgaris, renal function impairment, oral ulcerations, hypogeusia (25%-33%), hypoglycemia, hypersensitivity, skin rashes (44%-50%)
azathioprine	Leukopenia (28%) thrombocytopenia, severe bone marrow depression, infections, GI toxicity, hepatotoxicity, carcinogenesis
cyclosporine	Nephrotoxicity, hepatotoxicity, CNS toxicity (tremor, convulsions, confusion), carcinogenesis, hypersensitivity reactions, hypertension (26%), GI distress, hypomagnesemia, hirsutism
tacrolimus	Nephrotoxicity, hyperkalemia, neurotoxicity (tremor, headache), lymphomas, myocardial hypertrophy, hypersensitivity, renal/hepatic function impairment, carcinogenesis
etanercept	Infection (38%), injection site reactions (37%), headache (17%) CNS demyelinating disorders, pancytopenia, hypersensitivity, chest pain, stroke, paresthesias, GI distress, interstitial lung disease
infliximab	Demyelinating syndromes, TB reactivation, infections, exacerbation of CHF
anakinra	Infections (35%), decreased neutrophils, hypersensitivity, injection site reactions (28%), headache
leflunomide	Hypersensitivity, hepatotoxicity, renal function impairment, carcinogenesis, fetal harm, hypertension (10%), headache, alopecia (10%), GI distress

trexate (category D) can cause fetal harm. None of these products are recommended for use when a patient is pregnant or breast-feeding. Pregnancy should be ruled out before patients of childbearing age begin taking any of these medications.

PATIENT EDUCATION

Thorough patient education regarding potential adverse reactions and how to monitor for them is important because these medications can cause death. See Table 38-2 for the adverse reactions for each particular drug.

Specific Drugs

ANTINEOPLASTICS

methotrexate (MTX) sodium (Rheumatrex, Folex)

Contraindications

- Hypersensitivity
- Nursing mothers

Warnings

Toxic effects, potentially serious, have been seen at all doses. Deaths have occurred.

- Marked bone marrow depression may occur with resultant anemia, leukopenia, or thrombocytopenia.
- Coadministration of methotrexate with NSAIDs increases the risk of severe marrow suppression and GI toxicity.
- Close monitoring for toxicity is necessary. See *How to Monitor.*
- Liver: hepatotoxicity, fibrosis, and cirrhosis, usually after prolonged use. Acutely, liver enzyme elevations are frequent, usually transient and asymptomatic, and do not appear predictive of subsequent hepatic disease.
- Methotrexate-induced lung disease is a potentially dangerous lesion that may occur acutely at any time.
- Pregnancy: fetal death and congenital anomalies have occurred; do not use in women of childbearing potential unless benefits outweigh possible risks.
- Renal use: use methotrexate in patients with impaired renal function with extreme caution, and at reduced dosages, because renal dysfunction will prolong elimination.
- GI: diarrhea and ulcerative stomatitis require interruption of therapy; hemorrhagic enteritis and death from intestinal perforation may occur.
- Mutagenesis: causes embryotoxicity, abortion and fetal defects, impairment of fertility.

Precautions

- Use with extreme caution in the presence of active infection; usually contraindicated in patients with immunodeficiency syndromes.
- Neurologic: a transient acute neurologic syndrome with behavioral abnormalities; focal sensorimotor signs and abnormal reflexes have been observed in patients treated with high dosages.

Drug Interactions

! Methotrexate toxicity may occur when administered with protein-bound agents and with drugs that alter renal elimination, such as NSAIDs, sulfonamides (including trimethoprim/sulfamethoxazole), tetracycline, and chloramphenicol. Phenytoin and cyclosporine may also interfere with the elimination of methotrexate and vice versa; thus concomitant use of these two agents may lead to increased risk of toxicity.

Although there has been concern that vitamins containing folic acid or its derivatives may decrease the response of methotrexate, concomitant therapy with folic acid may reduce methotrexate toxicity without compromising its therapeutic effect.

Patient Education

- The patient should report immediately signs and symptoms of infection, bleeding, shortness of breath, or dysuria to the health care provider.
- Alcohol should be avoided while the patient is on methotrexate.
- The patient should avoid prolonged exposure to sunlight.
- Methotrexate must be stored at room temperature.

RESOURCES FOR PATIENTS AND PROVIDERS

Arthritis Foundation, www.arthritis.org.

Website for the Arthritis Foundation; can also be contacted at The Arthritis Foundation, 1330 West Peachtree Street, Atlanta, GA 30309; (800) 283-7800.

National Arthritis and Musculoskeletal and Skin Diseases Information Clearinghouse: NIAMS/National Institutes of Health, 1 AMS Circle, Bethesda, MD 20892-3675.

Call (301) 881-2731; using the phone on a fax machine, listen to the instructions, dial 01301 and a comprehensive booklet about arthritis for patients will print out on the fax machine.

BIBLIOGRAPHY

Bathon JM et al: A comparison of etanercept and methotrexate in patients with early rheumatoid arthritis, *N Engl J Med* 343:1586, 2000.

Callahan LF: The burden of rheumatoid arthritis: facts and figures, *J Rheumatol Suppl* 53:8, 1998.

Lipsky PE et al: Infliximab and methotrexate in the treatment of rheumatoid arthritis, *N Engl J Med* 343:1594, 2000.

Machold KP et al: Early arthritis therapy: rationale and current approach, *J Rheumatol Suppl* 53:13, 1998.

Schrand LM: Rheumatoid arthritis: update on the newest DMARDs and their potential place in therapy, *Formulary* 37:301-310, 2002.

van Everdingen AA et al: Low-dose prednisone therapy for patients with early active rheumatoid arthritis: clinical efficacy, disease-modifying properties, and side effects. A randomized, double-blind, placebo-controlled clinical trial, *Ann Intern Med* 136:1, 2002.

CHAPTER 39

Gout Medications

Christy L. Crowther

Drug Names

Class	Subclass	Generic Name	Trade Name
NSAIDs		indomethacin naproxen sulindac	Indocin Naprosyn Clinoril
Colchicine		colchicine	Generic, ColBenemid
Uricosuric agents		probenecid sulfinpyrazone	Benemid, ColBenemid Anturane
Xanthine oxidase inhibitors		(200) allopurinol	Zyloprim

(200), Top 200 drug.

General Uses

Indications

- Hyperuricemia
- Prophylaxis of gouty arthritis
- Acute gouty arthritis

Pharmacologic management of gout relies on nonsteroidal antiinflammatory drugs (NSAIDs) (see Chapter 37), colchicine, uricosuric agents (probenecid and sulfinpyrazone), and xanthine oxidase inhibitors (allopurinol).

DISEASE PROCESS

Gout is a term used to describe a collection of disorders caused by the deposition of monosodium urate crystals in body tissue. Gout can be classified as either primary or secondary. Primary gout, which affects males 10 times more often than females, is caused by an inborn error of purine metabolism that results in the overproduction or underexcretion of uric acid.

Secondary gout is associated with hyperuricemia resulting from other diseases or drugs that interfere with uric acid secretion. Secondary gout arises from a multitude of causes, including endocrine disorders, lead poisoning, high-dose salicylates (more than 3 g/day), myeloproliferative disorders, and chronic renal disease.

The basic pathology of gout is generally classified into one of two categories: either overproduction or underexcretion of uric acid. A 24-hour urine collection is used to differentiate overproducers from underexcreters of uric acid.

Four phases are generally recognized in the development of gout. The first is asymptomatic hyperuricemia, which, as the name implies, is not associated with any clinical symptoms. There is evidence that the higher an individual's serum uric acid level, the greater the likelihood that acute gout will develop. Acute gouty arthritis, the next phase, typically presents as a sudden, exquisitely painful monoarthropathy. Although any synovial joint can be affected, the most common site for this painful manifestation is the metatarsophalangeal joint of the great toe. The third phase, the intercritical period, is the period between acute attacks. Most individuals who develop gout have a second episode of gout within 6 months to 2 years of the first attack. Untreated gout tends to result in more frequent, severe attacks of longer duration. There are, however, some patients who will never have a second attack. Finally, chronic tophaceous gout can develop. Tophi tend to appear anywhere from 2 or 3 years to 10 years after the onset of gout. Tophi are sodium urate crystals that are deposited in the soft tissues and can occur in up to 50% of patients with gout. The most common locations for tophi are synovium, prepatellar, and olecranon bursae, the Achilles tendon, and the helix of the ear.

The predominant risk factor for development of gout is the presence of hyperuricemia. Hyperuricemia alone, however, is not diagnostic of gout, and gout can occur in patients having normal serum uric acid levels. Other risk factors for developing gout include age older than 60, family history, obesity, excessive alcohol consumption, lead exposure (patients who consume "moonshine" whiskey have an even greater risk because moonshine tends to have a high lead content), and hypertension. Conditions such as thyroid problems, kidney disease, anemia, hyperlipidemia, diabetes, vascular disease, trauma, surgery, and radiation treatment may also serve as triggers for gout.

Up to 90% of individuals with gout are underexcreters of uric acid. Normally the kidneys turn over approximately 700 mg/dl of uric acid per day. Of that amount, about 10% is excreted. Normal serum uric acid in males ranges from 2 to 7 mg/dl; the normal range for females is 2 to 6 mg/dl. Any factor that interferes with the glomerular and renal tubular reabsorption of uric acid can result in elevated serum uric acid levels.

Overproduction of uric acid is much less common. It is often the result of another disease, frequently one associated with excessive rates of cell turnover. Hemolytic anemias, myeloproliferative and lymphoproliferative diseases, and psoriasis are examples of processes causing secondary gout from overproduction of uric acid. Some inherited diseases and genetic abnormalities can cause primary gout due to overexcretion of uric acid.

The most important differential diagnosis to be made in a patient with gout is the exclusion of a septic joint. Synovial fluid aspiration and examination help confirm the diagnosis. Fluid is sent for white blood cell count (WBC) and differential, crystal analysis, and Gram stain with culture. Examination of joint fluid using a polarized microscope will determine the presence of crystals. The presence of birefringent crystals in the synovial fluid does not exclude the possibility of infection because gout and infection can coexist in a joint.

DRUG ACTION AND EFFECTS

Basically the following three mechanisms are utilized in the treatment of gout (Figure 39-1):

1. Increase the excretion of uric acid (uricosurics)
2. Decrease the synthesis of uric acid (allopurinol)
3. Decrease or stop the inflammatory response (NSAIDs, colchicine)

NSAIDs inhibit prostaglandin synthesis, thereby reducing the intensity of inflammation and pain in injured tissue. See Chapter 37 for a detailed discussion of prostaglandin inhibition.

Colchicine's exact mechanism of action is unknown. Colchicine affects leukocyte function to reduce lactic acid production. This results in a decreased deposition of uric acid and reduction of the inflammatory response. Colchicine has no effect on uric acid metabolism and it is not an analgesic.

Uricosuric agents (probenecid and sulfinpyrazone) are tubular blocking agents. They decrease serum uric acid levels by increasing urinary excretion of uric acid due to inhibition of tubular reabsorption of urate. During this process high concentrations of uric acid develop in the proximal renal tubules. This may predispose the patient to the development of urinary stones. For that reason, increased fluid intake is necessary and alkalinization of the urine is desirable when initiating uricosuric therapy. Probenecid also inhibits the tubular secretion of most penicillins and cephalosporins. This increases the effectiveness of the antibiotics.

Allopurinol inhibits xanthine oxidase, the enzyme that converts xanthine to uric acid. This reduces uric acid production by altering the breakdown of purines to produce xanthines rather than urates. Xanthines are much more soluble than uric acid and therefore have a much greater renal clearance. Unlike uricosuric agents, allopurinol does not promote uric acid secretion, so there is no increased level of uric acid in the renal tubules.

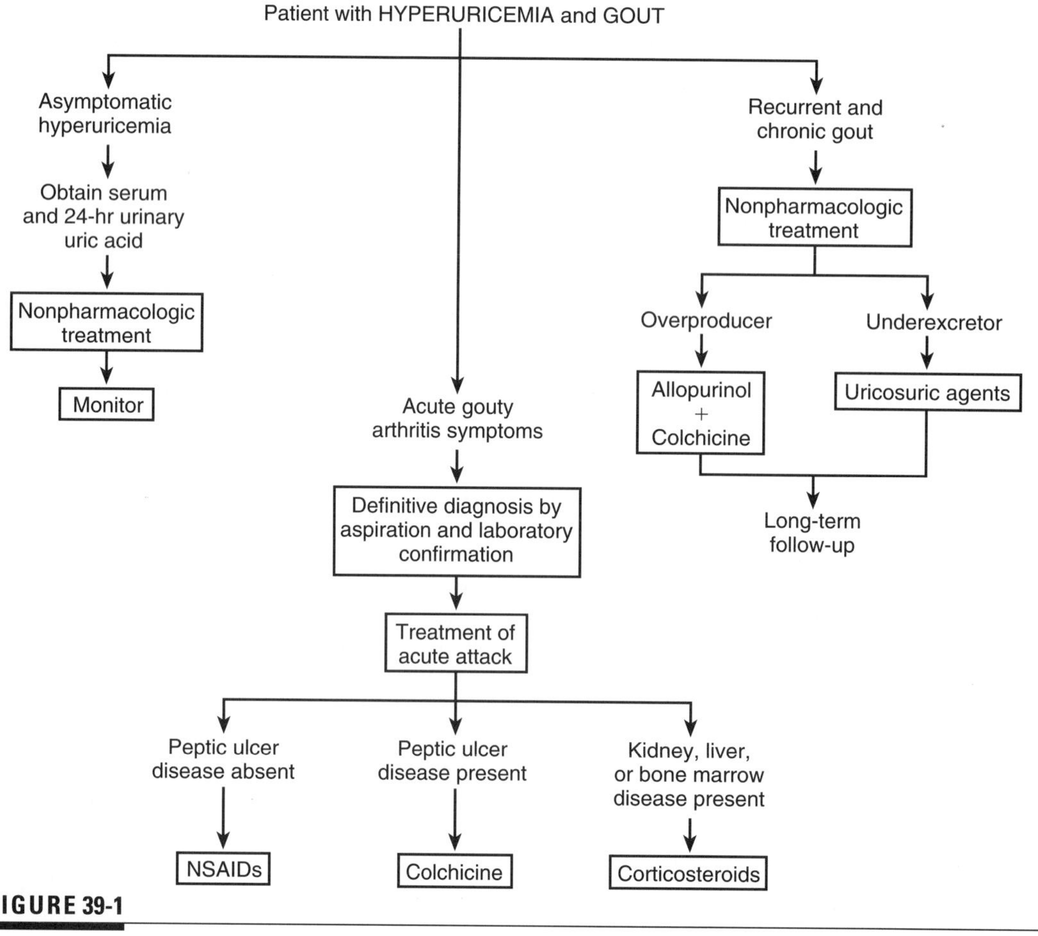

FIGURE 39-1

Suggested treatment algorithm for gout. (Modified from Gall EP: Hyperuricemia and gout. In Greene HL II, Johnston WP, Lemcke D, editors: *Decision-making in medicine*, ed 2, St Louis, 1998, Mosby.)

DRUG TREATMENT PRINCIPLES

Treatment decisions are based on the phase of gout being treated.

Asymptomatic Hyperuricemia

Although the treatment of asymptomatic patients is somewhat controversial, a blood uric acid level greater than 7 mg/dl may warrant treatment if the patient has multiple other risk factors. However most clinicians recommend *not* treating asymptomatic hyperuricemia.

Nonpharmacologic management of gout is generally attempted before or concurrently with medication. Adequate fluid intake is necessary. Acute gouty arthritis is treated with bed rest for the first 24 hours. Preventive measures include managed weight loss, primary prevention of hypertension, decreased alcohol consumption, and dietary modification to reduce purine intake. A low-purine diet restricts consumption of meat and prohibits alcohol, liver, kidney or sweetbreads, dried beans and peas, mushrooms, lentils, spinach, anchovies, sardines, and whole grain and bran breads and cereals.

Acute Gouty Arthritis

The goal is to decrease or stop the inflammatory response. Treatment of acute gout usually begins with NSAIDs; treatment of hyperuricemia must be started after the acute attack has subsided. Treatment should be initiated as soon as possible.

NSAIDs are the drugs of choice for reducing the inflammation and pain of acute gout. NSAIDs indicated for gout are indomethacin, naproxen, and sulindac, but all are probably effective. Indomethacin has traditionally been used most frequently. However it has a higher risk for adverse effects and the newer NSAIDs are probably equipotent. If the patient is high risk for gastrointestinal (GI) bleed, a COX-2 inhibitor may be appropriate. Naproxen is over the counter (OTC); sulindac is prescription only.

Colchicine, when initiated within the first 24 hours of an acute attack of gout, is effective in relieving pain and inflammation. Once the gold standard for acute gout, colchicine has become less commonly prescribed in recent years because of adverse effects such as nausea, vomiting, diarrhea, and abdominal pain. Colchicine has a fairly narrow therapeutic spectrum. If the patient has received IV colchicine, no more colchicine *(in any form)* should be given for at least 7 days.

Corticosteroids are very effective, but should be reserved for patients unable to take NSAIDs or colchicine. They are generally given by intraarticular injection. Pain may be treated with opioids if required; avoid aspirin.

The Intercritical Period

The goal is to increase the excretion of uric acid. and/or decrease the synthesis of uric acid to reduce the frequency and severity of acute attacks and to minimize urate deposition in tissues, the cause of chronic tophaceous arthritis. The decision to treat during the intercritical period is based on the likelihood of further attacks. Patients able to make significant lifestyle changes may not need medication. Patients at high risk for recurrences (e.g., on diuretics, elderly, mild renal failure) probably need treatment.

Colchicine may be sufficient prophylaxis. Because the primary mechanism of pain in an acute gout attack appears to be the inflammation resulting from granulocytes phagocytizing monosodium urate crystals, interference in this cycle will prevent an attack. It is also used as adjunctive therapy, to prevent acute attacks when starting uricosuric and allopurinol therapy. If an acute gout attack occurs while the patient is on colchicine, the drug should be continued or increased and another agent (such as an NSAID) should be added.

Reduction of the serum uric level is accomplished with uricosurics or allopurinol. Uricosurics are mainly used to prevent and treat tophi. However with colchicine, they help prevent acute attacks. One of these should be added to colchicine if colchicine alone is not sufficient. Probenecid should not be given within the first 2 to 3 weeks of an acute gout attack because it may intensify and prolong the inflammation. An increased frequency of attacks is fairly common during the first 6 to 12 months of therapy.

Allopurinol lowers uric acid levels in both underexcreters and overproducers. It is especially useful in overproducers, tophaceous gout, unresponsive patients, and patients with uric acid renal stones. Decreases of uric acid in both serum and urine are usually evident within 2 to 3 days after initiating therapy. Allopurinol should not be started during the acute phase of gout because the drug has no antiinflammatory or analgesic action, and it may prolong the acute phase of gout. It should not be used for treatment of asymptomatic hyperuricemia. As with probenecid, allopurinol has a tendency to increase the frequency of attacks during the first few months of therapy, so concurrent administration of colchicine is recommended.

Chronic Tophaceous Gout

Allopurinol is very effective in shrinking and eliminating tophi. A serum level of uric acid below 5 mg/dl may necessary. This can be accomplished with the addition of a uricosuric. Colchicine will not prevent the progression of tophaceous gouty arthritis.

HOW TO MONITOR

Perform baseline serum uric acid level, then monitor every 2 to 3 months. Normal serum uric acid levels in men range from 2 to 7 mg/dl. In women, normal serum uric acid levels are 2 to 6 ml/dl.

NSAIDs

- Obtain baseline kidney and liver function tests, especially in the elderly.
- Short-term use (i.e., until the attack subsides) is recommended.
- Monitor for adverse reactions.
- GI disturbances may occur in up to 60% of patients taking NSAIDs. The incidence of GI side effects increases with age.

colchicine

- With first-time administration of colchicine, the patient should be monitored weekly for signs of toxicity. These include weakness, nausea, vomiting, diarrhea, and anorexia.

- Periodic blood counts (every 3 to 6 months) should be performed if the patient is on long-term therapy.
- Colchicine can cause a reversible malabsorption of vitamin B_{12}; periodic monitoring may alert the clinician to potential deficiency.
- Monitoring of liver function tests and blood cell counts should be done every few months.

Uricosuric Agents

- Symptomatic reduction in gouty attacks.
- Baseline RBC, WBC, and platelet count should be obtained and monitored every 2 to 3 months.
- Baseline and periodic blood counts and serum uric acid levels should be done on patients receiving allopurinol. Serum uric acid is the best test to evaluate the efficacy of therapy.
- Renal function testing, especially BUN, creatinine, and creatinine clearance should be monitored in patients with renal disease or any other disease that can affect renal function.

PATIENT VARIABLES

Geriatrics

Elderly patients frequently have diminished renal function, and the risk of adverse renal effects is increased. Begin at the lowest recommended dosage. Monitor renal function.

- Colchicine adverse reactions have resulted in death. Gastrointestinal toxicity occurs in up to 80% of patients. Bone marrow suppression, blood dyscrasias, hepatic necrosis, and seizures are more common in the elderly.

Pediatrics

- Safety and efficacy not established: colchicine, sulfinpyrazone
- Probenecid is contraindicated in children younger than 2 years of age. It is used with penicillins and cephalosporins to prolong duration of action.
- Allopurinol should only be used in children with hyperuricemia secondary to malignancy or those with certain rare inborn errors of purine metabolism.

Pregnancy

- *Category B:* probenecid
- *Category C:* lactation not known: colchicine, allopurinol
- No information: sulfinpyrazone

PATIENT EDUCATION

- Maintain an adequate fluid intake.
- Take medication with food to prevent GI upset.
- Report any symptoms of GI distress.
- Lose weight slowly on an approved weight-loss diet. Quick weight loss may bring on a gout attack.

NSAIDs

- Notify the health care provider if increased swelling or pain develops.
- NSAIDs can mask symptoms of infection.
- Dizziness may occur when some NSAIDs are initiated. Engaging in tasks requiring mental alertness may be hazardous.

colchicine

- Advise the patient to begin colchicine at the first sign of an acute attack. The medication should be easily accessible to the patient. Discontinue medication as soon as gout pain is relieved or GI symptoms develop.
- Notify the practitioner if skin rash, sore throat, fever, unusual bleeding, bruising, tiredness, weakness, numbness, or tingling occurs.

Uricosuric Agents

- Avoid taking aspirin or other salicylates because these may cancel the efficacy of each drug.
- Increased fluid intake is necessary to prevent uric acid kidney stones. Patients should drink at least 6 to 8, 8-oz glasses of water a day. Drinking 10 to 12 glasses of water daily will help keep urine diluted.
- Notify the practitioner if a rash develops.

allopurinol

- May produce drowsiness. Use caution with tasks requiring alertness.
- Notify provider of skin rash, painful urination, blood in urine, irritation of the eyes, or swelling of the lips and mouth.
- Large doses of vitamin C may increase the possibility of kidney stone formation.
- Advise patient that acute attacks of gout may occur during the early stages of allopurinol therapy.
- Allopurinol is usually better tolerated if taken with food or milk. Fluid intake sufficient to produce urine output of at least 2 L per day is necessary to prevent formation of kidney stones.
- It may take 6 weeks to achieve optimal benefit from the drug; until then the patient needs to continue any other antigout medication that has been prescribed.

Specific Drugs

COLCHICINE

colchicine (generic, Colbenemid)

Contraindications

- Serious GI, hepatic, renal, or cardiac disease

Warnings/Precautions

Nausea, vomiting, abdominal discomfort, and diarrhea are early signs of toxicity. Colchicine should be discontinued if these signs appear, and the drug should not be reinstituted until the symptoms subside (usually within 24 to 48 hours).Death has occurred with ingestion of as little as 7 mg of colchicine, although patients have survived larger doses. Bone marrow suppression can occur with prolonged administration.

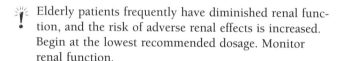

TABLE 39-1 Pharmacokinetics of Selected Drugs Used to Treat Gout

Medication	Time to Peak Concentration	Half-Life	Duration of Action	Protein Bound	Metabolism	Excretion
colchicine	30 min to 2 hr	20 min plasma; 60 hr leukocytes		NA	Liver	Liver; urine, 10%; other tissues
probenecid	2-4 hr	5-8 hr	NA	85%-95%	Kidneys	Kidneys
sulfinpyrazone	2.2-3 hr	1-6 hr; usually about 3 hr	Usually 4-6 hr; may be up to 10 hr	98%-99%	Kidneys, liver	Kidneys, 45% in first 48 hr
allopurinol	1.5-4.5 hr	allopurinol 1-2 hr	24 hr	0	Kidneys	Kidney, 70%; feces, 20%

TABLE 39-2 Common and Serious Adverse Effects of Gout Medications

Medication	Common Side Effects	Serious Adverse Effects
NSAIDs (indomethacin, naproxen, sulindac)	More frequent: GI upset, sodium and water retention, dizziness	More frequent: gastric/duodenal ulcers, reversible acute renal failure, hepatotoxicity, renal papillary necrosis, bronchospasm
colchicine	More frequent: nausea, vomiting, diarrhea, abdominal pain	Less frequent: severe diarrhea, hemorrhagic gastroenteritis, hepatocellular damage, bone marrow depression, seizures
probenecid	More frequent: headache, anorexia, nausea, vomiting, precipitation of acute gout	Less frequent: hypersensitivity reactions, development of uric acid renal stones
sulfinpyrazone	More frequent: nausea, dyspepsia, GI pain and blood loss, aggravation of peptic ulcers	Less frequent: blood dyscrasias, development of renal acid stones
allopurinol	More frequent: pruritic maculopapular rash, nausea, vomiting, drowsiness	Less frequent: reversible clinical hepatotoxicity, transient elevations in liver function tests; hypersensitivity reactions, including Stevens-Johnson syndrome, fever, chills, acute attacks of gout, granulocytosis, granulocytopenia

- If weakness, anorexia, nausea, or vomiting occurs, the dosage should be reduced or discontinued.
- Colchicine is rarely recommended as long-term prophylactic therapy.
- Chromosomal aberrations have been reported in some patients on long-term colchicine therapy.

Pharmacokinetics. See Table 39-1.

Adverse Effects. See Table 39-2. GI disturbances are the most common manifestations.

Drug Interactions. The effect of CNS depressants and sympathomimetic agents may be enhanced by colchicine. Colchicine may interfere with vitamin B_{12} absorption.

Dosage and Administration. Initially, dosage is 0.5 to 1.3 mg followed by 0.5 to 0.65 mg every 1 to 2 hours or 1 to 1.3 mg every 2 hours until the pain is relieved or until GI symptoms occur. Pain is usually much improved within 12 hours and is gone within 24 to 48 hours. For chronic use, the usual dose is 0.6 mg bid.

URICOSURIC AGENTS

probenecid (Benemid, ColBenemid)

Probenecid is frequently the uricosuric agent of choice because it seems to have fewer GI and hematologic side effects than sulfinpyrazone, but the latter is associated with fewer dermatologic and hypersensitivity reactions.

Contraindications

- Hypersensitivity to the product, blood dyscrasias, ongoing attack of acute gout, and presence of uric acid kidney stones.

Warnings/Precautions

- Probenecid may exacerbate or prolong acute gout; concurrent use of colchicine will reduce this risk.
- Salicylates antagonize the uricosuric effect of probenecid and should not be used. Probenecid should be discontinued if hypersensitivity reactions occur.
- Alkalinization of urine may prevent formation of uric acid stones, hematuria, and costovertebral pain associated with probenecid therapy.
- This drug must be used with caution in patients with a history of peptic ulcer.
- The false diagnosis of glycosuria may be made secondary to the presence of a reducing substance in the urine. Falsely elevated theophylline levels have occurred.

Pharmacokinetics. See Table 39-1.

Adverse Effects. See Table 39-2. Headache, dizziness, and precipitation of acute gouty arthritis are the most common reactions.

Drug Interactions. Plasma concentration of β-lactam antibiotics is increased, thus raising the risk of antibiotic-related side effects. The action or effect of oral sulfonylureas may be enhanced, causing hypoglycemia. Plasma concentrations of indomethacin, acetaminophen, rifampin, naproxen, ketoprofen, methotrexate, meclofenamate, lorazepam, and other drugs may be increased. Sulindac can reduce the uricosuric effect of probenecid, but its clinical significance has not been determined.

Dosage and Administration. Therapy should not begin until after the acute attack has subsided. If an acute attack of gout occurs during probenecid therapy, continue the drug and add therapeutic doses of colchicine or an NSAID.

Initial dosing is 0.25 g twice daily for 1 week, then 0.5 g twice daily. A maximum dose of 2 g a day, in four divided doses, may be necessary for some patients. If the patient has not had any attacks in at least 6 months and has a normal serum uric acid level, the daily dosage can be decreased by 0.5 g every 6 months.

sulfinpyrazone (Anturane)

Contraindications

- Active peptic ulcer disease, blood dyscrasias, hypersensitivity

Warnings/Precautions

- Renal function has been affected in patients receiving sulfinpyrazone. Monitor renal function periodically.
- Obtain periodic CBCs. Use with caution in patients with a history of peptic ulcer disease. There is increased risk of developing uric acid kidney stones; adequate hydration is mandatory. Alkalinization of the urine is recommended; this can be accomplished by using oral potassium citrate, sodium bicarbonate, or orange juice.

Drug Interactions

- Anticoagulant effect of warfarin is enhanced.
- Sulfinpyrazone can potentiate the effects of certain sulfonamides. As a result, diabetic patients on sulfonylurea hypoglycemic agents should have their serum glucose levels carefully monitored for hypoglycemia.
- Verapamil's clearance may be enhanced, thus decreasing its bioavailability.
- Salicylates decrease sulfinpyrazone's uricosuric effect.
- Concomitant use of insulin may increase hypoglycemic effect.

Dosage and Administration. Initially, give 200 to 400 mg daily in two divided doses, with meals. Gradually increase dosage over 1 week (as needed) to full maintenance dose of 400 mg to 800 mg daily in divided doses.

If the patient has previously been on other uricosuric therapy, he or she may be transferred to sulfinpyrazone therapy at its full maintenance dose. Medication should be continued without interruption even during acute exacerbations of gout, which can be treated concomitantly with colchicine or NSAID.

XANTHINE OXIDASE INHIBITORS

allopurinol (Zyloprim)

Contraindications

- Prior severe reaction to allopurinol

Warnings/Precautions

Allopurinol has caused hepatotoxicity. Hypersensitivity reactions, including Stevens-Johnson syndrome have occurred. Skin rash is one of the earliest signs of allergic reaction.

- Patients with impaired renal function require a reduction in dosage and careful monitoring of renal parameters.
- Acute attacks of gout may occur during the early stages of therapy. Colchicine should be given concurrently for the first 3 to 6 months of allopurinol therapy to decrease this risk.
- Bone marrow depression has occurred from 6 weeks to 6 years after initiation of therapy.
- Drowsiness may occur with allopurinol.

Pharmacokinetics. See Table 39-1.

Adverse Effects. See Table 39-2.

Drug Interactions. Potentiates oral anticoagulants, hypoglycemics, and theophylline. Uricosurics reduce effect of allopurinol. Incidence of rash is increased with ampicillin and amoxicillin. Avoid urinary acidifiers; monitor renal function with thiazides. Mercaptopurine and azathioprine doses should be decreased to reduce risk of side effects.

Concomitant administration of thiazides may induce hypersensitivity reactions in patients with diminished renal function. Dosages of mercaptopurine and azathioprine must be decreased. Use of iron preparations results in increased hepatic iron concentration. Half-life of theophylline is increased.

Dosage and Administration. Allopurinol dosage will vary according to the patient's serum uric acid level and symptoms of gout. Initial therapy should begin at 100 mg per day. It can be increased by 100 mg per week until the patient's serum uric acid is below 6 mg/dl. The usual effective range for allopurinol is 100 to 800 mg daily.

The effective range for patients with mild gout is usually 200 to 300 mg per day. Doses of 400 to 600 mg per day are appropriate for patients with moderately severe tophaceous gout.

Doses up to 300 mg may be given as a single dose; amounts greater than 300 mg should be in divided doses.

Normal serum urate levels are generally achieved in 1 to 3 weeks.

RESOURCES FOR PATIENTS AND PROVIDERS

Arthritis Foundation Fact Sheet, www.arthritis.org.
Medscape Internet Drug Information, www.Medscape.com.
Rheumatology, www.rheumatology.org.

BIBLIOGRAPHY

Arromdee E, Michet CJ, Crowson CS, O'Fallon WM, Gabriel SE: Epidemiology of gout: is the incidence rising? *J Rheumatol* 29(11):2403-2406, 2002.

Canoso O: *Rheumatology in primary care,* Philadelphia, 1997, WB Saunders.

Crowther CL: *Primary orthopedic care,* St Louis, 1999, Mosby.

Kamienski M: Gout: not just for the rich and famous! Every man's disease, *Orthop Nurs* 22(1):16-20, 2003.

Perez-Ruiz F, Calabozo M, Erauskin GG, Ruibal A, Herrero-Beites AM: Renal underexcretion of uric acid is present in patients with apparent high urinary uric acid output. *Arthritis Rheum* 47(6):610-713, 2002.

Perez-Ruiz F, Calabozo M, Pijoan JI, Herrero-Beites AM, Ruibal A: Effect of urate-lowering therapy on the velocity of size reduction of tophi in chronic gout, *Arthritis Rheum* 47(4):356-360, 2002.

Schlesinger N, Schumacher HR Jr: Update on gout, *Arthritis Rheum* 47(5):563-565, 2002.

Shekarriz B, Stoller ML: Uric acid nephrolithiasis: current concepts and controversies, *J Urol* 168(4 pt 1):1307-1314, 2002.

Yamamoto T, Moriwaki Y, Takahashi S, Tsutsumi Z, Ka T, Fukuchi M, Hada T: A simple method of selecting gout patients for treatment with uricosuric agents, using spot urine and blood samples, *J Rheumatol* 29(9):937-1941, 2002.

CHAPTER 40

Osteoporosis Treatment

Jan DiSantostefano

Drug Names

Class	Subclass	Generic Name	Trade Name
Hormones		(200) calcitonin	Miacalcin, Calcimar, Osteocalcin
	Parathyroid hormone	teriparatide	Forteo
Bisphosphonates		(200) alendronate sodium	Fosamax
		risedronate	Actonel
Selective estrogen receptor modulators (SERMs)		raloxifene hydrochloride	Evista

(200), Top 200 drug.

General Uses

Indications

- Treatment and prevention of osteoporosis in postmenopausal women and osteopenia
- Treatment to increase bone mass in men with osteoporosis
- Treatment of glucocorticoid-induced osteoporosis in men and women
- Treatment of Paget's disease in men and women (teriparatide excluded)

Calcitonin and the bisphosphonates are bone metabolism regulators. Calcitonin is a hormone that is naturally produced in the thyroid, and is a powerful inhibitor of osteoclastic activity. The bisphosphonates are primarily antiresorptive agents, and prevent or significantly slow the normal osteoclastic activity responsible for the resorption of bone. Raloxifene is a selective estrogen receptor modulator (SERM) and decreases resorption of bone and the rate of bone turnover and remodeling. Parathyroid is the primary regulator of calcium and phosphate metabolism in the bones. It stimulates new bone by both the number and action of bone-forming cells called osteoblasts. This chapter concentrates on the use of these medications for osteoporosis because this is the condition seen most commonly by the primary care provider.

Hormone replacement was the first-line therapy for osteoporosis prevention. But because a recent study associated it with increased risk of stroke, heart disease, and breast cancer, careful consideration must be made of alternatives.

The drugs in this chapter not only stop loss of bone but also can produce an increase in bone density. Thus they can be used for both preventing and treating osteoporosis. They also can be effective in controlling the bone pain experienced by many patients with severe osteoporosis.

DISEASE PROCESS

Osteoporosis is a serious health problem that affects both men and women, but the greatest burden is borne by postmenopausal women. It is associated with significant morbidity, reduced quality of life, and soaring medical costs. Each year an estimated 1.5 million women in the United States alone experience osteoporotic fractures. Up to 20% of women with a hip fracture die within a year of fracture, and more than half fail to regain prefracture mobility and independence. Experts estimate almost one third of hip fracture patients require placement in a nursing home due to temporary or permanent disability. Fracture of the spine may lead to crowding of internal organs, GI disorders, or restrictive lung disease. Increased mortality and morbidity are associated with limited physical activity, back pain, skeletal deformity, height loss, and kyphosis.

Women are more susceptible to osteoporosis because their peak bone mass tends to be 10% to 30% less than males. With the progressive aging of the world's population, this health problem will continue to escalate not only morbidity and mortality rates but also health care costs. Advancing age is a strong predictor for fracture risk; the incidence of fracture will inevitably rise as the U.S. population rises. Diagnostic evaluation of at-risk individuals and interventions to prevent osteoporotic fracture have the potential of great savings of both suffering and money.

The prevalence of osteoporosis in men increases after age 80. Men have a shorter life span than women, so they account for only 21% of hip fractures. By the age of 90, only 17% of men have had a hip fracture, compared with 32% of women.

Pathophysiology

The bony skeleton is made up of an outer shell of cortical dense bone surrounding an internal honeycomb-like structure of trabecular bone. Bone is composed of a protein framework that hardens when the minerals calcium and phosphorus are deposited on it. Without enough calcium, bones get weak.

Bone is constantly changing. This occurs in an ongoing cyclic pattern that allows both proper bone health and the appropriate use of calcium in the bones for other body functions such as maintaining a normal heart rhythm. Bone remodeling is a process in which old bone is removed and new bone is laid down. The two stages of bone remodeling are resorption and formation. The first stage of remodeling is bone breakdown or resorption, when old bone is removed. The osteoclasts scoop away the bone over a period of about 2 weeks and are replaced by osteoblasts. The calcium in the broken down bone tissue circulates throughout the body and is used for other key functions. The second stage, bone formation, follows when new bone fills in the spaces where the old bone was removed. When the bone is completely replaced, bone strength is maintained. In osteoporosis, too much bone is removed, too little bone is formed, or a combination of both occurs. This leads to a loss in bone amount and strength.

During childhood and through early adulthood, new bone is added to the skeleton faster than old bone is removed. As a result, bones become stronger, larger, and denser. Peak bone mass, the maximum amount of bone that a person can have, is reached between 20 and 30 years of age. After age 30, bone is removed faster than it forms. Osteoporosis may also be linked to chronic glucocorticoid use, including use of inhaled steroids for treatment of chronic obstructive lung disease. Table 40-1 lists risk factors associated with osteoporosis.

The Disease

According to the World Health Organization (WHO), osteoporosis is now widely recognized as a progressive systemic disease, characterized by low bone density (osteopenia) and microarchitectural deterioration in bone that predisposes patients to increased bone fragility and fracture. Fragility fractures result from trauma that would not cause normal bone to fracture due to decrease in bone mass.

Assessment

Bone loss does not show up on conventional x-ray films until one fourth or more of the bone's mineral content is gone. The most commonly used technique is central dual energy x-ray absorptiometry (DXA), which measures the spine, hip or total body. It is the most sensitive test and provides the most precise T-scores. Peripheral dual energy x-ray absorptiometry (pDXA) measures the wrist, heel, or finger. Quantitative computed tomography (QCT) measures the spine, hip, or total body. Ultrasonometry uses sound waves to measure density at the heel, shinbone and kneecap. This technique can easily be performed in the office setting, but is currently less sensitive than DXA.

Bone density testing is indicated for women and men with an increased risk for osteoporosis. If a woman is at least 5 years postmenopausal or has several risk factors, she should be strongly encouraged to have bone density testing and be placed on therapy if the testing is indicative of osteoporosis or osteopenia. See Box 40-1 for indications for bone mineral density (BMD) testing.

A T-score represents the number of standard deviations (SDs) above or below the mean BMD for the young healthy female population (women who are less than 35 years of age). A T-score of –1 signifies a 10% to 12% loss of bone mass, compared with mean values for young normal adults. According to recommendations of the WHO Task Force for Osteoporosis, osteoporosis is defined as a T-score of ≤2.5 in women without history of fragility fractures (Table 40-2). Treatment is generally indicated if the patient is 2 or more standard deviations below the normal premenopausal level.

TABLE 40-1 Risk Factors Associated with Osteoporosis

Potentially Modifiable	Nonmodifiable
Current cigarette smoking	Personal history of fracture
Diet low in calcium/vitamin D	First-degree relative with fracture
Use of glucocorticoids, anticonvulsants	Race (Caucasian or Asian)
Excessive alcohol intake	Elderly age
Sedentary lifestyle	Poor health
Body weight less than 127 lb	Dementia
Lack of estrogen	Hormonal disorders
Environmental risks (loose rugs, dark stairs, etc.)	Neoplastic disorders
Poor eyesight	Metabolic abnormalities
History of organ transplants	Connective tissue disorders

BOX 40-1

INDICATIONS FOR MEASURING BONE MINERAL DENSITY

- Postmenopausal women who are 2 years postmenopausal and have two or more risk factors
- Postmenopausal women who are 5 years postmenopausal without other risk factors
- Patients with osteopenia on plain radiographs
- Patients being treated for osteoporosis to monitor changes in bone mass
- Patients receiving long-term glucocorticoid therapy
- Patients with hyperparathyroidism or other diseases associated with high risk of osteoporosis
- Men with hypogonadism
- Patients with gastrointestinal disease, such as malabsorption and hemigastrectomy (10 years after surgery)
- Patients with prolonged immobilization
- Rheumatoid arthritis or ankylosing spondylitis
- Methotrexate use
- Prolonged use of thyroid replacement
- Anticonvulsant use for 5 years
- Previous fracture in adult years with minimal trauma or in classic fracture sites for osteoporosis (vertebra, wrist, hip, pelvis)
- Lifelong low calcium intake

TABLE 40-2 WHO Criteria for Diagnosis of Osteoporosis

T-Score*	Classification
≥–1	Normal
–1 to –2.5	Osteopenia
≤–2.5	Osteoporosis
≤–2.5 + fracture	Severe osteoporosis

*T-score indicates the number of standard deviations below the average peak bone mass in young adults.

DRUG ACTION AND EFFECTS

Calcitonin is a naturally occurring hormone produced by the C cells in the thyroid gland. Although its mechanism of action in osteoporosis is not fully delineated, calcitonin is known to block bone resorption through its potent inhibitory effects on osteoclasts. Calcitonin is a protein and therefore cannot be taken orally because it would be digested before it could work. Intranasal salmon calcitonin is 50- to 100-fold more potent than human calcitonin. Calcitonin lowers serum calcium concentration primarily by a direct inhibition of bone resorption. Osteoclasts are reduced in number and function, and osteocytic resorption is decreased. Calcitonin also has a direct effect on the kidneys. By inhibiting tubular reabsorption, there is increased excretion of calcium, phosphate, and sodium. However, urinary calcium is decreased rather than increased in some patients as calcitonin-induced inhibition of bone resorption has a greater effect on calcium excretion than does the drug's direct renal action. In the Prevent Reoccurrence of Osteoporosis Fractures (PROOF) study, treatment with nasal calcitonin produced a 1.2% increase in spinal BMD, with a 36% risk reduction for new vertebral fractures. Calcitonin also has an analgesic effect through mechanisms that may involve increased release of endorphins, and therefore produces beneficial pain relief after a fracture.

Bisphosphonates are nonhormonal agents that have an extremely high affinity for bone. Alendronate was the first of the newer bisphosphonates to be approved by the FDA for treatment and prevention of osteoporosis. Risedronate is the second bisphosphonate to be approved for the treatment of osteoporosis. Bisphosphonates are analogs of pyrophosphate that bind to hydroxyapatite and specifically inhibit bone resorption by inhibiting the activity of osteoclasts to normalize the rate of bone turnover. Both alendronate and risedronate are nitrogen-containing bisphosphonates and inhibit osteoclast-mediated bone resorption by inhibiting the mevalonate pathway and by inducing osteoclast apoptosis. The bisphosphonates are very specific to the skeleton; they reduce risk for both vertebral and nonvertebral fractures without demonstrating other benefits outside of the skeleton. Alendronate and risedronate are incorporated into bone matrix, but are not pharmacologically active thereafter. It is unknown if the incorporated bisphosphonates, when released by resorption, could eventually interfere with bone remodeling.

Another class of agents used in treating osteoporosis is the SERMs. Raloxifine is the only SERM in use for osteoporosis. It blocks estrogen receptors so that estrogen is unable to exert its effect. Raloxifene belongs to the benzothiophene class of compounds. It reduces resorption of bone and decreases overall bone turnover. Although raloxifene reduces the risk for developing vertebral fracture and increases hip and spine BMD, it has no significant effects on most nonvertebral fractures, including hip fracture. Raloxifene prevents endometrial thickening, reducing the risk of endometrial cancer, but does not relieve the vasomotor symptoms of menopause. It also reduces the risk of cardiovascular events in women with increased risk at baseline, and lowers low-density lipoprotein cholesterol levels. It seems to exert antiestrogenic effects on breast tissue, which theoretically might decrease the risk of breast cancer.

Tamoxifen is a SERM that blocks the estrogen receptors in breast tissue. However, it triggers cell proliferation in the lining of the uterus and can cause endometrial cancer. It is not used in osteoporosis. See Chapter 57 for more detailed discussion of tamoxifen.

Synthetic human parathyroid hormone (PTH), approved by the FDA in November 2002, is the first approved agent for the treatment of osteoporosis that stimulates new bone formation. Once-daily injections stimulate new bone formation on trabecular and cortical bone surfaces by preferential stimulation of osteoblastic activity over osteoclastic activity. This effect is manifested as an increase in skeletal mass and an increase in bone turnover markers. By increasing new bone formation, teriparatide improves bone mass and bone strength. PTH also acts on the kidneys by reducing renal clearance of calcium. Patients treated with PTH, along with calcium and vitamin D supplementation had statistically significant increases in bone mineral density (10% to 20% after 1½ years) at the spine and hip when compared with patients taking only calcium and vitamin D.

A new osteoporosis drug, zoledronic acid (Zometa), which requires a once a year infusion, is in clinical trials. It is currently used to treat complications of cancer that have spread to the bone. Zoledronic acid, an intravenous bisphosphonate, is generally well tolerated. The major side effects are low-grade fever, musculoskeletal pain, and nausea after the infusion. Researchers don't yet understand how a single, yearly dose can protect bone as well as daily or weekly therapy, but a greater understanding of the drug is expected to emerge during the 3-year study launched in November 2002.

DRUG TREATMENT PRINCIPLES

The first step in prevention and treatment of osteoporosis is nonpharmacologic (Figure 40-1). The patient must have an adequate calcium intake (1200 to 1500 mg daily), receive enough vitamin D (400 IUs or 10 minutes of sun exposure daily) and participate in weight-bearing exercise for at least 30 minutes three times weekly. See Table 40-3 for recommended daily requirements of calcium. Calcium supplementation is necessary if there is inadequate calcium in the diet. Calcium replacement and exercise will slow bone loss, but will not prevent it, or reverse it (see Table 40-3 for recommended daily requirements for calcium, and Table 40-2 for calcium levels in

TABLE 40-3 Women's Recommended Daily Requirements for Calcium

Lifestage	Daily Requirement
Adolescent girls, aged 9 to 17 years	1300 mg
Pregnancy, ≤18 years of age	1300 mg
Pregnancy, 19 to 50 years of age	1000 mg
Lactation, ≤18 years of age	1300 mg
Lactation, 19 to 50 years of age	1000 mg
Premenopausal women	1000 mg
Postmenopausal women on HRT	1000 mg
Postmenopausal women not on HRT	1500 mg

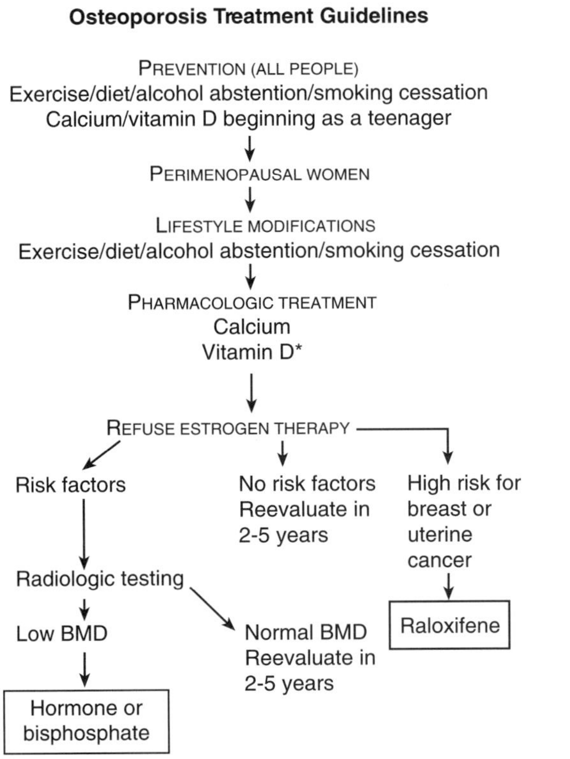

Osteoporosis Treatment Guidelines

PREVENTION (ALL PEOPLE)
Exercise/diet/alcohol abstention/smoking cessation
Calcium/vitamin D beginning as a teenager
↓
PERIMENOPAUSAL WOMEN
↓
LIFESTYLE MODIFICATIONS
Exercise/diet/alcohol abstention/smoking cessation
↓
PHARMACOLOGIC TREATMENT
Calcium
Vitamin D*
↓
REFUSE ESTROGEN THERAPY
- Risk factors → Radiologic testing
  - Low BMD → Hormone or bisphosphate
  - Normal BMD: Reevaluate in 2-5 years
- No risk factors: Reevaluate in 2-5 years
- High risk for breast or uterine cancer → Raloxifene

BMD, bone mineral density.
*Vitamin D: if vitamin D deficient, elderly, or institutionalized/housebound.

FIGURE 40-1

Osteoporosis treatment guidelines.

common foods). Both phosphorus and magnesium are also required.

Hormone replacement therapy (HRT) helps prevent osteoporosis, but recent studies have shown other health risks associated with combined therapy making HRT a less desirable option. Estrogen therapy alone has been shown to be effective, but continued studies regarding other health risks associated with estrogen are still being conducted.

Drug Choice

The bisphosphonates alendronate and risedronate have similar efficacy, side effects, and cost, although risedronate may be slightly less expensive. Both must be taken on an empty stomach first thing in the morning, and the patient must remain upright and not eat or drink anything for 30 minutes. Newer dosing regimens allow for the bisphosphonates to be taken once a week for ease of dosing. Effectiveness is greatly decreased if not taken correctly.

Calcitonin is made of salmon calcitonin. It is available as a nasal spray. The nasal spray is convenient (but expensive) and has few side effects except for occasional nasal irritation, but it is not as effective as the bisphosphonates. Calcitonin is not recommended in osteoporotic women during the first 5 years after menopause because there are few data to support its efficacy during this period.

Raloxifene is as effective as the bisphosphonates in promoting bone density. It has the added benefit of lowering low-density lipoprotein (LDL) cholesterol. Raloxifene does not increase risk of breast or uterine cancer. In women who suffer from hot flashes, it may increase the amount of hot flashes. Women treated with raloxifene have an increased risk of venous thromboembolism, deep vein, pulmonary, and superficial, with the greatest risk during the first 4 months of use. Because immobilization increases the risk of venous thromboembolic events independent of therapy, raloxifene is not indicated for women who are not fully ambulatory, and should be discontinued for women who undergo prolonged immobilization.

PTH appears to be a promising new drug for osteoporosis treatment, but because it was just introduced in November 2002, little information is available. Patients who are at risk for osteosarcoma should not take teriparatide (see listings under contraindication section). Safety and efficacy are not approved for use beyond 2 years of treatment.

HOW TO MONITOR

- The practitioner should monitor levels of serum calcium and phosphorus prior to initiating therapy and yearly thereafter.
- Lumbar vertebral bone mineral density testing should be measured by DXA to establish the diagnosis of osteoporosis prior to initiating treatment and every 2 years to monitor therapy.
- The rate of bone loss can be monitored with a urine test called NTx prior to initiating therapy, 3 months later, and yearly or whenever therapy is changed. This test measures urine levels of a compound linked to bone breakdown and should be collected as the second void of the day. Normal levels are less than 38 (values above the normal indicate a faster rate of bone loss). If therapy is effective, then subsequent tests will show decreased levels.
- Periodic nasal examinations observing for crusts, dryness, erythema, and irritation are recommended for patients receiving calcitonin nasal spray.

PATIENT VARIABLES

Geriatrics

No overall differences in efficacy or safety were observed between patients older than 65 and younger patients receiving any of these medications.

Pediatrics

Safety and effectiveness in patients younger than the age of 18 have not been evaluated in any of these medications. Teriparatide should not be used in pediatric populations and young adults with open epiphyses.

Pregnancy

Category C: raloxifene is contraindicated in women who are or may become pregnant. There are no studies in pregnant women with the other drugs in this category and they should be used during pregnancy only if the potential benefit justifies the potential risk to the mother and fetus. Calcitonin has been shown to cause a decrease in fetal birthweight in animals when given many times the normal dose. Calcitonin does not cross the placenta. High doses of alendronate have been shown to cause decreased birthweight, bone changes, and late pregnancy deaths in animal studies. Raloxifene and teriparatide are not indicated for premenopausal women.

Lactation

It is not known if alendronate, risedronate, raloxifene, and teriparatide are excreted in human breast milk. The impact of these drugs has not been studied in nursing women, so they are not recommended for nursing mothers. Calcitonin is distributed in breast milk. In animal studies, calcitonin has been shown to inhibit lactation. Raloxifene and teriparatide are only indicated for postmenopausal women.

Race

Pharmacokinetic differences due to race have been studied on a limited basis with no discernible differences. Osteoporosis is more common in Caucasians and Asians than members of other races. Darker-skinned races genetically are found to have denser bones.

Gender

Bioavailability and pharmacokinetics following oral administration of bisphosphonates are similar in men and women. Safety and effectiveness of bisphosphonates have been demonstrated in clinical studies in men for glucocorticoid-induced osteoporosis and Paget's disease, but no studies have been done for osteoporosis due to other causes and for weekly dosing. No significant differences were noted between age-matched men and women with raloxifene, but safety and efficacy have not been evaluated in men. Systemic exposure to teriparatide was approximately 20% to 30% lower in men than women.

PATIENT EDUCATION

- Advise patient to include adequate amounts of calcium (1000 to 1500 mg/day), vitamin D (400 IU), and general good nutrition in the diet. (See Tables 40-3 and 40-4.)
- Weight-bearing exercise, particularly walking, should be encouraged along with modification of other risk factors for osteoporosis, such as smoking and alcohol consumption.
- Calcitonin nasal spray: advise patient on pump assembly, pump priming, and use of pump. Any significant nasal irritation should be reported. Once the pump has been activated, the bottle may be maintained at room temperature for 2 weeks until the medication is finished. Explain the action of absorption through the mucosal membranes into the bloodstream to facilitate patient understanding of mechanism of action and compliance with medication. Calcitonin can be taken without regard to food or beverage intake.
- Alendronate and risedronate: these medications must be taken at least 30 minutes before eating the first food, beverage, or medication every day. To facilitate absorption, the bisphosphonates should be taken with a full glass (6 to 8 oz) of plain water and the patient should avoid lying down for 30 minutes thereafter to facilitate delivery to the stomach and reduce the potential for esophageal irritation.
- Raloxifene can be taken without regard to food intake.
- Teriparatide is administered by subcutaneous injection using a prefilled delivery device, and instructions should be given to inject once daily into the thigh or abdomen. It can be injected at any time of day. Teriparatide should be refrigerated at 36° to 46°F both before and after use. It should not be frozen and should be discarded if it has been frozen. Do not use teriparatide that is discolored or cloudy or that has particles in it or after the expiration date on the pen. One pen provides 28 days of medication. There are no restrictions on food, beverage, or activity when taking teriparatide. Data are not available on safety and efficacy after taking for more than 2 years.

TABLE 40-4 Calcium Content of Readily Available Foods

Food	Serving Size	Calcium (mg)
Sesame seed meats	1 cup	1080
Yogurt, unflavored	1 cup	415
Mackerel, canned	5 oz	400
Sardines, in oil	4 oz	400
Milk, skim, nonfat	1 cup	302
Milk, 1% low-fat	1 cup	300
Collard greens, frozen, cooked	1 cup	300
Salmon, baked, broiled	6 oz	300
Milk, 2% low-fat	1 cup	297
Milk, whole	1 cup	291
Cheese, Swiss	1 oz	272
Cheese, provolone	1 oz	214
Cheese, mozzarella (part-skim)	1 oz	207
Frozen yogurt	1 cup	200
Dried figs	10	200
Macaroni and cheese (box mix)	1 cup	199
Ice cream, plain	1 cup	176
Ice milk	1 cup	176
Cheese, American	1 oz	174
Cheese, mozzarella (whole-milk)	1 oz	163
Cottage cheese, 2%	1 cup	155
Bok choy	1 cup	150
Instant oatmeal	1 packet	150
Rhubarb, cooked with sugar	1/2 cup	150
Cottage cheese, 1%	1 cup	138
Broccoli, cooked	1 cup	136
Cottage cheese, regular	1 cup	130
Almonds	1.5 oz	100
Soybeans, cooked	1 cup	100
Turnip greens, frozen, cooked	1/2 cup	100
Baked beans	1/2 cup	50
Broccoli, kale, mustard greens	1/2 cup	50
English muffin, oatmeal muffin	1	50
Orange	1 medium	50
Orange juice	6 oz	50
Pita	1 small	50
Refried beans	1/2 cup	25

Specific Drugs

HORMONES

calcitonin (Miacalcin, Calcimar, Osteocalcin)

Indications. Helpful for bone pain.

Contraindications. Allergy/sensitivity to calcitonin or allergy to proteins.

Precautions. Because calcitonin is a polypeptide, the possibility of a systemic allergic reaction exists. Skin testing should be considered prior to treatment for patients with suspected sensitivity.

Pharmacokinetics. See Table 40-5. Calcitonin is destroyed in the GI tract and therefore must be administered either parenterally or intranasally. There is great variability in the data on bioavailability of calcitonin nasal spray.

Adverse Effects. See Table 40-6.

Drug Interactions. In the treatment of osteoporosis, calcium-containing preparations may be given 4 hours after calcitonin. No other significant drug interactions have been identified.

Dosage and Administration. Osteoporosis: 200 IU/day intranasally, alternating nostrils daily.

Parathyroid Hormone

teriparatide (Forteo)

Contraindications. Allergy/sensitivity to teriparatide or allergy to proteins. Avoid use in treatment of patients with a higher risk of osteosarcoma such as Paget's disease of the bone, unexplained high levels of alkaline phosphatase in the blood, pediatric population or young adult, and anyone who has ever been diagnosed with bone cancer or other cancers with metastasis to the bone, has had radiation therapy involving the bone, has a bone disease other than osteoporosis, or has a high level of calcium in the blood.

Precautions. Teriparatide may cause dizziness or tachycardia after an injection, so the injection should be given where there is availability for patient to sit or lie down. Transient episodes of orthostatic hypotension have been observed infrequently, but resolved spontaneously and did not preclude continued treatment. It should be used with caution in patients with active or recent urolithiasis because of the potential to exacerbate this condition.

Drug and Food Interactions. There are no food interactions. A dosage adjustment or special monitoring may be required if patient is also taking digoxin.

Overdosage. Symptoms of overdose may include nausea, vomiting, dizziness, and headache and require immediate medical attention.

Dosage and Administration. Osteoporosis: 20 µg once daily subcutaneously into the thigh or abdominal wall.

BISPHOSPHONATES

alendronate (Fosamax), risedronate (Actonel)

Contraindications

- Hypocalcemia, renal insufficiency, inability to stand or sit upright for 30 minutes, abnormalities of the esophagus that delay emptying such as stricture or achalasia

Precautions

- Patients need to have adequate nutrition, calcium, and vitamin D.

Nephrotic syndrome, mineralization deficits, and fracture have been reported with prolonged continuous treatment.

- Alendronate and risedronate are not recommended for patients with renal insufficiency (creatinine clearance <35 ml/min). Use with caution in patients with active upper GI problems, such as dysphagia, esophagitis, gastritis, duodenitis, ulcers, and symptomatic esophageal diseases. Hypocalcemia must be corrected before administration of bisphosphonates. Bisphosphonates are poorly absorbed, and food blocks their absorption altogether.

Drug and Food Interactions. Increased incidence of adverse GI events with aspirin. Calcium-, aluminum-, and magnesium-containing medications may interfere with absorption and should not be administered within 2 hours of dose.

Overdosage. Hypocalcemia, hypophosphatemia, and upper GI adverse events such as upset stomach, heartburn, esophagitis, gastritis, or ulcer may result from overdosage. Death is seen with significant overdosage of both alendronate and risedronate in rats.

Dosage and Administration

alendronate (Fosamax)

- Osteoporosis: 10 mg every morning or 70 mg once a week
- Osteopenia: 5 mg every morning

risedronate (Actonel)

- Osteoporosis: 5 mg every morning or 35 mg once a week. Take 30 minutes before the first food or drink of the day. Patient should be in upright position and not lie down for 30 minutes after taking medication.

SERMs

raloxifene hydrochloride (Evista)

Contraindications

- Active or past history of venous thromboembolic events, including deep vein thrombosis, pulmonary embolism, and retinal vein thrombosis. Prolonged immobilization.

Warnings/Precautions. The greatest risk for thromboembolic events occurs during the first 4 months of treatment. Raloxifene should be discontinued at least 72 hours prior to and during prolonged immobilization and should be resumed only after the patient is fully ambulatory. Patients should be advised to avoid prolonged restriction of movement during travel. There is no indication for premenopausal women. Safety and efficacy in women with severe hepatic insufficiency have not been established.

TABLE 40-5 Pharmacokinetics of Medications Used to Treat Osteoporosis

Drug	Absorption	Onset of Action	Time to Peak Concentration	Half-Life	Duration of Action	Metabolism	Excretion
calcitonin	Destroyed in GI tract			6-24 mo of continuous treatment	Nasal, 31-39 min	Primarily kidneys, some in blood and peripheral tissues	Renal
teriparatide	95%	Unknown	30 min	1 hr	Unknown	Believed to occur by nonspecific enzymatic mechanisms in the liver	Renal
alendronate	78% available after first pass	<6 hr		Terminal half-life: 10 yr ✱	78% protein-bound; not metabolized		Renal
risedronate	Rapid absorption within first hour	Unknown	Unknown	1.5 hr	Terminal exponential half-life of 480 hr	None	Urine, 50% excreted in 24 hr; unabsorbed drug is eliminated unchanged in feces
raloxifene	60%	Improvement in bone mass observed after 3 mo of treatment	27.7 hr	Unknown after discontinuing medication		>95% protein-bound; hepatic metabolism, but not CYP 450 pathway	Urine, 0.2%

✱ = for long acting meds such as risedronate & alendronate, the terminal ½ life, which reflects the prolonged activity of low levels of the drug, is clinically more significant than the commonly used ½ life.

TABLE 40-6 Most Common Adverse Effects

Medication	Adverse Effects
calcitonin nasal spray	Intranasal: rhinitis, nasal crusts, dryness, erythema, irritation, epistaxis
teriparatide	Dizziness and leg cramps
alendronate and risedronate	GI upset, diarrhea, nausea, musculoskeletal pain
raloxifene	Hot flashes, leg cramps, increased risk of venous thromboembolic events

Drug and Food Interactions. Cholestyramine causes a 60% reduction in the absorption and enterohepatic recycling of raloxifene and should not be coadministered. Coadministration with warfarin has not been observed under chronic conditions; however, 10% decreases in prothrombin time have been observed, and prothrombin time should be monitored. Raloxifene is highly bound to plasma proteins, and caution should be used when administered with other highly protein-bound medications such as clofibrate, indomethacin, naproxen, ibuprofen, diazepam, and diazoxide.

Dosage and Administration

- Osteoporosis: 60 mg daily. May be administered any time of day without regard to food.

RESOURCES FOR PATIENTS AND PROVIDERS

National Osteoporosis Foundation, www.NOF.org.
General information.
American Arthritis Foundation, www.Arthritis.org.
Specific programs and information related to arthritis and osteoporosis.

Websites maintained by pharmaceutical companies

Latest research findings included.
www.actonel.com
www.forteo.com
www.fosamax.com

BIBLIOGRAPHY

Campion JM, Maricie MJ: Osteoporosis in men, *Am Fam Physician* 67(7):1521-1526, 2003.

Davidson MR: Pharmacotherapeutics for osteoporosis prevention and treatment, *J Midwifery Womens Health* 48(1):39-54, 2003.

Davis L: Prevention of bone loss with alendronate in postmenopausal women under 60 years of age, *J Nurs Midwif* 43(5):395, 1998.

Eichner SF, Lloyd KB, Timpe EM: Comparing therapies for postmenopausal osteoporosis prevention and treatment, *Ann Pharmacother* 37(5):711-724, 2003.

Genant HK, Jergas M: Assessment of prevalent and incident vertebral fractures in osteoporosis research, *Osteoporos Int* (epub), March 12, 2003.

Hallworth RB: Prevention and treatment of postmenopausal osteoporosis, *Pharm World Sci* 20(5):198, 1998.

Laroche M et al: Beneficial effect on bone density in male osteoporosis of postmenopausal osteoporosis treatment, *Clin Exp Rheumatol* 16(6):760, 1998.

Levine JP: Long-term estrogen and hormone replacement therapy for the prevention and treatment of osteoporosis, *Curr Womens Health Rep* 3(3):181-186, 2003.

Ott K: Osteoporosis and bone densitometry, *Radiol Technol* 70(2):129, quiz 149-152, 1998.

Placide J, Martens MG: Comparing screening methods for osteoporosis, *Curr Womens Health Rep* 3(3):207-210, 2003.

Ragsdale AB et al: Alendronate treatment to prevent osteoporotic fractures, *Arch Fam Med* 7(6):583, 1998.

Sagraves R: Evaluating therapeutic modalities for prevention and treatment of postmenopausal osteoporosis, *Ann Pharmacother* 37(5):744-746, 2003.

Sedlak CA et al: Osteoporosis prevention in young women, *Orthop Nurs* 17(3):53, 1998.

Sickels JM, Nip CS: Risedronate for the prevention of fractures in postmenopausal osteoporosis, *Ann Pharmacother* 36(4):664-670, 2002.

Sparidans RW et al: Bisphosphates in bone diseases, *Pharm World Sci* 20(5):206, 1998.

Watts NB, Lindsay R, Li Z, Kasbhatla C, Brown J: Use of matched historical controls to evaluate the anti-fracture efficacy of once-a-week risedronate, *Osteoporos Int* April 29 (epub), 2003.

Woodhead GA, Moss MM: Osteoporosis: diagnosis and prevention, *Nurs Pract* 23(11):18, 1998.

CHAPTER 41

Muscle Relaxants

Drug Names

Class	Subclass		Generic Name	Trade Name
Centrally acting sedative/CNS depressants		(P) (200)	metaxalone	Skelaxin
			methocarbamol	Robaxin
			chlorzoxazone	Paraflex, Parafon Forte
		(200)	carisoprodol	Soma
Miscellaneous	TCA relative	(200)	cyclobenzaprine	Flexeril
	Benzodiazepine		diazepam	Valium
	GABA receptor stimulant		baclofen	Lioresal
	Centrally acting α_2-adrenergic agonist		tizanidine	Zanaflex

(200), Top 200 drug; (P), prototype drug.

General Uses

Indications

- Centrally acting sedatives: musculoskeletal conditions, as an adjunct to rest, physical therapy, and other measures for relief of discomfort associated with acute, painful musculoskeletal conditions.
- Cyclobenzaprine (Flexeril): musculoskeletal conditions
  Unlabeled use:
  Fibrositis syndrome
- Lioresal: used to alleviate spasticity resulting from multiple sclerosis. May be of some value in patients with spinal cord injuries and other spinal cord diseases
  Unlabeled use:
  Trigeminal neuralgia, tardive dyskinesia
- Tizanidine: increased muscle tone associated with muscle spasticity

These muscle-relaxant medications are chemically unrelated. For the purposes of this chapter, they are divided into two groups. The first group works by sedation of CNS depression. Although they do not have any direct relaxation effect upon muscles, they have many characteristics in common and are treated as a group. Metaxalone is treated as the prototype for this group because it is most commonly used. The second group is composed of medications not related by mechanism of action. Of these, only cyclobenzaprine is discussed in detail.

DISEASE PROCESS

Muscle spasms result from two very different mechanisms. The most common mechanism is a peripheral problem with a skeletal muscle. These are most often minor to moderate problems and acute in nature. Common problems with muscle spasms are seen with low back irritation, following motor vehicle accidents, and musculoskeletal injuries. If these are not treated adequately they can become a chronic problem with disability. Other causes of chronic skeletal muscle spasm are rheumatic disorders, stroke, cerebral palsy, and Parkinson's disease.

The second common mechanism of muscle spasms is due to a CNS problem. Examples are multiple sclerosis and spinal cord injuries and diseases. These are not commonly seen in primary care and are mentioned briefly.

DRUG ACTION AND EFFECTS

The centrally acting sedatives are CNS depressants. They act primarily on the CNS at the brainstem. The exact mode of action is unknown. These agents do not work directly on skeletal muscle or at the neuromuscular junction. These skeletal muscle relaxants achieve their effect on localized muscle spasms by producing sedation in the patient. This sedation causes a decrease in the facilitative and inhibitory neuronal activity, which affects the muscle stretch reflex. These agents do not have analgesic or antiinflammatory properties. These agents have been found to reduce the involuntary contractions or muscle spasms that result from skeletal muscle injuries. They are effective against peripherally caused muscle spasms. Centrally acting sedatives are ineffective at treating spasticity of muscles caused by a CNS disease.

The exact mechanisms of action of the miscellaneous group of relaxants are not precisely known. Cyclobenzaprine (Flexeril) is structurally related to the tricyclic antidepressants. It acts in the CNS to reduce tonic somatic motor activity. It has reserpine antagonism, norepinephrine potentiation, potent anticholinergic effects, and sedation. It is effective against peripherally caused muscle spasms.

Lioresal is effective only for muscle spasm caused by CNS disease. It inhibits monosynaptic and polysynaptic reflexes at the spinal level and is a structural analog of gamma-aminobutyric acid (GABA), the inhibitory neurotransmitter. Lioresal also causes CNS depression.

Diazepam and tizanidine are effective for both peripheral spasms and CNS-caused spasms. Diazepam (Valium) has direct skeletal muscle relaxant action at the spinal level, enhancing GABA-mediated presynaptic inhibition, and in the brainstem. Diazepam is used for both skeletal muscle strain and spasticity caused by upper motor neuron disorders.

Tizanidine is an imidazoline derivative, an α_2-adrenergic receptor agonist with centrally mediated myospasmolytic action. It has muscle relaxant, antinociceptive, and gastroprotective properties, lowering gastric acid secretion.

DRUG TREATMENT PRINCIPLES

This section is limited to the discussion of treatment of peripherally caused muscle spasms. Management of CNS spasm is beyond the scope of this book.

Nonpharmacologic

Treatment of acute injury consists of rest, ice, compression, and elevation (RICE). Ice is used for the first 24 to 48 hours; heat, or ice alternating with heat, may then be applied. Physical therapy may be indicated as the injury begins to heal. Chronic muscle spasm should also be treated with physical therapy.

Pharmacologic Treatment

Medication for acute muscle injury begins with nonsteroidal antiinflammatory drugs (NSAIDs). If these alone are ineffective in relieving pain or if muscle spasm is a significant component of the patient's complaints, a muscle relaxant may be considered. The use of skeletal muscle relaxants has been somewhat controversial over the years. When used for acute muscle spasm, these drugs are used as adjunctive therapy.

Recent research on low back pain suggests that patients who receive both NSAIDs and skeletal muscle relaxants have better outcomes than those who receive other medications or no medications, although the specific combinations of medications that are most effective are still under study.

Therapy with a muscle relaxant should be short term—from 2 to 8 weeks. Chronic muscle spasm may also be treated with short-term muscle relaxants to help break the cycle of muscle spasm and pain.

Drug Choice

The provider should become familiar with one or two of the sedative muscle relaxants; the ones most commonly used are metaxalone and methocarbamol. Cyclobenzaprine, having a different mechanism of action, is also useful. Carisoprodol is one of the top 200 drugs and is very similar to the prototype.

> ! Diazepam is the only benzodiazepine indicated for muscle relaxation, and is the only drug in this category with direct muscle-relaxant effect. It is very effective for short-term relief with severe muscle spasms. However, because of its abuse potential, its use should be limited to short term and the amount of medication closely monitored.

Other benzodiazepines have indirect effect as muscle relaxants. Their advantage is a shorter half-life with fewer adverse reactions. Baclofen is used for CNS disorders with muscle spasm. Discussion of this use is beyond the scope of this chapter. Tizanidine is a new medication; its role in management of muscle spasm has not yet been fully elucidated.

PATIENT VARIABLES

Geriatrics

- Elderly patients may be more susceptible to the sedative effects; thus these medications must be used very cautiously
- At increased risk for falls

Pediatrics

- Safety of use in children younger than the age of 12 years has not been established

Pregnancy

- Safety for use in pregnant women has not been established
- Lactation: not known

HOW TO MONITOR

- Reduction in severity and duration of muscle spasms
- Sedation or dizziness
- Liver function tests in patients at risk

PATIENT EDUCATION

- May cause sedation and decreased mental alertness; use caution when performing hazardous tasks
- Do not drink alcohol or take any other CNS depressants concomitantly with skeletal muscle relaxants because there are additive effects
- Notify provider if skin rash or jaundice occurs

Specific Drugs

SEDATIVE/CNS DEPRESSANTS

(P) Prototype Drug

metaxalone (Skelaxin)

Contraindications

- Hypersensitivity

Warnings

- Hepatic function impairment: administer with great care to patients with preexisting liver damage and perform serial liver function studies as required. Discontinue if signs or symptoms of liver dysfunction are observed.
- May impair mental or physical abilities. Patients should use caution while driving or performing other tasks requiring alertness, coordination, or physical dexterity.

Pharmacokinetics

See Table 41-1 for pharmacokinetic activity for all products.

TABLE 41-1 Pharmacokinetics of Selected Muscle Relaxants

Drug	Onset of Action	Half-life	Duration of Action	Metabolism	Excretion
metaxalone (Skelaxin)	1 hr	2-3 hr	4-6 hr	Liver	Metabolites in urine
methocarbamol (Robaxin)	30 min; peak levels in 2 hr	1-2 hr		Liver	Urine, inactive metabolites; small amount in feces
chlorzoxazone (Paraflex, Parafon Forte)	1 hr		3-4 hr	Rapidly in liver	Urine
carisoprodol (Soma)	30 min		4-6 hr	Liver	Urine
cyclobenzaprine (Flexeril)	Well absorbed orally but great deal of variance in serum levels	1-3 days		Highly protein-bound 1A2 2D6 3A4	Urine
baclofen (Lioresal)	Peak serum levels in 2 hr	3-4 hr			Excreted in urine unchanged
tizanidine (Zanaflex)	1-2 hr to peak Food increases rate to achieve peak concentration	2.5 hr	3-6 hr	Extensive first-pass metabolism in liver	Urine, 60%; feces, 20%

TABLE 41-2 Dosage and Administration Information for Selected Muscle Relaxants

Drug	Dosage and Administration
metaxalone (Skelaxin)	800 mg tid or qid daily
methocarbamol (Robaxin)	Give three 500-mg tablets qid or two 750-mg tablets qid; then decrease to two 500-mg tablets qid or two 750-mg tablets tid for maintenance
chlorzoxazone (Paraflex, Parafon Forte)	250 mg tid or qid or 500 mg tid-qid; up to 750 mg po tid-qid; reduce dose as symptoms improve
carisoprodol (Soma)	350 mg qid
cyclobenzaprine (Flexeril)	10 mg tid (maximum dose in 24 hr is 60 mg)
diazepam (Valium)	*Adults:* 2-10 mg po tid or qid *Geriatrics:* 2-2.5 mg po qd or bid
baclofen (Lioresal)	Start low, increase dosage gradually until effective Usually begin with 5 mg tid × 3 days; 10 mg tid × 3 days; 15 mg tid × 3 days; 20 mg tid × 3 days; maintenance dosage is usually 40-80 mg/day, not to exceed 80 mg daily
tizanidine (Zanaflex)	*Adults:* begin with 4 mg Increase dosage gradually 2-4 mg to maximum of 8 mg Dose can be repeated q6-8hr with maximum dosage 36 mg/day Little experience with doses >8 mg

Adverse Effects

- CNS: drowsiness, dizziness, headache, nervousness, irritability
- GI: nausea, vomiting, GI upset
- Miscellaneous: hypersensitivity (light rash with or without pruritus), leukopenia, hemolytic anemia, jaundice

Drug Interactions

- May enhance the effects of alcohol, barbiturates, and other CNS depressants

Drug Administration and Dosage

- See Table 41-2 for information on all drugs.

Other Drugs in Class

Other drugs in this class are similar to the prototype except as follows.

carisoprodol (Soma)

Contraindications

- Hypersensitivity

Warnings

- Use for short periods, usually 2 to 3 weeks. Drug has potential for abuse and habituation.

Precautions

- Somatic dysfunction during carisoprodol cessation suggests evidence for a carisoprodol withdrawal syndrome.

Drug Interactions
- Possible dangerous interaction of oxycodone (OxyContin) and carisoprodol.

OTHER CENTRALLY ACTING AGENTS

cyclobenzaprine (Flexeril)

Contraindications
- Hypersensitivity
- Concomitant use of monoamine oxidase inhibitors (MAOIs)
- Acute recovery phase of MI, patients with arrhythmias, heart block, or conduction disturbances or CHF
- Hyperthyroidism

Warnings
- Not effective in treatment of cerebral or spinal cord disease spasticity
- Use for short periods, usually 2 to 3 weeks
- Tricyclic antidepressants (TCAs): closely related, may cause same adverse reactions

Precautions
- Use cautiously in patients with urinary retention, angle-closure glaucoma, or increased intraocular pressure, and in patients taking anticholinergic medication.
- May impair mental or physical abilities. Patients should use caution while driving or performing other tasks requiring alertness, coordination, or physical dexterity.

Adverse Effects
- May have all of the adverse effects of TCAs. The most common adverse effects are drowsiness, dry mouth, dizziness, fatigue, nausea, constipation, asthenia, dyspepsia, unpleasant taste, headache, confusion, nervousness, and blurred vision.

Drug Interactions
- Cyclobenzaprine may interact with MAOIs and may enhance the effects of alcohol, barbiturates, or other CNS depressants. May have all of the drug interactions characteristic of TCAs.

BIBLIOGRAPHY

Argoff CE: Pharmacologic management of chronic pain, *J Am Osteopath Assoc* 102(9 suppl 3):S21-27, 2002.

Bailey DN, Briggs JR: Carisoprodol: an unrecognized drug of abuse, *Am J Clin Pathol* 117(3):396-400, 2002.

Caterino JM: Administration of inappropriate medications to elderly emergency department patients: results of a national survey, *Acad Emerg Med* 10(5):493-494, 2003.

Cherkin DC et al: Medication use for low back pain in primary care, *Spine* 23(5):607, 1998.

Reeves RR, Mack JE: Possible dangerous interaction of oxycontin and carisoprodol, *Am Fam Physician* 67(5):941-942, 2003.

Reeves RR, Parker JD: Somatic dysfunction during carisoprodol cessation: evidence for a carisoprodol withdrawal syndrome, *J Am Osteopath Assoc* 103(2):75-80, 2003.

UNIT 10

Central Nervous System Agents

Unit 10 deals with drugs that are used to treat central nervous system conditions seen in primary care. Some chapters are organized by the drug's mechanism of action and others are organized by the condition the drugs are used to treat.

- **Chapter 42** gives an overview of the anatomy and physiology of the CNS, which will be useful for understanding the following chapters.
- **Chapter 43** deals with stimulants and other cognitive function agents. Many new products for the demented patient have come into the market in the last few years. This chapter focuses on the use of methylphenidate and other drug treatment for attention deficit hyperactivity disorder (ADHD). The second section of the chapter discusses the use of cholinesterase inhibitors to treat Alzheimer's disease.
- **Chapter 44** on analgesics discusses the use of analgesics in pain management, emphasizing the use of opioid medications. This chapter uses morphine sulfate as the drug against which all other opioids are measured.
- **Chapter 45** discusses the management of migraines with a focus on medications used exclusively for migraines—the ergots and the triptans. The use of other medication is mentioned.
- **Chapter 46** discusses the standard nomenclature, theories, and treatment guidelines for anticonvulsant therapy of seizures.
- **Chapter 47** discusses drugs and accepted treatment protocols used in the management of Parkinson's disease.

The CNS problems represent serious pathology and perplexing symptoms. None of these medications are without substantial adverse effects. Some of these drugs have serious abuse potential and are misused to commit suicide. Vigilance is mandatory for the primary care provider when patients are taking these products. Although the patients with these various CNS problems are seen in primary care settings, often the prescription for many of these medications originates with a specialist. Periodic review of these medications by the primary care provider, in consultation with specialists, will lead to better coordinated care for the patient.

CHAPTER 42

Overview of the Nervous System

V. Inez Wendel and Maren Stewart Mayhew

The ability to understand the pharmacotherapy of the nervous system is highly dependent on the mastery by the clinician of basic concepts of anatomy and physiology of the nervous system. Information foundational to understanding central nervous system medications is presented here for easy review and retrieval.

NERVE CELL (NEURON) AND SYNAPTIC TRANSMISSION

The neurologic system is composed of the central, peripheral, and autonomic nervous systems. The *neuron* is the specialized cell of the nervous system. Neurons, or nerve cells, transmit an impulse from the body of the cell through the axon to the *synapse*. The axon may be covered with a myelin sheath, which increases conduction (Figure 42-1). A *Schwann cell* forms the myelin sheath around a single axon in the peripheral nervous system. The *node of Ranvier* is the unmyelinated portion of the axon between nodes. The myelin sheath increases conduction velocity by causing depolarization across one or more nodes. Each nerve cell is separated from the next cell by a space called the synapse.

Chemicals that transmit the signal from one neuron to the next are called *neurotransmitters*. They are synthesized in the cell body or nerve terminal of the presynaptic neuron (Figure 42-2). Neurotransmitters are released from the synapse and cross the synaptic cleft. The dendrite on the nerve cell body receives the signal. There are various receptors on the postsynaptic membrane of the dendrite that accept only certain neurotransmitters. The receptors are discussed in more detail in the section on the autonomic nervous system.

Modifying levels of neurotransmitters with medications is an important concept in the management of many neurologic diseases and conditions, including depression, dementia, Parkinson disease, and seizures. There are 30 different neurotransmitters in the brain classified as amino acids, amines, and neuropeptides. The amino acid neurotransmitters are glutamate, γ-aminobutyric acid (GABA), and glycine. Glutamate is an excitatory neurotransmitter. GABA and glycine are inhibitory neurotransmitters. GABA is the target for many anticonvulsants. The amines include the catecholamines: dopamine, norepinephrine, and epinephrine as well as serotonin, histamine, and acetylcholine. Most neuropeptide neurotransmitters are also hormones; these include vasopressin, oxytocin, insulin, somatostatin, gastrin, substance P, endorphin, and enkephalin. Other neurotransmitters are nitric oxide, carbon monoxide, adenosine triphosphate (ATP), and adenosine (see Table 42-1 for neurotransmitters and their synthesis, location, function, and receptors).

CENTRAL NERVOUS SYSTEM

The central nervous system consists of the brain and the spinal cord. It coordinates information that makes interaction with the environment possible.

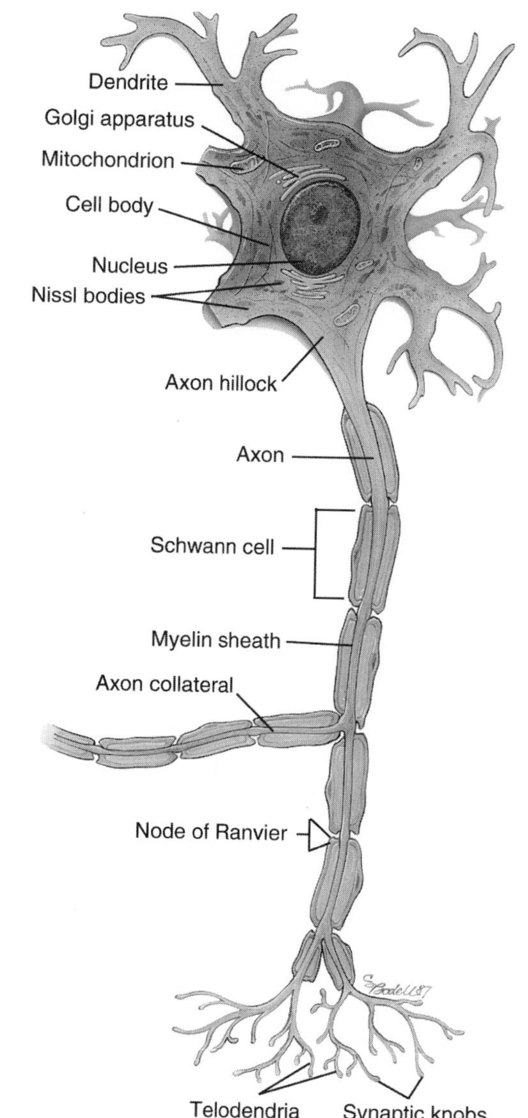

FIGURE 42-1

Structure of neuron. (From Thibodeau FA, Patton KT: *Anatomy and physiology*, ed 5, St Louis, 2003, Mosby.)

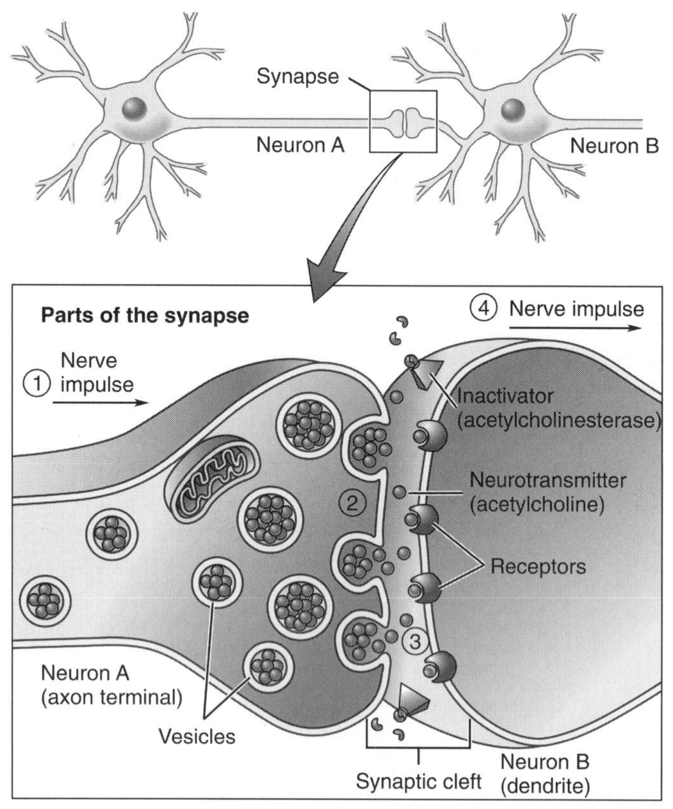

FIGURE 42-2

Structure of a synapse showing an axon terminal of a presynaptic neuron, a synaptic cleft, and a postsynaptic neuron with receptor sites. On the arrival of an action potential at a synaptic knob, neurotransmitter molecules are released from vesicles in the knob into the synaptic cleft. The combining of neurotransmitter and receptor molecules in the plasma membrane of the postsynaptic neuron initiates impulse conduction in the postsynaptic neuron. (From Lewis SM, Heitkemper MM, Dirksen SR: *Medical-surgical nursing,* ed 6, St Louis, 2004, Mosby.)

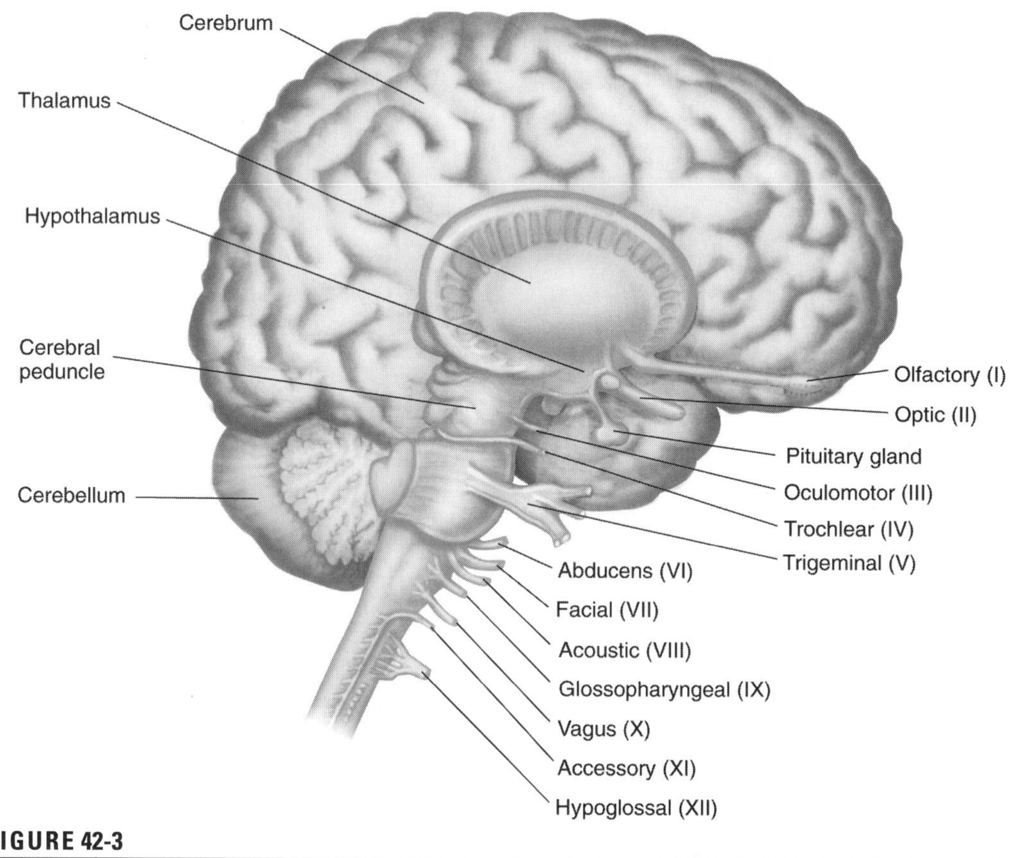

FIGURE 42-3

The brain, including major components of the cerebrum, diencephalons, and brainstem, as well as the cranial nerves. (From Rudy EB: *Advanced neurological and neurosurgical nursing,* St Louis, 1984, Mosby.)

Brain

The brain consists of the cerebrum, cerebellum, pituitary, diencephalon, and brainstem (Figure 42-3). Each part of the brain is responsible for specific functions.

The *cerebrum (cortex and corpus callosum)* is responsible for global function, which is measured by level of consciousness (LOC) and mental status (MS). LOC is the patient's ability to relate to himself or herself and to the environment. MS is mental function, intellectual abilities, memory, orientation, and judgment. The dementias are disorders of global impairment in cerebral function.

Specific areas of the brain are responsible for specific functions. The *frontal lobe* is responsible for complex problem solving, value judgments, language expression, and expression of emotions. The *parietal lobe* allows for voluntary interpretation of touch, pressure, temperature, and position sense. The *temporal lobe* is responsible for interpretation of sounds and comprehension of language. Seizures often originate here. The *occipital lobe* interprets visual images. The *motor cortex* lies anterior to the central fissure and extends laterally across the brain in an organized pattern. It is responsible for voluntary movements. The *sensory cortex* lies just posteriorly to the motor cortex and is responsible for conscious interpretation of sensation. The *basal ganglia* located in the subcortical gray matter surrounding lateral ventricles are responsible for modulation and integration of voluntary body movements. Parkinson's disease is associated with dysfunction of neurotransmitters in the basal ganglia.

The *cerebellum* is responsible for coordination of involuntary muscular activity, balance, timing, posture, and position in space. The *pituitary gland* supplies numerous hormones that govern many vital processes.

The *diencephalon* consists of the hypothalamus and thalamus. The *hypothalamus* controls the peripheral autonomic nervous system and endocrine processes and regulates body temperature, sleep, appetite, and emotions. The *thalamus* is a relay center for interpretation and integration of sensory impulses and complex reflex movements.

The *brainstem* consists of the midbrain, pons, and medulla. The brainstem is the origin of the cranial nerves. The *midbrain* is responsible for coordination of motor, sensory, and reflex functions. The *pons* coordinates movement and regulates respiratory rate. Heart rate, blood pressure, respiration, and swal-

TABLE 42-1 Neurotransmitters

Neurotransmitter	Synthesis	Inactivation	Location	Function	Receptors
Glutamate	Kreb cycle metabolite, α-ketoglutarate, and glutamine	Astrocytes	CNS	Excitatory	Ionotropic and metabotropic
GABA	Glutamic acid by glutamic acid decarboxylase	Reuptake into nerve terminals or glial cells	CNS	Inhibitory	$GABA_A$ and $GABA_B$
Glycine	Serine by serine hydroxymethyltransferase	Reuptake		Inhibitory	
Catecholamines	L-Tyrosine to	Uptake into nerve			
Dopamine	L-dihydroxyphenylalanine (DOPA) by tyrosine hydroxylase DOPA to dopamine by aromatic amino acid decarboxylase Dopamine to L-norepinephrine by dopamine	terminal with storage in synaptic vesicles or degradation by monoamine oxidase (MAO) and catechol-O-methyltransferase (COMT)	Substantia nigra	Control of movement	D_1 cause excitation D_2 cause inhibition
			Medial mesencephalic tegmentum	Control of primitive functions such as emotions and visceral function	
			Hypothalamus	Inhibits release of prolactin	
Norepinephrine (noradrenalin)	β-hydroylase L-norepinephrine to L-epinephrine by phenylethanolamine-*N*-methyltransferase	Uptake also occurs in glial cells and smooth muscle that contain MAO or COMT	Locus ceruleus	Memory, information processing, emotions, energy, psychomotor function, movement, blood pressure, heart rate, and bladder emptying	α-adrenergic receptors β-adrenergic receptors
			Ventral brainstem reticular formation	Attention	
Epinephrine (adrenaline)			Ventral pontine and medullary reticular formation	Blood pressure and heart rate, attention	

Continued

TABLE 42-1 Neurotransmitters—cont'd

Neurotransmitter	Synthesis	Inactivation	Location	Function	Receptors
Serotonin	L-tryptophan to L-5-hydroxytrytophan (5-HTP) by tryptophan hydroxylase. 5-HTP to L-5-hydroxytryptamine (5-HT or serotonin)	Degradation by glial cells with MAO and aldehyde dehydrogenase to 5-hydroxyindole-acetic acid (5-HIAA)	Pontomedullary caudal raphe nucleus Midbrain rostral raphe nuclei Gastrointestinal neurons	Stimulates release of growth hormone, adrenocorticotropic hormone (ACTH), and prolactin Regulates circadian rhythms Regulation of food intake, satiation Mood control Mostly associated with inhibitory responses	14 or more types of receptors, 5-HT_1, 5-HT_2, 5-HT_3, 5-HT_4 Also associated with various effector mechanisms, including G proteins, cAMP. cyclic guanosine monophosphate (cGMP), IP3, and gated channels
Histamine	L-histidine to histamine by histidine decarboxylase	Inactivated in glial cells by monoamine oxidase and histamine methyltransferase	Tuberal and mammillary regions of the hypothalamus	Arousal, biorhythms, pain control, temperature regulation, and food and water intake	H_1, H_2, H_3
Acetylcholine	Acetyl CoA and choline by choline acetyltransferase	Acetylcholinesterase breaks down to choline and acetic acid, reuptake of choline occurs	Neuromyal junctions Preganglionic sympathetic and parasympathetic axons Most parasympathetic and some sympathetic postganglionic axons in autonomic effect organs Basal nucleus of Meynert, hippocampus, and cerebral cortex	Voluntary movement Regulation of autonomic nervous system target organs (eye, salivary glands, heart, gastrointestinal tract, sweat glands) Memory	Nicotinic receptors in the peripheral nervous system Muscarinic in the brain and autonomic target organs
Neuropeptides (substance P, neurotensin, endorphin, enkephalin, vasopressin, oxytocin, insulin, gastrin, somatostatin, and others)	Processed in the cell body from a large precursor peptide molecule	Removed from the synaptic cleft by peptidase	Stored in vesicles in the nerve terminal	Modulate the release or action of neurotransmitters, or act as growth factors Involved in pain modulation, control of cardiovascular system, and stress responses	
Nitric oxide	Arginine and reduced nicotinamide-adenine dinucleotide phosphate (NADPH)		Hippocampus	Memory	
Adenosine triphosphate	Adenosine	Degradated by 5′ nucleotidases resulting in ADP, AMP, and adenosine	Synaptic vessels, coreleased with classic neurotransmitters	Mediates contraction of urinary bladder, vas deferens, and blood vessels and relaxation of intestines and some blood vessels Involved in nociceptive pain responses	Purinergic

lowing are regulated in the medulla. The *medulla* is where the motor tracts cross over, which accounts for contralateral control. The *reticular activating system* (RAS) controls consciousness, arousal from sleep, wakefulness, alertness or directions of attention, perceptual association, and direct introspection. It consists of neurons from brainstem and thalamus to the cerebral cortex and receives stimuli from the sensory system.

Spinal Cord

The spinal cord is a continuation of the medulla, and it connects the brain to the body (Figure 42-4). Nerves are grouped in bundles or tracts, with each tract performing specific functions (Table 42-2). The center *gray matter* contains cell bodies with projections to the periphery. The surrounding *white matter* contains myelinated axons of the ascending and descending tracts. The ascending tracts relay sensory impulses from the periphery to the brain. The descending tracts control voluntary and involuntary movement. The descending pathways are composed of the upper motor neurons, which originate and terminate within the central nervous system and modify spinal reflexes. Lower motor neurons originate in the gray matter of the anterior horn and terminate at the muscle fibers.

PERIPHERAL NERVOUS SYSTEM

The peripheral nervous system consists of cranial nerves and spinal nerves.

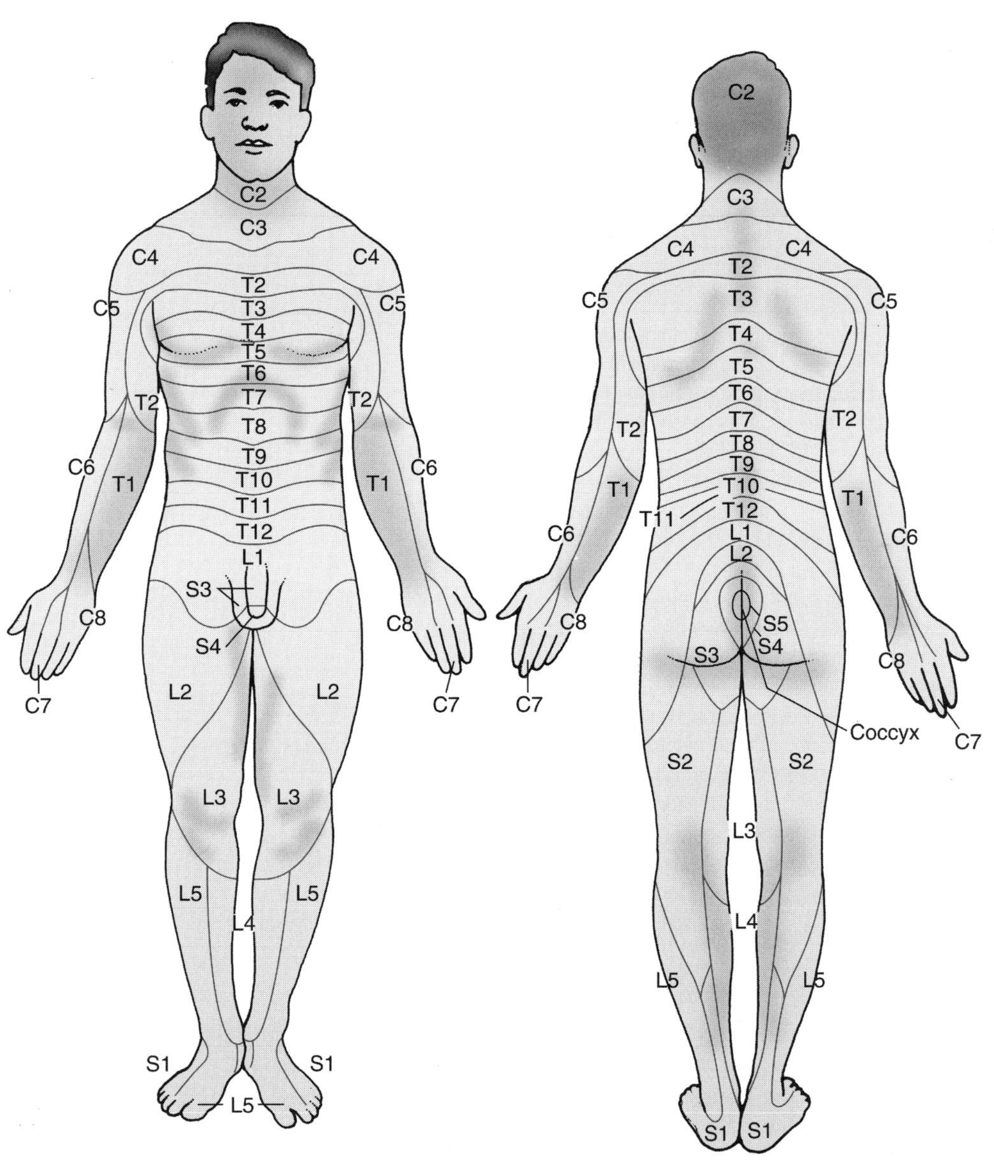

FIGURE 42-4

Spinal nerves. Location of exiting spinal nerves in relation to the vertebrae. (From Shpritz DW: Assessment of the nervous system. In Ignatavicius DD, Workman ML: *Medical-surgical nursing: critical thinking for collaborative care,* ed 4, vol 1, Philadelphia, 2002, Saunders.)

TABLE 42-2 Major Ascending Tracts of Spinal Cord

Name	Function	Location*	Origin	Termination†
Lateral spinothalamic	Pain, temperature, and crude touch opposite side	Lateral white columns	Posterior gray column opposite side	Thalamus
Anterior spinothalamic	Crude touch and pressure	Anterior white columns	Posterior gray column opposite side	Thalamus
Fasciculi gracilis and cuneatus	Discriminating touch and pressure sensations, including vibration, stereognosis, and two-point discrimination; also conscious kinesthesia	Posterior white columns	Spinal ganglia same side	Medulla
Anterior and posterior spinocerebellar	Unconscious kinesthesia	Lateral white columns	Anterior or posterior gray column	Cerebellum
Spinotectal	Touch related to visual reflexes	Lateral white columns	Posterior gray columns	Superior colliculus (midbrain)

From Thibodeau GA, Patton KT: *Anatomy and physiology*, ed 5, St Louis, 2003, Mosby.
*Location of cell bodies of neurons from which axons of tract arise.
†Structure in which axons of tract terminate.

TABLE 42-3 The Cranial Nerves and Their Functions

Cranial Nerves	Function
Olfactory (I)	Sensory: smell reception and interpretation
Optic (II)	Sensory: visual acuity and visual fields
Oculomotor (III)	Motor: raise eyelids, most extraocular movements
	Parasympathetic: pupillary constriction, change lens shape
Trochlear (IV)	Motor: downward, inward eye movement
Trigeminal (V)	Motor: jaw opening and clenching, chewing and mastication
	Sensory: sensation to cornea, iris, lacrimal glands, conjunctiva, eyelids, forehead, nose, nasal and mouth mucosa, teeth, tongue, ear, facial skin
Abducens (VI)	Motor: lateral eye movement
Facial (VII)	Motor: movement of facial expression muscles except jaw, close eyes, labial speech sounds (b, m, w, and rounded vowels)
	Sensory: taste—anterior two thirds of tongue, sensation to pharynx
	Parasympathetic: secretion of saliva and tears
Acoustic (VIII)	Sensory: hearing and equilibrium
Glossopharyngeal (IX)	Motor: voluntary muscles for swallowing and phonation
	Sensory: sensation of nasopharynx, gag reflex, taste—posterior one third of tongue
	Parasympathetic: secretion of salivary glands, carotid reflex
Vagus (X)	Motor: voluntary muscles of phonation (guttural speech sounds) and swallowing
	Sensory: sensation behind ear and part of external ear canal
	Parasympathetic: secretion of digestive enzymes; peristalsis; carotid reflex; involuntary action of heart, lungs, and digestive tract
Spinal accessory (XI)	Motor: turn head, shrug shoulders, some actions for phonation
Hypoglossal (XII)	Motor: tongue movement for speech sound articulation (l, t, n) and swallowing

Modified from Rudy EB: *Advanced neurological and neurosurgical nursing*, St Louis, 1984, Mosby.

Cranial Nerves

Cranial nerves I and II are integrated in the brain, and cranial nerves III to XII are integrated in the brainstem (see Table 42-3 for functions of the cranial nerves).

Spinal Nerves

There are 31 pairs of spinal nerves that run through intervertebral foramina: 8 cervical, 12 thoracic, 5 lumbar, 5 sacral, and 1 coccygeal. Each spinal nerve receives and supplies information to a specific region called a *dermatome* (see Figure 42-4).

AUTONOMIC NERVOUS SYSTEM

The autonomic nervous system controls involuntary (smooth) muscle and gland activity. This area is not assessed directly during the neurologic examination, although blood pressure, pulse, sweating, bladder, and rectal sphincter tone are regulated by the autonomic nervous system. Function of the heart, eye, uterus, urinary bladder, and gastrointestinal tract, from the salivary glands to the anal sphincter, is governed and maintained by the autonomic nervous system (Table 42-4).

TABLE 42-4 Actions of Autonomic Nervous System Neuroreceptors

Effector Organ or Tissue	Receptor	Adrenergic Effect	Cholinergic Effect
Eye, iris			
Radial muscle	α_1	Contraction (mydriasis)	—
Sphincter muscle		—	Contraction (miosis)
Eye, ciliary muscle	β_2	Relaxation for far vision	Contraction for near vision
Lacrimal glands	—	—	Secretion
Nasopharyngeal glands	—	—	Secretion
Salivary glands	α_1	Secretion of potassium and water	Secretion of potassium and water
	β	Secretion of amylase	—
Heart			
SA node	β_1	Increased heart rate	Decreased heart rate; vagus arrest
Atrial	β_1	Increased contractility and conduction velocity	Decreased contractility; shorten action potential duration
AV junction	β_1	Increased automaticity and propagation velocity	Decreased automaticity and propagation velocity
Purkinje system	β_1	Increased automaticity and propagation velocity	—
Ventricles	β_1	Increased contractility	—
Arterioles			
Coronary	α_1, β_2	Constriction, dilation	Dilation
Skin and mucosa	α_1, α_2	Constriction	Dilation
Skeletal muscle	α, β_2	Constriction, dilation	Dilation
Cerebral	α_1	Constriction (slight)	—
Pulmonary	α_1, β_2	Constriction, dilation	—
Mesenteric	α_1	Constriction	—
Renal	α_1, β_1, β_2, D	Constriction, dilation	—
Salivary glands	α_1, α_2	Constriction	Dilation
Veins, systemic	α_1, β_2	Constriction, dilation	—
Lung			
Bronchial muscle	β_2	Relaxation	Contraction
Bronchial glands	α_1, β_2	Decreased secretion; increased secretion	Stimulation
Stomach			
Motility	α_1, β_2	Decreased (usually)	Increased
Sphincters	α_1	Contraction (usually)	Relaxation (usually)
Secretion	—	Inhibition (?)	Stimulation
Liver	α, β_2	Glycogenolysis and gluconeogenesis	Glycogen synthesis
Gallbladder and ducts	—	Relaxation	Contraction
Pancreas			
Acini	α	Decreased secretion	Secretion
Islet cells	α_2, β_2	Decreased secretion; increased secretion	—
Intestine			
Motility and tone	α_1, β_1, β_2	Decreased	Increased
Sphincters	α_1	Contraction (usually)	Relaxation (usually)
Secretion	α_2	Inhibition (?)	Stimulation
Adrenal medulla	—	—	Secretion of epinephrine and norepinephrine (nicotinic effect)
Kidney			
Renin secretion	α_1, β_1	Decreased; increased	—
Ureter			
Motility and tone	α_1	Increased	Increased

From Sugerman RA: Structure and function of the neurologic system. In McCance KL, Heuther SE (eds): *Pathophysiology: the biologic basis for disease in adults and children,* ed 3, St Louis, 1998, Mosby.

AV, Atrioventricular; *D,* dopaminergic; *SA,* sinoatrial.

Continued

TABLE 42-4 Actions of Autonomic Nervous System Neuroreceptors—cont'd

Effector Organ or Tissue	Receptor	Adrenergic Effect	Cholinergic Effect
Urinary bladder			
Detrusor	β_2	Relaxation (usually)	Contraction
Trigone and sphincter	α_1	Contraction	Relaxation
Sex organs, male	α_1	Ejaculation	Erection
Skin			
Pilomotor	α_1	Contraction	—
Sweat glands	α_1	Localized secretion	Generalized secretion
Fat cells	α_2; β_1 (β_3)	Inhibition of lipolysis; stimulation of lipolysis	—
Pineal gland	β	Melatonin synthesis	—

The autonomic nervous system is a complex set of neurons originating in the hypothalamus and composed of two antagonistic systems, as follows.

Sympathetic

"Fight or flight" response prepares the body to spend energy. The neurotransmitter norepinephrine, also called adrenalin, is released at the postganglionic fibers. Therefore this system is also known as the *adrenergic system*. There are two types of adrenergic receptors, α and β, and these are further subdivided depending on their action.

Parasympathetic

Vegetative system prepares the body to conserve energy and uses acetylcholine as neurotransmitter. Anticholinergic medications block the action of acetylcholine and interfere with parasympathetic nervous system.

FUNCTION

Reflexes

The reflexes reflect the primitive system combining sensory and motor functions. A specific motor or efferent response occurs in response to sensory or afferent input. Reflexes regulate most bodily functions and homeostasis and occur without perception or input from the cerebrum (Figure 42-5).

Sensory System

Cell bodies of the afferent or sensory neurons are located in the dorsal or posterior horn of the gray matter of the spinal cord (Figure 42-6). The ascending spinothalamic tract is responsible for the primary sensations of crude touch, pressure, temperature, and pain. The spinocerebellar tract is responsible for discriminatory sensation—describing details about the stimulus and its location, or the position of the body in space.

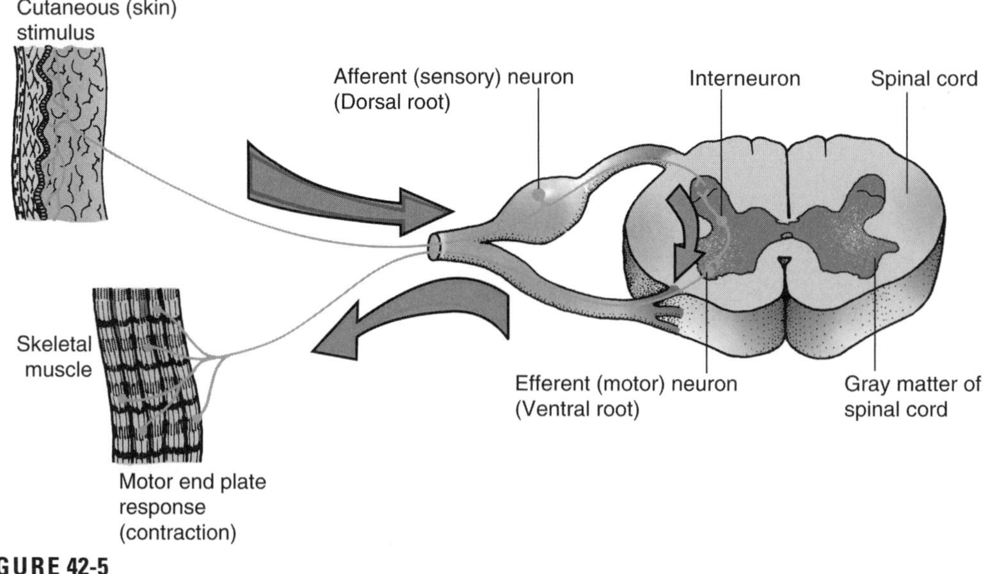

FIGURE 42-5

Cross section of spinal cord showing simple reflex arc. (From Shpritz DW: Assessment of the nervous system. In Ignatavicius DD, Workman ML: *Medical-surgical nursing: critical thinking for collaborative care,* vol 1, ed 4, Philadelphia, 2002, Saunders.)

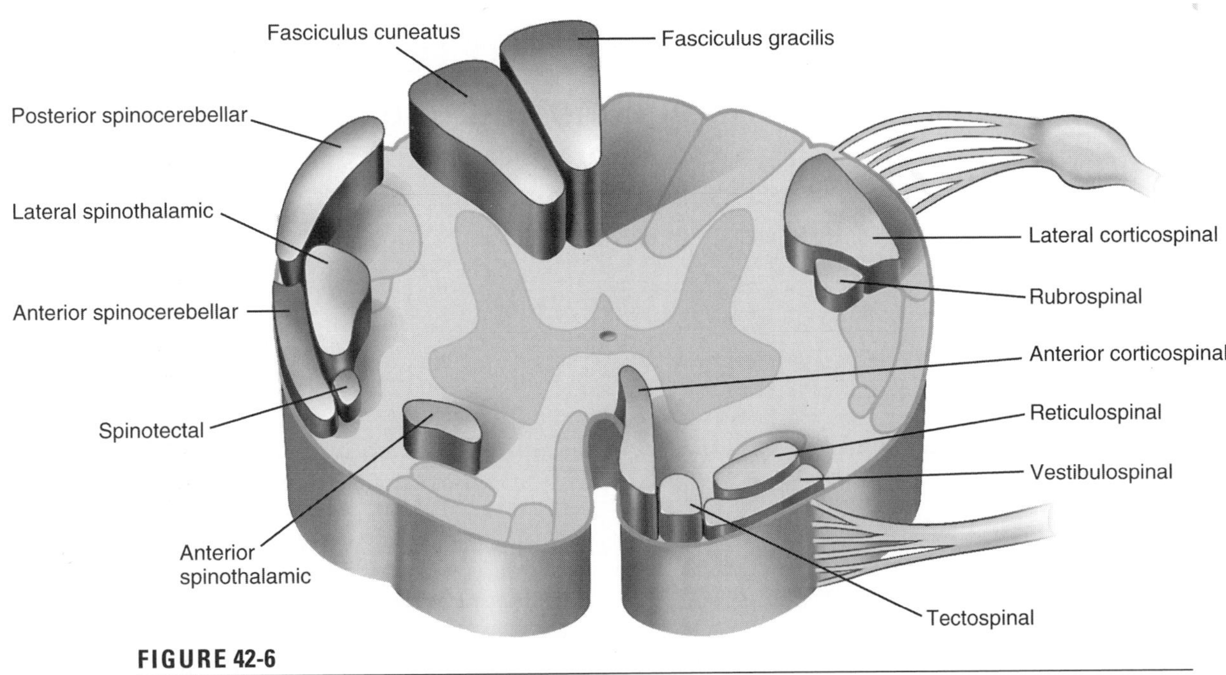

FIGURE 42-6

Spinal cord tracts. Cross section of upper thoracic cord showing tracts and their placement at various levels of the cord. (From Thibodeau FA, Patton KT: *Anatomy and physiology*, ed 5, St Louis, 2003, Mosby).

Motor System

The motor system controls skeletal muscle, somatic, and voluntary activity. The neurotransmitter used is acetylcholine. Two different pathways are involved in the motor system, as follows.

Corticospinal (also called pyramidal): upper motor neurons (central nervous system) from the motor cortex cross over in the brainstem to the spinal cord to synapse with lower motor neurons (peripheral nervous system) that run from the spinal cord to muscle. This pathway controls voluntary movements, integrates complex movements, and is a direct connection.

Extrapyramidal (affected in Parkinson's disease) is a complicated pathway with many interrelated neurons that provides background muscle control to allow voluntary movements, maintain muscle tone, control of body movements (especially gross automatic movements such as walking), and coordination of movements. There are two extrapyramidal pathways originating in the basal ganglia. The "direct" pathway facilitates movement through the D_1 dopamine receptors using GABA and substance P neurotransmitters. The "indirect pathway" inhibits movement through the D_2 dopamine receptor using GABA and enkephalin as neurotransmitters.

The *cerebellar area of the brain* coordinates muscular activity, maintains equilibrium, and controls posture.

CHAPTER 43

Central Nervous System Stimulants and Cognitive Function Drugs

V. Inez Wendel, Marilyn Winterton Edmunds, and Maren Stewart Mayhew

Drug Names

Class	Subclass		Generic Name	Trade Name
Analeptics			caffeine modafinil	Vivarin Provigil
Amphetamines	Short-acting		dextroamphetamine methamphetamine	Dexedrine Desoxyn
	Intermediate-acting	(200)	amphetamine/dextroamphetamine	Adderall
	Long-acting		amphetamine/dextroamphetamine	Adderall-XR
Amphetamine-like drugs	Short-acting	(P) (200)	methylphenidate	Ritalin
	Intermediate-acting	(P) (200)	methylphenidate	Ritalin SR; Metadate SR
	Long-acting	(P) (200)	methylphenidate SR dexmethylphenidate pemoline	Concerta Focalate Cylert
Norepinephrine reuptake inhibitor			atomoxetine	Strattera
Cognitive function	Cholinesterase inhibitors	(P)	donepezil rivastigmine galantamine	Aricept Exelon Reminyl
	NMDA receptor antagonist		memantine hydrochloride	Namenda

(200), Top 200 drug; (P), prototype drug.

Central Nervous System (CNS) Stimulants (Table 43-1)

General Uses

Labeled Uses

- Attention-deficit hyperactivity disorder (ADHD)
- Narcolepsy

Unlabeled Uses

- Depression in frail elderly, cancer, and post-stroke patients
- Improvement in pain control, sedation, or both in patients receiving opiates

• • •

This chapter discusses drugs used primarily in the treatment of ADHD and dementia of the Alzheimer's type. Both classes of medications act to alter levels of neurotransmitters in the brain and therefore modify behaviors and to improve and maintain function in patients with these two different but socially devastating conditions.

Analeptics are not discussed in detail. An *analeptic* is a drug that acts as a stimulant to the CNS. Caffeine is the only analeptic seen in primary care. It is used on an over-the-counter (OTC) basis as an aid to help people stay awake and to restore mental alertness and as an adjunct in analgesic formulations. It is a methylxanthine and is not discussed here in detail. Chapter 17 provides a discussion of the theophyllines, which are chemically related. Because modafinil has high potential for drug abuse, it is not in general use and will not be discussed in detail.

Amphetamines have very high potential for abuse. They are category II drugs and are prescribed or dispensed sparingly and used primarily for ADHD in primary care. They are not discussed in detail. Methylphenidate is similar to the amphetamines but has less abuse potential. Methylphenidate is frequently encountered. There are new formulations that make it easier to use.

TABLE 43-1 CNS Stimulant Indications and Unlabeled Uses

Class	Drug	Trade Name	Indications	Unlabeled Uses
Analeptics	caffeine	Vivarin	Fatigue, drowsiness, analgesia adjuvant	Atopic dermatitis (topical), obesity, headache (adjunct in migraine)
	modafinil	Provigil	Narcolepsy	
Amphetamine	amphetamine salt	Adderall	Narcolepsy, ADHD	
	dextroamphetamine sulfate	Dexedrine	Narcolepsy, ADHD, obesity	Cocaine dependence, autism
	methamphetamine	Desoxyn	ADHD, obesity	
Amphetamine-like drugs	dextromethylphenidate	Focalate	ADHD	
	methylphenidate	Ritalin, Concerta	ADD, ADHD, narcolepsy	Depression in medically ill, elderly; improvement in pain control, sedation, or both in patients receiving opiates
	pemoline	Cylert	ADHD	Narcolepsy, fatigue, excessive daytime sleepiness
Norepinephrine reuptake inhibitor	atomoxetine	Strattera	ADHD	

ADD, Attention-deficit disorder; *ADHD*, attention-deficit hyperactivity disorder.

DISEASE PROCESS

Pathophysiology

ADHD is a heterogeneous disorder of unknown cause. Studies on twins confirm a genetic etiology. Variation in basal ganglia symmetry and in the corpus callosum has been noted in some studies. Circuits connecting these areas help to control how the brain sustains or shifts attention in response to stimuli. Both dopamine and norepinephrine appear to be important in ADHD. Previously it was thought that ADHD primarily affected dopamine, but studies have also emphasized the importance of norepinephrine. ADHD affects the limbic system, causing changes in feelings and moods. The frontal lobe affects inhibition and impulse control and aggression. Stimulant drugs probably work by increasing "background" dopamine levels in the synapses.

Associated factors for ADHD include parental discord, low social class, low maternal education, parental criminality, and parental substance abuse. ADHD symptoms may lead to antisocial personality disorder. If patients are treated properly with medication and support, they usually do very well. There is a high comorbidity of ADHD with bipolar disorders.

The Disease

The diagnosis of ADHD in children is made by observation and history and requires documented history or inattention or hyperimpulsivity causing impairment in at least two settings (usually home and school) before the age of 7. Symptoms must have been prominent for at least 6 months. ADHD is common, affecting 3% to 8% of school-age children and 3% to 4% of adults. Childhood ADHD is a prerequisite for the diagnosis of ADHD in adults. The male/female ratio is 6:1 in children and 1:1 in adults. ADHD usually causes interference with social, academic, or occupational functioning.

There are at least three, and probably many more, subtypes of ADHD. Current diagnostic criteria recognize two major types. In one, inattention is the major problem. The child cannot focus on instructions or tasks, fails to finish schoolwork, cannot organize, and is forgetful and easily distracted. Another type of child, the hyperimpulsive, may get more attention because they fidget, cannot wait their turn, are constantly in motion, and talk and act impulsively. Some patients have both inattentiveness and hyperimpulsivity, or a "combined" type. ADHD is a dimensional, not a categorical, disorder with varying degrees of severity that blend into normal. In children hyperactivity usually predominates. Adolescents often display oppositional and restless behavior. Adults have more problems with attention. The five symptom clusters are as follows:

1. Activating/organizing for work
2. Sustaining attention and concentration
3. Sustaining energy and effort
4. Affective interface (shyness, temper)
5. Working memory impairment; decreased short-term memory or recall access, forgetting intentions, losing objects

Before diagnosing ADHD, other causes of impaired concentration and memory should be ruled out by a thorough organic work-up, including a neurologic and mental status examination. Laboratory studies should include CBC studies, comprehensive metabolic panel, thyroid function studied, serum B_{12}, serum heavy metal screen, and other tests as indicated by the history and physical examination.

DRUG ACTION AND EFFECTS

Amphetamines are sympathomimetic amines with CNS stimulant activity. Norepinephrine is released from central noradrenergic neurons. At high doses, dopamine may be released. The site of action for appetite suppression is thought to be the lateral hypothalamic feeding center. Peripheral α and β activity includes elevation of systolic and diastolic blood pressures and weak bronchodilator and respiratory stimulant actions.

Methylphenidate is a mild cortical stimulant with CNS actions similar to those of the amphetamines. The exact mechanism of action is not fully understood. It may activate the brainstem arousal system and cortex to produce its stimulant effect. In ADHD, neural transmission is slowed. The drug action is not a "paradoxical response." The drug stimulates norepinephrine and dopamine. In normal children as well as ADHD children, this causes a decrease in motor activity and an increase in attention and cognition.

Caffeine, a methylxanthine, competitively blocks adenosine receptors. It is a potent stimulant of the CNS. It also produces cardiac stimulation, dilation of coronary and peripheral blood vessels, constriction of cerebral blood vessels, skeletal muscle stimulation, augmentation of gastric acid secretion, and diuretic activity. It may produce tachycardia or premature ventricular contractions. The CNS-stimulating effects and constriction of cerebral blood vessels are effective as analgesic adjuncts. It also increases absorption of ergot alkaloids. Tolerance to these effects may develop.

The mechanism of action of modafinil is not known. It is not a direct- or indirect-acting dopamine or α_1-adrenergic receptor agonist.

The exact mechanism of atomoxetine action is not clear. It is a selective presynaptic norepinephrine reuptake inhibitor. It does not bind to monoamine receptors in the brain, which decreases the risk of adverse reactions compared with older norepinephrine reuptake inhibitors (see Chapter 48 for information on depression).

DRUG TREATMENT PRINCIPLES

Nonpharmacologic Treatment

Drug therapy is not indicated for all children with this syndrome. Stimulants are not intended for use in the child who exhibits symptoms secondary to environmental factors and/or primary psychiatric disorders, including psychosis. Appropriate educational placement is essential, and psychosocial intervention is generally needed.

Classes or counseling to teach parents techniques for changing behavior (such as point systems that allow children to earn rewards) are often considered an integral part of the treatment plan for ADHD.

Pharmacologic Treatment

When nonpharmacologic measures alone are insufficient, the decision to prescribe stimulant medication will depend on the clinician's assessment of the chronicity and severity of the child's symptoms.

Methylphenidate is usually the first-line drug of choice for ADHD. When giving medications to children, it is necessary to first obtain permission from the parents.

A medication challenge with methylphenidate should be administered in the office. The computerized continuous processing test called the Test of Variables of Attention (TOVA) can be administered. Obtain baseline measurement of the child's performance on the TOVA or an equivalent neurologic test of attention, impulsivity, response time, or variability of response time. Give the patient 5 to 10 mg methylphenidate and repeat the test after 90 minutes. A positive response is an improvement on the neurologic test. An adverse response would be increased inattention, impulsivity, agitation, aggression, emotional lability, or motor tics.

A once-a-day formulation of methylphenidate (Concerta) may be used to help children for whom multiple doses per day are difficult. The child should be well controlled with methylphenidate and then make the transition to the once-a-day formulation following the conversion guidelines.

If paradoxic aggravation of symptoms or other adverse effects occur, reduce dosage or, if necessary, discontinue the drug. The product should be periodically discontinued to assess the child's condition. Improvement may be sustained when the drug is either temporarily or permanently discontinued. In children, drug treatment should not and need not be indefinite and usually may be discontinued after puberty. However, a growing number of adults are finding that they have long-standing and untreated symptoms of ADHD that are helped by using the product.

If the patient does not respond to methylphenidate, other medications may be considered. Pemoline must be used with caution because of the risk of hepatotoxicity.

The amphetamines are more potent. Of them, the amphetamine salt is most commonly used for ADHD. Adderall contains both amphetamine and dextroamphetamine. In higher doses, the duration of action is prolonged.

Atomoxetine (originally called tomoxetine) is a new drug. Currently it is used as second-line option for patients who cannot tolerate CNS stimulants. In studies, it has been used for only 3 to 10 weeks. It is much more expensive than other treatment options, averaging about $6 a day.

The antidepressant venlafaxine has been shown to be effective. Venlafaxine blocks the reuptake of norepinephrine and serotonin, and dopamine at higher doses. The antidepressant bupropion also has been show to be effective. It affects dopamine.

Alternative therapies are antioxidants; vitamin and mineral preparations, especially copper, zinc, selenium, and B vitamins; and herbal extracts. Valerian root, kava kava, ginkgo biloba, and pycnogenol (pine bark extract) have been used. The safety and efficacy of the herbal extracts are unknown.

evolve For additional information, see the supplemental tables on the Evolve Learning Resources website.

HOW TO MONITOR

- Patients should be seen every 2 weeks during the dosage adjustment. Once patients are stable, they should be followed about once every 3 months.
- Periodic CBC, differential, and platelet counts are advised during prolonged therapy.
- Monitor blood pressure levels.

PATIENT VARIABLES

Geriatrics

Methylphenidate has an unlabeled use in the elderly population. It may increase mental alertness and stimulate appetite. Low dosages and careful monitoring are required. Monitor cardiovascular status closely. Many patients will be unable to tolerate the stimulant effect.

Pediatrics

Safety and efficacy in children under 6 years have not been established. Although a causal relationship has not been established, suppression of growth has been reported with the long-term use of stimulants in children.

Pregnancy

Adequate studies have not been conducted to determine safety; not recommended for women of childbearing age.

Specific Drugs

(P) Prototype Drug

methylphenidate (Ritalin); methylphenidate SR (extended-release tablet) (Concerta)

Contraindications

- Hypersensitivity
- Marked anxiety, tension, and agitation
- Glaucoma
- Motor tics or family history or diagnosis of Tourette syndrome

Preexisting severe GI disease such as esophageal motility disorders, small bowel inflammatory disease, and others.

Warnings

- *Drug dependence:* use with caution in emotionally unstable patients, history of drug dependence, alcoholism. Chronic abuse can cause frank psychotic episodes.
- There is some evidence that the product may lower the convulsive threshold in patients with prior history of seizures, with prior EEG abnormalities in absence of seizures, and, very rarely, in the absence of history of seizures and no prior EEG evidence of seizures. Safe use concomitant with anticonvulsants has not been established.
- Use cautiously in patients with hypertension. Blood pressure should be monitored at appropriate levels in all patients.
- Do not use methylphenidate for severe depression, prevention, and treatment of normal fatigue states or acute stress reactions.
- Visual disturbances have been encountered.

Precautions

Agitation may be exacerbated.

Pharmacokinetics

Observe children for at least 1 week before making any changes in dosage. Input should be sought from both parents and teachers whenever possible in making dosage change decisions.

Adverse Effects

Side effects may subside after the first few weeks of treatment. Nervousness and insomnia are the most common adverse effects and are usually controlled by reducing dosage and omitting the drug in the afternoon or evening. Common side effects include GI upset, nausea, abdominal cramps, anorexia, insomnia, and mild tachycardia. Less common side effects include headache, dizziness, nervousness, irritability, emotional lability, psychotic symptoms, and tics. Rare adverse effects include irregular heartbeat, palpitations, tachyarrhythmias, elevated blood pressure, hair loss, decreased white blood cell count, anemia, and rash. A rare hypersensitivity reaction consists of hives, fever, and susceptibility to bruising. Occasionally visual disturbances with difficulty accommodating and blurring have been reported. Psychologic adverse effects include dejection, lifelessness, tearfulness, oversensitivity or excitement, confusion, and withdrawal.

Chronic abusive use can lead to marked tolerance and psychic dependence with varying degrees of abnormal behavior. Frank psychotic episodes can occur.

Drug Interactions

- May decrease hypotensive effect of guanethidine. Use cautiously with pressor agents and monoamine oxidase inhibitors.
- May inhibit metabolism of coumarin anticoagulants, anticonvulsants (e.g., phenobarbital, diphenylhydantoin, primidone), and tricyclic drugs (e.g., imipramine, clomipramine, desipramine). Downward dosage adjustments of these drugs may be required when given with this product.

Dosage and Administration

Methylphenidate is usually initiated at 5 mg orally in the morning. Dosage and timing usually need to be adjusted. It has a short half-life (3 to 6 hours), so more frequent dosing (two to four per day) may be required. The sustained-release (SR) formulation may also be useful. Some children metabolize the psychostimulants more quickly than do others, and some children experience a "rebound" effect of increased impulsiveness and activity, requiring more frequent dosing. As children grow up, their need for medication changes.

Oral doses of methylphenidate do not reach peak concentrations in the brain until 60 minutes after ingestion. The fact that the medication taken orally is drawn so slowly into the brain is a likely reason why patients do not experience a high from it. In general, if brain concentrations of a substance peak quickly, the potential for abuse and addiction increases, as an individual experiences the drug more dramatically and, thus, is more likely to try to repeat the experience more frequently. This helps clarify why methylphenidate use rarely leads to abuse and addiction when taken properly as a treatment for ADHD.

Individualize dosage according to needs and responses of the patient.

Adults

Administer in divided doses two or three times daily, preferably 30 to 45 minutes before meals. The average dosage is 20 to 30 mg daily. Some patients may require 40 to 60 mg daily; in others, 10 to 15 mg is adequate. Patients who are unable to sleep if medication is taken late in the day should take the last dose before 6 PM.

SR tablets: SR tablets have a duration of action of approximately 12 hours. Tablets must be swallowed whole and never crushed or chewed.

Children 6 Years and Older
Initiate medication in small doses with gradual weekly increments. Daily dosage above 60 mg is not recommended. If improvement is not observed after appropriate dosage adjustment over a 1-month period, the drug should be discontinued.

Tablets (short acting): start with 5 mg twice daily (before breakfast and lunch) with gradual increments of 5 to 10 mg each week. Give the last dose before 6 PM to avoid insomnia. It is recommended but not necessary for the medication to be taken 30 to 45 minutes before meals.

SR tablets: for those who have never taken methylphenidate, start with 18 mg tablet every morning.

For those who are already taking methylphenidate:

- Concerta 18 mg every morning provides an initial dose of 4 mg plus and extended dose of 14 mg.
- Concerta 27 mg every morning provides an initial dose of 6 mg plus an extended dose of 21 mg.
- Concerta 35 mg every morning provides an initial dose of 8 mg plus an extended dose of 28 mg.
- Concerta 65 mg every morning provides an initial dose of 12 mg plus an extended dose of 42 mg.
- Tablets must be swallowed whole and never crushed or chewed.

Other Drugs in Class

Other drugs in this class are similar to the prototype except as follows.

pemoline

Administer as a single dose in the morning. Start with 37.5 mg/day and increase by 18.75 mg each week. The usual dose is 56.25 to 75 mg and the maximum dose is 112.5 mg. The full benefit may not be seen for 3 to 4 weeks.

atomoxetine

Pharmacokinetics. Drug is metabolized by the 2D6 enzyme system. Half-life is 19 hours in poor metabolizers (7% of population) and 4 hours in most patients. An active metabolite in excreted in the urine.

Adverse Effects. Atomoxetine causes more vomiting and somnolence than methylphenidate. Adverse effects with a frequency over 10% are headache, rhinitis, abdominal pain, pharyngitis, vomiting, increased cough, fever, accidental injury, flu syndrome, decreased appetite, nausea, nervousness, insomnia, pain, infection, allergic reactions, rash, and diarrhea. In adults, sexual dysfunction may be a problem. There is no evidence of QT prolongation. There were increases in blood pressure and heart rate.

Dosage and Administration. For children, start with 0.5 mg/kg/day. Titrate at 3 or more day intervals to 1.2 mg/kg/day. The maximum dosage is 1.4 mg/kg/day or 100 mg/day, whichever is less. It may be administered once a day without regard to meals.

Cognitive Function Drugs

General Uses

Medication treatment for Alzheimer's disease (AD) is an intensely researched area, limited by our understanding of the cause and pathology. Drug treatment is sought to increase cerebral metabolism and blood flow, prevent or reverse degeneration of neurons, and facilitate function in the remaining neurons that support memory and cognition. No drugs have been found that prevent or reverse degeneration of neurons.

Cholinesterase Inhibitors

Indications

- Management of mild to moderate Alzheimer's-type dementia

Unlabeled Uses

- Moderate to severe dementia of Alzheimer's type, vascular dementia, dementia with Lewy bodies (DLB), or mixed dementia to modify behaviors

NMDA Receptor Antagonists

- Moderate to severe dementia of Alzheimer's type

The three cholinesterase inhibitors are the medications currently available specifically for the treatment of mild to moderate dementia of the Alzheimer's type. The drugs do not cure the disease; they may slow the progression of the disease and at best may modestly improve function. These medications may be initiated by primary care practitioners in patients meeting the criteria for mild to moderate Alzheimer's-type dementia or may be initiated after consultation with a provider specializing in geriatrics or a neuropsychiatrist.

A new drug, memantine hydrochloride, is available for moderate to severe dementia. It is the first NMDA receptor antagonist, a new class of medications using a different mechanism of action.

DISEASE PROCESS

Anatomy and Physiology

Neuritic plaques composed of amyloid, neurofibrillary tangles, and neuronal loss occur to the greatest degree in the neocortex and hippocampus of patients with AD. There is a loss of cholinergic neurons. These regions are involved with memory and cognitive function.

Pathophysiology

There is a loss of neurons in the nucleus basalis of Meynert, the origin of the cholinergic neurons. There is a decrease in cholinergic activity due to loss of neurons as well as a decrease in choline acetyltransferase activity, the enzyme for synthesis of acetylcholine.

The Disease

Dementia is a syndrome of impaired cognition involving memory, language, and reasoning. AD is the most common cause of dementia. Multiinfarct dementia is the second most common cause of dementia (there are more than 50 causes of dementia). The incidence of AD varies from 5% of those over 65 years of age to 30% to 50% of those over 85. Diagnosis of AD is based on exclusionary and inclusionary data. The criteria for dementia are listed in the *DSM-IV*. Work-up includes CBC, chemistries, B_{12}, folate, thyroid profile, VDRL test, and computed tomography scans or magnetic resonance images to rule out correctable causes for impaired cognition.

DRUG ACTION AND EFFECTS

Mechanism of Action

The cholinesterase inhibitors act by reversible inhibition of acetylcholinesterase in the brain. They reduce acetylcholine reuptake, and thereby increase the availability of acetylcholine at the synapses in the brain. The effect is to diminish signs and symptoms of dementia and therefore may improve function and slow the progression of the disease, and possibly delay need for nursing home placement. The effectiveness of the drugs wears off as the disease progresses, and more neurons are destroyed. There is no evidence that they alter the disease process or cure the disease. While the drugs seem to diminish symptoms, when the medications are stopped, symptoms return and the patient may soon be as symptomatic as if they had never taken the drug.

Memantine is an *N*-methyl-D-aspartate (NMDA) receptor antagonist. It targets natural neurotransmitters—the excitatory amino acids such as glutamate—to correct a glutamate imbalance. β-Amyloid disrupts the transmission of glutamate. Elevated glutamate levels are associated with nerve cell death. Memantine blocks the excitotoxic effects associated with the abnormal transmission of glutamate. It improves overall function of the patient but there is no evidence it prevents or slows down neurodegeneration.

DRUG TREATMENT PRINCIPLES

Presence of depression and/or delirium should be identified and treated. Avoid medications with sedating or anticholinergic side effects. Avoid polypharmacy; use the least amount and smallest dose of medication, including OTC medications. Treat any metabolic disorders, infections, and comorbid illness. Advise patients with dementia to avoid alcoholic beverages. Educate caregivers regarding behavioral and environmental management, recommend caregiver support groups, and use community resources, including respite care. Some controversial studies suggest that patients with ASA or long-term nonsteroidal antiinflammatory use may have some reduction in the incidence of AD. Some evidence suggested that vitamin E slows the progression of Alzheimer's-type dementia by protecting cell membranes from the oxidative damage of free radicals. Although patients may believe ginkgo biloba or vitamin E may slow the progression of AD, the research does not support this. Other studies are examining whether diet might have a protective or harmful role in the etiology of Alzheimer's disease.

Candidates for these medications are patients diagnosed with Alzheimer's-type dementia with mild to moderate cognitive impairment. Evidence from various trials suggests the cholinesterase inhibitors stabilize cognitive and functional ability for about 1 year. Approximately one third of those treated will have a modest improvement in cognitive testing scores, function, and behavior; one third will have no change; and one third will not be able to tolerate the medication secondary to adverse effects.

Tacrine was the first drug of this class approved for treatment of dementia. However, it required dosing four times a day, had adverse hepatic effects, and required frequent monitoring of liver function. Tacrine is not widely prescribed now since the introduction of newer cholinesterase inhibitors. The newer drugs offers two main advantages over tacrine. They do not have adverse hepatic effects, do not require as frequent liver function monitoring as tacrine required, and can be given once or twice a day. All of these medications are metabolized by the cytochrome P450 hepatic enzyme system and have the potential for drug interactions. Interactions can occur with anticholinergic medications and cholinomimetics. These drugs must be used with caution if at all in patients with concomitant myasthenia gravis.

HOW TO MONITOR

A variety of cognitive assessment tools are available. The most commonly used standardized assessment tool is the Folstein Mini-Mental Exam. The Katz assessment of activities of daily living and instrumental activities of daily living (IADLs) is useful to monitor improvement or decline in function. Clinical evaluation and family observation of behaviors and function are also helpful.

Because these medications are metabolized in the liver, periodic monitoring of hepatic function may be justified, particularly in those receiving multiple medications or if symptoms suggesting hepatic dysfunction occur, including weight loss, anorexia or nausea, vomiting, and abdominal pain.

PATIENT VARIABLES

Pediatrics

Efficacy not established in any dementing conditions occurring in children.

Geriatrics

Age does not influence the metabolism or clearance of the cholinesterase inhibitors; galantamine should be used with caution in those with severe renal impairment.

Pregnancy and Lactation

- *Category C:* donepezil
- *Category B:* rivastigmine, galantamine, memantine
- There are no controlled studies of these drugs in pregnancy

- It is unknown whether these drugs are excreted in breast milk

Race/Gender

Plasma concentrations are found to be 50% higher in women.

PATIENT EDUCATION

- Do not change dose without consulting health care provider.
- Advise of initial and long-term/delayed side effects.
- Advise of purpose, expectations from treatment, and time frame to note improvement, not cure.
- Counsel regarding behavioral and environmental management of the disease.
- Advise regarding long-term care including in home services, adult day care, assisted living facilities, and nursing homes.

There are many excellent sources of education and support for patients and families. See Resources at end of the chapter.

Specific Drugs

Ⓟ **Prototype Drug**

donepezil (Aricept)

Contraindications

Known sensitivity or if the drug has previously caused an increase in bilirubin or caused jaundice.

Warnings/Precautions

- These drugs are cholinesterase inhibitors and may exaggerate succinylcholine-type muscle relaxation in anesthesia. Synergistic affects will also occur with cholinomimetics and other cholinesterase inhibitors such as bethanechol.
- Vagotonic effects on the heart rate may be provoked, causing bradycardia. Use with caution in patients with conduction abnormalities.
- Because of their cholinergic activity, these drugs may increase gastric acid secretion. Use with caution in patients at increased risk for developing ulcers, those with a history of ulcer disease or receiving nonsteroidal antiinflammatory drugs. Nausea, vomiting, and diarrhea can result.
- Genitourinary effects: may cause bladder outflow obstruction.
- Use caution in patients with a history of asthma.
- These drugs may have some potential to cause generalized convulsions. However, seizure activity may also be a symptom of AD.

Pharmacokinetics

Donepezil is completely absorbed and reaches peak levels in 3 to 4 hours with linear pharmacokinetics. Neither food nor time of administration influences the rate or extent of absorption. Half-life is about 70 hours, and steady state is reached within 15 days. Ninety-six percent of the drug is protein bound. Seventeen percent is excreted in urine intact. The drug is extensively metabolized in the liver by the P450 2D6 and 3A4 enzyme systems.

Adverse Effects

Donepezil is associated with nausea, vomiting, diarrhea, insomnia, fatigue, muscle cramps, and anorexia.

Drug Interactions

Donepezil interacts with other drugs highly bound to plasma proteins. It may also interact with other drugs metabolized by P450 3A4 or 2D6 enzyme systems.
No effect on the pharmacokinetics of theophylline, cimetidine, warfarin, and digoxin has been found.
It may decrease the effect of anticholinergic medications.

Overdosage

Cholinergic crisis may occur. Symptoms include severe nausea, vomiting, bradycardia, sweating, convulsions, collapse, and death if respiratory muscles are involved. Atropine is used as an antidote.

Dosage and Administration

The newer cholinesterase inhibitors, rivastigmine and galantamine, have a similar mechanism of action and adverse reaction profile. See Table 43-2 for specific dosing. Individual patients, however, may respond better or better tolerate a different agent. At this time these medications are not approved for combination therapy.

NMDA RECEPTOR ANTAGONISTS

memantine (Namenda)

Contraindications

- Hypersensitivity

Precautions

- Seizures occurred in a small number of patients. Consider dosage reduction in renal impairment.

Pharmacokinetics

- Well absorbed. Half-life 60-80 hr. Excreted unchanged in urine. CYP system plays no significant role.

Adverse Effects

- Hypertension, dizziness, headache, constipation, vomiting, back pain, confusion, somnolence, hallucination, cough

Drug Interactions

- Use caution with amatadine, ketamine, dextromethorphan

Dosage Administration. May take concurrently with cholinesterase inhibitors for better results. See Table 43-2.

TABLE 43-2 Dosage and Administration of Cognitive Function Drugs

Drug	Dosage	Administration
donepezil	5-10 mg qd	Administer at bedtime Increase to 10 mg after 4-8 wk at 5 mg; 10-mg dose may have improved effect at expense of increased cholinergic side effects
rivastigmine	1.5-6 mg bid	Administer with morning and evening meals Increase dosage by 1.5 mg bid q2wk If GI side effects occur, hold dose for several days and restart at lower dosage
galantamine	4-12 mg bid	Administer with morning and evening meals Increase dosage by 4 mg bid q4wk If treatment is interrupted, restart at lowest dosage and titrate up
memantine	10 mg bid	Start with 5 mg at 8 AM Increase in 5-mg increments to 5 mg bid, 5 in AM, 10 in PM; then 10 mg bid with 1-week interval between dosage increases Take with or without food

RESOURCES FOR PATIENTS AND PROVIDERS

Attention deficit hyperactivity disorder

American Academy of Child and Adolescent Psychiatry, www.aacap.org.
Professionals should type in "hyperactivity" for selection of articles and studies on ADD/ADHD.

American Academy of Family Physicians, www.aafp.org.
Website has patient information handouts, such as Does Your Hyperactive Child Have ADHD? *and* How to Take Medicine for ADHD? *Just type in the keyword "ADHD."*

American Psychiatric Association, www.psych.org/public info/child.html.
This site is good for parents. Provides definitions, list of resources for parents and health care providers.

Attention Deficit Disorder, www.ADD.idsite.com.
Practical information for parents and teachers of ADHD children. Lists 23 strategies to enhance self-esteem in ADHD children. Offers other ADHD links.

Weiss M, Bailey R: *Advances in the treatment of adult ADHD: landmark findings in nonstimulant therapy,* www.medscape.com/viewprogram/2530_pnt. (8/2003).

Alzheimer's disease

Alzheimer's Association, www.alz.org.
Latest research, extensive information.

BIBLIOGRAPHY

Attention deficit hyperactivity disorder

Biederman J, Spencer T: Methylphenidate in treatment of adults with attention-deficit/hyperactivity disorder, *J Atten Disord* 6(suppl 1):S101-S107, 2002.

Biederman J et al: Growth deficits and attention-deficit/hyperactivity disorder revisited: impact of gender, development, and treatment, *Pediatrics* 111(5 pt 1):1010-1016, 2003.

Donnelly CL: Pharmacologic treatment approaches for children and adolescents with posttraumatic stress disorder, *Child Adolesc Psychiatr Clin North Am* 12:251-269, 2003.

Gottesman MM: Helping parents make sense of ADHD diagnosis and treatment, *J Pediatr Health Care* 17:149-153, 2003.

Hale JB et al: Evaluating medication response in ADHD: cognitive, behavioral, and single-subject methodology, *J Learn Disabil* 31:595, 1998.

Kratochvil DM et al: Atomoxetine and methylphenidate treatment in children with ADHD: a prospective, randomized, open label trail, *J Am Acad Child Adolescent Psychiatry* 41:776-784, 2002.

Schnoll R et al: Nutrition in the treatment of attention-deficit hyperactivity disorders: a neglected by important aspect, *Appl Psychophysiol Biofeedback* 28:63-75, 2003.

Spencer T, Biederman J: Non-stimulant treatment for attention-deficit/hyperactivity disorder, *J Atten Disord* 6(suppl 1):S109-S119, 2002.

Strattera approved to treat ADHD, *FDA Consum* 37:4, 2003.

Swanson JM et al: Attention deficit hyperactivity disorder and hyperkinetic disorder, *Lancet* 351:429-433, 1998.

Zimmerman ML: Attention-deficit hyperactivity disorders, *Nurs Clin North Am* 38:55-66, 2003.

Cognitive function drugs

Bentue-Ferrer D et al: Clinically significant drug interactions with cholinesterase inhibitors: a guide for neurologists, *CNS Drugs* 17(13): 947-963, 2003.

Cummings JL et al: Reduction of behavioral disturbance and caregiver distress by galantamine in patients with Alzheimer's disease, *Am J Psych* 161(3):532-538, 2004.

DeLaGarza VW: Pharmacologic treatment of Alzheimer's disease: an update, *Am Fam Physician* 68(7):1365-1372, 2003.

Ibah B, Haen E: Acetylcholinesterase inhibition in Alzheimer's disease, *Curr Pharm Des* 10(3):231-251, 2004.

Jonsson L: Pharmacoeconomics of cholinesterase inhibitors in the treatment of Alzheimer's disease, *Pharmacoeconomics* 21(14):1025-2037, 2003.

Liston DR et al: Pharmacology of selective acetylcholinesterase inhibitors: implications for use in Alzheimer's disease, *Eur J Pharmacol* 486(1):9-17, 2004.

Lojkowska W et al: The effect of cholinesterase inhibitors on the regional blood flow in patients with Alzheimer's disease and vascular dementia, *J Neurol Sci* 216(1):119-126, 2003.

Nordberg A, Svensson AL: Cholinesterase inhibitors in the treatment of Alzheimer's disease: a comparison of tolerability and pharmacology, *Drug Safety* 19(6):465-480, 1998.

Ogura H et al: Comparison of inhibitory activities of donepezil and other cholinesterase inhibitors on acetylcholinesterase and butyrylcholinesterase in vitro, *Methods Find Exp Clin Pharmacol* 22(8):609-613, 2000.

Pakrasi S: Clinical predictors of response to acetyl cholinesterase inhibitors: experience from routine clinical use in Newcastle, *Int J Geriatr Psychiatry* 18(10):879-886, 2003.

Palmer AM: Cholinergic therapies for Alzheimer's disease: progress and prospects, *Curr Opin Investig Drugs* 4(7):820-825, 2003.

Quinn J et al: Antioxidants in Alzheimer's disease-vitamin C delivery to a demanding brain, *J Alzheimers Dis* 5(4):309-313, 2003.

Wu G et al: The cost-benefit of cholinesterase inhibitors in mild to moderate dementia: a willingness-to-pay approach, *CNS Drugs* 17(14):1045-1057, 2003.

CHAPTER 44

Analgesics

V. Inez Wendel

Drug Names

Class	Subclass	Generic Name	Trade Name
Opioid agonists	Phenanthrenes	(P) morphine sulfate (extended release)	MS Contin, Avinza
		morphine, morphine sulfate IR, short acting	(short acting)
		(200) codeine with acetaminophen	Tylenol #3
		(200) codeine with promethazine	
		(200) hydrocodone with acetaminophen	Lortab, Vicodin
		(200) hydrocodone with ibuprofen	Vicoprofen
		(200) oxycodone	Oxycontin
		(200) oxycodone with aspirin	Percodan
		(200) oxycodone with acetaminophen	Endocet, Percocet, Roxicet, Tylox
		hydromorphone	Dilaudid
	Phenylpiperidenes	meperidine	Demerol
		fentanyl	Sublimaze, Duragesic transdermal
	Diphenylheptanes	methadone	Dolophine
		propoxyphene	Darvon
Mixed agonist-antagonists		pentazocine	Talwin
		(200) tramadol	Ultram

(200), Top 200 drug; (P), prototype.

General Uses

Indications

- Symptomatic treatment of moderate-to-severe acute pain
- Relief of pain from acute coronary, pulmonary, hepatic, renal, or peripheral vascular origin
- Treatment of chronic, severe intractable pain of terminal illness
- Preoperative medication
- Postsurgical pain
- Severe diarrhea and cramping
- Dyspnea related to left ventricular failure or pulmonary edema
- Methadone only: detoxification of opioid addiction
- Codeine only: persistent cough

This chapter discusses pain management in the outpatient setting, including the use of drugs other than opioids, but it focuses on the use of opioids in pain management; only the drugs listed above are discussed in detail.

Endogenous opioids include three families: the enkephalins, the endorphins, and the dynorphins. Each family contains structurally similar peptides and has a characteristic anatomic distribution.

Natural opioids come from opium, which is obtained from unripe seed capsules of the poppy plant. Opium contains more than 20 distinct alkaloids. The main phenanthrenes are morphine, codeine, and thebaine. The benzylisoquinolines are papaverine (a smooth muscle relaxant) and noscapine. Heroin is diacetylmorphine, which breaks down into morphine.

Synthetic opioids have been developed. Many were developed in attempts to produce less addictive drugs but without success. They are, however, useful for pain management and as an opioid antagonist. There are many semisynthetic derivatives made by simple modifications of morphine or thebaine. Morphine is the precursor of the synthetic opioid analgesics, hydrocodone, hydromorphone, and oxycodone. Thebaine is the precursor of naloxone. The phenylpiperidines and diphenylheptanes are chemical classes that are structurally distinct but similar to morphine. These drugs have actions similar to morphine.

The opioids are classified as narcotics and thus are controlled substances according to abusive potential as mandated by the Controlled Substances Act of 1970. Clinicians should be familiar with regulations concerning the use and dispensing of narcotic analgesics. Methadone for the treatment of opiate detoxification and maintenance may be dispensed only by pharmacies and maintenance programs approved by the Food and Drug Administration and state authorities according to the requirements of the Federal Methadone Regulations. Methadone used for pain management may be prescribed by any provider with a DEA license to prescribe Schedule II drugs and is dispensed by any licensed pharmacy (see Chapter 11). Because of the potential for abuse, the health care provider must justify the use of opioid analgesics on an ambulatory basis.

Morphine is the standard opioid to which all others are compared. It is used extensively in acute care and in hospice settings. Codeine, hydrocodone, and oxycodone are frequently used in combination with acetaminophen in the primary care setting. Hydromorphone is very potent and is reserved for severe pain not relieved by morphine; primary care providers will generally not prescribe this drug. Opioid agonist-antagonists are also used. Agonist-antagonists may be preferred over agonist opioids for use in ambulatory patients because their potential for abuse is less. Tramadol is an agonist-antagonist in common use in primary care. However, pentazocine has limited use due to CNS toxicity.

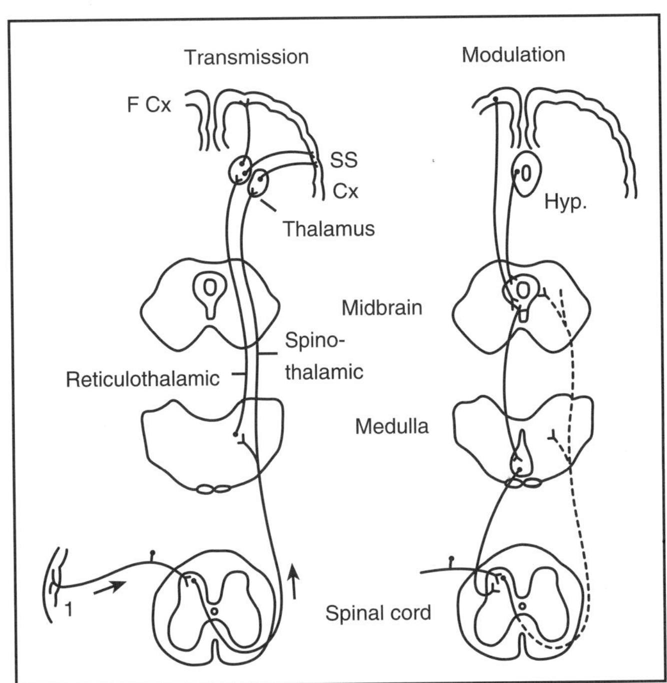

FIGURE 44-1

Pain transmission and modulation. (From Fields HL: *Pain*, New York, 1987, McGraw-Hill.)

DISEASE PROCESS

Anatomy and Physiology

Melzack and Wall's gate control theory of pain is the most comprehensive theory of pain proposed to date. They suggest that four processes are required for pain to occur: transduction, transmission, modulation, and perception. Sensory receptors, or nociceptors, that are sensitive to painful or tissue-damaging (noxious) stimuli are present in the skin, bone, muscle, connective tissue, and thoracic, abdominal, and pelvic viscera.

Transduction occurs when a noxious stimulus depolarizes peripheral nerve endings and sets off electrical activity. The nerve endings that transduce the noxious stimuli conduct electrical signals to the spinal cord using two types of nerve fibers: A delta fibers and C fibers. A delta fibers are myelinated, and their activation is associated with sharp, stinging sensations. C fibers are unmyelinated, and their activation is associated with vaguely localized pain that is dull or burning.

Next, transmission occurs whereby electrical impulses are carried throughout the peripheral and central nervous systems. Modulation is the central neural activity that controls the transmission of pain impulses. Finally, during perception, the neural activities involved in the transmission and modulation result in a subjective correlate of pain that includes behavioral, psychologic, and emotional factors (Figure 44-1).

The Disease

Pain is defined by the International Association for the Study of Pain (IASP) as "an unpleasant sensory and emotional experience associated with actual or potential tissue damage, or described in terms of such damage. Pain is always subjective."

All opioid drugs cause tolerance and dependence. This is not the same as abuse. *Tolerance* is a pharmacologic phenomenon that occurs in which there is decreasing drug effect over time. More drug is needed to have the same effect. *Dependence* is the physiologic development of abstinence syndrome or withdrawal symptoms when the drug is discontinued or antagonist is given. Slowly tapering the drug can eliminate withdrawal symptoms. Psychologic dependence, or *addiction*, is the overwhelming obsession with obtaining and using a drug for a nonmedically approved purpose. Tolerance and dependence are the consequence of regular use of an opioid for a certain length of time and are not a problem. Addiction is a problem; however, a patient in pain should not be deprived of adequate pain relief because of fear of addiction.

Acute pain is usually related to an identifiable injury such as recent surgery, trauma, or infection and resolves within a predictable and expected time interval. Chronic pain is any pain continuing beyond the usual course of an acute injury process. Persons with cancer-related pain account for the majority of people with chronic pain. In the person with cancer-related chronic pain, about 60% to 70% of pain is related to the tumor, 15% to 20% is related to diagnostic procedures or treatment of cancer, and finally 10% to 15% is completely unrelated to cancer or its treatment.

Pain can be classified as nociceptive or neuropathic (Table 44-1). Nociceptive pain is further divided into two categories: somatic and visceral. Nociceptive pain arises from the direct stimulation of afferent nerves in cutaneous or deep musculoskeletal tissues. It occurs in response to tissue injury or disease infiltration of the skin, soft tissue, or viscera. Somatic pain is well localized and often described as dull or aching. Visceral pain is poorly localized and often described as a continual aching or a deep, crampy, squeezing pain. Visceral pain may be referred to dermatomal sites that are distant from the source of pain. Visceral pain occurs in response to the

TABLE 44-1 Classification of Pain

Category	Characteristics	Example
NOCICEPTIVE		
Somatic	Well localized Dull, aching, or throbbing	Laceration, fracture, cellulitis, arthritis
Visceral	Poorly localized Continual aching Referred to dermatomal sites that are distant from the source of the pain	Subscapular pain arising from diaphragmatic irritation Right upper quadrant pain arising from stretching of liver capsule
NEUROPATHIC	Shooting or stabbing pain superimposed over a background of aching and burning	Post-herpetic neuralgia, post-thoracotomy neuralgia, post-stroke pain, trigeminal neuralgia, diabetic polyneuropathy

BOX 44-1

INITIAL PAIN ASSESSMENT

ASSESSMENT OF PAIN INTENSITY AND CHARACTER

- **Onset and temporal pattern** When did your pain start? How often does it occur? Has its intensity changed?
- **Location** Where is your pain? Is there more than one site?
- **Description** What does your pain feel like? What words would you use to describe your pain?
- **Intensity** On a scale of 0 to 10, with 0 being no pain and 10 being the worst pain you can imagine, how much does it hurt right now? How much does it hurt at its worst? How much does it hurt at its best?
- **Aggravating and relieving factors** What makes your pain worse? What makes your pain better?
- **Previous treatment** What types of treatments have you tried to relieve your pain? Were they and are they effective?
- **Effect** How does the pain affect physical and social function?

PSYCHOSOCIAL ASSESSMENT

The following should be included.

- Effect and understanding of the cancer diagnosis and cancer treatment on the patient and the caregiver
- Meaning of the pain to the patient and the family
- Significant past instances of pain and their effect on the patient
- Patient's typical coping responses to stress or pain
- Patient's knowledge of, curiosity about, preferences for, and expectations about pain management methods
- Patient's concerns about using controlled substances such as opioids, anxiolytics, or stimulants
- The economic effect of the pain and its treatment.
- Changes in mood that have occurred as a result of the pain (e.g., depression, anxiety)

PHYSICAL AND NEUROLOGIC EXAMINATION

- Examination of site of pain and evaluation of common referral patterns
- Pertinent neurologic evaluation
- Head and neck pain: cranial nerves and funduscopic evaluation
- Back and neck pain: motor and sensory function evaluation in limbs; rectal and urinary sphincter function

DIAGNOSTIC EVALUATION

- Evaluation of recurrence or progression of disease or tissue injury related to cancer treatment
- Tumor markers and other blood tests
- Radiologic studies
- Neurophysiologic (e.g., electromyography) testing
- Appropriate radiologic studies and correlation of normal and abnormal findings with physical and neurologic examinations
- Recognition of limitations of diagnostic studies
- Bone scan: false-negative results in myeloma, lymphoma, previous radiotherapy sites
- Computed tomography scan: good definition of bone and soft tissue but difficult to image entire spine
- Magnetic resonance imaging: bone definition not as good as computed tomography; better images of spine and brain

Modified from Jacox A et al: *Management of cancer pain,* Clinical Practice Guideline No. 9, AHCPR Publication No. 94-0592, Rockville, MD, 1994, Agency for Health Care Policy and Research, Public Health Service, US Department of Health and Human Services.

stretching, distention, compression, or infiltration of organs such as the liver.

Neuropathic pain results from injury to peripheral nerves or the CNS. Neuropathic pain is described as episodes of shooting or stabbing pain superimposed over a background of aching and burning. It is often associated with paresthesias and dysesthesias.

Assessment

It is important to determine the cause of the pain to eliminate it whenever possible. Do not simply treat pain without understanding the source of the particular pain. Even in a patient with terminal cancer, evaluate each new pain for proximate cause that may be specifically treated. For example, bone pain can be ameliorated by radiation.

Initial assessment of pain is done to characterize the pathophysiology of the pain, identify cause, determine the intensity, and its impact on the patient' s ability to function. Assessment should include a detailed history and physical examination, psychosocial and functional assessment, and diagnostic evaluation as indicated (Box 44-1). Associated findings of acute pain can include facial grimacing, tachycar-

TABLE 44-2 Action of Opioids on Pain Receptor Sites

Receptor	Primary Location	Function	Associated With	Opioids Involved
Mu	Supraspinal > spinal	Mediate somatic primarily, and visceral analgesia	Respiratory depression, euphoria, dependence, decreased GI motility, and miosis	morphine-like, endorphin
Kappa	Spinal > supraspinal	Mediate visceral pain	Sedation, miosis, dysphoria	pentazocine, morphine (slight), dynophin
Delta	Spinal > supraspinal	Antagonist activity	Tachycardia, tachypnea, dysphoria, hallucinations, mydriasis, hypertonia	Antagonists, enkephalins

dia, hypertension, pallor, diaphoresis, mydriasis, and nausea. Chronic pain may be accompanied by fatigue, depression, sleep disturbances, decreased appetite, increased irritability, and decreased libido. Visible facial expressions of pain are usually lacking, and there is an absence of physiologic signs because of adaptation. Patients can also have intermittent chronic pain such as recurrent episodes of neuralgia, headaches, or angina.

Because pain is a subjective experience, assessment must also include patient self-report, which includes a description of pain, onset, duration and diurnal variation, location and radiation of pain, intensity or severity, aggravating and relieving factors, and the patient' s goal for pain control.

Follow-up assessment of the outcome of pain management is required to assess the effectiveness of the intervention. Changes in pain pattern or the development of new pain should trigger reassessment and diagnostic evaluation, and modification of the treatment plan. Documentation of patient's compliance with regard to dosing and duration of prescriptions is essential in all pain management.

The Agency for Health Care Policy and Research (AHCPR) clinical practice guidelines include the following principles of pain assessment (A-A-B-C-D-E-E):

Ask about pain regularly.
Assess pain systematically. (Use pain intensity scales.)
Believe the patient and family in their reports of pain and what relieves it.
Choose pain-control options appropriate for the patient, family, and setting.
Deliver interventions in a timely, logical, and coordinated fashion.
Empower patients and their families.
Enable them to control their course to the greatest extent possible.

DRUG ACTION AND EFFECTS

Opioid Agonists

Opioid analgesics are thought to inhibit painful stimuli in the substantia gelatinosa of the spinal cord, brainstem, reticular activating system, thalamus, and the limbic system. Opiate receptors in each of these areas interact with neurotransmitters of the autonomic nervous system, producing alterations in reaction to painful stimuli. The opioid action of the drug is manifested by analgesia, sedation, euphoria, mental clouding, respiratory depression, miosis, decreased peristaltic motility, depression of the cough reflex, and orthostatic hypotension.

Opiate receptors in the CNS mediate analgesic activity. Opioid agonists occupy the same receptors as endogenous opioid peptides, and both alter the central release of neurotransmitters from afferent nerves sensitive to noxious stimuli.

Actions of opioid analgesics can be defined by their activity at three specific receptor types: mu, kappa, and delta. The mu receptors mediate morphine like supraspinal analgesia. The kappa receptors mediate spinal analgesia. The delta receptors mediate antagonist activity (Table 44-2). Morphine-like agonists have activity at the mu, kappa, and delta receptors. Mixed agonist-antagonist drugs such as pentazocine and tramadol have agonist activity at some receptors and antagonist activity at other receptors. The opioid antagonist naloxone does not have agonist activity at any opioid receptors.

The mechanism by which opioids produce euphoria is not clear. They alter the hypothalamic heat regulation such that body temperature often falls slightly. They also affect the hypothalamus to cause decreased levels of testosterone, cortisol, adrenocorticotropic hormone (ACTH), and β-endorphin. With chronic use, this effect diminishes. The miosis is caused by excitatory effects on the parasympathetic nerve, which causes constriction of the pupil.

The respiratory depression is caused by a direct effect on the brainstem respiratory centers. The brainstem becomes less responsive to carbon dioxide. Death from morphine overdose is usually the result of respiratory arrest. The cough reflex is depressed by a direct effect on the cough center in the medulla. This is separate from the respiratory depression.

Opioids produce nausea and vomiting by direct stimulation of the chemoreceptor trigger zone for emesis in the medulla. There is a vestibular component in the effect because the nausea and vomiting are more common in ambulatory patients than in patients on bed rest.

Opioids produce peripheral vasodilation, reduce peripheral resistance, and inhibit baroreceptor reflexes, causing orthostatic hypotension and fainting.

The effects of opioids on the GI system are many. They decrease gastric motility, prolonging gastric emptying time and increasing the likelihood of esophageal reflux. The absorption of other orally administered drugs is retarded. Opioids diminish biliary, pancreatic, and intestinal secretions. The sphincter of Oddi constricts and causes pressure in the common bile duct to rise, causing biliary colic. Opioids delay digestion of food in the small intestine. Propulsive peristaltic waves in the colon are diminished and tone is increased to the point of spasm. This delays the passage of stool and leads to constipation.

Opioids inhibit the urinary voiding reflex and may cause urinary retention. They may prolong labor. They cause dilation of cutaneous blood vessels, causing flushing. Some opioids—morphine and meperidine, but not methadone or fentanyl—cause histamine release. This may cause pruritus, sweating, and urticaria. The opioids affect the immune system. This is poorly understood, but they seem to cause suppression of natural killer cells.

Mixed Agonist-Antagonists

These products are potent analgesic agents that act through the CNS, possibly at the limbic system. They also antagonize the action of opioids. These drugs compete with the agonists at the mu receptors. They may be agonistic or antagonistic depending upon the receptor and the drug. Thus, they may produce withdrawal symptoms in patients with opioid dependency but are also less likely to be abused than pure opioid agonists.

DRUG TREATMENT PRINCIPLES

Chronic pain requires routine administration of drugs. Giving medications before pain is severe means that the patient will use less of the drug. The clinician should instruct that medication is to be given regularly, not waiting until the patient is in severe pain and begging for medication. Experts agree that addiction is generally not a concern, especially for patients with chronic pain or terminal illness. Primary care providers should be comfortable with managing patients who have chronic pain. Greater pain severity may be relieved by combining therapies. More severe pain may require the addition of an opioid preparation that is useful at higher dosages. Analgesic adjuvants may be useful. Frequent follow-up is needed to assess outcomes and side effects, provide reassurance, and establish goals. It is unrealistic to expect total relief in patients with chronic pain.

The variety of patients who present with pain is extensive and treatment should be individualized to the patient's response. Acute mild-to-moderate pain such as seen with strains and sprains is commonly managed in the primary care setting. Acute severe pain is usually managed in an acute care setting to address the underlying cause such as acute myocardial infarction or fractures. Chronic pain, both benign and malignant, is managed in primary care or by referral to specialty pain management clinics. Hospice referral is important for management of pain and other symptoms associated with terminal disease and dying. Because of reimbursement mechanisms and changes in practice, more of pain management is being moved from the area of the specialist to the primary care setting.

Patients with chronic pain can be very complex to manage. They have multiple problems, including psychiatric responses to chronic pain and other comorbid conditions. Simply prescribing a pill is not effective pain management. These patients require a comprehensive pain management program that includes the patient, family and caregivers, and all health care providers including specialists in the plan. The plan must be consistent from one health professional to the next. Primary care clinicians may need to refer patients to pain management clinics for evaluation and specialized treatments such as nerve blocks. Hospice referral must be considered for terminal conditions.

New drugs, new formulations of drugs, and new uses for old drugs are constantly being developed. Guidelines for the better management of patients with different types of pain have been developed and are being refined every year by various organizations. The clinical treatment guidelines for chronic and acute pain treatment developed and disseminated by the AHCPR in 1992 brought a good deal of attention to this area of practice. Most recently, the American Geriatric Society updated its guideline "The Management of Persistent Pain in Older Persons."

To adequately treat pain, the cause must first be identified and then management of the underlying disease must be maximized. Refer the patient to appropriate specialists and members of the interdisciplinary team for further evaluation and interventions such as orthopedics, neurosurgery, psychiatry, pain specialists, physical and occupational therapy, or hospice. Provide the patient with education regarding the nature of pain, assessment (through use of pain scales and pain diaries), and the purpose and expected results of nonpharmacologic and pharmacologic management. Allow the patient to have some control over the situation and make decisions when possible. This will reduce anxiety.

Nonpharmacologic treatment of pain can be used alone or in combination with medications. These include patient education, management of anxiety and depression, cognitive-behavioral therapy, and appropriate exercise and activity. Common cognitive behavioral interventions include distraction, meditation, and relaxation therapy. Complementary alternative medicine therapies may be helpful, although there is little scientific evidence to support the use of chiropractic manipulation, homeopathy, and spiritual healing. Heat, ice, massage, topical analgesics, acupuncture, and transcutaneous electrical nerve stimulation (TENS) may provide relief alone or in combination with analgesic medications.

Whenever possible, begin pharmacologic pain management with acetaminophen on an around-the-clock schedule. The maximum dose for patients without renal or hepatic dysfunction or alcohol use is 4000 mg/day in divided doses. If acetaminophen is not effective, a nonsteroidal antiinflammatory drug (NSAID) can be used. The combined use of NSAIDs and acetaminophen is unlikely to improve pain relief. NSAIDs have side effects of GI bleeding; in addition, they elevate blood pressure, cause fluid retention, and may provoke renal failure, particularly in the elderly.

If nonopioid medications are not effective or tolerated, opiates alone or with acetaminophen can be used for both nonmalignant and malignant pain. Fear of drug dependency or addiction does not justify withholding opiates or inadequate management of pain. Advise regarding side effects and driving. Prophylactically treat constipation.

Adjuvant drugs, which are medications developed for purposes other than analgesia, are used to alter pain perception. They are particularly useful for neuropathic pain alone or in combination with NSAIDs or opioids. Gabapentin and the

TABLE 44-3 Adjuvant Analgesics

Drug Class	Indication	Comment	Example
Anticonvulsants	Neuropathic pain from diabetic neuropathy, trigeminal neuralgia, post-herpetic neuralgia, glossopharyngeal neuralgia, and neuralgia from nerve trauma or cancer infiltration	Especially useful for episodic lancing or burning pain	carbamazepine clonazepam gabapentin phenytoin
Corticosteroids	Inflammatory diseases or tumor infiltration of nerves	Temporary use for management of a pain crisis Chronic use should be avoided	dexamethasone
Neuroleptics	Chronic pain syndromes, moderate-to-severe pain unrelieved by opioids, or the presence of severe side effects to opioids	Antiemetic and anxiolytic effects	methotrimeprazine
Tricyclic antidepressants	Neuropathic pain, including post-herpetic neuralgia and neuropathy	These drugs have innate analgesic properties and may potentiate the analgesic effects of opioids Anticholinergic side effects	amitriptyline nortriptyline

other newer anticonvulsants are good first-line choices with less side effects than the older tricyclic antidepressants (Table 44-3).

If opioids are to be used:

- Start at lowest possible dose
- If converting from one opioid to another, use equianalgesic dose
- Adjust dosage to achieve pain relief with acceptable level of adverse effects
- Titration rate depends on the half-life of selected opioid
- No ceiling effect to analgesia with pure opioid agonists, ceiling is limited only be side effects

Steps to Changing Opioids

- Calculate the 24-hour dose of current opioids, including around-the-clock and rescue doses
- Use equianalgesic table to convert dosage of current drugs to equivalent of new drug
- Adjust the dosage of new drug to accommodate patient variablity and to account for incomplete cross tolerance
- Determine dosing interval according to duration of action of new opioid
- Calculate rescue doses

Guidelines for Starting Doses of New Opioids

After determing 24-hour dosage of the new opioid:

- Reduce dosage by 25% to 50% based on:
  Patient age
  Pain intensity
  Renal/hepatic dysfunction
  Incomplete cross tolerance
- New dosage may have to be reduced by 75% when treating frail, elderly patients or in patients who have:
  Moderate pain
  Major organ dysfunction (renal/hepatic disease)
  History of adverse reactions to opioids

Rescue Doses

Administer rescue doses to patients to treat pain that breaks through their regularly scheduled around-the-clock drug regimen

- 5% to 15% of the 24-hour oral dose
- Administer oral rescue doses every 1 to 2 hours as needed
- Administer parenteral rescue doses every 15 to 60 minutes

HOW TO MONITOR

The severity of pain experienced by the patient determines which parameters to monitor. The initial database should be used to formulate treatment goals and monitor progress.

The patient taking opioids should be seen at least weekly until pain is controlled, and perhaps more frequently, depending on the nature of the condition. Once stable, the patient should be seen regularly.

Assess for therapeutic effect. Use a standard pain assessment tool.

Assess patient for presence of common side effects, dependency, and interference with activities of daily living or lifestyle patterns. Most patients on opioids become constipated. Monitor for nausea, especially when first starting on opioids.

Specific signs and symptoms to assess include the following:

- Vital signs, including orthostatic blood pressure
- Respiratory function: rate, breath sounds
- Cardiac heart sounds
- Abdomen: abdominal sounds, bowel and urinary functions

PATIENT VARIABLES

Geriatrics

Elderly patients are more susceptible to the CNS and constipation side effects of opioids. Usually they should be placed on bowel regimen when opioids are started. Use a lower dose of opioids. Avoid or use with caution propoxyphene, tramadol, and methadone in the elderly.

Pediatrics

Children experience pain in the same way as adults. Sometimes they have more difficulty communicating their pain, so providers need to be alert. A pain scale using smiling or frowning faces may help assess their pain. Use morphine, codeine, or meperidine; do not use oxycodone, propoxyphene, methadone, or pentazocine. The safety of hydromorphone is not established in children.

Pregnancy

Category C: maternal addiction and neonatal withdrawal occur after illicit use. Some association of first-trimester exposure and congenital defects has been shown with codeine. Although there may be no significant respiratory depression of the mother when morphine is administered before delivery, the neonate may exhibit respiratory depression because of an immature blood–brain barrier. The opioids cross the placental barrier and are excreted in breast milk.

PATIENT EDUCATION

- Take medications exactly as prescribed. It may be important to jot down times when medication was last taken to prevent overdosing.
- Work to taper doses if taken over a long time.
- Although this product has the potential for addiction, used properly, it should not be a problem.
- It is most effective when taken before severe pain is experienced.
- Use other methods for relieving pain whenever possible.
- Do not take any other medications without the knowledge of the health provider.
- Do not drink alcoholic beverages.
- Report to the health care provider any new or troublesome symptoms. Common side effects include constipation, suppression of cough reflex, dizziness, nausea, drowsiness, sweating, and flushing.
- Avoid operating heavy machinery, driving, or performing tasks requiring alertness after taking this medication.
- Urinate frequently and monitor bowel habits daily. Report any problems with constipation to health care practitioner.
- The patient should rise from lying or sitting positions slowly to minimize feelings of light-headedness and avoid standing in one position for long periods.
- During initial doses, the patient should lie down for short periods to avoid developing nausea.
- Family members should alert the health care practitioner if any of the following develop in the patient: presence of shallow, slow respiration; shortness of breath; pupil constriction; deep sleep; vomiting; abdominal pain; palpitations; and skin rash.
- Keep this medication out of the reach of children and all others for whom it is not prescribed. Dispose of all extra medication when there is no longer any need for it. Do not keep it for another time. Do not share this medicine with any other person.

Specific Drugs

OPIOID AGONISTS

Phenanthrenes

(P) Prototype Drug

morphine (MS Contin) (Schedule II Drug)

Other opioids are compared with morphine in terms of efficacy (Table 44-4). Morphine is the primary opioid analgesic used for relief of severe pain. It is classified as a Schedule II controlled substance. Morphine is more effective against dull continuous pain than sharp spasmodic pain.

Contraindications

- Hypersensitivity to opioids
- Acute bronchial asthma and/or upper airway obstruction
- Premature infants or during the delivery of a premature infant
- Epidural or intrathecal morphine should not be given in the presence of infection at the injection site or anticoagulation therapy or with any condition or medication therapy that would contraindicate epidural or intrathecal anesthesia
- Respiratory insufficiency, CNS depression, increased intracranial pressure, acute alcohol intoxication, convulsive disorders, heart failure secondary to chronic lung disease, and cardiac arrhythmias
- Patients taking monoamine oxidase inhibitors (MAOIs) or who have received MAOIs within 14 days

TABLE 44-4 Opioid Analgesic Doses Equivalent to morphine 10 mg IM

Medication	Oral Dose	Subcutaneous Dose
morphine	60 mg	10 mg
MS Contin	60 mg	ND
hydromorphone	7.5 mg	1.3 mg
fentanyl (Duragesic patch)*	ND	ND
codeine	200 mg	130 mg
hydrocodone	5-10 mg	ND
oxycodone	5-10 mg	ND
OxyContin	5-10 mg	ND
propoxyphene	65 mg	ND
tramadol	ND	ND
meperidine	300 mg	75 mg
methadone	20 mg	10 mg
pentazocine	180 mg	30-60 mg

Modified from Hardman JG, Limberd LW, editors: *Goodman and Gilman's pharmacological basis of therapeutics,* ed 9, New York, 1996, McGraw-Hill.
ND, Not determined.
*100 μg/hr = morphine 10 mg IM q4hr.

TABLE 44-5 Pharmacokinetics of Different Forms of Analgesic Medications

Drug	Availability after First Pass	Onset of Action	Time to Peak Concentration	Half-Life	Duration of Action	Metabolism (Primarily in Liver)
morphine, immediate release	25% (low lipid solubility)	15-60 min	0.5-1 hr	20-25 hr	3-7 hr	Extensive metabolism by 2D6
morphine, extended release	About 25%	10 min	30 min	12 min	24 hr	2D6
MS contin	25%		0.5 hr		24 hr	
avinza	About 25%	10 min	30 min	12 min	24 hr	2D6
codeine	60%; lipid soluble	10-30 min	0.5-1 hr	2-4 hr	4-6 hr	10% converted to morphine; 2D6
hydrocodone (Vicodin)		10-30 min	0.5-1 hr	4 hr	4-8 hr	2D6
oxycodone (Percodan)	About 60%-87%	15-30 min	1 hr	3 hr	3-6 hr	2D6
hydromorphone (Dilaudid)	Very highly lipid soluble; 62%	15-30 min	0.5-1 hr	2-3 hr	3-6 hr	
meperidine (Demerol)		10-45 min	0.5-1 hr	3-4 hr	2-4 hr	2D6
fentanyl (Duragesic transdermal)	Very highly lipid soluble	Hours	18-24 hr		3 days	Via CYP 3A4 in liver
methadone	About 80% (highly lipid soluble)	30-60 min	0.5-1 hr	15-40 hr	Pain: 4-7 hr Sedation: 24-48 hr	2D6
propoxyphene (Darvon)		30-60 min	2-2.5 hr	6-12 hr	4-6 hr	Liver
pentazocine (Talwin)		15-30 min	1-3 hr	4-5 hr	3-6 hr	
tramadol (Ultram)	75%	60 min	2 hr	6-7 hr	6 hr	20% protein bound; extensive metabolism by 2D6

Warnings/Precautions

- In cases of head injury and increased intracranial pressure, opioids may obscure the clinical picture
- In asthma and other respiratory conditions, use with extreme caution, as opioids depress the respiratory drive while increasing airway resistance
- These products may cause severe hypotension, especially in patients at risk for orthostatic hypotension
- These products given to patients with renal or hepatic dysfunction may produce a prolonged duration and cumulative effect, requiring a reduced dosage and longer intervals between doses
- Opioids may obscure diagnosis in acute abdominal conditions
- Use with caution in patients who are elderly, debilitated, hypoxic, or sensitive to CNS depressants or have hypercapnic cardiovascular disease, myxedema, convulsive disorders, increased ocular pressure, acute alcoholism, delirium tremens, cerebral arteriosclerosis, ulcerative colitis, fever, decreased respiratory reserve, hypothyroidism, kyphoscoliosis, Addison' s disease, prostatic hypertrophy, urethral stricture, CNS depression, coma, gallbladder disease, recent GI or genitourinary tract surgery, or toxic psychosis
- Use with caution in patients with supraventricular tachycardias; vagolytic action may increase the ventricular response rate
- Cough reflex is suppressed, and this may be a problem in patients with pulmonary problems
- Some products contain sulfites, which produce asthma-like symptoms in sensitive individuals
- May produce drowsiness or dizziness; observe caution while driving or performing other tasks requiring alertness or physical activity
- Monitor for drug abuse and dependence

Pharmacokinetics

Opioids are readily absorbed from the GI tract (Table 44-5). The more lipophilic opioids are absorbed through the nasal or buccal mucosa and through the skin. All are readily absorbed after subcutaneous or intramuscular injection. Oral opioids undergo a variable but significant first-pass effect, decreasing the bioavailability of oral preparations. Morphine is only about 25% bioavailable. The time-effect curve is prolonged with the oral route, lengthening the duration of action. Only about one third of the drug is protein bound. The opioid analgesics are metabolized by the liver, most by the cytochrome P450

TABLE 44-6 Common Adverse Effects of Opioid Analgesics

Body System	Adverse Effects
Body, general	Interference with thermal regulation, paresthesia, pain at injection site, local tissue irritation and induration after SC injection, particularly when repeated; facial flushing, chills, faintness, pruritus (not an allergic reaction)
Hypersensitivity	Pruritus, urticaria, other skin rashes, diaphoresis, laryngospasm, edema, hemorrhagic urticaria; anaphylactoid reactions after IV administration; morphine thrombocytopenia, flushing
Respiratory	Bronchospasm, depression of cough reflex, laryngospasm, respiratory depression, apnea, and respiratory arrest
Cardiovascular	Peripheral circulatory collapse, tachycardia, bradycardia, arrhythmia, palpitations, chest wall rigidity, hypertension, hypotension, orthostatic hypotension,* syncope, asystole, shock, coma
GI	Nausea,* vomiting, diarrhea, cramps, abdominal pain, taste alterations, dry mouth, anorexia, constipation,* biliary tract spasm; exacerbation of ulcerative colitis
Musculoskeletal	Muscular rigidity
CNS	Euphoria, dysphoria, delirium, insomnia, agitation, anxiety, fear, hallucination, disorientation, drowsiness,* sedation,* lethargy, impairment of mental and physical performance, skeletal or uncoordinated movements, mood changes, weakness, headache, mental cloudiness, tremor, convulsions, psychic dependence, toxic psychoses, depression, increased intracranial pressure, miosis, sweating headache, dizziness, lightheadedness, coma
Special senses	Blurred vision, visual disturbances, diplopia, miosis; hydromorphone-nystagmus
Hepatic	propoxyphene—reversible jaundice
Genitourinary	Ureteral spasm and spasm of vesical sphincters, urinary retention or hesitancy, oliguria, antidiuretic effect, reduced libido or potency

*Very common.

2D6 enzyme system, and excreted through the kidney in a conjugated form. Genetic variability produces wide differences in how quickly opioids are metabolized. All opioids are excreted in urine, some to a small extent in feces.

Adverse Effects

Most common adverse effects are constipation, dry mouth, headache, light-headedness, dizziness, sedation, nausea, vomiting, and sweating (Table 44-6).

Drug Interactions

With P450 2D6

See Table 44-7.

With Analgesics

In general, the CNS depressant effects may be potentiated by the concomitant use of other opioid analgesics, alcohol, antianxiety agents, barbiturates, anesthetics, nonbarbiturate sedative hypnotics, phenothiazines, sedative hypnotics, skeletal muscle relaxants, and tricyclic antidepressants. (Respiratory depression, hypotension, profound sedation, and coma may also result.) Opioid use with furosemide may aggravate or produce orthostatic hypotension. Concurrent use of opioids with anticholinergics may produce paralytic ileus. The phenothiazines enhance the sedative effects but antagonize the opioid analgesia. Plasma amylase or lipase levels may be unreliable for 24 hours after the administration of opioids.

With Warfarin

Morphine may potentiate the anticoagulation effect of warfarin.

Overdosage

Signs and symptoms include the following.

- *Acute:* profound respiratory depression, respiratory rate less than 12 breaths/min; irregular shallow respirations, deep sleep, stupor or coma, miosis, cyanosis, gradually decreasing blood pressure, oliguria, clammy skin, hypothermia.
- *Chronic:* constricted pupils, constipation, skin infections, mood changes, depressed level of consciousness; skin infections, itching, needle scars, abscesses when drug is abused.

Dosage and Administration

The dosage and formulation of opioid analgesic used depends on the severity of pain experienced by the patient, the response to the pain and the medication, the nature of the illness, and the route of administration. The route of administration for this category includes oral, rectal, sublingual, intramuscular, subcutaneous, and intravenous routes. The oral route is used most often in primary care except in the case of the terminal, dying patient. Oral, sublingual, or rectal route is still preferred over parenteral routes in these patients. Refer to hospice for assistance.

Morphine sulfate comes in immediate and extended release formulations. The immediate formulation, IR morphine, is given for breakthrough pain. IR Morphine comes in tablet and liquid formulations. Morphine oral concentrate is 20 mg/ml and can be used sublingually in patients who are unable to swallow.

ER formulations such as MS Contin and Avinza are used for routine administration in chronic pain. MS Contin is commonly used in hospice. Given twice a day, it provides around-the-clock pain control. MS Contin can be given rectally when the patient is unable to swallow.

The morphine sulfate extended-release capsules (Avinza) consist of two components: an immediate-release

TABLE 44-7 Drug Interactions with Analgesics

Drug	Increase Level	Decrease Level
morphine	amitriptyline Antihistamines Barbiturates chloral hydrate chlorpromazine cimetidine clomipramine furazolidone glutethimide MAOIs methocarbamol nortriptyline thioridazine	Agonist-antagonist analgesics
codeine	Barbiturates chlorpromazine furazolidone MAOIs thioridazine	Agonist-antagonist analgesics
hydrocodone	Barbiturates chlorpromazine furazolidone MAOIs Protease inhibitors thioridazine	Agonist-antagonist analgesics
oxycodone	Barbiturates chlorpromazine furazolidone MAOIs Protease inhibitors thioridazine	Agonist-antagonist analgesics
hydromorphone	Barbiturates chlorpromazine furazolidone MAOIs thioridazine	Agonist-antagonist analgesics
meperidine	Barbiturates chlorpromazine thioridazine MAOIs furazolidone cimetidine Hydantoins Protease inhibitors	Agonist-antagonist analgesics
fentanyl	Barbiturates chlorpromazine thioridazine MAOIs furazolidone diazepam droperidol nitrous oxide Protease inhibitors	Agonist-antagonist analgesics
methadone	Barbiturates chlorpromazine thioridazine MAOIs furazolidone cimetidine fluvoxamine Hydantoins Protease inhibitors	Agonist-antagonist analgesics rifampin
propoxyphene	Barbiturates chlorpromazine thioridazine MAOIs furazolidone Protease inhibitors	Agonist-antagonist analgesics Charcoal Cigarette smoking
pentazocine	Barbiturates	
tramadol	MAOIs	carbamazepine

MAOI, Monoamine oxidase inhibitors.

component that rapidly achieves plateau morphine concentrations and an extended-release component that maintains plasma concentrations throughout the 24-hour dosing interval. The amount absorbed is similar to other forms of oral morphine.

The extended-release formulation of morphine must be taken correctly: they must be swallowed whole, and not chewed, crushed, or dissolved. If crushed or dissolved, the patient may receive a fatal overdose. Avoid multiple dosing in chronic pain patient and allow the patient to get on with his or her life instead of counting the hours until the next analgesic dose. Patients can take one capsule in the morning and go out and function all day; they do not have to take the medication with them.

See Table 44-8 for dosage and administration information for all products.

Other Drugs in Class

Other drugs in this class are similar to the prototype except as follows.

codeine (Schedule II-III)

Codeine has two primary therapeutic effects: analgesic and antitussive. Ten percent of codeine is metabolized to morphine. Codeine is relatively less potent than morphine and does not have the drug abuse potential of morphine. It is more likely to cause constipation and nausea than other opioids. Codeine is often combined with nonopioid analgesics, centrally acting muscle relaxants, antihistamines, and decongestants. Noncombination forms of codeine are classified as Schedule II controlled substances. Codeine is as effective orally as it is parenterally.

Dosage and Administration. See Table 44-8.

TABLE 44-8 Dosage and Administration of Opioids

Drug	Dosage	Administration
morphine	5-30 mg 10-20 mg 10 mg (5-20 mg)/70 kg 2.5-15 mg/70 kg	5 L, PO q4hr PR q4hr SC or IM q4hr IV in 4-5 ml of sterile water over 4-5 min; have opiate antagonist immediately available during IV administration
morphine, controlled release	10-200 mg	PO q12 hr
codeine (pain relief)	Adult: 15-60 mg Child >1 yr: 0.5 mg/kg or 15 m^2 body surface area	PO, IM, SC, or IV q4hr PO, IM, SC q4hr; do not administer IV in children
codeine (antitussive)	Adult: 10-20 mg Child 6-12 yr: 5-10 mg Child 2-6 yr: 2.5-5 mg	PO q4-6hr; do not exceed 120 mg/24 hr PO 14-6hr; do not exceed 60 mg/24 hr PO q4-6hr; do not exceed 30 mg/24 hr
hydrocodone	5-10 mg	PO q4-6hr up to 8 tablets in 24 hr
oxycodone	5-30 mg Immediate release (OxyIR): 5 mg Controlled release (OxyContin) 10-160 mg	PO q4-6hr PO q6hr PO q12 hr
hydromorphone	Adult only: 2-4 mg 3 mg 1-2 mg	PO q4-6hr PR q8hr SC, IM, or slow IV q4-6hr
meperidine	Adult: 50-150 mg Child (1-1.5 mg/kg): up to 50-75 mg	PO, IM, or SC q3-4hr PO, IM, or SC q3-4hr
fentanyl	25-100 μg patch	Change patch every 3 days; see text discussion for details
methadone (pain relief)	2.5-10 mg	PO, SC, or IM q3-4hr
methadone (detoxification)	15-40 mg	PO (if possible); see text discussion for details
propoxyphene	65 mg	PO q4hr
pentazocine	>50 mg	IM q3-4 hr
tramadol	50-100 mg	PO q4-6hr, not to exceed 300-400 mg/24 hr; 300 mg/day in elderly

hydrocodone (Lortab, Vicodin) (Schedule III)

Hydrocodone is a semisynthetic opioid with primary actions that affect the CNS and organs composed of smooth muscle. The principal actions are analgesia and sedation. It is similar to codeine in that at least one half of the analgesic activity is retained in the oral form. It is used to treat moderate-to-severe pain of an acute nature or as an antitussive. It is available in combination only with acetaminophen, aspirin, or ibuprofen and with antihistamines, decongestants, and expectorants for cough suppression. Hydrocodone produces drug dependence similar to morphine. It should not be used in patients hypersensitive to any of the combination tablet ingredients. Hydrocodone preparations may be less constipating than codeine, especially in older adults.

oxycodone (Schedule II)

Oxycodone is similar to hydrocodone; it is a semisynthetic opioid. It is similar to codeine in that it retains at least one half of its analgesic activity in the oral form. The immediate-release form is used to treat moderate-to-severe pain of an acute nature.

The controlled-release form is indicated for chronic pain requiring continuing analgesia for an extended period only; they are not to be used on an as-needed basis.

They are not to be broken or chewed as this can lead to rapid release and absorption of a potentially lethal dose of oxycodone, particularly with the 80- and 160-mg tablets.

These high-dose tablets are to be used for those with opiate tolerance only, as they have become popular for drug abuse. Oxycodone is also available in combination with aspirin or acetaminophen. It produces drug dependence similar to morphine.

hydromorphone hydrochloride (Dilaudid) (Schedule II)

Hydromorphone is a very potent synthetic compound that maximizes analgesic effects and minimizes some of the common side effects of morphine. Hydromorphone has 7 to 10 times the analgesic action of morphine. Hydromorphone produces less sedation, nausea, vomiting, and constipation than its counterpart. The incidence of respiratory depression is marked, requiring close observation. Use the lowest dose possible to prevent this adverse effect. Rectal suppositories are particularly useful for producing a prolonged effect. It is a very desirable drug among intravenous drug abusers.

Phenylpiperidines

meperidine (Demerol) (Schedule II)

This is a synthetic opioid analgesic with less potency than morphine. It is used for the relief of moderate-to-severe pain, preoperative sedation, postoperative analgesia, obstetric anesthesia, and intravenous administration for supportive anesthesia. It causes less sedation and pruritus than morphine. The onset of action is more rapid but the duration of action is shorter than morphine. The major metabolite, normeperidine, can cause irritability, dysphoria, and seizures. Meperidine should not be used to treat chronic pain because of the high risk of seizure even in those with normal renal function. It should be used with particular caution, if at all, in the elderly. When administering with phenothiazine and many other tranquilizers, reduce the dosage of meperidine (Demerol) by 25% to 50% because they potentiate the action of meperidine. Each dose of syrup should be taken in one-half glass of water because, if undiluted, it can exert a topical anesthetic effect on mucous membranes. It is a drug of choice among drug abusers and must be used with extreme caution.

fentanyl (Sublimaze, Duragesic Transdermal) (Schedule II)

Intravenous fentanyl is a very potent short-acting opioid used for relief of moderate-to-sezvere pain and preoperative sedation and operative and postoperative analgesia. A 0.1-mg dose of fentanyl is equivalent to 10 mg of morphine. The respiratory depressant effects of fentanyl are particularly dangerous and mandate that the provider have resuscitative measures and opioid antagonists present, making it unacceptable for the outpatient setting.

Transdermal fentanyl is useful in the outpatient setting for long-term relief of pain, especially in a patient unable to take oral medications. It can be useful in tapering opioids. It is to be used only in patients with severe chronic pain who require continuing analgesia. Initiate therapy with the 25-µg patch, particularly in the elderly, who may have decreased fat stores and altered clearance. It is very lipid soluble with enhanced CNS penetration. Patient must have adequate fat stores. The patch strength is roughly equivalent to the 12-hour MS Contin dose. It has a depot or holding effect, is deposited in the skin, and will continue to be absorbed for hours after the patch is removed.

Dosage and Administration (Fentanyl Transdermal System)

1. *Initial Dose Selection.* Individualize dosage. If the patient is opioid naïve, start with the lowest dose, 25 µg/hr. Generally, however, this is not the first opioid the patient has used. The fentanyl patch should be used only in those with chronic pain who cannot be managed with short-acting narcotics. The usual use of fentanyl transdermal systems is to convert the patient from oral or parenteral opioids to the transdermal system, as follows:

- Calculate the previous 24-hour analgesic requirement.
- Convert this amount to the equianalgesic oral morphine dose (see Table 44-8).
- Convert from 24-hour morphine dose to transdermal fentanyl dose (Janssen Pharmaceutical Company provides a dosage conversion calculator).

2. *Apply Patch.* Apply to nonirritated skin on a flat surface of the upper torso. Clip, but do not shave, hair. Clean skin with clear water; do not use soaps, oils, lotions, alcohol, or any other agents that might irritate the skin or alter its characteristics. Allow the skin to dry completely before system application.

Apply patch immediately on removal from the sealed package. Press firmly with palm of hand for 10 to 20 seconds, making sure contact is complete, especially around the edges.

Each system works continuously for 72 hours. However, occasionally patients find they need to replace the system every 48 hours. Remove the old system, and apply the new system to a different skin site. Dispose of the old system carefully.

3. *Wearing the First System.* Because peak levels are not reached for 24 hours, the patient may need short-acting analgesics. After 24 hours, assess the efficacy of the system by counting the number of times the patients needs a rescue dose of short-acting analgesic.

4. *Titrate Dosage.* Titrate upward if necessary after the initial 3-day system. Because the conversion system from morphine to fentanyl is conservative, about half of the patients will need upward titration. If the patient is using rescue doses of analgesic equivalent to 90 mg/24 hr of morphine, increase the fentanyl system dose by 25 µg/hr.

After the first titration, then titrate upward every 6 days. For delivery rates in excess of 100 µg/hr, multiple systems may be used.

5. *Discontinue.* If the patient requires more than 300 µg/hr, change the patient to another method of opioid administration. Remember that it takes about 18 hours for the fentanyl concentration to decrease by 50% after removal of the system.

A fentanyl patch can be used to discontinue opioids by using the patch, then simply removing and allowing the concentration to gradually decrease.

Diphenylheptanes

methadone hydrochloride (Dolophine) (Schedule II)

Methadone hydrochloride is a synthetic opioid analgesic used primarily in the detoxification, treatment, and maintenance of narcotic addicts. It may be used orally for management of severe pain in patients unable to tolerate other narcotics. The drug is highly addictive. It is longer acting (36 to 48 hours) and tends to accumulate; therefore, use it with caution, if at all, in the elderly. Remember that the side effects have a longer duration than the analgesic effects due to extensive protein binding. Refer to pain specialists with experience using methadone. It is less sedating and euphoric than morphine. When used for heroin addicts for more than 3 weeks, methadone moves from a treatment phase to a maintenance phase. Respiratory depression and arrest remain one of its serious adverse effects. The regulations for its use for narcotic detoxification and maintenance are quite complicated.

Drug Interactions. Methadone increases blood levels of desipramine.

Dosage and Administration. See Table 44-8.

- *Opioid detoxification:* individualize treatment.
- *Adults:* specific to severity of withdrawal symptoms: 5 mg tid PO for 21 days with the dose gradually reduced every few days.
- *Opioid maintenance:* 40 to 120 mg or higher once daily PO.

propoxyphene (Darvon)

Propoxyphene HCl is a centrally acting opioid, structurally related to methadone. It is a weak analgesic with efficacy similar to acetaminophen or aspirin alone but has physical and psychological addictive properties. To improve its overall effect, the drug is often combined with nonopioid analgesics. It has a fairly long half-life. Drug accumulation can cause ataxia and dizziness contributing to falls, particularly in the elderly. However, many providers continue to use propoxyphene; alternative analgesic therapy may be safer and more effective, especially when initiating narcotic therapy in patients who have not used propoxyphene. A metabolite has cardiac conduction effects, increasing the PR and QRS intervals. Propoxyphene products in excessive doses, either alone or in combination with other CNS depressants (including alcohol), are a major cause of drug-related deaths. It is classified as a Schedule IV controlled substance.

Drug Interactions. Propoxyphene potentiates the effect of warfarin. Carbamazine toxicity may occur in patients taking propoxyphene; monitor serum carbamazine levels. See Table 44-7 for drug interactions with narcotics.

Dosage and Administration. See Table 44-8.

A dose of 100 mg propoxyphene napsylate is required to equal 65 mg of propoxyphene HCl due to differences in molecular weight.

MIXED AGONIST-ANTAGONISTS

pentazocine (Talwin)

Pentazocine is a synthetic opioid with weak opioid antagonist properties. It is used primarily for the relief of moderate-to-severe pain or as a preoperative or preanesthetic medication. It is a category IV narcotic.

Contraindications. Hypersensitivity

Warnings/Precautions. See also warnings and precautions for morphine.

Use with extreme caution in patients who are emotionally unstable and in patients with a previous history of drug abuse. As both psychologic and physiologic dependence may occur, this drug should be given under careful supervision and prescribed only in limited amounts.

Because the tablets are popular with drug addicts for intravenous injection, Talwin NX with naloxone was developed. When taken orally, the naloxone is not absorbed, allowing the pentazocine to exert its analgesic effect. When the drug is misused by injection, severe effects may occur, such as pulmonary emboli, vascular occlusion, ulceration and abscesses, and withdrawal symptoms in opioid-dependent individuals.

If patients receiving therapeutic doses demonstrate any evidence of hallucinations, confusion, or disorientation, medication should be discontinued.

In patients who have demonstrated dependence to opioids, it may produce withdrawal symptoms.

It has been known to provoke seizures, especially in those patients with known seizure disorders.

Adverse Effects. See adverse effects for morphine.

In addition, pentazocine causes the following effects:

- *Cardiovascular:* circulatory depression, shock
- *CNS:* agitation, clammy feeling, confusion, crying, dizziness, dysphoria, faintness, floating feeling, hostility, lethargy, light-headedness, nervousness, nystagmus, numbness, paresthesias, syncope, tingling, tinnitus, tremor, unreality, unusual dreams, vertigo
- *Dermatologic:* burning, edema of face, urticaria, rash, severe sclerosis, soft tissue induration, sting on injection, ulceration
- *Hematopoietic:* depression of white blood cells, transient eosinophilia
- *Other:* speech difficulty

Dosage and Administration. See Table 44-8.

tramadol (Ultram)

Tramadol is not a scheduled drug.

Warnings

- See warnings for morphine. Seizure risk exists, especially in patients with a history of seizures or on a medication that increases the risk of seizures.
- Anaphylactoid reactions have occurred.
- Use great caution in combination with MAOIs.

Adverse Effects. See adverse effects for morphine; the most common are dizziness/vertigo, nausea, constipation, and headache and somnolence.

Drug Interactions. Drug is metabolized by cytochrome P450 2D6 isoenzymes. Use with carbamazepine causes an increase in tramadol metabolism.

Dosage and Administration. See Table 44-8.

RESOURCES FOR PATIENTS AND PROVIDERS

Internet

American Academy of Pain Medicine, www.painmed.org.

American Chronic Pain Association, www.theacpa.org.

American Pain Society, www.ampainsoc.org.

Pain PDQ Supportive Care Health Professionals, cancernet.nci.nih.gov/clinpdq/supportive/Pain Physicians.html.

Comprehensive internet presentation of pain and its treatment.

Publications

Acute Pain Management Guideline Panel: *Acute pain management: operative or medical procedures and trauma,* Clinical Practice Guideline, AHCPR Publication No. 92-0032, Rockville, Md, 1992, Agency for Health Care Policy and Research, Public Health Services, U.S. Department of Health and Human Services.

It may be convenient to use one of these suggested pain intensive scales to provide easy ways to measure the effectiveness of pain treatment.

Kanner R: *Pain management secrets: questions you will be asked*, Philadelphia, 1997, Hanley & Belfus, Inc.

BIBLIOGRAPHY

Agency for Health Care Policy and Research: *Acute pain management: operative or medical procedures and trauma, clinical practice guidelines,* Publication No. 92-0032, Washington, DC, 1992, Department of Health and Human Services.

Agency for Health Care Policy and Research: *Management of cancer pain, clinical practice guidelines,* Publication No. 94-0592, Washington, DC, 1992, Department of Health and Human Services.

American Academy of Pain Medicine and the American Pain Society: *The use of opioids for the treatment of chronic pain (a consensus statement),* Washington, DC, 1997, American Academy of Pain Medicine/American Pain Society.

American Geriatrics Society Panel on Persistent Pain in Older Persons: The management of persistent pain in older persons, *J Am Geriatr Soc* 50:S205-S224, 2002.

American Pain Society: *Definitions related to the use of opioids for the treatment of pain,* Washington, DC, 2001, American Academy of Pain Medicine/American Pain Society/American Society of Addiction Medicine.

Aronson M: Nonsteroidal anti-inflammatory drugs, traditional opioids, and tramadol: contrasting therapies for the treatment of chronic pain, *Clin Ther* 19:422, 1997.

Brant JM: Opioid equianalgesic conversion: the right dose, *Clin J Oncol Nurs* 5:163-165, 2001.

Fleischman J, Galler D: Prescription for addiction? *Adv Nurse Pract* 9:27, 2001.

Marcus DA: Treatment of nonmalignant chronic pain, *Am Fam Phys* 61:1331-1338, 2001.

Phero JC, Becker D: Rational use of analgesic combinations, *Dent Clin North Am* 46:691-705, 2002.

Rapp CJ, Gordon DB: Understanding equianalgesic dosing, *Orthop Nursing* 19:65-71, 2000.

Regan JJ, Alderson A: OxyContin: maintaining availability and efficacy while preventing diversion and abuse, *Tenn Med* 96:88-90, 2003.

Zacny JP: Characterizing the subjective, psychomotor, and physiologic effects of a hydrocodone combination product (Hydocan) in non-drug-abusing volunteers, *Psychopharmacol* 165:146-156, 2003.

Migraine Medications

Drug Names

Class	Subclass	Generic Name	Trade Name
Abortive agents	Serotonin 5-HT_1 receptor agonist	(P) (200) sumatriptan	Imitrex
		naratriptan	Amerge
		rizatriptan	Maxalt
		zolmitriptan	Zomig
		almotriptan	Axert
		frovatriptan	Frova
	5-HT 1B/1D	eletriptan	Relpax
	Ergotamine derivatives	isometheptene mucate	Midrin
		(P) ergotamine tartrate	Cafergot
		dihydroergotamine (DHE)	DHE-45, Migranal
Prophylactic agents		methysergide	Sansert
		cyproheptadine	Periactin

(200), Top 200 drug; (P), prototype drug.

General Uses

Indications

- Acute treatment of migraines with or without aura
- Prophylaxis of migraines

A wide variety of drugs are used for the treatment of migraines. They are divided into preparations effective in acute treatment of migraine symptoms and preparations used for chronic prophylaxis. The most commonly used are the serotonin$_1$ (5-HT_1) receptor agonists, commonly known as the "triptans." Migraine-specific products are discussed in detail in this chapter. Drugs from many classes are used in the treatment of migraines. Abortive medications include acetaminophen, aspirin, and nonsteroidal antiinflammatory drugs (NSAIDs). Preventative medications include the β-blockers, calcium channel blockers, tricyclic antidepressants (TCAs), selective serotonin reuptake inhibitors (SSRIs), and anticonvulsants. Only their use in the treatment of migraines is discussed in this chapter.

DISEASE PROCESS

Pathophysiology

Migraines are a primary disorder of the brain. A strong genetic influence seems to be apparent in some patients. Neural events cause dilation of blood vessels, which causes pain and other nerve activation. The basic problem is in the dysfunction of an ion channel in brainstem neurons that normally modulate sensory input and exert neural influence on cranial vessels. The brain neurotransmitters involved are primarily from the serotonergic system. Serotonin receptor subtypes, including 1B, 1D, and 1F, play a role in cerebral vasodilation and trigeminal nerve activation, which are believed to be the precursors of migraine pain.

The Disease

Headaches are a very common complaint in primary care. They have many causes ranging in seriousness from stress to brain tumor; therefore the cause must be determined before effective therapy may be ordered.

Tension headache is the most common headache, generally described as vise-like pressure associated with stress and fatigue. They are usually generalized but may be worse in the area of the neck and back of head. These are generally treated with analgesics for mild-to-moderate pain. (See Chapter 44 for more information on pain management.) When analgesics fail, migraine agents may be used.

Approximately 23 million Americans are afflicted with migraine headaches: The onset of migraine headaches usually begins in young adulthood, peaking between the ages of 25 and 34. These headaches are a debilitating and costly medical problem. There also are a large group of patients who, for a variety of reasons, do not seek medical care for their migraines.

The symptomatology of migraines is variable. All migraines are paroxysmal in nature—clearly defined attacks separated by symptom-free intervals. Daily or continuous headaches usually

TABLE 45-1 Phases of a Migraine

Phase	Experienced by	Symptoms	Timing
Prodrome	50%	Increased/decreased perception, irritability or withdrawal, food cravings, yawning, speech difficulties	Starts 24 hr before overt migraine
Aura	20%	Visual disturbances (flashing lights, shimmering zigzag lines), numbness or tingling in hands, dysphagia	Starts 30-60 min before headache, lasts 5-60 min
Headache		Severe, pulsating, unilateral; accompanied by nausea and vomiting, photophobia or phonophobia; all reversible	Lasts 4-72 hr
Postdrome		Fatigue, aching muscles, or euphoria	Lasts up to 24 hr

are not migraines. Migraines can be classified as with aura or without aura and are graded as mild, moderate, or severe in intensity. Duration of the migraine is an important variable that helps guide treatment. Migraines go through specific phases (Table 45-1).

Complicated migraines are characterized by attacks in which neurologic symptoms last for the entire headache or for several days or weeks or, in some cases, leave a permanent neurologic deficit. Complicated migraines are divided into three subtypes. An *ophthalmoplegic* migraine affects the third, fourth, or sixth cranial nerve; permanent damage to the third nerve has been reported. *Hemiplegic* migraine is characterized by motor and sensory symptoms that are unilateral and last longer than the headache itself. Complete recovery many take weeks; permanent weakness can occur after multiple attacks. *Basilar artery* migraine is characterized by vertigo, diplopia, tinnitus, ataxia, and altered consciousness. Visual symptoms may be difficult to distinguish from a classic migraine aura, although basilar artery migraine is more likely to affect both visual fields.

A transformed migraine is a long-lasting headache from overuse of pain and/or migraine medications. The patient has rebound headache daily or nearly daily. Medications that can cause this are caffeine, acetaminophen, nonsteroidal antiinflammatory drugs (NSAIDs), barbiturates, sedatives, narcotics, ergots, triptans, and decongestants.

Assessment

The diagnosis of migraines is based on meeting specific criteria (Box 45-1). A diagnostic work-up should include a headache history that includes age of onset, duration of complaint, frequency and duration of each headache, site, quality, time of onset, associated phenomena, and aggravating and relieving factors. Physical examination, including neurologic examination, is typically normal. The Migraine Disability Assessment Scale (MIDAS) is a five-item questionnaire for use in practice (see Goadsby et al for questionnaire).

It is essential that adequate evaluation and diagnostic testing be completed to confirm the diagnosis of migraine. Some headaches that patients may call migraines are actually other pathologic conditions; some of these headaches represent significant problems that must not be ignored. Box 45-2 lists headache symptoms that warrant more detailed evaluation.

The patient must also be screened for concurrent illnesses, especially cardiovascular problems such as increased blood

BOX 45-1

DIAGNOSTIC CRITERIA FOR MIGRAINE

MIGRAINE WITHOUT AURA

A. At least five attacks fulfilling criteria B through D
B. Headache lasting 4 to 72 hours (untreated or unsuccessfully treated)
C. At least two of the following pain characteristics:
   1. Unilateral location
   2. Pulsating quality
   3. Moderate or severe intensity
   4. Aggravation by walking stairs or similar physical activity
D. During headache, at least one of the following:
   1. Nausea and/or vomiting
   2. Photophobia and phonophobia

MIGRAINE WITH AURA

A. At least two attacks fulfilling criterion B
B. At least three of the following characteristics:
   1. One or more fully reversible aura symptoms indicting focal cerebral cortical and/or brainstem dysfunction
   2. At least one aura symptoms develops gradually over more than 4 minutes, or two or more symptoms occur in succession.
   3. No aura symptoms lasts more than 60 minutes; if more than one aura symptoms is present, accepted duration is proportionally increased.
   4. Headache follows aura, with a free interval of less than 60 minutes (headache may also begin before or simultaneously with aura).

Adapted from Headache Classification Committee of the International Headache Society: Classification and diagnostic criteria for headache disorders, cranial neuralgias and facial pain, *Cephalalgia* 8(suppl 7): 1-96, 1988.

pressure and coronary artery disease (CAD). These will affect treatment options.

DRUG ACTION AND EFFECTS

Abortive Agents

See Box 45-3 for a list of abortive medications and Table 45-2 for drug effects on serotonin receptors.

All serotonin$_1$ (5-HT$_1$) receptor agonists (triptans) have a similar chemical structure and comparable mechanism of action. 5-HT$_{1B}$ and 5-HT$_{1D}$ receptors are located on the extracerebral, intracranial blood vessels that become dilated during a migraine attack and on nerve terminals in the trigeminal system. Therapeutic activity is caused by activation of these receptors, which results in cranial vessel constriction, inhibition of neuropeptide release, and reduced transmission in trigeminal pain pathways. Each product varies with regard to onset of action, duration of action, and incidence of recurrent headache.

Ergotamine derivatives have partial agonist or antagonist activity against tryptaminergic, dopaminergic, and α-adrenergic receptors depending on their site. They constrict peripheral and cranial blood vessels and depress central vasomotor centers, reduce extracranial blood flow and decrease hyperperfusion of the basilar artery area, and increase the force and frequency of uterine contractions.

Ergotamine tartrate is an α-adrenergic–blocking agent with direct stimulating effect on the smooth muscle of the peripheral and cranial vessels. Ergot drugs also produce an increase in central vasomotor center stimulation. Although dihydroergotamine (DHE) is an ergot, it is also a 5-HT$_{1B/1D}$ receptor agonist. It is not as selective as the triptans. DHE binds to nonepinephrine (noradrenaline) α_1, α_{2A}, and α_{2B} and dopamine D_{2L} and D_3 receptors. It is a stronger venoconstrictor and weaker arterial vasoconstrictor than ergotamine.

Isometheptene mucate is a sympathomimetic agent that acts as a vasoconstrictor of dilated cranial and cerebral arterioles. Midrin is a combination capsule. It contains 65 mg of isometheptene mucate, 325 mg of acetaminophen, which exerts an analgesic effect, and 100 mg of dichloralphenazone, a mild sedative that acts centrally to allay anxiety. Caffeine, which is added to many migraine combinations, helps promote constrictive properties and enhances absorption.

BOX 45-2

HEADACHE DANGER SIGNALS THAT WARRANT INVESTIGATION

- Sudden onset of new, severe headache
- Progressively worsening headache
- Onset of headache after exertion, straining, coughing, or sexual activity
- Presence of associated symptoms
- Onset of first headache after the age of 50 years

BOX 45-3

ABORTIVE MEDICATIONS

MILD TO MODERATE
acetaminophen
aspirin
caffeine-containing combination products
isometheptene
naproxen, ibuprofen, indomethacin

MODERATE TO SEVERE
Corticosteroids
dihydroergotamine
ergotamine
Opioids
Triptans

Prophylactic Agents

See Box 45-4 for a list of prophylactic medications. Methysergide is an ergot drug useful for prophylaxis. It acts as a 5-HT$_2$ receptor antagonist and/or 5-HT$_1$ agonist. It exerts central effects of vasoconstriction in the cerebral blood vessels. This action stabilizes the cerebral vascular system and reduces headache activity.

Cyproheptadine is an antihistamine, anticholinergic, and serotonin antagonist. It belongs to the nonselective

TABLE 45-2 Drug Effects on Serotonin (5-HT) Receptors

Drug	1	1A	1B	1D	1E	1F	2A/2C	5A	7	2 to 4
sumatriptan	High	Weak						Weak	Weak	None
naratriptan				High		Weak				None
rizatriptan		Weak	High	High	Weak	Weak			Weak	
zolmitriptan		Weak	High	High		Weak				
almotriptan		Weak	High	High		High			Weak	
frovatriptan			High	High						
eletriptan			High	High						
DHE		High		High			High			

BOX 45-4

PROPHYLACTIC MEDICATIONS

- β-Blockers: propranolol and timolol
- Calcium channel blocker: verapamil
- Anticonvulsants: divalproex, gabapentin, and topiramate
- Tricyclic antidepressants: amitriptyline, doxepin, nortriptyline, imipramine, protriptyline, and desipramine
- Selective serotonin reuptake inhibitors: fluvoxamine and paroxetine
- cyproheptadine
- methysergide

piperidine class and is generally used for hypersensitivity reactions.

The β-blockers are postulated to exert their antimigraine effect through stabilization of vascular tone. Inhibition of norepinephrine release by blocking prejunctional β-receptors, reduction in the enzyme activity (tyrosine hydroxylase) that is the rate-limiting step in norepinephrine synthesis, and the delayed reduction of locus ceruleus neuron firing are other postulated mechanisms. Blocking central β-receptors interferes with vigilance-enhancing adrenergic pathways important in headache prevention. Interaction with serotonin receptors by some β-adrenergic blockers may also stabilize vascular tone.

Calcium channel blockers regulate cellular function, including vascular smooth muscle contraction, neurotransmission, and hormone secretion enzyme activity. These products also block intracerebral vasoconstriction caused by vasoactive neurotransmitters such as 5-HT (serotonin) and norepinephrine. It has also been suggested that calcium channel blockers impede neurovascular inflammation and prevent hypoxia of cerebral neurons.

Tricyclic antidepressants act to reduce migraine activity by increasing availability of synaptic norepinephrine or serotonin "downregulation" of 5-HT receptors and β-receptor density. This enhances the opiate mechanism, provides inhibition of 5-HT and norepinephrine reuptake, while binding to receptors on platelets and neurons blocking 5-HT uptake. The net result is to increase the threshold for precipitation of a migraine attack in selected individuals.

SSRIs are potent-specific 5-HT receptor reuptake inhibitors that reduce migraine frequency and intensity. They act to prevent the vasoconstrictive effect of decreased serotonin levels during headache. Such constriction sets up a cascade of neuron inflammatory changes producing headache pain. Maintaining the serum level of 5-HT with SSRIs prevents initiation of this pathway, preventing migraine.

Anticonvulsants are believed to exert their antimigraine activity through their influence on cerebral arteries and circadian rhythms. They may also help regulate secretion of hormones from the anterior pituitary gland.

DRUG TREATMENT PRINCIPLES

The goal of migraine treatment is to decrease pain and associated symptoms, prevent recurrence, improve quality of life, and allow patient to maintain function. Treatment of migraine headache must be individualized for each patient. Some of the critical decisions that need to be made in determining treatment for a patient with migraine are illustrated in Figure 45-1.

Nonpharmacologic Treatment

The prevention of migraines includes healthy regular daily habits, including sleep, meals, and exercise. Patients should avoid peaks of stress and troughs of relaxation, because acute stress and the abrupt removal of stress are common triggers. Regularity of habits, rather than just searching for triggers, is the key to effective nonpharmacologic approaches.

The second step in the management of migraine headache is the avoidance of headache triggers. The patient must determine the factors responsible for initiating his or her headaches. Have the patient keep a diary that correlates the patient's activity, food, and stressful events with the migraines. Common migraine triggers include loud noise, strong smells (e.g., perfumes), flashing lights, changing time zones, weather and altitude changes, smoke, and menstruation. Food triggers include caffeine withdrawal, aged cheese, chocolate, monosodium glutamate (MSG), nitrate/nitrite-preserved foods, glutamate, excessive vitamin A, and alcohol. Triggers include oral contraceptives, nitroglycerin, histamine, reserpine, corticosteroid withdrawal, and hydralazine.

Treatment of the acute attack begins with resting in a quiet dark place; this will allow the medications to work better. It also reduces external stimuli and allows the patient to relax. Other effective techniques include local pressure, local application of cold, and sleep. These approaches are frequently not feasible when people are at work or have responsibilities they must meet.

Relaxation training, thermal biofeedback, and cognitive behavioral therapy may help prevent migraines. Alternative therapies include feverfew, riboflavin, and magnesium.

Pharmacologic Treatment

Factors to consider when determining drug therapy include frequency, duration, and severity of headaches; symptoms other than pain such as nausea; and previous therapies that have been tried. Complicated and transformed migraines should be managed by a specialist. Boxes 45-3 and 45-4 respectively list commonly utilized abortive and prophylactic migraine medications.

Abortive Treatment

All diagnosed migraineurs should have medication on hand in anticipation of an acute migraine attack. Abortive agents are used in the absence of prophylactic management in migraineurs who have less than four attacks a month. It is important that any abortive agent be administered no more than 2 days per week to avoid the possibility of rebound headache. Usually the patient will have headaches of a variable intensity, so varying options of intensity of treatment should be available to them. No drug works perfectly every time. Patients should try products at least twice before they determine that they are ineffective.

The major choice is between ergots and triptans. Triptans have become the first-line treatment for abortive treatment of

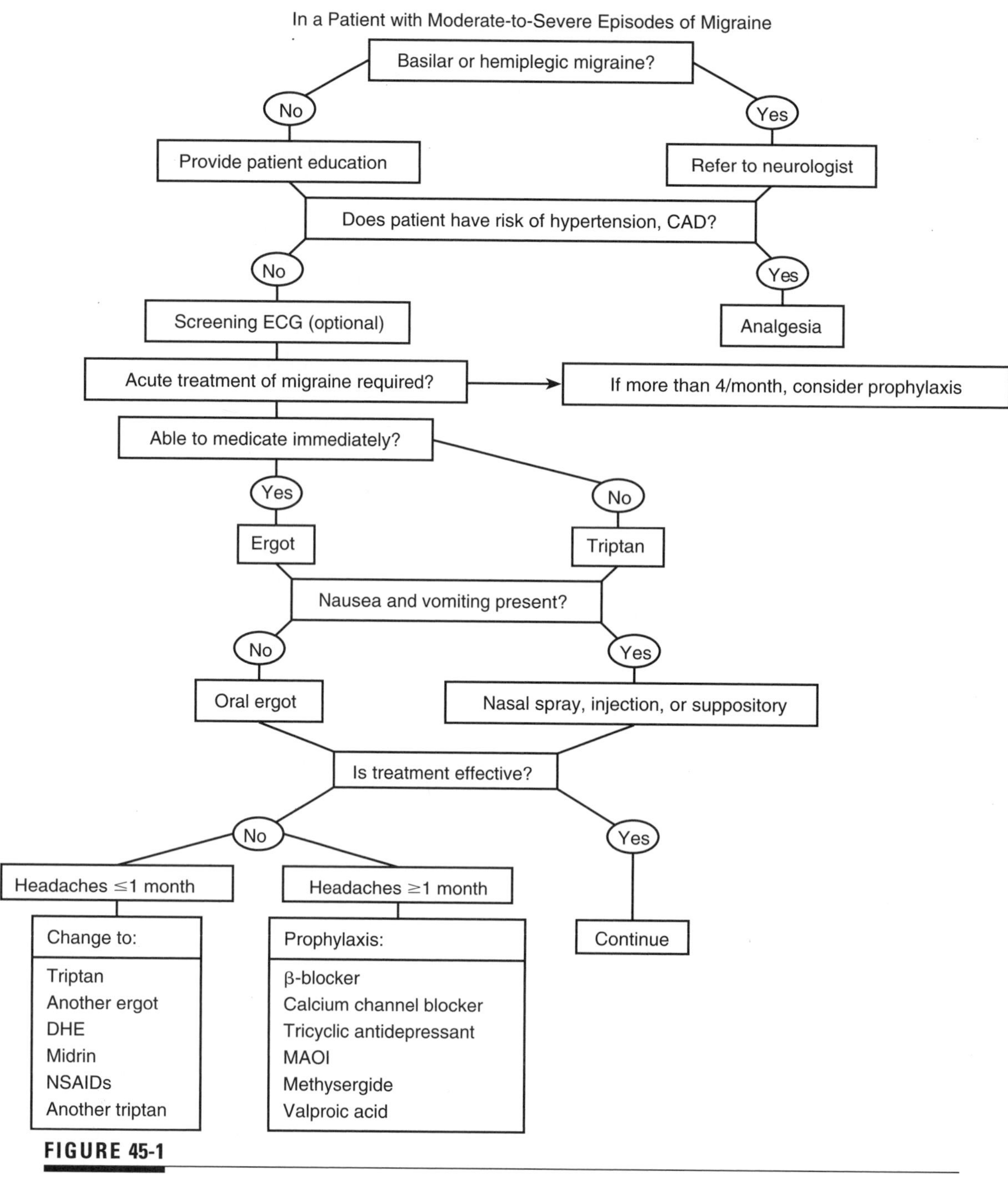

FIGURE 45-1

Critical decision making in the treatment of migraines.

migraines. In general, triptans have fewer adverse reactions. However, they are expensive. Ergotamine formulations are effective and cost less than the triptans. If the patient is able to take medication at the earliest onset of the headache, ergots will usually be effective. If a patient wakes up with the headache or has difficulty "catching the headache in time," a triptan will be more effective. All triptan and ergotamine drugs have the same cardiovascular cautions.

Although all triptans are similar, it is possible that there are differences in patient response. One might be more effective than another for a particular patient. Zolmitriptan and rizatriptan are lipid soluble, which facilitates its penetration of the blood-brain barrier. Duration of action may become an issue for patients with long-lasting or recurring migraines. Frovatriptan has a half-life of 26 hours and has a recurrence rate as low as 7%. Often, choice of formulation will determine the medication prescribed. Imitrex has a new formulation that, when swallowed whole, dissolves like Alka-Seltzer, and begins to work in 15 minutes.

Isometheptene is a mild ergotamine that is safe and effective for mild migraines. It is an over-the-counter (OTC) drug. It does not have the adverse effects commonly associated with ergotamines. Ergotamine tartrate is seldom used any more because of the increased risk of adverse reactions. It has been used for migraines of long duration, but newer triptans have a longer half-life. DHE is increasingly being used for severe migraines. It is safer because of the decrease in arterial vasoconstriction and produces relief reliably and quickly.

Mild-to-Moderate Migraines. Analgesics such as aspirin, NSAIDs, or a combination product are commonly used. Excedrin Migraine (aspirin, acetaminophen, and caffeine) is an approved migraine treatment drug available on an OTC basis. NSAIDs are commonly used. Naproxen and ibuprofen are effective; indomethacin is also highly effective.

Isometheptene is generally used on an OTC basis by patients who have not seen a primary care provider. It is found in an OTC combination product called Midrin (65 mg isometheptene, 100 mg dichloralphenazone, and 325 mg acetaminophen). It is not as effective as other OTC medications and has potentially serious adverse effects. Patients should be instructed to use drugs listed in the preceding paragraph.

Nausea and Vomiting. Administer migraine medication in nasal spray or injection formulation. Nasal spray is very easy to use and quite effective for mild to moderate migraines. Antiemetics commonly used include prochlorperazine (Compazine), promethazine (Phenergan), and trimethobenzamide (Tigan). Metoclopramide (Reglan) has the added effect of speeding up absorption of other drugs and is being used with aspirin for mild-to-moderate migraines. Although it appears to be the most effective antiemetic, it has potentially serious adverse reactions (see Chapter 31).

Moderate-to-Severe Migraines. Triptans are first-line drugs and are generally very effective. Ergotamine tartrate may be used if triptans are not effective. DHE is very effective for severe migraine and is available as nasal spray or intramuscular or subcutaneous injection for the treatment of moderate-to-severe migraine. It has a quick response and low recurrence rate. It should be tried if triptan drugs have not been adequate.

Migraine Recurrence. Migraines may recur within 24 hours after initial response to medication in 30% to 40% of patients. Consider giving a long-acting triptan such as frovatriptan.

Severe Migraine. Consider injection of a triptan or DHE; these are generally very effective. If these are not effective, there are rescue medications. Corticosteroids should be administered intravenously, intramuscularly, or orally at 2 to 4 mg bid for 2 days and tapered over 3 more days, one event per month. Opioids can be used for patients who have infrequent but severe migraines.

Prophylactic Medications

Prophylactic medications are typically used when sufferers experience more than two or three attacks each month that do not respond adequately to abortive medication. These products will not completely eliminate migraine headaches but will decrease their frequency, intensity, and duration.

Select a medication that has a low adverse effect profile and is compatible with the patient's coexisting conditions. Use once-daily dosage if possible to improve compliance. Start slowly and gradually increase dose until headaches are relieved or patient has adverse reaction. Give a drug an adequate trial of at least 2 to 6 months. Consider tapering medication if headaches are well controlled at 6 months.

First-line prophylactic agents in the treatment of migraine are β-blockers. These agents produce a reduction of headache frequency and severity in 60% to 80% of cases. Propranolol or timolol is most commonly used. Gradually increase dosages to minimize adverse reactions. Three to 4 weeks of therapy is required to evaluate effectiveness. These agents may aggravate neurologic symptoms associated with hemiplegic or basilar migraine.

Second-line agents include calcium channel blockers. They decrease headache frequency, intensity, and duration in 40% to 60% of migraineurs. Verapamil is most commonly used. Clinical improvement may not be seen for 4 to 6 weeks after initiation of therapy. Tolerance may develop. Calcium channel antagonists may be used in patients who cannot tolerate β-blockers or those who have complicated migraine.

The TCAs are also used in the prophylactic treatment of migraines. Amitriptyline is considered first line; the others are considered second line. They provide sedation and stabilization of the sleep cycle, a common problem with migraineurs. Amitriptyline, doxepin, nortriptyline, and imipramine are the more sedating TCAs. Less sedating TCAs include protriptyline and desipramine. Tricyclics are rapid acting, providing benefit to 60% of individuals in 10 to 14 days. Dosages required for migraine are lower than those needed for mood disorders.

SSRIs considered third-line treatment. They are less effective than TCAs. Fluvoxamine and paroxetine have been the most researched.

The anticonvulsants divalproex, gabapentin, and topiramate have been used. Divalproex has been the most researched. These are used for severe migraines.

Methysergide is fourth-line treatment because of its potential long-term fibroprolific side effects caused by fibroblastic activity in connective tissue. It is no longer in common use. This drug is helpful in approximately 60% of cases. Before initiation of therapy, patients require a thorough cardiovascular screening to rule out problems that would contraindicate use of the drug.

HOW TO MONITOR

Patient should keep a headache diary to document frequency and severity of headaches and to help identify triggers. This should be reviewed at regular intervals with the health care provider.

Monitor cardiovascular status when using triptans or ergots.

methysergide

Baseline cardiovascular assessment should be completed that includes assessment of blood pressure, peripheral pulses, heart and lung sounds, and ECG. Cardiovascular status should be reassessed at 1- to 2-month intervals for 6 months, followed by a month-long drug holiday. After 1 year of treatment, an echocardiogram and an abdominal computed tomography scan with and without contrast should be obtained to rule out the possibility of fibrotic changes of the heart valves or retroperitoneal fibrosis. Chest x-ray examination should also be performed to establish pulmonary fibrotic changes.

cyproheptadine

Liver function studies should be obtained at regular intervals. Patient's weight should be checked and monitored for abnormal weight gain. Questions concerning the anticholinergic side effects such as dry eyes, dry mouth, constipation, urinary retention, and excessive drowsiness should be included in general follow-up assessment. Effectiveness of cyproheptadine is apparent within 3 weeks after initiation of treatment.

PATIENT VARIABLES

Geriatrics

- Use all products with caution as the elderly are more susceptible to adverse effects than are younger patients.
- Migraines are very rare in geriatrics; suspect an intracranial lesion.

Pediatrics

- Children's migraines frequently last less than 2 hours.
- Safety and efficacy have not been established.
- Cyproheptadine is used for prophylaxis; use under age 2 is contraindicated.
- Sumatriptan has been used in children older than 5 years but does not have the indication.

Pregnancy

- *Category B:* cyproheptadine
- *Category C:* triptans; may be secreted in milk
- *Category X:* ergotamines, methysergide; these drugs should not be used in women who are likely to become pregnant.

Gender

- Two thirds of migraineurs are female; one third are male.
- The frequency and severity of migraines occasionally decrease in postmenopausal women.

PATIENT EDUCATION

Extensive education is necessary so these patients can make decisions and manage their headaches as they happen:

- Use a product no more than twice a week to avoid rebound headaches.
- Patient should be instructed on how to use the medication, particularly with nasal sprays and injections.
- Avoid alcohol with these medications.
- Report adverse symptoms.

Prophylactic Agents

Patients should take the product daily regardless of whether they have symptoms.

It often takes weeks to months to determine the efficacy of specific products.

Specific Drugs

ABORTIVE AGENTS

Triptans

Ⓟ Prototype Drug

sumatriptan (Imitrex)

Contraindications

- Hypersensitivity
- Significant cardiovascular disease: CAD, strokes, transients ischemic attacks, uncontrolled hypertension, peripheral vascular disease, ischemic bowel disease
- Basilar artery, hemiplegic, or complicated migraine
- Concomitant use of monoamine oxidase inhibitors, ergots, or SSRIs
- Individuals under 18 years of age
- Pregnancy

Warnings

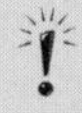

Risk of myocardial ischemia or infarction and other adverse cardiac events; these agents have a potential to cause coronary vasospasm. Do not give to patients with cardiac risk factors unless a cardiovascular evaluation shows no underlying disease. Give first dose in office with adequate medical equipment; consider obtaining an ECG during administration. Ventricular fibrillation/tachycardia and myocardial infarction have occurred.

- Cerebrovascular events and fatalities: cerebral hemorrhage, subarachnoid hemorrhage, stroke, and other cerebrovascular events have been reported
- Markedly increased blood pressure, including hypertensive crisis, has been reported
- Nasal spray may cause local irritation
- Hypersensitivity reactions are rare, but severe anaphylaxis reactions have occurred
- Renal function impairment: use rizatriptan and sumatriptan with caution
- Hepatic function impairment: administer with caution; dose may need to be decreased
- Carcinogenesis and impaired fertility have been observed in animal studies

Precautions

- Chest, jaw, or neck tightness has occurred after administration; monitor for angina
- Seizures have occurred rarely
- Ophthalmic effects: bind to melanin; can accumulate over time; causes corneal effects in animals
- Photosensitivity may occur

Pharmacokinetics

Table 45-3 compares all migraine products.

TABLE 45-3 Pharmacokinetics of Migraine Products

Drug	Absorption and Drug Availability	Onset of Action	Time to Peak Concentration	Half-Life	Duration of Action	Protein Bound	Metabolism	Excretion
sumatriptan								
Injectable (Imitrex)	97% Available	<2 hr	12 min	13-17 min	100-135 min	15%	Liver	Renal, 60%; feces, 40%
Oral	Rapid; 14% available	<2-2.5 hr	2.5 hr	2	Standard*	15%	Liver	Renal, 60%; feces, 40%
Nasal spray		15-30 min			Less	15%	Liver	Renal, 60%; feces, 40%
naratriptan (Amerge)	70% Available	2-3 hr	2 hr	5-6 hr	Longer	30%	Liver	Renal, 70%
rizatriptan (Maxalt/MLT)	40% Available	30-120 min	1 hr	2 hr	Longer	14%	Liver	Renal, 70%; feces, 30%
zolmitriptan (Zomig)	49% after first pass			2.8-3.7 hr		25%		Urine, 60%-80%; feces, 20%-40%
almotriptan	80%	<2 hr		3.5 hr	Longer			
frovatriptan	30%	2-3 hr		2.5 hr	Longest			
eletriptan (Relpax)	Well	<2 hr	1.5 hr	4 hr	24 hr			Renal; 70%
ergotamine tartrate								
Tablets	<1%	30 min	70 min		24 hr		Liver	Feces
Suppositories	Good			2 hr	24 hr		Liver	Feces
DHE 45								
Injection	50% Available	15-30 min		21-32 hr	3-4 hr	90%	Liver	Biliary, 90%; renal, 10%
Migranal	Variable	<2 hr		10		93%	Liver	Feces
methysergide (Sansert)		1-2 days		10 hr	1-2 days	13%-22%	Liver	Renal
cyproheptadine		30-60 min			8-12 hr			Renal, 65%-75%; feces, 25%-35%

*Standard: duration of action of triptans are compared to sumatriptan.

Adverse Effects

See Table 45-4.

Drug Interactions

- Cimetidine increases drug levels of zolmitriptan.
- Ketoconazole increases levels of almotriptan.
- Oral contraceptives increase levels of frovatriptan.
- Propranolol increases levels of rizatriptan and frovatriptan.
- Sibutramine increases levels of naratriptan, sumatriptan, zolmitriptan, and rizatriptan.
- Triptans increase levels of SSRIs.

Overdosage

Symptoms to be expected are hypertension and other more serious cardiovascular symptoms.

Dosage and Administration

See Table 45-5.

Patient should take initial dose at first sign of migraine. If first dose is not effective, patient may repeat dosage once, generally after 2 hours. Patient should repeat with same dosage as initial dose. With the next migraine, patient may start with higher dose if first dose was ineffective. No more triptan should be used within that 24-hour period.

TABLE 45-4 Common and Serious Adverse Effects of Migraine Medications

Drug	Common Minor Reactions	Serious Adverse Effects
Serotonin (5-HT_1) receptor agonists (triptans)	Dizziness, fatigue, pain, warm sensation, headache, flushing, hot or cold sensation, erythema, pruritus, chest or neck tightness, nausea, dry mouth, paresthesia, asthenia, somnolence	Chest pain, coronary artery vasospasm, MI, myocardial ischemia, ventricular fibrillation/tachycardia, agitation, TIA, seizure, elevated blood pressure
isometheptene	Transient dizziness and skin rash, drowsiness	Feeling of weakness
ergotamine tartrate	Localized edema, drowsiness, dry mouth, dizziness, nausea, vomiting	Peripheral vascular effects (numbness, tingling), tachycardia, weakness in legs
DHE	Dizziness, somnolence, paresthesia, nausea, vomiting *Nasal spray:* altered sense of taste, rhinitis	*Injection:* serious cardiac events including vasospasm, MI, ventricular fibrillation/tachycardia, fibrotic complications
methysergide	Nausea, vomiting, diarrhea, weight gain, insomnia, drowsiness, dizziness, abdominal pain	Arterial spasm, peripheral ischemia, possible MI, fibrotic complications, edema, claudication, seizure, hallucinations, severe myalgias
cyproheptadine	Sedation, weight gain, GI upset, palpitations, dryness of mucous membranes, dizziness	Hypotension, increased heart rate, urinary frequency or retention, restlessness

TABLE 45-5 Dosage and Administration Recommendations of Migraine Medications

Drug	Formulation	Dosage	Administration	Maximum Dosage in 24 hr
sumatriptan	Tablets: 25, 50, 100 mg Nasal spray: 5 mg/spray Injection	25, 50, 100 mg 5, 10, 20 mg 6 sq	q2hr One puff each nostril q2hr One injection, repeat in 1 hr	200 mg 40 mg 12 mg
naratriptan	Tablets: 1, 2.5 mg	2.5 mg	q4hr (May repeat ×1)	5 mg
rizatriptan	Tablets: 5, 10 mg Orally disintegrating tablets: 2.5, 5, 10 mg	5 mg 5 mg 2.5 mg	q2hr q2hr q2hr (May repeat ×1)	30 mg 30 mg 10 mg
zolmitriptan	Tablets: 2.5, 5 mg	2.5, 5 mg	q2hr (May repeat ×1)	10 mg
almotriptan	Tablets: 6.25, 12.5 mg	6.25 mg	q2hr (May repeat ×1)	25 mg
eletriptan	Tablets: 20, 40 mg	40 mg	q2hr (May repeat ×1)	80 mg in 24 hr
frovatriptan	Tablets: 2.5 mg	2.5 mg	q2hr (May repeat ×1)	7.5 mg
isometheptene	Caplets, combination Injection: 1 mg/ml	1-2 caplet(s) 1 ml IV, IM, SC	1 caplet qhr q1hr bid	5 caplets 3 mg IM or SC
ergotamine tartrate	Tablets, sublingual	2 mg	q30min bid	6 mg/day
DHE	Nasal spray: 4 mg/ml, 0.5 mg/spray	One spray each nostril	q15min	3 mg
methysergide	N/A			
cyproheptadine	Tablets: 4 mg 2 mg/5 ml solution	8 mg	2 μg bid-qid in divided doses	24 mg

Patients should administer a triptan no more than 2 days per week. There must be a 24-hour hiatus between the use of this medicine and an ergot or methysergide.

The most commonly used formulation is the tablet. Nasal spray will work if the patient has nausea and vomiting that interfere with absorption of a tablet. The orally disintegrating tablets dissolve on the tongue, requiring no water. This makes it a very convenient dosing system. Patients with severe migraines prefer injection formulation as it has the fastest onset of action. Injection is generally given in the thigh.

The initial dose, whether oral, nasal spray, or subcutaneous injection, should be administered in the office so that the provider can monitor blood pressure and pulse. The provider should also be present to answer questions about any side effects that may occur.

The newest drug, eletriptan, is a potent CYP 3A4 inhibitor. Concentration of eletriptan may increase up to fourfold if given with ketoconazole, itraconazole, clarithromycin, erythromycin, or nefazodone. Research suggests faster headache relief and less headache recurrence with this drug as compared to other triptans.

Ergots

Ⓟ Prototype Drug

ergotamine tartrate (Cafergot)

Contraindications

- Coronary heart disease or coronary artery vasospasm, uncontrolled hypertension, impaired hepatic or renal function, hemiplegic or basilar migraine, and concomitant use with peripheral and central vasoconstrictors.
- In pregnancy and in women who may become pregnant, uterine stimulant actions may cause fetal harm.
- Do not use ergots within 24 hours of using triptans or methysergide.

Warnings

- Possible vasospastic reaction may occur with the use of ergots; the clinician and patient should be aware of the signs and symptoms of such vascular changes.

! Overuse of ergot agents may lead to ergotism. Manifestations include symptoms of intense arterial vasoconstriction with evidence of peripheral vascular ischemia, headache, intermittent claudication, muscle pain, numbness, coldness, and pallor of the extremities. If the condition progresses, gangrene may occur.

- Vasospasm-related events include peripheral vascular ischemia and Raynaud's phenomenon.
- Increased blood pressure may occur.

Precautions

- Do not exceed recommended dosage.
- Drug abuse and dependence may occur with extended use.

Drug Interactions

- β-Blocker, nicotine, and sibutramine will increase adverse effects of ergots.
- Ergots will increase the effect of triptans and vasoconstrictors.

Overdosage

Most effects of overdose are related to ergotamine as opposed to caffeine. Effects include vomiting, numbness, tingling, pain or cyanosis of the extremities, decrease or absence of pulses, hypotension or hypertension, drowsiness, stupor, coma, or shock.

Dosage and Administration

See Table 45-5.

Have the patient self-administer the preparation in a lower-than-recommended dose when headache free. Dosing should be increased gradually to recommended levels until this dose is achieved or patients are troubled with side effects. The most common side effect is nausea.

Other Drugs in Class

Other drugs in this class are similar to the prototype except as follows.

isometheptene mucate (Midrin)

Contraindications. Glaucoma, severe renal disease, hypertension, organic heart disease, hepatic disease, and concomitant use with monoamine oxidase inhibitors

Warnings. *CNS effects:* The capsules contain 100 mg dichloralphenazone, which is structural similar to chlorohydrate. There is risk of CNS depressant effects. Caution patients to use caution in tasks requiring metal alertness. Caution about possible combined effects with alcohol and other CNS depressant drugs. There is a theoretical risk of dependence.

Precautions. Use with caution in patients with hypertension and peripheral vascular disease and after recent cardiovascular attacks.

Drug Interactions. Do not give with monoamine oxidase inhibitors because it could lead to hypertensive crisis.

dihydroergotamine (DHE-45, Migranal)

Contraindications. Life-threatening peripheral ischemia has been associated with the coadministration of DHE with potent CYP 3A4 inhibitors, including protease inhibitors, ketoconazole, and macrolide antibiotics. Concurrent use is contraindicated.

Warnings. Fibrotic complications: pleural and retroperitoneal fibrosis following prolonged daily use of injectable DHE.

Risk of myocardial ischemia and/or myocardial infarction and other adverse cardiac events: do not use in patient with documented ischemic or vasospastic CAD. Do not give to patients with cardiac risk factors unless a cardiovascular evaluation shows no underlying disease. Give first dose in adequately equipped office. Obtain ECG during administration.

Drug-associated cerebrovascular events and fatalities: cerebral hemorrhage, subarachnoid hemorrhage, stroke, and other cerebrovascular events have been reported.

Local irritation can occur.

Drug Interactions

- Metabolized by CYP 3A4 system, will interact with other drugs metabolized by the 3A4 system.
- Ingestion with grapefruit will increase the serum levels.
- DHE will decrease the therapeutic effect of nitrates.

Dosage and Administration. See Table 45-5.

Nasal treatment: prime pump before administration by squeezing four times. Discard unused drug in opened ampule after 8 hours.

PROPHYLACTIC AGENTS

methysergide (Sansert)

Contraindications. Uncontrolled hypertension; heart murmur; peripheral, cerebral, or cardiovascular disease; deep vein thrombosis; severe arteriosclerosis; renal/hepatic disease; previous fibrotic changes; pregnancy; and collagen diseases.

Warnings/Precautions

- Monitor for fibrotic changes through vigilant cardiovascular examination and diagnostic testing. Symptoms may include urinary tract obstruction, general malaise, and elevated erythrocyte sedimentation rate with low-grade fever.
- Patients should be seen by the health care provider regularly to monitor for the development of fibrotic or vascular complications.

Drug Interactions. Methysergide used with ergots or triptans may increase coronary vasospasm. Use with other vasoconstrictors will augment the effect. At least 24 hours should elapse between the last dose of methysergide and the institution of ergot or triptan therapy.

Overdosage. Symptoms include euphoria, hyperactivity, tachycardia, dilated pupils, and dizziness. Evidence of ischemia may be present.

cyproheptadine (Periactin)

Contraindications

- Contraindications include elderly, debilitated patients or those with angle-closure glaucoma, prostatic hypertrophy, stenosing peptic ulcer, or bladder neck obstruction
- Do not use in children under 2 years

Warnings/Precautions

- Overdose in children may produce hallucinations, CNS depression, convulsions, or death
- Sedation is common
- Children may experience excitement, restlessness, insomnia, and seizures
- The drug may produce an atropine-like action, so it must be used with caution in patients treated for bronchial asthma, increased intraocular pressure, hyperthyroidism, cerebral vascular disease, or hypertension

Drug Interactions. This product produces additive sedating effects with alcohol, other CNS depressants, hypnotics, sedatives, tranquilizers, or anxiolytic drugs. Monoamine oxidase inhibitors may intensify the anticholinergic effects of antihistamine.

Overdosage. Signs and symptoms may vary from CNS depression to stimulation, especially in children. A dry mouth, fixed dilated pupils, and GI symptoms are seen. Vomiting should be induced, followed by gastric lavage.

BIBLIOGRAPHY

Clinch CR: Evaluation of acute headaches in adults, *Am Family Physician* 63:685-692, 2001.

Church EJ, Odle TG: Diagnosis and treatment of migraines, *Radiol Technol* 74:281-314, 2003.

Cottrell C et al: Perceptions and needs of patients with migraine: a focus group study, *Headache* 43:428, 2003.

Deleu D, Hanssens Y: Eletriptan vs sumatriptan: a double-blind, placebo-controlled, multiple migraine attack study, *Neurology* 60:1221-1222, 2003.

Diener HC et al: A practice guide to the management and prevention of migraine, *Drugs* 56:811, 1998.

Fox A et al: Migraine management in primary care: focus on the triptans, *Clin News Suppl* March 2002.

Goadsby PJ et al: Drug therapy: migraine—current understanding and treatment, *N Engl J Med* 346:257-270, 2002.

Headache Classification Committee of the International Headache Society: Classification and diagnostic criteria for headache disorders, cranial neuralgias, and facial pain, *Cephalgia* 8(suppl 7):279, 1988.

Miller VA et al: Migraine headaches and sleep disturbances in children, *Headache* 43:362-368, 2003.

Rainero I et al: A comparison of familial and sporadic migraine in a headache clinic population, *Funct Neurol* 17:193-197, 2002.

Smith MS et al: Comparative study of anxiety, depression, somatization, functional disability, and illness attribution in adolescents with chronic fatigue or migraine, *Pediatrics* 111(4 pt 1):376-381, 2003.

Wenzel RG, Sarvis CA, Krause ML: Over-the-counter drugs for acute migraine attacks: literature review and recommendations, *Pharmacotherapy* 23:494-505, 2003.

CHAPTER 46

Anticonvulsants

V. Inez Wendel

Drug Names

Class	Subclass	Generic Name	Trade Name
Hydantoin		(200) phenytoin	Dilantin
Succinimide		ethosuximide	Zarontin
GABA analogs		(P)(200) valproic acid	Depakene
		divalproex sodium	Depakote
		felbamate	Felbatol
		(200) gabapentin	Neurontin
		lamotrigine	Lamictal
		tiagabine	Gabatril
		topiramate	Topamax
		zonisamide	Zonegran
Miscellaneous		carbamazepine	Tegretol
		oxcarbazepine	Trileptal
		levetiracetam	Keppra
Barbiturates		(P)(200) phenobarbital	Luminal
		primidone	Mysoline
Benzodiazepines		diazepam	Valium
		lorazepam	Ativan
		clonazepam	Klonopin
Diuretics		acetazolamide	Diamox

(200), Top 200 drug; (P), prototype drug.

General Uses

Indications (Table 46-1)

- Simple partial seizures
- Complex partial seizures
- Secondarily generalized seizures
- Generalized tonic-clonic seizures
- Absence seizures

There are four major classes of anticonvulsants. Anticonvulsants or *antiepileptic drugs* (AEDs) are terms for the medications used to control seizures. These classes include hydantoins, γ-aminobutyric acid (GABA) analogs, succinimides, and a miscellaneous class. Barbiturates, benzodiazepines, and the diuretic, acetazolamide, are also used adjunctively to manage seizures. These medications may be used alone or in combination. Some of the newer AEDs are approved for adjunctive use only. These medications are unrelated chemically. In general, neurologists manage seizure disorders. The primary care provider often monitors patients once they are stable. The newer anticonvulsants are increasingly being used for peripheral neuropathy and pain management.

Most anticonvulsants are cytochrome P450 inducers and, as such, are involved in many drug–drug interactions.

DISEASE PROCESS

The Disease and Pathophysiology

A *seizure* is an alteration in behavior, function, and/or consciousness that results from an abnormal electrical discharge of neurons in the brain. Epilepsy, or the term *seizure disorder*, is used to describe chronic recurrent seizures. Seizures are classified according to clinical presentation and electroencephalographic (EEG) characteristics. The International Classification of Seizures by the Commission on Classification and Terminology of the International League Against Epilepsy is summarized in Table 46-2. The treatment of seizure disorder depends on the type of seizure; thus the correct diagnosis of seizure disorder is imperative. Drugs appear in the table in the order usually initiated for the type of seizure.

A seizure is a symptom of an underlying brain disorder, not a disease itself. However, the etiology of most seizure disorders is unknown. Underlying pathologic conditions, such as tumor, subarachnoid hemorrhage, or hematoma, must be ruled out.

TABLE 46-1 Anticonvulsants and Their Uses

Drug	Approved Uses	Unlabeled Uses
phenytoin	Monotherapy and combination therapy for partial and generalized seizure Used parenterally for control of status epilepticus Prevention and treatment of seizures occurring during neurosurgery	Trigeminal neuralgia Parenterally for preeclampsia Antiarrhythmic
ethosuximide	Drug of choice for absence seizures	
valproic acid	Monotherapy or adjunctive therapy for absence and complex partial seizures Manic episodes associated with bipolar disorder Prophylaxis for migraine headaches	May be effective as monotherapy and combination therapy for all seizure types, including generalized Intractable status epilepticus
felbamate	Only in those with severe seizure for whom other therapies have failed Monotherapy or adjunctive therapy for partial seizures with or without generalization	Generalized seizure disorders
gabapentin	Adjunctive therapy for partial seizures with or without generalization in patients >12 yr Adjunctive therapy for partial seizures in children 3-12 yr	Neuropathic pain, peripheral neuropathy Bipolar disorder Migraine prophylaxis Tremors associated with multiple sclerosis
lamotrigine	Monotherapy and adjunctive therapy for partial seizure disorders in adults Patients with Lennox-Gestaut syndrome >2 yr	Generalized seizure disorders Neuropathic and chronic pain syndromes Bipolar disorder
tiagabine	Adjunctive therapy for partial seizures in patients >12 yr	
topiramate	Adjunctive therapy for partial and generalized seizure disorders for patients >2 yr	Neuropathic and chronic pain syndromes Weight loss Monotherapy for seizure disorders Cluster headaches
zonisamide	Adjunctive therapy for partial seizures in adults	Generalized seizure disorders
carbamazepine	Monotherapy and combination therapy for partial and general seizure disorders Trigeminal neuralgia Do not use in absence seizures	Chronic pain, restless leg syndrome, psychiatric disorders including bipolar disorder treatment of alcohol, benzodiazepine, or cocaine withdrawal
oxcarbazepine	Monotherapy and adjunctive therapy for partial seizure disorder in adults Adjunctive therapy for partial seizure disorder in children >4 yr	Atypical panic disorder Neuropathic and other chronic pain syndromes
levetiracetam	Adjunctive therapy for partial seizures in adults	
phenobarbital	Tonic-clonic and partial seizures often in combination with other anticonvulsants Prevention of febrile seizures in children	Not for myoclonic and generalized absence seizures
Benzodiazepines (lorazepam, diazepam)	IV for status epilepticus, acute seizure for drug overdose and poisons	

Not all behaviors that appear to be seizure activity are seizures. The differential diagnosis for the patient presenting with history of "seizure" is lengthy. The practitioner must consider systemic, neurologic, and behavioral conditions that may cause altered consciousness or behavior; this includes syncope, hypoglycemia, cardiac arrhythmias, transient ischemic attacks, narcolepsy, psychogenic seizures, and attention deficit disorder. New-onset idiopathic epilepsy would be unusual in the elderly; they are more likely to have an underlying pathologic condition or metabolic disorder. The most frequent presentation of a seizure is by a patient with a known seizure disorder who fails to take adequate suppressive medication.

Assessment

Make sure the episode is actually a seizure. Next, determine the cause of the seizure. Rule out metabolic disorders, trauma,

TABLE 46-2 Seizure Classification and Recommended Medication Therapy

Seizure Type	Description	Drug*
Simple partial	Focal motor or sensory symptoms, reflects area of brain affected; no change in consciousness	phenytoin carbamazepine valproic acid phenobarbital
Complex partial	Characterized by an aura, followed by impaired consciousness with automatisms, usually originating from temporal lobe	carbamazepine phenytoin phenobarbital valproic acid
Secondarily generalized	Simple or complex partial seizures that progress to generalized tonic-clonic seizures	phenytoin carbamazepine phenobarbital valproic acid
Generalized tonic-clonic	Formerly "grand mal"; sudden loss of consciousness with tonic-clonic motor activity, postictal state of confusion, drowsiness, and headache	phenytoin carbamazepine phenobarbital valproic acid
Absence	Formerly "petit mal"; brief (<30 seconds) episodes of unresponsiveness characterized by staring, blinking, or facial twitching	ethosuximide valproic acid clonazepam

* Listed in order recommended for use.

tumors or other space-occupying lesions, vascular disease, degenerative disorders, or infectious disease.

DRUG ACTION AND EFFECTS

For most of these drugs, the exact mechanism for reducing seizure activity is not clearly understood. They all increase the threshold of the central nervous system (CNS) to convulsive stimuli or inhibit the spread of seizure activity. Specific mechanisms of action are discussed for each class.

Hydantoins

The primary site of action appears to be the primary motor cortex, where spread of seizure activity is inhibited. Phenytoin prolongs the effective refractory period relative to the action potential duration. It stabilizes the threshold against hyperexcitability caused by excessive stimulation or environmental changes and reduces the maximal activity of brainstem centers responsible for the tonic phase of grand mal seizures. It also exhibits antiarrhythmic properties, similar to those of quinidine or procainamide. Although it has little effect on the electrical excitability of cardiac muscle, it decreases the force of contraction, depresses pacemaker action, and improves atrioventricular conduction, particularly when it has been depressed by digitalis glycosides.

GABA Analogs

The mechanism of action of valproic acid and the newer GABA analogs is not clearly understood. All of these drugs are chemically unrelated, but they all increase the brain level of GABA, an inhibitory neurotransmitter. They may inhibit the voltage-dependent sodium channel and thereby stabilize the neuronal membranes.

carbamazepine

Carbamazepine is chemically similar to the tricyclic antidepressants. It is unrelated structurally to the other anticonvulsants. Its action is similar to that of phenytoin; it limits seizure propagation by blocking postsynaptic transmission.

Barbiturates

The mechanism of action may be reduction of monosynaptic and polysynaptic transmission, resulting in decreased excitability of the entire nerve. Barbiturates also increase the threshold for electrical stimulation of the motor cortex. Primidone, an analog of phenobarbital, and its metabolites, phenobarbital and phenylethylmalonamide (PEMA), have anticonvulsant activity. PEMA may potentiate the activity of phenobarbital.

Benzodiazepines

Benzodiazepines suppress the spread of seizure activity but do not abolish the abnormal discharge from a focus. After termination of seizures, maintenance anticonvulsant therapy should be initiated.

DRUG TREATMENT PRINCIPLES

The decision to initiate anticonvulsant therapy must be made with consideration of several variables; most important are the consequences of seizure recurrence to the patient. These consequences are mainly psychosocial and may depend on age, employment, family responsibility, and access to transportation. The decision about drug therapy is best made in consultation with the primary care practitioner, the neurologist, the patient, and the family.

Discontinuation of anticonvulsant medication may be considered in patients who have been seizure free for longer than 2 years. An EEG should be obtained before withdrawal of medication. The recurrence rate is usually about 40%, with most seizures occurring in the first year after medication is discontinued. The same psychosocial factors and risks of seizure reoccurrence for the individual patient should be considered when withdrawing anticonvulsants as when initiating therapy.

There is no evidence that prophylactic anticonvulsant treatment prevents epilepsy. It is common practice to give an anticonvulsant, usually phenytoin, at the time of neurosurgery, and after head trauma. Most survivors of brain surgery or head trauma do not later develop epilepsy. The use of phenytoin at therapeutic doses during the week after severe head trauma does suppress seizures. This treatment is appropriate at that time when the brain is swollen and cerebral blood flow may be compromised. A seizure could further compromise cerebral blood and lead to increased swelling and intracranial pressure. The same can be applied to the perioperative period. However, there is no evidence that anticonvulsants prevent later epilepsy; therefore it is not necessary to maintain these patients on long-term anticonvulsants.

A seizure is usually self-limiting and generally causes no physical harm from the seizure activity itself. However, SE is a medical emergency; the primary practitioner must be prepared to recognize and manage this emergency. For practical purposes, SE is defined as two or more seizures without complete recovery of neurologic function between seizures or as continuous seizure activity for longer than 30 minutes. Therapy should be initiated for any generalized tonic-clonic convulsive seizure activity (formerly called grand mal). Most generalized convulsive seizures last less than 2 minutes. Thus the practitioner who witnesses generalized convulsive seizures for longer than 2 minutes should be prepared to initiate emergency procedures. This should include activating emergency medical services, such as calling 911, and protecting the airway. Emergency personnel should initiate intravenous access and administer intravenous benzodiazepines (lorazepam or diazepam) as protocols permit.

The goal of medical treatment is to control the seizures and allow patients to return to their usual activities. This should ideally be done with a single medication with no significant side effects. This is achieved with about two thirds of patients.

The medication to use depends on the type of seizure (see Tables 46-1 and 46-2). A neurologist generally makes this decision. The medication is started at a low dose and gradually increased until the seizures are controlled or the patient exhibits adverse effects. If the patient continues to experience seizures despite the highest tolerated dose, a second drug is added gradually. Then the first drug is gradually withdrawn.

Phenobarbital is effective for the prevention of febrile seizures in children, although long-term prophylactic treatment of febrile seizures is controversial. The risk/benefit ratio must be carefully assessed. In general, treatment is reserved for those children at greatest risk for future neurologic problems because of seizures; this includes children with febrile seizures before 18 months of age, those with neurologic dysfunction or severe developmental delays, and those with complex seizures or those who have seizures with a focal component that last longer than 15 minutes. Prophylactic treatment should also be considered for any child whose family member has a history of febrile seizures.

HOW TO MONITOR

The patient beginning anticonvulsant therapy must be monitored frequently to confirm drug is in the therapeutic range, for adverse events, and for seizure control. Therapeutic levels of different drugs are given in Table 46-3.

These drugs have individual therapeutic ranges, above which most patients will experience toxic effects. If the therapeutic range is too low, most patients will not have adequate seizure control. However, there will be individuals who may do better with drug levels above or below the therapeutic range. Monitoring of serum drug levels usually needs to be done yearly on the patient being maintained on an anticonvulsant. A serum level should be checked when there is an increase in seizure frequency, if compliance is an issue, or if the patient is exhibiting toxic signs. Many medications interact with the metabolism of the anticonvulsants; therefore a serum level of the anticonvulsant should be checked when there are medication changes. Ideally a trough level should be drawn for routine monitoring. A random level should be drawn when seizures occur. Anticonvulsant drugs have long half-lives, so once steady state is achieved on a maintenance dose, there should be little fluctuation in serum levels.

These antiseizure drugs are metabolized by the liver. Hepatic enzymes should be checked before initiating anticonvulsant therapy. It is common for hepatic enzymes to be mildly elevated in those on anticonvulsants. They should be monitored yearly and more frequently in patients with known hepatic dysfunction. Children under 10 years of age who are on valproic acid should be monitored closely for hepatotoxicity.

The practitioner must inform the patient and assess for adverse or toxic effects. The most common reactions are rash, visual disturbances, drowsiness, and ataxia. Adverse and toxic effects specific to the individual drugs are discussed later (Table 46-4).

Abnormal thyroid function tests have been reported in patients on anticonvulsants. The clinical significance of this is unknown.

Agranulocytosis is rare but has been associated with use of carbamazepine, ethosuximide, and felbamate. Baseline and periodic blood counts should be performed; the interval between checks can be less frequent when the dose is stable. If febrile illness or anorexia occurs, blood count and liver function should be assessed. This is especially important in children.

PATIENT VARIABLES

Geriatrics

There are no specific guidelines for the use of anticonvulsants in the elderly. All anticonvulsant therapy is individualized and must be carefully monitored when initiating therapy. Careful attention must be paid to those patients with hepatic or renal dysfunction. Lower, less-frequent doses are needed in those with hepatic or renal dysfunction or other concomitant disease. Because many anticonvulsants are involved in the cytochrome P450 enzyme system, care must be used in giving these products to patients who are taking multiple medications.

Pediatrics

Febrile seizures are treated with phenobarbital, benzodiazepines, or valproic acid. Phenytoin and carbamazepine are not effective for febrile seizures. Ethosuximide is the first-line medication of choice for childhood absence epilepsy. Valproic acid is the medication of choice for juvenile myoclonic epilepsy. A pediatric neurologist should be consulted before initiating anticonvulsant therapy. Risks of recurrent seizures vs. side effects of medications and compliance with long-term daily medication must be considered. The dosages of individual medications are based on the pediatric patient's weight and age.

Pregnancy

All anticonvulsants have been associated with an increase in birth defects.

In general, there is about two to three times the normal risk of birth defects in babies of epileptic mothers. There is an

TABLE 46-3 Pharmacokinetics of Selected Anticonvulsant Medications

Drug	Absorption	Drug Availability after First Pass	Onset of Action	Time to Peak Concentration	Half-Life	Protein Bound	Metabolism	Excretion	Therapeutic Level
phenytoin (Dilantin)	95%		3-6 hr	1.5-12 hr	7-42 hr	90%	1A2 inducer Liver 3A4 inducer 2C inducer	Urine, feces	10-20 ng/ml
valproic acid (Depakene, Depakote)				1-4 hr	6-16 hr	90%	Liver Kidney	Urine	50-100 ng/ml
gabapentin (Neurontin)		60%	2-3 hr	1.5-4.5 hr	5-8 hr	0%-5%	Urine		2-20 ng/ml
lamotrigine (Lamictal)			1-4 hr	1.4-4.8 hr	30 hr (monotherapy)	50%-55%	Liver	Urine, 94%; feces, 2%	1-12 ng/ml
topiramate (Topamax)	80%			2 hr	21 hr	13%-17%		Urine	
carbamazepine (Tegretol)			5-10 hr	2-6 hr	12-65 hr	70%-93%	90% liver 2D6 inducer 2C induces	Urine, 72%; feces, 28%	5-12 ng/ml
phenobarbital (Luminal)	Well		0.3-1 hr	8-12 hr	2-6 days	20%-45%	Liver	Urine	15-30 μg (children) 20-40 μg (adults)
primidone (Mysoline)	60%-80%		1.5-3 hr	0.5-9 hr PEMA 7-8 hr	3-24 hr PEMA 24-48 hr	phenobarbital 50%	Liver 3A4 inducer	Urine	5-12 ng/ml phenobarbital 15-40 ng/ml

TABLE 46-4 Common and Serious Adverse Effects of Anticonvulsants

Drug	Adverse Effects
phenytoin	Hypotension, atrial and ventricular conduction delay, ventricular fibrillation with IV administration, nystagmus, ataxia, slurred speech, confusion, drowsiness, gingival hyperplasia
ethosuximide	Appetite loss, ataxia, drowsiness, headache, nausea, hiccups, Steven-Johnson syndrome, systemic lupus erythematosus, blood dyscrasias, convulsions
valproic acid	GI disturbances, weight loss or gain, irregular menses, alopecia, pruritus, rashes, including erythema multiforme, photosensitivity
felbamate	Aplastic anemia, hepatic failure, GI disturbance, insomnia, headache
gabapentin	Drowsiness and ataxia dose-dependent adverse effects; weight gain can occur
lamotrigine	Rash, dizziness, headache, ataxia, visual disturbances, GI disturbances, drowsiness
tiagabine	Dizziness, drowsiness, depression, confusion
topiramate	Drowsiness, inattention, anorexia, weight loss, paresthesias
zonisamide	Drowsiness, dizziness, agitation and inattention, renal calculi
carbamazepine	Dizziness, drowsiness, ataxia, nausea, and vomiting; rashes, photosensitivity reactions, toxic epidermal necrolysis, and Stevens-Johnson syndrome, hypersensitivity (fever, rash, eosinophilia), pulmonary hypersensitivity (fever, dyspnea, pneumonitis)
oxcarbazepine	Dizziness, diplopia, ataxia, vomiting, nausea, drowsiness, headache, fatigue, rash, and hyponatremia most common reasons for discontinuing the drug
levetiracetam	Drowsiness, dizziness
phenobarbital/primidone	Drowsiness, confusion, dizziness, headache, nausea, vomiting, constipation

increased frequency of birth defects in untreated epileptic mothers, but there seems to be a higher frequency in mothers treated with AEDs. All epileptic women of childbearing age must be informed of the risks before pregnancy. Many serious defects occur in the first trimester. The most common defects are cleft lip and palate, cardiac septal defects, and neural tube defects. A neurologist specializing in seizure disorder should be consulted before pregnancy to determine the need for medications. The frequency of seizures may increase, decrease, or remain the same during pregnancy. Alterations in metabolism occur during pregnancy that affects serum drug levels of anticonvulsants. Monthly follow-up and monitoring is required. Ninety-five percent of babies born to mothers on anticonvulsants are normal. Seizures and treatment with anticonvulsants are not reasons to discourage pregnancy. The woman must be made aware of the potential risks and outcomes. Care must be coordinated between the patient, the primary care provider, the obstetrician, and the neurologist to help the patient make the right decision for herself and her unborn child.

Anticonvulsants, particularly barbiturates and hydantoins, have been associated with a coagulation disorder in the neonate. Bleeding may occur in the infant in the first 24 hours after birth. There are decreased levels of the vitamin K–dependent clotting factors, with a prolonged prothrombin time and/or partial thromboplastin time. It is recommended that vitamin K be given to the mother 1 month before and during delivery and to the infant immediately after birth.

Some of the anticonvulsants are excreted in breast milk. There is potential for serious adverse effects in the nursing infant. A decision must be made whether to discontinue the medication or discontinue nursing the infant.

Race

There are no special considerations for the use of anticonvulsants among the races; however, most of the participants in studies of anticonvulsants have been white. There may not be adequate data on the use of anticonvulsants in other races.

Gender

There are no specific differences in the metabolism and general use of anticonvulsants in male and female patients. There are a few special considerations in women of childbearing age; in some women, an increase in seizure activity is reported around the time of the menses. If this is a pattern, it may be helpful to increase the anticonvulsant dose at this time. All anticonvulsants except valproic acid may increase the metabolism of steroid hormones, thereby altering the effectiveness of birth control pills. This requires special attention in women taking birth control pills containing low concentrations of hormones.

PATIENT EDUCATION

- Do not abruptly discontinue seizure medication because this can precipitate SE.

- Advise patients of side effects and toxic effects and monitoring of medications.
- Anticonvulsants may reduce the effectiveness of birth control pills.
- Counsel women wishing to become pregnant about risks and outcomes. There is an increased risk of birth defects in babies of mothers with untreated seizure disorder as well as mothers taking anticonvulsant medications. Some anticonvulsant medications are excreted in breast milk.

! All seizure medications can cause drowsiness and impair concentration. Advise about not swimming alone and other situations that could be dangerous if the patient has an adverse medication event or seizure.

- Sleep deprivation, fever, stress, medications, and alcohol can lower seizure threshold.
- Wear a medical alert bracelet to identify seizure disorder.
- Advise the family how to protect the patient from injury during a seizure: help the patient to the floor, away from any objects he or she may bump; protect the airway from aspiration by using the left side-lying position if possible; do not place any objects in the patient's mouth, including fingers.
- Advise about driving regulations within the state. Most states require a seizure-free period before driving can be resumed. Health care providers should be familiar with their state regulations or have a contact at the Motor Vehicle Administration.
- Give information about national organizations and support groups.

Specific Drugs

HYDANTOINS

phenytoin (Dilantin)

Contraindications

- Pure absence (petit mal) seizures (because the drug may increase the frequency of these seizures), sinus bradycardia, sinoatrial block, second- and third-degree atrioventricular (AV) block, and Adams-Stokes syndrome (because of its effect on ventricular automaticity)

Warnings

! Phenytoin should be discontinued if skin rash appears. Scarlatiniform or morbilliform rash, sometimes accompanied by fever, may occur. Rarely, phenytoin has produced severe dermatologic reactions such as bullous, exfoliative, or purpuric dermatitis; lupus erythematosus; Stevens-Johnson syndrome; or toxic epidermal necrolysis. A few deaths have resulted.

- Acute alcoholic intake may increase phenytoin serum levels, whereas chronic alcoholic use may decrease levels.
- Serum levels sustained above the optimal range may produce delirium, psychosis, encephalopathy, or cerebellar dysfunction. Hypotension occurs if phenytoin is administered rapidly via the intravenous route. The intravenous rate of administration must not exceed 50 mg/min in adults.
- Occasionally, fever, lymphadenopathy, eosinophilia, arthralgias, and hepatic dysfunction, including jaundice, producing a syndrome resembling mononucleosis, have accompanied severe cutaneous reactions.
- Adverse hematologic effects include thrombocytopenia, leukopenia, granulocytopenia, agranulocytosis, and pancytopenia. Macrocytosis and megaloblastic anemia that responds to folic acid therapy may also occur.
- Osteomalacia can occur and may be related to phenytoin interference with vitamin D metabolism.

Precautions. Use with caution in patients with impaired liver function, elderly patients, or the gravely ill because they may show early signs of toxicity. May contribute to gingival hyperplasia, hirsutism, coarse features, and xanthemia.

Improper administration, including subcutaneous or perivascular injection, should be avoided to prevent soft tissue irritation, ranging from tenderness to necrosis, which has, in rare instances, led to amputation.

Pharmacokinetics. Phenytoin is metabolized by the CYP 450 enzyme system (see Table 46-3).

Phenytoin follows nonlinear pharmacokinetics. In general, therapeutic plasma phenytoin levels are reached after 1 week of therapy with an oral dose of 300 mg daily in adults. Rapid therapeutic concentrations can be achieved in adults in 2 to 24 hours by administering an initial oral loading dose of 1 g, followed by 300 to 500 mg daily. Therapeutic concentrations can be attained within 1 to 2 hours after an intravenous loading dose of 1 g (at a rate not exceeding 50 mg/min).

Adverse Effects. See Table 46-4 for common adverse effects of anticonvulsants.

Drug Interactions. See Table 46-5 for drug interactions with anticonvulsants.

Ingestion times of antacids containing calcium should be staggered to prevent absorption problems.

Overdosage. Most patients tolerate blood concentrations of less than 25 ng/ml. Initial symptoms of overdosage are nystagmus, ataxia, and dysarthria.

Other signs are tremor, hyperreflexia, lethargy, slurred speech, nausea, and vomiting. Extreme lethargy, hypertension, and comatose states occur with levels greater than 50 μg/ml. The lethal dose in adults appears to be 2 to 5 g. Death occurs because of respiratory and circulatory depression. There is no known antidote.

Dosage and Administration. Treatment of adults with SE: Loading dose of 10 to 15 mg/kg should be administered slowly intravenously at a rate not to exceed 50 mg/min, while monitoring for respiratory depression, hypotension, or ECG changes.

TABLE 46-5 Drug Interactions of Anticonvulsant Medications

Drug	Increase Level	Decrease Level
HYDANTOINS		
phenytoin*	alcohol amiodarone chloramphenicol chlordiazepoxide diazepam dicumarol disulfiram Estrogens H_2-antagonists halothane isoniazid methylphenidate Phenothiazines phenylbutazone Salicylates Succinimides Sulfonamides tolbutamide trazodone	carbamazepine Chronic alcohol abuse reserpine sucralfate
GABA ANALOGS		
valproic acid†	chlorpromazine cimetidine erythromycin felbamate Salicylates Antidepressants MAOIs	carbamazepine cholestyramine lamotrigine phenobarbital phenytoin
felbamate*†		carbamazepine phenobarbital phenytoin
gabapentin	cimetidine	Antacids
lamotrigine*	Folate inhibitors valproate acid	acetaminophen carbamazepine phenobarbital phenytoin primidone
tiagabine	Change in concentration and clearance when administered with valproate, carbamazepine, phenytoin, or phenobarbital; clinical implications of these interactions undetermined	
topiramate†		carbamazepine phenytoin valproic acid
zonisamide		carbamazepine phenobarbital phenytoin
MISCELLANEOUS		
carbamazepine	cimetidine danazol diltiazem erythromycin fluoxetine isoniazid nicotinamide propoxyphene troleandomycin verapamil	phenobarbital phenytoin primidone Succinimides theophylline valproic acid haldol warfarin
oxcarbazepine*		carbamazepine phenobarbital phenytoin valproic acid verapamil
levetiracetam	No clinically significant interactions with current anticonvulsant medications	

*Hepatic enzyme inducer.
†Hepatic enzyme inhibitor.

Maintenance doses may be given orally or intravenously at 3 to 5 mg/kg/day (approximately 100 mg every 8 hours).

Oral suspension must be shaken well before each dose is administered, or the amount of phenytoin in each milliliter will differ at various levels of the suspension.

Phenytoin should be given intramuscularly only as a last resort because it is erratically absorbed from intramuscular injection sites. When a patient is transferred from phenytoin to another anticonvulsant, the dosage of phenytoin should be gradually reduced over a period of 1 week while, at the same time, therapy is instituted with a low dose of the replacement drug. Orally, 100 mg of phenytoin has been given two to four times daily in the management of cardiac arrhythmias.

How to Monitor. Because of nonlinear kinetics, there is a poor correlation between dosage and serum level, and serum level may increase dramatically with a small increase in dose. It should be remembered that different formulations may have different bioavailability.

Patient Variables: Pregnancy. Safe use during pregnancy has not been established. Phenytoin should be used in pregnancy only when clearly needed. In addition to fetal hydantoin syndrome, there have been rare reports of malignancies in children whose mothers received phenytoin during pregnancy. If it is administered during pregnancy, serum phenytoin concentrations should be closely monitored and dosage adjusted. Because of altered absorption or metabolism during pregnancy, an increased frequency of seizures may occur in pregnant women receiving the drug.

Infant breast-feeding is not recommended for women taking this drug because phenytoin appears to be secreted in human milk.

SUCCINIMIDE

ethosuximide (Zarontin)

This drug is usually considered the drug of choice in the management of absence seizures, but is ineffective in treating most other types of seizures. It is administered orally and titrated up or down by patient response. Usual initial dosage is 250 mg orally for patients 3 to 6 years of age; 500 mg for those older than 6. May increase dosage by 250 mg every 4 to 7 days until seizures are controlled and side effects are minimized. Do not exceed 1.5 g daily.

GABA ANALOGS

(P) Prototype Drug

valproate, valproic acid, divalproex sodium (Depakene, Depakote)

Contraindications

- Hepatic disease or severe hepatic dysfunction; hypersensitivity to valproic acid

Warnings

Potential for fatal hepatotoxicity; children less than 2 years seem to be at increased risk, particularly those on multiple AEDs and those with severe seizure disorders, congenital metabolic disorders, mental retardation, or organic brain disease. In this group of pediatric patients, use as the only agent with extreme caution.

The incidence of fatal hepatotoxicity decreases progressively with increasing age. Hepatotoxicity usually occurs in the first 6 months of treatment.

Liver function tests should be performed before and at frequent intervals during therapy. Monitor patients closely; hepatotoxicity may be preceded by loss of seizure control, weakness, lethargy, edema, anorexia, or vomiting. Discontinue immediately if significant hepatic dysfunction is suspected.

Precautions

Valproic acid may cause thrombocytopenia and inhibition of platelet aggregation. Platelet counts and coagulation studies should be done before initiation of therapy, at regular intervals, and before any surgical procedure.

Any hemorrhage, bruising, or disorder of coagulation should be investigated, and the dosage reduced or valproic therapy withdrawn.

Hyperammonemia may occur with or without lethargy or coma; it may occur in the absence of elevated liver enzymes. The drug should be discontinued if this occurs. (Also see warning related to hepatotoxicity.)

May cause drowsiness, especially if the drug is taken with other anticonvulsants. Advise the patient to be cautious when driving, swimming, or in other potentially hazardous situations requiring mental alertness.

Pharmacokinetics

Valproate is the sodium salt of valproic acid. Divalproex sodium is a prodrug, a 1:1 compound of valproic acid and valproate in a delayed-release formulation. Valproic acid is rapidly and almost completely absorbed from the stomach. Valproate is converted to valproic acid in the stomach. Divalproex sodium dissociates into valproate in the upper small intestine. All forms of the drug are dosed as equivalent to valproic acid.

Adverse Effects

Valproic acid has most frequently been used in combination with other anticonvulsants; therefore it is not possible to determine whether the adverse reactions are the result of valproic acid alone or the combination of drugs.

The common initial GI side effects are usually transient and rarely requires discontinuation of the drug. Administering the drug with meals and starting with low doses and slowly increasing the dose can minimize these effects. Divalproex sodium may be better tolerated and reduce the gastrointestinal effects in some patients. Table 46-4 provides common adverse effects of anticonvulsants.

Abnormal thyroid function test results have been reported; the clinical significance of these abnormal findings is unknown.

Drug Interactions

Additive CNS depression may occur when valproic acid is administered with other CNS depressants, including other anticonvulsants and alcohol. Valproic acid and phenobarbital or primidone can produce severe CNS depression without significant increase in serum concentration of either drug. Patients on valproic acid and a barbiturate must be observed carefully for toxic signs, and serum levels of the barbiturate should be monitored and the dose adjusted as needed. Administration of valproic acid and clonazepam has produced absence status. It is recommended that this combination of drugs be avoided. Valproic acid has been associated with both increase and decrease in serum phenytoin level. It is important to monitor serum phenytoin levels when valproic acid is added or withdrawn. It is advisable to monitor serum concentrations of any concomitant anticonvulsants during initial valproic acid therapy.

Valproic acid may affect bleeding time; it should be used with caution in patients receiving drugs that affect coagulation, such as aspirin or warfarin. Salicylates may elevate valproic acid levels, which may lead to toxicity.

Concomitant use of cimetidine and valproic acid decreases the clearance and increases the half-life of valproic acid (see Table 46-5 for drug interactions with anticonvulsants).

Overdosage
Overdosage may result in coma and death. Valproic acid is absorbed very rapidly; therefore the efficacy of gastric lavage will vary with time since ingestion. Naloxone may reverse CNS depression but may also reverse anticonvulsant effects; use with caution.

Dosage and Administration
The initial dosage is 15 mg/kg/day; it may be increased at 1-week intervals by 5 to 10 mg/kg/day until seizures are controlled or side effects prevent further increase in dose. The maximum recommended daily dose is 60 mg/kg/day. If the total daily dose is greater than 250 mg, it should be administered in divided doses.

Bedtime administration may minimize CNS effects. It should be given with food to decrease gastrointestinal distress. Valproic acid capsules should be swallowed whole, not chewed, to prevent local irritation to the mouth and throat. Valproate sodium oral solution should not be given with carbonated drinks; the valproic acid will be liberated and cause local irritation and an unpleasant taste. Divalproex sodium (Depakote) may be better tolerated. It may be swallowed intact, or the entire contents of the capsule(s) may be sprinkled on 1 teaspoon of semisolid food such as applesauce or pudding just before administration. The mixture should not be chewed and should not be stored for future use.

How to Monitor
Valproic acid may interact with concomitant anticonvulsants. Serum levels of the anticonvulsants should be monitored when a new drug is added and periodically.

Patient Variables: Pregnancy
- *Category D:* there may be an increased incidence of neural tube defects in the fetuses of mothers receiving valproic acid in the first trimester.
- Concentrations of valproic acid in breast milk are 1% to 10% of the maternal serum concentration. The effect of this on the nursing infant is unknown. Use caution when administering valproic acid to a nursing woman.

Other Drugs in Class

Other drugs in this class are similar to the prototype except as follows.

gabapentin (Neurontin)

One of the new anticonvulsants, gabapentin is different from other anticonvulsants because it is primarily excreted by the renal system. Caution is needed when administering it to elderly patient with decreased creatinine clearance, decreased muscle mass, concomitant disease, and polypharmacy.

Gabapentin has no interaction with the common anticonvulsants.

Routine monitoring of clinical laboratory data is not indicated for the safe use of gabapentin. The use of monitoring serum concentrations has not been established. Gabapentin does not alter the metabolism of other anticonvulsants; therefore monitoring serum concentrations of gabapentin or other anticonvulsants is not necessary.

Dosage and Administration. Effective dose for patients more than 12 years of age is 900 to 1800 mg/day in divided doses; start at 300 mg tid.

In children 3 to 12 years of age give 10 to 15 mg/kg/day in three divided doses and titrate upward. Effective dose is usually reached in 3 days.

Gabapentin is emerging as first-line therapy for neuropathic pain in doses starting at 100 mg po at bedtime.

(See Tables 46-1, 46-4, and 46-5 for use, adverse events, and drug interactions.)

lamotrigine (Lamictal)

Contraindications, Warnings, Precautions. Serious rashes requiring hospitalization may occur. This seems to be more frequent with rapid introduction of lamotrigine.

Instruct patients beginning therapy to notify the provider if a rash occurs. The rash should be promptly evaluated and a decision made whether to continue treatment. If therapy is continued, the rash must be carefully monitored. Stevens-Johnson syndrome, epidermal necrolysis, and angioedema have occurred in association with lamotrigine therapy. Fatal or life-threatening hypersensitivity reactions have occurred with clinical features of multiorgan dysfunction and disseminated intravascular coagulation.

How to Monitor. The value of monitoring serum levels of lamotrigine has not been established. There may be pharmacokinetic interactions between lamotrigine and concomitant anticonvulsants. Serum levels of lamotrigine and the other anticonvulsants should be monitored, particularly when adjusting dosages.

Lamotrigine binds to melanin. It could cause toxicity in these tissues with extended use. One should be aware of the possibility of long-term ophthalmologic effects.

Photosensitization may occur; patients should be advised to protect against exposure to ultraviolet light or sunlight by using sunscreens and protective clothing.

Phenytoin and carbamazepine decrease the half-life of lamotrigine. Valproic acid increases the half-life of lamotrigine.

See Tables 46-1, 46-4, and 46-5 for use, adverse events, and drug interactions.

MISCELLANEOUS ANTICONVULSANTS

carbamazepine (Tegretol, Epitol)

Contraindications. Hypersensitivity to carbamazepine or any tricyclic antidepressant, concurrent use of monoamine oxidase (MAO) inhibitors (discontinue MAO inhibitors at least 14 days before initiating carbamazepine therapy), history of bone marrow depression.

Warnings. Aplastic anemia and agranulocytosis, although rare, have been reported in association with carbamazepine therapy.

A benign leukopenia is not uncommon. It is usually not progressive or associated with increased mortality from infection, and it is reversible and dose related. However, any patient with a history of adverse hematologic reaction to any drug should be considered at high risk. A complete blood cell count with white cell differential should be done before initiating treatment. This should be repeated every 3 months during the first year of treatment. For white cell counts less than 2500/mm, careful monitoring is required, and the drug may need to be discontinued.

Carbamazepine has mild anticholinergic activity; use with caution in patients with increased intraocular pressure.

Confusion or agitation may occur in the elderly because of the drug's relationship to the tricyclic compounds.

Carbamazepine produced a dose-related increase in the incidence of hepatocellular tumors in female rats and benign interstitial cell adenomas in male rats. It is not known how these findings relate to humans.

Precautions. Carbamazepine is ineffective for controlling absence seizures. Use with caution in patients with mixed seizure disorder. Carbamazepine has been associated with exacerbation of generalized seizures in these patients.

! Baseline and periodic liver function tests should be performed. Carbamazepine should be discontinued immediately if liver dysfunction occurs or acute liver disease is suspected.

Baseline and periodic urinalyses and blood urea nitrogen, and creatinine levels should be determined. Carbamazepine has been associated with the syndrome of inappropriate antidiuretic hormone (SIADH), water intoxication, and hyponatremia.

Baseline and periodic eye examinations should be performed. Lens opacities have occurred rarely in patients on carbamazepine.

Pharmacokinetics. Carbamazepine is adequately absorbed from the gastrointestinal tract. Carbamazepine suspension is absorbed more rapidly than the tablet. The liver metabolizes carbamazepine by the CYP 450 enzyme system. It can induce its own metabolism, which accounts for variability in the half-life. The initial half-life is 25 to 65 hours; after multiple dosing this decreases to 12 to 17 hours (see Table 46-3).

Adverse Effects. Initiation of carbamazepine therapy at low doses and increasing it slowly to an effective therapeutic dose can usually minimize gastrointestinal symptoms as well as dizziness and drowsiness (see Table 46-4).

Drug Interactions. The concomitant use of multiple AEDs (see Table 46-5) may decrease serum concentrations of carbamazepine. This is probably the result of induction of hepatic microsomal enzymes that metabolize the drugs. There may be no loss of seizure control because the anticonvulsant activity is added. Monitor serum concentrations of AEDs given in combination and adjust dosages accordingly. See also drug interaction discussion under the other individual anticonvulsants and Table 46-5.

Concomitant use of carbamazepine and verapamil or diltiazem may result in increased plasma concentrations of carbamazepine and lead to toxicity. The interaction does not appear to occur with nifedipine.

Fluoxetine (Prozac) may increase plasma carbamazepine concentrations.

Increased CNS toxicity may occur with concomitant use of lithium and carbamazepine. The patient and the serum levels of both drugs should be monitored closely.

Carbamazepine may increase the metabolism of acetaminophen, resulting in increased risk of hepatotoxicity, or it may decrease the efficacy of acetaminophen.

Concomitant use of carbamazepine and theophylline may decrease the effects of both drugs.

Carbamazepine may increase the risk of isoniazid-induced hepatotoxicity.

The half-life of doxycycline may be decreased when administered with carbamazepine. If possible, alternative antibiotic agents should be used in patients receiving carbamazepine.

Overdosage. Signs and symptoms of carbamazepine toxicity are declining mental status, ataxia, dizziness, abnormal movements, nausea, vomiting, nystagmus, and urinary retention.

Dosage and Administration. Individualize dosage; begin with a low daily dose and gradually increase. When adequate control is achieved, reduce the dose gradually to the minimum effective level. Administer with meals.

For management of epilepsy in adults and children older than 12 years, begin with 200-mg tablets twice daily or 100 mg suspension four times daily. Increase at weekly intervals up to 200 mg daily using a three- or four-times-daily regimen until the response is obtained. Dosage should not exceed 1000 mg/day in children 12 to 15 years or 1200 mg in those older than 15 years. Rarely, doses up to 1600 mg/day have been used in adults. Adjust maintenance dose to the minimal effective level, usually 800 to 1200 mg daily.

For children 6 to 12 years old, begin with 100-mg tablets twice daily or 50 mg suspension four times daily. Increase at weekly intervals by 100 mg/day, using a three- or four-times-daily regimen until an optimal response is obtained. Do not exceed 1000 mg/day. You may also calculate dose on basis of 20 to 30 mg/kg/day in divided doses three to four times daily. Adjust maintenance dose to minimal effective level, usually 400 to 800 mg/day.

For the symptomatic relief of pain associated with trigeminal neuralgia in adults, begin with 100-mg tablets twice daily or 50 mg four times daily of oral suspension on the first day. The dosage may be increased gradually up to 200 mg daily, using 100-mg increments every 12 hours with tablets or 50-mg increments four times daily for suspension until pain is relieved. The dosage needed to relieve pain may range from 200 to 1200 mg daily. The dose should not exceed 1200 mg/day. Control of pain can usually be maintained with 400 to 800 mg/day. An attempt should be made at least every 3 months to reduce the dose or discontinue use of carbamazepine.

Patient Variables

Pediatrics. Safety and efficacy for use in children under the age of 6 years have not been established.

Pregnancy

- *Category C:* adverse effects have been observed in animal studies.
- The concentration of carbamazepine in breast milk is approximately 60% of the maternal plasma concentration. There is a potential for serious adverse effects in the infant. A decision must be made to discontinue nursing or discontinue the drug, considering the importance of the drug to the mother.

BARBITURATES

Ⓟ Prototype Drug

phenobarbital (Luminal)

Contraindications

- Hypersensitivity to barbiturates, preexisting CNS depression, severe respiratory depression/disease, uncontrolled pain, porphyria, pregnancy, and lactation

Warnings/Precautions

Use with caution in patients with cardiac, renal, or hepatic impairment; hypovolemic shock; congestive heart failure; chronic or acute pain syndrome; or history of psychologic or physical drug dependence. Recommend cautious use in the elderly because of long half-life. This drug may cause paradoxical excitement in children. It cannot be withdrawn abruptly; abrupt withdrawal may cause withdrawal symptoms or SE in persons with epilepsy.

Drug Interactions

Benzodiazepines, CNS depressants, propoxyphene, valproic acid, methylphenidate, chloramphenicol, and phenytoin increase the effect of phenobarbital.

Anticoagulants, β-blockers, doxycycline, metronidazole, quinidine, verapamil, theophylline, anticonvulsants, corticosteroids, estrogens, and oral contraceptives decrease the effect of phenobarbital.

Overdosage

Confusion, hypothermia, hypotension, slurred speech, unsteady gait, jaundice, respiratory depression, or coma can result.

Dosage and Administration

The usual oral dosage of phenobarbital is 100 to 300 mg/day for adults, administered in a single dose at bedtime. Phenobarbital has a long half-life, so there is no benefit to divided doses. For the prevention of febrile seizures in children, the usual maintenance dosage is 3 to 4 mg/kg/day.

Other Drugs in Class

Other drugs in this class are similar to the prototype except as follows.

primidone (Mysoline)

Contraindications

- Porphyria and hypersensitivity to phenobarbital

Warnings. Abrupt withdrawal of primidone or any anticonvulsant may precipitate SE. It takes several weeks to fully assess the therapeutic efficacy of primidone.

Patient Variables

Pregnancy. The effects of primidone in pregnancy are unknown. Primidone and the barbiturates have been associated with coagulation defects in the newborn infant.

Lactation. Primidone is excreted in breast milk in significant quantity. It is recommended that if increasing drowsiness occurs in the nursing infant of mothers taking primidone, a decision should be made to discontinue nursing.

Precautions. The manufacturers recommend a complete blood cell count and chemistry panel be performed every 6 months on patients receiving primidone.

Adverse Effects. Primidone is less sedating than phenobarbital; therefore less impairment of cognitive function is seen. Psychotic reactions are rarely seen with primidone. Nausea, vomiting, drowsiness, ataxia, and vertigo are common dose-related side effects that usually disappear with continued therapy or reduction in initial dosage.

Megaloblastic anemia is a rare idiosyncrasy that may occur with primidone therapy.

Drug Interactions. Primidone, phenobarbital, and PEMA concentrations may be increased when hydantoins are administered with primidone.

Concomitant use of carbamazepine and primidone may result in decreased primidone and phenobarbital levels and higher carbamazepine levels.

Primidone levels may increase when isoniazid or nicotinamide are given concomitantly.

Concomitant use of primidone and acetazolamide may result in decreased primidone levels.

Concomitant use of primidone and the succinimides may result in decreased primidone and phenobarbital levels.

Overdosage. Symptoms are similar to acute barbiturate overdosage. CNS depression that can progress to coma with severe respiratory depression and even death may occur.

Dosage and Administration. Primidone is given orally. When initiating therapy, slowly increase the dose to meet the individual's requirements. When primidone is replacing another anticonvulsant, the anticonvulsant should be decreased slowly as the primidone is being increased over at least 2 weeks.

To initiate primidone therapy in adults and children over 8 years old, begin with 100 to 125 mg at bedtime for 3 days, 100 to 125 mg twice daily for 3 days, 100 to 125 mg three times daily for 3 days, and then a maintenance dose of 250 mg three times daily. The maximum dose is 2000 mg in divided doses.

For children younger than 8 years, begin with 50 mg at bedtime for 3 days, 50 mg twice daily for 3 days, 100 mg twice daily for 3 days, and then a maintenance dose of 125 to 250 mg three times daily. Do not exceed dose of 500 mg four times a day (2 g/day).

RESOURCE FOR PATIENTS AND PROVIDERS

Epilepsy Foundation of America and National Epilepsy Library, 4351 Garden City Drive, Landover, MD 20785; telephone: (800) EFA-4050.

BIBLIOGRAPHY

American Academy of Neurology: Practice parameter: evaluating a first nonfebrile seizure in children. Report of the Quality Standards Subcommittee of the American Academy of Neurology, the Child Neurology Society, and the American Epilepsy Society, *Neurology* 55:5, 2000.

American Academy of Neurology: Practice parameter: anticonvulsant prophylaxis in patients with newly diagnosed brain tumors. Report of the Quality Standards Subcommittee of the American Academy of Neurology, *Neurology* 54:10, 2000.

American Academy of Neurology: Practice parameter: management issues for women with epilepsy. Report of the Quality Standards Subcommittee of the American Academy of Neurology, *Neurology* 51:4, 1998.

Anderson GD, Miller JW: The newer antiepileptic drugs: their collective role and defining characteristics, *Formulary* 36, 2001.

Commission on Classification and Terminology of the International League against Epilepsy: Proposal for revised clinical and electroencephalographic classification of epileptic seizures, *Epilepsia* 22:8, 1981.

Commission on Classification and Terminology of the International League against Epilepsy: Proposal for revised classification of epilepsies and epileptic syndromes, *Epilepsia* 30:4, 1989.

Deckers C et al: Selection criteria for the clinical use of the newer antiepileptic drugs, *CNS Drugs* 17:405-421, 2003.

Gatti G et al: The new antiepileptic drugs: pharmacological and clinical aspects, *Curr Pharm Des* 6:839-860, 2000.

Hachad H, Ragueneau-Majlessi I, Levy RH: New antiepileptic drugs: review on drug interactions, *Ther Drug Monit* 24:91-103, 2002.

King M: The new patient with a first seizure, *Aust Fam Physician* 32:221-228, 2003.

Pelleck JM: Treatment of epilepsy in the new millennium, *Pharmacotherapy* 20:129S-138S, 2000.

Perucca E: Clinical pharmacology and therapeutic use of the new antiepileptic drugs, *Fundam Clin Pharmacol* 15:405-417, 2001.

Perucca E: Marketed new antiepileptic drugs: are they better than old-generation agents? *Ther Drug Monit* 24:74-80, 2002.

Prego-Lopez M, Devinsky O. Evaluation of a first seizure, *Postgrad Med* 111:1, 2002.

CHAPTER 47

Antiparkinson Agents

V. Inez Wendel

Drug Names

Class	Subclass	Generic Name	Trade Name
Dopamine precursors		(P) carbidopa/levodopa Controlled-release carbidopa/levodopa	Sinemet Sinemet CR
Monoamine oxidase-B inhibitor		selegiline	Eldepryl
Dopamine agonists		amantadine bromocriptine pergolide pramipexole ropinirole	Symmetrel Parlodel Permax Mirapex Requip
Anticholinergic agents		benztropine trihexyphenidyl	Cogentin Artane
COMT inhibitor		tolcapone entacapone	Tasmar Comtan

(P), Prototype drug.

General Uses

Indications

- Idiopathic Parkinson's disease (PD)
- Management of symptoms related to parkinsonism—tremor at rest, bradykinesia, rigidity, and postural instability

Unlabeled Use

- Sinemet and the dopamine agonists are used for management of the symptoms of restless leg syndrome.

DISEASE PROCESS

Anatomy and Physiology

The neurotransmitters, acetylcholine and dopamine, and others in the neurons of the substantia nigra modulate movement. Damage to these neurons by amyloid result in excess acetylcholine and diminished dopamine in the basal ganglia. Replacement and regulation of the neurotransmitters with exogenous medications represent the hallmark of Parkinson's disease (PD) management; however, these medications must be able to cross the blood-brain barrier without being metabolized in the periphery to improve symptoms and avoid side effects.

Synthesis and Metabolism of Dopamine in the Nerve Terminals. Tyrosine is converted to levodopa (L-dopa) by tyrosine hydroxylase. L-Dopa is then enzymatically decarboxylated by L-amino acid decarboxylase (L-AAD) to form dopamine. Dopamine is stored in synaptic vesicles until needed and then is released into the synapse and activates D receptors. The action of dopamine is terminated by reuptake into presynaptic vesicles or metabolism via monoamine oxidase-B (MAO-B) or catechol-*O*-methyl-transferase (COMT). This results in the formation of hydrogen peroxide, which is then metabolized to water by glutathione. If glutathione is deficient or a surplus of hydrogen peroxide exists, hydroxyl free radicals are formed, causing lipid peroxidation and cell membrane damage.

Pathophysiology

The etiology of PD is categorized as (1) primary, or idiopathic, (2) secondary, or acquired, parkinsonism, (3) heritable parkinsonism, or (4) multisystem parkinsonism. For purposes of this text, only idiopathic PD is discussed. Practitioners are urged to consult differential diagnostic references to distinguish among the types of parkinsonism, including drug-induced cases.

PD results from a relative excess of cholinergic activity and a deficiency of dopaminergic activity in the basal ganglia. Lewy bodies (amyloid inclusion bodies) in the neurons of the pars compacta region of the substantia nigra are common in the pathophysiology of parkinsonism. Damage to these dopaminergic neurons causes the loss of dopamine at their terminal projections in the caudate nucleus and putamen. Dopamine normally inhibits the action of acetylcholine in the striatum; therefore decreased concentrations of dopamine caused by neuronal degeneration result in unopposed acetylcholine. This manifests as tremors in the patient. Clinical signs and symptoms of parkinsonism develop after the loss of approximately 80% of dopaminergic neurons.

Some understanding of the etiology of idiopathic PD was gained when several intravenous drug abusers developed PD after injecting a meperidine analog, methylphenyltetrahydropyridine (MPTP). The MPP^+ ion that was formed after oxidative metabolism of MPTP by MAO-B was found to be neurotoxic to melanin-containing neurons in the substantia nigra. Inhibition of MAO-B by selegiline prevented the formation of the MPP^+ ion and the development of idiopathic PD. Epidemiologic studies have shown an increased risk of developing PD with rural living and exposure to well water, pesticides, herbicides, and wood pulp mills. Discovery of a gene that could be responsible for a certain type of familial PD has brought hope for further research in the mechanism and prevention of the disease, perhaps through the use of stem cells.

The Disease

Dr. James Parkinson first described paralysis agitans, or shaking palsy, in 1817. Today we know this condition as PD, Parkinson's syndrome, or parkinsonism. The age at onset of signs and symptoms varies; the majority of patients experience symptoms between the ages of 50 and 69. Up to 30% of patients develop symptoms before age 50. Patients present with one or more of four typical clinical symptoms: tremor at rest, bradykinesia, rigidity, and postural instability. Younger patients with IPD may present with only a resting tremor of 4 to 7 cycles/sec as the principal symptom. These patients usually experience a slower progression of disease and little mental status change. Patients presenting with postural instability and gait difficulty, however, often have a more rapid disease progression that includes dementia and bradykinesia. Early research suggests that NSAIDs may protect against the development of PD.

Assessment

Clinically, idiopathic PD progresses slowly. Early signs and symptoms include paresthesias, pain, and numbness, which progress to the classic clinical features of tremor, bradykinesia, rigidity, and postural instability. Other typical problems include micrographia, hypophonia, shuffling or festinating gait, lack of facial expression (masked facies), drooling, decreased blinking, and decreased dexterity. PD patients may experience difficulty initiating movements, may freeze or be unable to move when they walk in confined spaces, or may exhibit pill-rolling movements of their hands, jaw, or legs. The tremors and pill-rolling subside on initiation of voluntary movement and do not occur during sleep. Cogwheel-like rigidity, dystonic postures, and postural instability are causes of significant morbidity in PD patients because they can lead to falls. PD patients also exhibit autonomic nervous system dysfunctions such as excessive sweating, constipation, and postural hypotension. Neuropsychologic disorders such as dementia and depression may occur.

DRUG ACTION AND EFFECTS

Drug treatment of PD has centered on increasing dopamine's availability in the CNS, inhibiting the effects of acetylcholine, and preventing further cell membrane damage. The D_2 receptor subtype is the primary modulator of both clinical improvement and adverse reactions such as dystonias and hallucinations. Increasing levodopa precursors and synthesis cofactors has not been found to be effective.

Levodopa has been the single most important drug in the antiparkinson armamentarium. Levodopa administered orally enters the blood after it is absorbed from the GI tract, and 95% of levodopa is converted to dopamine by L-AAD. The action of this enzyme can be blocked by the antagonist carbidopa, which does not cross the blood-brain barrier; therefore levodopa in the CNS will follow the synthetic path to dopamine formation and storage. Combining carbidopa with levodopa results in increased concentrations of levodopa in the CNS and decreased conversion of L-dopa to dopamine in the periphery, where it causes adverse effects.

Selegiline, an MAO-B inhibitor, is used early in the management of idiopathic PD in an attempt to prevent further neuronal degeneration. Selegiline's mechanism of action is not fully understood; however, selective MAO-B inhibition irreversibly blocks the metabolism of dopamine in the brain, where MAO-B is the major subtype and extends the duration of action of L-dopa. Selegiline often permits dose reductions of L-dopa and increases the duration of effect by 1 or more hours in patients who experience "wearing-off" effects of L-dopa. Selegiline may delay the use of levodopa/carbidopa in the early stages of PD via the same mechanism. Selegiline may be neuroprotective by shunting dopamine's metabolic path away from free radical production and oxidative stress. This beneficial effect lasts about 1 year and only partially protects against the progression of PD. Selegiline also may interfere with dopamine reuptake at the synapse, thus prolonging its action at the receptor. Some of the actions of selegiline may be the result of the actions of the three active metabolites (see Table 47-3). Another selective MAO inhibitor (MAOI) (lazabemide) and several dopamine agonists (cabergoline, lisuride, apomorphine) are also being evaluated for use in treating idiopathic PD.

Dopamine agonists are used in the treatment of IPD to increase the availability of dopamine in the CNS. These drugs work at the presynaptic and postsynaptic dopamine receptors in the nigrostriatal system by inhibiting dopamine reuptake, increasing its release, and stimulating dopamine receptors. They are being used more frequently in early parkinsonism to avoid using high doses of levodopa and in late stages of the disease to aid in the management of levodopa dose-response fluctuations.

Anticholinergic agents are used to control tremors caused by excess, unopposed acetylcholine. They suppress central cholinergic activity and may inhibit reuptake and storage of dopamine in CNS, thus prolonging action of dopamine. They also reduce the incidence and severity of akinesia, rigidity, and tremor by about 20%, and they reduce drooling.

COMT inhibitors are central and/or peripheral blockers of dopamine metabolism. These drugs are used as adjuvants with levodopa to increase the availability of levodopa in the brain.

The function of COMT is to eliminate biologically active catechols (dopamine, norepinephrine, epinephrine, and their hydroxylated metabolites). COMT is the major enzyme for levodopa metabolism. The mechanism of action of tolcapone is probably related to its ability to inhibit COMT and alter the plasma pharmacokinetics of levodopa. The administration of tolcapone in conjunction with levodopa and carbidopa produces more sustained plasma levels of levodopa than does the administration of levodopa and carbidopa alone. These sustained plasma levels may result in increased therapeutic effects on the symptoms of PD as well as increased adverse effects. A decrease in the levodopa dose may be required.

DRUG TREATMENT PRINCIPLES

Parkinsonism is a chronic, debilitating disease with no known cure. Current therapies are strictly palliative, and the goal of treatment is to relieve the symptoms of the disease and maintain the patient's independence and mobility. Management of parkinsonism should include programs to optimize the patient's general health, nutrition, emotional, and neuromuscular status. Table 47-1 provides a treatment algorithm. The patient should be referred to a neurologist to confirm the diagnosis and for guidance with medical management.

Disease staging is an important tool in determining drug and supportive therapy. The following scale of Hoehn and Yahr is recommended:

Stage I: unilateral involvement

Stage II: bilateral involvement but no postural abnormalities

Stage III: bilateral involvement with mild postural imbalance; the patient leads an independent life

Stage IV: bilateral involvement with postural instability; the patient requires substantial help

Stage V: severe, fully developed disease; the patient is restricted to bed and chair

The timing of treatment initiation in PD is controversial. Some clinicians prefer to initiate early treatment to maximize clinical benefits. Others prefer to delay treatment initiation to avoid complications of levodopa metabolism and the risk of accelerating the disease progression. Functional status impairment is usually a hallmark sign of the need for treatment. Factors useful in assessing the need to start treatment include which hand is affected (dominant or nondominant), the patient's employment status, specific Parkinson's symptoms (bradykinesia is more disabling than tremor), the individual patient's sentiments, and the individual prescriber's philosophy.

Most experts agree that neuroprotection is the first issue that should be considered when a patient is newly diagnosed with early PD and that selegiline is the agent of choice. There is considerable controversy in the literature as to the timing of levodopa initiation versus dopamine agonists versus COMT inhibitors, alone or in combination. Many experts favor initiating symptomatic treatment with a dopamine agonist rather than levodopa with consideration for factors such as age, cognitive impairment, disease severity, employment status, cost, and combined therapy.

TABLE 47-1 Treatment Algorithm for Parkinson's Disease

Stage or Problem	Therapeutic Alternatives
Mild disease (stage I and II)	selegiline for neuroprotection Anticholinergics if tremor predominant amantadine Group support, exercise, education, nutrition
Functionally impaired (stage III)	
Age <60 yr	Tremor predominant: Anticholinergics Functional disability: Sustained-release carbidopa/levodopa (lowest dose possible) Dopamine agonists
Age >60 yr	Sustained-release carbidopa/levodopa
Stage IV or V	Immediate-release carbidopa/levodopa Dopamine agonists
Poor symptom control	Increase carbidopa/levodopa dose Add or increase dopamine agonist dose Add COMT inhibitor
Suboptimal peak response	Begin combination therapy Add levodopa to dopamine agonist Add dopamine agonist to levodopa Increase dose of levodopa/carbidopa or dopamine agonist Add COMT inhibitor as levodopa adjunct Switch dopamine agonists
Wearing off	Begin combination dopaminergic therapy Add levodopa to dopamine agonist Add dopamine agonist to levodopa Increase frequency of levodopa dosing Increase dose of levodopa/carbidopa (sustained- or immediate-release) Add COMT inhibitor and decrease levodopa dose Change to sustained-release carbidopa/levodopa Add liquid levodopa/carbidopa Add selegiline if not already taking
On-off	Begin combination dopaminergic therapy Add levodopa to dopamine agonist Add dopamine agonist to levodopa Add COMT inhibitor Modify distribution of dietary protein
Freezing	Increase or decrease carbidopa/levodopa dose Add dopamine agonist Increase or decrease dopamine agonist dose Discontinue selegiline Gait modification, assistance device
No "on" time	Manipulate time and dose of levodopa Add COMT inhibitor Avoid dietary protein Increase GI transit time

Age. Patients less than 70 years of age should be started with a dopamine agonist, whereas older patients should be started with levodopa/carbidopa. The older patients are less likely to develop levodopa-related motor problems. Anticholinergics are contraindicated in older patients because of increased risk of cognitive impairment, blurred vision, and dry mouth.

Cognitive Impairment. Treatment with levodopa/carbidopa should be initiated and polypharmacy eliminated by gradually discontinuing drugs in the following order: sedative medications, anticholinergics, amantadine, selegiline, dopamine agonists.

Disease Severity. It is controversial whether to start with levodopa/carbidopa or dopamine agonists. Further studies are needed.

Employment Status. Dopamine agonists could be used first, especially in younger patients who are at greater risk for developing motor complications. Other experts advocate starting with levodopa/carbidopa.

Cost. When financial realities outweigh the potential for future benefits, treatment should be initiated with the least expensive medications.

Combined Therapy. When patients treated with single agents (either levodopa/carbidopa or dopamine agonists) require additional treatment, most experts agree that the patient should receive combination therapy rather than pushing the dose of the current drug.

levodopa Management Problems

Approximately 50% of patients treated with levodopa will experience fluctuations in their response to the drug within 6 years. These fluctuations include "wearing-off," "on-off" effects, dyskinesias, and dystonias.

A therapeutic controversy in the treatment of IPD revolves around the initiation and duration of levodopa therapy. Some practitioners believe levodopa therapy is useful for only approximately 5 years and should be withheld until disabling symptoms appear. Others believe there is insufficient evidence to support these beliefs and withholding levodopa therapy deprives patients of the benefits of the drug. Most do agree that levodopa should be added to a patient's treatment when the disease affects activities of daily living or job performance.

The sustained-release formulation of carbidopa/levodopa may provide a more physiologic replacement of dopamine than other regimens (e.g., alternate-day, pulse-, or as-needed dosing) that attempt to reduce total levodopa exposure. An immediate-release dose may be added to the morning dose if the patient experiences late onset or an inadequate peak response. The occurrence of blepharospasm or involuntary movements signify a dose reduction is needed.

As PD progresses, neurons lose their storage capabilities for dopamine and patients are dependent on the rate of levodopa administration for a therapeutic response. Patients experiencing "wearing-off" of therapeutic effect after 1.5 to 2 hours require more frequent doses of levodopa or a sustained-release formulation to alleviate this problem. Dopamine agonists and COMT inhibitors may also be beneficial.

Patients experiencing choreiform dyskinesias during their peak levodopa effect may benefit from substituting an immediate-release for a sustained-release product, or the opposite. Another alternative includes discontinuing selegiline, lowering individual doses of levodopa/carbidopa, and then adding a dopamine agonist as levodopa/carbidopa doses are decreased. Dystonias occurring at the end of the dosing cycle may benefit from more frequent doses of levodopa/carbidopa or from adding or increasing the dose of a dopamine agonist. Restricting levodopa/carbidopa to several early to midday doses may also be of benefit.

Early-morning foot dystonias may benefit from nocturnal administration of sustained-release levodopa/carbidopa. If that is not successful, a nocturnal dopamine agonist could be used or early morning levodopa/carbidopa. Dystonias occurring at the peak dose time may benefit from lowering the dose of levodopa/carbidopa or adding or increasing the dopamine agonist dose.

If patients have a delayed onset of action, levodopa may be given on an empty stomach before meals and crushed or chewed and taken with a full glass of water.

HOW TO MONITOR

In general, there are no laboratory tests that are used to monitor the efficacy of antiparkinson drugs. Exceptions are discussed in the specific drug sections.

Patients' responses to therapy are monitored by assessment of their functional and clinical status, using physical assessment measures of neurologic function. The following should be assessed regularly: facial appearance, salivation, seborrhea; speech; tremor; rigidity/dyskinesia; finger/foot tapping; rapid alternating movement; standing up from chair without assistance of arms/hands; posture; stability; gait; handwriting; and intellectual and psychiatric assessment.

The most common adverse effects of antiparkinson drugs are nausea, hypotension, and psychiatric problems; these symptoms should be continually monitored (Table 47-2).

PATIENT VARIABLES

Pregnancy

Most antiparkinson drugs are either pregnancy category C or unknown; pergolide is category B. Excretion in breast milk is either unknown or does occur; therefore none of the antiparkinson drugs should be used during pregnancy or lactation.

Pediatrics

Safety in children younger than 12 years of age has not been established.

PATIENT EDUCATION

Support of emotional needs for both patients and caregivers is essential. Patients, families, and significant others should be educated about realistic expectations from various treatments. Encourage patients and their families to adhere to their treatment regimens and keep a diary of their symptoms and daily medication administration times.

TABLE 47-2 Adverse Drug Effects of Antiparkinson Drugs

Drug	Adverse Effects*	More Frequent	Less Frequent
levodopa	After >1 yr, patient may experience on-off phenomenon or start hesitation Neuroleptic malignant syndrome upon abrupt discontinuation	Difficult urination, dizziness, orthostatic hypotension, irregular heartbeat, depression, mood changes, nausea, vomiting, unusual body movements, anxiety, confusion, nervousness	Blepharospasm, duodenal ulcer, hemolytic anemia, hypertension, anorexia, diarrhea, dry mouth, flushing, headache, insomnia, muscle twitching, unusual tiredness, weakness
carbidopa	No ability to produce adverse drug effects; allows CNS adverse effects of levodopa because of increased CNS levodopa See levodopa entry		
selegiline	With doses >10 mg daily: bruxism, muscle twitches, myoclonic jerks	Dyskinesia, mood or other CNS changes, abdominal pain, dizziness, dry mouth, insomnia, nausea, vomiting	Angina, arrhythmias, asthma, bradycardia, edema, extrapyramidal effects, GI bleeding, hallucinations, headache, hypertension, orthostatic hypotension, prostatic hypertrophy, tardive dyskinesia, anxiety, apraxia, blepharospasm, diplopia, body aches, bradykinesia, chills, constipation, diarrhea, diaphoresis, drowsiness, headache, heartburn, impaired memory, urination difficulty, irritability, loss of appetite, palpitations, circumoral paresthesias, photosensitivity, tinnitus, taste changes, euphoria, tiredness, weakness
amantadine	Convulsions, leukopenia	Nausea, dizziness, insomnia	Depression, anxiety, irritability, hallucinations, confusion, dry mouth, constipation, livedo reticularis, peripheral edema, orthostatic hypotension
bromocriptine	Pulmonary infiltrates on long-term, high-dose therapy (20-100 mg daily) have occurred and slowly resolve after therapy was discontinued; rare: MI, stroke	Hypotension, nausea	Confusion, dyskinesia, hallucinations, constipation, diarrhea, drowsiness, dry mouth, nocturnal leg cramps, loss of appetite, depression, stomach pain, stuffy nose, Raynaud's phenomenon, vomiting
pergolide	10% experience orthostatic hypotension (tolerance develops); CNS symptoms, hallucinations, confusion caused discontinuation most frequently	CNS effects (dyskinesia, hallucinations, insomnia), hypertension, nausea, constipation, diarrhea, dyspepsia, dry mouth, dysphagia, flu-like symptoms, rhinitis, weakness, anemia, peripheral edema, twitching, myalgia, sweating, diplopia, urinary frequency	
pramipexole	Hallucinations, dizziness, somnolence, extrapyramidal symptoms, headache, confusion, nausea	Nausea, dizziness, somnolence, insomnia, constipation, asthenia, hallucinations, accidental injury, dyspepsia, general edema	Malaise, fever, anorexia, dysphagia, decreased weight
ropinirole	Nausea, dizziness, aggravated Parkinson's, hallucinations (dose related), somnolence, vomiting, headache	Fatigue, syncope, dizziness, dyspepsia, nausea, vomiting, somnolence	Constipation, pain, increased sweating, asthenia, leg edema, orthostatic symptoms, abdominal pain, pharyngitis, confusion, hallucinations, abnormal vision

*Adverse effects that led to discontinuation of treatment during clinical trials or occurred in more than 2% of patients.

Continued

TABLE 47-2 Adverse Drug Effects of Antiparkinson Drugs—cont'd

Drug	Adverse Effects*	More Frequent	Less Frequent
Anticholinergic agents	Anhidrosis, hyperthermia Withdrawal symptoms: anxiety, extrapyramidal symptoms, tachycardia, orthostatic hypotension	Anticholinergic effects: blurred vision; constipation; decreased sweating; difficulty urinating; drowsiness; dry mouth, nose, or throat; nausea; vomiting; sensitivity to light	Euphoria, headache, memory loss, muscle cramps, nervousness, numbness in hands or feet, orthostatic hypotension, sore mouth and tongue, stomach pain, unusual excitement
tolcapone	Diarrhea; hallucination (>75 yr); dystonia (<75 yr); somnolence (females > males)	Abdominal pain, anorexia, diarrhea, dizziness, dyskinesia, dystonia, hallucinations, headache, insomnia, nausea, orthostatic complaints, somnolence, syncope, upper respiratory tract infection, vomiting, urine discoloration	Chest pain, dyspnea, fatigue, falling, hematuria, hyperkinesia, influenza-like symptoms, loss of balance control; rare incidence of agitation, arthritis, burning of feet, chest discomfort, hyperactivity, hypotension, irritability, mental deficiency, muscle cramps, neck pain, paresthesia, sinus congestion, stiffness, urinary tract infection, rhabdomyolysis

Specific Drugs

DOPAMINE PRECURSORS

(P) Prototype Drug

carbidopa/levodopa (Sinemet, Sinemet CR)

Indications

Treatment of IPD: Used in combination because carbidopa inhibits peripheral decarboxylation of levodopa and allows higher CNS concentrations of levodopa. Allows smoother, more rapid titration, reduces nausea and vomiting, allows concurrent pyridoxine (vitamin B_6) when needed.

Unlabeled use: Management of postherpetic neuralgia and restless leg syndrome.

Contraindications

- Discontinue MAOI 2 weeks before initiation of levodopa.
- Narrow-angle glaucoma.
- Undiagnosed skin lesions or history of melanoma as levodopa may activate malignant melanoma.

Risk-benefit assessment should be made if the following medical problems exist:

- *Major significance:* bronchial asthma, emphysema, severe pulmonary disease; severe cardiovascular disease; angle-closure glaucoma; melanoma (history or suspected); history of myocardial infarction with arrhythmias; history of peptic ulcer disease; psychosis; renal dysfunction; urinary retention.
- *Slightly less significance:* history of convulsive disorder, diabetes mellitus, endocrine disease, open-angle glaucoma, hepatic dysfunction.

Warnings

- Use with caution in patients with severe cardiovascular, pulmonary, renal, hepatic, or endocrine disease.
- Use in patients with previous myocardial infarction with residual arrhythmias should only take place in a coronary or intensive care unit.
- Possibility of upper gastrointestinal bleeding in patients with history of peptic ulcer disease.
- Observe patients for depression, suicidal ideation. Use cautiously in psychotic patients.
- Ten to 25 mg pyridoxine (vitamin B_6) inactivates the effects of levodopa. Patients taking carbidopa/levodopa products will not experience this inactivation as carbidopa inhibits this action of vitamin B_6.
- Neuroleptic malignant syndrome may develop if drug is withdrawn abruptly.
- Dyskinesias may occur at lower doses with coadministration of carbidopa/levodopa and may require dose reduction. Occurs because more levodopa is available to the CNS.

Precautions

- Evaluate hepatic, hematopoietic, cardiovascular, and renal function periodically.
- Monitor patients with wide-angle glaucoma carefully for increases in intraocular pressure.
- Monitor patients on antihypertensive drugs cautiously. May require lower antihypertensive dose because of hypotensive effects of levodopa.

Drug Interactions

Antacids increase levodopa bioavailability. Anticholinergics, benzodiazepines, hydantoins, methionine, papaverine, pyridoxine, and tricyclic antidepressants decrease levodopa effectiveness. MAOIs increase the effect of levodopa and may precipitate hypertensive reactions.

Tricyclic antidepressants have caused hypertension and dyskinesia.

Dietary note. Levodopa competes directly with amino acids for absorption across the GI membrane and with amino acid transport mechanisms into the CNS. Patients should take levodopa initially with food to avoid GI adverse effects. Tolerance usually develops to these effects. Patients may eat 15 minutes after taking levodopa if they tolerate the GI effects. Patients experiencing suboptimal response to levodopa should limit their protein intake at their morning and noon meals to increase absorption and bioavailability of the drug.

Dosage and Administration
carbidopa/levodopa Dosage
Initiation. Individualize and titrate dosage. Start with one tablet of 10:100 carbidopa/levodopa three or four times daily or one tablet of 25:100 three times daily. Dosage may gradually be increased every 1 to 2 days as needed and tolerated.

Prior levodopa therapy. Levodopa must be discontinued at least 8 hours before initiation of carbidopa/levodopa therapy.

Patients requiring less than 1.5 g levodopa daily: same as no prior levodopa therapy.

Patients requiring more than 1.5 g levodopa daily: 25 mg carbidopa/250 mg levodopa three or four times daily initially. May gradually increase dosage per day at 1- to 2-day intervals as needed and tolerated. The initial carbidopa/levodopa dose should provide 25% of the total levodopa daily dose previously required.

carbidopa/levodopa Extended-Release Dosage
Initial, no prior levodopa: in mild-to-moderate disease, initiate therapy with 50 mg carbidopa, 200 mg levodopa twice daily at least 6 hours apart.

Initiating, currently receiving carbidopa/levodopa: dosage of extended-release product should be substituted so it will provide 10% higher levodopa doses than with the previous combination product. This may need to be increased to doses that provide 30% more levodopa/day.

Total Daily levodopa Dose	carbidopa/levodopa Extended Release
300 to 400 mg	200 mg twice daily
500 to 600 mg	300 mg twice daily
200 mg	Three times daily
700 to 800 mg	800 mg in three or more divided doses (300 mg in AM and early PM, 200 mg late PM)
900 to 1000 mg	1000 mg in three or more divided doses (400 mg AM and early PM, 200 mg late PM)

Patient Variables
Geriatrics. Older adult patients have an age-related decrease in dopa-decarboxylase; therefore they may require a lower dose.

MAO-B INHIBITOR

selegiline (Eldepryl)

Contraindications
- Meperidine or other opioids

Warnings
- Do not exceed 10 mg per day.

Precautions. Exacerbation of levodopa adverse effects because of increased concentrations of dopamine acting on supersensitive dopamine receptors.

Observe patients for atypical responses as the MAO system of enzymes is not completely understood, and the quality of enzymes may vary from patient to patient.

Drug Interactions. Interactions occur with fluoxetine and meperidine.

Overdosage. Hypotension and psychomotor agitation can occur. Doses greater than 10 mg/day are likely to inhibit both MAO-A and MAO-B, and patients may experience a hypertensive crisis similar to the tyramine or "cheese-effect" crisis.

Dosage and Administration. Parkinsonian patients receiving levodopa/carbidopa who demonstrate a deteriorating response to this treatment should take 10 mg/day in divided doses (5 mg at breakfast and lunch).

Attempt to reduce the levodopa/carbidopa dose after 2 to 3 days of selegiline therapy; 10% to 30% reductions are typical, and further reductions should be individualized.

Patient Variables
Stage of PD: selegiline may delay the need for carbidopa/levodopa by 1 year and prolong a patient's ability to remain employed full-time.

Advanced PD patients may benefit from selegiline's relief from "wearing-off" and fluctuations of L-dopa.

Patient Education
- Patients should not exceed the recommended daily dose of 10 mg to avoid a hypertensive crisis. Describe the tyramine reaction to both patients and their families.
- Patients should immediately report any sudden, severe headache or other unusual symptoms they have not previously experienced.

DOPAMINE AGONISTS

amantadine (Symmetrel)

This antiviral agent was discovered to have antiparkinson activity also (see Chapter 70 for antiviral use).

Warnings. Prescriptions should be written for the smallest quantity needed. Suicidal ideations and successful suicides have occurred in patients with and without prior history of psychiatric illness. Use caution in prescribing amantadine to patients taking other drugs with CNS effects.

Increased seizure activity is possible in patients who have a history of epilepsy.

Amantadine has been implicated in causing chronic heart failure and peripheral edema; therefore patients with these conditions should be monitored closely on initiation of amantadine.

Precautions

- Do not discontinue abruptly or parkinsonian crisis may be precipitated.
- Neuroleptic malignant syndrome may occur with decreases in dosage or discontinuation of therapy.
- Adjust dose of amantadine in elderly and in patients with renal dysfunction (see chart in Dosage and Administration section).
- Monitor patients with liver dysfunction closely. Elevated concentrations of liver enzymes have occurred, which are reversible on discontinuation of the drug.

Drug Interactions. Thioridazine has reportedly caused worsening tremor in elderly patients. It is unknown if other phenothiazines may cause the same reaction.

Dyazide (triamterene/hydrochlorothiazide) administered with amantadine caused elevated amantadine concentrations.

Overdosage. Deaths have occurred at 2-g doses of amantadine. Serious cardiac, respiratory, renal, and CNS toxicity has occurred with overdoses. Treatment in a hospital emergency department is necessary.

Dosage and Administration. Give 100 mg twice daily when used alone. The initial dose is decreased to 100 mg daily in patients with serious associated medical illnesses or patients receiving high doses of other antiparkinson agents. Onset is usually within 48 hours. Increase to 100 mg twice daily after 1 to several weeks. Some patients benefit from doses up to 400 mg daily; however, close monitoring is required. Patients who initially respond to amantadine therapy may experience decreased efficacy after several months. They may benefit from increasing doses to 300 mg daily or by discontinuing for several weeks and then restarting amantadine therapy.

Rapid therapeutic benefit can be attained when amantadine is started with levodopa. The dose of amantadine should be held steady at 100 to 200 mg daily while the levodopa dose is increased.

Amantadine added to optimal levodopa therapy may yield additional benefit such as less fluctuation. Patients who require their levodopa dose to be decreased because of adverse effects may regain some benefit by adding amantadine to their regimen.

Dosage in renal impairment: adjustments in dosage are required based on degree of impairment. See package insert.

bromocriptine mesylate (Parlodel)

Contraindications

- Sensitivity to ergot alkaloids

Warnings. Hypotension, hypertension, seizures, stroke, and acute myocardial infarctions have occurred. Use with caution in patients on other antihypertensive medications. Monitor patients carefully.

Precautions. Safety for longer than 2 years is unknown. Periodic monitoring of hepatic, hematopoietic, cardiovascular, and renal function is recommended. High doses can cause confusion and mental disturbances. Hallucinations usually remit on dosage reduction or discontinuation.

Drug Interactions. Dopamine antagonists (neuroleptics, metoclopramide) can diminish the effectiveness of bromocriptine.

Use with caution with other highly protein-bound drugs.

Dosage and Administration. *Initiation:* start with 1.25 mg twice daily with meals. Assess response every 2 weeks to ensure maximum response from minimum dose. If necessary, increase dosage by 2.5 mg per day every 2 to 4 weeks, taken with meals. If adverse reactions require dosage reduction, do so gradually and in 2.5-mg increments. The usual dosage range is 10 to 40 mg per day. The safety of doses greater than 100 mg daily has not been demonstrated. Avoid alcohol intake.

pergolide (Permax)

Warnings. Symptomatic orthostatic hypotension and hallucinations may occur.

Precautions. Use with caution in patients who are prone to arrhythmias.

Drug Interactions. Dopamine antagonists (neuroleptics, metoclopramide) diminish the effectiveness of pergolide.

Use with caution with other highly protein-bound drugs.

Overdosage. Symptoms include nausea, vomiting, convulsions, decreased blood pressure, and CNS stimulation. Supportive care and monitoring blood pressure in a hospital are required.

Dosage and Administration. *Initiation:* use 0.5 mg for first 2 days. Gradually increase dose by 0.1 or 0.15 mg a day every third day over the next 12 days of therapy. Dosage may then be increased by 0.25 mg/day every third day until optimal therapeutic response is achieved.

Administer in divided doses three times daily. Decrease carbidopa/levodopa dosage cautiously during pergolide dose titration period. Mean daily dosage is 3 mg/day. Dosage above 5 mg/day has not been studied.

pramipexole (Mirapex)

A nonergot dopamine agonist with high relative in vitro specificity and full intrinsic activity at the D_2 dopamine receptors. It binds with higher affinity to D_3 than to D_2 or D_4 receptor subtypes. The relevance of D_3 receptor binding in PD is unknown.

Pharmacokinetics. Pramipexole is renally eliminated and is secreted by renal tubules via the organic cation transport

TABLE 47-3 Pharmacokinetics of Antiparkinson Drugs

Drug	Absorption	Onset of Action	Time to Peak Concentration	Half-Life	Duration of Action	Metabolism	Elimination	Protein Binding
levodopa	Rapid, complete	2-3 wk; up to 6 mo	0.5 hr	1 hr	0.5 hr	Extensive	Renal	
carbidopa	Rapid, complete		0.7 hr	1-2 hr			Renal	
carbidopa/levodopa	Released over 4-6 hr; 70%-75% bioavailable		2.4 hr	2 hr				
selegiline active metabolites						(Metabolites)		
N-desmethyldeprenyl						2		
L-amphetamine						17.7		
L-methamphetamine						20.5		
amantidine	Rapid, complete	48 hr	2-4 hr	11-15 hr	—	None	Renal	
bromocriptine	28% of oral dose	1-1.5 hr	1-2 hr	Initial: 6-8 hr Terminal: 50 hr		Complete	Biliary	90%–96%
pergolide						Hepatic	Renal	90%
pramipexole	Rapid, 90% bioavailable		2 hr	8 hr in young; 12 hr in elderly			Renal	15%
ropinirole	Rapid, 55% bioavailable		1-2 hr	6 hr		Extensive, inactive	Renal	40%
Anticholinergics	Well absorbed							
benztropine		1-2 hr			24 hr			
biperiden		IM 10-30 min	1-1.5 hr	18-24 hr 4-15 hr	1-8 hr			
diphenhydramine			2-4 hr					
ethopropazine		1 hr			4 hr			
procyclidine			1.1-2 hr	11.5-12.6 hr	4 hr			
trihexyphenidyl			1-1.3 hr	5.6-10 hr	6-12 hr			
tolcapone	Rapid, 65% bioavailable		2 hr	2-3 hr		Extensive, inactive metabolites	Renal, 0.5%	99.9%

system; therefore dose adjustment is required in renal insufficiency (see Dosage and Administration following). See Table 47-3.

Contraindications

- Hypersensitivity to the drug or its ingredients

Warnings/Precautions. Carefully monitor patients starting pramipexole therapy or undergoing a dose escalation for signs and symptoms of orthostatic hypotension.

There is an age-related risk of hallucinations attributed to pramipexole. The risk is 1.9 times greater than placebo in early Parkinson patients less than 65 years of age and 6.8 times greater than placebo in patients older than 65. The risk increase compared with placebo in advanced Parkinson patients was 3.5 in patients younger than 65 years of age and 5.2 in patients older than 65.

One case of rhabdomyolysis occurred in a 47-year-old man with advanced disease. Symptoms resolved after pramipexole was discontinued.

Caution should be exercised when prescribing pramipexole to patients with renal insufficiency.

Pramipexole may cause or exacerbate dyskinesias when used in conjunction with levodopa. Decreasing the levodopa dose may ameliorate this side effect.

Drug Interactions. Carbidopa/levodopa does not influence the pharmacokinetics of pramipexole. However, pramipexole increases the levodopa C_{max} by 40% and decreases the T_{max} from 2.5 to 0.5 hour.

Cimetidine causes a 50% increase in pramipexole area under curve (AUC) and a 40% increase in half-life. Coadministration of drugs that are secreted by the cationic transport system (e.g., cimetidine, ranitidine, diltiazem, triamterene, verapamil, quinidine, quinine) decreases the oral clearance of pramipexole by about 20%. Drugs secreted by the anionic transport system (e.g., penicillins, indomethacin, hydrochlorothiazide, chlorpropamide) have little effect on the oral clearance of pramipexole. Pramipexole does not inhibit cytochrome P450 (CYP) enzymes, and inhibitors of CYP enzymes do not affect pramipexole elimination.

It is possible that dopamine antagonists such as neuroleptics may diminish the effectiveness of pramipexole.

Overdosage. There is no clinical experience with massive overdosage. One case of a patient taking 11 mg/day resulted in no adverse effects. Blood pressure remained stable while pulse rate increased to 100 to 120 beats/min.

Dosage and Administration. Consult a neurologist. Pramipexole should be titrated gradually in all patients. The dosage should be increased to achieve a maximum therapeutic effect, balanced against the principal side effects of dyskinesia, hallucinations, somnolence, and dry mouth.

Patients with normal renal function: starting dose of 0.375 mg/day given in three divided doses. Do not increase more frequently than every 5 to 7 days. The following ascending dosage schedule of pramipexole was used in clinical trials and is suggested for use.

Week	Dosage (mg)	Total Daily Dose (mg)
1	0.125 tid	0.375
2	0.25 tid	0.75
3	0.5 tid	1.5
4	0.75 tid	2.25
5	1.0 tid	3.0
6	1.25 tid	3.75
7	1.5 tid	4.5

When pramipexole is used in conjunction with levodopa, a reduction of the levodopa dosage should be considered. In one controlled study in advanced PD, the levodopa dosage was reduced an average of 27% from baseline.

Patients with renal impairment: adjustments in dosage are required based on degree of impairment. See package insert.

Discontinuation: gradual discontinuation over a period of 1 week is recommended. However, abrupt discontinuation can be uneventful.

For restless leg syndrome, 0.125 to 0.375 mg at bedtime or up to 1.5 mg in divided doses two or three times a day for daytime symptoms, increase by 0.125 mg every 3 days until satisfactory management of symptoms or intolerable side effects or no relief occurs.

ropinirole hydrochloride (Requip)

This drug is a nonergot dopamine agonist with high relative in vitro specificity and full intrinsic activity at the D_2 and D_3 dopamine receptors. It binds with higher affinity to D_3 than to D_2 or D_4 receptor subtypes. The relevance of D_3 receptor binding in PD is unknown.

Pharmacokinetics. Ropinirole has a 55% absolute bioavailability, indicating a first-pass effect. Food does not affect the extent of absorption; however, the T_{max} is increased by 2.5 hours when the drug is taken with a meal. See Table 47-3.

No dosage adjustment is necessary based on gender, weight, age, or moderate renal impairment (creatinine clearance, 30 to 50 ml/min). Ropinirole has not been studied in patients with severe renal impairment.

Contraindications

- Hypersensitivity to the drug or its ingredients.

Warnings/Precautions. Syncope, sometimes associated with bradycardia, was observed in association with ropinirole in both early PD without concomitant levodopa and advanced PD patients with concomitant levodopa.

Carefully monitor patients starting ropinirole therapy or undergoing a dose escalation for signs and symptoms of orthostatic hypotension.

Hallucinations occurred in 5.2% of Parkinson's patients without concomitant levodopa compared with 1.4% of placebo-treated patients. In advanced Parkinson's patients receiving both ropinirole and levodopa, 10.1% of ropinirole-treated patients experienced hallucinations compared with 4.2% in the placebo group.

Ropinirole may potentiate the dopaminergic side effects of levodopa and may cause and/or exacerbate dyskinesias. Decreasing the dose of levodopa may ameliorate this side effect.

Drug Interactions. CYP 1A2 is the major isoenzyme responsible for metabolism in the line; therefore there is the potential for substrates or inhibitors of this enzyme to alter the clearance of ropinirole when coadministered. Adjustment of the ropinirole dosage may be required. Coadministration of theophylline (a CYP 1A2 substrate) did not alter the steady state pharmacokinetics of ropinirole. Coadministration of ciprofloxacin (a CYP 1A2 inhibitor) increased the AUC of ropinirole by 84% and the C_{max} by 60%.

Estrogens reduce the oral clearance of ropinirole by 36%. Dosage adjustment may not be needed for ropinirole in patients on estrogen therapy because patients must be carefully titrated with ropinirole to tolerance or adequate effect. However, if estrogen therapy is stopped or started during treatment with ropinirole, adjustment of the ropinirole dose may be necessary.

Overdosage. Side effects from inadvertent overdosage include mild orofacial dyskinesia, intermittent nausea, agitation, increased dyskinesia, grogginess, sedation, orthostatic hypotension, chest pain, confusion, vomiting, and nausea.

Dosage and Administration. Ropinirole should be titrated gradually in all patients. The dosage should be increased to achieve a maximum therapeutic effect, balanced against the principal side effects of nausea, dizziness, somnolence, and dyskinesia.

Ropinirole may be taken with or without food. Taking ropinirole with food decreases the C_{max}; therefore patients taking ropinirole with food may experience less nausea.

The recommended starting dose is 0.25 mg three times daily. Dosage may be titrated according to patient's individual response in weekly increments as described in the following ascending dose schedule of ropinirole. After week 4, if necessary, daily dosage may be increased by 1.5 mg/day on a weekly basis up to a dose of 9 mg/day and then by up to 3 mg/day weekly to a total dosage of 24 mg/day. Doses greater than 24 mg/day have not been tested in clinical trials.

Week	Dosage (mg)	Total Daily Dose (mg)
1	0.25 tid	0.75
2	0.5 tid	1.5
3	0.75 tid	2.25
4	1.0 tid	3.0

When ropinirole is administered as adjunctive therapy with levodopa, the dose of levodopa may need to be decreased gradually as tolerated. During clinical trials, the levodopa dose was reduced by 31% in ropinirole-treated patients.

Ropinirole should be discontinued gradually over a 7-day period. The frequency of administration should be reduced from three times daily to twice daily for 4 days. For the remaining 3 days, the frequency should be reduced to once daily before complete withdrawal of ropinirole.

Restless leg syndrome: for nocturnal symptoms, the initial dose is 0.25 mg at bedtime, for daytime symptoms, use 0.25 mg two or three times daily. Dose may be doubled weekly until symptoms are managed or intolerable adverse events occur. The average dosage is 3.5 mg/day. Consult a neurologist.

ANTICHOLINERGIC AGENTS

Synthetic agents that have more selective CNS activity have replaced the use of naturally occurring belladonna alkaloids. Peripheral anticholinergic effects may be the dose-limiting factors. Antihistamines also have central anticholinergic effects and have a lower incidence of peripheral adverse effects than the natural or synthetic alkaloids. Trihexyphenidyl and benztropine are the two agents most frequently used as adjunctive therapy for PD, but little evidence exists to support the use of one agent over the others. If a patient does not respond to one anticholinergic, another may be tried.

Patient Variables

Geriatrics. Elderly patients may show an increased sensitivity to anticholinergic drugs, thus requiring strict dosage adjustment and monitoring. CNS adverse events may develop.

Stage of PD. This drug is only helpful in patients presenting with tremor. Patients in early stages of PD who function well may not require medication. Consider adding anticholinergics as disease progresses.

How to Monitor

Periodic intraocular pressure determinations should be made.

Patient Education

- Patients may take with food if gastrointestinal upset occurs.
- Drowsiness, dizziness, and blurred vision may be caused; caution is required while driving or performing tasks requiring alertness.
- Avoid alcohol and other CNS depressants.
- Dry mouth may be caused. Sucking hard candy, adequate fluid intake, or good oral hygiene may relieve symptoms. Constipation or difficulty urinating may occur; stool softeners may relieve constipation. Alert health care provider if effects persist.
- Notify health care provider of rapid heartbeat, confusion, eye pain, or rash.
- Use caution in hot weather. Susceptibility to stroke increased.

Contraindications

Glaucoma, especially angle-closure; pyloric or duodenal obstruction; stenosing peptic ulcers; prostatic hypertrophy or bladder neck obstruction; achalasia; myasthenia gravis; and megacolon.

Warnings

- *Ophthalmic:* incipient narrow-angle glaucoma may be precipitated.
- *Elderly:* increased sensitivity to anticholinergic drugs requires strict dosage adjustment. CNS adverse events may develop.

Precautions

- Use with caution in patients with tachycardia, cardiac arrhythmias, hypertension, hypotension, prostatic hypertrophy (particularly in elderly), urinary retention, liver or kidney disorders, and gastrointestinal or genitourinary obstructive disease.
- Mental or physical abilities may be impaired; caution is required when performing tasks that require alertness.
- If discontinuation of drug is required, do so gradually to avoid acute exacerbations of PD.
- Anhidrosis may occur during hot weather. Decrease dose so thermal-regulating ability is not impaired.
- Dry mouth may cause difficulty swallowing or speaking and loss of appetite. Reduce dose or discontinue temporarily.
- Abuse potential exists. Cannabinoids, barbiturates, opiates, and alcohol have additive effects with anticholinergics.

Drug Interactions

- *Amantadine, other anticholinergics, MAOIs:* anticholinergic adverse effects may be increased; they disappear when dose is decreased.
- *Digoxin:* serum levels increased when slow-dissolution oral tablet is administered.
- *Haloperidol:* worsening schizophrenia, decreased haloperidol concentrations, and tardive dyskinesias may develop.
- *Levodopa:* decreased levodopa activity because of decreased gastric motility and increased gastric deactivation of levodopa.
- *Phenothiazines:* pharmacologic and therapeutic actions of phenothiazines reduce effects of anticholinergics and increase anticholinergic adverse reactions.
- *Antidiarrheals:* adsorbent produces decreased effects of anticholinergics because of drug adsorption. Separate administration by 1 to 2 hours.

Overdosage

Serious cardiac, respiratory, or CNS symptoms, including circulatory collapse, may develop.

benztropine (Cogentin)

Dosage and Administration

- Administer 1 to 2 mg per day (range 0.5 to 6 mg/day), orally or parenterally.
- *PD:* Start with 0.5 to 1 mg at bedtime; 4 to 6 mg/day may be required. Reduce or discontinue other antiparkinson drugs gradually.

trihexyphenidyl (Artane, Artane Sequels)

Dosage and Administration. *Initiation of therapy:* start with 1 to 2 mg the first day; increase by 2-mg increments at intervals of 3 to 5 days until a total of 6 to 10 mg is given daily (maximum benefit seen in many patients at these doses). Administer in three divided doses at mealtimes. High doses may be divided by 4 and administered at mealtimes and bedtime.

With levodopa: dose of each may need to be reduced; adjust doses carefully depending on adverse effects and degree of symptom control. Total daily doses of 3 to 6 mg are usually adequate.

Concomitant use with other anticholinergics: substitute in whole or in part for other anticholinergics. Substitute partially at first; then gradually reduce the other anticholinergic while increasing trihexyphenidyl dose.

Sustained-release: not for initial therapy. Patients on stable therapy may be switched to the sustained-release dosage form on a milligram-per-milligram basis. Administer as a single dose after breakfast or in two divided doses every 12 hours. Some patients may experience Parkinson exacerbations and require supplemental doses of tablets or elixir.

COMT INHIBITOR

entacapone (Comtan)

Contraindications

- Hypersensitivity to the drug or its ingredients

Warnings. MAO and COMT are the two major enzymes that metabolize catecholamines. Patients should not be treated concomitantly with entacapone and a nonselective MAOI (e.g., phenelzine, tranylcypromine) because this combination could result in inhibition of the majority of the pathways responsible for normal catecholamine metabolism.

Coadministration of entacapone with drugs metabolized by COMT, including epinephrine, norepinephrine dopamine, dobutamine, methyldopa, and apomorphine, may result in increased heart rate, arrhythmias, and fluctuation in blood pressure.

Precautions. Entacapone enhances the bioavailability of levodopa; therefore the possibility of orthostatic hypotension induced by excess dopaminergic activity is possible. Syncope has also been reported.

Ten percent of entacapone-treated patients in clinical trials experienced diarrhea; 1.7% discontinued the entacapone due to diarrhea.. The diarrhea generally resolved on discontinuation of the drug; however, it did lead to hospitalization in two patients. Diarrhea typically presents 4 to 12 weeks after entacapone is started, but it may appear as early as 2 weeks and as late as many months after treatment initiation.

Hallucinations may present shortly after initiation of therapy, typically within the first 2 weeks. The hallucinations may be responsive to levodopa dose reduction of 20% to 25% after the onset of hallucinations.

Entacapone may cause or exacerbate preexisting dyskinesia. Many patients in clinical trials continued to experience frequent dyskinesias despite a reduction in their levodopa dose.

Rhabdomyolysis has been reported with entacapone. This may be related to prolonged motor activity associated with dyskinesia.

Ergot-derived dopaminergic agents have been reported to cause neuroleptic malignant syndrome, retroperitoneal fibrosis, pulmonary infiltrates, pleural effusion, and pleural thickening. These complications may or may not resolve when the drug is discontinued. It is not known if other drugs affecting dopamine neurotransmission (e.g., entacapone) can also cause these symptoms.

Adverse Reactions. Dyskinesia, nausea, urine discoloration, diarrhea, and abdominal pain are the most frequent adverse events.

Drug Interactions. MAOIs and entacapone given concomitantly can inhibit catecholamine metabolism. Selegiline, a selective MAO-B inhibitor, may be given concomitantly.

Drug interfering with bile excretion such as probenecid, cholestyramine, erythromycin, rifampicin, ampicillin, and chloramphenicol may increase the availability of entacapone.

See warnings for concomitant use with drugs metabolized by COMT.

Overdosage. COMT inhibition is dose dependent; therefore major overdose of entacapone could inhibit COMT and prevent metabolism of catechols.

Dosage and Administration. As an adjunct to levodopa/carbidopa therapy, administer one 200-mg entacapone tablet with each levodopa/carbidopa up to 8 times a day or 1600 mg/day.

RESOURCES FOR PATIENTS AND PROVIDERS

National Parkinson Foundation, www.parkinson.org.

Parkinson disease gene discovery.

Perkin GD, Hochberg FH, Miller DC: *Atlas of clinical neurology,* St Louis, 1996, Mosby, CD-ROM.

Olanow CW, Koller WC: An algorithm (decision tree) for the management of Parkinson's disease: treatment guidelines, *Neurology* 50(suppl 3):S1, 1998.

The practitioner is referred to an excellent review of PD that includes extensive treatment algorithms for the management of IPD and problems encountered in later stages (e.g., dysautonomias, falls, motor problems, neuropsychiatric problems, sleep disorders, etc.).

The Activities of Daily Living (ADL) Scale of the Unified Parkinson Disease Rating Scale (UPDRS)

This is a good practitioner's guide to consistency in evaluating patients' symptoms over time. The Mini-Mental State Examination can be used to measure cognitive impairment.

Organizations

The American Parkinson Disease Association, Inc, 1250 Hylan Boulevard, Suite 4B, Staten Island, NY 10305, (800) 223-2732.

National Parkinson Foundation, Inc, 1501 NW 9th Avenue NW, Bob Hope Road, Miami, FL 33136-1494, (800) 433-7022.

Parkinson's Disease Foundation, 710 W 158th Street, New York, NY 10032, (800) 457-6676.

The Parkinson Action Network, 818 College Avenue, Suite C, Santa Rosa, CA 95404, (707) 544-1994.

BIBLIOGRAPHY

LeWitt P: *Management of Parkinson's disease,* St Louis, 1998, Martin Dunitz.

MacMahon DG: The initial drug treatment of older patients with Parkinson's disease—consider an agonist but don't demonize dopa, *Age Ageing* 32:244-245, 2003.

Martin WR, Wieler M: Treatment of Parkinson's disease, *Can J Neurol Sci* 30(suppl 1):S27-S33, 2003.

Olanow CW, Koller WC: An algorithm (decision tree) for the management of Parkinson's disease: treatment guidelines, *Neurology* 50(suppl 3):S1, 1998.

Siderowf A, Stern M: Update on Parkinson disease, *Ann Intern Med* 138:651-658, 2003.

Uitti RJ: Medical treatment of essential tremor and Parkinson's disease, *Geriatrics* 53:46, 1998.

Weimerskirch PR, Ernst ME: Newer dopamine agonists in the treatment of restless legs syndrome, *Ann Pharmacother* 35:2001.

UNIT 11

Psychotropic Agents

The rapid diffusion of new research findings and new products has revolutionized the treatment of mood disorders and psychiatric problems. Many of the beliefs once held about how drugs work on mood disorders and the appropriate use of medications has undergone substantial change. These medications now are used more extensively and for a greater variety of indications. The recognition of the importance of drug interactions caused by the P450 enzyme system also requires that clinicians stay up to date on the latest findings and recommendations. **Unit 11** includes the following four chapters:

- **Chapter 48** discusses antidepressants, providing the underlying physiology for how many medications affect the CNS. The specific treatment profiles of the different medications are presented with updated indications.
- **Chapter 49** deals with antianxiety agents. Expanded knowledge about treatment of panic attacks and other anxiety disorders has coincided with a variety of new products. Each new agent brings its own set of unique characteristics.
- **Chapter 50** discusses antipsychotics. A gradually increasing arsenal of medications gives new hope to seriously psychotic patients, allowing them to live in the home or community. Use of antipsychotics to treat acute agitation in the elderly is also mentioned. These products are often some of the most dangerous medications ordered and have substantial adverse effects and drug interactions, to which the primary care provider must be alert.
- **Chapter 51** outlines substance abuse treatment. New therapies are beginning to appear for the treatment of alcoholism. Drugs used to treat opioid addition are mentioned but not discussed in detail. This small group of drugs is taking on growing importance for its treatment potential as treatment of addictions moves into primary care.

The CNS and the drugs used to treat mood and psychiatric disorders are complex. Patients with mood disorders are among the most difficult to treat and there is risk for misuse of the medications. The FDA has requested that all drug manufacturers place a special warning on all antidepressant medications to monitor patients for the risk of suicide. As patients who are severely depressed start feeling better, they often regain enough energy to plan and implement a suicide. Thus, these patients require special attention. Often the initial use of all of the agents in the primary care area should be determined by or in consultation with a specialist.

CHAPTER 48

Antidepressants

Drug Names

Class	Subclass	Generic Name	Brand Name
Monoamine oxidase inhibitors (MAOIs)		phenelzine tranylcypromine	Nardil Parnate
Tricyclic antidepressants (TCAs)		(P) (200) nortriptyline (200) amitriptyline desipramine doxepin imipramine	Pamelor Elavil Norpramin Sinequan Tofranil
Selective serotonin reuptake inhibitors (SSRIs)		(P) (200) fluoxetine (200) citalopram (200) sertraline (200) paroxetine fluvoxamine escitalopram	Prozac SR, generic Celexa Zoloft, generic Paxil Luvox Lexapro
Serotonin/norepinephrine reuptake inhibitors (SNRIs)		(200) venlafaxine SR	Effexor SR
Norepinephrine reuptake inhibitors (NRIs)		reboxetine	Not available in USA
Serotonin 2 agonist/blocker/serotonin reuptake inhibitors (SARIs/SSRIs)		(200) trazodone (200) nefazodone	Desyrel Serzone
Norepinephrine/dopamine reuptake inhibitors (NDRIs)		(200) bupropion	Wellbutrin SR
α_2-Noradrenergic antagonists		(200) mirtazapine	Remeron

(200), Top 200 drug; (P), prototype drug.

General Uses

Indications

- Major depression (except fluvoxamine)
- Dysthymia

Other Indications

Selective serotonin reuptake inhibitors (SSRIs)

- Fluvoxamine: obsessive-compulsive disorder (OCD)
- Fluoxetine: bulimia nervosa, panic disorder, premenstrual dysphoric disorder (PMDD), OCD
- Sertraline: panic disorder, PMDD, post-traumatic stress disorder (PTSD), social phobia, OCD in adults and children
- Bupropion: smoking cessation
- Venlafaxine: generalized anxiety disorder
- Paroxetine: generalized anxiety disorder, panic disorder, PTSD, OCD, social phobia

Unlabeled Uses

- Tricyclic antidepressants (TCAs): adjunct treatment of pain, panic disorder, irritable bowel syndrome
- Bupropion: neuropathic pain, attention-deficit hyperactivity disorder (ADHD), enhance weight loss
- Trazodone: aggressive behavior, panic disorder, insomnia, cocaine withdrawal

• • •

There are many types of depressive disorders, but major depressive disorder forms the basis for the discussion in this chapter. Antidepressants are the medications of choice for the pharmacotherapy of patients with mood disorders.

Monoamine oxidase inhibitors (MAOIs) are used as third-line agents for cases of refractory and atypical depression. This chapter mentions MAOIs briefly but does not discuss them in detail because they are generally prescribed by a psychiatrist, not a primary care provider. There are also many TCAs, but this chapter mentions only a few. These agents still provide excellent results in patients who have not responded to one of the newer antidepressants. They are also used when cost is a concern and as an adjunct treatment of depression and pain.

The SSRIs are the most commonly used first-line therapy. They provide excellent response with a good safety profile. The other antidepressants demonstrate a trend toward more specifically tailored mechanisms of action. Their use varies with the clinician's familiarity with the medication. Venlafaxine and bupropion are commonly used in primary care, whereas the others are generally prescribed by psychiatrists.

This chapter discusses the forms in common use. Many of these drugs come in both short- and long-acting forms; racemic variations of the drug are being developed. Citalopram (Celexa) has been largely replaced by escalitopram (Lexapro). Paxil is increasingly being used in its long-acting form. Although the NRI reboxetine is not currently available in the United States, atomoxetine (Strattera) has the same mechanism of action and is indicated for ADHD (see Chapter 43).

DISEASE PROCESS

Anatomy and Physiology

Monoaminergic Neurons and Their Neurotransmitters. There are three important types of monoaminergic neurons in the brain that modulate mood. The first group includes the noradrenergic neurons, which use norepinephrine as their neurotransmitter. Noradrenergic is an old name for norepinergic but the term has remained in use. The second group includes the dopanergic neurons, which use dopamine as their neurotransmitter. The third monoaminergic neuron group contains the serotonergic neurons, which use serotonin as their neurotransmitter.

The monoamine transmitters are subclassified as the catecholamines norepinephrine (NE, also called noradrenaline) and dopamine (DA); and the indolamine serotonin (5-HT).

Monoamine Neurons. See Chapter 42 for review of the anatomy and physiology of neurons. Table 42-1 on neurotransmitters is particularly useful. Although monoamine neurons have the same structure as all neurons, the critical difference between neurons is the neurotransmitter they use.

Monoamine Neurotransmitter Synthesis. All three monoamine neurotransmitters are synthesized by enzymes in the cell body or nerve terminal of the nerve cell. Catecholamine synthesis begins with the amino acid tyrosine, which is made into dihydroxyphenylalanine (DOPA). DOPA is then converted into dopamine. Dopamine is converted into norepinephrine by the enzyme dopamine beta-hydroxylase (DBH).

Synthesis of the indolamine serotonin begins with the amino acid tryptophan. Enzymes convert tryptophan into 5-hydroxytryptophan (5-HT).

Monoamine Neurotransmitter Inactivation. Neurotransmitters can be inactivated by destruction or by removing the neurotransmitter from the synapse, which is their site of action. All three neurotransmitters can be destroyed by the enzyme MAO. The catecholamines norepinephrine and dopamine can also be destroyed by the enzyme catechol-O-methyltransferase (COMT).

All three neurotransmitters can be inactivated by being removed from the synapse. This is accomplished by presynaptic transport pumps, also called reuptake pumps. The neurotransmitter can then be stored for reuse.

Neurotransmitter Action on Neuron Receptors. All receptors are specific; they only recognize certain transmitters. This is how different neurons can have different functions. Various receptors on the postsynaptic neuron mediate different functions.

The neurotransmitter passes the nerve impulse from one cell to the next by being released from one cell and attaching to a receptor (a postsynaptic receptor) on the next cell. Once attached, the neurotransmitter can excite or inhibit the activity of the cell. Postsynaptic receptors recognize a particular neurotransmitter and start the process of impulse transmission in the postsynaptic neuron.

The neurotransmitter can also attach to a receptor on the same cell it was released from (a presynaptic receptor) and affect the activity of that cell. These presynaptic receptors act as autoreceptors. They recognize when a sufficient amount of neurotransmitter is present in the synapse and inhibit further release of the neurotransmitter, operating as a brake. This works as a negative feedback system that regulates the amount of neurotransmitter in the synapse. If the presynaptic receptor is blocked, the receptor will keep the brake from functioning, allowing enhanced release of the neurotransmitter.

The receptors can be blocked by an agent that occupies the receptor site but does not act on the site. This prevents the normal neurotransmitter from doing what it usually does.

Noradrenergic Neurons. Noradrenergic neurons are primarily located in the part of the brain stem called the locus coeruleus. The main function of the noradrenergic neurons is attention. They also have a role in control of memory, information processing, emotions, energy, psychomotor function, movement, blood pressure, heart rate, and bladder emptying.

Although noradrenergic neurons have many receptors for NE, there are three key classes: β_1, α_1, and α_2. Other classes of NE receptors include β_2.

Dopanergic Neurons. Dopanergic neurons are located in the substantia nigra, medial mesencephalic tegmentum, and hypothalamus. They control movement, primitive emotions, and visceral functions. Dopanergic neurons have at least five types of receptors, of which D_2 receptors are the most studied. The D_2 receptor is important in Parkinson's disease and schizophrenia. D_1 through D_4 receptors are affected by some of the atypical antipsychotic drugs. The newer antipsychotics affect mainly D_2 receptors.

Serotonergic Neurons. Serotonergic neurons are located mainly in the area of the brain stem called the raphe nucleus. They regulate anxiety, movements, obsessions and compulsions, appetite and eating behavior, sleep, sexual response, and GI motility.

The two major presynaptic serotonergic neuron receptors are 5-HT_{1A} and 5-HT_{1D}. There are six major serotonergic postsynaptic receptors: 5-HT_{1A}, 5-HT_{1D} (the same as presynaptic), 5-HT_{2A}, 5-HT_{2C}, 5-HT_3, and 5-HT_4. There are many more postsynaptic receptors, with new ones being discovered.

Stimulation of HT_{1A} (desirable) receptors improves mood and decreases eating disorders. HT_{2A} (undesirable) receptors are associated with anxiety, agitation, panic, decreased libido, sexual dysfunction, myoclonus, impaired sleep, and apathy. Stimulation of 5-HT_{2C} receptors causes anxiety, agitation, and panic. 5-HT_3 and 5-HT_4 receptors are located in the gut where they control tone and motility and their stimulation may cause nausea, vomiting, increased bowel motility, cramps, and diarrhea.

Serotonergic neurons also have postsynaptic autoreceptors, 5-HT_{1A}, unlike the catecholamines norepinephrine and dopamine. Serotonergic neurons also have receptors on the cell bodies that enhance serotonin release. Norepinephrine can function as a brake for serotonin release by acting on the NE α_2 receptors that are on serotonin neurons as well as on adrenergic neurons.

Other Neurons and Their Neurotransmitters. Many other neurotransmitters are affected by antidepressant medications, causing numerous side effects. To understand the process, it is necessary to remember the other neurotransmitters and their effects (Table 48-1). The muscarinic system has two branches, the nicotinic and the cholinergic. Of the two, the cholinergic is by far more important. Cholinergic neurons use acetylcholine. The terms muscarinic and cholinergic are often used interchangeably. The histaminergic, α_1-adrenergic, and α_2-adrenergic systems are also important.

Pathophysiology

There have been many theories regarding the cause of depression. The monoamine hypothesis of the pathophysiology of depression states that depression is caused by a deficiency of the monoamine neurotransmitters, mainly norepinephrine and serotonin. Neurotransmitters become depleted by stress, drugs, or an unknown process. This is an overly simplistic explanation. If it were correct, the depression would be relieved as soon as the levels of the neurotransmitters are raised; however, antidepressants take weeks to have an effect.

The neurotransmitter receptor dysfunction theory states that the receptors are not working properly. This receptor dysfunction may be caused by neurotransmitter depletion, as discussed above. There is evidence of down-regulation of receptors with treatment. Although there is some evidence of receptor abnormalities in depression, there is no clear evidence of receptor dysfunction accounting for depression.

The next hypothesis is called the monoamine hypothesis of gene expression. Neurons communicate with each other by other signaling molecules in addition to neurotransmitters. These signaling molecules are called neurotrophic factors. One of these is called brain-derived neurotrophic factor (BDNF), which supports nerve survival and growth. Under stress the gene responsible for BDNF is repressed, leading to a decreased level of BDNF, which results in further atrophy of neurons (causing fewer synapses), thus causing impaired neuronal firing. Antidepressants increase the availability of neurotransmitters at receptor sites. This changes the expression of the genes responsible for the production of BDNF. The BDNF causes the neurons to develop more synapses, which improves neuronal transmission. Positron emission tomography (PET) has demonstrated changes in neuronal firing in patients who have depression. Clinical neuroimaging has demonstrated decreased brain volume of the hippocampus of depressed patients.

An even newer hypothesis for the pathophysiology of depression is the neurokinin hypothesis, which involves peptide neurotransmitters (neurokinins). One of the neurokinins is substance P. Neurokinins are located in peripheral tissues, the spinal cord, and areas of the brain such as the amygdala and the brain stem where the monoamine transmitters are located. Substance P is released from neurons in peripheral tissues in response to inflammation, causing swelling and pain. Substance P is also present in spinal pain pathways. Experiments with substance P antagonists for treatment of migraine pain were not successful in reducing the pain, but seemed to improve the subject's mood. Antagonists for all neurokinins, especially substance P, are currently being formulated and tested.

To conclude, researchers still do not know what causes depression.

TABLE 48-1 Adverse Effects of Neurotransmitters

Neurotransmitter	Adverse Effects
Serotonin	Anxiety, agitation, anorexia, GI distress, headache, hypotension, sexual dysfunction
Norepinephrine	Tachycardia, tremors, sexual dysfunction, augments sympathomimetics
Dopamine	EPS, ↑ prolactin levels, psychosis, insomnia, anorexia, psychomotor activation
Acetylcholine	Memory dysfunction, tachycardia, blurred vision, dry mouth, urinary retention, constipation
Histamine	Sedation, hypotension, weight gain, allergy
α_1-adrenergic	Orthostatic hypotension, dizziness, cardiac conduction disturbance
α_1-adrenergic	Priapism

The Disease

Major depression is a very common, vastly under-treated, and potentially fatal disease. Depression is a heterogeneous disorder with a wide variety of presentations. Many concepts of how to categorize depression have been proven incorrect, including categorization based on biologic versus nonbiologic, endogenous versus reactive, melancholic versus neurotic, acute versus chronic, and familial versus nonfamilial.

There are many mood disorders to distinguish among. See Box 48-1 for the *Diagnostic and Statistical Manual of Mental Disorders* (DSM-IV) diagnostic criteria for major depression and Box 48-2 for risk factors for depression. A person with adjustment disorder with depressed mood has depressive symptoms accounted for by bereavement but persisting for longer than 2 months or accompanied by severe symptoms. Dysthymia has the same symptoms as major depression but milder symptoms and longer duration. Melancholia is a severe form of major depression with a preponderance of somatic symptoms. Depression with psychotic features is a major depression with hallucinations or delusions.

BOX 48-1

THE DSM-IV CRITERIA FOR DIAGNOSIS OF MAJOR DEPRESSIVE DISORDER

At least five of the following symptoms should be present nearly every day, continuously over 2 weeks. One of the symptoms must be either depressed mood or anhedonia.

- Depressed mood most of the day
- Anhedonia: lack of interest or pleasure in normal activities
- Appetite change or weight change
- Insomnia or hypersomnia
- Psychomotor agitation or retardation
- Fatigue, loss of energy
- Feeling worthless or excessive or inappropriate guilt
- Diminished ability to think or concentrate, indecisiveness
- Recurrent thoughts of death, suicidal ideation

BOX 48-2

RISK FACTORS FOR DEPRESSION

- Female sex
- Ages 20 through 40, then elderly
- Family history
- Marital status: unmarried men, married women
- Postpartum, within 6 months
- Negative life events, major psychosocial stressors, family distress
- Pain

Other forms of depression include atypical depression, catatonic depression, comorbid anxiety disorder, depression with cognitive dysfunction (especially in the elderly), and seasonal affective disorder (SAD). (See Tables 48-2 and 48-3 for types of depressions and their different symptoms.) Other diagnoses to consider include depression with alcohol or substance abuse or dependence, prenatal and postpartum depression, comorbid personality disorder, and the depressive phase of bipolar disorder.

Severity of major depression is classified by mild, moderate, or severe. Mild means the patient has symptoms enough to qualify for the diagnosis but has little functional impairment. Moderate means the patient has a greater degree of symptoms as well as functional impairment. Severe means the patient has excess symptoms along with severe impairment of function.

The natural history of untreated depression is that of recurrences. Untreated depression may resolve on its own, but recurrences are common. Risks for recurrence include severity

TABLE 48-2 Types of Symptoms in Depression

Mood	Cognitive	Vegetative	Physical	Behavioral	Emotions
Quality	Memory	↓↑ Sleep	Fatigue	Social withdrawal	Feelings of worthlessness
Severity	Attention, inability to concentrate	↓↑ Appetite	Muscle tension	Loss of interest in usual activities	Suicidal ideation or behavior
Duration	Frustration tolerance	↓↑ Weight	Pain, especially head and stomach	Crying, weeping	Disappointment with self
	Indecisiveness	↓ Sexual function	↓ Sex drive	↓ Frustration, tolerance	Hopelessness, helplessness
	Negative thinking	↓↑ Psychomotor movement	Weakness	Agitation	Anxiety, nervousness
				Irritability	Delusions or hallucinations
					Guilt

TABLE 48-3 Symptoms of the Various Types of Depression

Types of Depression	Mood	Cognitive Symptoms	Vegetative	Physical	Behavioral
Atypical	Mood, reactivity, sensitivity		Increased sleep, appetite, and weight	Fatigue	Phobic
Catatonic		Extreme negativism		Motor immobility, abnormal movements	Extreme agitation
Cognitive dysfunction		Thoughts slowed, ↓ memory, attention, concentration			Poor attention to self-care, complaints about memory
SAD	Manic or hypomanic episodes		Hypersomnia, overeating		Onset in fall/winter with ↓ light

TABLE 48-4 Illness Commonly Co-occurring with Depression

System	Examples
Autoimmune disease	Rheumatologic disorders
CNS disease	Stroke Dementia
Endocrine system disease	Diabetes Thyroid disorder
Heart disease	Chronic heart failure Myocardial infarction
Malnutrition	Vitamin deficiency Protein/calorie deficiency
Mood disorders and psychiatric conditions	Bipolar disorders Alcohol/drug dependency Eating disorders Obsessive-compulsive disorders Anxiety disorders Somatization disorders Personality disorders Psychosis
Other medical problems	Oncologic/hematologic disease Chronic fatigue syndrome Infectious disease

TABLE 48-5 Drug Classes Producing the Side Effects of Depression

Drug Class	Specific Examples
Antihypertensives	Calcium channel blockers (diltiazem), methyldopa, nifedipine, thiazide diuretics, verapamil
Hormones	estrogen, progestins (Norplant), corticosteroids (prednisone, cortisone, ACTH), dapsone
$Histamine_2$ receptor blockers	famotidine (Pepcid), cimetidine, metoclopramide, nizatidine
Anticonvulsants	Barbiturates, carbamazepine, clonazepam, phenytoin, valproic acid
Antiparkinsonian drugs	levodopa
Cardiac medications	digitalis glycosides, HMG-COA reductase inhibitors (statins)
Antiinfectives	fluoroquinolone antibiotics, isoniazid, metronidazole, sulfonamides
Sedative-hypnotic agents	Benzodiazepines
Antineoplastics	vinblastine
Antiinflammatory agents and analgesics	ibuprofen, indomethacin, naproxen, sulindac

and duration of the depression, psychotic symptoms, incomplete recovery in between episodes, and prior episodes of depression. If a patient has had three or more episodes of depression, there is a more than 90% chance of a relapse.

Assessment

A complete history and physical examination are essential for the differential diagnosis of depression and for selecting the best medication for the patient. The discussion below is a brief review. It is crucial to assess the patient for the risk of suicide.

Although many patients react to bad health or chronic illness with depression, some medical illnesses contribute directly to development depression (Table 48-4). Many medications also are associated with symptoms of depression (Table 48-5).

Various assessment tools are useful in the diagnosis of depression. The Beck Depression Scale is popular, as is the Geriatric Depression Scale (GDS) for geriatric patients. The five-item GDS has been shown to be a good screening tool with geriatric patients. The Hamilton Depression Score is used by researchers. There are many other good assessment tools, including the Zung depression tool.

DRUG ACTION AND EFFECTS

All currently marketed antidepressant medications increase the levels of neurotransmitters. Each category has a major mechanism of action in common. There may be slight variations within a drug category. Table 48-6 shows the antidepressants classified according to mechanism of action. The medications are discussed in order of introduction, in part because the mechanism of action becomes more specific with each new class of medication.

Monoamine Oxidase Inhibitors (MAOIs)

The monoamine neurotransmitters (e.g., epinephrine, norepinephrine, serotonin) are broken down by the enzyme monoamine oxidase (MAO) in the process known as oxidation. MAOIs are the medications that block this breakdown, causing increased levels of these three neurotransmitters. The earliest MAOIs were irreversible but very new ones are reversible inhibitors of MAO, known as reversible inhibitor monoamines (RIMAs). These are associated with a lower risk of severe hypertensive episodes.

The enzyme MAO exists in two subtypes: A and B. Both are equally affected by the MAOI medications. The A form of the MAO is the enzyme involved in depression. It breaks down the neurotransmitters serotonin, norepinephrine, and dopamine. Remember that norepinephrine is also linked to control of blood pressure. This is why a potentially fatal hypertensive crisis can be caused by ingesting too much food containing tyramine. The B form of MAO is the enzyme that breaks down amines into toxins that may damage neurons. MAO B inhibition (selegiline [Eldepryl]) is associated with slowing certain neurodegenerative processes such as Parkinson's disease.

Tricyclic Antidepressants (TCAs)

The tricyclics are named for their chemical structure, which contains three rings. TCAs exert their therapeutic effect by blocking (inhibiting) reuptake of norepinephrine and serotonin at the presynaptic neurons. They also block the reuptake

TABLE 48-6 Antidepressant Classification Based on Neurotransmitter

Neurotransmitter	Tricyclics	SSRIs*	MAOIs	Trazodone	Bupropion	Nefazodone	Venlafaxine	Mirtazapine
Norepinephrine uptake inhibition	+++	0	++	0	+	++	++	++
5-HT serotonin uptake inhibition	++	+++	++	++	+	+++	+++	++
Cholinergic inhibition	+++	0*	0	+	0	0	0	0
Histaminergic inhibition	++	0	0	+	0	0	0	0
α_1-Adrenergic inhibition	++	+	0	++	0	+	0	0
α_2-Adrenergic inhibition	+	+	0	++	0	0	00	++
Dopaminergic inhibition	0	0	++	0	++	0	+	0

0, No activity; +, weak activity; ++, moderate activity; +++, high activity.
*citalopram, fluoxetine, fluvoxamine have weak cholinergic inhibition.

TABLE 48-7 Recommendations to Minimize Common Adverse Effects

Adverse Effect	Antidepressant	Recommendation
Dryness of eyes and mouth	TCA	Natural tears, increase fluid intake, pilocarpine oral rinse, suck on sugar-free sour candy
Sexual dysfunction	Most	sildenafil
Sedation	trazodone, TCA, SARI mirtazapine	Do not perform dangerous tasks; take at bedtime
Insomnia	SSRI, venlafaxine, bupropion	Take in morning
Constipation	TCA	Increase fiber and fluid in diet; get regular exercise
Weight gain	TCA, MAOI, mirtazapine	Avoid snacking, exercise regularly; switch to SSRI, venlafaxine, bupropion
Orthostatic hypotension	TCA, SARI, MAOI	Change position slowly; add salt to diet; prescribe fludrocortisone

of dopamine to a lesser degree. Some TCAs block serotonin 2A receptors, an added therapeutic action. In addition they block cholinergic, histamine, and α_1-adrenergic receptors; this effect is associated with the many side effects of TCAs. And TCAs block sodium channels in the heart and brain, which can cause cardiac arrhythmias and seizures.

Selective Serotonin Reuptake Inhibitors (SSRIs)

All SSRIs exhibit selective serotonin inhibition. However, they are each chemically different and exhibit significant variation in action among the five (see Table 48-7 for the differences).

The SSRIs work presynaptically by blocking the reuptake of serotonin. They also block serotonin reuptake on the dendrites of the cell body. This causes down-regulation (desensitization) of the serotonin 1A autoreceptors on the dendrites, which stops the inhibition of sending the impulse through the neuron. This in turn causes the neuron to release more serotonin at the axon. This down-regulation also is a source of reduced side effects as the patient develops tolerance.

There are at least 14 different postsynaptic serotonin receptors in humans. Each of these receptors controls a different physiologic and/or psychiatric function. The action of the SSRIs is related to which postsynaptic receptor is stimulated. The 5-HT_{1A} receptors are responsible for the antidepressant effect. The other receptor subtypes may be responsible for some of the side effects of SSRIs. Serotonin acts as an important neurotransmitter involved in a variety of physiologic functions ranging from control of thermoregulation, cardiovascular function, and spinal regulation of motor function. It can also cause psychotic behavior and hallucinatory states.

New research suggests an SSRI increases survival when given to patients with recent CVA.

There is no good evidence that one SSRI is better than another for treatment of depression or any of the other indications for which these drugs are used, regardless of the FDA approval for different problems. Some patients fail to respond to one SSRI but may respond to another. This may be due to differences in tolerability.

Selective Noradrenergic Reuptake Inhibitors (NRIs)

Reboxetine is a noradrenergic reuptake inhibitor that increases norepinephrine in all noradrenergic pathways. The NRIs increase NE only in the pathways the overlap with serotonin pathways. Reboxetine causes increased activity from the locus coeruleus to the frontal cortex and the limbic cortex.

Serotonin/Norepinephrine Reuptake Inhibitors (SNRIs)

Venlafaxine blocks the presynaptic reuptake of both serotonin and norepinephrine. It is, however, more potent as a serotonin reuptake blocker than as a norepinephrine reuptake blocker. It also blocks dopamine reuptake. Thus it acts on all three of the monoamine neurotransmitters, as do the TCAs. Unlike the TCAs and similar to the SSRIs, venlafaxine has virtually no affinity for muscarinic, histaminergic, or α_1-adrenergic receptors. Its side-effect profile is thus closer to the SSRIs than the TCAs.

Serotonin 2 Agonist/Serotonin Reuptake Inhibitor (SARIs)

These agents block serotonin 2A receptors and serotonin reuptake pre- and postsynaptically. Their most powerful action is to block the serotonin 2A receptors. This is called serotonin 2A antagonism. They block serotonin reuptake, as do the SSRIs, but this is a less potent action. They are weak α_1-adrenergic blockers.

Nefazodone is also a weak blocker of norepinephrine reuptake inhibitors. It has virtually no affinity for cholinergic, α_2-, or β-adrenergic, dopamine D_1, D_2, or histamine receptors.

Trazodone also blocks histamine-1 (H_1) receptors, which causes sedation.

Norepinephrine and Dopamine Reuptake Inhibitor (NDRI)

Bupropion is metabolized into a more active metabolite that is concentrated in the brain. It is a norepinephrine and dopamine reuptake blocker. It does not have any serotonin activity.

Noradrenergic Antagonists

Mirtazapine is an α_2 antagonist, it blocks the α_2 receptors on the adrenergic neurons. The α_2 receptors are noradrenergic receptors that act as presynaptic autoreceptors. When they detect adequate levels of norepinephrine, they stop norepinephrine release. An α_2 antagonist will block the negative feedback loop, raising norepinephrine levels. This same mechanism will also stop norepinephrine from blocking serotonin release, thus raising serotonin levels. It blocks three serotonin receptors (i.e., 5-HT_{2A}, 5-HT_{2C}, 5-HT_3) and has antihistaminergic properties.

DRUG TREATMENT PRINCIPLES

The American Psychiatric Association has published guidelines on management of patients who have major depressive disorder. These guidelines will be included as appropriate in the discussion of these drug treatment principles. They can be accessed at www.psych.org. However, they are targeted at psychiatrists, and the focus of this chapter is on primary care, so many other resources are used. Depression is a very common illness and is generally treated in the primary care setting. Patients who should be referred to a psychiatrist include those who fail to achieve remission, have symptoms of psychosis or severe symptoms, or have depression with other comorbid psychiatric illness. Life-threatening situations such as the risk of suicide must be referred to the emergency department. Patients who are not eating or drinking should be urgently sent to psychiatry for consideration of electroconvulsive therapy (ECT). Children and adolescents often present with complex situations; all should be referred to a specialist.

Acute Treatment Phase

The acute phase of treatment begins when the diagnosis is established. The acute phase lasts at least 6 to 8 weeks. Remission is the goal. A remission is defined as a return to baseline level of symptoms and severity.

Most antidepressants must be started at a low dosage and gradually increased, to minimize adverse effects. Most patients experience side effects as their dosage is being increased. Monitor the patient closely to prevent him or her from discontinuing the medication. Help the patient cope with the side effects (see Table 48-7 for recommendations). Adjust the dosage, based on the patient's tolerance of the drug, at intervals until therapeutic remission is achieved, patient has bothersome side effects, or the maximum dosage is given. If the patient shows a partial response in the first weeks of the trial, continue the trial of that medication. Effectiveness cannot be evaluated until the patient has been on the same dosage for 2 to 6 weeks, depending on the medication.

Patients often fail to achieve remission but do achieve a response. A significant response is defined as having a reduction of signs and symptoms by more than 50% from baseline. It is important to continue to adjust treatment to achieve remission instead of response. This is because patients who achieve remission feel better and have fewer recurrences than those patients who just achieve a response. Venlafaxine appears to have a higher rate of remission instead of response when compared with other antidepressants. A patient may still have symptoms of apathy or anxiety. An apathetic responder may continue to have lack of pleasure, decreased libido, and lack of energy. An anxious responder may continue to have anxiety, excessive worry, insomnia, and somatic symptoms.

If the patient has no response from the first medication chosen, discontinue the drug and select a second drug, usually from a different category. In general, the first drug should be tapered quickly if the patient has not been on the drug for long; taper the dosage more slowly if he or she has taken the drug for a while. Once the patient is on a low dosage or has discontinued the first drug, start gradually increasing the dosage of the second drug.

If a partial response is achieved with one drug, consider adding a second medication. Continue to adjust mediations until remission is achieved. If several trials have failed, refer the patient to a psychiatrist for further evaluation and treatment.

Continuation Phase

Once the patient achieves remission, the continuation phase begins, which lasts 16 to 20 weeks. During the continuation phase, treatment is continued. The goal is to preserve remission and prevent relapse. Relapse is defined as reemergence of significant symptoms following a remission. The patient needs close monitoring during this phase.

Maintenance Phase

If the patient completes the continuation phase without remission, the maintenance phase is entered. The goal here is to prevent recurrence. The duration of treatment depends on many factors. The initial treatment of a patient who has simple depression in remission usually lasts for 1 year. Maintenance generally consists of continuing the medication prescribed during the treatment phase. Dosage reduction is generally not recommended. Those who will probably require an indefinite pharmacologic treatment maintenance phase include those who have a response but not remission, more than one episode of depression, the elderly, those with symptoms of psychosis, depression of long duration, and severe depression. If treatment is stopped, regular follow-up with the patient continues to be necessary to monitor for relapse. In general, depression is a lifelong chronic recurrent illness that will require lifelong treatment.

Treatment Modality Decision

Patient preference is a major factor in the decision of which treatment medications to use. Compliance is enhanced if the patient is included in the decision making. There are many modalities for treatment of depression, including medications, psychotherapy, ECT, light therapy, and herbs. These may be used alone or in combination. Medications may be used alone or in combination with nonpharmacologic treatment.

Nonpharmacologic treatment of depression is important in primary care. The primary care provider can often teach simple procedures that make important contributions to recovery, such as relaxation techniques, exercise, diet, and sleep hygiene. The patient needs to be instructed to get up in the morning, attend to personal hygiene, and dress completely. Exercise is especially important. Guidance on a daily routine may help get the patient moving. These requirements may be written on a prescription pad or established through a contract with the patient if the provider believes it will be helpful in having the patient take them seriously.

Psychotherapy may be considered alone as initial therapy. Initial therapy may also include psychotherapy plus medication. Therapy is especially helpful for patients with psychosocial stressors, interpersonal difficulties, and other psychiatric illness. Psychotherapy should be recommended to all depressed patients. Often they will refuse because of the social stigma or lack of insurance reimbursement, but studies show that psychotherapy and medications work best when used together. Occasionally patients are more receptive to psychotherapy after the antidepressant has started working. ECT is useful for patients who have severe functional impairment, such as those with catatonia, those who refuse to eat, drink, or take medications, and those with symptoms of psychosis.

Medications are particularly helpful for initial therapy for patients who had prior response to antidepressants, or have symptoms of sleep or appetite disturbances or anxiety. All medications have about the same response rate. About two thirds will respond, with one third nonresponders. Keep in mind that one third will respond to placebo. All medications will also decrease the risk of relapse. A difficulty with treatment of depression is the "poop out" phenomenon, which is the failure to maintain the response to the medication. This phenomenon may be associated with patients who did not achieve remission, and it is also seen in patients treated with SSRIs. SSRIs, like other antidepressants, may cause mania when used to treat depression in patients who have bipolar disorder. Because bipolar disorder is often unrecognized, mood switching should be monitored.

DRUG SELECTION

See Box 48-3.

BOX 48-3

DRUG CHOICE

First-line drugs: SSRIs, except fluvoxamine, SNRIs (venlafaxine), NDRIs (bupropion)
First line in certain conditions: TCAs, mirtazapine
Second-line drugs: SARIs: trazodone
Third-line drugs: MAOIs, nefazodone

BOX 48-4

FACTORS TO CONSIDER IN CHOOSING A FIRST-LINE ANTIDEPRESSANT MEDICATION

Safety and tolerability
Anticipated side effects (see Table 48-6)
History of prior response in patient or family member
Patient preference
Dosage schedule
Cost
Medical conditions (see Table 48-8)
Patient variables: Age, gender, see Patient Variables

Adapted from American Psychiatric Association: Practice guideline for psychiatric evaluation of adults, *Am J Psychiatry* 152(suppl):63-80, 1995.

Dosage Forms

The long-acting formulation of paroxetine, venlafaxine, and bupropion are commonly used because the short-acting formulations have a higher risk of causing side effects and are less efficacious. Citalopram has come out with a racemic isomer, escitalopram (Lexapro) that is identical to citalopram, but without the inactive isomer. Escitalopram may have lower incidence of side effects and is being phased in as the drug of choice.

Factors to Consider

Each neurotransmitter regulates different functions important to mood. To summarize briefly, *NE* regulates alertness, energy, vigilance, and interaction with the environment; *dopamine* regulates motivation, pleasure, and reward; and *serotonin* regulates inner equilibrium, anxiety, obsessions, and compulsions.

Drug selection is not a clear-cut decision. Box 48-4 lists factors to consider in choosing a first-line antidepressant medication. When selecting a drug, consider the mechanism of action of the drug and the therapeutic effect of the neurotransmitters affected. Compare the action of the drug to patient's symptoms and condition and weigh the impact of the drug on the patient. Review the patient's complete history and physical examination for factors that will influence choice. See Table 48-8 for consideration of medical conditions when selecting an antidepressant.

Consider also the side effects associated with those neurotransmitters. Examine the adverse effects of each drug; some have more serious potential side effects than others. For example, certain drugs such as TCAs are more lethal in a suicide attempt. Others have common minor side effects that

TABLE 48-8 Considerations of Medical Conditions in the Treatment of Depression

Medical Condition	Drug	Implications
Asthma	MAOI	Interactions with sympathomimetics; other antidepressants are safe
Cardiac disease	All	Consult with cardiologist; monitor for cardiac symptoms, especially orthostatic hypotension
Arrhythmia: ventricular, sinus node dysfunction, conduction defects, prolonged QT interval, recent history of MI	TCAs trazodone	Can cause; not recommended May induce ventricular arrhythmias
Ischemic heart disease	Most	Use with caution Do not use after acute MI
Hypertension	TCAs, trazodone TCAs TCAs, trazodone venlafaxine SSRIs, bupropion	Drugs that block α receptors (prazosin, etc) intensify effect Antagonize guanethidine, clonidine, or α-methyldopa Interact with diuretics to induce orthostatic hypotension May cause usually mild, dose-dependent elevations, monitor Appear safer
Dementia	Drugs with anticholinergic action bupropion, fluoxetine, sertraline, trazodone	Cause ↓memory and attention, sedation Recommended
Epilepsy	 bupropion	Monitor for drug interactions Caused seizures in patients with eating disorders
Glaucoma	Drugs with anticholinergic action bupropion, sertraline, fluoxetine, and trazodone	Precipitate acute narrow-angle glaucoma in susceptible patients Are safe
Obstructive uropathy	Drugs with antimuscarinic effects trazodone and MAOIs SSRIs, bupropion, desipramine	Contraindicated May retard bladder emptying Recommended
Parkinson's disease	bupropion SSRIs	Has beneficial effect on Parkinson's symptoms, but may produce psychotic symptoms Increased risk of serotonin syndrome

may cause the patient to discontinue the medication, for example, an SSRI causing sexual dysfunction in a sexually active patient. One issue is that most antidepressants can produce different side effects in different patients, for example, many drugs can cause either insomnia or sedation. Table 48-9 lists general considerations of drug desirability for a patient.

Dosing can be a major factor in drug choice. The dosing schedule must be one with which the patient will comply. Dosage frequency used to be a major concern, but now most antidepressants are taken once a day. Whether to take one in the morning because patients are tired, or one in evening because they have insomnia often becomes an important factor.

Cost is often important to the patient. Patients are often more unwilling to pay for antidepressants than other drugs, such as antihypertensives. Generic versions are generally less expensive. However, the SSRI generics available so far do not offer much price reduction, compared with TCAs.

Augmentation for Partial Responders

Partial responses can generally be divided into two categories, which affects the choice of augmentation. An apathetic responder may continue to have lack of pleasure, decreased libido, and lack of energy. An anxious responder may continue to have anxiety, excessive worry, insomnia, and somatic symptoms. Lithium, estrogen, risperidone, and clozapine may be used for either category. Bupropion, SSRI, methylphenidate (Ritalin), and thyroid may be used for apathetic responders. Trazodone, TCAs, mirtazapine, sedating antihistamines, and sedatives may be used for partial responders who remain anxious.

Specific Drug Categories

Monoamine Oxidase Inhibitors. MAOIs are not discussed in detail because they are not generally prescribed by primary care providers. The broad spectrum of action is inevitably associated with a broad spectrum of adverse reactions, including hypertensive crisis, which can be fatal. A hypertensive crisis can occur within several hours after ingesting a substance containing tyramine. Tyramine releases norepinephrine and other sympathomimetic amines, raising the blood pressure. Early symptoms include occipital headache, palpitations, stiff neck, nausea, vomiting, and sweating. There is a long list of medications that can release this response (especially other

TABLE 48-9 Considerations of Drug Desirability for a Patient

Drug	Effective For	Not Effective for, or Likely to Cause Adverse Reaction	Cause Symptoms that Are Good or Bad, Depending on the Patient
FIRST LINE			
NDRI: bupropion	Overweight, psychomotor retardation, sexually active	Seizure, eating disorder, atypical, anxiety	Weight loss Nonsedating
SNRI: venlafaxine	Difficulty taking medications OCD, bulimia nervosa Anxiety, insomnia Many types of patients; pain	Anxious, insomnia, hypertension	
SSRIs	Atypical, bipolar, social phobia, bulimia		
fluoxetine	Healthy, young, severe, anxious, melancholic	Cardiac, thyroid, seizure	
fluvoxamine	Pain		
paroxetine	Atypical, anxiety, many types of patients	Can cause anxiety; sexually active	Weight loss at first then weight gain, sedation
FIRST OR SECOND LINE			
α-NDRI: mirtazapine	Underweight, insomnia, agitation, anxiety	Psychomotor retardation	Weight gain
TCAs	Healthy, young, severe, anxious, melancholic	Cardiac, thyroid, seizure	Sedation
amitriptyline	Pain		
SECOND LINE			
SARIs			
nefazodone	Disturbed sleep patterns, sexually active, anxiety, agitation		Weight neutral
trazodone	Insomnia	Cardiac	Sedation
THIRD LINE			
MAOIs	Nonresponsive to other treatments, anxious, atypical, bipolar, social phobia, bulimia	Inability to follow strict diet	

antidepressants). And there is a long list of foods (especially cheese and alcohol) that contain dangerous amounts of tyramine. The patient should seek emergency department help during such an episode. Any change of medication to or from an MAOI absolutely must have a wash-out period.

Tricyclic Antidepressants. TCAs are usually used as second-line agents, although they can be considered for first-line treatment in certain circumstances. Consider TCAs when cost is an important factor; the TCAs are available in generic form and are much less expensive than SSRIs, even those coming out in generic formulations. Their use is generally limited by side effects, although tolerance may develop over time. TCAs improve sleep continuity, but may cause a daytime hangover effect.

TCAs slow cardiac conduction, which may lead to heart block or arrhythmia. They are used with caution in patients who have any preexisting cardiac dysfunction. TCAs are potentially lethal when taken in overdose because of their cardiac and CNS effects. They should be tapered over a couple weeks to avoid any uncomfortable rebound cholinergic side effects.

TCAs are very effective and are commonly used as an adjunct therapy for pain (see Chapter 44 on pain management). The mechanism of action is thought to be NE reuptake blockade. Amitriptyline is the TCA of first choice in pain relief. Other TCAs are also effective and have fewer side effects. The initial dose of TCA for neuropathic pain is 10 to 25 mg at bedtime. Increase the dosage by 10 to 25 mg every 2 to 3 days. Analgesic effects are usually evident within about 1 week after reaching an effective dosage. Patients should be informed of this delay in analgesic effects.

Selective Serotonin Reuptake Inhibitors. The SSRIs are the most commonly used first-line drug therapy for depression. They are generally very safe and effective, although there are two major considerations: discontinuation syndrome and serotonin syndrome.

SSRIs are not effective for pain relief. Venlafaxine and nefazodone also affect norepinephrine; research is starting to show their effectiveness in treating pain, although they are not commonly used for that purpose.

Since all SSRIs in adequate doses are similarly efficacious, the choice among them often comes down to drug interactions, cost, and adverse effects experienced by the patient.

Discontinuation Syndrome. Abrupt SSRI discontinuation can lead to withdrawal, characterized as "flu-like" symptoms. Taper the drug dosage over a couple of weeks, as tolerated by the patient.

Serotonin Syndrome. Serotonin syndrome is caused by overstimulation of 5-HT receptors, which can be caused by coadministration of any drug that increases serotonin, including MAOIs, bupropion, lithium, dopamine agonists, tryptophan, amphetamines, and psychostimulants. Symptoms include hyperactivity, tachycardia, hypertension, tremulousness, GI distress, sweating, altered mental states, fever, agitation, tremor, myoclonus, hyperthermia, and death by cardiovascular collapse.

Most side effects seen with SSRIs usually subside with continued use. Patients on SSRIs are more likely to attempt suicide than patients on TCAs because of their activating effects. Some patients develop tolerance to the initial dosage of SSRIs and lose their initial positive response within several months to a year. Increase the dosage, augment with a second medication, or switch to a different category of drug. Sexual dysfunction can occur in 30% to 40% of patients, the highest incidence seen in antidepressants.

Serotonin and Norepinephrine Reuptake Inhibitors. Venlafaxine is also a common first-line medication. It is very effective as a second-line drug should the patient fail to respond to SSRIs. Venlafaxine at low doses increases serotonin levels only, like the SSRIs. At doses greater than 300 mg/day, it increases norepinephrine levels. Severe nausea may be avoided by starting at a lower dosage and titrating up. High dosages have caused elevated blood pressure. All patients should have their blood pressures measured at regular intervals because this effect may be seen later in therapy. It is recommended that venlafaxine be tapered off over a 2-week period for patients who have been on it at high dosages for more than 3 weeks. The short-acting form of the drug is associated with a much higher incidence of side effects, especially cognitive symptoms, and is seldom used.

Serotonin 2A Antagonist and Serotonin Reuptake Inhibitors. Trazodone and nefazodone are both in this class, and have similar mechanisms of action. However, they are used very differently. Trazodone is very sedating and is generally used for treatment of insomnia and to augment drug therapy for patients who have a partial response but remain anxious.

Nefazodone is generally reserved as a third-line drug for those who fail to respond to first-line therapy. Although many of the first-line drugs are activating, nefazodone has a more calming effect (with less sedation than TCAs) and is very helpful for patients who have sleep disorders. Sleep disorders and depression are so closely linked that it is theorized that the sleep disorder may be a central part of the depression. Nefazodone is generally safe in cardiac patients, and has a very low incidence of sexual side effects. Photosensitivity and hepatic toxicity may occur.

Norepinephrine and Dopamine Reuptake Blocker. Bupropion is becoming increasing popular as a first-line drug, partly because of the lack of risk for sexual dysfunction. It is quite activating, helping with motivation. Although increased risk for seizures is a potential effect of bupropion, most seizures occur in patients who have a significant predisposing factor (e.g., history of head trauma, prior seizure, CNS tumor, concomitant medications that lower seizure threshold, eating disorder) or with the short-acting formulation.

α_2-Noradrenergic Antagonists/Mixed Serotonin Blockers. Mirtazapine (Remeron) is used as a first-line treatment for certain patients. It is commonly used in geriatric patients. It is very effective in alleviating depression while increasing appetite and eliminating insomnia. The anxiolytic and sleep improvements are reported to occur as early as 1 week after starting the drug, although the full antidepressant response may take several weeks as with other antidepressants. Its use in younger patients is limited by the sedation and weight gain.

HOW TO MONITOR

The patient should be seen weekly for the first few weeks to months until improvement is seen, and then monthly until remission occurs and periodically thereafter. Monitor for therapeutic effect and adverse reactions.

The chances that the patient will successfully commit suicide are highest during the first few months of a depressive episode.

When the medication starts to work, the patient may be energized enough to follow through on a plan. At first limit the quantity of medication prescribed and do not use the refill option, to avoid giving the patient a method for suicide by drug overdose.

See Table 48-10 for laboratory values that need to be monitored for the specific drugs.

PATIENT VARIABLES

Geriatrics

Elderly patients have more vegetative and cognitive symptoms and complain less of mood problems. Drug selection is often limited by medical conditions such cardiac conditions and stroke. Dehydration may lead to toxicity from antidepressants even if low dosages are used. The elderly often have subclinical renal and hepatic dysfunction that will slow drug metabolism and excretion, raising drug levels. This is why lower dosages are usually required. Side effects are more frequent and less well tolerated, especially histaminic and anticholinergic effects. Elderly white single males have the highest risk of suicide of all patients.

TABLE 48-10 Baseline and Periodic Tests Recommended

Drug	Test	Look For
All antidepressants	Weight, as indicated	Loss/gain
TCAs	ECG CBC Liver function studies Blood sugar	QT prolongation Bone marrow dysfunction ↑ AST and ALT ↑↓ Blood sugars
SSRIs	CBC, as indicated Electrolytes, as indicated	↓ Platelets ↓ Sodium SIADH
SNRIs: venlafaxine	Blood pressure Electrolytes, as indicated	Hypertension ↓ Sodium SIADH
SARIs trazodone nefazodone	 CBC, as indicated LFTs	 Low WBCs Hepatotoxicity
bupropion	LFTs, as indicated	Toxic in ↓ liver function
NDRI: mirtazapine	CBC with differential as indicated	Agranulocytosis (rare)

LFTs, Liver function tests.

Pediatrics and Adolescents

Depression occurs in children and adolescents. Presentation can be very different than in the adult, and it varies with age. Younger children have behavioral problems such as social withdrawal, aggressive behavior, apathy, sleep disruption, and weight loss. Adolescents have somatic complaints, self-esteem problems, rebelliousness, poor performance in school, or risky or aggressive behavior. Risk of suicide is relatively high, especially when accompanied by alcohol or other substance abuse.

Evidence to guide treatment decisions is lacking. However, some antidepressants are being used in children for more serious disorders such as obsessive-compulsive disorder (OCD) and are establishing data on drug safety that will be useful. Counseling should be an important component of treatment. There is better evidence of the safety and efficacy of antidepressants in adolescents than in children. Increased vigilance in detection and treatment of depression in adolescents is encouraged. Depression should be treated by a pediatric specialist.

The US Food and Drug Administration (FDA) specifies the following:

- TCAs: use in children older than 12 years
- SSRIs: use in patients older than 18 years (has been used in children ages 6 to 18 for other conditions)
- Others: use in patients older than 18 years

Pregnancy and Lactation

The risks of the depression, which include suicide and impaired function (e.g., lack of self-care, lack of care of the fetus, ability to care for other children) are significant. The risks of using antidepressants include intrauterine death, teratogenicity, and growth impairment, depending on the agent. Antidepressants should not be administered during pregnancy unless absolutely necessary. Depression may follow childbirth and is both common and serious.

Category B: bupropion
Category C: SSRIs, venlafaxine, trazodone, nefazodone, mirtazapine
Category D: TCAs
Lactation (excreted in milk): TCAs, SSRIs, venlafaxine, trazodone, bupropion, mirtazapine
Unknown: nefazodone

Gender

Men are at risk of priapism if given trazodone. Elderly men may have prostate hypertrophy, making them at risk for anticholinergic effects on urination. Men are at risk of experiencing ejaculatory dysfunction with drugs that cause sexual dysfunction.

Culture

Culture may hamper the diagnosis and hinder treatment. Many cultures do not recognize depression as an illness. The patient may have a difficulty expressing his or her feelings. The depression may manifest as physical, somatic, and psychomotor symptoms. Language may be a barrier. The patient may often be reluctant to take medication.

PATIENT EDUCATION

Tell primary care provider of all other medications or herbs you are taking.

It may take 4 to 6 weeks before benefits are seen.

Avoid alcohol and sedatives when taking antidepressants.

Many antidepressants can cause sedation; caution patients to avoid tasks requiring alertness or coordination until they know how the medication will affect them.

Notify primary care provider if you experience adverse effects.

Notify physician if you intend to or become pregnant or are breast-feeding.

Suggest to the patient ways to minimize adverse effects (see Table 48-7 for recommendations).

! A withdrawal syndrome may be experienced if the antidepressant is abruptly discontinued.

Notify the patients of the following specific risks:

- TCAs: seizures, photosensitivity
- SSRIs: rash, hives or allergic phenomena, photosensitivity; swallow controlled release form whole
- Venlafaxine: rash, hives, or allergic phenomena; swallow controlled release form whole
- Trazodone: take with food; priapism in males
- Nefazodone: liver abnormalities; can cause death; rash, hives, or allergic phenomena, visual disturbances, photosensitivity
- Mirtazapine: agranulocytosis; notify care provider if symptoms of infection

Specific Drugs

TRICYCLIC ANTIDEPRESSANTS

(P) Prototype Drug

nortriptyline (Pamelor)

Nortriptyline has lower anticholinergic and cardiovascular side effects than TCAs.

Contraindications
- Hypersensitivity
- Status post–acute MI
- Concomitant use with MAOIs

Warnings
- Seizure disorder: TCAs may lower seizure threshold; use with caution in patients with a history of seizures or predisposing conditions
- Anticholinergic effects: use with caution in patients at risk for urinary retention and glaucoma
- Cardiovascular disorders: use with extreme caution in patients with cardiovascular disorders, especially arrhythmias and angina; orthostatic hypotension may occur. Obtain ECG before prescribing
- Hyperthyroid patients: monitor for cardiovascular toxicity
- Psychiatric: worsening of psychosis; possibility of suicide
- Mania/hypomania may occur, especially in patients with cyclic disorders
- Rash: drug fever, may be severe, discontinue if rash appears
- Renal/hepatic function: Use with caution and with reduced doses
- Elderly: low dosage; monitor for anticholinergic effects

Precautions
- Monitor baseline and periodic leukocyte and differential counts and LFTs. Fever or sore throat may signal serious neutrophil depression; discontinue therapy.
- Monitor ECG before therapy and at appropriate intervals.
- ECT with TCAs may increase hazards of therapy.
- Elective surgery: discontinue TCA for as long as possible before elective surgery.
- Blood sugar levels: elevated and lowered blood sugar levels have occurred.
- Weight gain has been observed.
- Serotonin syndrome may be caused by amitriptyline.
- Hazardous tasks: use caution.
- Photosensitivity may occur; have patient take protective measures.

Pharmacokinetics
See Table 48-11.

Adverse Reactions
See Table 48-12.

Drug Interactions
See Table 48-13.

Overdosage
Overdosage is more serious in children.

Any overdose is serious and potentially fatal. Early signs include confusion, agitation, hallucinations, and coma. Cardiotoxicity depresses myocardial contractibility and causes arrhythmias.

Dosage and Administration
See Table 48-14. For additional information on indications, administration, and dosages for various antidepressants, see the supplemental tables on the evolve Evolve Learning Resources website.

Other Drugs in Class

Other drugs in this class are similar to the prototype except as follows.

amitriptyline
- Has more side effects than other TCAs
- Better studied than others in treatment of pain

desipramine
- Less sedating than other TCAs

SELECTIVE SEROTONIN REUPTAKE INHIBITORS

(P) Prototype Drug

fluoxetine HCl (Prozac)

Contraindications
- Hypersensitivity
- Concomitant use with MAOIs

Warnings
- Periodically reevaluate the SSRIs to determine long-term usefulness.
- Monitor for altered platelet function.
- Rash and accompanying events: approximately 7% of patients taking fluoxetine have developed a rash or urticaria. Events associated with rash include fever, leukocytosis, arthralgias, edema, carpal tunnel syndrome, respiratory distress, lymphadenopathy, proteinuria, and mild transaminase elevation. Most improve quickly when drug is discontinued. Systemic events, possibly related to vasculitis, have developed in patients with rash. These are rare but can be serious, involving lung, kidney, or liver. Death has occurred. Anaphylactoid events have occurred with fluoxetine. Pulmonary events have occurred rarely. Discontinue if rash appears.
- Renal function impairment: use lower or less-frequent dosage.

TABLE 48-11 Pharmacokinetics of Antidepressant Medications

Drug	Absorption	Drug Availability (After First Pass)	Onset of Therapeutic Action	Time to Peak Concentration	Half-Life	Protein Bound	Metabolism	Excretion	Therapeutic Serum Level
TRICYCLIC ANTIDEPRESSANTS									
nortriptyline	Good	Significant first-pass effect	2-4 wk for therapeutic action	2-4 hr	18-44 hr	>90%	Extensive in liver; 2D6 substrate	Metabolites in urine	50-150 mg/ml
amitriptyline	Good	Significant first-pass effect	2-4 wk	2-4 hr	31-46 hr	>90%	1A2, 2C, 2D6 and 3A4 substrate	Metabolites in urine	100-250 mg/ml
desipramine	Good	Significant first-pass effect	2-4 wk	2-4 hr	12-24 hr	>90%	1A2 substrate 2D6 substrate and inhibitor	Metabolites in urine	125-300 mg/ml
SELECTIVE SEROTONIN REUPTAKE INHIBITORS									
fluoxetine	72%	N/A	4 wk	6-8 hr	1-16 days	95%	2C substrate 2D6 substrate and inhibitor 3A4 inhibitor		
citalopram	Well absorbed; unaffected by food	N/A	1-4 wk	4 hr	33 hr	80%	Liver, by 3A4 and 2C19	Renal, 35%; fecal, 65%	
sertraline	44%		1-4 hr	4-8 hr	1-4 days	98%	2C substrate 3A4 substrate and inhibitor	Renal, 50%; fecal, 50%	
paroxetine	64%	100%	1-4 hr	3-8 hr	10-24 hr	95%	1A2 inhibitor 2D6 substrate and inhibitor	Renal metabolites, 64%; fecal, 36%	

fluvoxamine	Decreased by food	53%	1-4 wk	3-8 hr	15.6 hr nonlinear kinetics	80%	Extensively metabolized 1A2 inhibitor (potent) 2C9 inhibitor (potent) 3A4 inhibitor Weak 2D6	Urine, 95%	
SEROTONIN/NOREPINEPHRINE REUPTAKE INHIBITORS									
venlafaxine	92%	100%		1-2 hr	5 hr	20%-30%	2D6 substrate	Urine, 87%	
SARIs/SSRIs									
trazodone	60%-80%		2-4 wk	1-2 hr	4-9 hr	89%-95%	2D6 substrate	Urine; feces, 1% unchanged	900-2100 mg/ml
nefazodone	100%	20%		1-3 hr	11-24 hr nonlinear kinetics	99%	Extensive hepatic 3A4 substrate and inhibitor 2D6 substrate	Urine, 55% as metabolites; feces, 30%	
NDRIs									
bupropion	80%	5%-20%		1-3 hr	10-21 hr	80%	Extensive hepatic 2D6 substrate	Urine metabolites, 87%; feces, 10%	50-100 mg/ml
α_2-NORADRENERGIC ANTAGONISTS									
mirtazapine	Well absorbed		2-4 wk	5 days	20-40 hr; longer in women than men	85%	Hepatic 2D6, 1A2, and 3A4	Urine, 75%; feces, 15%	

TABLE 48-12 Common and Serious Adverse Reactions to Antidepressants

Drug	Common Minor	Serious Adverse Reactions
MAOIs	Weight gain, sedation, postural hypotension	Hypertensive crisis
TCAs	Dry mouth, constipation, blurred vision from dry eyes, sedation, urinary retention, weight gain, orthostasis, precipitation of narrow-angle glaucoma, sexual dysfunction.	Cardiac arrhythmias, lower seizure threshold, psychotic symptoms, rash, bone marrow suppression
nortriptyline	Less anticholinergic than amitriptyline	
amitriptyline	Most anticholinergic	
desipramine	Less sedating than other TCAs	
SSRIs	Headache, nausea, insomnia, anorexia, weight gain, sexual dysfunction, restlessness and anxiety	Serotonin syndrome, withdrawal syndrome, cardiac effects
paroxetine SR	Anticholinergic properties, sedating	
fluvoxamine		Tardive dyskinesia, CNS depression, psychotic symptoms
SNRIs: venlafaxine XR	Anxiety, insomnia, anorexia, nausea, constipation, sexual dysfunction	Hypertension, seizures
SARIs	Sedation, dizziness, nausea, insomnia	
trazodone	Fatigue headache, nervousness, dry mouth, blurred vision	Priapism
nefazodone	Confusion, dry mouth, constipation, dyspepsia, diarrhea, photosensitivity	Hepatic failure, cardiac effects
NDRI: bupropion SR	Restlessness, anxiety, insomnia, weight loss, dry mouth	Agitation, seizure, hepatotoxicity, psychotic symptoms, cardiac effects, SIADH
α_2-NE: mirtazepine	Dizziness, sedation, nervousness, dry mouth, weight gain	Agranulocytosis, cardiac effects

- Hepatic function impairment: SSRIs are extensively metabolized by the liver. Use with caution in patients who have severe liver impairment.

Precautions

- Anxiety, nervousness, and insomnia occur frequently.
- Altered appetite and weight: weight loss may occur, especially in underweight patients; after prolonged treatment, patients tend to gain weight.
- Activation or mania/hypomania occur infrequently.
- Seizures have occurred.
- Hyponatremia has occurred because of syndrome of SIADH.
- Photosensitivity may occur.
- Have patient use caution when performing hazardous tasks

Pharmacokinetics

Fluoxetine has the longest half-life of any SSRI (with repeated administration, half-life of 2 to 7 days). This results in persistence of adverse effects after the drug is discontinued, but also allows for missed doses and minimization of discontinuation symptoms. The drug is now available in a timed-release formulation that requires only weekly administration. It is also available generically.

Dosage and Administration

Fluoxetine is the only SSRI approved by the FDA for treatment of depression in children.

Drug Interactions

Fluoxetine is metabolized by 2D6 and is a potent inhibiter of 2D6. It has many more drug interactions than most other SSRIs.

Overdosage

SSRIs are relatively safe drugs.

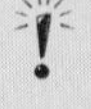

Overdosage is less likely to cause death than TCAs. However, patients on SSRIs are more likely to attempt suicide. Nausea and vomiting often prevent absorption.

TABLE 48-13 Drug Interactions with Antidepressants

Antidepressant	Effect on Other Drugs
TCAs	↑ carbamazepine, anticholinergic, clonidine, dicumarol, quinolones, grepafloxacin, sparfloxacin
	↓ guanethidine, levodopa, sympathomimetics
SSRIs	↑ Sympathomimetics, warfarin
fluoxetine	↑ hydantoin, benzodiazepines, buspirone, carbamazepine, clozapine, cyclosporine, haloperidol, phenytoin, pimozide
	↓ Digoxin
	↑↓ Lithium
sertraline	↑ hydantoin, benzodiazepines, clozapine, tolbutamide
paroxetine SR	↑ Phenothiazines, procyclidine, sumatriptan, theophylline
	↓ Digoxin
fluvoxamine	↑ Nonsedating antihistamines, cisapride, benzodiazepines, β-blockers, buspirone. carbamazepine, clozapine, diltiazem, haloperidol, methadone, sumatriptan, tacrine, theophylline
	↑↓ lithium
citalopram	↑ β-blockers, carbamazepine
	↑↓ lithium
SNRIs: venlafaxine XR	↑ desipramine, haloperidol, trazodone, sibutramine, sumatriptan
SARIs	↑ phenytoin
trazodone	↑↓ warfarin
nefazodone	2D6: ↑ benzodiazepines, buspirone, atorvastatin, simvastatin
NDRI: bupropion SR	↑ nefazodone, 2D6
α_2-NE: mirtazapine	↑ diazepam

Other Drugs	Effect on Antidepressant
Barbiturates, carbamazepine, charcoal, rifamycins	↓ TCAs
bupropion, cimetidine, haloperidol, histamine H_2 antagonists, SSRIs, valproic acid	↑ TCAs
venlafaxine	↑ desipramine
Barbiturates, cimetidine, L-tryptophan	↑ SSRIs
cyproheptadine, phenytoin	↓ SSRIs
cyproheptadine	↓ fluoxetine
Barbiturates	↑ paroxetine
cyproheptadine, phenytoin	↓ paroxetine
lithium	↑ fluvoxamine
Azole antifungals, erythromycin	↑ citalopram
cimetidine	↑ venlafaxine
carbamazepine	↑ trazodone
SSRIs, venlafaxine	↑ serotonin syndrome
sibutramine, sumatriptan, carbamazepine, cisapride, cyclosporine, digoxin	↑ nefazodone
carbamazepine	↓ bupropion
amantadine, levodopa, ritonavir	↑ bupropion

Other Drugs in Class

Other drugs in this class are similar to the prototype except as follows.

paroxetine

Paroxetine (Paxil) has some antihistamine actions that can cause sedation, more than other SSRIs. Paroxetine appears to cause more weight gain, sexual effects, and discontinuation symptoms than other SSRIs; also has many drug interactions.

fluvoxamine

Do not use fluvoxamine with cisapride.

citalopram (Celexa)

- New form of Lexapro
- Has the lowest incidence of side effects

SEROTONIN/NOREPINEPHRINE REUPTAKE INHIBITORS

venlafaxine hydrochloride (Effexor SR)

Contraindications
- Hypersensitivity
- Concomitant use with MAOIs

Warnings
- Sustained hypertension has occurred in patients on venlafaxine; effect is dosage dependent; monitor blood pressure.
- Renal/hepatic function impairment: use with caution; lower dosage; monitor for effectiveness in long-term use.

Precautions
- Anxiety, insomnia, and nervousness are commonly reported.
- Appetite/weight changes: anorexia is commonly reported. Weight loss often occurs in underweight patients.

TABLE 48-14 Dosage and Administration Recommendations for Antidepressants

Drug	Starting Dose	Administration	Dosage Titration	Usual Dosage	Maximum Dose
TCAs					
nortriptyline	25 mg	qHS	25 mg qwk	100 mg	150 mg/day
amitriptyline	75 mg	Divided/qhs	25 mg qwk	100-150 mg	300 mg/day
desipramine	75-100 mg	Divided/qAM	50 mg qwk	100-200 mg	300 mg/day
SSRIs		With/without food			
fluoxetine	20 mg	qAM	↑ 10 mg q2wk	20-40 mg	80 mg/day
sertraline	50 mg	qAM	↑ 25 mg qwk	50-150 mg	200 mg/day
paroxetine	20 mg	qPM	↑ 10 mg qwk	20-60 mg	50 mg/day
fluvoxamine	50 mg	qHS	↑ 50 mg q4-7 days	50-100 mg	300 mg/day
citalopram	20 mg	qd	20 mg/day qwk	20-40 mg	60 mg/day
SNRIs: venlafaxine XR	37.5 mg	Divided in AM	To 75 mg, then ↑ by 75 mg q4 days	150-225 mg	375 mg/day
SARIs					
trazodone	25-50 mg	qHS, after food	↑ 50 q3-4 days	75-300 mg	300 mg/day
nefazodone	100 mg bid	May change to qHS	↑ qwk	300-600 mg	600 mg/day
bupropion	150 mg	qAM/divide; allow 8 hr between doses, swallow whole	↑ 100 mg/day q3 days, gradual has less risk of seizure		
NDRI: mirtazapine	15 mg	qHS, as orally disintegrating tablet, with/without water; do not split tab	↑ q1-2wk	30 mg	45 mg/day

- Mania/hypomania may occur.
- Hyponatremia and SIADH may occur.
- Mydriasis may occur; monitor patients who have increased intraocular pressure or glaucoma.
- Seizures have been reported, especially at higher dosages.
- Abnormal bleeding, especially ecchymosis has been associated with venlafaxine.
- Concomitant illness: use with caution in conditions that could affect hemodynamic responses or metabolism.
- Have patient use caution when performing hazardous tasks.

Drug Interactions
- Drugs that use cytochrome P450 2D6

SEROTONIN 2 AGONIST/SEROTONIN REUPTAKE INHIBITOR

Trazodone and nefazodone are very different and are discussed separately.

trazodone (Desyrel)

Contraindications
- Hypersensitivity
- Recovery phase of MI
- Concomitant use with MAOIs

Warnings
- Preexisting cardiac disease: trazodone may produce arrhythmias in some patients; monitor cardiac patients closely.
- Priapism: may require emergency treatment.

Precautions
- Hypotension, including orthostatic hypotension and syncope may occur.

Overdosage
- Symptoms: CNS depression, seizures, and ECG changes. Death may occur when ingesting trazodone with other drugs. Hospitalize for treatment.

nefazodone (Serzone)

Contraindications
- Coadministration with cisapride, pimozide, or carbamazepine
- Liver disease
- Hypersensitivity to nefazodone or other phenylpiperazine antidepressants
- Concomitant use with MAOIs

Warnings
- Hepatotoxicity: may cause liver disease, ranging from mild elevations of LFTs to death. Hepatic disease increases levels of nefazodone and its metabolites. Use lower dosages in patients with liver impairment. Rates of hepatic failure are four times that anticipated.
- Do not use with MAOIs.

Precautions
- Do not use in patients who have cardiac disease
- May cause postural hypotension

- Mania/hypomania may occur; use with caution in patients who have a history of mania
- Seizures occur rarely.
- Visual disturbance: blurred vision, scotoma, and visual trails occur.
- Photosensitivity can occur.

Overdosage
- Symptoms of nausea, vomiting, and somnolence. Treatment is symptomatic. No deaths reported in overdosage.

NOREPINEPHRINE AND DOPAMINE REUPTAKE BLOCKERS

bupropion (Wellbutrin)

Contraindications
- Hypersensitivity
- Seizure disorder
- With current or prior diagnosis of bulimia or anorexia nervosa (seizure risk)
- In combination of Zyban (contains same ingredient)
- Withdrawal from alcohol or sedatives
- Concomitant use with MAOIs

Warnings
- Patients with a drug abuse history may experience a mild amphetamine-like effect
- Hepatotoxicity: rare elevations in liver function test
- Renal/hepatic function impairment: bupropion is metabolized in the liver and excreted by the kidneys. Use with caution in patients with renal or hepatic insufficiency

Precautions
- CNS: symptoms may occur, including restlessness, agitation, anxiety, and insomnia
- Neuropsychiatric signs and symptoms, including delusions, hallucination, psychotic episodes, difficulty concentrating, confusion, and paranoia; can precipitate manic episode in bipolar disorder
- Weight loss is common
- Cardiac effects: can cause hypertension; use with caution in cardiac patients

Overdosage
- Symptoms include seizures, hallucinations, loss of consciousness, and tachycardia. Deaths have been reported rarely. Treatment requires hospitalization.

α_2 NORADRENERGIC ANTAGONISTS

mirtazapine (Remeron)

Contraindications
- Hypersensitivity
- Concomitant use with MAOIs

Warnings
- Agranulocytosis may occur, monitor for signs of infection.
- Seizures are very rare; have only occurred in patients who are at increased risk for seizures.
- Cardiovascular effects: use with caution in patients with cardiac disease.
- Renal function impairment slows clearance of the drug; use lower dosage.
- Hepatic function impairment slows metabolism of the drug; use lower dosage.

Precautions
- Somnolence occurs in about half of patients.
- Dizziness may occur.
- Increased appetite/weight gain is observed in many patients.
- Elevated cholesterol/triglycerides have been seen.
- Orthostatic hypotension infrequently occurs.

Overdosage
- Limited experience with this drug. Symptoms were disorientation, drowsiness, impaired memory, and tachycardia.

RESOURCES FOR PATIENTS AND PROVIDERS

Depression Guideline Panel: *Depression in Primary Care, Clinical Practice Guideline (Detection and Diagnosis,* vol 1, *Treatment of Major Depression,* vol 2)

This booklet was developed with support from the AHCPR to assist primary care providers (e.g., general practitioners, family practitioners, internists, nurse practitioners, registered nurses, mental health nurse specialists, physician assistants) in the diagnosis of depressive conditions and the treatment of major depressive disorder. The panel hopes that the general principles embodied in these guidelines will also provide a framework for other medical and nonmedical practitioners who assume responsibilities for the recognition and care of depressed persons.

National Institutes of Health AHCPR, www.text.nlm.nih. gov/ahcpr/dep/www/dep2cg.html.

NIH information on depression medications. Look under "Clinical Information" for new reports.

National Institute of Mental Health (NIMH), www.thebody/com/nimh/nimhix.html.

Full text reports on depression, panic, bipolar disorders, stress, and anxiety.

National Library of Medicine, text.nlm.nih.gov/ahcpr/dep/www/clcover.html.

Comprehensive listing of medications used in treating depression.

Associations

American Psychiatric Association, Division of Public Affairs, Department HM-2 1400, K Street NW, Washington, DC 20005; (202) 682-6220.

Depression and Related Affective Disorders Association, Johns Hopkins Hospital, Meyer 3-181 600 N Wolfe Street, Baltimore, MD 21287-7381; (410) 955-4647.

National Alliance for the Mentally Ill, (800) 950-6264.

National Depressive/Manic Depressive Association, (800) 826-3632.

National Institute of Mental Health Public Inquiries Branch, 5600 Fishers Lane #7C02, Rockville, MD 20857; (301) 442-4513.

National Mental Health Association, 1021 Prince Street, Alexandria, VA 22314-2971; (800) 969-6642.

BIBLIOGRAPHY

American Academy of Child and Adolescent Psychiatry: Practice parameters for the assessment and treatment of children and adolescents with depressive disorders, Washington, DC., 1998, American Academy of Child and Adolescent Psychiatry.

American Psychiatric Association: Practice guideline for psychiatric evaluation of adults, *Am J Psychiatry* 152 (Nosuppl):63-80, 1995.

American Psychiatric Association: Diagnostic and statistical manual of mental disorders, ed 4, Washington, DC, 1994, American Psychiatric Association.

Bailey RE, Johnson KM III: Low-dose tricyclics effective for depression, *J Fam Pract* 52 (5):356-357, 2003.

Davis KM, Mathew E: Pharmacologic management of depression in the elderly, *Nurs Pract* 23(5):16, 1998.

Ershefsky L et al: Antidepressant drug interactions and the cytochrome P450 system, *Clin Pharmacokinet* 29(suppl 1):10, 1995.

Fave M et al: Comparison SSRI efficacy, *J Clin Psychopharmacol* 22:137, 2002.

Hegarty K et al: Use of antidepressant medications in the general practice setting: a critical review, *Aust Fam Physician* 32(4):229-234, 236-237, 2003.

Kroenke K et al: Efficacy of SSRIs, *JAMA* 286:2947, 2001.

Lam RW: Review: antidepressants and psychotherapy may be equally effective for promoting remission in major depressive disorder, *Evid Based Ment Health* 6(2):45, 2003.

Lauber C, Nordt C, Rossler W: Patients' attitudes toward antidepressants, *Psychiatr Serv* 54(5):746-747, 2003.

McIntyre RS et al: What to do if an initial antidepressant fails? *Can Fam Physician* 49:449-457, 2003.

Moret C et al: The role and therapeutic potential of 5-HT-moduline in psychiatry, *Semin Clin Neuropsychiatry* 8(2):137-146, 2003.

Muldrow CD: *Treatment of depression: new pharmacotherapies, summary,* AHCPR Publication No. 99-E013, Washington, DC, 1999, Agency for Health Care Policy and Research, HHS.

Prozac for pediatric use, *FDA Consum* 37(2):3, 2003.

Ruhe H: Review: low dose tricyclic antidepressants may be effective for adults with acute depressive disorder, *Evid Based Ment Health* 6(2):46, 2003.

Some drugs that cause psychiatric symptoms, *Med Lett* 40(1020):21, 1998.

Which SSRI? *Med Lett* 45(1170):93-95, 2003.
Newsletter.

CHAPTER 49

Antianxiety and Insomnia Agents

Drug Names

Class	Subclass	Generic Name	Trade Name
Barbiturates		(P) phenobarbital	Luminal
		amobarbital	Amytal
		butabarbital	Butisol
		pentobarbital	Nembutal
		secobarbital	Seconal
		thiopental	Pentothal
Medications similar to barbiturates		chloral hydrate	Noctec
		ethchlorvynol	Placidyl
		meprobamate	Equanil, Miltown
Benzodiazepines		(P) diazepam	Valium
		(200) alprazolam	Xanax
		chlordiazepoxide	Librium
		(200) clonazepam	Klonopin
		clorazepate	Tranxene
		estazolam	ProSom
		halazepam	Paxipam
		flurazepam	Dalmane
		(200) lorazepam	Ativan
		oxazepam	Serax
		quazepam	Doral
		(200) temazepam	Restoril
		triazolam	Halcion
Other antianxiety		buspirone hydrochloride	BuSpar
Insomnia		(200) zolpidem	Ambien
		zaleplon	Sonata

(200), Top 200 drug; (P), prototype drug.

General Uses

Indications

- Anxiety
- Insomnia
- Barbiturates: anticonvulsant
- Benzodiazepines: anxiety, insomnia (also see Table 49-1)
- Clonazepam: seizures (i.e., petit mal, petit mal variant, akinetic, myoclonic)

Unlabeled Uses

- Benzodiazepines: restless leg syndrome, multifocal tic disorders, neuralgia, Parkinsonian dysarthria, adjunctive therapy for schizophrenia, acute manic disorders, neuralgias, anxiety/agitation of dementia
- Buspirone: anxiety
- Zolpidem, zaleplon: short-term treatment of insomnia

The use of these drugs in the treatment of anxiety and insomnia will be discussed in this chapter. Antidepressants have become a major category of drug treatment of anxiety. Their use in treatment of anxiety is included in this chapter. See Chapter 48 for detailed discussion of these medications.

In the past, barbiturates and medications similar to barbiturates were used to treat anxiety and for insomnia. However, they should no longer be used for these purposes because of tolerance, addiction, and seizures upon withdrawal. Of these drugs, only phenobarbital has a clear indication, which is for seizures (see Chapter 46).

Benzodiazepines are still commonly used, but their use for anxiety and insomnia should be strictly limited because of the potential for adverse effects. They remain an important class of medications and will be discussed in detail in this chapter.

Two newer drug classes have improved safety profiles: buspirone is used for anxiety, and zolpidem and zaleplon are used for insomnia.

TABLE 49-1 Indications and Unlabeled Uses of Benzodiazepines

Drug	Indication	Unlabeled Use
diazepam (Valium)	Anxiety, acute alcohol withdrawal, muscle relaxant, anticonvulsant, preoperative relief of anxiety	Panic attacks, IBS
alprazolam (Xanax)	Anxiety, panic, agoraphobia	Social phobia, PMS, panic attacks
chlordiazepoxide (Librium)	Anxiety, acute alcohol withdrawal, preoperative apprehension and anxiety	IBS
clonazepam (Klonopin)	Seizures	Periodic leg movements, Parkinsonian dysarthria, manic episodes in bipolar disorder, multifocal tic disorders, adjunct in treatment of schizophrenia, neuralgias
clorazepate (Tranxene)	Anxiety, acute alcohol withdrawal, partial seizures	IBS
estazolam	Insomnia	
flurazepam	Insomnia	
lorazepam (Ativan)	Anxiety	Status epilepticus, chemotherapy-induced nausea and vomiting, acute alcohol withdrawal, psychogenic catatonia, chronic insomnia, IBS
oxazepam (Serax)	Anxiety, alcohol withdrawal	IBS
quazepam	Insomnia	
temazepam	Insomnia	
triazolam	Insomnia	

IBS, Irritable bowel syndrome; *PMS,* premenstrual syndrome.

DISEASE PROCESS

Anatomy and Physiology

Fear is a normal and useful emotion when an individual is confronted with perceived danger. The sympathetic adrenergic nervous system discharges while the parasympathetic nervous system is inhibited. Adrenaline and other catecholamines are released. Physiologic changes include mydriasis, pallor, increased respiratory, cardiac, basal metabolic rate, increased blood sugar, decreased bladder, bowel and genital functioning, and increased blood flow to muscles.

The Disease

Anxiety. Anxiety is fear without a cause. It is a normal reaction and a positive motivating factor in many situations. Anxiety becomes a problem when it interferes with everyday personal, social, and/or occupational functions or with adaptive behavior. It may cause physical symptoms and psychologic distress that are incapacitating.

Anxiety may be a symptom of an underlying disorder, such as a medical or a psychologic problem (Box 49-1).

Therapeutic pharmacologic intervention should be considered only after the practitioner has eliminated other treatable causes and has concluded that nonpharmacologic methods are insufficient.

The practitioner must obtain a comprehensive history and perform a complete physical examination of the patient to assess the possible causes and effects of the anxiety. The symptoms of anxiety vary with the subtype of anxiety experienced. The physical symptoms of anxiety are listed in Box 49-2.

Elements of the history that are particularly important in evaluating anxiety include the following:

- Somatic complaints that defy remedy
- Substance use disorders
- Complaints of a lump in the throat
- Inability to fall asleep at night

There are five major subtypes of anxiety: generalized anxiety disorder, panic disorder, phobias, obsessive compulsive disorder, and post-traumatic stress disorder.

Generalized Anxiety Disorder. Generalized anxiety disorder (GAD) is defined as excessive anxiety and worry about life circumstances that are difficult to control. The anxiety is unrealistic, generalized, and persistent. It is present on more days than not for longer than 6 months. The patient often complains of somatic symptoms, including restlessness, fatigue, difficulty concentrating, irritability, muscle tension, and sleep problems. These patients are in distress and experience social and vocational impairment.

Panic Disorder. A panic attack is an unexpected severe, acute exacerbation of psychic and somatic anxiety symptoms accompanied by intense fear or discomfort that is not triggered by a particular situation, and which the individual cannot "sit out." It starts abruptly and reaches a peak within 10 minutes, with at least four of the following symptoms: palpitations, tachycardia, sweating, shaking or trembling, shortness of breath, choking, chest pain or discomfort, nausea or abdominal distress, dizziness or faintness, feeling unreal or detached from

BOX 49-1

CONDITIONS THAT CAN CAUSE ANXIETY SYMPTOMS

MEDICAL CONDITIONS

Respiratory
COPD
Pulmonary embolism
Asthma
Hypoxia
Pulmonary edema

Cardiovascular
Angina pectoris
Arrhythmias
Chronic heart failure
Hypertension
Hypotension
Mitral valve prolapse

Neurologic
Delirium
Dementia
Benign essential tremor
Parkinson's disease
Akathisia
Postconcussion syndrome
Temporal lobe epilepsy
Vertigo

Endocrine
Hyperthyroidism
Hypercortisolism
Pheochromocytoma
Hypoglycemia

Metabolic
Hypercalcemia
Hyperkalemia
Hyponatremia

DRUGS
caffeine
amphetamine
methylphenidate
theophylline
phentermine
pseudoephedrine

Anticholinergics
dopaminergics
cocaine

Drug Withdrawal
alcohol
narcotics
benzodiazepines
barbiturates

Other Psychologic Disorders
Psychosis
Manic depression
Depressive disorder

BOX 49-2

PHYSICAL SYMPTOMS OF ANXIETY

RESPIRATORY
Chest pressure
Choking
Sighing
Dyspnea

CARDIOVASCULAR
Tachycardia
Palpitations
Chest pain
Faintness

AUTONOMIC
Dry mouth
Sweating
Headaches
Hot flushes

MUSCULOSKELETAL
Aches and Pains
Twitching
Stiffness
Fatigue

GENITOURINARY
Frequency
Urgency
Sexual dysfunction
Menstrual problems

GASTROINTESTINAL
Swallowing difficulties
Abdominal pain
Nausea
Irritable bowel
Lump in throat

NEUROLOGIC
Dizziness
Numbness or tingling
Visual disturbance
Weakness
Tremor

oneself, fear of going crazy, fear of dying, paresthesias, and chills or hot flashes. Typical presentations are cardiovascular symptoms (40%), neurologic symptoms (40%) or GI symptoms (30%). Panic attacks become a panic disorder when the patient worries about having another attack and what will happen if that should occur.

Phobic Disorders. A patient who has a phobia is afraid of a clearly definable situation or object. Exposure to the feared stimulus results in intense anxiety and avoidance that interferes with the patient's life. There are three main groups of phobic disorders:

1. Agoraphobia is a fear of experiencing distress if one leaves home.
2. Social phobia is a fear of being with people.
3. Simple phobia is fear of specific objects.

Specific phobias can be normal in children and many persist in a mild form in adults. Incapacity depends on the frequency with which the situation is encountered and the amount of interference with function that results.

Obsessive-Compulsive Disorder. Obsessive-compulsive disorder (OCD) is a situational preoccupation with thoughts or acts despite the patient's efforts at resistance. Obsessions are persistent thoughts, ideas, or images that intrude into conscious awareness. Compulsions are urges or impulses for repetitive intentional behaviors, performed in a stereotyped manner, in an attempt to reduce anxiety. The patient realizes these are senseless and intrusive but is unable to stop. Insight and resistance may not be present in children who have OCD.

Post-Traumatic Stress Disorder. The patient with post-traumatic stress disorder (PTSD) has recurrent anxiety precipitated by exposure to or memory of some past traumatic situation. They may have recurrent dreams or suddenly act or feel as if the event is recurring. They have a sense of numbness and emotional blunting, which acts as an attempt to avoid reminders of the trauma The patient may also have increased arousal and hypervigilance, with an enhanced startle reaction and insomnia. These patients have experienced a catastrophic event that would be clearly distressing to anyone. The onset follows the trauma with a latency period of a few weeks to months, but not more than 6 months, and the condition lasts for at least 1 month.

Insomnia. As many as 30% of adults report problems with sleep. Sleep disorders are a symptom and not a diagnostic entity, and thus require a comprehensive review of the patient's history and a thorough physical examination to rule out all possible causes of the sleep disturbance.

Sleep disorders are categorized into the following four groups to better facilitate diagnosis and management:

1. Insomnia disorders of initiating and maintaining sleep
2. Hypersomnia: disorders of excessive somnolence
3. Disorders of the sleep-wake cycle
4. Parasomnias: sleepwalking, sleep tremors, enuresis

Insomnia may be associated with depression, manic disorders, alcohol or other drug abuse, heavy smoking, caffeine use, an adverse effect of many drugs, and medical conditions.

Medications contributing to insomnia include the psychotropic drugs and CNS stimulants such as OTC cold medicines and theophylline. Medical conditions associated with insomnia include delirium, respiratory distress, pain, and hyperthyroidism. Certain sleep disorders such as sleep apnea are made worse with insomnia medications. The only sleep disorder discussed in this chapter will be insomnia because it is the one disorder these medications are used to treat. Insomnia is generally classified as short term, 7 to 10 days, and long term.

The practitioner must rule out all possible causes of a sleep disorder and determine the type of disorder present before prescribing any type of medication.

DRUG ACTION AND EFFECTS

Barbiturates and Similar Drugs

Barbiturates block the impulse transmission of the cerebral cortex and inhibit the reticular activating system. Phenobarbital has an anticonvulsant effect by increasing the threshold for motor cortex stimuli. CNS depression can range from light sedation to deep coma, depending on the dosage, route of administration, drug tolerance, and level of CNS excitability. Initial use of barbiturates suppresses rapid eye movement (REM) sleep.

Drugs similar to barbiturates cause CNS depressant action similar to barbiturates by acting on multiple CNS sites to block corticothalamic impulses. They have no effect, however, on the medulla, reticular formation, or autonomic nervous system. They also suppress REM sleep.

Benzodiazepines

Benzodiazepines act by potentiating the action of gamma-aminobutyric acid (GABA), an amino acid and an inhibitory neurotransmitter, which results in an increased neuronal inhibition and CNS depression. They bind to specific benzodiazepine receptor sites (i.e., BZ1, BZ2). BZ1 is involved in sleep; BZ2 is involved in memory, motor, sensory, and cognitive functions. Inhibition of benzodiazepine receptors located in the spinal cord causes muscle relaxation; in the brain stem it acts as an anticonvulsant; in the cerebellum it causes ataxia; and in the limbic and cortical area it effects emotional behavior. Anxiolytic effects are distinct from the nonspecific consequences of CNS depression (i.e., sedation ,motor impairment). Benzodiazepines act as a sedative hypnotic by acting on the limbic system and the subcortical CNS. They shorten REM sleep and stage 4 sleep but increase the total sleep time.

Clonazepam suppresses neural discharge in the patient during seizures. Seizure activity is inhibited by depressing nerve transmission in the motor cortex and suppressing the spike-and-wave discharge in absence seizures.

buspirone

The exact mechanism of action of buspirone is unknown. It is not chemically related to the benzodiazepines, barbiturates, or any other anxiolytic agents. It has a high affinity for serotonin receptors and a lesser affinity for dopamine receptors. It does not have muscle relaxation or anticonvulsant properties and is nonsedating.

The antianxiety effect is achieved via a selective antagonistic effect on the CNS serotonin 5-HT_{1A} receptors without affecting the benzodiazepine GABA receptors or causing CNS depression. There is also a possible down-regulation of postsynaptic 5-HT_2 receptors. Buspirone increases norepinephrine metabolism.

zolpidem

The chemical structure of zolpidem is dissimilar to the benzodiazepines and other sedative hypnotics. It appears to act through the potentiation of GABA on benzodiazepine receptors, especially omega-1 receptors. It is primarily used for its sedative effect. Zolpidem has some anxiolytic action, but has little effect on skeletal muscle or seizure thresholds. Zolpidem appears to have minimal disruptive action on the normal sleep cycle, preserving deep sleep (stages 3 and 4). It has shown no potential for causing addiction.

zaleplon

Zaleplon is also dissimilar to the benzodiazepines and other sedative hypnotics. It modulates the GABA benzodiazepam receptor complex; specifically it binds to the brain omega-1 receptor on the alpha subunit of the GABA A receptor complex.

DRUG TREATMENT PRINCIPLES

Anxiety

The initial step in treatment is patient education. Usually patients need to be reassured that they do not have some terrible disease such as heart disease or cancer. Once patients understand the nature of their disorder, they can start learning to control the anxiety. Relaxation exercises and breathing exercises can be useful and can be taught by the primary care provider. Meditation also can be helpful.

Psychotherapy is an important component of the treatment of anxiety disorders and should be considered for every patient. The type of anxiety disorder often determines the approach used. The patient should be referred to a specialist for determination of the appropriate psychotherapy.

Benzodiazepines may cause retrograde amnesia that will interfere with the patient's ability to learn adaptive behavior, defeating the purpose of the psychotherapy.

Pharmacologic treatment of anxiety depends on the subtype of anxiety. It is frequently necessary to treat the acute problem with benzodiazepines, which calm the patient within an hour or so. However, it is important to start the patient on a long-term medication with the goal to eliminate the use of short-term benzodiazepines. GAD is generally treated with any one of the SSRIs. If this is not effective, nefazodone may be used. Buspirone can be used to augment the other medications but is seldom effective on its own.

Panic disorder requires short-term use of benzodiazepines and long-term management, often using SSRIs. The benzodiazepine clonazepam can be used for long-term treatment.

Phobic disorders are usually treated with short-term use of benzodiazepines and long-term management with SSRIs. β-Blockers, lithium, and valproate can be used to augment the SSRIs.

OCD is usually treated with fluvoxamine, although other SSRIs may be used. The TCA clomipramine is also effective. Buspirone has been used to augment the action of these medications.

PTSD is usually treated with SSRIs; nefazodone or venlafaxine are also effective.

Insomnia

Treatment of insomnia begins with sleep hygiene. It is important that the patient follow the regimen provided in Box 49-3. The patient must have reasonable expectations. Overcoming insomnia is a gradual process with no overnight success. One can move up the time of onset of sleep by only 15 minutes every 3 to 4 days.

If these measures are ineffective, a medication may be considered. It should be used in conjunction with the sleep hygiene program and should be given for a limited time to help the patient reestablish a regular sleep pattern. These medications usually move up sleep onset by 10 to 30 minutes and increase total sleep time by 20 to 40 minutes. Although the practitioner may not think this is much progress, the benefit perceived by the patient is substantial.

Benzodiazepines have been used for many years in the short-term treatment of insomnia. Used properly, they are safe and effective and less expensive than zolpidem or zaleplon. However, the potential for abuse and addiction is high. Many patients become dependent on the benzodiazepine to fall asleep and withdrawal can be very difficult. Benzodiazepines must be used only for a limited time and only to treat appropriate sleep disorders. Benzodiazepines are contraindicated in patients who have sleep apnea and the other hypersomnias.

Zolpidem and zaleplon are used frequently for short-term treatment of insomnia. Zolpidem is used for patients who have difficulty sleeping through the night. Zaleplon is more useful for onset insomnia,. especially in patients who have occasional difficulty falling asleep because of time zone change or a stressful event.

Treatment of long-term insomnia is a therapeutic dilemma. No drug has been determined to be safe and effective for long-term problems. Sleep hygiene remains the mainstay. A sedative antidepressant may be considered in cases that do not respond to the standard regimen.

BOX 49-3

SLEEP HYGIENE

Develop a regular bedtime with lights out or dimmed.
Develop a regular waking time and avoid sleeping longer than usual.
Adjust total sleep time to fit your needs.
Avoid routine daytime naps.
Exercise regularly but not within 1 hour of bedtime.
Sleep in a cool room.
Avoid alcohol 3 to 4 hours before bedtime.
Avoid stimulants such as caffeine 8 hours before bedtime.
Avoid stressful topics, arguments before bedtime.
Try a warm bath.
Try warm milk.
Use bed only for sleeping and making love. Avoid reading, watching TV.
Learn and practice relaxation techniques.

Benzodiazepines

There are many medications in the benzodiazepine class; diazepam (the prototype) was the first. Benzodiazepines share a common mechanism of action and thus have the same therapeutic effects and adverse reactions. Despite many claims by the manufacturers, there is no evidence that these drugs, other than clonazepam, have different effects. The drugs differ mainly by duration of action, and the desired duration of action is an important consideration in drug selection. Benzodiazepines are classified as short-acting, intermediate-acting, and long-acting. Table 49-2 compares the pharmacokinetics of the anxiolytics. The short-acting benzodiazepines are used for medical procedures and are not included in this chapter. Long-acting benzodiazepines are used for the treatment of alcohol withdrawal and anxiety symptoms; the intermediate-acting ones are used for insomnia and in the elderly. Choose a few benzodiazepines to prescribe, include intermediate-, and long-acting ones. Alprazolam, lorazepam, and diazepam are commonly used.

Clonazepam has completely different uses from the other benzodiazepines; it is not used for anxiety or insomnia. It is used for certain specific psychiatric disorders and for seizures.

Benzodiazepines have a strong risk for causing physiologic and psychologic dependency.

The maximum therapeutic effect may take 1 to 2 weeks to achieve, and tolerance develops in 6 to 8 weeks. Benzodiazepine use must be tapered gradually to avoid a withdrawal syndrome. Patients who have a history of addiction, depression, or psychosis are not good candidates for the use of benzodiazepines. Potential side effects must be carefully considered, especially in elderly patients and in those who have a history of cardiorespiratory problems, addiction, depression, or suicidal tendencies because of the risk of lethal respiratory depression.

HOW TO MONITOR

Benzodiazepines

- Periodic laboratory work to monitor liver and renal function (LFTs, BUN, CR); CBC and urinalysis.
- Monitor for side effects such as dizziness, "hangover" effect, daytime sleepiness, ataxia, and slurred speech.
- Monitor for signs of dependence such as increased requests for medication or increased refills on prescriptions.
- Perform routine review of all medications, including OTC medications, before prescribing and at each visit.

buspirone

- Monitor for increase in LFTs, eosinophilia, leukopenia, thrombocytopenia.

zolpidem

- Monitor for increase in LFTs, BUN

zaleplon

- Monitor for anemia, leukocytosis.

PATIENT VARIABLES

Geriatrics

Elderly, debilitated patients and those who have impaired liver and renal function require dosage reduction and cautious monitoring.

TABLE 49-2 Pharmacokinetics of Antianxiety Agents

Drug	Absorption	Drug Availability (After First Pass)	Onset of Action	Time to Peak Concentration	Half-Life	Duration of Action	Protein Bound	Metabolism	Excretion
Benzodiazepines	Rapid, well absorbed in 1-3 hr			For parent compound	Parent compound/metabolites		70%-99%	Extensively metabolized by the liver; most 3A4	
diazepam			Very fast	0.5-2 hr	20-80 hr	Long	98%	Long-acting metabolite	
alprazolam			Fast	1-2 hr	6.3-26.9 hr	Intermediate	70%	Short-acting metabolite	
chlordiazepoxide			Intermediate	0.5-4 hr	5-30 hr	Long		Long-acting metabolite	
clonazepam			Intermediate	1-2 hr	18-50 hr	Long		5 metabolites	
clorazepate			Fast	1-2 hr	40-50 hr	Long		Long-acting metabolite	
estazolam			Intermediate	2 hr	8-28 hr	Long	93%	No long-acting metabolites	Urine, unchanged, <5%
flurazepam			Fast	0.5-1 hr; metabolite 10 hr	47-100 hr	Long	97%	Long-acting metabolite	Urine, unchanged, <1%
halazepam			Slow	1-3 hr	14 hr		97%	Long-acting metabolite	
lorazepam			Intermediate	2-4 hr	10-20 hr	Intermediate	85%	Metabolized to inactive	
oxazepan			Slow	2-4 hr	5-20 hr	Intermediate	87%	Metabolized to inactive	
quazepam			Intermediate	2 hr	47-100 hr	Long	>95%	Long-acting metabolite	Trace excreted unchanged
temazepam			Fast	1.2-1.6 hr	9-15 hr	Intermediate	96%	No long-acting metabolites	0.2% excreted unchanged
triazolam			Fast	1-2 hr	1.5-5.5 hr	Short	78%-89%	No long-acting metabolites	2% excreted unchanged
buspirone	Rapid	Extensive	7-10 days		2-3 hr, nonlinear		95%	Oxidation	
zolpidem	Rapid		Fast	1.6 hr	2.6 hr	6 hr	92.5%	To inactive metabolites	Renal
zaleplon	Rapid, complete	30%	Fast	1 hr	1 hr	2 hr	60%	Metabolized by liver, some 3A4	Inactive metabolites in urine

! The use of benzodiazepines or barbiturates in the elderly increases the risk of oversedation and ataxia and increases the risk of falls. The risk of orthostatic hypotension is also increased and may lead to increased episodes of falling.

Barbiturates should not be used in elderly patients. When it is necessary to use a benzodiazepine in an elderly patient, the lowest dose of a short-acting drug is tolerated best; the use of long-acting benzodiazepines should be avoided. Chloral hydrate is occasionally used but it is not recommended. Buspirone and zolpidem are relatively safe when used in the geriatric population. Zolpidem for insomnia is possibly the best tolerated with the least risk of side effects. Because of the risks associated with polypharmacy, the practitioner must examine all medications for the possibility of drug-drug interactions.

Pediatrics

Phenobarbital is often used as an anticonvulsant in children and during episodes of status epilepticus. With phenobarbital, a child may exhibit a paradoxical reaction, with excitement and agitation rather than sedation.

The safety and efficacy of buspirone, zolpidem, and zaleplon in children under the age of 18 years has not been established.

Benzodiazepines suitable for use in children include the following:

chlordiazepoxide: children >6 years
clorazepate: children >9 years
diazepam: children >6 months
lorazepam: children >12 years
Other benzodiazepines: persons over age 18 years

Pregnancy

- *Category B:* buspirone and zolpidem; breastfeeding should be avoided.
- *Category C:* zaleplon
- *Category D:* barbiturates. Fetal abnormalities occur when barbiturates are given during pregnancy. Women of childbearing age should be cautioned to use effective contraception when taking benzodiazepines or barbiturates.
- *Category D/X:* benzodiazepams can cause fetal damage; benzodiazepines are excreted in breast milk.

PATIENT EDUCATION

Benzodiazepines and Barbiturates

- May cause drowsiness, dizziness, and fatigue and should be used with caution when driving or operating machinery that requires alert mental status.
- Do not use alcoholic beverages or other CNS depressants while taking these medications.
- Dependency can be a problem.
- Do not stop the medication suddenly. Withdrawal symptoms (sweating, vomiting, muscle cramps, tremors, and seizures) may occur. Dosage must be reduced gradually under the supervision of the practitioner.
- Do not take any medications, including OTC preparations, without the knowledge of your provider.
- Report the following symptoms to the provider: tremor, seizures, ataxia, dizziness, difficulty breathing, or chest tightness.
- Rise slowly from lying or sitting positions, because orthostatic hypotension caused by the medication may result in dizziness.

Specific Drugs

BENZODIAZEPINES

(P) Prototype Drug

diazepam (Valium)

Contraindications

- Hypersensitivity to other benzodiazepines
- Psychoses
- Acute narrow-angle glaucoma
- Concurrent use with other drugs mediated by CYP 450 3A: ketoconazole, itraconazole, and nefazodone
- Clonazepam: significant liver disease

Warnings

- Psychiatric disorders: not intended for use in patients who have a primary depressive disorder or psychosis
- Long-term use (>4 months): effectiveness has not been assessed
- Dependence: prolonged use of therapeutic dosages can lead to dependence. Withdrawal syndrome has occurred in patients after as little as 4 to 6 weeks.
- Retrograde amnesia of varying severity and paradoxical reactions have occurred
- Renal/hepatic function impairment: observe for excess sedation or impaired coordination
- Abnormal liver function tests and blood dyscrasias have been reported

Precautions

- Depression: administer with caution, may intensify depression
- Rebound sleep disorder: insomnia, worse than before treatment, may occur after withdrawal.
- Respiratory depression and sleep apnea: use with caution; has occurred in patients who have respiratory disease, respiratory depression, and/or sleep apnea.
- Drug abuse and dependence: high risk of dependence with prolonged use; withdrawal symptoms ranging from mild dysphoria to abdominal and muscle cramps, tremor and convulsions. To avoid withdrawal symptoms, taper drug dosage
- Hazardous tasks: use caution while driving or performing tasks requiring alertness. Be aware of potential impairment of the performance of such activities the day following ingestion.
- Amnesia, paradoxical reactions (excitement, agitation) and other adverse behavioral effects may occur unpredictably.

Pharmacokinetics

See Table 49-2.

TABLE 49-3 Adverse Effects of Benzodiazepines by Body System

Body System	Common Minor Effects	Serious Adverse Effects
Body, general	Fever, increase or decrease in body weight, dehydration, lymphadenopathy	Behavior problems, hysteria, psychosis
Skin, appendages	Dermatitis, hair loss, hirsutism, ankle and facial edema, diaphoresis	Urticaria, pruritus, skin rash, including morbilliform, urticarial, and maculopapular
Hypersensitivity	Skin rash	
Respiratory	Nasal congestion	Respiratory depression
Cardiovascular	Palpitations, edema	Bradycardia, tachycardia, cardiovascular collapse, hypertension, hypotension
GI	Constipation, diarrhea, dry mouth, coated tongue, sore gums, nausea, anorexia, change in appetite, increased salivation, gastritis, hiccoughs	Vomiting, difficulty in swallowing
Hemic and lymphatic		Leukopenia, blood dyscrasias including agranulocytosis, anemia, thrombocytopenia, eosinophilia
Metabolic and nutritional	Gynecomastia, galactorrhea	
Musculoskeletal	Muscular disturbance, joint pain	
Nervous system	CNS sedation and sleepiness, depression, lethargy, apathy, fatigue, hypoactivity, lightheadedness, headache, vertigo, dizziness, nervousness, difficulty concentrating, agitation, inability to perform complex mental functions, hypotonia, unsteadiness, weakness, vivid dreams, psychomotor retardation, glassy-eyed appearance,	Memory impairment; disorientation, retrograde amnesia, restlessness, confusion, crying, delirium, slurred speech, aphonia, dysarthria, stupor, seizures, coma, syncope, rigidity, tremor, dystonia, euphoria, irritability akathisia, hemiparesis, ataxia, incoordination extrapyramidal symptoms, paradoxical reactions, paresthesias, suicide tendencies
Special senses	Depressed hearing, auditory disturbances	Visual disturbances, diplopia, nystagmus
Hepatic		Elevated LFTs, hepatic dysfunction, hepatitis and jaundice
Genitourinary	Incontinence, changes in libido, menstrual irregularities	Urinary retention

LFTs, Liver function tests.

Adverse Reactions
See Table 49-3.

Drug Interactions
- Alcohol/CNS depressants, cimetidine, disulfiram, isoniazid, probenecid increase the effects of benzodiazepines
- Rifampin, smoking, theophyllines, antacids decrease the effect of benzodiazepines
- Benzodiazepines increase the level of digoxin, phenytoin; increase action of alcohol/CNS depressants
- Benzodiazepines decrease the level of levodopa
- Ranitidine decreases the effect of diazepam
- Macrolides increase the effect of triazolam
- Scopolamine increases the effect of lorazepam
- Oral contraceptives decrease the effects of lorazepam, oxazepam.
- Oral contraceptives increase the effects of alprazolam, chlordiazepoxide, clorazepate, diazepam, halazepam
- Cimetidine, disulfiram, fluoxetine, isoniazid, ketoconazole, metoprolol, propoxyphene, propranolol, valproic acid may increase the effect the effect of alprazolam, chlordiazepoxide, clorazepate, diazepam, and halazepam.

Overdosage
Confusion, hypoactive reflexes, impaired coordination, slurred speech; cardiac suppression hypotension, circulatory collapse, respiratory depression, respiratory arrest; and CNS depression somnolence, coma, death.

Dosage and Administration
See Table 49-4.

Other Drugs

buspirone HCl (BuSpar)

Contraindications
- Hypersensitivity

TABLE 49-4 Dosage and Administration Recommendations for Antianxiety and Insomnia Agents

Type of Anxiety	Drug Category	Drug	Usual Dosage	Administration	Maximum Dose
GAD					
Acute treatment	Benzodiazepine	alprazolam	0.5 mg	bid or tid	4 mg
		diazepam	2-5-15 mg		30 mg
		lorazepam	2-4 mg		4 mg
		clonazepam	1-2 mg		10 mg
Long-term treatment	SSRIs		Usual dose, antidepressant		
	SNRI	venlafaxine	Usual dose, antidepressant		
	Miscellaneous	buspirone	10-20 mg	bid	
PANIC DISORDER					
Acute treatment	Benzodiazepine	alprazolam	0.5-1 mg	PRN	
		lorazepam	0.5-2 mg		
Long-term treatment	SSRIs	paroxetine	10 mg	qd	
		sertraline	25-50 mg	qd	
	Benzodiazepines	alprazolam	0.25-0.5 mg	tid	
		clonazepam	0.125-0.25 mg	bid	
	Other (augment)	lithium, β-blocker, valproate			
PHOBIC DISORDERS					
Acute treatment	Benzodiazepines	As above			
Long-term treatment	SSRI		Usual dose, antidepressant		
	β-blocker,	propranolol	20-40 mg	PRN	
OBSESSIVE-COMPULSIVE DISORDER	SSRI	fluoxetine	50-100 mg	qHS	100-300 mg
		fluvoxamine	up to 80 mg	qd	
		paroxetine	up to 80 mg	qd	
		sertraline	up to 200 mg	qd	
	TCA	clomipramine	up to 250 mg	qd	
	Other (augment)	buspirone	15-60 mg	qd	
POST TRAUMATIC STRESS DISORDER	SSRIs	fluoxetine	20 mg	qd	
		nefazodone or venlafaxine	Usual doses, antidepressant		

Warnings

- Do not use for treatment of psychosis
- Physical and psychological dependence: no potential has been seen. However, monitor patients for misuse.
- Renal/hepatic function impairment: do not use

Precautions

- Monitoring: effectiveness for more than 3 to 4 weeks has not been demonstrated in controlled trials. However, patients have been treated for several months without ill effect. If used for extended periods, periodically reassess the usefulness of the drug.
- Interference with cognitive and motor performance: buspirone is less sedating than benzodiazepines and does not produce significant functional impairment. However, its CNS effect may not be predictable. Use with caution.
- Withdrawal reactions: will not block withdrawal syndrome seen with benzodiazepines and other sedative/hypnotic drugs.
- Dopamine receptor binding: buspirone binds to central dopamine receptors and has the theoretical potential to cause dystonia, parkinsonism, akathisia, tardive dyskinesia. However, this has not been seen in patients.

Adverse Effects. See Table 49-5.

Drug Interactions

- Erythromycin, itraconazole, and nefazodone can increase the effect of buspirone.
- Buspirone can increase the effect of haloperidol and MAO inhibitors.

TABLE 49-5 Common and Serious Adverse Effects of Other Anxiety and Insomnia Medications

Drug	Common Minor Effects	Serious Adverse Effects
buspirone	CNS disturbance (dizziness, insomnia, nervousness, drowsiness, lightheadedness, GI (nausea), fatigue, headache, galactorrhea, urinary frequency	Chest pain, syncope, hypotension, hypertension, depersonalization, akathisia, hallucinations, seizures, involuntary movements, blood dyscrasias
zolpidem	Headache, drowsiness, dizziness, nausea, diarrhea, dyspepsia lethargy, URI, dry mouth	Myalgia, dysarthria, back pain, allergy, anaphylactic shock hypertension, arrhythmia, hypertension, ataxia, confusion, agitation, autonomic symptoms, anemia, elevated LFTs, BUN, asthenia
zaleplon	Amnesia, anxiety, dizziness, paresthesia, somnolence, tremor, migraine, rash, constipation, dry mouth	Angina pectoris, arrhythmia, hyper or hypotension, syncope, postural hypotension, depression, hypertonia, agitation, ataxia, confusion, anemia, leukocytosis, elevated LFTs, arthritis

Overdosage
- Symptoms of overdosage include dizziness, nausea, vomiting, drowsiness, pinpoint pupils. There is no known antidote for buspirone overdosage

zolpidem (Ambien)

Contraindications. None known.

Warnings
- Limit therapy to 7 to 10 days
- Do not use for insomnia associated with a psychiatric or physical disorder
- Abrupt discontinuation: withdrawal symptoms may occur
- CNS-depressant: do not engage in hazardous occupations requiring complete mental alertness, motor coordination, or physical dexterity
- Renal function impairment: use with caution
- Hepatic function impairment increases half life
- Carcinogenesis has occurred in rates and mice

Precautions
- Respiratory depression: has not been observed, but use with caution
- Depression: use in depression may worsen the depression
- Drug abuse and dependence: there is no evidence that zolpidem leads to abuse and dependence; but use with caution

Drug Interactions
- Increased effect: CNS depressants, ETOH

Overdosage
- Hypotension, coma

zaleplon (Sonata)

Contraindications. None known.

Warnings
- Duration of therapy: use only for 7 to 10 days. If insomnia persists, evaluate for psychiatric or medical illness.
- Efficacy: zaleplon decreased the time to sleep onset for 28 days. It has not been shown to increase total sleep time or decrease the number of awakenings.
- Abnormal thinking/behavior changes: a variety of abnormal thinking and behavior changes have been reported to occur in association with sedatives/hypnotics. Use with caution.
- Rapid dose decrease/discontinuation: there have been reports of signs and symptoms similar to withdrawal.
- CNS effects: has CNS depressant effects, do not engage in hazardous tasks.
- Renal function impairment: no adjustment of dosage required.
- Hepatic function impairment: clearance is reduced in cirrhotic patients, reduce dose. Do not use in patients with severe hepatic impairment.

Precautions
- Timing of administration: take immediately before bedtime or after going to bed and experiencing difficulty falling asleep. Taking zaleplon while ambulatory may result in short-term memory impairment, hallucinations, impaired coordination, dizziness, and lightheadedness.
- Concomitant illness: use with caution in patients who have diseases or conditions that could affect metabolism or hemodynamic responses.
- Respiratory effects: no respiratory depressant effect at normal dose in healthy subjects. Use with caution if patient has compromised respiratory function.
- Depression: use with caution.
- Drug abuse and dependence: may have abuse potential similar to benzodiazepine.
- Tolerance: no development of tolerance was observed for time to sleep onset over 4 weeks.

Drug Interactions
- CYP 3A4 is a minor metabolizing enzyme of zaleplon.
- Drugs that induce CYP 3A4 may reduce zaleplon levels.
- Drugs that inhibit CYP 3A4 are not expected to affect zaleplon levels.
- Cimetidine increases the drug level of zaleplon.
- A high-fat meal may prolong drug absorption.

Overdosage
- Signs and symptoms of CNS depressant overdose.

RESOURCES FOR PATIENTS AND PROVIDERS

National Institute of Mental Health, www.thebody/com/nimh/nimhix.html.
Full-text reports on depression, panic, bipolar disorders, stress, and anxiety.

The Guide to Psychotropic Agents.
Free handbook published every 2 years by Pocket Prescribing, Inc., One Harmon Meadow Blvd, Secaucus, NJ 07094.Panic Disorder Information Helpline: 1 (800) 64-PANIC.

BIBLIOGRAPHY

Ballenger JC, et al: Consensus statement on social anxiety disorder from the Internal Consensus Group on Depression and Anxiety, *J Clin Psychiatr* (Suppl 17):54-60, 1998.

Brady K et al: Efficacy and safety of sertraline treatment of post traumatic stress disorder, *JAMA* 284:1837, 2000.

Benzodiazepines are the right choice in certain anxiety disorders: a recent report from the WHO confirms the evidence-based experience, *Lakartidningen* 95(35):3696, 1998.

Gorman JM. New molecular targets for antianxiety interventions, *J Clin Psychiatry,* 64 Suppl 3: 28-35, 2003.

Hohagen F: Cognitive-behavioral therapy and integrated approaches in the treatment of obsessive-compulsive disorder, *CNS Spectrums* 5:35, 1999.

National Heart, Lung, and Blood Institute: Insomnia: assessment and management in primary care, NIH Publication No. 98-4088, Washington, DC, 1998, National Institutes of Health.

Pimlott NJ, Hux JE, Wilson LM, et al: Educating physicians to reduce benzodiazepine use by elderly patients: a randomized controlled trial, *CMAJ,* 168(7): 835-839, 2003.

Panic-disorder treatment guidelines published, *Am J Health Syst Pharm* 55(13):1352, 1998.

Tonks A: Treating generalised anxiety disorder. *Br Med J*, 326(7301): 700-702, 2003.

CHAPTER 50

Antipsychotics

Drug Names

Class	Subclass	Generic Name	Trade Name
FIRST GENERATION			
Phenothiazine	Aliphatic	(P) chlorpromazine	Thorazine
	Piperazine	fluphenazine	Prolixin
		perphenazine	Trilafon
		prochlorperazine	Compazine
		trifluoperazine	Stelazine
	Piperidine	mesoridazine	Serentil
		thioridazine	Mellaril
Thioxanthenes		thiothixene	Navane
Phenylbutylpiperadine	Butyrophenone	haloperidol	Haldol
Dihydroindolones		molindone	Moban
Dibenzepine	Dibenzoxazepine	loxapine	Loxitane
SECOND GENERATION			
Dibenzepine	Dibenzodiazepine	clozapine	Clozaril
Benzisoxazole		(200) risperidone	Risperdal
	Thienbenzodiazepine	(200) olanzapine	Zyprexa
	Dibenzothiazepine	quetiapine	Seroquel
		ziprasidone	Geodon
Quinolinone	Dopamine system stabilizer	aripiprazole	Abilify

(200), Top 200 drug; (P), prototype drug.

General Uses

Indications

- Management of psychotic disorders: schizophrenia
- Antiemetic (see Chapter 31)

Unlabeled Uses

- Behavioral/psychologic symptoms of dementia (BPSD):
- Parenteral antipsychotics for combative patients or other serious manifestations of acute psychosis
- Control of severe nausea and vomiting, intractable hiccups

• • •

Antipsychotics, also known as major tranquilizers or neuroleptics, are commonly used in the treatment of psychotic disorders. Their use in schizophrenia and in the management of behavioral and psychologic symptoms in geriatric patients is discussed in this chapter. A psychiatrist generally treats psychosis. Primary care providers see these patients for other medical problems and should be familiar with these drugs. Providers who see geriatric patients, especially in a nursing care facility, should be prepared to use this category of drugs.

The first antipsychotic was chlorpromazine, which was introduced in the early 1950s. This is the prototype of the phenothiazine antipsychotic agents. Currently antipsychotics are divided into two generations. The first generation are the older, "typical" drugs that treat the positive but not the negative symptoms. The second-generation drugs have much fewer extrapyramidal symptoms (EPS) and tardive dyskinesia (TD), and treat both positive and negative symptoms of schizophrenia. With the exception of risperidone, they are prolactin sparing.

Extrapyramidal Symptoms

The most important adverse effects with antipsychotic drugs are EPS, which can be irreversible. EPS include parkinsonian syndrome, akathisia, dystonia, neuroleptic malignant syndrome, and TD.

TD (permanent abnormal involuntary movements) may be progressive and irreversible, even after discontinuing the drug. It is characterized by rhythmic involuntary movements of the tongue, face, mouth, or jaw (e.g., protrusion of tongue, puffing of cheeks, puckering of mouth, chewing movements). These may be accompanied by involuntary movements of extremities. TD has been the major limitation of first-generation antipsychotics because the symptoms of TD can be disabling, preventing the patient from returning to society even if the schizophrenia is controlled.

Neuroleptic malignant syndrome (NMS): symptoms usually occur weeks after initiation of treatment with antipsychotics. NMS is idiosyncratic, and symptoms typically develop over a period of hours to days and are life threatening. Major symptoms include fever, catatonic stupor, muscle rigidity, autonomic instability, tachycardia, delirium, and myoglobinemia.

Parkinsonian symptoms typically occur more commonly in the elderly and with higher-potency antipsychotics, except risperidone. Symptoms include masked facies, tremor, bradykinesia, rigidity, cogwheeling, drooling, and festination.

Akathisia may be difficult to differentiate from anxiety because they appear so similar. Symptoms are an intensely unpleasant need to move, restlessness, and agitation. Because of the discomfort felt, akathisia is often a big factor in noncompliance regarding medications.

Acute dystonia: symptoms include muscular rigidity, usually of the tongue, neck, face, or trunk. It is most likely to occur within the first week of antipsychotic drug treatment. Acute dystonia can be frightening, extremely uncomfortable, and life threatening if laryngeal dystonia occurs.

BOX 50-1

SYMPTOMS OF CLINICAL PSYCHOSIS

POSITIVE AXIS	NEGATIVE AXIS
Delusions	Deficits of attention
Depersonalization	Lack of grooming
Hallucinations	Impoverished thought
Illusions	Anhedonia
Loss of reality	Lack of initiative
Paranoia	Alogia (absence of speech due to confusion)
Thought disorder	Blunted affect

DISEASE PROCESS

Psychosis is a gross impairment of reality testing. It has many causes. Box 50-1 lists symptoms of clinical psychosis. Table 50-1 shows the most common medical disorders that may present with psychiatric symptoms. There are a large number of diverse medications that can cause psychiatric symptoms. Table 50-2 lists some of more common drugs that can cause psychiatric symptoms. Table 50-3 lists different psychiatric disorders that may present with psychosis.

TABLE 50-1 Medical Causes of Psychiatric Symptoms

Causes	Example
Metabolic and endocrine	Addison's disease Calcium imbalance Carcinoid syndrome Cushing's syndrome Electrolyte abnormalities Hepatic failure Hyperparathyroidism Hyperthyroidism Hypoglycemia Hypothyroidism Hypoxia Magnesium imbalance Pheochromocytoma Porphyria Renal failure Serotonin syndrome Wilson's disease
Electrical	Complex partial seizures
Peri-ictal states (depression, hallucinations)	Postictal states (depression, dissociation, or disinhibition) Temporal lobe status epilepticus
Neoplastic	Carcinoid syndrome Carcinoma of the pancreas
Metastatic brain tumors	Primary brain tumors Remote effects of carcinoma
Arterial	Arteriovenous malformations Hypertensive lacunar state Inflammation (cranial arteritis, lupus) Migraine
Multi-infarct states	Subarachnoid bleeds Subclavian steal syndrome Thromboembolic phenomena Transient ischemic attacks
Mechanical	Concussion Normal pressure hydrocephalus Subdural or epidural hematoma Trauma
Infectious	Abscesses AIDS Hepatitis Meningoencephalitis (including tuberculosis, fungal, herpes) Multifocal leukoencephalopathy Subacute sclerosing panencephalitis Syphilis
Nutritional	Vitamin B_{12} deficiency Folate deficiency Niacin deficiency Pyridoxine (vitamin B_6) deficiency Thiamine deficiency
Degenerative and neurologic	Aging Alzheimer's disease Heavy metal toxicity Huntington's disease Jakob-Creutzfeldt disease Multiple sclerosis Parkinson's disease Pick's disease

Modified from Goldberg RJ: *Practical guide to the care of the psychiatric patient,* ed 2, St. Louis, 1998.

TABLE 50-2 Medications That Can Cause Psychotic Symptoms

acyclovir	Cephalosporins
amantadine	Corticosteroids
Amphetamine-like drugs	Dopamine receptor agonists
Anabolic steroids	fluoroquinolone antibiotics
Anticholinergics and atropine	Histamine H_1 receptor blockers
Anticonvulsants	Histamine H_2 receptor blockers
Antidepressants, all	HMG-CoA reductase inhibitors (statins)
baclofen	NSAIDs
Barbiturates	Opioids
Benzodiazepines	Procaine derivatives
β-Adrenergic blockers	Salicylates
Calcium channel blockers	Sulfonamides

Data from Some drugs that cause psychiatric symptoms, *Med Lett* 44:1134, 2002.

TABLE 50-3 Psychiatric Disorders That May Present with Psychosis

Type of Psychiatric Disorder	Examples
Chronic psychosis (severe)	Schizophrenia Schizoaffective disorder, bipolar type (with prominent episodes of mania) Schizoaffective disorder, depressed type (with prominent depressive episodes) Schizophreniform (<6 months' duration)
Chronic psychosis (less severe or bizarre)	Delusional disorder Shared psychotic disorder
Episodic psychosis	Depression with psychotic features Bipolar disorder (manic or depressed) Brief psychotic disorder

Modified from Cassem NH et al: *Massachusetts General Hospital handbook of general hospital psychiatry*, ed 4, St Louis, 1997, Mosby.

Schizophrenia

Schizophrenia is a disease that is heterogeneous and complex. The pathophysiology of schizophrenia is poorly understood. Early theories involved the dopaminergic system. Recently serotonergic pathways have been implicated. Newer theories are focusing on the interplay between the dopaminergic and serotonergic systems with the involvement of muscarinic, α-adrenergic and histaminergic systems.

Assessment

Schizophrenia is a diagnosis made by history after evaluating the patient in three areas:

1. Characteristic symptoms: two of more of the following:
   a. Positive symptoms
      Delusions
      Hallucinations
      Disorganized speech (e.g., incoherence)
      Grossly disorganized or catatonic behavior
   b. Negative symptoms
      Impoverished thought
      Deficits of attention
      Blunted affect
      Lack of initiative
2. Social or occupational dysfunction, notably problems with work, school, interpersonal relations, or self-care
3. Duration of symptoms 6 months or more

Antipsychotic drugs should not be used unless the practitioner has performed a thorough physical and psychiatric assessment, the diagnosis is ascertained, and other therapy is ruled out. The key diagnostic questions to ask include the following:

1. Has a reversible, organic cause been ruled out?
2. Are cognitive deficits prominent? (delirium or dementia)
3. Is the psychotic illness continuous or episodic? Have psychotic symptoms (active phase) been present for at least 4 weeks? Has evidence of the illness been present for at least 6 months? Is there evidence of a decline in level of functioning? Are negative symptoms present?
4. Are mood episodes prominent? Have there been episodes of major depression or mania? Do psychotic features occur only during affective episodes?

Before starting antipsychotic drugs, take baseline vital signs. Baseline laboratory tests to be completed include liver function tests, CBC, ECG, and UA. These tests should be repeated periodically. Special consideration should be given if the patient is taking clozapine.

History of previous responses to medication, especially antipsychotics, should be noted.

Geriatric Patients with Dementia and Delirium

Geriatric patients with dementia or delirium exhibit behavioral and psychologic symptoms. Symptoms commonly encountered include agitation, physical aggression, delusions, and hallucinations. Others include refusing personal care, inability to communicate or function, wandering, restlessness, and self-destructive behavior.

DRUG ACTION AND EFFECTS

The exact mechanism of antipsychotic drug action is unknown. These drugs are thought to work by blocking postsynaptic dopamine receptors in the hypothalamus, basal ganglia, limbic system, brainstem, and medulla and to some extent serotonin receptors. Much work has been done to elucidate what receptors each drug affects. How this receptor blocking causes the specific changes in behavior and cognition is not known. See Table 50-4 for specific neurotransmitter receptor blocking action of the individual medications. Each neurotransmitter is associated with specific side effects. However, the correlation between the two is not perfect. This is because this is a very complicated and overlapping set of mechanisms that interact to produce a wide variety of effects. Another complication is these drugs cause different effects in different patients. Most cause sedation in some people and agitation in others (Box 50-2).

TABLE 50-4 Comparison of Mechanism of Action and Associated Adverse Reactions

Drug	Potency	D_1	D_2/EPS Prolactin	D_4	5-HT_2/ Weight Gain	Anti-cholinergic	α_1/ Orthostasis	α_2	Histamine H_1/Sedation
FIRST GENERATION									
chlorpromazine (Thorazine)	Low	++	++ / ++		+ / 0	++	+ / +++	+	+ / +++
fluphenazine (Prolixin)	High	+	+ / +++		++ / 0	+	+ / +	+++	+ / +
perphenazine (Trilafon)	Low	0	++ / ++		+ / 0	+	+ / +	++	0 / ++
prochlorperazine (Compazine)	Low		++ / +++			+	/ +		/ ++
trifluoperazine (Stelazine)	High		/ +++			+	/ +		/ +
mesoridazine (Serentil)		0	++ / +		+ / 0	+++	0 / ++	0	0 / +++
thioridazine (Mellaril)	Low	+	++ / +	+	+++ / 0	+++	+ / +++	0	0 / +++
thiothixene (Navane)	High	+++	+ / +++	+++	+++ / 0	+	+ / ++	++	+ / +
haloperidol (Haldol)	High	++	+ / +++	+	+++ / 0	+	+ / +	+++	+++ / +
molindone (Moban)		0	+++ / ++	0	++++ / 0	+	+++ / +	++	+++ / ++
loxapine (Loxitane)	High	0	+++ / ++	+	+ / 0	+	++ / +	+++	+ / +
SECOND GENERATION									
clozapine (Clozaril)	High	+	+ / +	+++	+ / +	+++ / ++	+ / ++	++	+ / +++
risperidone (Risperdal)	High		++ / ++		++ / 0	0	/ +	++	/ +
olanzapine (Zyprexa)	High	+	++ / +	++	+ / +++	+++ / ++	+ / ++	++	+ / +++
quetiapine (Seroquel)	High	+++	+++ / +	+++	+++ / +	0 / ++	++ / ++	+++	+ / ++
ziprasidone (Geodon)	High	+++	+ / ++	+++	+	+++	+	0	++ /
aripiprazole (Abilify)	High	0	Partial +++/0	D3 +++	Partial 1 and 2A +++; 2c and 7 ++	+/+	+/+		+/+

BOX 50-2

NEUROTRANSMITTER AND ADVERSE EFFECTS

Antidopamine D_2: EPS, prolactin release
Anticholinergic: blurred vision, urinary retention constipation, dry mouth
Antihistaminic: sedation
Antiserontonergic: weight gain
Anti–α_1-adrenergic: orthostatic hypotension, reflex tachycardia

Antipsychotics are beneficial because they slow down the thought processes so the patient may regain reality without changing intellectual functioning.

First Generation

The typical antipsychotic drugs are potent antagonists of D_2 dopamine receptors, more than the D_1 receptors. They have a varying degree of selectivity among the dopamine tracts. They also have effects on cholinergic, α_1-adrenergic, and histaminic receptors.

Psychotropics are also classified as high or low potency. Low-potency typical antipsychotic drugs have relatively small effect on dopamine receptors but are potent antagonists of muscarinic, α-adrenergic, and histamine H_1 receptors, resulting in side effects such as dry mouth, constipation, orthostatic hypotension, and sedation. High-potency antipsychotics have a higher effect on dopamine receptors, which causes more EPS than low-potency drugs. But they do have fewer muscarinic, α-adrenergic and histamine effects. High-potency drugs, in general, also have fewer cardiac, sedative, seizure-promoting, and skin reactions. High-potency drugs tend toward diarrhea, whereas low-potency tends toward constipation.

The drugs that affect dopamine, D_2, receptors act as an inhibitor of the synthesis and release of prolactin, thereby causing hyperprolactinemia. However the correlation between the drugs' effect on the D_2 receptor and the frequency of causing galactorrhea is imperfect (see Box 50-2).

Second Generation

The newer antipsychotics affect different receptor sites than the first-generation antipsychotics. They bind dopamine, including the D_1, D_2, D_4, and D_5 receptors, with selectivity for limbic dopamine receptors. They have an increased affinity for serotonin (5-HT_2, 5-HT_6, and 5-HT_7) receptors compared with D_2 receptors. In addition, they bind acetylcholine at α-adrenergic receptors, muscarinic, histamine H_1, and nicotinic receptors. They have decreased ability or inability to induce EPS. A recent warning has been issued regarding the incidence of hyperglycemia, obesity, and diabetes mellitus seen in patients taking second-generation drugs, especially olanzapine.

Aripiprazole is the first of a new class of antipsychotic agents called dopamine system stabilizers or dopamine partial agonists. It combines the actions of D_2 and serotonin 5HT2A receptor antagonism.

Clozapine is specific for limbic receptors and not striated (muscle) receptors, which explains the low incidence of EPS and TD.

DRUG TREATMENT PRINCIPLES

Psychosis

Each patient is individual in therapeutic response and development of adverse effects to these drugs. There is no basis for choosing the drug to use according to target symptoms. Response or lack of response to one drug does not predict the response to another drug. Therapeutic effect is determined by the patient's increase in functional abilities and decrease of psychotic symptoms.

It generally takes weeks to achieve the full therapeutic benefits of antipsychotic drugs. Even with initially responsive patients, relapse is possible because of drug tolerance, physical illness, comorbid conditions, or changing life circumstances.

Gradually increase dosage to achieve therapeutic levels. Once therapeutic effect is established, attempt to decrease dosage for long-term maintenance. Allow sufficient time between dosage adjustment to assess effectiveness. Drug holidays are no longer recommended as they were not effective in minimizing development of TD.

The formulation used is frequently determined by the patient's willingness to take the medication. If the patient is not willing, it may be necessary to give the medication as a colorless, odorless liquid mixed with a beverage or as an IM injection. Once the medication reaches therapeutic levels, it may then be possible to switch to an oral tablet formulation. Depot preparations are administered by injection, may be effective for up to 4 weeks, and are useful in the long-term management of the patient unwilling to take daily oral medications.

First-generation antipsychotics tend to have a greater effect on decreasing positive symptoms, with negative symptoms tending to be more chronic and refractory in nature. The second-generation agents may be more effective against the negative symptoms. Trends in psychotropic use for chronic conditions are toward the second-generation drugs. The first-generation drugs are available in generic form and are significantly less expensive than the newer drugs. There are many drugs in development.

Symptom Management in Geriatric Patients

The American Psychiatric Association has written guidelines (see Bibliography for reference).

Nonpharmacologic management is the initial approach. Evaluate the safety of the patient and others around him or her. Evaluate for a medical, psychiatric, or psychosocial problem causing the behaviors. The environment must be modified to minimize triggers. Discussion of the many behavior modification techniques is beyond the scope of this book.

The use of psychotropics in geriatric dementia patients is a common practice, but these drugs do not have FDA approval for this use. Recent studies using risperidone and zyprexa showed increased risk of heart disease and stroke; the manufacturers released statements declaring they are not safe and effective in the elderly population. Whether this finding can be generalized and how the studies should affect clinical practice is not known at this time. Psychotropics are useful in treating some psychiatric symptoms of dementia including agitation, hyperactivity, hallucination, suspiciousness, hostility, and uncooperativeness. They have done much to improve the quality of life in demented elderly. However, they do not improve memory loss and may impair cognitive function. As always, use the lowest dose for shortest duration possible.

For short-term treatment of an aggressive dangerous patient or a geriatric patient with delirium or dementia with agitation, haloperidol or chlorpromazine can be used IM, with results in 15 to 20 minutes. Use 1 mg of haloperidol for geriatric patients and 2 to 5 mg for young adults. The dose may be repeated in 20 minutes. There is no atypical antipsychotic for treatment of acute aggressive behavior at this time.

Antipsychotics are used for the long-term management of behavioral/psychologic symptoms of dementia and delirium resistant to behavioral therapy. Benzodiazepines are useful for patients who have predominant anxiety. They are also useful on an as-needed (prn) basis when the distressing event cannot be avoided (e.g., bath, dentist visit, etc). The second-generation antipsychotics are frequently used to avoid EPS symptoms. Extremely low doses should be used, often starting with the lowest dose possible. Risperidone, olanzapine, and quetiapine are commonly used in geriatric patients. The other new antipsychotics have not been studied in geriatric patients.

HOW TO MONITOR

- Monitor liver functions, CBC for blood dyscrasias, cholesterol
- Clozapine: monitor weekly CBC with differential, following the manufacturer's protocol
- Assess for extrapyramidal symptoms at each patient encounter. Use of the Abnormal Involuntary Movement Scale (AIMS) is recommended (for scale see Goldberg reference in Bibliography).

- Monitor blood glucose monthly for onset of diabetes mellitus
- Follow weight

PATIENT VARIABLES

Geriatrics

Elderly patients have slower hepatic metabolism as well as increased sensitivity to dopamine antagonism. This makes them susceptible to extrapymamidal symptoms. Lower doses of antipsychotic drugs should be used. In general use one quarter the normal dosage. Longer waiting periods should be used before increasing doses to achieve therapeutic levels. The newer antipsychotics have been used with good results.

Pediatrics

In general, antipsychotics are not recommended for children younger than 12 years old. Antipsychotic drugs for use in children younger than age 12 include chlorpromazine, chlorprothixene (>6 years), thioridazine, triflupromazine (low potency), prochlorperazine, trifluoperazine (>6 years), and haloperidol (high potency). Chlorpromazine should not be used in children younger than 6 months of age except when potentially lifesaving. Prochlorperazine should not be used in pediatric patients less than 20 pounds or younger than 2 years of age. Thioridazine may be used in children older than 2 years of age.

Antipsychotic drugs should be used only for the treatment of acute psychosis or explosive, hyperexcitable behavior. Low doses should be used with long waiting periods before increasing doses to achieve therapeutic levels. Children are prone to developing EPS. Children tend to metabolize these drugs faster than adults.

Pregnancy

Antipsychotic drugs should be avoided during pregnancy, especially during the first trimester, because significant levels of the medications are found in both the fetus and amniotic fluid. The teratogenicity of antipsychotics is unclear. Infants have been born with EPS when antipsychotic drugs have been administered to severely psychotic pregnant mothers. Breastfeeding should also be discouraged because of the risks involved.

Category B: clozapine

Category C: first and second generation

Race

Current research has not shown that any particular race has a greater benefit from antipsychotic drugs than another. There have been no documented differences in side effects or adverse effects, although elderly black women appear to be at greater risk for TD.

Gender

It has been found that young men (<40 years) and elderly women are at increased risk for development of EPS, especially akathisia, and acute dystonia. Drug therapy should be approached cautiously and monitored carefully in those patients when they are placed on antipsychotic drugs.

PATIENT EDUCATION

- Hypotensive effects may be experienced during titration of dose.
- Use caution when driving or operating dangerous machinery due to drowsiness caused by the drug.
- Inform patient of risk of EPS including irreversible TD.
- Use sunscreen and wear hats or protective clothing to avoid sunburn, rashes, and skin pigmentation because antipsychotics may increase skin pigmentation and photosensitivity.
- If patients experience dry mouth, encourage them to drink more fluids, chew gum, or suck on hard candy.
- Any spilled medication (liquid concentrate) should be washed off the skin immediately to avoid contact dermatitis.
- Smoking increases the metabolism of antipsychotic drugs and may require a dosage adjustment.
- Alcohol should be avoided when taking antipsychotics because it potentiates the drug effects and may lead to symptoms of overdosage.
- Advise the patient to take missed doses only if remembered within 1 hour after the time the dose was due.
- The provider should be consulted if the patient takes any over-the-counter medications concurrently with antipsychotic drugs.
- The patient may experience less GI upset if antipsychotics are taken with food, juice, or milk.
- Antacids may interfere with drug metabolism and should not be ingested within 1 hour after the antipsychotic drug has been taken.

Specific Drugs

PHENOTHIAZINES

(P) Prototype Drug

chlorpromazine (Thorazine)

Contraindications

- Hypersensitivity to any of these agents; there is evidence of cross-sensitivity
- Coma, severe CNS depression, subcortical brain damage, concomitant use with other CNS depressants
- Bone marrow suppression, blood dyscrasias, myeloproliferative disorders
- Severe cardiovascular disease, cerebral arteriosclerosis, coronary artery disease, severe hypotension or hypertension
- Liver disease
- Thioxanthenes: circulatory collapse
- Haloperidol: Parkinson's disease

Warnings

TD may occur with these drugs and may be irreversible. Approximately 15% to 20% of patients who are on first-generation antipsychotic drugs long term develop TD. Symptoms may appear while the patient is on antipsychotics or may become apparent when the drug is discontinued. The only prevention is low-dose antipsychotics, administered only when necessary.

! Neuroleptic malignant syndrome. Symptoms occur weeks after initiation of treatment with antipsychotics. NMS is idiosyncratic, and symptoms typically develop over a period of hours to days and are life threatening.

CNS effects may impair mental or physical abilities and cause drowsiness.

Antiemetic effects: drugs with an antiemetic effect can obscure signs of toxicity of other drugs or mask symptoms of disease. They can suppress the cough reflex; aspiration of vomitus is possible.

Pulmonary: CNS depression may lead to decreased fluid intake, dehydration, and bronchopneumonia, which can be fatal.

Cardiovascular: use with caution in patients with cardiovascular disease or mitral insufficiency. Increased pulse rate often occurs. Orthostatic hypotension may occur. The increased activity as the result of therapy may exacerbate CAD.

The phenothiazines are direct myocardial depressants and effects may include cardiomegaly, congestive heart failure, and refractory arrhythmias, some fatal. Quinidine-like ECG changes (increased QT interval, ST depression, and changes in AV conduction) and a variety of nonspecific ECG changes may occur; these are usually reversible and their relationship to myocardial damage has not been confirmed.

Carcinogenesis: first-generation drugs (except promazine and risperidone) elevate prolactin levels. Breast cancers may be prolactin dependent.

Use with caution in patients who have a history of glaucoma because of the anticholinergic effects.

These drugs may lower seizure threshold.

Adynamic ileus occasionally occurs.

Sudden deaths due to cardiac arrest or asphyxia or pneumonia have occurred.

Hyperprolactinemia: drugs that antagonize dopamine D_2 receptors elevate prolactin levels.

Jaundice is considered a hypersensitivity reaction. Monitor hepatic function due to possibility of liver damage. Use with caution in patients with liver disease.

Use with caution in patients with renal function impairment. Monitor renal function.

Abnormal sperm has occurred in rodents.

Thioridazine: pigmentary retinopathy occurs most frequently in patients receiving thioridazine.

Precautions

Anticholinergic effects: all first-generation antipsychotics have anticholinergic effects; they are strongest in the low-potency drugs.

Cholesterol: some of these drugs elevate cholesterol; others decrease cholesterol; monitor cholesterol levels.

Concomitant conditions: use with caution.

Hematologic: various blood dyscrasias have occurred.

Hyperpyrexia: a significant rise in body temperature may indicate intolerance to antipsychotics. Discontinue.

Abrupt withdrawal: these drugs are not known to cause psychic dependence and do not produce tolerance or addiction. However, the patient may experience symptoms upon abrupt withdrawal.

Suicide attempt is a possibility in schizophrenia. Do not give large quantities of medication to patients at risk for suicide.

Pigment changes and photosensitivity have occurred but are rare.

Tartrazine sensitivity and sulfite sensitivity: some of these drugs contain these ingredients.

Pharmacokinetics

They are lipophilic and achieve high CNS concentrations (Table 50-5).

Adverse Effects

See Table 50-6 for antipsychotic drug side effects and adverse effects.

Drug Interactions

Many; see Table 50-7.

Overdosage

For all antipsychotics, overdosage may lead to increased CNS depression with resultant respiratory arrest.

Dosage and Administration

Dosage must be individualized (Table 50-8). Liquid form is usually better absorbed than tablets.

Other Drugs in Class

Other drugs in this class are similar to the prototype except as follows.

fluphenazine (Prolixin, Permitil)

Start treatment with oral formulation to determine effectiveness and dosage. General conversion rate is 0.5 ml (12.5 mg) IM every 3 weeks for every 10 mg PO.

prochlorperazine (Compazine)

Commonly used for nausea and vomiting.

OTHER FIRST-GENERATION ANTIPSYCHOTICS

haloperidol (Haldol)

- Very similar to phenothiazines; high potency

TABLE 50-5 Pharmacokinetics or Antipsychotics

Drug	Absorption	Time to Peak Concentration	Half-Life	Duration of Action	Protein Bound	Metabolism	Excretion
chlorpromazine (Thorazine)	Erratic, variable	2-4 hr	24 (8-35)	Up to 12 hr	91%-99%	Extensive 2D6	Renal, 1%
fluphenazine (Prolixin) po	Same	2-4 hr	18 (14-24)		91%-99%	2D6	
perphenazine (Trilafon)	Same		12 (8-21)	6-12 hr		2D6	
prochlorperazine (Compazine)	Same						
trifluoperazine (Stelazine)	Same		18 (14-24)				
mesoridazine (Serentil)	Same		30 (24-48)				
thioridazine (Mellaril)	Same		24 (6-40)	8-12		2D6	
thiothixene (Navane)	Same		34	34 hr			
haloperidol (Haldol)	Same		24 (12-36)	Up to 12 hr		2D6	
molindone (Moban)	Same		12 (6-24)	36 hr			
loxapine (Loxitane)	Same		8 (3-12)	12 hr			
risperidone (Risperdal)			20-24			2D6	
ziprasidone (Geodon)	60%, increased with food	6-8 hr	7 hr		99%	Extensive liver 3A4 and 1A2	Urine, 1%; unchanged feces, 66%
clozapine (Clozaril)			12 (4-66)			2D6 1A2	
olanzapine (Zyprexa)			30 (20-54)			1A2	
quetiapine (Seroquel)			6			3A4	
aripiprazole (Abilify)	Good	3-5 hr	75-94		99%	3A4 2D6	

TABLE 50-6 Adverse Reactions by Body System for First-Generation Antipsychotics

Body System	Common Minor Effects	Serious Adverse Reactions
Body, general	Enlarged parotid glands, polydipsia, systemic lupus erythematosus-like syndrome	Sudden death, heatstroke/hyperpyrexia
Skin	Pigment changes and photosensitivity have occurred but are rare	
Hypersensitivity	Pruritus, dry skin, seborrhea, erythema	Urticarial (5%), maculopapular hypersensitivity reactions, angioneurotic edema, papillary hypertrophy of the tongue, photosensitivity, eczema, asthma, laryngeal edema, anaphylactoid reactions, rashes, including acneiform, hair loss, exfoliative dermatitis
Respiratory	Increased depth of respiration	Laryngospasm, bronchospasm, dyspnea, suppression of cough reflex
Cardiovascular	Hypotension, postural hypotension, hypertension, tachycardia, bradycardia, light-headedness, faintness, dizziness	Cardiac arrest, circulatory collapse, syncope, myocardial depressant, quinidine-like effect (increased QT interval, ST depression, and changes in AV conduction)
GI	Dyspepsia, increased appetite and weight, antiemetic	
Hemic and lymphatic		Agranulocytosis (most occur wk 4-10), eosinophilia, leukopenia, leukocytosis, anemia, lymphomonocytosis, thrombocytopenia, granulocytopenia, aplastic anemia, hemolytic anemia, thrombocytopenic or nonthrombocytopenic purpura, pancytopenia

Continued

TABLE 50-6 Adverse Reactions by Body System for First-Generation Antipsychotics—cont'd

Body System	Common Minor Effects	Serious Adverse Reactions
Endocrine	Lactation and breast engorgement in females, galactorrhea, mastalgia, amenorrhea, menstrual irregularities, changes in libido, hyperglycemia or hypoglycemia, glucosuria, raised cholesterol levels	SIADH, hyponatremia
Central nervous system	Headache, weakness, tremor, twitching, tension, jitteriness, fatigue, slurring, insomnia, vertigo, drowsiness (80%, lasts 1 wk), CNS depression, drowsiness	NMS (0.5%-1%) with fatalities; TD, EPS: pseudoparkinsonism (4%-40%), akathisia (7%-20%), dystonias (2%-50%), cerebral edema, staggering gait, ataxia, seizures
Autonomic	Dry mouth, nasal congestion, nausea, vomiting, paresthesia, anorexia, pallor, flushed facies, salivation, perspiration, constipation, diarrhea, frequency or incontinence, polyuria, enuresis, priapism, ejaculation inhibition, male impotence	Obstipation, fecal impaction, atonic colon, adynamic or paralytic ileus, urinary retention, bladder paralysis
Hepatic		Liver dysfunction
Behavioral effects		Exacerbation of psychotic symptoms including hallucinations, catatonic-like states, lethargy, restlessness, hyperactivity, agitation, nocturnal confusion, toxic confusional states, bizarre dreams, depression, euphoria, excitement, paranoid reactions

TABLE 50-7 Drug Interactions with Antipsychotics

Antipsychotic	Drugs Affected
All	↑↓ phenytoin
chlorpromazine	↓ epinephrine, norepinephrine
clozapine	↑ risperidone
olanzapine, quetiapine, risperidone	↓ Dopamine agonists, levodopa
phenothiazines	↑ propranolol
phenothiazines	↓ Amphetamines, bromocriptine, barbiturates
phenothiazines, haloperidol	↑ TCAs
phenothiazines, haloperidol, thioxanthenes	↓ guanethidine
pimozide	↑ Phenothiazines, TCAs, antiarrhythmics
quetiapine	↑ lorazepam
thioridazine	↓ quetiapine

Drug	Antipsychotic Affected
Aluminum salts, charcoal	↓ Phenothiazines
Anticholinergics	↓ Phenothiazines
Barbiturates, meperidine, metrizamide, propranolol	↑ Phenothiazines
Barbiturates	↓ Phenothiazines, haloperidol
carbamazepine	↓ haloperidol, olanzapine, risperidone
cimetidine	↑ quetiapine
fluoxetine	↑ haloperidol
lithium	↑ phenothiazines, haloperidol
methyldopa	↑ haloperidol, trifluoperazine
phenytoin	↓ quetiapine, thioridazine, haloperidol
3A4, 2D6 inducers	↓ aripiprazole
3A4, 2D6 inhibitors	↑ aripiprazole

SECOND GENERATION

clozapine (Clozaril)

Indications

- For treatment of patients who are severely ill, with refractory (to at least two other drugs) chronic schizophrenia
- The most efficacious antipsychotic

Contraindications

- Hypersensitivity to clozapine or any other component of the drug
- Uncontrolled epilepsy
- Myeloproliferative disorders, history of clozapine-induced agranulocytosis or severe granulocytopenia, simultaneous administration with other agents having a well-known potential to cause agranulocytosis or otherwise suppress bone marrow function
- Severe CNS depression or comatose states from any cause

Warnings

- Clozapine presents a significant risk for agranulocytosis, a life-threatening adverse event. Monitor leukocyte count

TABLE 50-8 Dosage and Administration Recommendations for Antipsychotics

Drug	Use	Initial Dosage (mg)	Dosage, Geriatric	Adjust Dosage/ Usual Dosage	Maximum Daily Dose (mg)
FIRST GENERATION					
chlorpromazine (Thorazine)	Acute, long term	25 IM 10 tid-qid	Not used	May repeat in 1 hr ↑ by 20-50 mg q2wk	1000
fluphenazine (Prolixin)	Oral IM/SC	2.5-10 qd, q6-8 hr 12.5-25 q3-6wk	1-2.5 mg qd	prn ↑ 12.5 mg	100
perphenazine (Trilafon)	Oral	4-8 tid	Not used	prn	
prochlorperazine (Compazine)	Psychiatric, nausea and vomiting	5-10 bid-tid Oral: 5-10 tid-qid Rectal: 25 bid	Not used	prn	
trifluoperazine (Stelazine)		2-5 bid	Lower dose		
mesoridazine (Serentil)		50 tid	Not used	100-400 mg qd	
thioridazine (Mellaril)		50-100 tid		200-800 mg qd	800
thiothixene (Navane)		2 mg tid	Not used	↑ to 15 mg qd prn	
haloperidol (Haldol)	IM acute moderate symptoms, severe symptoms	2-30 0.5-2 bid-tid 3-5 bid-tid	0.5-2 mg	qhr	100
molindone (Moban)		50-75 qd	Not used	↑ to 100 mg qd in 3-4 days	225
loxapine (Loxitane)		10 bid	Not used	50 mg qd, increase in 7-10 days	100
SECOND GENERATION					
clozapine (Clozaril)		12.5 qd-bid	Not used	Daily dosage: increments of 25-50 mg qd to target of 300-450 mg qd in 2 wk	900
risperidone (Risperdal)		1 mg bid	0.25 mg qHS	3 mg bid by day 3, then qwk, to 4-8 mg qd	16
olanzapine (Zyprexa)		5-10 qd	2.5-5 mg	Target dose 10 mg qd within several days	20
quetiapine (Seroquel)		25 bid	Lower dosage, slower titration	↑ Daily 25-50 mg bid	800
ziprasidone (Geodon)		20 bid with food	Not used	20-100 mg	80 bid
aripiprazole (Abilify)		10-15 qd	Not used	10-30 mg	

before starting treatment, every week during treatment, and weekly for at least 4 weeks after discontinuation. Clozapine is available only through a distribution system that ensures monitoring of white blood cell (WBC) counts according to schedule.

- Seizures have been associated with the use of clozapine
- Myocarditis: clozapine is associated with an increased risk of fatal myocarditis.
- Orthostatic hypotension with or without syncope can occur. Collapse can be profound and accompanied by respiratory and or cardiac arrest. It is also associated with chest pain/angina, hypertension, hypotension, and tachycardia

(P) Prototype Drug

risperidone (Risperdal)

- Second only to clozapine as most efficacious antipsychotic (along with olanzapine)

Contraindications

- Hypersensitivity
- Patients with prolonged QT intervals, arrhythmias

Warnings
- Risperidone has an antiemetic effect in animals, which may occur in humans.
- All second-generation antipsychotics may cause hyperglycemia and diabetes mellitus.
- Risperidone and ziprasidone lengthen the QT interval, ziprasidone more than risperidone. Other drugs that prolong the QT level have been associated with the occurrence of torsades de pointes and sudden death.
- Priapism: one patient developed priapism.

Precautions
- A single case of thrombotic thrombocytopenic purpura (TTP) occurred.
- Evaluate for signs of risperidone misuse or abuse in patients with a history of drug abuse.
- Use with caution in patients with known cardiovascular disease or in patients at risk for hypotension.
- Use lower doses in patients with renal or hepatic impairment.
- Use with caution in patients who will be exposed to extreme heat.
- May have antiemetic effect.

Adverse Effects
See Table 50-9.

Drug Interactions
- Risperidone is metabolized by the P450 system 2D6.

Other Drugs in Class

Other drugs in this class are similar to the prototype except as follows.

olanzapine (Zyprexa)

- Second only to clozapine as most efficacious antipsychotic (along with risperidone).

TABLE 50-9 Adverse Effects (incidence in percentages) by Body System for Second-Generation Antipsychotics

Body System	risperidone	clozapine	olanzapine	quetiapine	aripiprazole
General	Fever, 2	Fever, 5	Fever, 5	Fever, 2	Fever
Skin	Rash, 3 Photosensitivity	Rash, 2	Rash, 2	Rash, 4	Rash, 6
Respiratory	Cough, 3 Rhinitis, 10		Cough, 5 Rhinitis, 10	Cough, 3	
Cardiovascular	Lengthen QT interval Chest pain/angina, 3 Tachycardia, 4	Fatal myocarditis Chest pain/angina, 1 Hypertension, 5 Hypotension, 10 Tachycardia, 25	Chest pain/angina, 5 Hypotension, 2 Tachycardia, 5	Chest pain/angina, 3 Tachycardia, 5	
Gastrointestinal	Abdominal pain, 3 Constipation, 10 Dyspepsia, 5-10 Nausea, 5	Constipation, 15 Dyspepsia, 4 Nausea, 5	Abdominal pain, 5 Constipation, 10	Abdominal pain, 3 Constipation, 10 Dyspepsia, 5	Nausea, 14 Vomiting, 12 Constipation, 10
Heme	None	Agranulocytosis	None	None	
Liver	Liver dysfunction	Liver dysfunction	Liver dysfunction	Liver dysfunction	
Endocrine	Galactorrhea	None	None	None	
CNS	Agitation, 25 Anxiety, 15 Dizziness, 5 Headache, 15 Insomnia, 25 Drowsiness, 5 Seizure, 0.3	Agitation, 5 Akathisia, 3 Dizziness, 20 Headache, 5 Seizures, 3 Somnolence, 40 Syncope, 5 Tremor, 5	Agitation, 25 Akathisia, 5 Anxiety, 10 Dizziness, 10 Headache, 15 Drowsiness, 25 Insomnia, 20 Tremor, 5	Dizziness, 10 Headache, 20 Drowsiness, 20 Insomnia, 24 Somnolence, 11 Akathisia, 10 Tremor, 3	Headache, 32 Asthenia, 5
Other					Blurred vision

- Agranulocytosis and seizures have not been noted.
- Metabolized by CYP 1A2 system.
- Weight gain is common. Most likely to cause diabetes mellitus.
- EPS low frequency, mild.

quetiapine (Seroquel)

- Causes less weight gain than clozapine or olanzapine.
- Cataracts have occurred in dogs, but not in humans.
- Priapism: one patient receiving quetiapine has developed priapism.
- Extensively metabolized in liver; have seen liver function test (LFT) elevations.
- Quetiapine oral clearance is induced by the prototype cytochrome P450 3A4 inducer, phenytoin. Use caution with potent enzyme inhibitors of cytochrome 3A.

ziprasidone (Geodone)

- Seldom causes weight gain
- More likely to cause QT interval prolongation than other second-generation antipsychotics
- Causes EPS in 5% of patients

aripiprazole (Abilify)

- May be taken without regard to food
- Does not increase QT interval
- Has little or no effect on weight

BIBLIOGRAPHY

Bailey KP: Aripiprazole: the newest antipsychotic agent for treatment of schizophrenia, *J Psychosocial Nursing* 41(2):14-18, 2003.

Beninger RJ et al: Typical and atypical antipsychotic medications differentially affect two nondeclarative memory tasks in schizophrenic patients: a double dissociation, *Schizophr Res* 61(2-3):281-192, 2003.

Blanchet PJ: Antipsychotic drug-inducted movement disorders, *Can J Neurol Sci* 30(suppl 1):S101-107, 2003.

Buckley PE: Aripiprazole: efficacy and tolerability profile of a novel acting atypical antipsychotic, *Drugs Today* 39(2):145-151, 2003.

Choice of an antipsychotic, *Med Lett* 45(1172):102-104, 2003. *Newsletter.*

Goldberg RJ: *Practical guide to the care of the psychiatric patient,* ed 2, St Louis, 1998, Mosby.

Gothelf D et al: Olanzapine, risperidone and haloperidol in the treatment of adolescent patients with schizophrenia, *J Neural Transm* 110(5):545-560, 2003.

Lalonde P: Evaluating antipsychotic medications: predictors of clinical effectiveness. Report of an expert review panel on efficacy and effectiveness, *Can J Psychiatry* 48(3suppl 1):3S-12S, 2003.

Menzin J et al: Treatment adherence associated with conventional and atypical antipsychotics in a large state medicaid program, *Psychiatr Serv* 54(5):719-717, 2003.

Some drugs that cause psychiatric symptoms, *Med Lett* 40(1020):21-24, Feb 13, 1998.

Velligan DI et al: Psychopharmacology: perspectives on medication adherence and atypical antipsychotic medications, *Psychiatric Serv* 54(5):665-667, 2003.

Ziegler DM, Peachey TJ : A study of treatment outcomes from atypical antipsychotic medications in the Virginia public system of community care, *Community Ment Health J* 39(2):169-182, 2003.

CHAPTER 51

Substance Abuse

Drug Names

Class	Subclass	Generic	Trade
Antialcoholic		disulfiram topiramate	Antabuse Topamax
Opioid antagonists		naloxone naltrexone nalmefene	Narcan ReVia Revex
Opioid		methadone	Dolophine
Opioid agonist-antagonist		buprenorphine buprenorphine and naloxone	Subutex Suboxone

General Uses

Indications

- Alcohol: disulfiram, naltrexone, topiramate
- Opioid: naloxone, naltrexone, nalmefene, buprenorphine

This chapter discusses drugs used to treat alcohol and opiate abuse. Alcohol abuse is discussed briefly. However, a discussion of opiate dependency is beyond the scope of this book.

Drug dependency is a general term. It is important to distinguish the type of dependency. There is psychologic and physiologic dependence. Tolerance is not a dependency. Psychologic dependence means the patient has a craving for a drug, with behavior revolved around procurement of the drug. Physiologic dependence is a physical addiction, with withdrawal symptoms on discontinuance. Tolerance is simply the need to increase the dose to obtain the desired effects, with no psychologic symptoms.

DISEASE PROCESS

Alcoholism is a serious disease, causing significant morbidity and mortality. It is a common problem; and it is very difficult to treat. Features of alcoholism are physiologic dependency, including withdrawal symptoms; tolerance to the effects of alcohol; alcohol-associated illness; continued drinking despite contraindications and impairment in functioning.

Assessment

All patients should be screened both for extent of alcohol use and any problem they may have with alcohol. One drink is equal to 12 ounces of beer, 5 ounces of wine, or 1.5 ounces of liquor. Most alcoholics understate the amount of alcohol they consume.

Use the CAGE questionnaire to evaluate the extent of problems with alcohol:

- Have you ever felt that you should *C*ut down on your drinking?
- Have people ever *A*nnoyed you by criticizing your drinking?
- Have you ever felt *G*uilty about your drinking?
- Have you ever had a drink (*E*ye opener) first thing in the morning to steady your nerves or get rid of a hangover?

Positive answers to any of these questions should prompt further discussion about alcohol.

Assess for use of medications that interact adversely with alcohol: H_2-blockers, aspirin, benzodiazepines, antidepressants, narcotics, barbiturates, antihistamines, NSAIDs, metronidazole, sulfonamides, reserpine, methyldopa, nitroglycerin, acetaminophen, isoniazid, antihypertensives, antidiabetic agents, warfarin, propranolol, and drugs used for ulcers, gout, and heart failure.

The physical examination may show alcohol odor on the breath, flushed face, scleral injection, tremor, bruising, and peripheral neuropathy. There may be injuries from accidents. Smokers may have cigarette burns on the hands or chest.

Laboratory tests should include CBC, liver function tests (LFTs), serum uric acid, and triglycerides. The earliest lab tests to show excessive chronic alcohol use are elevated GGT or MCV. A blood alcohol level may be indicated if you suspect the patient is inebriated.

Classification of the Patient's Drinking. *Light, safe drinking:* less than one drink/day, less than seven drinks/week, less than three drinks on any occasion, 0 CAGE score, no dysfunction related to drinking, *and* not using medications that interact adversely with alcohol.

Heavy and/or risky drinking: more than one drink/day, or more than seven drinks/week, more than three drinks/occasion, score of more than 1 on CAGE, evidence of drinking-related dysfunction, or using alcohol and medications that might adversely interact with alcohol.

Dependence (DSM-IV): more than three of the following: tolerance, withdrawal, drinking more than intended, persistent desire to drink or unsuccessful efforts to cut down or control drinking, increased time spent in activities related to alcohol, giving up important activities because of drinking, drinking despite knowledge of problems caused or worsened by alcohol.

Abuse: more than one of the following recurring situations: drinking resulting in failure to fulfill major obligations, drinking in hazardous situations, alcohol-related legal problems, continued drinking despite persistent problems caused or worsened by alcohol.

Alcohol Withdrawal

Mild symptoms include anxiety, decreased mental function, tremor, and elevated vital signs. Seizures may occur. Delirium tremens is an acute organic psychosis with mental confusion, tremor, sensory hyperacuity, visual hallucinations, autonomic hyperactivity, diaphoresis, dehydration with hypokalemia, hypomagnesemia, seizures, and cardiovascular symptoms. Withdrawal often occurs when a patient is removed from home to the hospital or nursing home. Withdrawal symptoms generally begin about 8 hours after the last drink. Seizures occur within the first 24 to 38 hours. Delirium tremens usually occurs about 24 to 72 hours after the last drink.

DRUG ACTION AND EFFECTS

Disulfiram: After alcohol is ingested, it is oxidized to acetaldehyde acetate and then to acetic acid. Disulfiram blocks oxidation of alcohol at the acetaldehyde stage by inhibiting the enzyme, aldehyde dehydrogenase. The accumulation of acetaldehyde causes numerous unpleasant symptoms that last from 30 minutes to 2 hours. The intensity of the reaction varies, depending on the amount of alcohol ingested, the dose of disulfiram, and the time between the two.

The theory behind disulfiram use in the treatment of alcoholism is based on aversion. The ingestion of alcohol becomes so uncomfortable that patients elect not to drink. Disulfiram plus alcohol causes the patient to feel an extremely unpleasant sensation manifested by flushing, dyspnea, nausea, thirst, abdominal and chest pains, palpitations, vertigo, hyperventilation, tachycardia, vomiting, hyperhidrosis, hypotension, syncope, and confusion. Acute reactions may be fatal.

Naloxone. A relatively minor change in the structure of the opioid produces naloxone, which is devoid of agonistic actions and interacts with all types of opioid receptors. It binds to opioid receptors and reverses the effects of opioid drugs. Naloxone precipitates a withdrawal syndrome in people who are dependent on opioids. Naloxone rapidly reverses the respiratory depression.

Naltrexone is a pure opioid antagonist that reversibly blocks the subjective effects of IV opioids and blocks the physical dependence. It is related to naloxone. Naltrexone has little effect on cravings, but the alcohol intake is less for individuals on this drug. The mechanism of action for alcohol withdrawal is not understood. It is through the endogenous opioid system that it probably has its effect on alcohol consumption. It does not cause the adverse effects that disulfiram does.

Topiramate is an antiepileptic drug that has recently been recognized to have some ability to help curb craving for alcohol. Researchers have found that those given this drug were six times more likely than those taking a placebo to abstain from alcohol for a month. The drug acts by reducing excess dopamine released by alcohol consumption. Initial studies suggest that the action of topiramate might be stronger than naltrexone or other drugs available in Europe in treating alcoholism. One of the main advantages of the drug is that it may be taken while people are still drinking. Even if it reduces the alcohol intake rather than leading to abstinence in confirmed drinkers, it would make a significant contribution to treatment options.

DRUG TREATMENT PRINCIPLES

Alcohol Abuse

Counsel all patients about safe drinking.

Nonpharmacologic treatment is the foundation of any therapy. Self-help groups such as Alcoholics Anonymous have the best success rate. Professional counseling may also help. Hospitalization is usually not necessary.

Pharmacologic treatment has limited success. Medications are used in conjunction with supportive treatment of patients who want to maintain their sobriety and have been unable to do so using traditional approaches. The patient must be compliant with strict instructions and able to completely stop drinking. Disulfiram has dangers inherent in its use and has a low success rate. However, it may be useful in certain situations. See Chapter 46 for more information on topiramate.

Naltrexone, an opiate antagonist has been helpful. It is useful as an adjunct to psychosocial therapy and is safer to use than disulfiram if the patient experiences a relapse. It works by decreasing alcohol cravings and can be used long term. It is also used in opiate addiction.

Benzodiazepines are not recommended because the patient will become addicted to both. Used together they worsen the problem. For alcohol withdrawal, benzodiazepines may be used acutely for delirium tremens. For milder symptoms, clonidine, carbamazepine, and atenolol have been used successfully.

Opiate Abuse

Because its duration of action is short (45 minutes, but dose dependent), naloxone is given either subcutaneously (SQ) or intramuscularly (IM) repeatedly or by continuous infusion. This is generally done in the emergency department setting because these patients are experiencing respiratory depression and may need resuscitation.

Naltrexone is considerably more active than naloxone. The duration of opiate antagonist activity is dose related. A single 50-mg oral dose of naltrexone effectively antagonizes the pharmacologic effect of 25 mg IV heroin for up to 24 hours.

Nalmefene is indicated for the reversal of opioid effects and for opioid overdose. Nalmefene is a narcotic antagonist, structurally related to naltrexone. Nalmefene prevents or reverses the effects of opioids, including respiratory depression, sedation, and hypotension. It has a longer duration of action than naloxone at fully reversing doses.

Methadone is dispensed only by pharmacies and maintenance programs approved by the US Food and Drug Administration (FDA) and designated state authorities. There are strict requirements for use stipulated in Federal Methadone Regulations (21 CFR 291.505). Methadone, used as an analgesic, may be dispensed in any licensed pharmacy (see Chapter 44).

Buprenorphine is usually used in combination with naloxone; it is started when the patient is experiencing signs of withdrawal.

HOW TO MONITOR

disulfiram

- CBC, SMA-12, and liver enzymes should be drawn before therapy is instituted and every 6 months thereafter.
- Liver enzymes should be checked after 10 to 14 days of treatment. Continually monitor for jaundice.
- Monitor for symptoms of optic neuritis, for example, eye pain or visual disturbances.
- Assess for tingling and numbness in hands and feet, which would indicate peripheral neuritis.
- Monitor for headaches, drowsiness, and psychotic reactions.
- Assess compliance to drug therapy, abstinence from alcohol use, and progress of therapy.

naltrexone

- Monitor kidney and liver function.
- Monitor response to therapy and abstinence from alcohol.
- Risk of suicide is often increased in those with substance abuse problems.

PATIENT VARIABLES

Geriatrics

- disulfiram: Of limited benefit in geriatric patients because of cardiac risks.
- naltrexone: Relatively effective

Pediatrics

- disulfiram: Safety and efficacy are not established.
- naltrexone: Use in those younger than 18 years of age has not been established.

Pregnancy

- disulfiram: Use in pregnancy has not been established. Use only if assumed benefits outweigh the risks.
- naltrexone: Category B. It is not known if medication is secreted in breast milk or affects labor and delivery; caution is advised.

PATIENT EDUCATION

disulfiram

Instruct patient to not take this medication if unwilling to make the commitment to avoid alcohol.

Tell patients to wear a Medic-Alert bracelet and notify any health care provider that they are taking this medication.

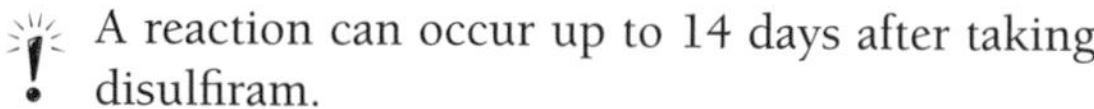

A reaction can occur up to 14 days after taking disulfiram.

Notify health care provider immediately if patient experiences chest pain, respiratory difficulty, jaundice, or drinks alcohol.

naltrexone

Tell patients to wear a Medic-Alert bracelet or carry ID and to notify any health care provider that they are taking this medication.

Tell patients that if they take heroin or other narcotics with this drug, they may die or sustain other serious injury, including coma.

They should monitor for signs of liver toxicity such as abdominal pain, white bowel movements, dark urine, or yellowing of eyes.

Specific Drugs

ANTIALCOHOLIC AGENTS

disulfiram (Antabuse)

Contraindications

- Concomitant use with alcohol
- Severe myocardial disease or coronary occlusion
- Psychosis
- Hypersensitivity to disulfiram or to other thiram derivatives used in pesticides and rubber vulcanization
- Patients who have recently received metronidazole, paraldehyde, alcohol, or alcohol-containing preparations such as cough syrups, candy containing liqueurs, alcohol-based flavoring extracts

Warnings. Disulfiram should *never* be administered to anyone under the influence of alcohol without patient's full knowledge and consent.

A disulfiram-alcohol reaction produces an extremely unpleasant reaction that can be severe. In vulnerable patients it may even provoke respiratory depression, cardiovascular collapse, arrhythmias, myocardial infarction, acute CHF, unconsciousness, convulsions, and death.

Use with caution in patients with diabetes mellitus, hypothyroidism, epilepsy, cerebral damage, chronic/acute nephritis, hepatic cirrhosis or insufficiency, or in pregnancy.

Patients with a history of rubber contact dermatitis should be evaluated for hypersensitivity to this medication.

Pharmacokinetics. Seventy percent to 90% of the dose is rapidly absorbed. The time to peak serum concentration is 1 to 2 hours. Half-life data are not available for all metabolites, but inhibition of aldehyde dehydrogenase develops slowly up to 12 hours and is reversible. Twenty percent of the dose remains in the body for 1 week or more. The lungs excrete carbon disulfide, and other metabolites are excreted via the kidneys. Five percent to 20% of each dose is excreted

BOX 51-1

DRUG INTERACTIONS WITH DISULFURIM

Drug	Possible Effect and Management
Anticoagulants	Increased anticoagulant effect; adjust dosage, monitor
phenytoin	Increased effect of phenytoin; adjust dosage, monitor
isoniazid (INH)	Increased CNS effects; lower disulfiram dosage; monitor
metronidazole	Avoid this combination; confusion and psychosis may occur
paraldehyde	Increased levels of acetaldehyde occur; not recommended

unchanged in the feces. Persistent effects are felt up to 2 weeks after discontinuing the drug.

Adverse Effects. Drowsiness is the most common side effect. Others include fatigue, headache, impotence in men, acne, metallic or garlic taste in mouth, psychotic reaction, neuropathies, or hepatotoxicity. Emergency medical intervention is necessary to treat severe effects.

Drug Interactions. See Box 51-1.

Dosage and Administration. Abstain from alcohol for at least 12 hours before beginning product. Initial dose is 250 mg daily (maximum dose is 500 mg) as a loading dose for 1 week.

Maintenance dose is 250 mg daily, with a range of 125 to 500 mg. May be taken for months to years. Tolerance does not develop, but the patient becomes more sensitive to disulfiram the longer the therapy is instituted.

OPIOID ANTAGONISTS

naltrexone HCl (ReVia)

Contraindications
- Hypersensitivity

Warnings
- Drug dependence: administer cautiously to persons who are know or suspected to be physically dependent on opioids. Reversal of narcotic effects will precipitate acute abstinence syndrome.
- Patients may require repeat doses as necessary if the opioid the patient took has a longer half-life than naltrexone.
- Not effective against respiratory depression due to nonopioid drugs.

Precautions. Cardiovascular effects: there have been several instances of hypotension, hypertension, pulmonary edema, and ventricular tachycardia and fibrillation have been reported in postoperative patients. A causal relationship is not established. Use with caution in patients with cardiovascular disease.

Pharmacokinetics. Product has 96% absorption from the GI tract with peak serum levels within 1 hour. There is significant first-pass effect. Product is excreted primarily by the kidneys.

Adverse Effects. Clinical studies have shown a 5% to 7% incidence of depression, and 2% suicide ideation. Other adverse effects include nausea, headache, dizziness, nervousness, fatigue, insomnia, vomiting, anxiety, and somnolence.

Drug Interactions
- Interacts with opioid-containing products
- Thioridazine levels increase

Dosage and Administration
- For treatment of alcoholism: 50 mg daily is recommended. A higher dose of 100 mg may be given on weekends.
- naloxone (Narcan): pure opioid antagonist. Rapidly inactivated after oral dosage. Plasma half-life 60 to 90 minutes after injection. Used for opiate-induced respiratory depression.
- Nalmefene (Revex): give IV, IM, or SC. Usual initial dose is 0.25 μg/kg given at 2- to 5-minute intervalus until desired response occurs.

BIBLIOGRAPHY

Drugs approved for opiate dependence, *FDA Consum* 37(1):6, 2003.

Fleming MF et al: Brief physician advice for problem alcohol drinkers: a randomized, controlled trial in community-based primary care practices, *JAMA* 277:1039, 1997.

Garbutt JC et al: Pharmacologic treatment of alcohol dependency: a review of the evidence, *JAMA* 281:1318, 1999.

Malcolm RJ: GABA systems, benzodiazepines, and substance dependence, *J Clin Psychiatry* 64(suppl 3):36-40, 2003.

National Consensus Development Panel of Effective Medical Treatment of Opiate Addiction: effective medical treatment of opiate addiction, 280:1936, 1998.

Resnick RB: Food and Drug Administration approval of buprenorphine-naloxone for office treatment of addiction, *Drug Alcohol* 69(1): 1-7, 2003.

Sinclair JD: Evidence about the use of naltrexone and different ways of using it in the treatment of alcoholism, *Alcohol Alcohol* 36:2, 2001.

Stotts AL, Schmitz JM, Grabowski J: Concurrent treatment for alcohol and tobacco dependence: are patients ready to quit both? *Ann Intern Med* 138(4):360, 2003.

Swift RM: Drug therapy for alcohol dependence, *N Engl J Med* 340:1482, 1999.

UNIT 12

Endocrine Agents

Unit 12 discusses the many conditions involving endocrine hormones. The drugs discussed in this unit are agents used to modulate intrinsic hormones. The conditions discussed are not necessarily diseases but may reflect physiologic dysfunction or attempts to alter physiologic function to achieve a particular goal. This section focuses on how these medications are used in primary care.

- **Chapter 52** focuses on the oral adrenal corticosteroids used to treat various conditions. Special attention must be paid to dosage and administration of these products.
- **Chapter 53** discusses the products used to treat hypothyroidism and hyperthyroidism. Products in this area have remained remarkably stable throughout the last decade.
- **Chapter 54** discusses the treatment of type 1 and type 2 diabetes, including the use of insulin and oral antidiabetic medications. New products have influenced treatment guidelines dramatically over the past few years.

CHAPTER 52

Glucocorticoids

Susan D. McConnell and Barbara E. Pokorny

Drug Names

Class	Subclass	Generic Name	Trade Name
Adrenocortical steroids		(P) hydrocortisone	Cortef, Hydrocortone
		(200) prednisone	Deltasone, Sterapred
		prednisolone	Delta-Cortef, Prelone
		triamcinolone	Aristocort, Kenacort
		(200) methylprednisolone	Medrol
		dexamethasone	Decadron
		betamethasone	Celestone

(200), Top 200 drug; (P), prototype drug.

General Uses

Indications

Glucocorticoids are used to treat numerous disorders, primarily for their antiinflammatory and immunosuppressive actions. In addition they are used as replacement therapy in adrenal insufficiency (Table 52-1).

Diagnostic Purposes. Long-acting glucocorticoids, particularly dexamethasone and betamethasone, are used to suppress adrenocorticotropic hormone (ACTH) production and allow measurement of plasma cortisol levels at specific intervals after administration. The results are useful in the diagnosis of Cushing syndrome and in the differentiation of excess glucocorticoid secretion from a pituitary versus an adrenal or ectopic source.

Other. Glucocorticoids are used in nephrotic syndrome to induce diuresis; in autoimmune thrombocytopenic purpura and certain hemolytic anemias; and in overwhelming infection, particularly gram-negative sepsis, to reduce inflammation. Glucocorticoids are used posttransplant for immune suppression.

Unlabeled uses with application to the primary care practitioner include the prevention of acute mountain sickness, treatment of the inflammatory exophthalmos of Graves' disease, and treatment of chronic obstructive pulmonary disease (COPD).

This chapter addresses the use of glucocorticoid therapy in the treatment of inflammatory disease.

DISEASE PROCESS

Anatomy and Physiology

The adrenal cortex synthesizes and secretes several hormones. Among them are the glucocorticoid cortisol, the mineralocorticoid aldosterone, and a small amount of the sex steroid androgen. Aldosterone, under the influence of the renin-angiotensin system and other metabolic pathways, regulates salt and water retention in the body. Cortisol has a powerful antiinflammatory effect, modifies the body's immune response, and influences metabolic processes. The production of cortisol is controlled by a negative feedback loop involving the hypothalamus-anterior pituitary-adrenal cortex (HPA) axis (Figure 52-1). A low level of plasma cortisol stimulates the anterior pituitary to increase production of ACTH, which in turn stimulates the adrenal cortex to increase cortisol secretion. Similarly a high level of circulating cortisol prompts a downregulation of ACTH production and resulting decrease in adrenal cortex production of cortisol.

Cortisol is naturally secreted in an uneven pattern over 24 hours, totaling 10 mg/day in normal adults. It is highest during the early morning hours, 2:00 to 7:00 AM, and lowest in the evening, 6:00 PM to midnight.

DRUG ACTION AND EFFECTS

Glucocorticoids affect the metabolism of carbohydrates, proteins, and fats. They have direct and indirect effects on immune response, modulate inflammatory response, and play a role in the body's response to stressful stimuli. All drugs in this class are remarkably similar and may be discussed as a group; the most important differences between the drugs are duration of

TABLE 52-1 Common Disorders Treated with Glucocorticoids

Disorder	Examples
Allergic conditions	Seasonal or perennial allergic rhinitis Serum sickness Drug hypersensitivity reactions
Dermatologic	Contact dermatitis Psoriasis Seborrheic dermatitis Pemphigus Erythema multiforme Stevens-Johnson syndrome Mycosis fungoides
Respiratory	Bronchial asthma Sarcoidosis Aspiration pneumonia
GI	Ulcerative colitis Regional enteritis
Endocrine	Adrenocortical insufficiency Congenital adrenal hyperplasia Nonsuppurative thyroiditis
Collagen, vascular	Systemic lupus erythematosus Acute rheumatic carditis Polymyositis Polymyalgia rheumatica Temporal arteritis
Rheumatic	Rheumatoid arthritis Psoriatic arthritis Ankylosing spondylitis Acute bursitis Acute gouty arthritis Post-traumatic osteoarthritis
Neurologic	Multiple sclerosis Cerebral edema Acute stroke and spinal cord injury
Ophthalmic	Allergic conjunctivitis Uveitis Optic neuritis Herpes zoster ophthalmicus

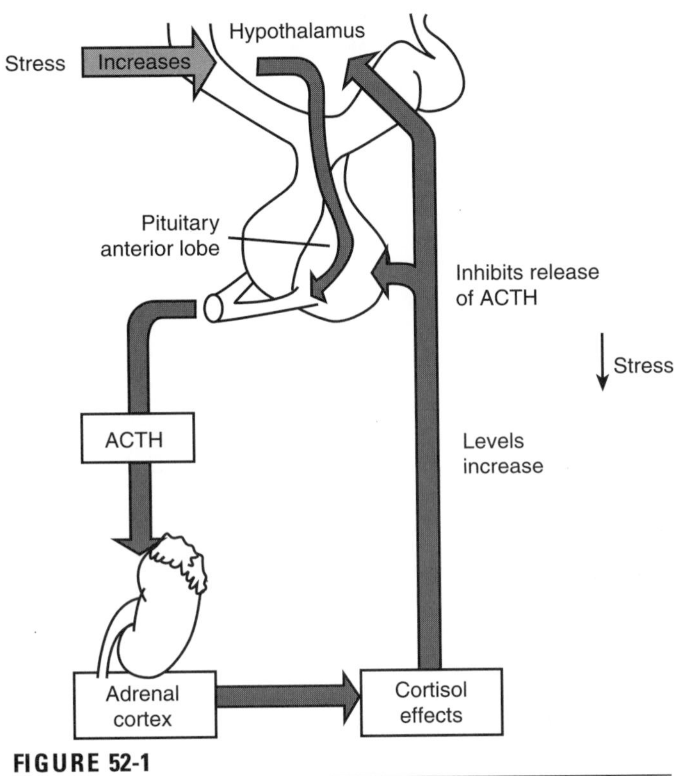

FIGURE 52-1

Adrenal-pituitary axis. (From McKenry LM, Salerno E: *Pharmacology in nursing*, ed 22, St Louis, 2002, Mosby.)

action and degree of inherent mineralocorticoid activity, which causes salt and fluid retention (Table 52-2). Mineralocorticoid activity is needed in adrenal insufficiency but not severe inflammation. Cortisone and hydrocortisone have both glucocorticoid and mineralocorticoid properties. Their synthetic analogs prednisone, prednisolone, and methylprednisolone have both effects as well, though glucocorticoid effects predominate. By contrast, triamcinolone, dexamethasone, and betamethasone have exclusively glucocorticoid antiinflammatory activity.

Carbohydrate and Protein Metabolism

Glucocorticoids maintain an adequate level of serum glucose by stimulating gluconeogenesis in the liver and inhibiting peripheral glucose use. They also stimulate protein breakdown, which results in an increase in plasma amino acid levels. In the liver, amino acids enhance enzymatic activity, which in turn supports increased glycogen deposition and decreased glycolysis. This action, intended to support homeostasis in the healthy body, can result in a diabetogenic state when large doses of exogenous steroids are used. Serum glucose rises in the fasting state; glucose tolerance decreases; insulin resistance develops; and glucosuria may be present. The result may be the clinical expression of latent diabetes or simply relative glucose intolerance while on steroid therapy.

Increased protein breakdown mobilizes amino acids from muscle, bone, skin, and lymph tissue. Muscle atrophy, osteoporosis, impaired wound healing, and thinning of the skin can result. In children growth can be impaired.

Lipid Metabolism

Glucocorticoids affect the mobilization of fats from areas of deposition. Increased lipolysis occurs in areas of adipose accumulation, and serum fatty acid concentration increases. Chronic use of steroid therapy may result in increased deposition of adipose tissue in the back of the neck and the supraclavicular area, sometimes described as a buffalo hump, and in the cheeks and face, referred to as a moon facies. A relative loss of subcutaneous fat in the extremities may be noted.

Immune Response

Glucocorticoids mask the manifestations of both cellular and humoral immunity. Humoral immunity involves the action of B lymphocytes in interaction with macrophages and helper

TABLE 52-2 Pharmacokinetics of Selected Glucocorticoids

Drug	Absorption	Onset of Action	Time to Peak Concentration	Duration of Action	Metabolism	Excretion
hydrocortisone	GI	1 hr	8-12 hr	30-36 hr	Hepatic	Renal
prednisone	GI	1-2 hr	18-36 hr	30-36 hr	Hepatic 3A4	Renal
prednisolone	GI	1-2 hr	18-36 hr	30-36 hr	Hepatic	Renal
triamcinolone	GI	1-2 hr	18-36 hr	52 hr	Hepatic	Renal
methylprednisolone	GI	1-2 hr	18-36 hr	30-36 hr	Hepatic	Renal
dexamethasone (PO)	GI	1-2 hr	36-54 hr	66 hr	Hepatic	Renal
betamethasone	GI	1-2 hr	36-54 hr	3.25 days	Hepatic	Renal

T lymphocytes to create antibodies. Steroids do not cause a decrease in the level of circulating antibodies but may inhibit antibody creation by interfering with macrophage function and the production and activation of lymphokines. Cellular immunity is mediated primarily by T lymphocytes. Steroids block several steps in the cascade of T-cell activation and thereby impede their ability to mount an effective cellular immune response. This action is used therapeutically to block rejection after transplant.

In addition, steroid administration has a direct effect on circulating white blood cells, causing a prompt drop in the number of lymphocytes, monocytes, and eosinophils in circulation and an increase in the number of circulating neutrophils. Lymphocytes are sequestered in lymph tissue, with T cells decreasing in relatively greater numbers than B cells. Neutrophils are released from the marrow in greater numbers and removed from circulation more slowly under the influence of exogenous steroids. The net result is a redistribution of white blood cell types rather than a true leukopenia.

Antiinflammatory Action

Lymphocytes, macrophages, and lymphokines all play a role in the modulation of the body's inflammatory response as well. Thus the impact of exogenous steroids is an interactive one between the immune response and the inflammatory response. By many of the pathways mentioned above, glucocorticoids inhibit both the early manifestations of inflammation, such as local edema, capillary dilation, migration and activation of white blood cells, and phagocytosis, and the later effects, including proliferation of capillaries and collagen deposition.

It is the simultaneous inhibition of inflammation and immune response that accounts for the effectiveness of glucocorticoids in circumstances such as acute asthma and acute allergic reactions. However, the practitioner must remain cognizant of the attendant risks of such suppression. Serious infection or illness may be masked by the absence of the characteristic signs of inflammation or immune system activation.

Stress Response

Stressful stimuli, such as surgery, fright, and abrupt physiologic challenge, prompt increased release of glucocorticoids from the adrenal cortex and the release of epinephrine and norepinephrine from the adrenal medulla. The steroids potentiate the effect of the catecholamines to raise heart rate, blood pressure, and blood glucose in the activation of the "fight-or-flight" response.

Other Effects

Glucocorticoids have several indirect effects on the central nervous system (CNS). Changes in mood, sleep pattern, and motor activity are seen. The typical mood change is an upregulation, or euphoria, but occasional anxiety and depression result for some patients. Rarely a so-called steroid psychosis occurs, which resolves with discontinuation of the medication. The precise mechanisms underlying these effects are unknown.

Glucocorticoids increase hemoglobin concentration and increase the number of circulating red blood cells.

Glucocorticoids impede the rate of growth in children. Many developing tissues, including brain, lung, liver, skin, and the epiphyses of long bones, are affected by an inhibition of cell division and cell growth.

DRUG TREATMENT PRINCIPLES

Critical decisions in the use of steroids revolve around length of therapy and how steroid use is stopped. The goal of treatment with glucocorticoids, other than as replacement therapy, is to control symptoms of inflammation and prevent organ damage while minimizing serious adverse effects. When possible, steroids should be added to other forms of therapy rather than given alone.

Most primary care uses of steroids call for short-term therapy (2 weeks or less). Steroid administration can suppress the hypothalamic-pituitary axis (HPA), leaving the body compromised during periods of physiologic stress due to complete or partial dependence on exogenous steroids.

TABLE 52-3 Glucocorticoids: Relative Potency, Equivalent Dose, Duration

Drug	Antiinflammatory Potency	Sodium-Retaining Potency	Equivalent Dose	Duration of Action
SHORT ACTING				
hydrocortisone	1	1	20 mg	8-12 hr
MEDIUM ACTING				
prednisone	4	0.8	5 mg	18-36 hr
prednisolone	4	0.8	5 mg	18-36 hr
methylprednisolone	5	0.5	4 mg	18-36 hr
triamcinolone	5	0	4 mg	18-36 hr
LONG ACTING				
dexamethasone	25	0	0.75 mg	36-54 hr
betamethasone	25	0	0.6-0.75 mg	36-54 hr

Use of oral or intramuscular steroids for less than 2 weeks, even in high doses, does not require gradual decrease in dosage to discontinue. However, 2- to 3-week courses are usually tapered to prevent symptom recurrence.

Longer courses require a gradual dosage reduction to avoid abrupt onset of the symptoms of adrenal insufficiency.

Recovery after HPA suppression can take up to 12 months. The use of a short-acting agent and an alternate-day dosage regimen should be considered for long-term therapy. The administration of a double dose every other morning has been found to cause less suppression of the HPA axis and less growth suppression in children. However, daily therapy is indicated for acute exacerbations of disease, and for a limited number of conditions such as temporal arteritis and pemphigus vulgaris.

Therapeutic administration is least likely to interfere with natural hormone production when given at the time of natural peak activity. It is generally recommended to administer the full daily dose before 9 AM. Large doses may need to be divided. Oral steroids are usually given with meals to limit GI irritation.

Prednisone is the drug of choice for most disorders seen in primary care, because of its short duration, minimal mineralocorticoid effect, and low cost. The initial dosage may need to be high for rapid control of symptoms, especially in life-threatening disease. To determine the minimal dose during long-term therapy, the dose should be tapered periodically to the point of worsening symptoms.

Oral preparations are the cheapest formulations, although convenience packs are available, the higher costs may not warrant their prescription. As true "miracle drugs," these products are remarkably inexpensive relative to many products on the market. Table 52-3 compares the potency of different steroid preparations.

HOW TO MONITOR

Short courses of therapy usually do not require laboratory tests. For long-term therapy, determination of baseline weight, blood pressure, serum glucose, and serum potassium levels is recommended.

Monitor for edema, weight gain, negative nitrogen balance, electrolyte imbalance, increased blood pressure, and other adverse effects as listed in Table 52-4.

Monitor for signs and symptoms of disease exacerbation.

Patients whose medication is being tapered after long-term therapy should be monitored for symptoms of steroid withdrawal and adrenal insufficiency (see Adverse Effects, below).

Children on chronic therapy should be closely followed for changes in rate of growth and continued attainment of developmental milestones.

PATIENT VARIABLES

Geriatrics

Because the elderly are more prone to certain potential adverse effects of steroid therapy, caution is needed with this population. Osteoporosis, susceptibility to compression fractures, thinning of the skin, and atrophy of subcutaneous fat are often seen with aging; steroid therapy may cause additive risks in these areas. Practitioners should use the lowest effective dose for the shortest effective time in the elderly.

Pediatrics

The potential for growth suppression is the greatest concern with use of glucocorticoids in children. Alternate-day dosing of intermediate-acting preparations may minimize suppression of activity of the HPA axis. A short course does not result in growth suppression.

Pregnancy and Lactation

Studies have not been done in humans to fully determine the level of safety in pregnancy. Glucocorticoids cross the placenta and appear in breast milk. Long-term use in the

TABLE 52-4 Adverse Effects of Oral and Intramuscular Glucocorticoids

System	Adverse Effects
Dermatologic	Acne, striae, urticaria, ecchymoses, erythema, thinning of skin, impaired wound healing
Cardiovascular	Hypertension, cardiac rupture following recent MI, thrombophlebitis, thromboembolic events
GI	Peptic ulcer, pancreatitis, ulcerative colitis, perforated viscus
Endocrine	Menstrual changes, decreased carbohydrate tolerance, hyperglycemia, increased insulin need in diabetics, hirsutism, decreased responsiveness of HPA axis
Musculoskeletal	Loss of muscle mass, weakness, tendon rupture, osteoporosis, necrosis of femoral and humeral heads, spontaneous fractures (long bones, vertebral compression fractures)
Neurologic	Vertigo, headache, seizure, paresthesias, steroid psychosis, pseudotumor cerebri (usually after abrupt halt to therapy)
Fluid and electrolyte	Hypokalemia, hypocalcemia, sodium and fluid retention, metabolic alkalosis
Miscellaneous	Insomnia, fatigue, hypersensitivity reactions, leukocytosis, altered manifestations of infection, posterior subcapsular cataracts

first trimester has been associated with a 1% incidence of cleft palate. Women who have taken large doses of steroids during pregnancy should be advised to avoid breast-feeding; their infants should be closely monitored for evidence of hypoadrenalism. Doses of prednisone or prednisolone of 20 mg/day or less or methylprednisolone of 8 mg/day or less for short periods may not cause harm to the infant. Waiting 3 to 4 hours after ingestion before breast-feeding has also been recommended.

PATIENT EDUCATION

- Take oral steroids with food to minimize GI upset.
- Take single daily or alternate-day doses before 9:00 AM to coincide with timing of peak endogenous adrenal cortical activity.
- Self-monitor for signs of adverse effects and notify practitioner if observed.
- Anticipate certain common side effects that can be troubling but not serious. These include changes in mood, insomnia, and increased appetite.
- Do not discontinue therapy abruptly without consulting practitioner.
- Taper dosage as directed.
- While on chronic therapy, carry a wallet card specifying drug and dosage. When therapy is over, indicate date of discontinuance on the card and carry it for an additional year to indicate the possible need for supplementation during times of severe physiologic stress.
- Learn the signs of adrenal insufficiency and report to practitioner if noted as dosage is tapered or after medication is discontinued. Signs include fatigue, weakness, nausea, anorexia, weight loss, diarrhea, dyspnea, and dizziness.
- Diabetic patients need to closely monitor serum glucose; changes in dosage of insulin or oral agent may be needed.
- Avoid immunizations with live virus such as smallpox, or close contact with people who have had recent live-virus vaccinations.

Specific Drugs

(P) Prototype Drug

hydrocortisone (Cortef, Hydrocortone)

Hydrocortisone, a naturally occurring glucocorticoid, is the drug prototype for this class of drugs. All other drugs are compared with hydrocortisone in terms of activity. It has both glucocorticoid and mineralocorticoid activity, making it most useful as replacement therapy or supplementation for patients with adrenal suppression during times of physiologic stress, such as surgery.

Contraindications

- Known hypersensitivity
- Systemic fungal infections
- Recent myocardial infarction (due to an association between corticosteroid use and left ventricular rupture)
- Intramuscular use of corticosteroids is contraindicated in immune thrombocytopenic purpura (ITP)

Warnings

Increased susceptibility to infection and potentially impaired host defense mechanisms necessitate a high index of suspicion for infection and prompt initiation of specific antiinfective therapy.

In patients with class II tuberculosis, observe closely for reactivation of active infection. Latent amebiasis can also be activated. It may be prudent to exclude amebiasis in the patient with undiagnosed diarrhea before initiating steroid therapy.

TABLE 52-5 Corticosteroid Drug Interactions

Drug	Potential Effect of Interaction
Oral contraceptives, estrogens	Steroid half-life and concentration increased; clearance decreased
Barbiturates, hydantoins, rifampin	Steroid clearance may be increased, resulting in decreased therapeutic effect of the steroid preparation
Oral anticoagulants	Steroid may oppose or potentiate the anticoagulant effect; careful monitoring of prothrombin time is required
digitalis	Increased potential for digitalis toxicity related to hypokalemia
Diuretics	Increased potential for electrolyte disturbance, particularly hypokalemia with potassium-depleting agents
isoniazid	Decreased concentration of isoniazid
Salicylates	Decreased concentration of salicylate; decreased therapeutic effectiveness
theophylline	Variable effect on the activity of both agents
ketoconazole	Steroid clearance decreased

The use of live-virus vaccines is contraindicated in patients receiving long-term steroid therapy because of concerns about ineffective antibody response and the potential risk of neurologic complications.

Patients on long-term supraphysiologic doses of steroids (or whose medication has been discontinued within the past year) who anticipate a period of increased physiologic stress (e.g., surgery) may need supplementation with a glucocorticoid that also has mineralocorticoid activity. The competency of the HPA axis can be evaluated by several outpatient laboratory tests.

Precautions

Corticosteroids should be used cautiously in the following conditions, with careful risk/benefit assessment and close monitoring during therapy: hypertension, CHF, peptic ulcer disease, GI tract infection, diabetes, osteoporosis, seizure disorders, hepatic cirrhosis, metastatic carcinoma, Cushing syndrome, and resistant infections.

Pharmacokinetics

The glucocorticoids, both natural and synthetic, are well absorbed from the GI tract (see Table 52-2). Intramuscular preparations are used when oral intake is contraindicated or sustained action needed. In general the sodium esters (phosphate and succinate) are rapidly absorbed parenterally; the acetate preparations are more slowly absorbed. Glucocorticoids are reversibly bound to both an albumin and a globulin, predominantly the latter. It is the unbound portion that is metabolically active. The liver metabolizes hydrocortisone and its synthetic analogs; hepatic enzyme induction increases their clearance. Prednisone is a P450 3A4 substrate. Excretion is via the kidneys; increased plasma levels result in increased renal clearance.

Relative potencies, dose equivalencies, and duration of action of the various agents are summarized in Table 52-3.

Adverse Effects

Adverse effects vary in intensity and severity. Controlling factors include both dosage and length of therapy, as well as underlying physiologic factors in the patient. The decision to stop treatment versus decrease the dosage must be individualized in each case. Prolonged use of glucocorticoids can result in a characteristic cushingoid state. Stigmata include truncal obesity, moon facies, hirsutism, abdominal striae, acne, and the presence of a buffalo hump. Additional common adverse effects to oral and intramuscular glucocorticoids are listed in Table 52-4.

Sudden discontinuation or rapid tapering of steroids in patients who have developed adrenal suppression can precipitate symptoms of adrenal insufficiency, including nausea, weakness, depression, anorexia, myalgias, hypotension, and hypoglycemia.

Interactions

Many potential drug-drug interactions are common to all corticosteroids. They are listed in Table 52-5.

Dosage and Administration

Hydrocortisone is used for oral administration only. Initial adult dosage range is 20 to 240 mg/day. Pediatric dosage is 0.5 to 4 mg/kg/day, usually divided into three or four doses. Dosage varies widely depending on disease and patient variables.

Other Drugs in Class

Other drugs in this class are similar to the prototype except as follows.

prednisone (Deltasone, Sterapred)

Indications. Prednisone is the most commonly prescribed glucocorticoid. It has four times as much antiinflammatory potency as hydrocortisone, and minimal mineralocorticoid activity, making it the drug of choice for most disorders treated with systemic steroids in primary care.

Pharmacokinetics. Prednisone is an inactive substance and must be metabolized in the liver to prednisolone. This activity may be impaired in patients with liver disease.

Dosage and Administration. Prednisone is administered orally only. Dosage varies widely depending on the indication and patient variables. Initial dosage may range from 5 to 60 mg/day in adults. In children dosage may range from 0.5 to 2 mg/kg/day, with a daily maximum of 60 mg/day. Dosage may be once daily or divided into two, three, or four daily doses.

prednisolone (Delta-Cortef, Prelone)

Pharmacokinetics. Prednisolone sodium phosphate oral liquid produces a 20% higher peak plasma level than tablet forms; that peak occurs approximately 15 minutes earlier than with oral tablets.

Dosage and Administration. Prednisolone is administered orally, in doses of 5 to 60 mg/day. Pediatric dosage is 1 to 2 mg/kg/day, to a daily maximum of 60 mg/day. As with all glucocorticoids, dosage must be individualized.

triamcinolone (Aristocort, Kenacort, Atolone)

Dosage and Administration. A variety of preparations are used for intraarticular, oral, topical, and inhalation therapy. The usual oral starting dose varies based on therapeutic indication, from 4 to 60 mg/day. Slightly higher doses are used in palliative treatment of acute leukemia and lymphoma. The maximum daily dosage to avoid suppression of HPA axis is 8 mg.

methylprednisolone (Medrol)

Pharmacokinetics. When given concurrently with the macrolide antibiotics, methylprednisolone clearance is slowed, so a smaller dose of methylprednisolone is needed. Methylprednisolone sodium succinate has a more rapid onset of action when given IM than the acetate salt. Methylprednisolone acetate is less soluble and therefore has a longer duration of action.

Dosage and Administration. Oral and injectable forms are long-acting. Usual initial oral dose is 4 to 48 mg/day. Usual pediatric dose is 0.16 to 0.8 mg/kg/day.

dexamethasone (Decadron)

Indications. Dexamethasone is often used in acute allergic disorders. It is used to confirm the diagnosis of Cushing syndrome and to distinguish excess glucocorticoid secretion of pituitary origin from that of adrenal or ectopic origin. It has several unlabeled uses, including the prevention and treatment of acute mountain sickness and as an antiemetic, and has been reported to decrease the incidence of hearing loss in bacterial meningitis.

Pharmacokinetics. Dexamethasone is well absorbed after oral administration. The acetate salt is used intramuscularly for prompt onset with a longer duration of effect.

Drug Interactions. Ephedrine interacts with dexamethasone to decrease the half-life and increase the clearance of dexamethasone. Aminoglutethimide potentially reverses the adrenal suppression of dexamethasone.

Dosage and Administration. Dosage varies widely and must be individualized. The usual initial adult dosage of oral dexamethasone is 0.75 to 9 mg/day. Usual pediatric dosage for airway edema is 0.5 to 1 mg/kg/day.

betamethasone (Celestone)

Dosage and Administration. Usual oral dosage is 0.6 to 7.2 mg/day. As with all glucocorticoids, dosage must be individualized.

BIBLIOGRAPHY

Douglas LO: Glucocorticoids and antibiotics in preterm PROM, *J Fam Pract* 47(3):175, 1998.

Goroll AH, May LA, Mulley AG, editors: *Primary care medicine*, ed 4, Philadelphia, 2000, Lippincott Williams & Wilkins.

Hardman JG, Limbird LE, editors: *Goodman & Gilman's the pharmacological basis of therapeutics*, ed 10, New York, 2001, McGraw-Hill.

Kirwin JR et al: Systemic glucocorticoid treatment in rheumatoid arthritis: a debate, *Scand J Rheumatol* 27(4):247, 1998.

Maccari S et al: Prenatal stress and long-term consequences: implications of glucocorticoid hormones, *Neurosci Biobehav Rev* 27(102):119-127, 2003.

Volcheck GW et al: Anti-inflammatory drugs for controlling asthma, *Postgrad Med* 104(3):127, 1998.

CHAPTER 53

Thyroid Medications

Susan D. McConnell

Drug Names

Class	Subclass	Generic Name	Trade Name
Thyroid supplements		(200) levothyroxine sodium (synthetic T_4) liothyronine (synthetic T_3) liotrix (T_4:T_3 = 4:1)	Synthroid, Levoxyl, Levothyroid Cytomel Thyrolar, Euthroid
Thyroid suppressants		propylthiouracil (PTU) methimazole	Generic Tapazole
Adjunctive diagnostic tool for thyroid cancer		thyrotropin	Thyrogen

(200), Top 200 drug.

Thyroid Supplements

General Uses

Indications

- Hypothyroidism as replacement therapy
- Pituitary thyroid-stimulating hormone (TSH) suppression, in treatment or prevention of euthyroid goiters and in the management of thyroid cancer

Unlabeled Use

- Obesity, but it is not considered to be safe or effective

Thyroid hormones are used as replacement or supplemental therapy in chronic hypothyroidism of any etiology. Thyroxine (T_4) is usually used only to treat uncomplicated hypothyroidism. Triiodothyronine (T_3) is usually only used in suppression treatment of thyroid cancer. Treatment for hypothyroidism generally requires lifelong replacement of the thyroid hormone.

DISEASE PROCESS

Anatomy and Physiology

Regulation of a basal metabolism is achieved through the complex coordination of the hypothalamic-pituitary-thyroid negative feedback control system (Figure 53-1). T_4 and T_3 are released from the thyroid gland in response to circulating serum levels of thyroid-stimulating hormone (TSH) and thyroid-releasing hormone (TRH). The feedback mechanism creates an inverse relationship between serum levels of T_3-T_4 and TSH-TRH. When T_3 and T_4 serum levels rise, TSH and TRH secretion is suppressed. TRH and TSH levels can be measured directly. An elevated TSH is diagnostic of primary hypothyroidism. A low TSH accompanied by low T_4 and T_3 is characteristic of secondary hypothyroidism. TRH is measured if tertiary hypothyroidism is suspected.

The thyroid gland releases T_4 (90%), T_3 (10%), and reverse T_3 (rT_3) (<1%). Elevated rT_3 may be an indication of euthyroid sick syndrome. This test is usually reserved for when standard thyroid function tests (TFTs) give inconclusive results.

T_3 and T_4 have a high affinity for protein. T_3 is 99.7% protein-bound, where T_4 is 99.97% protein-bound. Only the unbound portion is metabolically active. In the peripheral tissue, T_4 is converted to T_3 by the removal of iodine. Therefore in the majority of cases it is necessary to administer only T_4 because the body will produce T_3 from the T_4. The physiologic effects of thyroid hormones can be attributed to the peripheral T_3.

The thyroid hormones exert their effect through a variety of mechanisms. Basal metabolic rate is regulated by thyroid hormones. They affect every organ system. They increase oxygen consumption; respiratory rate; body temperature; cardiac output; heart rate; blood volume; and rate of fat, protein, and carbohydrate metabolism; enzyme system activity; and growth and maturation. They regulate catecholamine effects. They are especially important in CNS development.

Pathophysiology

In children thyroid hormones are essential for overall normal growth and development. Without thyroid hormone,

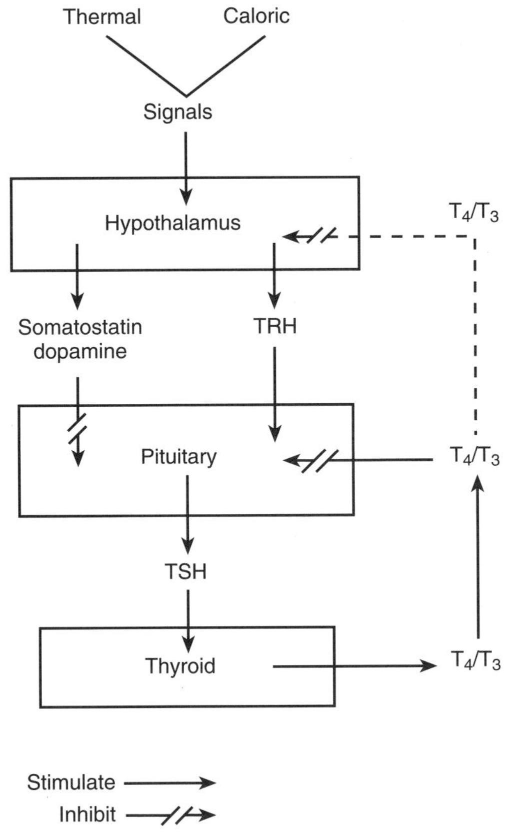

FIGURE 53-1

Regulation of thyroid-stimulating hormone (TSH) secretion. Thyroxine (T_4) and triiodothyronine (T_3) from the thyroid gland exert negative feedback on the pituitary by blocking the action of thyroid-releasing hormone (TRH). Negative feedback of T_4 and T_3 at the level of the hypothalamus is less well established. Somatostatin and dopamine each inhibit TSH secretion tonically. (From Berne RM, Levy MN: *Physiology,* ed 4, St Louis, 1998, Mosby.)

development of the central nervous system is impaired. Undetected deficiency of thyroid hormone may begin to affect children shortly after birth (as evidenced by cretinism).

Adults may also develop numerous problems related to a decreased metabolic rate. Cardiovascular, gastrointestinal, musculoskeletal, and neurologic function may be impaired as a result of inadequate thyroid hormones.

Primary hypothyroidism, the most common form of hypothyroidism, is caused by a failure within the thyroid gland. Secondary hypothyroidism is caused by the lack of TSH secretion from the pituitary. Tertiary hypothyroidism is caused by lack of TRH secretion from the hypothalamus.

There are a variety of causes of primary hypothyroidism. One common cause is iatrogenic, the result of therapy for hyperthyroidism, or other drugs such as lithium. Other causes include thyroid atrophy, autoimmune destruction of the thyroid, chronic thyroiditis such as Hashimoto's disease, and postpartum hypothyroidism.

The Disease

Hypothyroidism is the metabolic state resulting from deficient thyroid hormones. In adults it is most common in women and is characterized by disease in basal metabolic rate, tiredness and lethargy, sensitivity to cold, and menstrual disturbances. If untreated it progresses to full-blown myxedema, with characteristic appearance and physical symptoms, especially of the skin. Table 53-1 lists altered laboratory findings in thyroid dysfunction. The TSH is the most sensitive useful test in the diagnosis of hypothyroidism. T_4 and T_3 are also useful.

DRUG ACTION AND EFFECTS

A thyroid supplement serves to replace inadequate levels of endogenous T_3 and T_4. If an exogenous thyroid hormone is given in a euthyroid patient, endogenous secretion of TSH and TRH will be suppressed, therefore suppressing the body's production of T_3 and T_4.

Basal metabolic rate and metabolism of carbohydrates, proteins, and fats are increased by thyroid supplements. These drugs also exert a direct effect on tissue (e.g., increased myocardial contraction).

Thyrogen is a new drug indicated for adjunctive use for serum thyroglobulin testing with or without radioiodine imaging in the follow-up of patients with well-differentiated thyroid cancer. Patients who have had partial or total removal of their thyroid gland must take thyroid hormone supplements

TABLE 53-1 Altered Laboratory Findings in Thyroid Dysfunction

Dysfunctional States	TSH	T_4/Free T_4	T_3/Free T_3	Free Thyroxin Index (FTI)	T_3-Uptake	rT_3
HYPOTHYROID STATES						
Primary	Increased	Decreased	Decreased	Decreased	Not useful	Normal
Secondary	Normal or decreased	Decreased	Decreased	Decreased	Not useful	Normal
Subclinical hypothyroidism	Increased	Normal to decreased	Normal	Normal	Not useful	Normal
HYPERTHYROID STATES						
Primary	Decreased	Increased	Increased	Increased	Increased	Normal
Secondary	Increased	Increased	Increased	Increased	Increased	Normal
EUTHYROID						
Sick syndrome	Normal or decreased	Normal	Decreased	Increased	Not useful	Increased

TABLE 53-2 Laboratory Evaluation of Thyroid Disorders

Test	Hormone Evaluated	Interpretation of Test Results
TRH (thyrotropin)	Thyrotropin-releasing hormone	Assesses the function of the hypothalamic-pituitary-thyroid axis. Most useful when other tests are inconclusive
TSH	Thyroid-stimulating hormone	Assesses the function of the hypothalamic-pituitary-thyroid axis
TBG (thyroglobulin)	Thyroxine-binding globulin	As the primary protein for hormone binding, it is most useful for evaluating discrepancies in clinical findings and other serum hormone levels
T_4 (T_4 RIA, thyroxine)	Tetraiodothyronine, thyroxine	Concentration of bound and unbound thyroid hormone (T_4) in the serum
FT_4	Free thyroxine, free T_4	Concentration of unbound thyroid hormone (T_4) in the serum. It is most helpful for diagnosis when there is an abnormal TBG level
T_3 (T_3 RIA)	Triiodothyronine	Concentration of bound and unbound thyroid hormone (T_3) in the serum
FT_3	Free triiodothyronine, free T_3	Concentration of unbound, active T_3 in the serum
T_3-U (T_3 RU)	Resin T_3 uptake	Indirectly measures the concentration of thyroglobulin (TBG) by measuring the empty TBG binding sites in serum. Direct measurement of TBG may be more useful
rT_3	Reverse T_3	A T_3 antagonist, rT_3 can be increased in euthyroid sick syndrome
FTI (F T_4-I, T_7, T_{12})	Free T_4 index	Derived by multiplying T_4 and T_3-U, it reflects the free (unbound) T_4 in serum. This test has essentially been replaced by direct FT_3 and FT_4 measurements
LATS	Long-acting thyroid stimulator	A positive test supports the diagnosis of Graves' disease
Antithyroid antibodies	Antithyroglobulin antibodies Antimicrosomal antibodies	Useful in detecting autoimmune causes of thyroid disease

to maintain their metabolism and to suppress endogenous levels of TSH. However, a high level of TSH in a patient's bloodstream is necessary for radioiodine imaging to detect remnant thyroid tissue or metastatic disease and for achieving optimal sensitivity of serum thyroglobulin testing. In the past, patients had to stop taking their hormone supplements for 2 to 6 weeks prior to testing, causing them to experience symptoms of thyroid deficiency. Thyrogen, which is a recombinant form of TSH, allows the patients to avoid hormone withdrawal and its debilitating effects while undergoing diagnostic testing.

DRUG TREATMENT PRINCIPLES

Dosage of all thyroid medication must be individualized. Dosage is based on laboratory findings and the patient's clinical response. Generally therapy is started at a low dose and increased every 4 to 6 weeks until a normal TSH is obtained. Administer thyroid hormone as a single daily dose, preferably before breakfast.

Treatment of choice for hypothyroidism is T_4. It has a relatively slow onset of action, and the effects are cumulative over a period of several weeks. T_3 has a more rapid onset of action and dissipation of action. T_3 may be preferable to rapidly correct a hypothyroid state, in radioisotope scanning procedures, and in thyroid cancer.

The American Association of Clinical Endocrinologists (AACE) emphasizes that there are many brands of levothyroxine and they are not compared against a levothyroxine standard. Bioequivalence of levothyroxine preparations is based on total T_4 measurement and not TSH levels; therefore bioequivalence is not the same as therapeutic equivalence. This means that the patient should receive the same brand of levothyroxine throughout treatment. In general, desiccated thyroid hormone, combinations of thyroid hormones, or triiodothyronine should not be used as replacement therapy.

The mean replacement dosage of levothyroxine is 1.6 μg/kg of body weight per day, although the appropriate dosage varies among patients. The pace of treatment depends on the duration and severity of hypothyroidism and on whether there are other associated medical problems. The patient should undergo reassessment and therapy should be titrated after an interval of at least 6 weeks following any change in levothyroxine brand or dose.

Levothyroxine doses are commonly measured in micrograms rather than milligrams to avoid confusion regarding the dosage. A correct dose is 75 μg, which is the equivalent of 0.075 mg. The usual starting dose in treatment of hypothyroidism is levothyroxine (T_4) 25 to 75 μg. The usual maintenance dose is 75 to 150 μg po daily.

HOW TO MONITOR

See Tables 53-2 and 53-3.

The test for T_4 measures the total thyroxine, both bound and unbound in the serum. Free thyroxine (FT_4) measures only unbound T_4. Normally only the T_4 needs to be measured; thyroid-binding globulin is the protein thyroid hormones are bound to. It can be directly measured by the thyroid-binding globulin (TBG) test. The resin T_3 uptake (T_3 RU) is an indirect measure that is no longer used. If the patient has an abnormal TBG, free T_4 may need to be evaluated.

Usually measuring the TSH in 4 to 6 weeks is sufficient. T_4, T_3, and TSH can be monitored weekly for the first 4 weeks after initiation of therapy. Full therapeutic effectiveness may not be achieved for 4 to 6 weeks. TSH is usually monitored monthly until normal and stable. Annual evaluation is recommended

TABLE 53-3 Normal Range for Thyroid Function Laboratory Tests

Name of Test	Normal Range for Values
TRH (thyroid-releasing hormone)	Males: 14-24 μU/ml Females: 16-26 μU/ml
TSH (thyroid-stimulating hormone)	Newborn: <20 μU/ml Adult: 0.30-5.5 μU/ml
TBG (thyroglobulin)	16-34 μU/ml
T_4 (thyroxine)	Newborn: 6.4-23.2 μg/ml Child (1-10 yr): 6.4-15 μg/ml Adult: 5-12 μg/ml
FT_4 (free thyroxine)	0.9-1.7 ng/dl
T_3 (triiodothyronine)	Newborn: 32-250 ng/ml Child (1-10 yr): 94-269 ng/ml Adult: 95-190 ng/ml
FT_3 (free triiodothyronine)	0.2-.52 ng/dl
T_3-U (resin T_3 uptake)	25%-35%
rT_3 (reverse T_3)	
FTI (free thyroxine index)	1.3-4.2
Antithyroid antibodies: anti-TBG antimicrosomal	Negative or titer <1:100
LATS (long-acting thyroid stimulator)	Negative

once maintenance therapy is achieved. Levels should also be evaluated whenever patients experience signs and/or symptoms that could be related to underdosage/overdosage.

Children younger than 3 years old should be maintained on the upper end of T_4 therapeutic range with a normal serum TSH. It is recommended that children have laboratory assessment of medication effectiveness every 1 to 2 months for the first year, 2 to 3 months from 1 to 3 years old, and every 3 to 12 months thereafter.

PATIENT VARIABLES

Geriatrics

Hypothyroidism is common in the elderly. Atypical presentation includes CHF. Administration of thyroid hormone may exacerbate cardiovascular disease, particularly angina, in elderly patients. It is advisable to start low (25 μg) and gradually increase the dosage. Dosage adjustments may also be required as absorption may be increased with aging.

Pediatrics

Thyroid function is paramount for normal growth and development, especially for the central nervous system in children. Neonates at risk should have a screening T_4 and TSH as soon as possible after birth. Diagnosis and treatment of congenital hypothyroidism are essential to prevent cretinism. It is expected that children will require higher doses of medication to meet the metabolic demands of growth and development in the first 3 years of life. In congenital hypothyroidism, therapy may be stopped for 2 to 8 weeks after the client reaches 3 years old. If the TSH levels remain normal, thyroid supplementation may be permanently discontinued.

Pregnancy

- *Category A:* There is minimal excretion of thyroid medications in breast milk.

PATIENT EDUCATION

- Response to this medication is not immediate. Symptoms should improve within 2 weeks.
- Thyroid deficiency generally requires lifelong therapy. Taking the medication and compliance with therapy are extremely important.
- Do not alter doses or abruptly stop the medication unless directed by the primary care provider.
- It is recommended that patients do not alter the brand of medication they use because of a potential variability in the bioequivalence between manufacturers.
- Medications should be taken at approximately the same time each day. The preferable time of day is before breakfast or on an empty stomach to increase absorption. If it is taken too late in the day, it may make it difficult to go to sleep.
- Report signs and symptoms of overdosage (hyperthyroidism) or underdosage (hypothyroidism) to health care provider promptly. See Table 53-4 for symptoms.

Specific Drugs

levothyroxine sodium (T_4) (Synthroid, Levothroid, Levo-T)

Contraindications. Untreated thyrotoxicosis, uncorrected adrenal insufficiency (may precipitate adrenal crisis), or hypersensitivity to any of the medication components

Warnings/Precautions

- It is inappropriate to use any thyroid supplement for the management of obesity or fertility.
- Patients with known cardiovascular disease should be carefully monitored while taking levothyroxine. Problems may also occur in cases of occult cardiovascular disease. Therefore it should be cautiously administered to patients with the potential for undiagnosed disease. Start with a low dose, 25 to 50 μg and increase dose slowly.
- Diabetes mellitus and diabetes insipidus may also be aggravated by initiation of levothyroxine.

Because preparations vary, make certain to write prescription so that the patient will receive the same brand of medication throughout treatment.

Pharmacokinetics. See Table 53-5. T_4 absorption from the gastrointestinal tract is poor (50% to 80%). It may be increased with fasting and decreased further with malabsorption syndromes. A higher affinity for serum protein increases the half-life of T_4 as compared with T_3.

Adverse Effects. See Table 53-6. Thyroid hormone absorption may be affected by malabsorptive states and patient age.

TABLE 53-4 Clinical Presentation of Thyroid Dysfunctions

Type of Signs/Symptoms	Hyperthyroidism	Hypothyroidism
INITIAL Most frequent concerns that prompt medical care and evaluation	Amenorrhea/oligomenorrhea Diarrhea Goiter Nervousness/irritability Palpitations (tachycardia) Sleep disturbance (insomnia) Unexplained weight loss Vision changes (exophthalmos)	Cold intolerance Depression and loss of concentration Dry skin (pruritus) Menorrhagia Myalgias Somnolence and fatigue
LATER May be evidenced at the initial evaluation but usually develop with prolonged disease	Dependent edema Dyspnea Impaired mentation (confusion) Muscle weakness and fatigue Tremor	Constipation Goiter Memory loss/impairment Myxedema Unexplained weight gain
INCIDENTAL May be identified on physical examination but may not be offered as a complaint by the patient unless asked directly	Diaphoresis Heat intolerance Increased appetite	Anorexia Bradycardia Habitual abortion/sterility Impotence

TABLE 53-5 Pharmacokinetics of Thyroid Supplements

Drug	Absorption	Onset of Action	Time to Peak Concentration	Half Life	Duration of Action	Protein Bound	Metabolism
levothyroxine	Variable in GI (50%-80%)	1-3 wk	IV: 24 hr 6-7 days	1-3 wk		99%	Biliary
liothyronine	Complete in GI (95% in 4 hr)	12-36 hr	24-72 hr	2-3 days	3-5 days	99%	Biliary/renal
liotrix	Variable in GI but $T_3 > T_4$	T_3: 12-36 hr T_4: unknown	T_3: 24-72 hr T_4: 1-3 wk	T_3: 2-3 days T_4: 6-7 days	T_3: 3-5 days T_4: 1-3 wk	99%	Biliary/renal

TABLE 53-6 Adverse Effects of Thyroid Supplements

System	liothyronine	levothyroxine	liotrix
Dermatologic	Alopecia (children) Diaphoresis	Diaphoresis	Alopecia (children) Diaphoresis
Cardiovascular	Angina Arrhythmias Tachycardia	Angina Arrhythmias Palpitations	Angina Arrhythmias Tachycardia
GI	Abdominal cramps Diarrhea Nausea/vomiting	Abdominal cramps Diarrhea Nausea/vomiting	Abdominal cramps Diarrhea Nausea/vomiting
Endocrine	Irregular menses	Hyperglycemia Hypocholesterolemia Irregular menses	Hyperglycemia Hypocholesterolemia Irregular menses
Metabolic	Heat intolerance Weight loss	Heat intolerance Weight loss	Heat intolerance Weight loss
CNS	Insomnia Irritability Nervousness	Headache Insomnia Nervousness	Insomnia Irritability Nervousness

TABLE 53-7 Dosage and Administration of Thyroid Supplements

Thyroid Supplements	Hypothyroidism	Thyroid Suppression
INFANT (0-6 MONTHS)		
liothyronine	Initial: 5 μg/day; increase by 3-4 μg/day as needed	
levothyroxine	10-15 μg/kg/day	
liotrix	No information	
INFANT (6-12 MONTHS)		
liothyronine	20 μg/day is usual maintenance	
levothyroxine	6-8 μg/kg/day	
liotrix	No information	
CHILD (1-5 YEARS)		
liothyronine	50 μg/day is usual maintenance	
levothyroxine	5-6 μg/kg/day	
liotrix	Initial: ½ tablet every day; increase at 2-3 week intervals as needed	Calculate T_4 dose to equal 1.56 μg/kg/day for 7-10 days
CHILD (6-12 YEARS)		
liothyronine	Give usual adult dose	
levothyroxine	4-5 μg/kg/day	
liotrix	Initial: ½ tablet every day; increase at 2-3 week intervals as needed	Calculate T_4 dose to equal 1.56 μg/kg/day for 7-10 days
ADULTS		
liothyronine	Initial: 25 μg/kg/day; increase by 12.5-25 μg/day every 1-2 weeks as needed	75-100 μg/day for 7 days
levothyroxine	Initial: 1.6 μg/kg/day; increase by 12.5-25 μg/day every 2-6 weeks as needed	2 μg/kg/day titrate to desired level of suppression
liotrix	Initial: ½ tablet every day; increase by a ¼-½ tablet every 2-3 weeks as needed	Calculate T_4 dose to equal 1.56 μg/kg/day for 7-10 days

Because levothyroxine has a narrow therapeutic range, small differences in absorption may result in subclinical or clinical hypothyroidism or hyperthyroidism.

Drug Interactions. Certain drugs, such as cholestyramine, colestipol, ferrous sulfate, sucralfate, calcium, and some antacids containing aluminum hydroxide interfere with levothyroxine absorption. Some anticonvulsants affect thyroid hormone bindings. Rifampin and sertraline hydrochloride may accelerate levothyroxine metabolism and necessitate a higher replacement dose.

Oral anticoagulants may have an increased effect related to vitamin K metabolism.

Androgens and estrogens may reduce protein binding and decrease the medication effectiveness.

Insulin and oral hypoglycemic agents may be less effective with initiation of therapy. Therefore dosage adjustments may be required to maintain blood glucose levels.

β-blockers and digitalis preparations may become less effective as the hypothyroid patient's condition improves.

Overdosage. Toxicity is evidenced by signs and symptoms of hyperthyroidism and may mimic thyrotoxicosis. Decrease or temporarily discontinue levothyroxine for approximately 5 to 7 days, and then resume at a lower dose.

Dosage and Administration. See Table 53-7.

liothyronine (T_3) (Cytomel, Triostat)

Indications. Liothyronine effectively treats hypothyroidism from any cause other than transient thyroiditis. The most common use is for thyroid suppression therapy to evaluate and treat euthyroid goiter, nodular thyroid, and thyroid cancer.

liotrix (Thyrolar, Euthyroid)

Indications. Any form of hypothyroidism may be effectively treated with liotrix. Myxedema and thyroid suppression therapy (used in euthyroid goiter and nodular thyroid) are other common uses.

Thyroid Suppressants

General Uses

Indications

Hyperthyroidism: Long-term use may lead to disease remission. Used when surgery is contraindicated. Also used to ameliorate hyperthyroidism before subtotal thyroidectomy or radioactive iodine therapy.

Unlabeled Use

Propylthiouracil (PTU) may be useful in alcoholic liver disease by reducing the hepatic hypermetabolic state induced by alcohol.

DISEASE PROCESS

Pathophysiology

Hyperthyroidism (thyrotoxicosis) is the clinical state resulting from an excess of thyroid hormone. The most common causes of hyperthyroidism are Graves' disease, toxic nodular goiter, thyroiditis, and iodide-induced hyperthyroidism. An autoimmune process causes Graves' disease, also known as diffuse toxic goiter. Toxic nodular goiter is due to a hyperfunctioning multinodular goiter. In thyroiditis, hyperthyroidism is usually transient. Exposure to iodide is iatrogenic.

The Disease

The presentation of hyperthyroidism is highly variable. See Table 53-4 for symptoms of hyperthyroidism.

Excessive synthesis of thyroid hormone increases the individual's basal metabolism to potentially fatal levels. Cardiovascular and neurologic function may be markedly stimulated, resulting in systemic collapse.

Diagnosis is based on symptoms, physical findings, and laboratory findings. The TSH will be suppressed, and T_3 and T_4 will be increased. See Table 53-1 for altered laboratory findings in thyroid dysfunction.

DRUG ACTION AND EFFECTS

Mechanism of Action

By diverting iodine, thyroid hormone synthesis is inhibited. PTU, but not methimazole, also inhibits the conversion of T_4 to T_3 in the tissue.

By reducing the absorption of iodine, thyroid hormone synthesis is diminished. As the thyroid gland becomes depleted of hormones, tissue concentrations drop and the metabolic rate decreases. However, the medications do not inhibit stored or circulating levels of T_3 or T_4. Thyroid suppressant agents do not affect oral and parenteral thyroid supplements. Normal thyroid hormone synthesis resumes rapidly with cessation of therapy. PTU also inhibits conversion of T_4 to T_3 in peripheral tissues, unlike methimazole. This will speed conversion to a euthyroid state. Methimazole has the advantage of being longer acting and requiring a less frequent dosage schedule, which may increase compliance.

DRUG TREATMENT PRINCIPLES

Rest, adequate diet, and avoidance of occupational and domestic stress are also useful modalities of therapy.

Antithyroid drugs have been used since the 1940s and are prescribed in an attempt to achieve remission of symptoms. Remission rates are variable and relapses are frequent. The patients in whom remission is most likely to be achieved are those with mild hyperthyroidism and small goiters. Elderly or cardiac patients may require "pretreatment" with antithyroid drugs before radioiodine therapy. Some endocrinologists prefer antithyroid drug therapy in childhood Graves' disease. Hyperthyroidism during pregnancy is one clear indication for antithyroid drug treatment.

These drugs will control excessive production of thyroid hormone in almost all cases of hyperthyroidism. About one half or less will result in a permanent remission. Half of these will become hypothyroid. Relapses are uncommon but do occur. Antithyroid drugs will restore a euthyroid state in 4 to 8 weeks, although symptoms will improve sooner, usually in 1 to 2 weeks. The patient should be euthyroid before surgery. Antithyroid drugs are also useful before and after radioiodine therapy.

Titration of dosage to gain maximal therapeutic response with the lowest dosage is the objective. Generally therapy is maintained for 12 to 24 months. Once the patient has been euthyroid for 6 to 12 months, a decision may be made to reduce dosage and ascertain whether a remission has occurred. If remission is achieved, therapy is discontinued. Consultation and referral to a physician is warranted during the initiation and decision to maintain or end therapy.

β-adrenergic blocking drugs such as propranolol can control the signs and symptoms of hyperthyroidism that are related to sensitization of the sympathetic nervous system (see Chapter 21).

HOW TO MONITOR

Laboratory bloodwork should be done before initiating antithyroid therapy and periodically once the patient is on a maintenance dose. Serum T_4 and T_3 levels are monitored initially and after 2 weeks of therapy until a euthyroid state is achieved, usually in 3 to 5 months. Once clinical evidence of hyperthyroidism has been resolved, an elevated TSH level indicates a need to lower the dosage.

Before initiating therapy, a white blood cell (WBC) count with differential is done and then repeated with any sign of infection. Some recommend routine monitoring of the WBC for at least the first 3 months of therapy. Monitor prothrombin time during therapy, especially before surgical procedures.

With the potential for hepatotoxicity, AST, ALT, alkaline phosphatase, LDH, bilirubin, and prothrombin time (PT) may also be evaluated.

During each visit monitor for signs and symptoms of infection, as well as correction of the hypermetabolic state: decreased pulse, decreased blood pressure, weight gain, elimination of nervousness, and tremor. Evaluate for hepatitis, agranulocytosis, and GI irritation (see Tables 53-2 and 53-3).

PATIENT VARIABLES

Geriatrics

Elderly individuals are less likely to experience hyperthyroidism than hypothyroidism. Hyperthyroidism in the elderly may have an atypical presentation, with atrial fibrillation as a presenting symptom.

Pediatrics

PTU hepatotoxicity has occurred; discontinue immediately if signs and symptoms of hepatic dysfunction develop.

Pregnancy

- *Category D*: thyroid suppressants cross the placenta and can induce goiter or cretinism. PTU is generally preferred if a drug is necessary. They can be effective if used judiciously. In many pregnant women hyperthyroidism diminishes as the pregnancy proceeds, making dosage reduction or discontinuation of the drug possible. An endocrinologist usually follows the patient.

TABLE 53-8 Pharmacokinetics of Thyroid Suppressants

Drug	Absorption	Onset of Action	Time to Peak Concentration	Half-Life	Duration of Action	Protein Bound	Metabolism	Excretion
methimazole	Rapid, good in GI	1 wk	4-10 wk	5-6 hr	Weeks	Minimal	Hepatic	Renal
propylthiouracil	Rapid, good in GI	10-21 days*	6-10 wk	1-2 hr	Weeks	80%	Hepatic	Renal

* However, thyroid hormone may begin to increase as soon as 1 hr after dose is given.

Lactation

Thyroid suppressants should not be given while the patient is breast-feeding.

PATIENT EDUCATION

Avoid ingestion of substances containing iodine (e.g., seafood, iodized salt).

Patients should be advised to notify their practitioner of any illness or unusual signs or symptoms immediately. Report fever, sore throat, malaise, unusual bleeding or bruising, headache, skin rash, or enlargement of cervical lymph nodes to health care provider.

Specific Drugs

propylthiouracil (PTU) (Generic)

Contraindications. Hypersensitivity to any of the medication components.

Warnings/Precautions. Agranulocytosis is potentially the most serious side effect. Bone marrow function should be monitored because agranulocytosis may occur up to 4 months post therapy. Leukopenia, thrombocytopenia, and aplastic anemia may also occur.

Discontinue the drug in the presence of agranulocytosis, aplastic anemia, hepatitis, fever, or exfoliative dermatitis.

Use with caution in patients more than 40 years old. Use with caution in combination with other agranulocytosis-precipitating medications.

Carcinogenesis: carcinoma formation has been seen in laboratory animals treated with PTU for more than 1 year.

Pharmacokinetics. See Table 53-8.

Adverse Effects. See Table 53-9. Antithyroid drug treatment is not without the risk of adverse reactions, including minor rashes and, in rare instances, agranulocytosis and hepatitis. The success of this therapy depends on a high degree of patient adherence to recommendations.

Drug Interactions. Oral anticoagulants may have a decreased effect. Digoxin levels may rise (especially as the patient becomes euthyroid). Thyroid uptake to ^{131}I may be reduced. Amiodarone, iodine, potassium iodide, and iodinated glycerol may decrease the medication efficacy.

TABLE 53-9 Adverse Effects of Thyroid Suppressants

System	methimazole	propylthiouracil
Dermatologic	Pruritus Rash Urticaria	Rash Skin discoloration Urticaria
GI	Hepatitis (potentially fatal) Nausea/vomiting	Diarrhea Diminished taste Hepatitis (potentially fatal) Nausea/vomiting
CNS	Headache Paresthesia Vertigo	Drowsiness Headache Vertigo
Musculoskeletal	Arthralgia	Arthralgia
Hematologic	Agranulocytosis Aplastic anemia Hypoprothrombinemia Leukopenia Thrombocytopenia	Agranulocytosis Aplastic anemia Hypoprothrombinemia Leukopenia Thrombocytopenia

Overdosage. Symptoms include nausea, vomiting, epigastric distress, headache, fever, arthralgia, pruritus, edema, pancytopenia, and agranulocytosis. More rare are exfoliative dermatitis, hepatitis, neuropathies, or CNS stimulation or depression.

Dosage and Administration

Adult

- Initial: 300 to 400 mg/day
- Maintenance: 100 to 150 mg/day

Child

- Initial: 50 to 150 mg/day (<10 years), 150 to 300 mg/day (>10 years)
- Maintenance: based on patient's response to therapy

methimazole (Tapazole)

Dosage and Administration

Adults

- Initial: 15 mg/day (mild disease), 30 to 40 mg/day (moderate disease), 60 mg/day (severe disease) divided into three doses and given every 8 hours
- Maintenance: 5 to 15 mg/day in three divided doses

Children
- Initial: 4 mg/kg/day in three divided doses
- Maintenance: approximately half of the initial dose in three divided doses

Adjunctive Diagnostic Tool for Thyroid Cancer

Specific Drugs

thyrotropin (Thyrogen)

Indications. In postsurgical evaluation of patients requiring follow-up for remnant thyroid tissue, thyroid cancer recurrence, or metastases. Used in conjunction with or without radioiodine imaging.

Mechanism of Action. Significantly enhances the sensitivity of thyroglobulin testing in patients maintained on thyroid hormone therapy. Allows thyroid cancer patients to avoid the debilitating effects of hypothyroidism when undergoing radioiodine imaging scans.

Adverse Effects. Nausea, headache, mild reactions of hypersensitivity: urticaria, rash. In clinical studies, no patients have developed antibodies to thyrotropin after either single or repeated use of the product.

RESOURCES FOR PATIENTS AND PROVIDERS

Organizations

National Graves' Disease Foundation, 2 Tsitsi Court, Brevard, NC 28712 www.glandcentral.com.

The Thyroid Foundation of America, Ruth Sleeper Hall, RSL 350 40 Parkman Street, Boston, MA 02114-2698.

The Thyroid Society for Education and Research, 7515 S. Main Street, Suite 545, Houston, TX 77030; (800) THYROID.

BIBLIOGRAPHY

Cassio A et al: Treatment for congenital hypothyroidism: thyroxine alone or thyroxine plus triiodothyronine? *Pediatrics* 111(5 Pt 1):1053-1060, 2003.

Ineck BA, Ng TM: Effects of subclinical hypothyroidism and its treatment on serum lipids, *Ann Pharmacother* 37(5):725-730, 2003.

Kabadi UM: Influence of age on optimal daily levothyroxine dosage in patients with primary hypothyroidism grouped according to etiology, *South Med J* 90(9):920, 1997.

Mori T et al: Recent trends in the management of Graves' hyperthyroidism in Japan: opinion survey results, especially on the combination therapy of antithyroid drug and thyroid hormone, *Endocr J* 44(4):509, 1997.

Sauvage MF et al: Relationship between psychotropic drugs and thyroid function: a review, *Toxicol Appl Pharmacol* 149(2):127, 1998.

Schindler AE: Thyroid function and postmenopause, *Gynecol Endocrinol* 17(1):79-85, 2003.

Wallace K et al: Thyroid dysfunction: how to manage overt and subclinical disease in older patients, *Geriatrics* 53(4):32, 1998.

Wilson N et al: *Williams textbook of endocrinology,* ed 10, Philadelphia, 2002, WB Saunders.

CHAPTER 54

Diabetes Mellitus Agents

Cheryl Pandolf Schenk and Maren Stewart Mayhew

Drug Names

Class	Subclass	Generic	Trade
Insulin	Rapid acting	lispro	Humalog
		aspart	Novolog
	Short acting	regular	
	Intermediate acting	(200) NPH	Humulin N
		lente	
	Long acting	ultralente	
		glargine	Lantus
	Mixtures	(200) 70/30 (70% NPH, 30% regular)	Humulin 70/30
		50/50 (50% NPH, 50% regular)	
		75/25 humalog (75% lispro protamine, 25% lispro)	
ORAL MEDICATIONS			
Second-generation sulfonylureas		(200) glyburide	Micronase, DiaBeta, Glynase
		(P) (200) glipizide	Glucotrol, Glucotrol XL
		(200) glimepiride	Amaryl
Biguanides		(200) metformin	Glucophage, Glucophage XR and XL
Thiazolidinediones		(P) (200) rosiglitazone	Avandia
		(200) pioglitazone	Actos
Meglitinides (secretagogues)		(P) nateglinide	Starlix
		repaglinide	Prandin
α-Glucosidase inhibitors		(P) acarbose	Precose
		miglitol	Glyset
Combination therapies		metformin/rosiglitazone	Avandament
		(200) metformin/glyburide	Glucovance
		metformin/glipizide	Metaglip

(200), Top 200 drug; (P), prototype drug.

General Uses

Indications

- Diabetes, types 1 and 2

Pharmacologic agents are used in conjunction with diet and exercise to control blood glucose in those with diabetes. These agents include various insulins and five classes of oral agents. Type 1 diabetes requires the use of insulin. Type 2 diabetic patients are usually started on oral medication. Insulin is added if oral medications provide inadequate control. The American Diabetes Association (ADA) diagnostic and treatment criteria are used in these guidelines.

DISEASE PROCESS

Anatomy and Physiology

The pancreas is a gland with both endocrine and exocrine functions. The islets of Langerhans, which comprise only 1% to 2% of the gland, contain more than 1 million cells. Eighty percent of these cells are β cells that produce insulin. Alpha cells, also part of the islets, produce glucagon, a potent hormone that promotes glycogenolysis and gluconeogenesis in the liver. The pancreas and liver are the primary organs of glucose regulation via a negative feedback mechanism. When blood glucose rises, the β cells are stimulated by the elevated glucose and release insulin. Insulin allows the muscle and liver to use glucose and to store it as glycogen in the liver. Insulin also facilitates fat storage in adipose tissue and facilitates the uptake and conversion of amino acids into protein. As blood glucose levels fall, the α cells are stimulated to release glucagon, resulting in glycogenolysis and gluconeogenesis in the liver. Glycogenolysis, the conversion of glycogen into glucose, and gluconeogenesis, the production of glucose from lactate and amino acids, result in increased serum glucose level.

Insulin lowers blood glucose by enhancing glucose transport by facilitated diffusion into target tissues. Insulin binds to and stimulates receptors on each cell that in turn fosters transport of glucose though the cell wall. Tissue insensitivity to insulin can occur when there are defects in receptors or defects in receptor response to insulin. Insulin also inhibits the lipoprotein lipase, thereby preventing the release of fatty acids into the blood. Insulin promotes the transport and storage of glucose as triglycerides in fat cells.

Pathophysiology

The onset of diabetes involves a relative or absolute lack of insulin, and/or insulin resistance and impaired or insufficient target cell receptors. These effects cause a lack of available glucose for cellular metabolism, resulting in glycogenolysis, lipolysis, and gluconeogenesis. Glucose uptake by the liver is impaired with resultant increase in circulating glucagon. There is decreased protein storage. There is an overproduction of free fatty acids by fat cells as well. Elevated plasma free fatty acid levels increase hepatic glucose production by stimulating gluconeogenesis.

Type 2 diabetes is a disease of insulin resistance and hyperinsulinemia. The cause of type 2 diabetes is unknown, but certain factors increase the risk of development of the disease. With type 2 diabetes, there is impaired insulin secretion, increased hepatic glucose production, and insensitivity to insulin in the tissues. An altered β-cell response to glucose with an absolute or relative lack of circulating insulin occurs. There is also an increase in glycogenolysis and glycogenolysis in the liver. The rate of hepatic glucose production is often responsible for elevated fasting glucose levels. If the tissue is insensitive or resistant to insulin, there continues to be a rise in blood glucose. This action is most evident with postprandial hyperglycemia. Most likely this occurs as a result of a postreceptor defect at the cell site. Increased levels of insulin are necessary to overcome this resistance, and often those newly diagnosed with type 2 diabetes have elevated insulin levels in an attempt to overcome resistance. This is often a process that begins years prior to diagnosis of type 2 diabetes. There may eventually be an absolute insulin deficiency as β cells continue to be affected and insulin production decreases.

Autoimmune destruction of the β cells is implicated in the diagnosis of type 1 diabetes. Environmental and genetic predisposition may also play a role. Onset of type 1 diabetes may occur suddenly such as the onset of diabetic ketoacidosis or slowly with less risk of ketoacidosis.

The Disease

Testing for diabetes should be considered in all adults age 45 years and older particularly if overweight. Testing should be repeated every 3 years. According to the American Diabetes Association (ADA), risk factors for the development of diabetes that should alert the provider to screen for diabetes are as follows:

- Age ≥45 years
- Overweight (body mass index [BMI] ≥25 kg/m^2)
- Family history of diabetes (i.e., parents or siblings who have diabetes)
- Habitual physical inactivity
- Race/ethnicity (e.g., African Americans, Hispanic, Native American, Asian Americans, and Pacific Islanders)
- Previously identified impaired fasting glucose (IFG) or impaired glucose tolerance (IGT)
- History of gestational diabetes mellitus (GDM) or delivery of a baby weighing >9 pounds
- Hypertension ≥140/90 mm Hg in adults
- HDL cholesterol ≤35 mg/dl and/or triglyceride level ≥250 mg/dl
- Polycystic ovary syndrome

History of Vascular Disease. The Expert Committee of the Diagnosis and Classification of Diabetes under the sponsorship of the ADA modified criteria for diagnosis in 1998. These criteria were adopted by the ADA and represent current guidelines for diagnosis (Box 54-1).

Complications of diabetes include microvascular disease (nephropathy, retinopathy), macrovascular disease (coronary artery disease, peripheral vascular disease, cerebrovascular disease) and neuropathic disease (autonomic and peripheral). Vascular and neuropathic disease contributes to the increased risk of amputation. Multiple studies, such as the Diabetes Mellitus Control and Complications trial Research Group (DCCT) and the United Kingdom Prospective Diabetes Study (UKPDS) continue to prove that intensive glucose control to goal or below goal HgA_{1c} prevents and/or delays the onset of complications.

Assessment

Obtaining a thorough history and physical examination enables the provider to obtain a baseline evaluation, determine

BOX 54-1

CRITERIA FOR THE DIAGNOSIS OF DIABETES MELLITUS

Symptoms of diabetes plus casual plasma glucose concentration 200 mg/dl. Casual is defined as any time of day without regard to time since last meal. The classic symptoms of diabetes include polyuria, polydipsia, and unexplained weight loss.

or

Fasting plasma glucose (FPG): 126 mg/dl. Fasting is defined as no caloric intake for at least 8 hours. (Prediabetes level is 100 mg/dl.)

or

2-hour plasma glucose (PG): 200 mg/dl during an oral glucose tolerance test (OGTT). The test should be performed as described by WHO, using a glucose load containing the equivalent of 75 g anhydrous glucose dissolved in water.

TABLE 54-1 ADA Recommended Glycemic Goals

	Normal	Goal	Additional Action Suggested
Plasma values			
Average preprandial glucose (mg/dl)	<110	90-130	<90 or >150
Average bedtime glucose (mg/dl)	<120	110-150	<110 or >180
Peak postprandial glucose		<180	
Whole blood values			
Average preprandial glucose (mg/dl)	<100	80-120	<80 or >140
Average bedtime glucose (mg/dl)	<110	100-140	<100 or >160
A_{1C} (%)	<6	<7	>8

early effects and complications of diabetes, and, together with the patient, determine individual glycemic goals. The ADA Clinical Practice Recommendations lists the following:

History includes skin, visual problems (history of retinopathy; last examination), thyroid (history of hypo- or hyperthyroid disease), cardiac arrhythmias, hypertension, lipid abnormalities, history of CAD, and/or CHF, hematologic, pulmonary, GI (chronic diarrhea, constipation, early satiety, liver disease), GU (urinary tract infections, difficulty voiding, incontinence, erectile dysfunction), gynecologic (history of gestational diabetes, anticipation of pregnancy, contraceptive use), neurologic (weakness, wasting, paresthesias, hyperesthesia, hypoglycemic unawareness); and vascular (leg pain, transient ischemic attacks).

The physical examination should include assessing height, weight, and BMI, BP, eye, mouth, thyroid, heart, lungs, abdomen (hepatic enlargement), bruits, pulses, hands, feet, skin (acanthosis nigricans, inflammation or infection), nervous system (reflexes, sensory examination of feet).

Laboratory evaluation includes CBC, CMP (including creatinine, BUN, TSH, Hbg, fasting lipid profile, urinalysis, test for microalbuminuria), and ECG in adults. The HgA_{1c} reflects the state of glycemia for the past 8 to 12 weeks.

DRUG ACTION AND EFFECTS

See Tables 54-1 and 54-2.

Pharmacologic Treatment

Insulin. Insulins are proteins that bind to cell wall receptors to allow cellular utilization of glucose. Insulin lowers blood glucose levels by stimulating peripheral glucose uptake, particularly by skeletal muscle and fat and by inhibiting hepatic glucose production. An adequate supply of insulin is needed for transport of glucose across the cell membrane to sustain life.

Most insulin used today is produced by deoxyribonucleic acid (DNA) recombinant technology and is synthesized in a nonpathogenic strain of *Escherichia coli* bacteria or *Saccharomyces cerevisiae* fungus. The advantage to using synthetic human insulin is a decrease in the production of insulin antibodies and diminished risk for the development of lipodystrophy at the injection site.

Sulfonylureas. Because first-generation sulfonylureas are no longer used, this chapter will refer to second-generation sulfonylureas simply as sulfonylureas. Sulfonylureas enhance insulin secretion primarily by binding to receptor sites on β cells. This causes a decrease in potassium permeability and membrane depolarization. This then causes an increase in intracellular calcium ions that cause exocytosis of insulin from secretory granules. They also suppress hepatic glucose production by entry of insulin into the portal vein, and increase muscle glucose uptake via elevated insulin levels.

Biguanides. Metformin enhances insulin sensitivity in both the liver and peripheral tissues. It also decreases hepatic glucose production and intestinal absorption of glucose. Increased insulin sensitivity means increased peripheral glucose uptake and utilization. It has no direct effect on the pancreas. Metformin has also been shown to decrease triglycerides, decrease LDL, and increase HDL.

Triazolidinediones. Rosiglitazone and pioglitazone improve glycemic control and reduce circulating insulin levels. They

TABLE 54-2 Mechanism of Action of Diabetic Medications

Drug	Insulin Secretion from Pancreas	Hepatic Glucose Production	Peripheral Insulin Sensitivity	Glucose Absorption from GI tract
Insulin	Decrease	Decrease	Increase	None
Sulfonylureas	Increase	Slight decrease	Slight increase	None
Thiazolidinediones	No change	Decrease	Increase	None
Meglitinides	Increase	No change	No change	None
α-Glucosidase	No change	No change	No change	Delays
metformin	No change	Decrease	Increase	None

require functioning β cells for the medication to work. They improve sensitivity to insulin in muscle and adipose tissue and inhibit hepatic gluconeogenesis. They are agonists for peroxisome proliferator–activated receptors-γ (PPAR-γ), which are found in adipose tissue, skeletal muscle, and liver. Activation of PPAR-γ receptors regulates the insulin-responsive genes involved in the control of glucose production, transport, and utilization and participates in the regulation of fatty acid metabolism.

Meglitinides. Repaglinide and nateglinide lower blood sugar by stimulating the release of insulin from the pancreas. The patient must have functioning β cells for the medication to work. They bind receptor sites to close ATP-dependent potassium channels in the β cell membrane. This leads to opening of calcium channels causing an influx of calcium, which induces insulin secretion.

α-Glucosidase Inhibitors. Acarbose and miglitol act through inhibition of pancreatic α-amylase and membrane-bound intestinal α-glucoside hydrolase enzymes. These enzymes are responsible for metabolizing complex starches to oligosaccharides and the breakdown of other saccharides to glucose and other monosaccharides. This enzyme inhibition delays glucose absorption and lowers postprandial hyperglycemia. They do not enhance insulin secretion.

TABLE 54-3 Making Treatment Decisions in Type 2 Diabetes

BLOOD SUGARS MILDLY ELEVATED	
Trial of diet, exercise, and weight loss (if obese). If goals not reached, see below.	
NORMAL RENAL FUNCTION	
Nonobese	metformin
	Thiazolidinediones
	Second-generation sulfonylureas
	Nonsulfonylurea secretagogues (if erratic meals)
Obese	*Elevated Fasting Blood Sugar*
	metformin
	Thiazolidinediones
	Second-generation sulfonylureas
	Elevated Postprandial Blood Sugar
	Nonsulfonylurea secretagogues
	α-Glucosidase inhibitors
	Second-generation sulfonylureas
IMPAIRED RENAL FUNCTION	
Nonobese	Second-generation sulfonylureas
	Nonsulfonylurea secretagogues (if erratic meals)
	Thiazolidinediones
Obese	α-Glucosidase inhibitors
	Thiazolidinediones
	Sulfonylureas

Adapted from Dube D et al: Concise update in management of diabetes, *South Med J* 95(1):4-9, 2002.
Start at beginning dosages and titrate every 2 to 4 weeks by monitoring pre- and postprandial blood glucose; thiazolidinediones may take several weeks to reach maximum effectiveness; Add second and third agent to achieve goal glycemic control.
If poor control with three agents, or medical problems preclude the use of oral medications, consider insulin.
Because diabetes is progressive, more medications and higher dosages will be needed to maintain control.

DRUG TREATMENT PRINCIPLES

Importance is placed on maintaining optimal control to lessen the vascular and neurologic complications of the disease. The ADA guidelines (mentioned in assessment) also discuss treatment options.

Establish Goals

The first step is to establish glycemic goals for the individual patient. The patient's age, ability for self-care, other medical problems, social support, and financial issues all play a role in determining individual glycemic goals. (See Table 54-1 for the ADA-recommended glycemic goals.) The American Association of Clinical Endocrinologist Medical Guidelines for the Management of Diabetes Mellitus: the AACE System of Intensive diabetes Self Management—2003 update recommends a preprandial blood sugar goal of less than 100; a 2-hour postprandial blood sugar goal of less than 140; and a HgA_{1c} goal of 6.5.

For patients who have type 2 diabetes, an initial physician referral or collaboration may be needed, especially if the patient's condition is compromised. Patients with type 1 diabetes usually require a referral.

The second step focuses on nonpharmacological therapeutic techniques.

Type 2 Diabetes

Start Medications. The third step in treatment is oral medications. Medication decisions are based on the mechanism of action of the drug and on patient characteristics (see Table 54-3 for treatment decision guidelines). All oral medications are indicated as first choices depending on patient characteristics. Traditionally a sulfonylurea has been the first choice. However metformin or a thiazolidinedione is now frequently used as a first-line choice. Sulfonylureas, metformin, and thiazolidinediones reduce overall blood sugars and are used to provide 24-hour control. Their full effect may take several weeks. Meglitinides and α-glucosidase inhibitors act short term to reduce postprandial glucose.

Sulfonylureas. Sulfonylureas work best early in diabetes, while the pancreas is still responsive to stimulation. They generally lose their effectiveness as the diabetes progresses and so are discontinued. Glyburide (Micronase) is stronger than glipizide and more likely to cause hypoglycemia. Start with long-acting glipizide (Glucotrol XL). If this is not strong enough, consider glyburide. Glimepiride may cause less weight gain and hypoglycemia than other sulfonylureas.

metformin. Of the oral agents, metformin is the most potent in reducing hepatic glucose production. It is especially useful in patients who are obese or not responding to sulfonylureas. It improves fasting, postprandial glucose, and triglycerides. It does not promote weight gain.

TABLE 54-4 Therapeutic Combinations: Indicated and Unlabeled

Drug	Sulfonylurea	Metformin	Thiazolidinediones	Meglitinides	α-Glucoseidase Inhibitors
Insulin	Approved	FDA indication	Weight gain; pioglitazone: FDA indication; rosiglitazone: edema	Not indicated, use short-acting insulin	Not indicated, use short-acting insulin
Sulfonylureas		X	X	X	X
Thiazolidinediones	FDA indication, low risk of hypoglycemia, weight gain	FDA indication combination product		X	X
Meglitinides	NI	FDA indication	FDA indication		X
α-Glucosidase inhibitors	FDA indication, beneficial	Approved but both cause GI distress	NI	No added benefit expected	
metformin	FDA indication, combination product		X	X	X

X, Not indicated.

Thiazolidinediones. Thiazolidinediones address insulin resistance. They sensitize peripheral tissues to insulin, causing the body to better utilize the insulin that it is making. This makes them of particular benefit in patients with the metabolic syndrome (syndrome X). A fear of liver toxicity has slowed their acceptance.

Meglitinides. Meglitinides are short acting and are used to decrease postprandial blood sugars. Meglitinides are taken before meals to control postprandial blood sugars. When taken correctly, the risk of hypoglycemia is very low. They are especially useful in patients who had fairly low fasting blood glucose level, but high postprandial glucose level. Although they are relatively safe, they are rather weak and are used in mild diabetes and as an adjunct. Repaglinide has a longer duration than nateglinide.

α-Glucosidase Inhibitors. α-Glucosidase inhibitors are short acting and are used to decrease postprandial blood glucose levels. Hypoglycemia is rare with monotherapy. Because α-glucosidase inhibitors prevent or delay the absorption of sucrose, hypoglycemia must be treated with glucose or lactose and not sugar. Acarbose has fewer problems with systemic absorption than miglitol.

Adjust Medications. If glycemic goals are not attained after an adequate trial of one medication, add a drug with a different mechanism of action (see Table 54-2). A third drug may be added if necessary. Combination therapy is usually required (Table 54-4). An example is thiazolidinedione (decreases fasting blood sugars) plus a meglitinide to decrease postprandial blood sugars. If fasting blood sugars are not controlled by a sulfonylurea, the addition of acarbose will improve control and diminish the insulinotropic and weight-increasing effects of sulfonylureas. All combination pills combine metformin with a sulfonylurea or thiazolidinedione.

Consider Insulin. If glycemic goals are not reached with two or three oral medications, consider the addition of insulin. All oral medications may be used with insulin. Because of disease progression, treatment often requires progressing to high doses of medications and the addition of other medications for control. Insulin is required if there is an allergy, side effect, or contraindication to oral agents. Pregnancy requires the use of insulin as oral agents are contraindicated. In times of physiologic stress such as trauma or surgery, insulin is often used for glycemic control.

If a patient who has type 2 diabetes is symptomatic and/or has persistent blood glucose levels >300, insulin is generally recommended as initial treatment rather than oral medications. If good control is established with low doses of insulin in these patients, some may eventually be able to discontinue insulin and use oral medications.

When an endocrinologist initiates insulin in type 2 diabetes, one of the following regimens is usually ordered:

1. Start with glargine (Lantus) insulin 10 units at bedtime. Increase dosage 2 to 4 units every 3 to 5 days to achieve fasting blood sugar goal.
2. Start with NPH insulin 10 units at bedtime. Increase dose by 1 to 2 units every 3 to 5 days to achieve fasting blood sugar goal.
3. Start with 70/30 insulin at supper or NPH/Regular insulin at supper. This is a good combination if bedtime and fasting blood glucose levels are elevated. Increase dose by 10% to 20% every 3 to 5 days to achieve blood sugar goals.
4. Use NPH/Regular insulin before breakfast and before dinner.
   a. Use 0.5 to 1 unit per kilogram of patient's weight as total daily insulin dose.
   b. Divide dose so that two thirds of total dose is in the morning and one third of the total dose is before dinner.
   c. Divide each morning and dinner dose so that two thirds of dose is NPH and one third is Regular.
5. Use a basal/bolus insulin as discussed below.

A new preprandial inhaled insulin via AERx Insulin diabetes management system has been shown as effective as preprandial subcutaneous insulin in patients with type 2 diabetes and may be a new treatment option in the future.

Common Problems

When a patient who is stabilized on a diabetic regimen is exposed to stress such as fever, infection, trauma, or surgery, a temporary loss of glycemic control may occur. On occasion it is necessary to discontinue oral medications such as metformin. It is often necessary to temporarily administer insulin. Restart oral medications when condition is resolved.

When corticosteroids are administered, they can precipitate or worsen diabetes mellitus. Monitor glucose levels closely during steroid treatment and adjust diabetic medications as needed.

Insulin Therapy for Type 1 Diabetes

All patients with type 1 diabetes and some with type 2 diabetes need insulin. Treatment incorporates the use of long-acting or intermediate-acting insulin to provide daily basal coverage and rapid-acting or Regular insulin to provide bolus coverage for meals. Multiple daily insulin injections are often used. Open-loop insulin pumps as well as continuous subcutaneous insulin delivery devices are also used to simplify insulin administration. By use of multiple daily injection programs and pumps, insulin can be administered to better mimic normal physiology.

There are individual differences in action of insulin and times may vary according to injection techniques, care of insulin, and site of injection.

General dosage theory of regular insulin prior to meals assumes that 1 unit of Regular insulin will cover 10 to 15 g of carbohydrate. Endocrinologists beginning insulin therapy for a person who has type 1 diabetes might start with one of the following regimens:

In initiating long-acting and rapid-acting insulin:

Lantus insulin (long acting):

- Used once a day, usually at bedtime
- Usually start with 50% of total daily insulin dose

Or

Ultralente (long acting):

- Usually used every 12 hours
- One quarter of the daily total insulin dose is given every 12 hours

Aspart and Humalog:

- 50% of total insulin requirement is divided by 3 for each pre-meal bolus
- Premeal dosing will vary with carbohydrate intake, so there must be a determination of carbohydrate grams or servings per unit of insulin.

Currently, the use of long-acting insulin once a day or twice a day to provide basal coverage with rapid-acting insulin used premeals as bolus coverage is the most promising for good control. If the patient does not eat a meal, the rapid-acting insulin should not be taken. Long-acting insulin is taken regardless of meals (Table 54-5). Have "sick day rules" to guide dose.

TABLE 54-5 Insulin Characteristics and Duration of Action

Insulin	Color	Onset	Peak	Duration
RAPID ACTING				
lispro (Humalog)	Clear	15 min	30-90 min	4-6 hr
aspart (Novolog)	Clear	15 min	45 min	3-5 hr
SHORT ACTING				
Regular (R)	Clear	30-60 min	2-3 hr	6-8 hr
INTERMEDIATE ACTING				
NPH (N)	Cloudy	2-4 hr	6-10 hr	14-18 hr
lente (L)	Cloudy	3-4 hr	6-12 hr	16-20 hr
LONG ACTING				
ultralente (U)	Cloudy	6-10 hr	10-16 hr	14-20 hr
glargine (Lantus)	Clear	2 hr	None	24 hr
MIXTURES				
70/30	Cloudy	30 min	2-12 hr	24 hr
50/50	Cloudy	30 min	3-5 hr	24 hr
Humalog 75/25	Cloudy	15 min	30-90 min	24 hr

Determine correct basal dosing by monitoring the blood glucose level. If all blood glucose levels are elevated throughout the day or if the fasting blood glucose level is elevated, the basal insulin dose should be increased. Determination of correct premeal or bolus insulin is best determined by pre- and postmeal monitoring of blood sugars. For instance, if before-lunch blood glucose levels are high, then increasing pre-breakfast insulin might be indicated. If 2-hour postprandial supper blood glucose level is low, then a before-supper bolus of quick-acting insulin may need to be decreased. Consistent hypoglycemia presupper may be an indication that the pre-lunch bolus needs to be decreased.

HOW TO MONITOR

- Follow the patient closely. Patient should be seen at least weekly for the first month. After the first month, examine at monthly intervals or as indicated. Uncooperative individuals may be unsuitable for treatment with oral agents, but may not do well with insulin either.
- Patient should monitor fingerstick blood sugars at home. Monitor pre- and postprandial blood glucose levels to determine dose adjustments.
- HgA_{1c} baseline and periodically to determine overall control. Measurements more frequently than every 3 months are generally not useful.
- Monitor urine for microproteinuria.

Sulfonylureas

- Baseline and at least annual renal function. Assess more frequently if patient is at risk for development of renal impairment.
- Monitor CBC initially and periodically. If abnormalities are noted check vitamin B_{12} levels.

metformin

Test for lactic acidosis if patient develops laboratory abnormalities or clinical illness (especially vague and poorly defined illness). Tests should include measuring electrolytes, ketones, and blood glucose. Consider monitoring blood pH, lactate, pyruvate, and metformin levels.

Thiazolidinediones

- Check LFTs before administration. Do not use in patients with increased baseline liver enzyme levels (ALT more than 3.5 times normal).
- Patients who have mildly elevated enzyme levels should be evaluated every 2 months during the first year of treatment and periodically after.
- Monitor for symptoms suggesting hepatic dysfunction such as unexplained nausea, vomiting, abdominal pain, fatigue, anorexia, and dark urine; check enzyme levels.
- Monitor for signs and symptoms of CHF, especially edema.

α-Glucosidase Inhibitors

Monitor LFTs every 3 months during the first year of treatment and periodically thereafter.

PATIENT VARIABLES

Geriatric

- Sulfonylureas: decrease dosage in renal and hepatic impairment to avoid risk of hypoglycemia
- Meglitinides increase risk of hypoglycemia
- Biguanides should be used with caution because of the risk of accumulation with renal insufficiency with the increased risk of lactic acidosis
- Meglitinides: variable response in the elderly

Pediatric

- Sulfonylureas, thiazolidinediones (under age 18), meglitinides, α-glucosidase inhibitors not recommended
- Biguanides (children ages 10 to 16): metformin 500 mg bid (regular-release tablets only); maximum oral dose is 2000 mg only

Pregnancy and Lactation

- *Category B:* biguanides, α-glucosidase inhibitors
- *Category B:* the sulfonylureas glynase and micronase
- *Category C:* sulfonylureas, thiazolidinediones, meglitinides
- It is recommended that women who intend to become pregnant switch to insulin. Fetal mortality and major congenital anomalies generally occur three or four times more often in offspring of diabetic mothers
- Presence in breast milk is unknown; use not recommended in breast-feeding mothers

PATIENT EDUCATION

Patient education is essential to diabetes control. Patients must understand how to take their medications correctly to avoid hypoglycemia and how to adjust medications as needed (e.g., sick days).

Avoid herbal products such as bitter melon, fenugreek, and St. John's wort.

Diet and Exercise

Diet and exercise are cornerstones of Step 2 treatment. Self-management of the disease is crucial. Patients who have diabetes need to know how to care for themselves, how to best monitor and care for individual problems, and when to call a provider for assistance. Meal planning, exercise, home blood glucose monitoring (HBGM), hypoglycemia recognition and management, hyperglycemia management, sick day rules, weight management, and foot care are important. Referrals to a registered dietitian and a diabetes educator are mandatory for information and self-care. If a patient is unable to achieve a glycemic goal with diet and exercise, medication is prescribed.

Specific Drugs

SULFONYLUREAS

Ⓟ **Prototype Drug**

glipizide (Glucotrol, Glucotrol XL)

Contraindications
- Hypersensitivity
- Ketoacidosis

Warnings
- Cardiovascular risk: the administration of oral hypoglycemic drugs has been associated with increased cardiovascular mortality as compared with treatment with diet alone or diet plus insulin. The interpretation of this study using a first-generation sulfonylurea has been controversial.
- Renal/hepatic function impairment: oral hypoglycemic agents are metabolized in the liver. The drugs and most of their metabolites are excreted by the kidneys. Hepatic impairment may result in inadequate release of glucose in response to hypoglycemia and renal impairment may cause decreased elimination of sulfonylureas, leading to hypoglycemia. Use these drugs with caution.

Precautions
- Monitor closely; see *How to Monitor*
- Hypoglycemia may be severe

Pharmacokinetics
See Table 54-6.

Adverse Effects
See Table 54-7.

Drug Interactions
See Table 54-8.

Dosage and Administration
See Table 54-9. Patients on immediate-release glipizide may be switched to the extended release once a day at the same total daily dose.

TABLE 54-6 Pharmacokinetics of Oral Hypoglycemic Agents

Drug	Absorption	Drug Availability	Onset of Action	Time to Peak Concentration	Half-life	Duration of action	Protein Bound	Metabolism	Excretion
glyburide (Micronase)	Not affected by food	Unknown	<1 hr	2-4 hr	5-10 hr	Up to 24 hr	>99%	Liver	Urine 50%; active metabolites; feces
glipizide (Glucotrol)	Delayed by food	100%	30 min	2-3 hr	2-4 hr	6-12 hr	>98%	Liver CYP 450	Urine, 80%; no active metabolites
glipizide (Glucotrol ER)	Not affected by food	100%	2-3 hr	6-12 hr	8-12 hr	Up to 24 hr	>90%	Liver	Urine 80%; no active metabolites
glimepiride (Amaryl)	Not affected by food	100%	1 hr	2-3 hr	5-9 hr	Up to 24 hr	>99%	Liver	Urine, 60%; active metabolites; feces
metformin (Glucophage)	Delayed by food	50%-60%	4-8 hr	1-3 hr	2 hr	1.5-6 hr	Negligible	None	Urine, unchanged
rosiglitazone (Avandia)	Not affected by food	99%	15-30 min	1 hr	3-4 hr	24 hr	99.8%	Liver 3A4 2C8 1A1	Urine, 64%; feces, 23%
pioglitazone (Actos)	Not affected by food	Unknown		2-4 hr	3-7 hr	24 hr	99%	Liver 3A4 2C8 1A1	Urine, 20%; feces
nateglinide (Starlix)	Not affected by food	75%	15 min	0.5-2 hr	1.25-3 hr	1.5 hr	99%	Liver 3A4, 30% 2C9, 70%	Urine/feces
repaglinide (Prandin)	Completely absorbed	56%	15-30 min	<1 hr	1 hr	3 hr	>98%	Liver 3A4, oxidation	Urine/feces
acarbose (Precose)	<2%	2%	1 hr	2 hr	3 hr	4 hr	0%	Intestines	Feces- not absorbed; urine, trace
miglitol (Glycet)	50%-100%	Dose dependent		2-3 hr	2 hr	4 hr	Negligible	None	Urine, unchanged

TABLE 54-7 Adverse Reactions to Diabetic Medications

Body System	Sulfonylureas	Biguanides	Thiazolidinediones	Meglitinides	α-Glucosidase Inhibitors	Insulin
Body, general	Chills, fatigue, weakness, malaise, edema, weight gain	Chills, sweating, flushing, no weight gain	Edema, weight gain, fluid retention	Weight gain	No weight gain	Weight gain
Skin, appendages	Rash, eczema, pruritus, erythema multiforme, sweating, exfoliative dermatitis, photosensitivity	Rash, nail disorder				Rash, injection site dystrophy
Hypersensitivity	Skin reactions, urticaria					
Respiratory	Dyspnea	Dyspnea, flu syndrome		URI		
Cardiovascular	Arrhythmia, hypertension	Chest discomfort, palpitation	↑CHF			
GI	Anorexia, nausea, indigestion, diarrhea, GI pain, constipation, vomiting, hunger, flatulence cholestatic jaundice	Diarrhea, nausea, vomiting, flatulence, cramping, indigestion, abdominal discomfort, abnormal stools, anorexia	Nausea, vomiting, diarrhea, elevated liver function tests	Nausea, vomiting, diarrhea	Flatulence, diarrhea, abdominal pain, rare paralytic ileus, nausea, gas,	
Hemic and lymphatic	Leukopenia, thrombocytopenia, aplastic anemia, agranulocytosis, hemolytic anemia, pancytopenia, eosinophilia	B_{12} deficiency	Anemia (rosiglitazone)			
Metabolic and nutritional	Hypoglycemia, syndrome of inappropriate antidiuretic hormone (SIADH)	Lactic acidosis, hypoglycemia, metallic taste, vitamin B_{12} deficiency	Hypoglycemia (0.6%), Rosiglitazone: ↑ LDL and HDL	Hyperglycemia, hypoglycemia; nateglinide has less hypoglycemia than repaglinide	Hypoglycemia (less than with other drugs)	Hypoglycemia
Musculoskeletal	Arthralgia, myalgia, leg cramps	Myalgia	Myalgia	Arthropathy		
Nervous system	Drowsiness, asthenia, nervousness, tremor, pain, insomnia, anxiety, depression, hypoesthesia, hypertonia, confusion, somnolence, abnormal gait, migraine, paresthesia, dizziness, vertigo, headache	Headache, asthenia, light-headedness	Headache	Dizziness		
Special senses	Tinnitus, blurred vision, retinal hemorrhage	Taste disorder				
Hepatic	Hepatitis, hepatic porphyria		↑ LFTs		↑ LFTs	
Genitourinary	Decreased libido, polyuria					
Other	Disulfiram-like reaction, hyponatremia			↑ Uric acid		

TABLE 54-8 Drug Interactions of Oral Hypoglycemic Agents

Increase Drug levels	Decrease Drug levels
SULFONYLUREAS	
Increase sulfonylureas: cause hypoglycemia: androgens, anticoagulants, azole antifungals, chloramphenicol, clofibrate, gemfibrozil, Hx antagonists, magnesium salts, methyldopa, MAOIs, probenecid, salicylates, sulfinpyrazone, sulfonamides, tricyclic antidepressants (TCAs), urinary acidifiers ciprofloxacin ↑ glyburide sulfonylureas ↑ digoxin glyburide ↓↑ warfarin	Decrease sulfonylureas: decrease effectiveness of drug: β-blockers, calcium channel blockers, cholestyramine, corticosteroids, diazoxide, estrogens, hydantoins, isoniazid, nicotinic acid, oral contraceptives, phenothiazines, rifampin, sympathomimetics, thiazide diuretics, thyroid agents, urinary alkalinizers, charcoal
BIGUANIDES	
Alcohol, amiloride, digoxin, morphine, procainamide, quinidine, quinine, ranitidine, triamterene, trimethoprim, vancomycin, cimetidine, furosemide, iodinated contrast material, nifedipine ↑ metformin	metformin ↓ glyburide, furosemide
THIAZOLIDINEDIONES	
pioglitazone possible interaction with cyproheptadine and other CYP 3A4 drugs	troglitazone ↓ oral contraceptives
MEGLITINIDES	
3A4 inhibitors , β-blockers, NSAIDs, probenecid, MAOIs, salicylates, sulfonamides, estrogen, simvastatin ↑ repaglinide repaglinide ↑ estrogen	3A4 inducers, calcium channel blockers, corticosteroids, estrogens, isoniazid, nicotinic acid, OCPs, phenothiazines, phenytoin, sympathomimetics, diuretics, thyroid products ↓ repaglinide
α-GLUCOSIDASE INHIBITORS	
	Digestive enzymes, charcoal ↓ α-inhibitors acarbose ↓ digoxin miglitol ↓ digoxin, glyburide, metformin, propranolol, ranitidine

TABLE 54-9 Dosage (in mg) and Administration Recommendations for Oral Hypoglycemic Agents

Drug	Starting Dose	Administration and Titration	Usual Dose	Maximum Dose
glyburide	1.25-2.5 to 5 qd with first meal	Single or divided dose; ↑ 2.5 or less q wk	1.25 to 20 qd	20
glyburide, micronized	0.75-1.5 to 3 qd with first meal	Single or divided dose (>6/d); ↑ 1.5 or less q wk	0.75-12/d	12
glipizide	5 before first meal	30 min before meal; single or divided doses; ↑ 2.5-5 q2-3 d	5 qd	10 mg tid AC
glipizide ER	5 with first meal	↑ 5 q3 mo	5-10	20
glimepiride	1-2 with first meal	↑ 1-2 q1-2 wk	1-4	8
metformin	500 bid *or* 850 qd with meals	Divided dose up to tid, ↑ 500 q2 wk	500 tid-850 bid	Child 2000; adult 2550
metformin ER	500 qd with evening meal	↑ 500/wk	500-1000	2000
rosiglitazone	2-4 qd without regard to meals	Single or divided dose; ↑ q8-12 wk	4-8	8
pioglitazone	15-30 qd without regard to meals	↑ to 45	30	45
nateglinide	60-120 tid	1-30 min before meals	60-120 tid	60-120 tid
repaglinide	0.5-2 tid	1-30 min before meals; ↑ qw	0.5-4 tid	16
acarbose	25 qd-tid with first bite	↑ by 50 q4-8 wk	50-100 tid	100 tid
miglitol	25 qd-tid with first bite	↑ by 25 tid q4-8 wk	50 tid	100 tid

BIGUANIDES

metformin (Glucophage, Glucophage XR and XL)

Contraindications
- Hypersensitivity
- Renal disease or dysfunction (creatinine ≥1.4 in women; ≥1.5 in men)
- Metabolic acidosis including ketoacidosis or patient who is at risk
- CHF requiring pharmacologic treatment
- Withhold therapy when iodinated contrast media are used

Warnings
- Lactic acidosis is rare (about 0.03%), but serious metabolic complications can occur with metformin accumulation. It is fatal in about half of cases.
- Renal function impairment: metformin is substantially excreted by the kidney. Accumulation may occur with renal function impairment, which will increase the risk of lactic acidosis.
- Hepatic function impairment: avoid metformin with hepatic impairment because of increased risk of lactic acid acidosis.

Precautions
- Hypoxic states: cardiovascular collapse, acute CHF, acute MI, and other conditions have been associated with lactic acidosis.
- Hold metformin for surgical procedures. Resume when oral intake is resumed and renal function is normal.
- A decrease to subnormal levels of vitamin B_{12} was observed in about 7% of patients.
- Hypoglycemia does not occur under normal circumstances but could occur with deficient caloric intake, strenuous exercise not compensated by caloric supplementation, alcohol use, or during concomitant use with other glucose-lowering agents such as sulfonylureas and insulin.

Other Drugs in Class

Other drugs in this class are similar to the prototype except as follows.

THIAZOLIDINEDIONES

Ⓟ Prototype Drug

rosiglitazone (Avandia)

Contraindications
- Hypersensitivity

Warnings
- Hepatotoxicity: available clinical data show no evidence that pioglitazone and rosiglitazone induced hepatotoxicity or LFT elevations. However they are structurally related to troglitazone, which was removed from the market because of hepatotoxicity. Use with caution and monitor liver enzymes.
- Cardiac effects can cause fluid retention, which could exacerbate or cause heart failure. Do not use in New York Hospital Association Class 3 and 4 cardiac status.
- Ovulation: may result in resumption of ovulation in premenopausal anovulatory patients and cause risk for pregnancy.
- Carcinogenesis: increase in incidence of adipose hyperplasia in mice.
- Fertility impairment: rosiglitazone reduced fertility in rats.

Precautions
- Hypoglycemia: may be at risk for hypoglycemia.
- Hematologic: may cause decreases in hemoglobin and hematocrit.
- Weight gain has been seen, probably due to fluid retention and fat accumulation.

MEGLITINIDES

Ⓟ Prototype Drug

nateglinide (Starlix)

Contraindications
- Hypersensitivity
- Ketoacidosis

Warnings
- Renal insufficiency: use is safe in mild renal insufficiency but should not be used with severe renal failure.
- Renal failure on dialysis exhibited reduced overall drug exposure (not true of repaglinide).
- Hepatic insufficiency will cause increased concentration. Use lower dosages with caution.

Precautions

Hypoglycemia is a risk. Give before a meal. If patient skips a meal that dose of meglitinide should not be taken.

Other Drugs in Class

Other drugs in this class are similar to the prototype except as follows.

repaglinide (Prandin)

- Increased incidence of carcinogenesis (e.g., benign adenomas of thyroid) in rats.

α-GLUCOSIDASE INHIBITORS

Ⓟ Prototype Drug

acarbose (Precose)

Contraindications
- Hypersensitivity
- Ketoacidosis
- Cirrhosis

- Bowel disease such as inflammatory bowel disease, colonic ulceration partial, or complete or predisposition to intestine obstruction

Warnings
- Renal function impairment causes increased levels of the drug
- Carcinogenesis. Increase in incidence of renal tumors in kidney

Precautions
- Hypoglycemia

Pharmacokinetics
See Table 54-6. Because these drugs act locally in the GI tract, low systemic bioavailability is therapeutically desired.

RESOURCES FOR PATIENTS AND PROVIDERS

American Diabetes Association, www.diabetes.org.
Information for patient and professional.
CDC Diabetes and Public Health Resource, www.cdc.gov/diabetes/.
National Diabetes Education Initiative, www.ndei.org.
Information for professionals.

BIBLIOGRAPHY

The American Association of Clinical Endocrinologists Medical Guidelines for the Management of Diabetes Mellitus: the AACE System of Intensive Diabetes Self-Management—2002 Update, *Endocrine Prac* 8(suppl)1, 2002.
American Diabetes Association: Clinical Practice Recommendations 2003, *Diabetes Care* 6(suppl):1 2003.
Defronzo R: Pharmacological therapy for type 2 diabetes mellitus, *Ann Intern Med* 131:4, 281-303, 1999.
Drugs for diabetes, *Treat Guidelines Med Lett* 1(1):1-6, 2002.
Dube D et al: Concise update in management of diabetes, *South Med J* 95(1):4-9, 2002.
Economic costs of diabetes care in the United States in 2002, *Diabetes Care* 26:917-933, 2003.
Herbst K: Insulin strategies for primary care providers, *Clin Diabetes* 20(1):11-17, 2002.
McNeely M: Case study: atypical antipsychotic use associated with severe hyperglycemia, *Clin Diabetes* 20(4):195-196, 2002.
Metaglip and Avandament for type 2 diabetes, *Med Lett* 44(1146):107-110, 2002.
White J: Recent developments in pharmacological reduction of blood glucose in patients with type 2 diabetes, *Clin Diabetes* 19(4):153-199, 2001.

UNIT 13

Female Reproductive System Drugs

Unit 13 focuses on the utilization of reproductive hormones to either enhance the physiology of the female body or to prevent conception. The products represent some of the most commonly prescribed products in primary care practice. New research that has dramatically changed the way postmenopausal women are treated has also caused confusion among many primary care providers. This unit incorporates the latest findings into the treatment recommendations and guidelines.

- **Chapter 55** discusses the prevention of pregnancy through the use of hormones. New products just entering the market are included.
- **Chapter 56** discusses the short-term and long-term consequences of menopause and the current treatment recommendations for postmenopausal treatment of major symptoms described.
- **Chapter 57** includes a breast cancer drug and medications used to treat vaginitis.

Female Reproductive System Drugs

CHAPTER 55

Contraceptives

Drug Names

Class	Subclass	Generic Name	Trade Name
Combination	Monophasic	ethinyl estradiol and norethindrone	Ovcon 50
			Nortrel 1/35
			Norinyl 1+35
			Ortho Novum 1/35
			Brevicon 21
			Modicon 28
			Nortrel 0.5/35
			Ovcon 35
			Loestrin 1.5/30
			Loestrin FE 1.5/30
			Loestrin 1/20
			(200) Loestrin FE 1/20
		ethinyl estradiol and levonorgestrel	Portia
			Nordette
			Levlen
			(200) Alesse 21
			Aviane 21
			Lessina 28
			Levlite 28
			Ovral
			Ogestrel
		ethinyl estradiol and norgestrel	Cryselle
			Lo/Ovral
		ethinyl estradiol and ethynodiol diacetate	Demulen 1/50
			Demulen 1/35
		ethinyl estradiol and desogestrel	Apri
			Desogen
			Ortho-Cept
			Cyclessa
		ethinyl estradiol and drospirenone	Yasmine 28
		ethinyl estradiol and norgestimate	(200) Ortho-Cyclen
		mestranol and norethindrone	Demulen 1/50
			Demulen 1/35
	Biphasic	ethinyl estradiol and norethindrone	Jenest-28
			Ortho-Novum 10/11
		ethinyl estradiol and desogestrel	Kariva 28
			(200) Mircette 28
	Triphasic	ethinyl estradiol and norethindrone	Tri-Norinyl
			(200) Ortho-Novum 7/7/7
			Estrostep Fe
		ethinyl estradiol and norgestimate	(200) Ortho Tri-Cyclen
			Ortho Tri-Cyclen Lo
		ethinyl estradiol and levonorgestrel	Enpresse
			Tri-Levlen
			(200) Triphasil
			(200) Trivora-28

(200), Top 200 drug.

Continued

Drug Names—cont'd

Class	Subclass	Generic Name	Trade Name
Combination—cont'd	Extended cycle CCP	levonorgestrel/ethinyl estradiol	Seasonale
	Emergency contraception	ethinyl estradiol and levonorgestrel	Preven
		levonorgestrel	Plan B
	Progestin only	norethindrone	Micronor
			Nor-QD
		norgestrel	Ovrette
	Transdermal system	ethinyl estradiol and norelgestromin	Ortho Evra
	Vaginal	ethinyl estradiol and etonogestrel ring	Nuva Ring
	Intrauterine	progesterone IUD	Progestasert
		levonorgestrel IUD	Mirena
	Injection	medroxyprogesterone	Depo-Provera
	Subdermal implants	etonogestrel	Implanon

General Uses

Indications

- Prevention of pregnancy
- Acne: Ortho Tri-Cyclen, Estrostep
- Emergency contraception: Plan B, Preven

Unlabeled Uses

- Anemia prevention/improvement
- Amenorrhea
- Cycle control
- Endometriosis
- Dysfunctional uterine bleeding (DUB)
- Premenstrual syndrome (PMS) symptoms
- Benign breast disease
- Dysmenorrhea
- Mittelschmerz (ovulation pain)
- Hirsutism
- Rheumatoid arthritis control
- Perimenopausal symptom control
- Acne vulgaris
- Female hypogonadism
- Menorrhagia
- Emergency contraception

• • •

This class of medications includes combined hormonal contraceptive agents that contain a combination of synthetic progestin and estrogen, and progestin-only agents. Combined hormonal contraceptives are formulated for oral, transdermal, and intravaginal routes of administration. Progestin-only agents may be administered orally, intramuscularly, or intrauterine. Oral contraceptives (OCs) are commonly known as "birth control pills," or "the pill."

OC pills were first developed in the 1950s and originally contained only progestin in high amounts. One problem with these early pills was break-through-bleeding (BTB). Pure progesterone was difficult to manufacture and during synthesis became "contaminated" with estrogen. The women on the "contaminated" pills had less BTB, so the estrogen was left in. The first birth control pill, Enovid, containing 150 µg of mestranol and 9.85 mg of norethynodrel, was released in 1960.

In the 1970s, researchers first noticed a dose-response relationship between high estrogen pills and the risk of venous thromboembolism. This effect is due to the action of oral estrogen on hepatic induction of fibrinogen, thus increasing the tendency to form blood clots. The pill formulations in the 1960s and early 1970s had roughly three times more estrogen and greater than nine times the progestin dose in pills available today. As doses of estrogen have been decreased below 50 µg of ethinyl estradiol (EE), thrombus risk has also markedly diminished. All sub-50 µg EE pills are considered equally safe.

Over the years, several changes have taken place in the quest to develop safer, more tolerable hormonal contraceptives. The original hormonal contraceptives were monophasic (same daily dose) estrogen and progestin pills. Progestin-only pills and phasic preparations (estrogen and/or progestin doses change during the 21-day cycle in an attempt to mimic the "normal" menstrual cycle) were introduced in the 1970s. The longer acting progestin-only methods (medroxyprogesterone, a 3-month injectable progestin-only contraceptive, and Norplant, a 5-year implanted rod system) were approved for the U.S. market in the 1980s. Norplant was taken off the market because of adverse publicity over litigation regarding dose standardization and removal problems. Implanon is a single-rod implant containing etonogestrel, a desogestrel metabolite that is less androgenic and has more progestational activity than levonorgestrel. It is designed to provide a more stable release of hormone than Norplant. Insertion and removal take about 2.5 minutes and 1 minute, respectively. In the first 70,000 cycles studied, so far, no pregnancies have occurred. Implants prevent pregnancy through several different mechanisms. Implants cause thickening of cervical mucus, making it impenetrable to sperm. Progestins also act on the pituitary and the hypothalamus to suppress release of follicular-stimulating hormone (FSH) and suppress release of luteinizing hormone (LH). In addition, prolonged use of progestins suppresses the endometrium, making it inhospitable for implantation.

In 2000, a monthly combination injectable drug (Lunelle) was introduced but has since been removed from the market. The trend for new contraceptives continues with introduction of more combination OCs with lower estrogen levels and one pill with a new progestin, drospirenone, which is derived from the diuretic spironolactone rather than testosterone. In 2002, a transdermal and vaginal delivery system were approved.

The ring (Nuva-Ring) contains ethinyl estradiol and etonogestrel and is correlated with a pregnancy rate of 1 to 2 pregnancies per 100 women-years. The transdermal contraceptive system contains ethinyl estradiol and norelgestromin and is assocated with approximately 1 pregnancy per 100 women-years of use.

Seasonale, a levonorgestrel/ethinyl estradiol tablet, is an extended-cycle contraceptive consisting of 84 pink active tablets (each containing the active product) and 7 white inert tablets. Women on this product will only experience four menstrual cycles per year.

REPRODUCTIVE ANATOMY AND PHYSIOLOGY

The Menstrual Cycle

The ovaries are the female gonads. As such, they are responsible for secretion of the sex steroid hormones estrogen, progesterone, and testosterone. They are also the storage facility for ovarian follicles, which in turn are the home of oocytes. When a woman is born, her ovaries contain approximately 2 million follicles and, by puberty, 300,000 remain to carry her to menopause. Only about 500 follicles ovulate during the reproductive years.

The menstrual cycle is a classic negative feedback loop composed of the hypothalamus, the anterior pituitary gland, and the ovaries. The average length of the normal menstrual cycle is 28 days. Day 1 of the cycle is the first day of menses. Menses begins because estrogen and progesterone levels are very low, and the unsupported endometrium sheds. At the end of a menstrual cycle in which a pregnancy has not occurred and during the first half of the cycle, called the *follicular* or *proliferative phase,* low levels of estrogen and progesterone produced by the ovary stimulate the hypothalamus to secrete gonadotropin-releasing hormone (GnRH). GnRH stimulates the anterior pituitary gland to secrete hormonal messengers, follicle-stimulating hormone (FSH) and luteinizing hormone (LH) that stimulate the ovaries to begin the ovulation cycle anew.

FSH stimulates follicular growth and development in the ovary. In each cycle, 18 to 20 follicles are stimulated, but by cycle day 5, one dominant follicle develops and the other follicles eventually die off. The function of the dominant follicle is to produce estrogen and to promote an environment favorable to healthy development of the follicle and its oocyte, preparing for eventual ovulation. The dominant follicle enlarges as it fills with estrogen-rich follicular fluid, causing estrogen levels to gradually increase. Around day 12 to 13, estrogen blood levels reach a critical level (>200 pg/ml) that sends a hormonal message to the pituitary gland that the follicle is mature and that ovulation is imminent. The pituitary gland responds by sending out another hormonal messenger, LH. The midcycle surge in LH induces ovulation the follicle, now a "bubble" on the side of the ovary, bursts, releasing the egg into the ampulla of the fallopian tube. At the site of ovulation, the remains of the follicle form a cyst, called the corpus luteum cyst. At this time, estrogen levels drop sharply and then stabilize as the corpus luteum assumes the role of hormone production, producing progesterone in a larger quantity than estrogen.

Progesterone dominates in the second half of the cycle, or *luteal phase.* Progesterone levels are very low during the first half of the cycle but climb sharply after ovulation, with the appearance of the corpus luteum. The corpus luteum cyst, maintained by LH, is a "hormone factory," producing large amounts of progesterone. The corpus luteum remains functional in the normal woman for 12 days. If there is no further hormonal message (e.g., fertilization and implantation), the corpus luteum dies and collapses on day 26 of the cycle. With the demise of the corpus luteum, blood progesterone levels drop dramatically. By day 28, baseline progesterone and estrogen levels signal the hypothalamus to start a new menstrual cycle.

Endometrial Changes. Endometrial, or uterine lining, thickness parallels the changing hormone levels. The endometrium sheds at the beginning of the cycle, day 1 through about day 5, back to almost basement lining. Increasing estrogen levels in the first half of the cycle stimulates endometrial growth and thickness. This proliferative endometrium period parallels the increasing levels of estrogen. Progesterone, produced in large amounts by the corpus luteum in the second half of the cycle, stabilizes the endometrium by increasing endometrial blood supply and glycogen stores, producing a secretory endometrium that is receptive to implantation. Under the influence of progesterone, the endometrium ceases to grow in thickness but becomes significantly more dense. Without the stabilizing influence of progesterone, the endometrium would continue to thicken but, unsupported by an adequate blood supply, would shed irregularly. This condition is seen in the woman with anovulatory cycles: because she does not ovulate, she does not produce progesterone and has unpredictable, often heavy, noncyclic bleeding. Similarly, unopposed progesterone produces a thin endometrium that is not receptive to implantation. The proliferative effects of estrogen must be present in the first half of the cycle for progesterone to produce a secretory endometrium.

If fertilization occurs and the egg implants, the placenta begins producing human chorionic gonadotropin (hCG), which maintains the corpus luteum cyst for about 100 days until the placenta is advanced enough to produce its own progesterone. After 100 days the corpus luteum declines.

In summary, the uterine lining is a mirror image of rising estrogen levels in the first half of the cycle. In the second half of the cycle, progesterone maintains a secretory endometrium. At the end of the menstrual cycle, as progesterone and estrogen levels drop off, the uterine lining sheds for lack of support (Figure 55-1).

Hormone Physiology. A *hormone* is a substance that has an action on a specific organ or tissue. It is a chemical messenger that travels through the bloodstream from a gland to a distant site where it exerts its effect. Estrogen and progesterone are steroid hormones produced in the human body. Estrogens and progestins used in hormonal contraceptive agents are synthesized in the laboratory from either chemical or natural compounds.

The normal human ovary produces all three classes of sex steroid hormones: progestins, androgens, and estrogens.

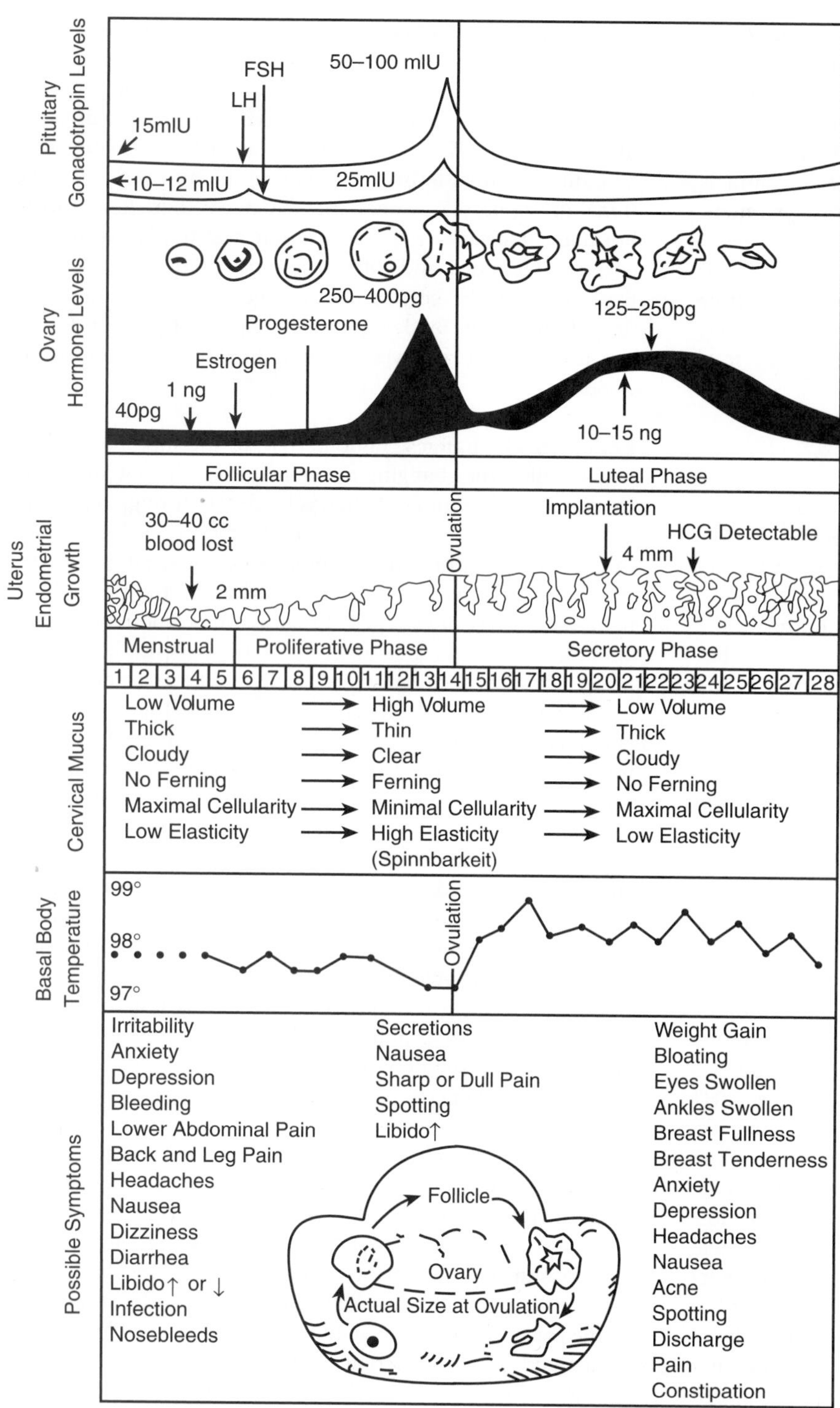

FIGURE 55-1

Menstrual cycle events: hormone levels, ovarian and endometrial patterns, and cyclic temperature and cervical mucus changes. (From Hatcher RA et al: *Contraceptive technology,* ed 16, New York, 1994, Irvington.)

Steroid hormones are derived from cholesterol. Sex-steroid hormones can be synthesized in the ovaries in situ or by blood cholesterol that enters the ovaries. There are several steps in the steroid biosynthesis pathway. Through a series of intermediary steps, cholesterol (a 27-carbon molecule) is broken down to progestins (21-carbon molecules), then androgens (19-carbon molecules), and finally to estrogens (18-carbon molecules). During steroidogenesis, the number of carbon atoms can be reduced but never increased. Therefore the metabolic breakdown of progestins can have progestational, androgenic, and estrogenic actions; the metabolic breakdown of androgens can have androgenic and estrogenic actions; but the metabolic breakdown of estrogens will have only estrogenic actions.

In women, the principal circulating sex hormones are the estrogen, estradiol, and the androgen, testosterone. Most estradiol and testosterone (69%) is bound to sex hormone–binding globulin (SHBG), a protein carrier. Roughly 30% is loosely bound to albumin, leaving only 1% unbound and free. It is this free 1% that determines the biologic effects of estradiol and testosterone. Estrogen administration increases SHBG levels, thereby decreasing the amount of free, or active, sex steroids. Progestins and androgens decrease SHBG increasing the amount of free sex steroids. All combined oral contraceptive pills (COCPs) increase SHBG, although some more than others depending on the progestin component and the ratio of estrogen to progestin. Because all COCPs increase SHBG, free testosterone is always decreased by some degree.

Progestins. Progesterone is the most important progestin. Progesterone is secreted in significant amounts (20 to 30 mg/day) in the second half of the normal menstrual cycle by the corpus luteum. During the first half of the cycle, estrogen dominates and progesterone is secreted in minute amounts (2 to 3 mg/day) by the ovaries and adrenals. During pregnancy, the placenta secretes very large amounts of progesterone.

The plasma half-life of progesterone is only 5 to 10 minutes, after which it is degraded to other steroids that have no progestational effect. The major end product of progesterone degradation is pregnanediol that is excreted in the urine. Progesterone in its natural state cannot be used in oral form because of its rapid breakdown by the liver, so chemical modifications of synthetic progestins in hormonal contraceptives were made to deliberately slow down liver metabolism, making it possible to use the oral route.

Progesterone's effects in the body are limited, seen primarily in the reproductive tract, the breast, and on metabolism. Progesterone is the hormone of pregnancy, producing a secretory endometrium, decreasing uterine contractions, and stimulating alveolar epithelial growth in the breast. Norethindrone, the original progestin used in OCs, was derived from ethisterone, an orally active form of testosterone. Removal of the 19-carbon molecule from ethisterone, forming norethindrone, changed the major effect from that of an androgen to that of a progesterone. Because the androgenic component was not totally eliminated, the potential for anabolic and androgenic effects remains. See Table 55-1 for biologic effects of progestins and estrogen and Table 55-2 for the androgenic effects of progestins.

Estrogens. The human body produces three estrogens: estradiol, estrone, and estriol. The major estrogen is estradiol. It is 12 times more potent than estrone and 80 times more potent than estriol. The primary source of estrogen in the normally cycling woman is estradiol secreted by the ovary. The ovarian follicle secretes 100 to 300 μg of estradiol daily, depending on the phase of the menstrual cycle. Estradiol levels of greater than 200 μg are required for ovulation to occur. The ovary also secretes small amounts of estrone, but most come from adrenal androgens that are converted to estrone in peripheral tissues, such as adipose, skin, and muscle. Estriol is a metabolite of estrone and estradiol.

Estrogens are conjugated in the liver to form glucuronides and sulfates. About one fifth of these conjugated products are excreted in the bile and the rest by the kidneys. Synthetic estrogens, such as EE, are degraded very slowly in the liver and other tissues, which result in their high intrinsic potency.

Estrogens are important in the development and maintenance of the female reproductive tract. Estrogen has effects throughout the body, most notably on the breasts, bones, liver, and urogenital structures. See Table 55-1 for estrogen effects on the body.

DRUG ACTION AND EFFECTS

Hormonal contraceptive agents interfere with the hypothalamic-pituitary-ovarian negative feedback loop to inhibit ovulation. Constant, low levels of estrogen and/or progestin have suppressive effects at both the hypothalamus and the pituitary, inhibiting GnRH, FSH, and LH. Suppression of FSH and LH inhibit ovulation. Additional contraceptive effects stem from actions on the cervical mucus (thickening, to prevent passage of sperm) and the endometrium (providing a lining that is hostile to implantation). Hormonal contraceptives are not considered abortifacients because an existing pregnancy will not be disrupted by their administration.

The primary contraceptive action of progestin in hormonal contraceptives is suppression of the surge of LH, thereby inhibiting ovulation. When given in supraphysiologic doses, progestins produce a decidualized endometrial bed with atrophied glands that is not receptive to implantation, thick cervical mucus, which hampers sperm transport, and may impair ovum transport by slowing peristalsis and decreasing secretions in the fallopian tubes.

The contraceptive action of estrogens in hormonal contraceptives is primarily due to suppression of FSH. Without FSH, no dominant follicle emerges, and ovulation is inhibited. Estrogen contributes to endometrial stability and avoidance of irregular shedding and/or bleeding. Estrogen increases intracellular progesterone receptors, making the given dose of progestin more effective.

The FDA recently approved a monophasic, continuous, 84-day active pill/7-day placebo pill regimen containing 150 μg levonorgestrel and 30 μg EE. The drug, named Seasonale is as effective in preventing pregnancy as conventional 21/7-day regimens. Withdrawal bleeding was comparable between the two regimens, with frequency of unscheduled bleeding episodes initially higher with Seasonale, then declining over time. No endometrial pathology was found, and the side-effect profile was similar in extended and conventional regimens. This drug is predicted to be attractive to women who will only have four menstrual periods a year.

Emergency contraceptives are thought to interfere with ovulation. Other possible actions include disruption of the endometrium to inhibit implantation and alteration in tubal transport of sperm or ova to prevent fertilization. ECs are not effective if there is an existing pregnancy.

DRUG TREATMENT PRINCIPLES

The goal of all of these medications is prevention of pregnancy. Because there are so many different products on the market, clinicians will want to become very familiar with one or two products in each contraceptive category. Learn common side effects for these products and how to make alterations in drug

TABLE 55-1 Biologic Effects of Estrogens and Progestins

Organ and/or System Effects	Estrogenic Effects	Progestational Effects
Adrenal gland	Increases cortisol-binding globulin (transcortin) Increases free cortisol	Increases free cortisol
Bone	Promotes bone formation Stimulates osteoblasts Increases efficiency of calcium absorption Promotes calcitonin synthesis	
Breast	Stimulates ductal growth Promotes growth of estrogen receptor–positive cancers	Stimulates glandular growth Inhibits proliferation decrease in fibrocystic disease
CNS	Improves quality of sleep Antidepressant Vasomotor stability	Sedation
Gallbladder	Alteration in composition of gallbladder bile increased cholesterol saturation Increases gallstones in women already at risk during first 2 years of estrogen use	
Hematologic effects	Increases fibrinogen; clotting factors VI, VII, IX, X, and prothrombin; ESR; transferrin Decreases antithrombin III	Increases hematocrit; fibrinolytic activity
Liver/serum lipids	Influence synthesis of hepatic DNA and RNA, hepatic cell enzymes, serum liver enzymes, and plasma proteins Increases HDL Increases triglycerides Decreases ratio of total cholesterol to HDL	Decreases HDL Increases ratio of total cholesterol to HDL
Metabolic effects	Fluid retention (breast discomfort, headaches) Maintenance of muscular strength Nausea Increases prolactin	Glucose intolerance (increases peripheral resistance to insulin action) Anabolic weight gain Increases appetite Depression, fatigue
Reproductive tract		
Uterus	Proliferative endometrium: endometrial growth due to gland maturation and enlargement; stromal development, capillary proliferation Primes progesterone receptors	Secretory endometrium: restrained growth endometrium becomes thicker, more dense; progressive tortuosity of glands; glands become secretory
Fallopian tubes	Increases secretions, ciliary activity, and peristalsis to improve ovum transport	Slows peristalsis and decreases secretions
Cervical mucus	Increases amount, spinnbarkeit, permeability to sperm	Thick, impermeable to sperm
Miscellaneous		Increases candidiasis Cervicitis
Skin	Increases secretions, lubrication Increases elasticity Chloasma (patchy increase in facial pigment)	
Thyroid	Increases T_3, thyroxine-binding globulin, total T_4 Normal free T_4	
Summary: combined effects of estrogen and progesterone	Increases angiotensin I and II, total iron binding capacity (TIBC) due to increased globulins; vitamin A (nonharmful) Decreases prothrombin time, B_6 (pyridoxine), B_{12}, folic acid, ascorbic acid	

TABLE 55-2 Androgenic Effects of Progestins

System	Effect
General body	Weight gain, nervousness
Skin	Oily skin, acne, sebaceous cysts, pilonidal cysts, hirsutism
Lipids	↓ HDL, ↑ LDL

prescribed to more closely approximate a woman's own menses.

Estrogen

There are two estrogenic compounds used in COCPs in the United States: EE and mestranol. Mestranol is considered pharmacologically weaker because it must first be converted to EE. Therefore, unconjugated EE is the active estrogen in the blood in both mestranol and EE. All of the low-dose (≤35 μg) pills contain EE. Mestranol is available in only a few pills in a 50 μg dose, which is roughly equivalent to 35 μg EE. A relatively safe dose of EE is 35 μg or less. EE 50 μg should be used under special circumstances, and will not generally be used in primary care. COCPs in this chapter are assumed to contain 35 μg or less of EE (see Table 55-3).

Progestin

There are many different progestins on the market in the United States used for hormonal contraception (Table 55-4). Progestins retain androgenic effects to a varying degree. This is a dose–effect relationship: the lower the dose, the lesser is the androgenic effect, At today's very low doses of progestin in COCPs, clinical effects are usually negligible. As with estrogens, serious side effects, especially adverse serum lipid changes, have been associated with high doses of progestins; therefore the lowest effective doses available should be used. Through the years, changes have been made in the chemical structure of progestins in the quest to produce new progestins that have more potent progestational activity without the lower androgenic side effects.

TABLE 55-3 Medications with Dosages

Generic Name	Trade Name	Estrogen (μg)	Progestin (mg)
COMBINATION			
Monophasic			
ethinyl estradiol and norethindrone	Ovcon 50	50	1
	Nortrel 1/35	35	1
	Norinyl 1+35		
	Ortho Novum 1/35		
	Brevicon 21	35	0.5
	Modicon 28		
	Nortrel 0.5/35		
	Ovcon 35		
	Loestrin 1.5/30	30	1.5
	Loestrin FE 1.5/30		
	Loestrin 1/20	20	1
	Loestrin FE 1/20		
ethinyl estradiol and levonorgestrel	Portia	30	0.15
	Nordette		
	Levlen		
	Alesse 21	20	0.1
	Aviane 21		
	Lessina 28		
	Levlite 28		
	Ovral	50	0.5
	Ogestrel		
ethinyl estradiol and norgestrel	Cryselle	30	0.3
	Lo/Ovral		
ethinyl estradiol and ethynodiol diacetate	Demulen 1/50	50	1
	Demulen 1/35	35	1
ethinyl estradiol and desogestrel	Apri	30	0.15
	Desogen		
	Ortho-Cept		
	Cyclessa	25	0.15

Continued

TABLE 55-3 Medications with Dosages—cont'd

Generic Name	Trade Name	Estrogen (μg)	Progestin (mg)
ethinyl estradiol and drospirenone	Yasmine 28	30	3
ethinyl estradiol and norgestimate	Ortho-Cyclen	35	0.25
mestranol and norethindrone	Demulen 1/50 Demulen 1/35	50 35	1 1
Biphasic			
ethinyl estradiol and norethindrone	Jenest-28	35 35	0.5 × 7 d then 1 × 14 d
	Ortho-Novum 10/11	35 35	0.5 × 10 d then 1 × 11 d
ethinyl estradiol and desogestrel	Kariva 28 Mircette 28	20 10	0.15 × 21 d then 0 × 5 d
Triphasic			
ethinyl estradiol and norethindrone	Tri-Norinyl	35 35 35	0.5 × 7 d then 1 × 9 d then 0.5 × 5 d
	Ortho-Novum 7/7/7	35 35 35	0.5 × 7 d then 0.75 × 7 d then 1 × 7 d
	Estrostep Fe	20 30 35	1 × 5 d then 1 × 7 d then 1 × 9 d
ethinyl estradiol and norgestimate	Ortho Tri-Cyclen	35 35 35	0.18 × 7 d then 0.215 × 7 d then 0.25 × 7 d
	Ortho Tri-Cyclen Lo	25 25 25	0.18 × 7 d then 0.215 × 7 d then 0.25 × 7 d
ethinyl estradiol and levonorgestrel	Enpresse Tri-Levlen Triphasil Trivora-28	30 40 30	0.05 × 6 d then 0.075 × 5 d then 0.125 × 10 d
levonorgestrol and ethinyl	Seasonale	0.03 mg	0.15 mg
EMERGENCY CONTRACEPTION			
ethinyl estradiol and levonorgestrel	Preven	0.05	0.25; two tablets × 2, 12 hours apart
levonorgestrel	Plan B	0	0.75 × 2, 12 hours apart
PROGESTIN ONLY			
norethindrone	Micronor Nor-QD	0	0.35
norgestrel	Ovrette	0	0.075
TRANSDERMAL SYSTEM			
ethinyl estradiol and norelgestromin	Ortho Evra	0.02/24 hr	0.15/24 hr qwk × 3, then no patch × 1 wk
VAGINAL			
ethinyl estradiol and etonogestrel ring	Nuva Ring	0.015/24 hr	0.12/24 hr for 3 wk, then off 1 wk, self-inserted
INTRAUTERINE			
progesterone IUD	Progestasert		38 q1yr
levonorgestrel IUD	Mirena		52 q5yr
INJECTION			
medroxyprogesterone	Depo-Provera		150 q3mo

TABLE 55-4 Synthetic Progestins and Their Characteristics

Generation	Class	Description	Specific Drug	Comments	Progestin	Estrogen	Androgen
First	Estranes	Equivalent in actions and potency	norethindrone	Most commonly used	++	++	+++
			norethindrone acetate	Converted into norethindrone	++	++	+++
			ethynodiol diacetate	Converted into norethindrone	++	++	+++
Second	Gonanes	Gonanes have longer half-lives than the estranes, which may translate into better cycle control	norgestrel		+++	0	++
			levonorgestrel	Second generation	+++	0	++
			norgestimate	In newest COCPs, converted into levonorgestrel	++	0	+
			desogestrel	In newest COCPs	+++	0	+
Third		More selective in progestational effects Raise the SHBG more than older progestins, thereby decreasing the amount of free testosterone	etonogestrel	In-vaginal ring Active metabolite of desogestrel	+++	0	+
			norelgestromin	In transdermal system Active metabolite of norgestimate	+++	0	+
Novel		Not a testosterone derivative	drospirenone	Antialdosterone activity	+++	0	0

Treatment Guidelines

Choosing a hormonal contraceptive must be individualized. Consider prior medical history, past experience on hormonal contraceptives, concomitant medications, and preferred mode of administration. Contraindications, with the exception of the intrauterine systems, are the same. Choose a method that is most likely to encourage compliance. Refer to the algorithm in Figure 55-2 for guidelines in making the choice. Table 55-5 compares hormonal methods, and Table 55-6 reviews clinical considerations in contraceptive choice.

Combined Oral Contraceptive Pills. COCPs have the following benefits:

- Dysmenorrhea improvement
- Menstrual cycle regulation
- Improvement in iron deficiency anemia due to lighter and shorter periods
- Decreased risk for benign breast disease. COCPs do not protect against premalignant ductal atypia
- Decreased ectopic pregnancy because COCPs prevent ovulation
- Acne and hirsutism improvement due to lower circulating testosterone levels (all COCPs)
- Decreased functional ovarian cysts by 80% to 90% over nonusers

COCPs can be divided into monophasic and multiphasic pills. Monophasic pills contain identical amounts of estrogen and progestin in all 21 active pills. Multiphasic pills vary the amount of estrogen, progestin, or both over the 21 active pill days in an attempt to mimic the normal menstrual cycle or minimize side effects. Because all women metabolize contraceptive hormones at different rates, "constant" hormone levels are more of an ideal than a reality.

First-Day Start. Start COCPs within 24 hours of period onset. This affords the best contraceptive effect. Backup contraception is not necessary.

Sunday Start. Start COCPs the Sunday after period onset. If the period starts on a Sunday, start that day. Backup contraception for 7 days is necessary. The only advantage of the traditional Sunday start is avoidance of periods on the weekend.

If the patient wants to adjust the time of menses, or eliminate menses, instruct her to take packs of pills "back-to-back," omitting the 7-day break. Breakthrough spotting or bleeding may occur but that is a normal side effect. This regimen is recommended only for monophasic COCPs.

When to Take the Pill. Take one pill every day at the same time. If using a 28-day pill pack, start the next pack as soon as the last pack is finished. If using a 21-day pill pack, stop pills for 7 days, then start the next pack the next day. If nausea occurs, switch to opposite time (morning to evening) or take with food.

Missed pills, especially at the beginning or the end of the pack, may allow ovulation and unintended pregnancy to occur. Increasing the pill-free interval (the period of time between active pills) increases risk of ovulation. Encourage associating pill-taking with a daily routine, such as brushing teeth or

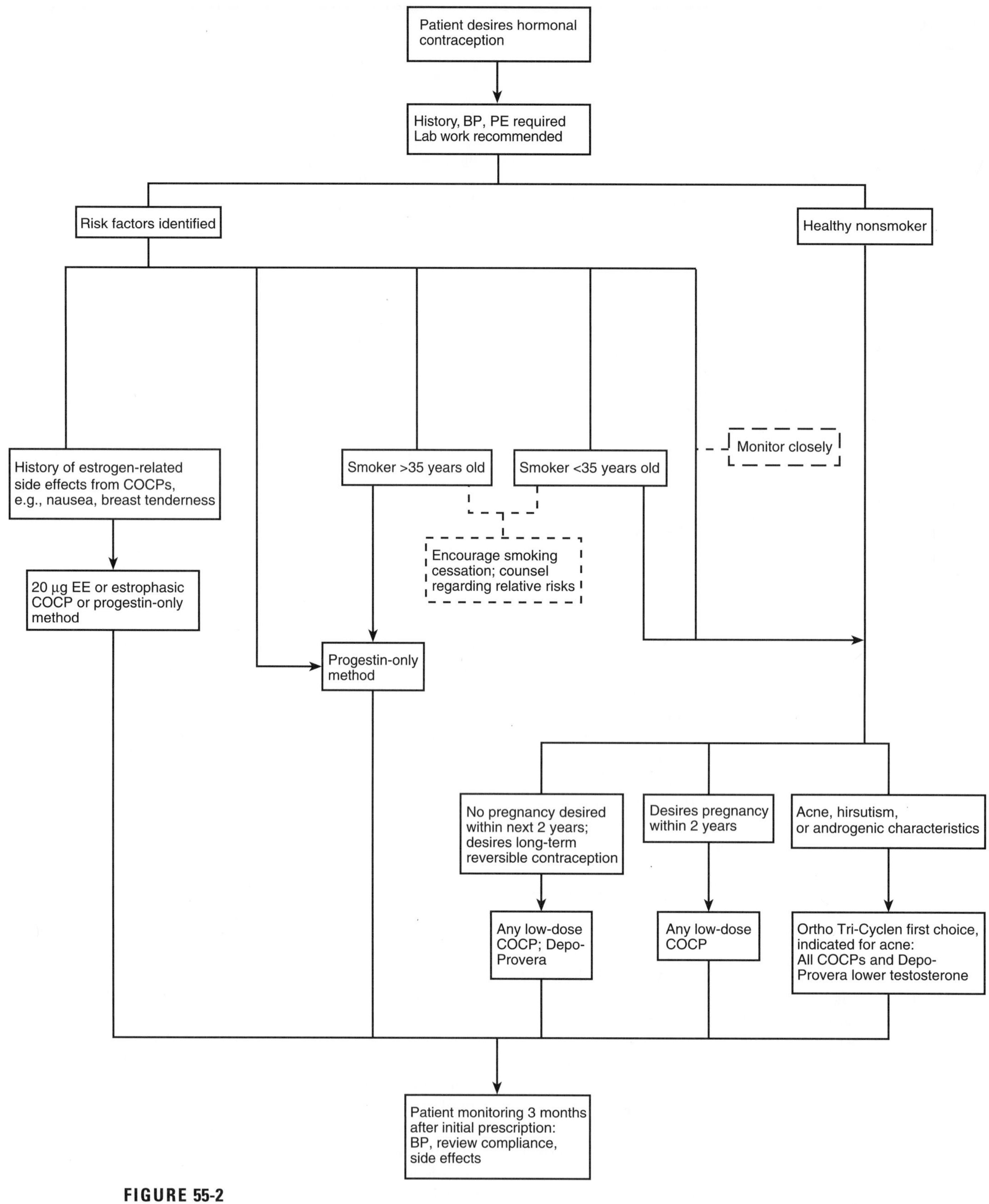

FIGURE 55-2

Algorithm for choice of a hormonal contraceptive.

TABLE 55-5 Comparison of Hormonal Methods

	Progestin-Only Methods		
	DMPA Injection	Progestin-Only Pill (POP)	Combined OC (COCP)
ADMINISTRATION			
Frequency	Every 3 months	Daily	Daily
Progestin dose	High	Ultra low	Low
Blood levels	Initial peak then decline	Rapidly fluctuating	Rapidly fluctuating
Fist pass through liver	No	Yes	Yes
MAJOR MECHANISMS OF ACTION			
Ovary: decreased ovulation	+++	+	+++
Cervical mucus: decreased sperm penetrability	Yes	Yes	Yes
Endometrium: decreased receptivity to blastocyst	Yes	Yes	Yes
FIRST-YEAR FAILURE RATE			
Perfect use	0.3%	0.5%	0.1%
Typical use		1%-13%	
MENSTRUAL PATTERN			
Typical	Very irregular	Often irregular	Regular
Amenorrhea during use	Very common	Occasional	Rare
REVERSIBILITY			
Immediate termination possible	No	Yes	Yes
By woman herself at any time	No	Yes	Yes
Median time to conception from first omitted dose, removal	6 months	<3 months	3 months

Modified from Hatcher RA, et al: *Contraceptive technology*, ed 16, New York, 1994, Irvington.

TABLE 55-6 Clinical Considerations in Contraceptive Choice

Condition	Considerations	Solution	Suggested Contraceptive
Age over 40	Increased cardiovascular risk	35 μg or less of EE or POP	Most COCP, transdermal or vaginal ring, POP
Adolescent	Risk for noncompliance	Individualize to patient's needs	Most COCP, transdermal, vaginal ring, medroxyprogesterone
Arthritis	Often take NSAID	Drospirenone contraindicated	Other methods
Cardiovascular risk	Assess risk factors, asymptomatic disease	COCP safe with superficial varicosities Mitral valve prolapse	Low-dose COCP
Diabetes mellitus	Estrogen ↓ glucose tolerance Progestins ↑ glucose resistance	COCP safe with no end stage disease	Low-dose COCP, low progestin; no POP
Coagulation disorders	Estrogen increases coagulability	Safe if treated with anticoagulants COCPs contraindicated	POP, Medroxyprogesterone
Dysmenorrhea	Estrogens increase dysmenorrhea, flow	Low or no estrogen	POP, continuous COCP, transdermal or vaginal ring
Hyperlipidemia	Estrogen ↑ HDL, ↓ LDL Progestin ↓ HDL, ↑ LDL	Estrogen beneficial overall, progestins are not; monitor lipids closely	Ortho-Cyclen, Apri, Desogen, Ortho-Cept
↑ Triglycerides	Estrogen ↑ triglycerides Progestin ↓ triglycerides	Triglycerides may precipitate pancreatitis	POP, medroxyprogesterone

Continued

TABLE 55-6 Clinical Considerations in Contraceptive Choice—cont'd

Condition	Considerations	Solution	Suggested Contraceptive
Hypertension, uncontrolled	OC ↑ blood pressure ↑ risk for MI and stroke	COCPs contraindicated	POP, medroxyprogesterone
Hypertension, controlled	With no end organ damage, nonsmoker	Low-dose COCP or POP	Ortho-Cyclen, Ortho Tri-Cyclen, Desogen, Ortho-Cept, POP, medroxyprogesterone
Headaches			
Migraines without aura, tension	Begin during or immediately before menses due to decreased estrogen levels	Continuous OCs, contraindicated if patient smokes	Monophasic COCP; 21-day pack × 3 or more packs then 7-day break; repeat Seasonale
Migraine with aura	Increased risk for stroke with COCPs (estrogen)	COCPs contraindicated	Barrier or IUD
Postpartum			
Less than 6 weeks	Increased risk of thrombosis	Progestin only	POP, medroxyprogesterone
More than 6 weeks, not breast-feeding	Ovulation usually 6-8 weeks postpartum	Any hormonal method, if not contraindicated for other reasons	OCP, POP, medroxyprogesterone
More than 6 weeks, breast-feeding	Estrogen may decrease quality and quantity of milk Progestins promote milk production	Progestin only	POP, medroxyprogesterone
More than 14 weeks	Theoretic risk of thrombosis	Low-dose estrogen	Low-dose COCP, POP, medroxyprogesterone
Seizure disorder	Anticonvulsants are enzyme inducers that may increase failure rate of OCs	Medroxyprogesterone	Medroxyprogesterone
Sickle cell anemia	Theoretic risk of thrombosis progestins stabilize the red blood cell membrane Medroxyprogesterone improves the oxygen carrying capacity of RBCs and decreases the risk of sickle cell crisis	Progestin only	POP, medroxyprogesterone
Smoking			
Less than or equal to 35 years	Potential increased risk for thrombosis, ↑ with heavy smoking	Low-dose estrogen or progestin only	Low-dose COCP, POP, medroxyprogesterone
More than 35 years	Greatly increased risk for vascular disease, including heart attack and stroke	Progestin only	POP, Medroxyprogesterone
System lupus erythematosus	Possible increased lupus flares with COCPs Vascular disease associated with lupus contraindicates estrogen	Progestin only	POP, medroxyprogesterone

mealtime, to avoid missed pills. See Box 55-1 for instructions for what the patient should do if they miss pills.

Seasonale. A new fixed-combination, extended-cycle oral contraceptive is available as a 91-day dosage preparation containing 84 hormonally active tablets and 7 inert tablets. Women on this regimen will have four menstrual cycles per year. Seasonale should be reserved for women who are consistent in taking pill every day.

Emergency Contraceptives. Emergency contraceptives (ECPs) are also known as "morning after pills." Treatment initiated within 72 hours of unprotected intercourse reduces the risk of pregnancy by at least 75%. Following EC use, the next menstrual period may start a few days earlier or later than usual. There may be some spotting before the next period. If the period does not start within 3 weeks, the patient should contact her health care provider for an examination and pregnancy test.

BOX 55-1

INSTRUCTIONS FOR PATIENTS WHO MISS PILLS

Do the following if pills are missed:

One pill: Take the missed pill as soon as possible. Take the next pill at the regular time. If the forgotten pill is not discovered until the next pill is due, take both pills at the same time. Use of backup contraception for 7 days is optional.

Two pills in a row: Take two pills as soon as possible. Take two pills the next day. Use a backup method for 7 days.

Three or more missed pills: For first-day starters, throw out the rest of the pack and start a new one that same day. For Sunday starters, take one pill every day until Sunday. On Sunday throw out the remaining pills from that pack and start a new pack that same day. The patient may or may not have a period that month. Order a sensitive pregnancy test if two periods are missed. Use backup contraception for 7 days after the missed pills.

Two or more missed pills at the beginning or end of a pack (total of nine or more missed pills during pill-free interval): Use emergency contraceptive pills, then restart new pill pack; use backup method for 7 days.

Backup method: All patients should have a backup method of contraception available, such as condoms and/or spermicide. Sunday starters need to use a backup method for the first 7 days during their first pack of pills. First-day starters do not need a backup method during the first cycle. The backup method should be readily available in case of missed pills, vomiting or diarrhea, or discontinuation due to serious pill warning signs. New starts may be instructed to use backup for the entire first cycle while side effects, such as nausea, and missed pills are more common.

The progestin-only emergency contraceptives are effective and have a low rate of side effects. There are two products marketed for emergency contraception. Plan B contains the progestin levonorgestrel only. Preven contains levonorgestrel and EE. Before these products were available, Ovral 4 tablets (0.25 mg levonorgestrel and 50 μg EE) was commonly used. The estrogen causes nausea and vomiting, including vomiting up the pills. If you use an OC, use a 21-day package and use monophasic pills to avoid confusion with dosage and placebo pills.

Administer first dose as soon as possible within 72 hours of unprotected intercourse; repeat in 12 hours. Take the first dose at a time that will make it convenient to take the second dose; for example, if the first dose is taken at 3 PM, the second dose would have to be taken at 3 AM. Taking additional ECPs will probably not decrease the risk of pregnancy any further and will increase the risk of nausea.

Progestin-Only Pills (Minipills). The benefits of progestin-only pills (POPs) include the following:

- Immediate return to fertility on discontinuation
- Avoidance of estrogen-related side effects
- Safe and effective for the lactating woman; may be started immediately postpartum
- Decreased anemia
- Decreased dysmenorrhea
- Decreased risk of endometrial and ovarian cancer
- Decreased risk of pelvic inflammatory disease (theoretic)
- Safe for patients with contraindications to estrogen

Also called minipills, POPs are used primarily in breast-feeding women and women with estrogen contraindications. In lactating women, POPs are nearly 100% effective. Advise the lactating woman to notify you when she stops nursing so she may be switched to COCPs. There is no increase in the risk for cerebral thromboembolic events.

Counseling may help prevent pill discontinuation. Explain that the more disrupted the bleeding pattern, the more likely it is that ovulation is inhibited. POPs are more effective when they inhibit ovulation. If the patient cycles regularly, she is probably ovulating and needs to use a backup method of contraception. The patient should report prolonged episodes of bleeding, amenorrhea, or severe abdominal pain.

Start pills on the first day of menses. Use a backup method the first 7 days.

Take pills at the same time each day. If more than 3 hours late taking a pill, a backup method must be used for the next 48 hours.

There is no pill-free interval. When one 28-day pack is finished, another pack is started the next day. All of the pills in the pack are active pills.

If changing from COCPs to POPs, omit the pill-free week and start POPs immediately after active COCPs.

Transdermal System. The transdermal system bypasses the liver eliminating the first pass effect. It has the benefit of being convenient, requiring weekly administration instead of daily. The main disadvantage is the frequency of skin irritation from the patch. It has a 99% effectiveness rate when used correctly. It has a lower incidence of side effects than OCs. The transdermal system has a higher contraceptive rate in women who weigh less than 90 kg.

A patch is applied once a week for 3 weeks. Apply to a different area of skin at each application. Then discontinue wearing a patch for 1 week. Repeat cycle. Apply to skin on buttock, abdomen, upper outer arm, or upper torso where it will not be rubbed by tight clothing. Skin must be healthy, clean, and free of any topical preparations before applying. If the patch becomes partly or completely detached on the first day of application, it should be reapplied or a new patch applied. Do not reapply a patch if it is no longer sticky; do not use supplemental adhesive. Single replacement patches are available from pharmacies. If the patch has been on more than one day, patient may not be protected from pregnancy; use alternative form of contraception until after the first week of the next patch. Stop current cycle and start a new cycle immediately. Switch from an OC by beginning the patch on the first day of withdrawal bleeding.

Vaginal Ring. The intrauterine ring is placed in the vagina by the patient. Its advantage is that it requires only monthly administration. Of the self-administered methods, this one is very convenient and very private. Again, any delivery system that avoids the first-pass phenomenon will need a lower dose and will have less risk of adverse reactions.

The user compresses the ring and inserts into the vagina. The exact position in the vagina is not critical. Remove 3 weeks later by hooking the index finger under the forward rim or by grasping the ring by hooking the index finger under the forward rim or by grasping the rim between the index and middle finger and pulling it out. Place in foil pouch and discard; do not flush. Switch from a combination OC by inserting the ring within 7 days after the last active OC tablet and no later than the day on which the new cycle of pills would have started. No backup method is needed. Switch from a progestin-only method by starting on the same day the previous method is stopped. Use an alternate method of contraception for the first 7 days.

Intrauterine Device. This method has additional contraindications in addition to those for OCs. See specific drug information. These must be inserted by a specially trained health care provider.

Subdermal Implant. Implanon, unlike Norplant, is designed to inhibit ovulation during the entire treatment period. Although its use is approved for 3 years, there is good evidence that Implanon may provide contraceptive protection up to 5 years. Follicular activity without ovulation, in the presence of near normal estradiol levels, has been seen with Norplant and Implanon. Because of this, women may develop palpable, but seldom symptomatic, physiologic ovarian cysts, which usually resolve spontaneously and do not require intervention. There have been no long-term effects on fertility in implant users. After removal of Implanon, concentrations of etonogestrel are undetectable within 1 week.

Advantages of implants include their high-efficacy, long-term action; ease of use; rapid onset of action; protection against ectopic pregnancy; low relative cost; and possible protection against upper genital tract infection. Possible disadvantages include menstrual irregularities, which usually improve over time; provider-dependent placement and removal; lack of protection against sexually transmitted infections; and side effects for some women, including headaches, acne, breast tenderness, weight and mood changes, ovarian cyst formation, and galactorrhea (breast milk expression).

Contraindications for contraceptive implants are the same as to OCPs: include acute thrombophlebitis or thromboembolic disease, undiagnosed genital bleeding, acute liver disease, benign or malignant liver tumors, and known or suspected breast cancer.

Implants, however, are an important option for women in whom combined OC hormones may not be indicated, such as cigarette smoking in a woman older than 35 years; diabetes mellitus with vascular disease; hypertriglyceridemia; history of stroke, heart attack, or deep venous thrombosis; gallbladder disease; vascular headaches or migraine headaches with neurologic symptoms; and depression.

medroxyprogesterone Injection (MPA) (Depo-Provera). Medroxyprogesterone is a long-acting injectable contraceptive. Medroxyprogesterone may be especially useful in the patient who has any condition worsened by the menstrual cycle, such as anemia, dysmenorrhea, or menstrual migraines. Some clinicians find it helpful in management of fibroid tumors because of its potential to suppress estrogen. Because medroxyprogesterone patients have less bleeding (many are amenorrheic), it is an excellent choice for the anemic patient. Benefits include convenience and ease of compliance. It has been used in mentally ill or retarded women. However, hygiene may be an issue because of bleeding irregularities.

- There are few drug interactions: medroxyprogesterone is not affected by medications that induce liver metabolism.
- Estrogen in contraindicated in patients with heart disease, smokers over age 35, and patients with a history of thromboembolism.
- Drug is useful in patients with sickle cell anemia, seizure disorders, and an increased risk of endometrial cancer and ovarian cancer. There is an increased risk of pelvic inflammatory disease or ectopic pregnancy.
- Medroxyprogesterone is available in vials of 150 mg/ml and prefilled 150-mg/ml syringe. Each 150-mg injection is administered deep intramuscularly by Z-track technique into the gluteus maximus or deltoid muscle every 11 to 13 weeks. The area of the injection should not be massaged because this can lower the effectiveness of medroxyprogesterone. Although contraceptive efficacy can be ensured only if injections are given every 3 months, medroxyprogesterone acetate (MPA) may remain in the bloodstream for 6 to 9 months. The initial injection should be given during the first 5 days of menses to ensure that the patient is not pregnant.

Timing of Injections. Injections must be given every 12 weeks (3 months). Although side effects of MPA may last for 6 to 9 months after the last injection, contraceptive efficacy cannot be guaranteed if an injection is given late. If it is inconvenient for the patient to come at the scheduled interval, it is safe to give the injection earlier than 12 weeks. The injection may be given up to 13 weeks after the last injection. A pregnancy test should be administered if more than 13 weeks has elapsed since the last injection.

Backup Method. If MPA is given during the first 5 days of menses, no backup method is necessary. If given at any other time in the cycle, backup is necessary for the first 2 weeks.

Modifying Treatment

Changing the specific medication ordered or adjust the dosage according to the symptoms experienced by the patient. Table 55-7 summarizes common problems with contraceptive use and their solutions.

HOW TO MONITOR

- The initial visit should include weight, blood pressure, clinical breast examination, Pap smear, and pelvic examination. STD testing should be performed for patients considered at risk for STD as part of the annual screening gynecologic examination, but is not necessary for monitoring.
- Follow-up visits in 3 months to check weight and blood pressure and to review side effects and warning signs.
- Yearly monitoring to include weight, blood pressure, clinical breast examination, Pap smear, pelvic examination, and STD testing as indicated.

TABLE 55-7 Contraceptive Use: Problems and Solutions

Problem	Considerations	Solution	Suggested Contraceptive
Androgenetic symptoms	Acne, weight gain, and others	COCP with low androgen activity	Orth-Cyclen, Apri, Desogen, Ortho-Cept
Amenorrhea	Risk of pregnancy Normal on many OCs Common with medroxyprogesterone Treat if patient is uncomfortable	Increase endometrial activity of COCP Change to progestin with higher endometrial activity Change to COCP with higher estrogen dose for a few cycles Change COCP with lower progestin dose	Desogen, Ortho-Cept, Ortho Tri-Cyclen, Ortho Cyclen, Ovcon 35, Brevicon, or Modicon
Break-through bleeding: OCs	Risk of pregnancy Normal in first 3 months More frequent with POPs Often due to missed pills	Reassurance during first 3 months Change to pill with greater endometrial activity, more potent progestin If on POP, add estrogen	Lo/Ovral, Nordette, Levlen, Desogen, Ortho-Cept, Ortho-Cyclen, Ortho Tri-Cyclen
Break-through bleeding: medroxyprogesterone	Atrophy of endometrium due to hypoestrogenic state	Stabilize the endometrium with short course of exogenous estrogen	Estradiol 2 mg qd × 7 or days, may repeat once
Estrogen sensitivity	Estrogenic effects such as nausea, edema, hypertension, heavy menses, migraines	Decrease estrogen in COCP or use progestin-only method	Loestrin 1/20, Desogen, Levlen, Loestrin 1.5/30, Lo/Ovral, Nordette, Ortho-Cept, medroxyprogesterone, POP
Decreased libido	Decreased free testosterone levels	Pill with increased androgenicity	Loestrin 1.5/30, Triphasil, Tri-Levlen

- Patients at high risk for heart disease (personal or family history) should have a baseline lipid profile and fasting glucose at the initial examination and yearly thereafter.

medroxyprogesterone Injection (Depo-Provera)

Monitor immediately after injection for 15 to 20 minutes for anaphylaxis.

PATIENT VARIABLES

Age Over 35 Years

OCPs are appropriate throughout the reproductive years. Nonsmoking women may continue on any COCP containing 35 μg or less EE until menopause. Perimenopausal women, in particular, are good candidates for COCPs because of their noncontraceptive benefits. COCPs help prevent some of the adverse sequelae associated with sporadic ovulatory events that occur in the perimenopause, such as endometrial hyperplasia, hot flushes, and vaginal atrophy.

It is important to determine when a woman has gone through menopause and can switch from COCPs to hormone replacement therapy (HRT) because even the very lowest dose COCPs have approximately four times the estrogen of HRT. Beginning at age 50, FSH levels should be drawn on day 5 to 7 of the pill-free week as part of the annual examination. If FSH is greater than 20 IU/L, the patient can be considered menopausal and switch to an HRT regimen.

Pregnancy

Category X

Lactation

Estrogen decreases the quality and quantity of milk and is not recommended for lactating women. Progestins promote breast milk production. Progestin-only methods are recommended for lactating women who desire hormonal contraception. If COCPs are used, they should not be introduced until at least 6 weeks postpartum.

PATIENT EDUCATION

Combined Oral Contraceptive and Progestin-Only Pills

Demonstrate use of the pill package. Have the patient give a return demonstration.

- Pills must be taken exactly as directed.
- Use a backup method when a progestin-only OC is taken more than 3 hours late.
- For COCPs, see the drug treatment principles.

The pill does not protect against STDs or human immunodeficiency virus (HIV). Stress use of latex male condoms or female condoms with every act of intercourse that may pose a risk of STD.

Instruct the patient to stop taking pills immediately and to contact her health care provider if any serious adverse reactions occur.

Specific Drugs

Combined Oral Contraceptive Pills

Contraindications

- Hypersensitivity
- Thrombophlebitis, thromboembolic disorders
- History of deep vein thrombophlebitis
- Cerebral vascular disease
- Myocardial infarction, coronary artery disease
- Known or suspected breast carcinoma or estrogen-dependent neoplasia
- Carcinoma of endometrium

- Hepatic adenomas/carcinomas
- Acute liver disease
- Undiagnosed abnormal genital bleeding
- Known or suspected pregnancy
- Cholestatic jaundice of pregnancy/jaundice with prior pill use
- Hypersensitivity

Warnings

! Smoking: cigarette smoking increases the risk of serious cardiovascular side effects from OCs. This risk increases with age and with heavy smoking and is quite marked in women over 35 years of age. Women who use OCs should not smoke.

! *Risks of OC Use:* The use of OCs is associated with increased risk of thromboembolism, stroke, MI, hypertension, hepatic neoplasia, and gallbladder disease, although risk of serious morbidity or mortality is very small in healthy women without underlying risk factors. Risk of morbidity/mortality increases significantly in the presence of other underlying risk factors such as hypertension, hyperlipidemias, obesity, and diabetes.

Mortality associated with all methods of birth control is low and below that associated with childbirth with the exception of women over age 35 who smoke and women over age 40. Weigh the risk of pregnancy versus risk of adverse reactions when prescribing OC use in healthy nonsmoking women over 40 years of age and prescribe the lowest effective dose.

- Thromboembolism: be alert to the earliest symptoms of thromboembolic and thrombotic disorders.
- Cerebrovascular diseases: OCs increases the risk of cerebrovascular events (thrombotic and hemorrhagic strokes) and vascular disease. A decline in HDL and increase in triglycerides have been seen.
- Ocular lesions: retinal thrombosis has occurred. Monitor for unexplained loss of vision, onset of proptosis, or diplopia, papilledema, or retinal vascular lesions.
- Carcinoma: increased incidence of breast, endometrial, ovarian, and cervical cancer has been seen.
- Hepatic lesions with benign and malignant have been associated with the use of OCs but this is rare.
- Gallbladder disease: this risk has decreased since the dosage of estrogen and progestin have been decreased.
- Carbohydrate metabolism: glucose tolerance may decrease related to estrogen dose. Progestins can create insulin resistance.
- Elevated blood pressure usually begins within a few months of beginning use.
- Headaches: onset of exacerbation of migraine or development of headache with focal neurologic symptoms of a new pattern that is recurrent, persistent, or severe requires OC discontinuation.
- Bleeding irregularities: BTB and spotting are sometimes encountered in OC patients, especially during the first 3 months of use.
- Ectopic pregnancy may occur in contraceptive failures, especially with progestin-only OCs.

Precautions

- Fluid retention: OCs may cause fluid retention. Use with caution in patients who have conditions that might be aggravated by fluid retention such convulsive disorders, migraine syndrome, asthma, cardiac, hepatic, or renal dysfunction.
- Contact lenses: changes in vision or lens tolerance may develop; refer to ophthalmologist.
- Serum folate levels may be decreased by OCs. Women who become pregnant shortly after stopping therapy may have a greater chance of birth defects.
- Acute intermittent porphyria: OCs may precipitate attacks of acute intermittent porphyria. Use with caution.
- Vomiting or diarrhea may cause OC failure. If significant GI distress occurs, use a back-up method of contraception for the remainder of the cycle

Pharmacokinetics. There is considerable individual variation in circulating levels of estrogen and progestin. EE and most oral progestins undergo a first-pass effect. A variety of factors, such as body weight, drug interactions, and timing of medications, also affect individual variability in bioavailability.

Estrogen and progestins are rapidly absorbed from the stomach. Both undergo first-pass hepatic degradation. Peak blood levels usually occur in 1 to 2 hours. Estrogen is 98% protein bound. Progestins are about 79% to 95% protein bound and bound to SHBG (except drospirenone). The elimination half-life for the progestins is usually about 8 to 9 hours, but it varies (Table 55-8). The half-life of the metabolites is usually several days. Some metabolites are active, others are not. Progestin metabolites are excreted in the urine. Progestin-only administration results in lower serum progestin levels and a shortened half-life than when administered with estrogens.

Adverse Reactions

- Most side effects, such as breakthrough bleeding, headaches, nausea, and breast tenderness, are most common during the first 3 months of use and should improve without intervention. Persistent problems beyond the initial 3 months of use may require a changing to a different COCP. Prolonged bleeding should always be investigated.
- Review of serious pill warning signs: a good acronym to help remember warning signs is ACHES.
  A: Severe *A*bdominal pain
  C: Severe *C*hest pain, cough, shortness of breath
  H: Severe *H*eadache, dizziness, weakness, or numbness
  E: *E*ye problems (vision loss or blurring), speech problems
  S: *S*evere leg pain (calf or thigh)
- Irregular vaginal bleeding, breakthrough bleeding usually improves after the first 3 months of use, although it may persist or occur after long period of use and necessitate a change to a different COCP formulation.
- Weight gain is largely a function of diet and exercise and not COCPs. Rarely, weight gain may be due to fluid retention

TABLE 55-8 Pharmacokinetics of Contraceptive Medications

Drug	Absorption	Drug Availability (After First Pass)	Time to Peak Concentration	Half-Life	Metabolism	Excretion
ethinyl estradiol	Rapid	50%	2 hr	13-27 hr	Liver	Urine
norethindrone	Rapid, complete	65%	30 min-4 hr	6.5 hr	Conjugation	Urine
levonorgestrel	Rapid, complete	100% active isomer of norgestrel	30 min-2 hr	15 hr	Conjugation	Urine
norgestrel				15 hr	Liver	Urine
desogestrel	Rapid, complete	84% converted into active metabolite	1.4 hr	12 hr	Liver	Urine
norgestimate	Well	Converted into levonorgestrel	2 hr	15 hr	Liver	Urine
norethynodrel and ethynodiol diacetate						Urine
norelgestromin	Transdermal	Active metabolite of norgestimate		29 hr	3A4	
etogestrel	Intrauterine	Active metabolite of desogestrel			Liver	
drospirenone			1-3 hr		Liver	Urine

(estrogen or progestin effect), increased subcutaneous fat (estrogen effect), or increased appetite (androgen effect).

- Nausea (estrogen effect) usually occurs during the first few pills in each cycle or the first few cycles of pill use.
- Amenorrhea or missed periods may occur.
- Chloasma/melasma that may persist after COCP discontinuation.
- Depression, decreased libido, hair loss, breast tenderness, increased breast size, and mastalgia may occur.

Drug Interactions

Drugs that Reduce Efficacy of Combined Oral Contraceptive Pills

- Cytochrome P450 enzyme inducers: drugs that induce cytochrome P450 3A4 enzymes, causing the rapid breakdown of estrogen and progestin, may decrease the effectiveness of COCPs. Patients on the following medications should use medroxyprogesterone or a reliable nonhormonal method of contraception.
- Anticonvulsants: phenobarbital, phenytoin (Dilantin), primidone (Mysoline), carbamazepine (Tegretol), ethosuximide. Note: patients on anticonvulsants who wish to continue on COCPs should be switched to valproic acid, if possible. Valproic acid does not interact with COCPs.
- Antituberculosis: rifampin
- Antifungals: griseofulvin

Drugs that May Reduce Efficacy of Combined Oral Contraceptive Pills

! Antibiotics, namely tetracycline and ampicillin, may decrease the amount of hormone absorbed from the intestine or interfere with enterohepatic recirculation. Patients should be cautioned to use a barrier method during a COCP cycle when antibiotics are taken.

Drugs that May Increase Estrogen Effects. High-dose vitamin C has been shown to increase the amount of circulating EE by inhibiting the liver enzymes that metabolize the steroids. Women taking 1000 mg or more of vitamin C per day who are taking low-dose COCPs are in effect getting high-dose-pill estrogen. When the patient stops taking vitamin C, she may experience spotting as estrogen levels decrease. Taking vitamin C either 4 hours before or after COCP administration will not affect EE dose.

Drugs that May Have Altered Pharmacokinetics with Concomitant Combined Oral Contraceptive Pill Administration. COCPs may decrease clearance of benzodiazepines, corticosteroids, theophylline, and aminophylline. Lower doses of these medications may be indicated. The effect of tricyclic antidepressants, β-blockers, and alcohol may be increased. Analgesics, such as acetaminophen, may have decreased pain-relieving effect.

Dosage and Administration. OCPs should be taken at the same time every day. The risk of pregnancy increases with each missed dose.

Other drugs in this class share the same characteristics except as follows.

ethinyl estradiol and drospirenone (Yasmin)

Yasmin contains drospirenone, a novel progestin and the only progestin that is not a testosterone derivative. It is chemically related to spironolactone and has antimineralocorticoid effects and antiandrogenic effects similar to progesterone. The 3-mg dose of drospirenone in the OC Yasmin is equivalent to 25 mg of spironolactone and may cause potassium retention. Caution should be used in women taking potassium-sparing diuretics, ACE inhibitors or ARBs, other aldosterone antagonists, heparin, or chronic NSAIDs. A serum potassium level should be checked during the first month of therapy in patients taking any of these drugs. With all of the other hormonal contraceptive choices available, it would be best to avoid drospirenone-containing products for women on these drugs. Drospirenone is contraindicated in women with renal, hepatic, or adrenal insufficiency.

Contraindications

- Renal insufficiency, hepatic dysfunction, adrenal insufficiency, heavy smoking (15 or more cigarettes per day), and age over 35 years

Warnings

Hyperkalemia. Drospirenone has antimineralocorticoid activity, including the potential for hyperkalemia in high-risk patients, comparable to a 25-mg dose of spironolactone.

! Yasmin should not be used in patients with conditions that predispose to hyperkalemia (e.g., renal insufficiency, hepatic dysfunction, adrenal insufficiency). Women receiving daily long-term treatment for chronic conditions or diseases with medications that may increase serum potassium should have their serum potassium level checked during the first treatment cycle. Drugs that may increase serum potassium include ACE inhibitors, angiotensin II receptor blockers, potassium-sparing diuretics, heparin, aldosterone antagonists, and NSAIDs.

Emergency Contraception

Contraindications

- Pregnancy
- Coronary artery disease
- Clotting disorders
- History of venous thromboembolism.

The Preven emergency contraceptive kit contains a pregnancy test.

Progestin-Only Oral Contraceptives

Adverse Effects. The most common complaint with POPs is irregular bleeding. Irregular bleeding may range from spotting to breakthrough bleeding to amenorrhea. This is expected and normal. The more irregular the bleeding is, the less likely it is that the patient is ovulating. Upfront counseling may help prevent pill discontinuation. Explain that the more disrupted the bleeding pattern, the more likely it is that ovulation is inhibited. POPs are more effective when they inhibit ovulation.

! If the patient cycles regularly, she is probably ovulating and needs to use a backup method of contraception. The patient should report prolonged episodes of bleeding, amenorrhea, or severe abdominal pain.

Other side effects include edema, abdominal bloating, anxiety, irritability, depression, and myalgia.

Drug Interactions. Drugs that induce liver enzymes will decrease efficacy of POPs. Patients on the following medications should use backup method or change to a different method: rifampin, phenobarbital, phenytoin (Dilantin), primidone (Mysoline), and carbamazepine (Tegretol).

Transdermal System

There is an increased risk of skin irritation, redness, or rash.

Vaginal Ring

There is an increased risk of vaginitis and vaginal discomfort.

Device-related events include foreign body sensation, coital problems, and device expulsion.

Intrauterine Devices

Additional Contraindications. Additional contraindications include congenital or acquired uterine anomaly including fibroids if they distort the uterine cavity; acute PID; postpartum endometriosis or infected abortion in the past 3 months; known or suspected uterine or cervical neoplasia or unresolved Pap smear; untreated acute cervicitis or vaginitis; woman or her partner with multiple sexual partners; conditions associated with increased susceptibility to infections with microorganisms including but not limited to leukemia, AIDS, and IV drug abuse; and history of ectopic pregnancy or condition that would predispose to ectopic pregnancy.

medroxyprogesterone Injection (Depo-Provera)

Warnings. Because of strong progestational effects on the endometrium, irregular bleeding and/or spotting is fairly common in the early months of use, and amenorrhea is fairly common with continued use. Unlike COCP users, medroxyprogesterone patients do not have regular menstrual patterns; there is no cyclic withdrawal bleeding. Any bleeding will always be unpredictable. Bleeding may be heavy and prolonged initially but is usually light and sporadic. At least 50% of users will become amenorrheic after the first year of use, some after the first injection. Thorough counseling regarding irregular bleeding pattern may improve method continuation.

Low estrogen levels associated with medroxyprogesterone use are a risk factor for osteoporosis. Medroxyprogesterone users should be instructed to supplement with calcium and to start or continue weight-bearing exercise programs. Medroxyprogesterone-induced bone loss is thought to be reversible. There is concern about bone loss in young adolescents on medroxyprogesterone. The risk of pregnancy-associated bone loss in this population must be weighed against medroxyprogesterone–associated bone loss.

Precautions

- Pregnancy planned in the near future: median time to conception after last injection is 10 months with a range of 4 to 31 months. A patient who desires a more rapid return to fertility should choose a different method of contraception.
- Concern over weight gain: average weight gain after 1 year is 5.4 lb; after 2 years, 8.1 lb; after 4 years, 13.8 lb; and after

6 years, 16.5 lb, according to the package insert. Increased appetite coupled with poor eating habits may account for even larger weight gain.

- Lipid effects: medroxyprogesterone is thought to negatively affect lipid profiles, but the extent is still unclear. Progestins tend to lower HDL cholesterol and increase the ratio of total cholesterol to HDL cholesterol. Obtain baseline lipid profile and reevaluate yearly or as clinically indicated.

Adverse Effects. Other common adverse effects include depression, breast tenderness, weight gain, allergy, headache, nervousness, dizziness, weakness, and fatigue.

Less common adverse effects include decreased libido or anorgasmia, vaginitis, leg cramps, alopecia, bloating, edema, rash, insomnia, acne, nausea, hot flashes, leukorrhea, and anaphylaxis.

Drug Interactions. Antibiotics and anticonvulsants that induce liver enzymes do not affect medroxyprogesterone. Aminoglutethimide (Cytadren), a drug given for Cushing syndrome, does lower serum concentrations of DMPA and may affect medroxyprogesterone's efficacy.

RESOURCES FOR PATIENTS AND PROVIDERS

For the provider

Major pharmaceutical companies that produce hormonal contraceptives have comparison charts, calendars, patient teaching handouts, videos, and texts. Ortho McNeil, Berlex, and Wyeth-Ayerst field representatives, in particular, have speakers' bureaus and are willing to provide lecturers for professional meetings on topics related to their products.

In addition, the following professional organizations have relevant information for providers:

National Association of Nurse Practitioners in Reproductive Health, 503 Capital Court NE Suite 300, Washington, DC 20002, (202) 543-9693.

Association for Reproductive Health Professionals, Washington, DC (202) 466-3825.

Provider and patient education materials, conferences.

Planned Parenthood Federation of America (212) 541-7800.

Provider and patient education materials, conferences, nurse practitioner program, postgraduate education.

The Association of Women's Health, Obstetric, and Neonatal Nurses, Washington, DC, (202) 261-2400.

Annual conference, continuing education materials.

The American College of Obstetrics and Gynecology, Washington, DC, (202) 638-5577.

Annual conference, continuing education geared toward physicians, patient education materials.

Patient education materials

Preparing for a Pelvic Exam, U.S. Health and Human Services, Public Health Service, National Institutes of Health, Clinical Center.

Family Health International, PO Box 13950, Research Triangle Park, NC 27709, (919) 544-7040.

Catalogue of publications on teaching about contraception and family planning,

Contraceptive Technology is an annual conference held on both coasts each spring. It provides an update on women's health issues. Call (510) 828-7100.

For the patient

Educational materials given at the time of the office visit are always helpful. Patients interested in additional resources often go to the Internet. Warn patients that not all websites are reliable. Many are there to express personal experience and are not scientifically based or even factual. Some excellent, reliable websites include

Emergency Contraception Website. Available at opr.princeton.edu/ec/%.

American Social Health Association (ASHA). Available at www.sunsite.unc.edu/ASHA/%.

The Mayo Clinic. Available at www.mayohealth.org.

Planned Parenthood. Available at www.plannedparenthood.org.

The JAMA Women's Health Information Center. Available at www.amaassn.org/contraception; www.ama-assn.org/std.

Hotlines

Emergency Contraception Hotline. Available at (888) NOT-2-LATE

The Centers for Disease Control National STD Hotline. Available at (800) 227-8922

The ASHA Herpes Hotline. Available at (919) 361-8488

Some oral contraceptive pills, particularly Organon products (Desogen, Mircette), can be purchased at a discount. Femscript: (800) 511-1314.

BIBLIOGRAPHY

Apgar B, Greenberg D: Using progestins in clinical practice, *Am Family Physician* Oct 15, 2000.

Collaborative Group on Hormonal Factors in Breast Cancer: Breast cancer and hormonal contraceptives: collaborative re-analysis of individual data on 53,297 women with breast cancer and 100,239 women without breast cancer from 54 epidemiological studies, *Lancet* 347:1713, 1996.

Dunn N et al: Oral contraceptives and myocardial infarction: results of the MICA case control study, BMJ 318:1579-1583, 1999.

Hatcher RA et al: *Contraceptive technology,* ed 17, New York, 1998, Arcent Media, Inc.

Kim C et al: Oral contraceptive use and association with glucose, insulin, and diabetes in young adult women: The CARDIA study. Coronary Artery Risk Development in Young Adults, *Diabetes Care* 25:1027-1032, 2002.

Levi F et al: Oral contraceptives and colorectal cancer, *Dig Liver Dis* 35:85-87, 2003.

Rosen MP, Breitkopf DM, Nagamani M: A randomized controlled trial of second- versus third- generation oral contraceptives in the treatment of acne vulgaris, *Am J Obstet Gynecol* 188:1158-1160, 2003.

Shulman LP et al: Oral contraceptives and venous thromboembolic events, *J Reprod Med* 48:306-307, 2003.

Sicat BL: Ortho Evra, a new contraceptive patch, *Pharmacotherapy* 23:472-480, 2003.

Yasmin—an oral contraceptive with a new progestin, *Med Lett* 44:55-57, 2002.

CHAPTER 56

Hormone Replacement Therapy

Maren Stewart Mayhew, Margaret Dean, and Linda L. Bransgrove

Drug Names

Class	Subclass		Generic Name	Trade Name
Estrogens	Combined estrogen	(P)(200)	conjugated equine estrogen	Premarin
		(200)	esterified estrogens	Estratab, Menest
	Natural		estradiol	Estrace, Climara, Vivelle
			estrone	Kestrone, Estrone (inj)
			estropipate (estrone)	Ogen (po)
			estriol	
	Synthetic		ethinyl estradiol	Estinyl, FemHrt
			synthetic conjugated	Cenestin
			estradiol hemihydrate	Vagifem
Progestins		(P)(200)	medroxyprogesterone acetate	Provera, Cycrin, Amen
			micronized progesterone	Prometrium
			norethindrone acetate	Aygestin
Combination agents		(200)	conjugated estrogen/medroxyprogesterone	PremPro, PremPhase
			acetate estradiol/norethindrone acetate	Combipatch
Androgens			methyltestosterone	Combination: Estratest, Estratest HS

(200), Top 200 drug; (P), prototype drug.

General Uses

Indications

Hormone replacement therapy (HRT)

- Short-term symptom relief
- Prophylaxis against long-term hypoestrogenic effects
- Dysfunctional uterine bleeding
- Secondary amenorrhea
- Primary ovarian failure and/or premature oophorectomy
- Prostatic cancer
- Certain breast cancers (palliative treatment)

Androgens

- Metastatic cancer

Unlabeled Uses

- Treatment of severe hot flashes
- Diminished libido in menopause
- Promotion of weight gain in underweight patients

• • •

Their use in HRT is the only indication discussed in this chapter. There are a variety of estrogen and progestin formulations. New products are available as hormones are reformulated, combined, and recombined.

Estrogen and progestins treat the short-term symptoms of menopause (hot flashes and atrophic vaginitis) and prevent the long-term complication of osteoporosis. Many patients feel subjectively that HRT improves quality of life but research has not confirmed this. At the time of press, many formerly agreed-on benefits are being challenged.

Results from the Women's Health Initiative (WHI) (2002) have changed the approach to prescribing estrogen and progestin. The WHI randomized controlled trial was halted in those women taking opposed therapy (PremPro) because of increased numbers of CHD, stroke, and thromboembolic disease, plus confirming an increase in invasive breast cancer and gallstones. The research with the estrogen-only group continues with no indications of risks not previously listed in literature. This study used conjugated equine estrogens, not natural estrogen. They did not address quality-of-life issues. The Women's HOPE (Health, Osteoporosis, Progestin, Estrogen) study suggests that lower doses of both estrogen and progestin will effectively decrease the vasomotor symptoms yet not raise the risk of CHD. These are just two of a large number of studies that have been conducted and have reached conflicting conclusions. Further research is required to determine exactly the relationship between HRT and cardiovascular health.

At the time of publication of this text, recognized sources for guidelines for HRT have not agreed on the conclusions to be drawn from this study. The American College of Obstetricians and Gynecologists (ACOG) recommends that the menopausal woman should take the lowest effective dose HRT to control menopausal symptoms for the shortest duration

with at least an annual review by her provider. The U.S. Preventive Services Task Force updated their guidelines on October 11, 2002. They now recommend against the routine use of estrogen and progestin for the prevention of chronic conditions in postmenopausal women. The North American Menopause Society concluded that it is not possible to generalize the current data on continuous oral PremPro to other estrogens and progestins, routes of administration, dosages, and regimens. They agreed on the short-term use of HRT and HRT for osteoporosis for women who cannot tolerate other therapy. Most benefits from HRT seems to occur in the first 7 years with no current recommendations to continue therapy beyond that time. Although HRT is effective in the prevention and treatment of osteoporosis, other medications are available and should be considered (see Chapter 40). HRT should not be used for primary or secondary prevention of coronary heart disease.

Additionally, the Women's Health Initiative Memory Study (WHIMS), a substudy of the WHI, suggests that women taking combination estrogen plus progestin therapy had an increased relative risk of developing probable dementia compared to women taking placebo in all age groups. Absolute risk was highest in the oldest group studied (women age 75 and older).

Many providers believe it is "prudent" to stop long-term treatment with combined estrogen and progestin in postmenopausal women but believe that therapy decisions should be individualized for each patient. Many others are switching patients on PremPro to other formulations and using the lowest dosage that controls menopausal symptoms. Many patients are using over-the-counter (OTC) and herbal remedies that have potential dangerous adverse effects. Consult up-to-date resources for the latest information on this topic.

DISEASE PROCESS

Anatomy and Physiology

See Chapter 55 for discussion of hormones during the reproductive years.

Menopause is a normal, universal occurrence for women. *Menopause* is defined as cessation of menses for 1 year. Perimenopause is the period before menopause where symptoms associated with decreasing levels of estrogen and progestin occur. Menopause is not a disease but a normal condition whose symptoms may require therapy. It is predicted that half of the women alive today at age 50 will live to the age of 90. For most women, their perception of general health as they become older may be substantially affected by whether they receive HRT.

The perimenopausal years usually occur between the ages of 45 and 55. For several years before menopause, the frequency of ovulation decreases. Hot flashes occur intermittently. Stress incontinence may be a problem. Premenstrual syndrome may intensify, and the menstrual cycles become unpredictable. Unplanned pregnancy is a risk.

Menses completely terminates at an average age of 51. Ovarian production of estrogen ceases. The low plasma estradiol concentration that remains comes from peripheral conversion of androgen precursors that are secreted predominately by the adrenal glands. The estrogen in plasma becomes estrone rather than estradiol. The conversion of androgen precursors to estrone occurs in adipose tissue; therefore obese women tend to have higher serum levels of estrone and a later onset of menopause. The adrenals provide a very small amount of progesterone.

During the perimenopausal period, as ovarian sensitivity to follicle-stimulating hormone (FSH) stimulation decreases, plasma levels of FSH and luteinizing hormone (LH) increase. Once menopause occurs, the loss of the negative feedback from ovarian production of estradiol causes the FSH and LH levels to increase to about 4 to 10 times the levels seen during the normal follicular phase. Pulsatile secretion may persist.

The Effects of Menopause

Immediate-Onset Effects. Some symptoms develop soon after estrogen levels drop. Vasomotor flushes are most problematic in the short term, but they can persist for years. Vaginal atrophy starts early and persists throughout menopause, causing a number of problems.

Vasomotor Tone Instability. Short-term, vasomotor changes resulting from hormonal changes can cause hot flashes, also called *vasomotor flush*. The skin temperature rises, the peripheral blood vessels dilate, electrical resistance in the skin changes, and the heart rate increases. These vasomotor flushes typically affect the face and neck, occasionally spreading to the chest. They may be accompanied by dizziness, nausea, headaches, palpitation, or sweating. They vary in duration and intensity, lasting from 1 to 4 minutes. They appear to be triggered by decreases in the level of estrogen rather than lack of estrogen. They can be triggered by emotional stress, excitement, fear, or anxiety. They often occur during the night, called *night sweats*, and interrupt sleep. The exact causal mechanisms are not known. They can be the source of much discomfort and loss of sleep in the perimenopausal period.

Vaginal Atrophy. In the postmenopausal woman, the vaginal pH increases from about 5.0 to 7.0, making the tissue more susceptible to infection. Definitive changes take place at the cellular level: the cervix atrophies, the cervical os decreases in size, the vaginal epithelium atrophies, the labia majora and minora shrink, and urethral tone decreases. Muscle tone throughout the pelvic area decreases; this may lead to urinary tract infections and incontinence. The ovaries decrease in size; the uterus also atrophies and decreases in size. The vagina shortens, narrows, and loses some of its elasticity. Vaginal walls do not lubricate as quickly. This predisposes the patient to urinary tract infections, vaginal prolapse, dyspareunia, and other conditions.

Long-Term Effects. These do not appear immediately but appear years after menopause.

Cardiovascular. Women begin to develop atherosclerosis immediately on the cessation of estrogen production and in 5 to 10 years have the same incidence of cardiovascular disease as men. Estrogen stimulates enzyme production that affects cholesterol metabolism. Estrogen deficiency leads to decreased breakdown of low-density lipoprotein (LDL) cholesterol and a decreased production of high-density lipoprotein (HDL) cholesterol, producing a lipid profile that contributes to the development of atherosclerosis.

Breast. Breast mass is decreased. Glandular breast tissue is replaced with fat deposits and connective tissue. The breast tissue decreases in size and firmness. With increased age, the risk of breast cancer increases.

Bone Density. Loss of bone density is associated with menopause. Bone density peaks in the early 30s and then begins to decline with a loss of 1% to 2% each year after menopause. This loss of bone mass leads to increased fragility of bone, or osteoporosis. Osteoporosis predisposes women to fractures and is a major cause of morbidity and mortality in the elderly. See Chapter 40, *Osteoporosis Treatment,* for further discussion.

Brain. Estrogen and progestin have poorly understood biochemical, neurophysiologic, and structural effects on the brain. For example, progestin affects the regulation of GABA (an important inhibitory neurotransmitter) receptor sites.

Other. Menopause is associated with many complaints such as dry skin, fatigue, insomnia, and decreased quality of life. Although these are documented to occur, their cause remains controversial.

Assessment of Menopause

Monitoring the FSH levels 7 to 10 days after menses confirms the diagnosis of menopause. Because FSH secretion is pulsatile, it is important to know the phase of the menstrual cycle (if any) when the FSH is drawn. If the woman is perimenopausal, several FSH levels may need to be drawn because of the irregularity of her cycles. If the woman is on low-dose oral contraceptive pills (OCPs), the FSH level should be checked on the sixth to seventh day of the placebo week during oral contraceptive use.

The FSH should be checked annually at age 50. It is recommended that HRT be started or OCP be changed to HRT when the FSH is greater or equal to 30 IU/L. If the FSH level does not increase, estradiol levels should be monitored. The estradiol level should remain less than 25 IU/L if the patient is menopausal.

DRUG ACTION AND EFFECTS

There are three classes of estrogen formulations: natural, combined, and synthetic. Equine and synthetic estrogens stimulate hepatic globulins and the renin-angiotensin system more than the natural estrogens. Studies have demonstrated no clinical difference between classes, but natural estrogens may be preferable. For drug action, see Anatomy and Physiology.

Estrogen exists in the body in three main forms: estrone (E_1), estradiol (E_2), and estriol (E_3). The active form of the most prevalent estrogen, 17β-estradiol, is not well absorbed when taken by mouth. The liver rapidly metabolizes the drug that is absorbed to inactive substances before it enters the bloodstream (first-pass phenomenon). Thus different methods of getting estrogen into the body have been devised by using either alternative compounds of estrogen or alternative methods of delivery.

In 1970, conjugated estrogens were officially defined as a mixture of sodium estrone sulfate and sodium equilin sulfate. The most commonly used form of estrogen is the conjugated estrogen, such as Premarin. Premarin is derived from the urine of pregnant mares and contains a number of different estrogens, including sodium estrone sulfate (50% to 65%) and sodium equilin sulfate (20% to 35%), and unidentified others. It received Food and Drug Administration (FDA) approval in 1942, before extensive testing was required. Exactly what Premarin contains and how it works remains a mystery. This makes generic equivalents of Premarin problematic.

Progestins include progesterone, which is naturally occurring, and a number of synthetic compounds. Two major classes of synthetic progestins are the 21-carbon progesterones, which are very similar to the endogenous hormone. The second major class is the 19-nortestosterone compounds, which have both progestin effects and a variety of androgenic side effects. Progestins are lipophilic. They bind to progesterone receptors in the female reproductive tract, breast, central nervous system, and pituitary. See Chapter 55 for more information on progestins.

Some androgens have predominately androgenic properties, whereas other have primarily anabolic characteristics. Those androgens with highly androgenic properties are used for treatment of ailments that are hormonal in nature. Methyltestosterone is highly androgenic. Those with mainly anabolic effects are used to promote weight gain or to stimulate red blood cell production in certain forms of anemia.

Drug Effects in Menopause

The effects of estrogens and progestins must be clearly separated. Estrogen has been the most researched. The effects of progestin are less well studied.

Vasomotor Effects. Estrogen effectively treats hot flashes, decreasing frequency, and severity.

Vaginal Atrophy. Use of intravaginal estrogen cream has been shown to decrease atrophic vaginitis and decrease the incidence of urinary tract infections.

Cardiovascular. Findings from the WHI study indicate a higher incidence of coronary heart disease (CHD), stroke, and pulmonary emboli risk in women taking estrogen plus progestin. This effect was not found in women on estrogen only. Earlier studies found cardiovascular benefits. Estrogen, in doses in OCPs, is known to increase the risk of thromboembolic disease.

Breast Cancer. Estrogen replacement increases the risk of breast cancer. No change in mortality has been observed. There is evidence progestin may also increase risk of breast cancer. Some postulate that HRT or estrogen only speeds up the development of breast cancer in patients who would have developed cancer at a later date. Estrogen also makes the breast tissue denser and causes increased false-positive and false-negative readings on mammograms.

Bone Density. HRT is well documented to slow or halt the progression of osteoporosis. It decreases the risk of fractures from osteoporosis.

Brain. The effect of HRT on brain function in Alzheimer's disease is an area of current research. One study showed that HRT may increase the risk of Alzheimer's disease in women. However, further research needs to be conducted in this area.

Endometrial Cancer. It is well established that unopposed estrogen in postmenopausal women with an intact uterus increases the risk of endometrial cancer. Progestins change the endometrium from constant proliferation to secretory, preventing endometrial hyperplasia associated with unopposed estrogen and decreasing the risk of endometrial cancer.

Gastrointestinal. HRT predisposes users to cholecystitis and other gallbladder problems.

Recent studies suggest HRT may reduce colorectal cancer risk in postmenopausal women.

Overall Effects of Hormone Replacement Therapy. HRT is a very controversial prescribing issue. The benefits are that HRT improves the short-term effects of menopause, prevents osteoporosis, and probably reduces the risk of colon cancer. The agreed-on risks are that HRT increases the risk of breast cancer and gallstones. It appears that women without a uterus may safely take estrogen. The confusion lies in prescribing for women with an intact uterus. Controversy exists over the effects on the cardiovascular system, coronary artery disease, stroke, thrombophlebitis, and pulmonary emboli. Clinicians have been advised to work with each patient to individualize their recommendations about continuing or suspending HRT.

DRUG TREATMENT PRINCIPLES

Nonpharmacologic Treatment

Lifestyle modifications are important to the management of the symptoms and long-term complications of estrogen deficit. Dietary changes include decreased fats, cholesterol, animal protein, alcohol, caffeine, sugar, salt, and overall calories and increased fiber, soy, fluids, calcium, and other vitamins.

Exercise is important for general well-being. Also, weight-bearing exercise is necessary to promote bone strength and prevent osteoporosis. Walking is generally recommended as a safe and effective exercise. It is recommended that all postmenopausal women engage in at least 30 minutes of weight-bearing exercise at least 3 times a week.

There are many alternative approaches to management of menopause that are being looked at much more carefully due to the results of the WHI study. None of these has been approved. Soy protein contains natural plant estrogens. Promensil is a natural estrogen sold OTC. None of these products has been scientifically studied. Herbal products and food supplements are considered foods and do not have to meet FDA requirements. Many herbs, such as black cohosh, dong quai, wild yam root, and motherwort, are used for the treatment of menopausal symptoms. Herbal products often contain impurities, and the dosages are unreliable. Recent studies have documented that black cohosh can cause serious liver damage (see Chapter 75 for more information on alternative therapies).

Pharmacologic Treatment

Varying medication regimens may affect patients differently, necessitating an individualized approach to selection of therapy. Medication delivery systems such as the vaginal ring and transdermal and intranasal routes are being studied to determine if they contribute to the development of CHD and breast cancer risk factors that are a concern to the menopausal woman.

There is some interest from clinicians in using selective estrogen receptor modulators (SERMs) to control symptoms in the postmenopausal patient. Two examples of this group of drugs that also promise to decrease some risks of HRT are tamoxifen and raloxifene. Endometrial cancer does not seem to be a factor with these drugs, although the risk for thromboembolism remains the same as that of estrogen.

Oral Contraceptives During Perimenopause. The clinician and the patient should make the decision together on the best treatment plan for menopausal symptoms, considering risks and benefits in view of the patient's personal medical and family health history. Informed consent is imperative.

As the woman undergoes the transition to menopause, her medication should be periodically adjusted to meet her needs. During the perimenopausal years, some women may need relief from the symptoms of menopause and often needs protection against pregnancy. Low-dose OCPs can be given during the perimenopausal years to decrease the symptoms of menopause while providing contraception and decreasing abnormal menstrual bleeding. The dose of estrogen in low-dose OCPs is approximately 4 times greater than that of standard HRT.

Low-dose OCTs during the perimenopausal years are contraindicated in smokers (Box 56-1) due to an increased risk of DVT. There is no increased risk of stroke. Ovarian cancer and endometrial cancer risk is decreased. The effect of OCP on breast cancer is unknown (see Chapter 55 for more information).

Short-Term Use. In general, HRT should be started as soon as the women experiences menopause. HRT is used in the short

BOX 56-1

CONTRAINDICATIONS TO USE OF ORAL CONTRACEPTIVE PILLS IN WOMEN OVER 35 YEARS OLD

- Estrogen-dependent neoplasm
- Smoking (>15 cigarettes/day)
- Suspected pregnancy
- Untreated hypertension
- History of DVT, pulmonary embolism, stroke ischemic heart disease
- Undiagnosed abnormal genital bleeding
- Diabetes with neuropathy, retinopathy, nephropathy, or vascular disease
- Active viral hepatitis, severe cirrhosis, benign or malignant liver tumors

term for the relief of menopausal symptoms, which are most problematic during early menopause. If given for relief of symptoms, HRT should be given for 2 to 3 years and then tapered as tolerated.

Long-Term Use. When started with the first symptoms of menopause, HRT is most effective in preventing the long-term consequences of such chronic complications such as osteoporosis. The main risk in starting HRT for women who are many years past menopause is in aggravating silent heart disease. One should not give estrogen to women at high risk of having a heart attack.

Cyclic Therapy. Cyclic HRT of some sort is usually the first choice for HRT for women willing to continue having periodic bleeding. This bleeding will be regular, predictable, and smaller in amount than regular menstrual periods. There are many variations of the cyclic regimen (Table 56-1).

1: Basic Cycle—Estrogen and then Progestin. Start with the basic cycle. This most closely mimics the physiologic cycle. Bleeding will usually occur on days 25 to 31 (when off hormones).

Days 1 to 25: Estrogen conjugated 0.625 or equivalent
Days 15 to 25: Progestin 5 mg
Days 26 to 31: Nothing

Start with 0.625 mg of conjugated estrogen or equivalent and 5 mg of progestin. Unless the patient is very young and has had a hysterectomy, more than 5 mg of progestin may be associated with depression and mood swings. Some patients experience fewer symptoms with estradiol 1 mg and micronized progesterone 100 mg.

With symptomatic, nonmenstruating women, start treatment with the first day of the calendar month. Remind them that they may experience withdrawal bleeding after the progestin.

2: Continuous Estrogen with Intermittent Progestin. If the patient has symptoms of estrogen deficiency (usually hot flashes) during days 25 to 30/31, switch to continuous estrogen with intermittent progestin. Bleeding will usually occur after the tenth day of progestin and last less than 1 week.

Days 1 to 31: Estrogen 0.625
Days 15 to 25: Progestin 5 mg

TABLE 56-1 Standard Dosing Regimens for Hormone Replacement Therapy (HRT)

Name	Dose	Pattern
Continuous	0.625 mg CEE or equivalent	Daily
	2.5 mg MPA or equivalent	Daily
Cyclic	0.625 mg CEE	Daily
	5-10 mg MPA (10-12 days/month)	Daily, day 1-10, or day 16-25
	0.625 mg CEE (25 days/month)	Daily, day 1-25
	5-10 MPA (10 days/month)	Daily, day 16-25

CEE, Conjugated equine estrogen; *MPA,* medroxyprogesterone acetate.

If the patient has adverse symptoms of progestin, change from Provera to micronized progesterone or switch to the cyclic estrogen with progestin every 3 months. Bleeding will occur after the progestin and last about a week. It may be heavier than with monthly progestin.

Days 1 to 25: Estrogen
Every 3 months, days 15 to 25: Progestin

If the patient is unable to tolerate progestin even once every 3 months, consider intramuscular progesterone injections. Rarely consider estrogen-only therapy with close monitoring for endometrial cancer such as periodic sonograms or endometrial biopsies. Bleeding is unpredictable, and the patient should be followed by a gynecologist.

3: Cyclic Estrogen Only

Days 1 to 25: Estrogen *or*
Days 1 to 31: Estrogen

Continuous Therapy

Continuous Estrogen and Progestin. If patients are adamant that they no longer will tolerate periodic bleeding or if they have difficulty remembering to take the medication on a cyclic pattern, consider continuous therapy. They will usually have irregular bleeding for the first 6 to 9 months with no bleeding thereafter. Some may elect endometrial ablation.

Every Day: Estrogen and Progestin (Continuous). Warn patients of the potential for 3 to 6 months of irregular spotting with this option even if they are already amenorrheic. Spotting that continues beyond 6 months warrants further investigation with either an endometrial biopsy or a pelvic ultrasound. Most practitioners do not choose continuous therapy as their first line of treatment because of the spotting. Increasing the progestin may stabilize the endometrium and help with the spotting. Another option is adding increased progestin for one or two cycles, creating a combination continuous and cyclic regimen.

Continuous Estrogen Only. If the patient has had a hysterectomy, there is no requirement for progestin and the patient can be placed on a continuous estrogen regimen. There will be no bleeding. Women experiencing a premature surgical menopause will need a higher daily dose of estrogen initially. They should be started at 1.25 mg or 0.9 mg and titrated down over 6 to 12 months, or they will likely experience rather severe menopausal symptoms.

Days 1 to 31: Estrogen. If the patient does not wish to take oral medication or has side effects from estrogen (nausea, worsening migraines, hypertension, history of DVT), the transdermal patches, vaginal cream, and vaginal ring may be considered. The disadvantage to these is that blood levels of estrogen are not reliably produced.

Adjust Dosage as Necessary. Recheck patients after 3 months of initial therapy. Titrate doses as needed. If the woman still reports symptoms, increase the estrogen to the next higher dose (e.g., increase to 0.9 mg of estrogen). Lower the progestin if progestational effects are reported and are intolerable. Evaluate again at 6 months for appropriate symptom relief.

Adding Androgens to Hormone Replacement Therapy. The androgens are classified as Schedule III drugs because of misuse by athletes and others wishing to enhance muscle mass and athletic performance. They are controlled under the Anabolic Steroids Control Act of 1990, and prescription and/or distribution of these drugs for nonindicated reasons can result in criminal penalties.

There is growing interest in the use of testosterone in women. In the area of women's health, the only approved indication for androgens is for treatment of severe hot flashes. The formulation used is in combination with estrogen that protects against misuse as well as assists with compliance. A popular unlabeled use of the combined product is to improve a woman's overall feeling of emotional well-being and to increase libido and energy. Some women do have a relative lack of androgen when they go through menopause, and androgens may decrease with vasomotor instability and hair loss. Androgens can lessen facial hair growth, lessen coarsening of the skin, and prevent vaginal dryness. Use testosterone with caution in patients with cardiac, renal, or hepatic disease. It is unclear if androgens affect cardiac risk or osteoporosis, however, androgens have the potential for adverse effects on the patient's lipid profile. Testosterone gel 1% has also been used on a short-term basis for complaints of diminished libido. The control of menopausal symptoms should be evaluated periodically because some of the known side effects of androgens include the symptoms the patient desires to be controlled.

HOW TO MONITOR

- Determine levels of FSH/LH if menopause is suspected (see assessment of menopause for details).
- Review bleeding patterns at each visit. Withdrawal bleeding should not begin before the eighth dose of progestin in either the sequential or cyclic regimen. No bleeding or spotting should occur with the continuous regimen after 6 months. Unplanned bleeding signals the need for consultation with a gynecologist.
- Schedule yearly physical examinations once the dose is stable (e.g., blood pressure, weight and height, thyroid, heart and lungs, breasts, abdomen, and complete pelvic and rectal examination).
- *Androgen therapy:* monitor hepatic function, hemoglobin, hematocrit, blood chemistry, and cholesterol. Do age-appropriate risk assessments, annual mammograms starting with age 40, and indicated laboratory work (Pap smear, sexually transmitted disease screening, cholesterol, thyroid function).

PATIENT VARIABLES

Geriatrics

Early studies favored starting HRT within 7 years of menopause and using it for short-term symptom relief only. The newest studies suggest use of the lowest dose of HRT to control symptoms for the shortest period of time. The geriatric woman may benefit from the positive effects of estrogen on the bladder and urethra.

Pediatrics

HRT is not indicated in pediatrics.

Pregnancy

Category X: Contraindicated.

Race/Gender

No race effect has been reported. Except for their use in the treatment of prostatic cancer, estrogen and progestin remain female-gender specific.

PATIENT EDUCATION

- Discuss the risks versus benefits and obtain informed consent.
- The effects of HRT may take 2 to 4 weeks, and sometimes longer, to be noticed. Dose titration requires time.
- Side effects that may appear with the initiation of HRT (nausea and breast swelling and/or tenderness).
- Take oral preparations with food or at bedtime.
- The patient should be advised to report any signs of thromboembolic events (warm, red tender area on leg, sudden onset of chest or abdominal pain, blurred vision) or abrupt changes in headache patterns.
- It is essential that the patient receive routine monitoring, including Pap smear from the heath care provider.
- Perform monthly breast self-examination, and obtain yearly mammogram.
- Patients on androgen replacement should be counseled on potential virilizing effects.

Specific Drugs

ESTROGENS

(P) Prototype Drug

conjugated equine estrogen (Premarin)

Contraindications

- *Absolute contraindications:* Estrogen-dependent neoplasia (especially breast and endometrial), pregnancy (possible or confirmed), undiagnosed abnormal vaginal bleeding, severely impaired liver function, active thrombophlebitis/DVT. Progestin therapy is not recommended as a preventative for heart disease.
- *Relative contraindications:* History of reproductive cancer, history of stroke, CAD, history of DVT (superficial or deep), liver disease, hypertriglyceridemia, heavy cigarette smoking, endometrial hyperplasia, pancreatitis, fibroids, endometriosis, uncontrolled hypertension, uncontrolled diabetes, severe varicosities, and gallbladder disease.

Pharmacokinetics

Table 56-2 provides pharmacokinetic information.

Adverse Effects

Table 56-3 lists side effects of HRT.

TABLE 56-2 Pharmacokinetics HRT Delivery Systems

Drug	Absorption	Drug Availability (After First Pass)	Onset of Action	Time to Peak Concentration	Half-Life	Duration of Action	Protein Bound	Metabolism	Excretion
ESTROGEN									
Oral	Rapid	50% +/−13%	Rapid 0.5-3 hr	4-5 hr	6-20 hr	12-24 hr	50%-80%	Liver	Bile, urine
Transdermal	Slow/site-dependent: 100% abdomen, 85% thigh			Variable	1 hr	3-4 days	50%-80%	Liver	Bile, urine
Vaginal	Variable		3 hr	6 hr		24 hr	50%-80%	Liver	Bile, urine
PROGESTIN									
Oral	Rapid	65%		0.5-4 hr	5-14 hr	Prolonged	50%-80%	Liver	Bile, urine
ANDROGEN									
Oral	Well absorbed, undergoes first-pass effect				10-100 min		98%	Liver, to active and inactive metabolites	Renal

TABLE 56-3 Adverse Effects of Estrogen, Progestin, and Androgens

Body System	Estrogen	Progestin	Testosterone
Body, general	Fluid retention		Sodium and fluid retention
Skin	Chloasma or melasma	Patchy alopecia, skin rash	Hirsutism, acne
GI	Nausea, vomiting, abdominal cramps, bloating, cholestatic jaundice, gallbladder disease	Nausea, weight gain or loss	Nausea, vomiting
Hematologic and lymphatic	Aggravation of porphyria, alteration of clotting factors	Thromboembolism	Polycythemia
Metabolic and endocrine	Induction of breast cancer, breast tenderness, breast enlargement, change in libido, increase or decrease in weight, reduced carbohydrate tolerance	Decreased glucose tolerance	Hypercalcemia, hyperlipidemia
Nervous system	Headache, migraine, dizziness, mental depression	Mental depression, insomnia, somnolence	Mental depression, headache
Special senses	Steepening of corneal curvature, intolerance of contact lenses		
Genitourinary	Abnormal uterine bleeding, induction of endometrial cancer (without progestin)	PMS symptoms, withdrawal bleeding	Virilization

Drug Interactions

- Some classes of drugs can decrease the effectiveness of estrogen (primarily due to increased hepatic clearance): anticonvulsant drugs (phenytoin, primidone, barbiturates, carbamazepine), rifampin.
- Estrogen exerts a decreasing effect on warfarin while increasing the effects of hydrocortisone. Estrogens can decrease antithrombin III. Triglycerides, prothrombin, and factors VII, VIII, IX, and X can all increase under the effects of estrogen. Impairment of glucose tolerance may occur.

Dosage and Administration

Table 56-4 compares different drug administration routes, and Table 56-5 provides dosage and administration information.

PROGESTINS

(P) Prototype Drug

medroxyprogesterone acetate (Provera, Cycrin, Amen, Premetrium)

Contraindications

- Do not use in patients with a history of cerebral hemorrhage, undiagnosed vaginal bleeding, pregnancy, history of thrombotic disorders.
- Use with caution in patients with liver impairment.

Drug Interactions

Aminoglutethimide may increase metabolism of medroxyprogesterone, thus decreasing its therapeutic effects.

See Chapter 56 for more information on progestins.

TABLE 56-4 Comparison of Routes of Estrogen Administration

Route	Advantages	Disadvantages
Oral	Easy to titrate dose, easy to use divided doses	Nausea, requires daily dosing
Transdermal	Simple application, enhances compliance, sustained blood levels	Irritation at site of patch, replacement of lost patches increases cost, may still require oral dosing with a progestin
Parenteral	Once-a-month dosing, prolonged blood levels	Pain at injection site, extra charge for injection, may necessitate office visit, may still require oral dosing with a progestin
Vaginal	Allows local treatment	Unreliable blood levels, messy application, may still require oral dosing with a progestin

TABLE 56-5 Specific Dosage and Administration Information for Estrogens, Progestins, and Methyltestosterone

Name	Composition	Strength	Dosage and Administration	Prescribing Information
TRANSDERMAL ESTROGEN SYSTEM				
Alora	estradiol	0.05 mg/day	Apply new patch twice/week	Dispensed as patient calendar pack
		0.075 mg/day 0.1 mg/day	Start at 0.05 mg/day	
Climara	estradiol	0.025 mg/day	Apply new patch once/week	Dispensed as individual carton of four systems
		0.05 mg/day 0.075 mg/day 0.1 mg/day		
Estraderm	estradiol	0.05 mg/day	Apply new patch twice/week	Dispensed as patient calendar pack
		0.1 mg/day	Start at 0.05 mg/day	
Fempatch	estradiol	0.025 mg/day	Apply new patch once/week	Dispensed as carton of four systems
Vivelle and Viville Dot	estradiol	0.0375 mg/day 0.05 mg/day 0.075 mg/day 0.1 mg/day	Apply new patch twice/week	Dispensed as patient calendar pack
TRANSDERMAL COMBINATION ESTROGEN/PROGESTIN SYSTEM				
Combipatch	estradiol and norethindrone	0.05/0.14 mg/day 0.05/0.25 mg/day	Apply new patch twice/week Start at 0.05/0.14 mg/day	Dispensed as eight systems

Continued

TABLE 56-5 Specific Dosage and Administration Information for Estrogens, Progestins, and Methyltestosterone—cont'd

Name	Composition	Strength	Dosage and Administration	Prescribing Information
ORAL ESTROGENS				
Estrace	estradiol	0.5 mg 1 mg 2 mg	Start with 1 mg	
Estinyl tablets	ethinyl estradiol	0.02 mg 0.05 mg 0.5 mg	Start with 0.02 mg	
Estratab tablets	esterified estrogen	0.3 mg 0.625 mg 1.25 mg 2.5 mg	0.3-1.25 mg/day	
Menest tablets	esterified estrogen	0.3 mg 0.625 mg 1.25 mg 2.5 mg	0.3-1.25 mg/day	
Ogen tablets	estropipate	0.625 mg (0.75 mg estropipate) 1.25 mg (1.5 mg estropipate) 2.5 mg (3 mg estropipate)	Start with 0.625 mg	
Ortho-Est tablets	estropipate	0.625 mg (0.75 mg estropipate) 1.25 mg (1.5 mg estropipate)	Start with 0.625 mg	
Premarin tablets	conjugated estrogens	0.3 mg 0.625 mg, 0.9 mg 1.25 mg 2.5 mg	Start with 0.625 mg	
Cenestin	synthetic conjugated estrogens	0.625 mg 0.9 mg	Start with 0.625 mg	
VAGINAL ESTROGENS				
Estrace cream, 1%	estradiol	0.1 mg/g	Start with 2-4 g/day	Apply topically
Estring	estradiol	2 mg/ring	1 ring q3 mo	
Ogen cream	estropipate	1.5 mg/g	2 to 4 g daily	
Premarin cream	conjugated estrogens	0.625 mg/g	0.5 to 2 g daily	
Ortho Dienestrol cream	dienestrol	0.01%		
PROGESTINS				
Amen tablets	medroxyprogesterone	10 mg	2.5-10 mg cyclic with estrogen	Comes in dispensing packets
Cycrin tablets	medroxyprogesterone	2.5 mg 5 mg 10 mg	2.5-10 mg cyclic with estrogen	
Provera tablets	medroxyprogesterone	2.5 mg 5 mg 10 mg	2.5-10 mg cyclic with estrogen	
Aygestin tablets	norethindrone	5 mg		
Prometrium capsule	progesterone	100 mg 200 mg	200 mg cyclic	Can be given vaginally

TABLE 56-5 Specific Dosage and Administration Information for Estrogens, Progestins, and Methyltestosterone—cont'd

Name	Composition	Strength	Dosage and Administration	Prescribing Information
PROGESTINS—cont'd				
Crinone vaginal gel	progesterone	4% 8%	Use 1-3 times/wk	Use depends on severity of symptoms
COMBINATION ORAL				
Prempro	conjugated estrogens and medroxyprogesterone	0.625 mg/2.5 mg	One tablet/day Start with 0.625/25 mg	
		0.625 mg/5 mg	One tablet/day	
Premphase	conjugated estrogens and medroxyprogesterone	0.625 mg/5 mg	One tablet/day	
Femhrt	ethinyl estradiol and norethindrone	5 mg/1 mg	One tablet/day	
Activella	estradiol and norethindrone	1 mg/0.5 mg	One tablet/day	
Ortho-Prefest	estradiol and norgestimate	1 mg/0.09 mg	One tablet/day	
Estratest HS	esterified estrogens and methyltesterone	0.625 mg/ 1.25 mg	Start with Estratest HS, increase to Estratest if needed	
Estratest	esterified estrogens and methyltesterone	1.25 mg/2.5 mg	One tablet/day	

ANDROGENS

methyltestosterone (Combination: Estratest, Estratest H.S.)

Contraindications
- Hypersensitivity
- Pregnancy and lactation
- Serious cardiac, hepatic or renal disease

Warnings
- Hepatic effects: Use of long-term androgens is associated with risk of developing hepatocellular neoplasms. Patients should be monitored for signs and symptoms of liver compromise (nausea, vomiting, jaundice, clay-colored stools, upper abdominal pain, abnormal liver function tests). Discontinue drug immediately if any of these signs or symptoms occur.
- Methyltestosterone can cause cholestatic hepatitis and jaundice and relative low doses.
- Breast cancer, androgen therapy, and immobilization may cause hypercalcemia.
- Hypercalcemia may develop in immobilized patients.
- Edema with or without CHF may be a serious complication.

Precautions
- Virilization may occur (deepening voice, hirsutism, mild scalp hair loss, facial acne, clitoromegaly, menstrual irregularities, and breast regression). Discontinue drug.
- Hypercholesterolemia: serum cholesterol may be altered.

Drug Interactions
Androgens may increase sensitivity to oral anticoagulants, requiring reduction in dose of warfarin. Diabetics may require a decrease in dose of insulin because of the metabolic effects of androgens.

RESOURCES FOR PATIENTS AND PROVIDERS

American College of Obstetricians and Gynecologists (ACOG), www.acog.org.
Up-to-date information on the health care issues for women.

Agency for Healthcare Research and Quality, www.ahrq.gov.
Information for health professionals on HRT and breast cancer.

American Heart Association, www.americanheart.org.
Information on the HRT issue as well as menopause recommendations for the professional and patient.

American Medical Association, www.jama.ama-assn.org.
Current articles for health professionals.

National Institutes of Health, www.nih.gov.
Excellent resource for information on health that includes a section on the latest resources for hormone therapy–related topics.

National Women's Health Resource Center, www.healthywomen.org.
Female patient information.

OBGYN, www.obgyn.net.
Physician-reviewed site that offers journal review, discussion groups, and resources for medical professionals.

The National Women's Health Information Center, www.4woman.gov.
Information for the female patient.

Women's Health Interactive, www.womenshealth.com.
Guide to help women with mid-life health issues.

Wyeth, www.wyeth.com.
Series of pamphlets and videotapes on HRT.

BIBLIOGRAPHY

American College of Obstetricians and Gynecologists, ACOG News Release, January 31, 2000.

American College of Obstetricians and Gynecologists, ACOG News Release, August 31, 2001.

American College of Obstetricians and Gynecologists, ACOG News Release, February 28, 2002.

American College of Obstetricians and Gynecologists, ACOG Questions and Answers on Hormone Therapy, August 2002.

American College of Obstetricians and Gynecologists, ACOG News Release, November 29, 2002.

Andrews W: Advances in prevention and treatment of osteoporosis, *Patient Care Nurse Pract* December 21-28, 2002.

Buist DS et al: Are long-term hormone replacement therapy users different from short-term and never users? *Am J Epidemio* 149:292, 1999.

Burki R: Menopause management, part 2: maintaining late menopausal health, *Clin Advisor* March 2002, pp 31-45.

Cholerton L et al: Estrogen and Alzheimer's disease: the story so far, *Drugs Aging* 19:405-427, 2002.

Creasman WT: Is there an association between hormone replacement therapy and breast cancer? *J Womens Health* 7:123, 1998.

Dickerson V: Contraception in the perimenopause, *Female Patient* August 2001, pp 12-16.

DiPiro JT, editor: *Pharmacotherapy: a pathophysiologic approach*, ed 5, New York, 2002, McGraw-Hill.

Fletcher S, Colditz G: Failure of estrogen plus progestin therapy for prevention, *JAMA* 288(3):366-368, 2002.

Grady D et al: Effect of postmenopausal hormone therapy on cognitive function: the Heart and Estrogen/progestin Replacement Study, *Am J Med* 113:543-548, 2002.

Kravitz H et al: Sleep difficulty in women at midlife: a community survey of sleep and the menopausal transition, *Menopause* 10:10-28, 2003.

Lange-Collett J: Promoting health among perimenopausal women through diet and exercise, *J Am Acad Nurse Pract* 14:172-179, 2002.

Maloney C: Estrogen and recurrent UTI in postmenopausal women, *Am J Nursing* 102(44-53, 2002.

Maruo T et al: Vaginal rings delivering progesterone and estradiol may be a new method of hormone replacement therapy, *Fertil Steril* 78:1010-1016, 2002.

Nolan T: The role of HRT and SERMs: evidence-based medicine, *Female Patient Suppl* 3-4, March 2002.

Phillips O: SERMs in preventive health care, *Female Patient Suppl* pp 15-16, November 2002.

Romero M: Bioidentical hormone replacement therapy, *Adv Nurse Pract* 47-52, November 2002.

Seibert C et al: Prescribing oral contraceptives for women older than 35 years of age, *Ann Intern Med* 138:54-64, 2003

Thacker H: The case for hormone replacement: new studies that should inform the debate, *Cleveland Clin J Med* 69:670-685, 2002.

U.S. Preventive Services Task Force: *Recommendations and rationale—hormone replacement therapy for primary prevention of chronic conditions,* October 2002, U.S. Preventive Services Task Force, Washington, DC.

Wattanakumtornkul S et al: Intranasal hormone replacement therapy, *Menopause* 10:88-98, 2003.

Writing Group for the Women's Health Initiative Investigators: Risks and benefits of estrogen plus progestin in healthy postmenopausal women—principal results from the Women's Health Initiative randomized controlled trial, *JAMA* 288(3):321-333, 2002.

Wysocki S: HRT decisions need to be made on an individual basis, *Women's Health Care: A Practical Journal for Nurse Practitioners* 1:32-33, 2002.

Zandi P et al: Hormone replacement therapy and incidence of alzheimer disease in older women: the Cache County Study, *JAMA* 288:2123-2129, 2002.

Other Gynecologic Agents

Drug Names

Class	Subclass	Generic Name	Trade Name
Breast cancer drug		(200) tamoxifen	Nolvadex
Antifungals		(P) clotrimazole miconazole butoconazole terconazole tioconazole fluconazole nystatin	Gyne-Lotrimin, Mycelex (OTC and Rx) Monistat (OTC and Rx) Femstat Terazol Vagistat Diflucan Mycostatin
Antibiotics		clindamycin phosphate	Cleocin cream, 2%
Antiprotozoals		(200) metronidazole	MetroGel vaginal gel, 0.75%

(200), Top 200 drug; (P), prototype drug.

Breast Cancer Drug: Tamoxifen

General Uses

Tamoxifen is indicated for the treatment of breast cancers in the following situations: when the axillary node is negative after total or partial mastectomy or radiation in tumors over 1 cm, for treatment of node-positive breast cancer in postmenopausal women after total mastectomy or after radiation, and in advanced estrogen receptor–positive metastatic disease in men or women. Women with tumors that are estrogen receptor positive are more likely to respond.

An important indication for the use of tamoxifen is to reduce the incidence of breast cancer in women at high risk for the disease. Tamoxifen has been shown to reduce the risk of noninvasive breast cancer by 50% and to reduce the risk of cancer in women with a history of lobular carcinoma in situ or atypical hyperplasia. Tamoxifen reduced the occurrence of estrogen receptor–positive tumors by 69% but had no effect on the occurrence of estrogen receptor–negative tumors. Tamoxifen had no effect on ischemic heart disease. It did, however, reduce fractures associated with osteoporosis. It has a black box warning due to the risk of increased endometrial cancer, stroke, pulmonary embolism, and deep venous thrombosis.

Patients who should be considered for preventive use of tamoxifen are women aged 35 or older who have a history of lobular carcinoma in situ or an increased risk of breast cancer based on the following factors:

- Number of first-degree relatives with breast cancer
- History and number of breast biopsies
- History of atypical hyperplasia
- Age at menarche
- Age at first live birth or nulliparity

The breast cancer risk assessment tool calculates a specific patient's risk of developing breast cancer and should be used as an aid in assessing the risk vs. benefit of tamoxifen therapy. It is based on the Gail model, the only validated model available for assessing breast cancer risk. It calculates a patient's 5-year absolute risk of developing breast cancer. It is available free at www.cancertrials.nci.nih.gov or by calling (800) 4-CANCER. AstroZeneca Pharmaceuticals will provide a free copy and has extensive information on tamoxifen.

DRUG ACTION AND EFFECTS

Tamoxifen is a nonsteroidal antiestrogen that competes with estradiol at binding sites in the cell nucleus in breast tissue, altering gene transcription and protein synthesis. This inhibits the growth of estrogen-dependent tumor cells. Tamoxifen acts as an estrogen agonist with a favorable effect on plasma lipid levels and bone mineral density. However, it has an unfavorable effect on endometrial malignancy and thromboembolism.

Specific Drugs

tamoxifen (Nolvadex)

Contraindications

Contraindication is known sensitivity to the drug.

Warnings

Thromboembolic effects: There is increased incidence of thromboembolic events, including deep venous thrombosis and pulmonary embolism.

- *Carcinogenesis:* Increased frequency of endometrial cancer is found. Increased hepatocellular carcinoma may also be seen.
- *Visual disturbances*, including corneal changes, cataracts, and retinopathy, have occurred.
- *Hypercalcemia* has occurred in patients with bone metastases.
- *Hepatic effects:* Elevated liver enzymes, hepatitis, and hepatic necrosis have occurred. Perform periodic LFTs.
- Increased *bone* and *tumor pain* may occur.

Precautions
- Leukopenia and thrombocytopenia may occur. Perform periodic CBCs.
- Hyperlipidemias have occurred infrequently. Consider monitoring.

Pharmacokinetics. The drug is extensively metabolized after oral administration and is primarily excreted in the feces. After initial therapy, steady state concentrations for tamoxifen are reached in 4 weeks. Half-life of the drug is 14 days.

Patient Variables
Pediatrics
- Tamoxifen is not indicated in children.

Pregnancy
- *Category D:* it may cause fetal harm. It is not known if the medication is excreted in breast milk; therefore the decision to continue breastfeeding should depend on the importance of the drug to the mother.

Race/Gender
- Tamoxifen is used to treat breast cancer in both men and women.

How to Monitor
- Patients taking tamoxifen should receive routine gynecologic care.
- Patients need routine eye care to monitor for cataracts and retinopathy.
- Monitor liver enzymes for elevation and perform blood counts for leukocytopenia and thrombocytopenia. Monitor lipids in patients at risk for elevated lipids.

Patient Education
- Report immediately abnormal vaginal bleeding or change in vaginal discharge.
- Report any change in vision.
- Routine gynecologic care is essential.
- Patients should not become pregnant; this medication may cause fetal harm.
- Regular blood work is important, including liver function tests and total blood counts.

Adverse Effects. Hot flashes, nausea/vomiting, weight gain or loss, fluid retention, vaginal discharge, irregular menses, skin rash, and headaches are seen. Infrequent adverse reactions include hypercalcemia, erythema multiforme, Stevens-Johnson syndrome, bullous pemphigoid, and hypersensitivity. Changes in liver enzymes are an important adverse reaction.

Drug Interactions. Tamoxifen is a substrate of the cytochrome P450 3A4 enzyme system. If taken with warfarin, an increase in prothrombin time occurs. Bromocriptine and cytotoxic agents may elevate serum tamoxifen levels. Medroxyprogesterone and rifamycin may decrease serum levels.

Overdosage. Overdosage has not been reported. Very high doses cause neurotoxicity and prolongation of QT interval, which abates when the drug is discontinued.

Dosage and Administration
- In men and women with breast cancer, the dosage is 20 to 40 mg/day. Give doses larger than 20 mg in divided doses twice a day.
- For prevention, give 20 mg qd × 5 years.
- There is no indication that doses over 20 mg/day are beneficial.

Vaginal Antiinfectives

General Uses

Indications
- Vaginal antifungals are used in the treatment of *Candida albicans*.
- Clindamycin is used in the treatment of bacterial vaginosis.
- Metronidazole is used for the treatment of *Trichomonas*.

DISEASE PROCESS
Candida, T. vaginalis, and *Gardnerella* are the most frequent causes of vaginitis, vaginal discharge, or vulvar itching and irritation. *Neisseria gonorrhoeae* can also cause a vaginal discharge. *T. vaginalis* and *N. gonorrhoeae* are generally transmitted sexually; *Candida albicans* and *Gardnerella* (most common cause of bacterial vaginosis) are not.

On physical examination, erythema of the vulva and evidence of scratching may be seen. The vaginal canal and vault may be swollen and erythematous and contain copious amounts of discharge. An obvious odor may be present. Examination of vaginal pool discharge in sterile saline or KOH may reveal fungus or *Trichomonas*. At times there may be no obvious symptoms, but Papanicolaou (Pap) smear reports document the presence of infection. KOH or saline smears and/or cultures should confirm the diagnosis. Often, a presumptive diagnosis can be made based on symptoms. However, unless the presentation is obviously classic, a physical examination with appropriate tests is necessary.

Candida Infections
A fungus known as *Candida* causes fungal infections of the vagina, which are commonly referred to as *yeast infections*. *Candida* is part of the normal flora of the vagina and is usually held in check by the acidic environment of the vagina. When there is overgrowth by the organism, it causes symptoms.

Many factors allow overgrowth, including change in diet, poor nutrition, sleep deprivation, diabetes, antibiotics, pregnancy, corticosteroids, oral progestin–dominant contraceptives, and decreased host immunity (e.g., HIV infection). *Candida* may be passed between sexual partners.

Symptoms. *Candida* infection usually presents with intense pruritus and burning and copious discharge that is malodorous, white, and curdlike. Candidiasis can also cause vaginal soreness, dyspareunia, and external dysuria.

Diagnosis of candidiasis is made by microscopic examination with 10% KOH showing filaments and spores. Cultures may be used when *Candida* is suspected but not seen on microscopic examination.

A patient who has recurrent or chronic candidiasis should be evaluated for risk factors such as diabetes mellitus or HIV infection.

Bacterial Vaginosis

Bacterial vaginosis is often an overgrowth of one or more bacteria and is not sexually transmitted. Often, the predominant organism is *Gardnerella.* The symptoms are a grayish, sometimes frothy, "fishy" smelling discharge. Vulvitis or vaginitis may be present. On saline wet mount, epithelial cells are covered with bacteria to such an extent that cell borders are obscured (clue cells). Vaginal cultures are generally not helpful.

A clinical diagnosis of bacterial vaginosis is defined by the presence of a homogeneous vaginal discharge that:

1. Has a pH of greater than 4.5
2. Emits a "fishy" amine odor when mixed with 10% KOH solution
3. Contains clue cells on microscopic examination

On laboratory examination, a Gram stain of vaginal secretions diagnostic of bacterial vaginosis will show:

1. Markedly reduced or absent *Lactobacillus* morphology
2. Predominance of *Gardnerella* morphotype
3. Absent or few white blood cells

Rule out other pathogens commonly associated with vulvovaginitis, including *Chlamydia trachomatis, Neisseria gonorrhoeae, C. albicans,* and herpes simplex virus.

Trichomonas

Trichomonas vaginalis is a protozoal flagellate that can infect the vagina, Skene's ducts, and lower urinary tract in women and the lower genitourinary tract in men. It is sexually transmitted. Trichomoniasis is usually asymptomatic in men, or they have nongonorrheal urethritis. Women have pruritus; malodorous frothy, yellow-green discharge; diffuse vaginal erythema; and red macular lesions on the cervix in severe cases. Diagnosis is made by saline wet mount showing motile organisms with flagella. *Trichomonas* is often noted on Pap smear.

DRUG ACTION AND EFFECTS

- Azoles break down the cell walls of the fungus and cause it to dissolve.
- Clindamycin inhibits bacterial protein synthesis by action at the bacterial ribosome.
- Metronidazole's mechanism of action is unknown. It interacts with bacterial DNA.

DRUG TREATMENT PRINCIPLES

The critical decision in appropriate therapy for vaginal infections depends upon accurate diagnosis of the responsible organism. A systematic format for assessment and treatment is included in the treatment algorithm found in Figure 57-1. The specific treatment regimens are listed in Table 57-1.

Candida Vaginitis

Many patients now self-treat with one of the many OTC preparations before calling their health care provider. The symptoms are often so intense that patients are in a hurry to be treated. It is safe and effective for a patient to use OTC preparations without being examined by a health care provider if she has previously been diagnosed with a candidiasis infection and is having the exact same symptoms. Women should notify their health care provider if they are having recurrent or chronic infections.

Initial therapy of a candidiasis infection should be one of the many azole topical medications, with treatment lasting either 3 or 7 days.

TABLE 57-1 Recommended Treatment of Vaginitis

Medication	Dosage and Administration
CANDIDA	
clotrimazole cream, 1%	5 g intravaginally × 7-14 days 100-mg vaginal tablet × 7 days, two tablets × 3 days 500-mg tablet, one tablet in a single application
miconazole cream, 2%	5 g intravaginally × 7 days One 100-mg vaginal suppository, once daily × 7 days One 200-mg vaginal suppository, qd × 3 days
butoconazole cream, 2%	5 g intravaginally × 3 days
butoconazole	One sustained-release, single intravaginal application
terconazole cream, 0.4%	5 g intravaginally × 7 days
terconazole cream, 0.8%	5 g intravaginally × 3 days One 80 mg vaginal suppository × 3 days
tioconazole ointment, 6.5%	5 g intravaginally in one application
BACTERIAL VAGINOSIS (*GARDNERELLA*)	
metronidazole	500 mg po bid × 7 days 2 g po as a single dose Gel (0.75%) 5 g qd × 7 days
clindamycin vaginal cream, 2%	5 g qd × 7 days 300 mg po bid × 7days
TRICHOMONAS	
metronidazole	500 mg po bid × 7 days 2 g single dose Treatment failure: 500 mg bid × 7 days

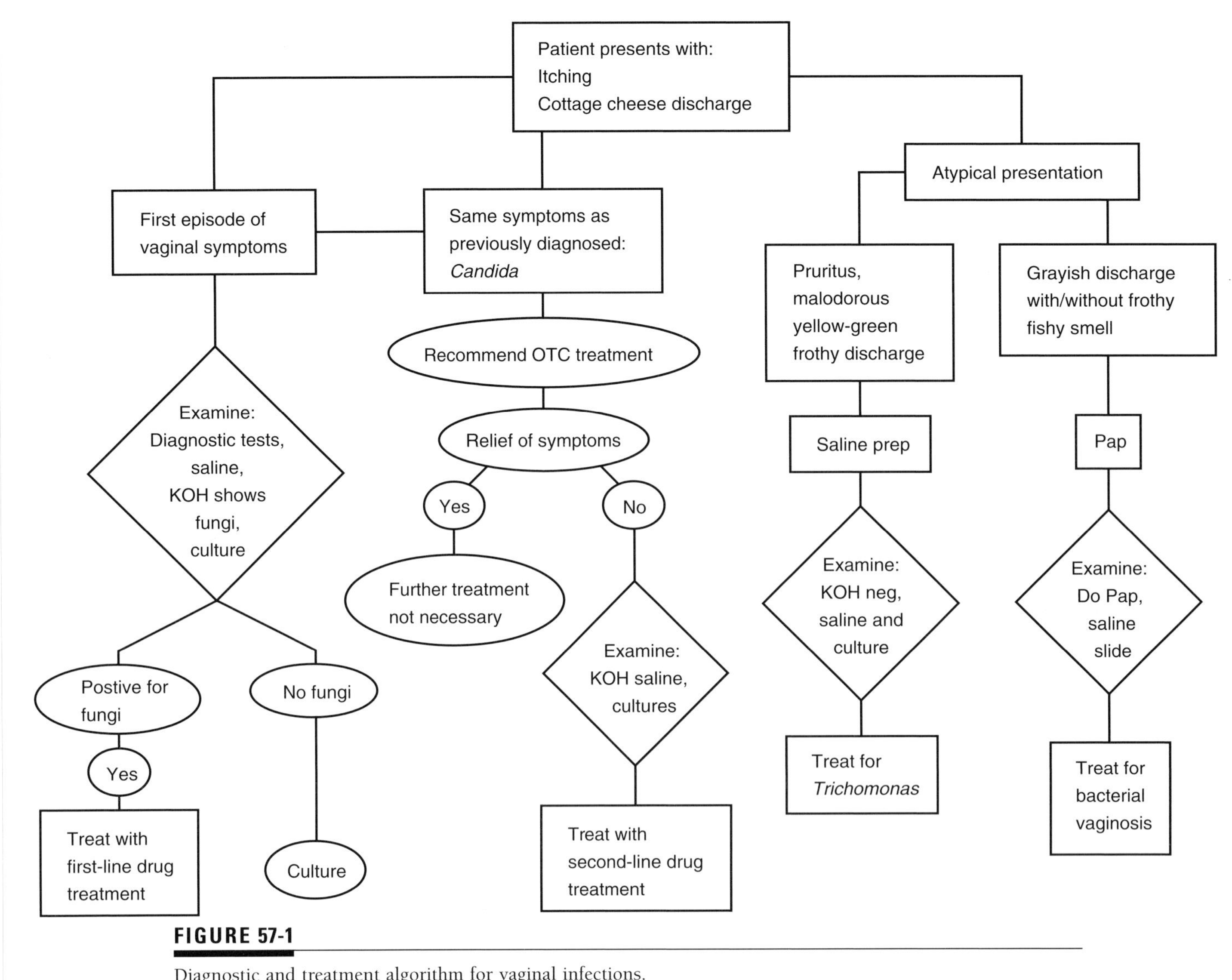

FIGURE 57-1

Diagnostic and treatment algorithm for vaginal infections.

Oral treatment consisting of one fluconazole tablet is very attractive to many women. The oral formulation takes about 2 to 3 days to start working. Application of a topical medication provides more immediate relief of symptoms than the oral medication. Oral treatment may be used if the patient has an aversion to vaginal products or if she is about to start her menstrual period. In general, the patient should be examined before prescribing the oral medication. The oral formulation may be used in conjunction with an azole or a hydrocortisone cream for more immediate relief of symptoms. Severe infections may be treated both orally for 1 to 2 days, plus a 7-day azole regimen.

Azole treatment duration of 1 day is often less effective than the longer-duration regimens. Azole treatment is usually either 3 or 7 days in duration.

For mild-to-moderate symptoms, a 3-day regimen is usually sufficient. The health care provider may order a refill in case a 3-day treatment does not eliminate the symptoms.

For a more severe infection, 7 or more days of treatment will be necessary. If the patient is having chronic symptoms, give a terconazole 7-day regimen with one repeat for a total of 14 days of continuous treatment.

Candida may become resistant to common treatments, especially from over-the-counter products. If the patient experiences a treatment failure, the health care provider should switch to a more potent preparation.

Vaginal antifungals come in a bewildering array of creams, applicators, tablets, and more. What is considered a prescription drug and an OTC drug is changing rapidly; more formulations are becoming OTC. If the patient has a prescription plan, a prescription medication may be less expensive for her. If she pays out of pocket, an OTC preparation is usually less expensive.

Short-course topical regimens effectively treat uncomplicated candidiasis. The azole drugs are more effective than nystatin. There is one effective oral agent. See Chapter 68 for a discussion of fluconazole. Self-medication with OTC preparations should be advised only for women who have been diagnosed with candidiasis and have a recurrence.

Bacterial Vaginosis

Bacterial vaginosis is most often caused by *Gardnerella* organisms. However, it can be caused by overgrowth of other anaerobes.

A variety of treatment options are available. The recommended regimen is metronidazole 500 mg bid oral × 7 days. A single oral 2-g dose is slightly less efficacious but may be indicated if compliance is doubtful. This may be especially important if the patient uses alcohol regularly, because metronidazole has a disulfiram-like effect. If the patient drinks alcohol while taking metronidazole, she may have psychosis, nausea, and vomiting.

Trichomonas

Both sex partners must be treated simultaneously, usually with the same product.

Specific Drugs

ANTIFUNGALS

Ⓟ Prototype Drug

clotrimazole (Gyne-Lotrimin, Mycelex)

Clotrimazole is the drug prototype for the azole derivative class of drugs. Azoles are broad-spectrum antifungal agents that inhibit the growth of pathogenic yeasts. They are fungicidal against *C. albicans* and other *Candida* species. Azoles are used in the treatment of vulvovaginal candidiasis.

Contraindications

- Hypersensitivity to any component in the preparation

Warnings/Precautions

- For vaginal use only; do not use in mouth or eyes.
- If irritation or sensitization occurs, discontinue use. Chronic or recurrent candidiasis may be a symptom of unrecognized disease such as diabetes mellitus or HIV infection.
- Recurrent candidiasis may be due to reinfections; evaluate sources of infection. It may be necessary to treat the patient's sexual partner.
- In patients with refractory cases, repeat cultures to confirm diagnosis before repeating therapy.

Adverse Effects

- Irritation, rash, and erythema are possible

Patient Variables

Geriatrics

- These preparations are generally safe and effective.

Pediatrics

- Safety and efficacy of these drugs have not been established in children.

Pregnancy

- *Category A:* nystatin
- *Category B:* clotrimazole
- *Category C:* butoconazole, terconazole, and tioconazole

No adverse effects or complications have been reported in infants born to women treated with these agents. During pregnancy, use of a vaginal applicator may be contraindicated; manual insertion of tablets may be preferred. Use only on advice of health care provider. Because small amounts of these drugs may be absorbed from the vagina, use category A and category B drugs only during the first trimester and only when essential.

Lactation

- It is not known whether these drugs are excreted in breast milk. Safety has not been established.

How to Monitor

- Reexamine patients treated for vaginal infection after the course of therapy has ended. Evaluate for therapeutic effect and development of adverse effects.

Patient Education

- Use this medication at bedtime.
- Be certain to use all the medication even if symptoms disappear and patient feels better.
- If any irritation, itching, or increase in vaginal discharge develops, patient should return to the health care provider for evaluation.
- Read the patient instructions enclosed with the product.
- Clean applicator after use with mild soap; rinse thoroughly.
- Insert medication high into the vagina except during pregnancy.
- Use continuously, do not skip because of menstrual period.
- Refrain from sexual intercourse.
- Use sanitary napkin to prevent staining of clothing. Do not use a tampon.
- Do not use with latex condoms or diaphragms because the base in these products may weaken latex.
- For prevention of *Candida* infections, the patient should do the following:
  1. Wear loose fitting clothing.
  2. Wear underwear and pantyhose with cotton crotches.
  3. Remove wet bathing suits promptly.
  4. Gently dry genital area after bathing.
  5. Avoid deodorant tampons and douches that may disrupt vaginal chemical balance.
  6. Eat yogurt containing active lactobacilli culture.
  7. Avoid processed sugar and alcohol.

See Chapter 68 for further details.

TOPICAL ANTIBIOTICS

clindamycin phosphate (Cleocin Cream, 2%)

Contraindications

- Hypersensitivity to product components, regional enteritis, ulcerative colitis, and "antibiotic-associated" colitis are contraindications to clindamycin use.

Warnings/Precautions

- Pseudomembranous colitis, which is caused by *Clostridium difficile,* can be caused by clindamycin even if given vaginally.
- The product contains mineral oil that may weaken latex or rubber in condoms or diaphragms. Do not use within 72 hours of each other.
- This product is for intravaginal use only. Avoid contact with the eyes.

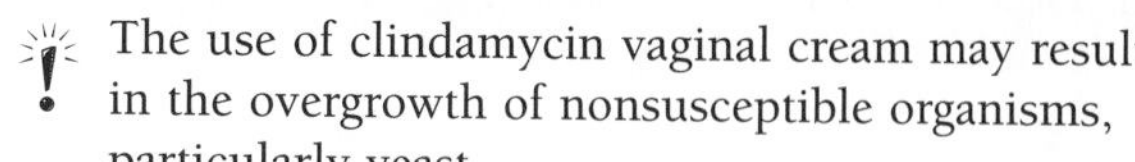
The use of clindamycin vaginal cream may result in the overgrowth of nonsusceptible organisms, particularly yeast.

Pharmacokinetics. Approximately 5% of the clindamycin dose is systemically absorbed from the vagina.

Adverse Effects

- Symptomatic cervicitis/vaginitis caused by *Candida* are reported in 11% of patients. Six percent of patients report vulvar irritation.
- GI symptoms, dizziness, and rash are rare adverse effects.

Patient Variables

Pediatrics

- Safety and efficacy in children have not been established.

Pregnancy

- *Category B*

Lactation

- It is not known if clindamycin is excreted in breast milk after vaginal administration. However, 5% of the drug is systemically absorbed.

How to Monitor

- Evaluate for side effects and therapeutic effect.
- If diarrhea develops, evaluate patient for *C. difficile* colitis.

See Chapter 14 for more details.

ANTIPROTOZOALS

metronidazole (Metrogel Vaginal G, 0.75%)

Contraindications

- Hypersensitivity.

Warnings/Precautions

- Oral use of the drug may cause seizures and peripheral neuropathy.
- Administer with caution in patients with hepatic function impairment.
- Carcinogenesis has been seen in animal trials.

Adverse Effects

- *Candida* cervicitis/vaginitis has been reported in 6.1% of patients using this product.
- Vaginal, perineal, or vulvar itching has been reported by 1.4%.

Patient Variables

Pregnancy

- *Category B*

Lactation

- Metronidazole is excreted in breast milk.

How to Monitor

- Monitor for therapeutic effect and side effects.
- Monitor for emergence of pathogens resistant to metronidazole.

Patient Education

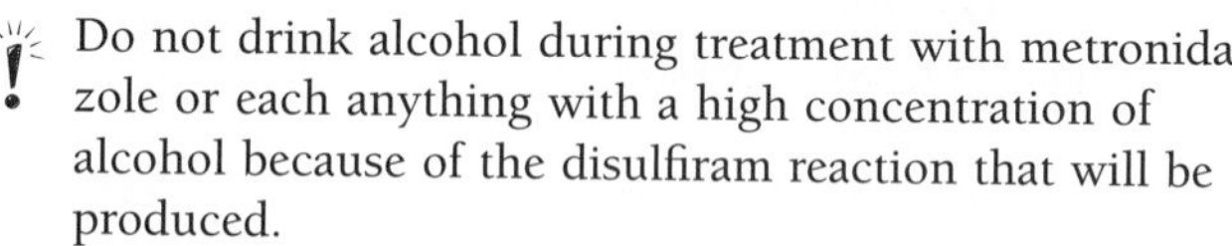
Do not drink alcohol during treatment with metronidazole or each anything with a high concentration of alcohol because of the disulfiram reaction that will be produced.

- Avoid sexual intercourse during treatment.

See Chapter 68 for more details.

RESOURCES FOR PATIENTS AND PROVIDERS

National Alliance of Breast Cancer Organizations, www.nabco.org.

BIBILIOGRAPHY

Burstein GR, Murray PJ: Diagnosis and management of sexually transmitted disease pathogens among adolescents, *Pediatr Rev* 24:75-82, 2003.

Egan ME: Diagnosis of vaginitis, *Am Fam Physician* 62:1095, 2000.

Hainsworth T: Diagnosis and management of candidiasis vaginitis, *Nurs Times* 98:30-32, 2002.

Karasz A, Anderson M: The vaginitis monologues: women's experiences of vaginal complaints in a primary care setting, *Soc Sci Med* 56:1013-1021, 2003.

Leitich H et al: Antibiotic treatment of bacterial vaginosis in pregnancy: a meta-analysis. *Am J Obstet Gynecol* 188:752-758, 2003.

Nyirjesy P: Diagnosis of bacterial vaginosis: pathways to effective treatment, *Clin Rev Therap Spotlight* suppl March 2003.

UNIT 14

Antiinfectives

Unit 14 discusses the use of antiinfectives to treat bacterial, fungal, retroviral, viral, and protozoal infections. The chapters dealing with antibiotics are divided according to class of antibiotic used, except for the medications used to treat tuberculosis. The last three chapters are organized by the type of infective agent.

- **Chapter 58** is a very important chapter, which should be read before any of the other chapters in this section. It provides general treatment principles applicable to most infections. It discusses selection of an antibiotic.
- **Chapter 59** discusses the treatment of common infections by site: respiratory tract, GI, GU, and skin and soft tissue.
- **Chapter 60** outlines penicillins, the first antibiotics of widespread use.
- **Chapter 61** discusses three generations of cephalosporins along with the pros and cons of their use.
- **Chapter 62** covers tetracyclines for adults.
- **Chapter 63** focuses on macrolides, including erythromycin.
- **Chapter 64** describes fluoroquinolones.
- **Chapter 65** describes aminoglycosides that, although important, are not commonly used in primary care.
- **Chapter 66** evaluates the important sulfonamides used to treat infections.
- **Chapter 67** discusses antibiotics used to treat tuberculosis.

The last three chapters discuss products for nonbacterial infections.

- **Chapter 68** discusses products to treat fungal infections.
- **Chapter 69** discusses antiretroviral medications.
- **Chapter 70** discusses products for viral and protozoal infections.

CHAPTER 58

Principles for Prescribing Antiinfectives

General Uses

This chapter discusses general treatment principles applicable to most infections, with an emphasis on those of bacterial origin. Although these general guidelines cover the most common first-line primary care drugs, there are many exceptions to these recommendations. Remember to consider each patient with an infection as an individual case. Patterns of resistance change constantly, and guidelines for treatment are updated at least yearly. Although these recommendations were the most current on publication, do not fail to consult the newest information from state and federal sources. The emphasis in this unit is on typical oral treatment for common primary care problems. The only exception is for single IM injections used primarily in treating sexually transmitted diseases.

DISEASE PROCESS

Anatomy and Physiology

The taxonomy of bacteria is undergoing changes to reflect the new body of information about genetic components of the bacteria. See Table 58-1 for the bacteria that are important pathogens. Bacteria are one-cell organisms with a primitive nucleus and rigid cell walls that are porous and permeable to substances of low molecular weight. Gram-negative bacteria have a more complex cell wall than gram-positive bacteria. They are called gram negative or positive because of the Gram stain used in laboratory testing. The difference in their cell walls is an important factor in an antibiotic's ability to penetrate the bacteria's cell wall and kill the bacteria. Another variable that is important in decision making is if the bacteria are aerobic or anaerobic (i.e., whether or not they need oxygen). This will determine where in the body the organism will grow best.

Bacteria (including rickettsia and spirochetes), protozoa (chlamydia, others), fungi, viruses, and retroviruses cause infections. Rickettsia such as *Borrelia burgdorferi* (Lyme disease) is a small gram-negative obligate intracellular bacterium. Spirochetes such as *Treponema pallidum* (syphilis) are highly coiled bacteria. The focus of the first nine antiinfective chapters is on bacteria. Viruses and protozoa are discussed in Chapter 70; fungi are discussed in Chapter 68.

Pathophysiology

Infections are among the most common reasons for primary care visits. Respiratory tract infections include acute upper respiratory infections (URIs), bronchitis, pneumonia, chronic sinusitis, acute pharyngitis, and otitis media. Other infections common in primary care are urinary tract infections (UTIs) and skin infections such as cellulitis, impetigo, and acne.

About 150 million prescriptions for oral antibiotics are written each year in the United States. Rates of prescription antimicrobials are highest in children. Among all types of health care providers, antibiotics rank as one of the most frequently prescribed products. Whereas their efficacy in decreasing mortality and morbidity is unquestioned, the overuse and abuse of these products has led to drug resistance and raised the specter of returning to a time when clinicians are powerless to cure patients with virulent infections.

To summarize the most important general information clinicians need to know in using different types of antibiotics, a brief review of relevant information is provided here rather than with each antibiotic chapter. Mastery of this foundational material will facilitate accurate decision making. More difficult or detailed clinical problems may require the clinician to review additional anatomic, physiologic, or microbiologic texts before making treatment decisions.

Accurate identification of the offending organism is the most critical clinical decision that must be made with any infection. This is often possible through simple laboratory tests, such as Gram stains, which many clinicians are able to perform in their offices. Some organisms require more extensive testing in commercial laboratories, and results may not be available fast enough to be helpful in the initial treatment decisions. Knowledge of which organisms are endemic in the community during that season and which organisms seem to have developed resistance to different drugs is also important for the clinician.

Assessment of Infection

Take a thorough history, especially concerning allergies and other drugs the patient is taking and previous antibiotic treatment. If the patient has had previous allergic reactions, determine the type of reaction. If the infection is in the respiratory tract, inquire about smoking. Look for concomitant illness and other complicating factors.

Before placing a patient on an antibiotic, confirm the diagnosis of bacterial infection. Infections caused by a virus should not be treated with an antibiotic.

At least 90% of URIs are viral. When treating infection, assess whether there are any symptoms or signs that indicate a bacterial infection. If none exist, consider culturing and waiting to treat until the culture results are available. If the patient has signs and symptoms that indicate probable bacterial infection, consider empiric treatment until culture results are available. The signs and symptoms that indicate bacterial infection are not always obvious and clearcut. Generally they may include fever higher than 102° F, lymphadenopathy, swelling, and pain. There may also be organ-specific signs and symptoms indicating a bacterial infection of particular tissue. No formula can be given that

TABLE 58-1 Important Pathogens

	Morphology	Aerobe vs Anaerobe	Organism	Most Important Pathogen	Disease Caused
BACTERIA					
Gram positive	Cocci		*Staphylococcus*	*S. aureus*	Skin and soft tissue infective endocarditis
					Osteomyelitis, bacteremia, toxic shock syndrome
			Streptococcus	*S. pyogenes group* A β-hemolytic (GABH)	Pharyngitis/rheumatic fever
					Impetigo
				S. viridans	Endocarditis
			Enterococcus	*E. faecalis*	Wound, UTI, endocarditis
			Pneumococcus	*S. pneumococcus*	Pneumonia
					Meningitis
	Rods		*Bacillus*	*B. anthracis*	Anthrax
		Anaerobe	*Actinomyces*	*A. israelii*	Cervicofacial
				A. haemolyticum	Pharyngitis
			Corynebacterium	*C. diphtheriae*	Diphtheria
		Aerobe	*Listeria*	*L. monocytogenes*	Listeriosis
		Anaerobe	*Clostridium*	*C. perfringens*	Gas gangrene
				C. difficile	Enteritis
				C. tetani	Tetanus
				C. botulinum	Botulism
Gram negative	Cocci	Aerobe	*Neisseria*	*N. gonorrhoeae*	Gonorrhea
				N. meningitidis	Meningitis
		Aerobe	*Moraxella*	*M. catarrhalis*	Otitis media, sinusitis, pneumonia
	Bacilli	Aerobe	*Pseudomonas*	*P. aeruginosa*	Bacteremia
ENTEROBACTERIA			*Escherichia*	*E. coli*	Gastroenteritis
			Shigella	*S. dysenteriae*	Shigellosis dysentery
			Salmonella	*S. typhi*	Typhoid fever
				S. enteritidis	Gastroenteritis
			Klebsiella	*K. pneumoniae*	UTI, various
			Proteus	*P. mirabilis*	UTI, various
				P. vulgaris	UTI, various
			Yersinia	*Y. pestis*	Plague
			Enterobacter	*E. cloacae*	
			Serratia	*S. marcescens*	
			Citrobacter	*C. freundii*	
			Morganella	*M. morgani*	
			Vibrio	*V. cholerae*	Cholera
			Helicobacter	*H. pylori*	Gastritis, PUD
	Small bacilli		*Haemophilus*	*H. influenzae*	Sinusitis, otitis, bronchitis, pneumonia
			Bordetella	*B. pertussis*	Whooping cough
			Pasteurella	*P. tularensis*	Tularemia
				P. multocida	Animal bite infections
			Campylobacter	*C. jejuni*	Gastroenteritis
			Gardnerella	*G. vaginalis*	Vaginitis
			Legionella	*L. pneumophila*	Legionnaire's pneumonia
		Aerobe	*Nocardia*	*N. asteroides*	Pulmonary endocarditis, systemic infection
		Anaerobe	*Bacteroides*	*B. fragilis*	
			Prevotella (formerly *Bacteroides*)	*P. melaninogenica*	URIs
Acid fast			*Mycobacterium*	*M. tuberculosis*	Tuberculosis
				M. avium	Bronchitis, etc
				M. leprae	Leprosy

TABLE 58-1 Important Pathogens—cont'd

	Morphology	Aerobe vs Anaerobe	Organism	Most Important Pathogen	Disease Caused
ENTEROBACTERIA—cont'd					
Mycoplasma			*Mycoplasma*	*M. pneumoniae*	Atypical pneumonia
				M. hominis	
			Ureaplasma	*M. urealyticum*	
Spirochetes			*Treponema*	*T. pallidum*	Syphilis
				T. pallidum sub	Yaws
			Borrelia	*B. burgdorferi*	Lyme disease
Rickettsia			*Rickettsia*	*R. rickettsia*	Rocky Mountain spotted fever, typhus
PROTOZOA			*Chlamydia* (closely related to Gram bacteria)	*C. trachomatis*	Lymphogranuloma venereum, urethritis, and cervicitis
				C. psittaci	Psittacosis
				C. pneumoniae	Pneumonia
			Trichomonas	*T. vaginalis*	Trichomonas vaginitis
			Entamoeba	*E. histolytica*	Amebiasis colitis
			Cryptosporidium (spore forming)	*C. parvum*	Diarrhea
		Flagellate	*Giardia* (cyst forming)	*G. lamblia*	Diarrhea
			Leishmania	Many species	Skin lesions
			Plasmodium	*P. falciparum*	Malaria
				P. vivax	Malaria
				P. malariae	Malaria
				P. ovale	Malaria
			Toxoplasma	*T. gondii*	Toxoplasmosis
HELMINTHIC	Trematode				Schistosomiasis
	Cestode				
	Nematode				Anisakiasis
				A. lumbricoides	Ascariasis
					Enterobiasis
			Trichinella	*T. spiralis*	Trichinosis

says if x, y, and z are present, it is always a bacterial infection. Having a high index of suspicion, doing the appropriate testing, and being able to recognize when a patient is really ill requires a blend of both art and science.

Some of the red flags that serious bacterial infection may be present include the following:

- Loss of appetite: in the presence of fever this can signal the presence of a significant infection. Maintenance of appetite with fever is a more reliable indicator for localized or limited infection.
- Symptoms of dehydration: ask about fluid intake. Consider dehydration even if illness seems minor. Look for dizziness when standing, unsteady walk, orthostatic changes of vital signs, urine concentration of 1.025 to 1.030, and dry mucous membranes.
- Absence of fever: especially in patients with diabetes or in the extremes of life, when the immune system may not cause adequate release of pyrogens, this does not exclude serious infection. High or persistent fever in children is often a sign of serious illness and requires a more comprehensive search for the cause.

Although minor infections make up the bulk of most primary care practices, always consider referral to a specialist for unusual symptoms or unusual responses to treatment. Hospital-based infectious disease specialists are highly attuned to knowledge of community-acquired infections and their treatment as well as to the more exotic presentations. Simple localized infections may progress to septic shock within hours, and the clinician must not discount the ominous symptoms of shaking chills and soaring temperatures that require emergency attention.

Overuse of antibiotics and resulting drug resistance not only affect the individual patient but also leads to the development of resistant strains of bacteria that are then spread throughout the community. Resistant bacteria cause infections that are harder to treat, last longer, and require hospitalization. Future infections may also prove resistant to antibiotics. As a result, the patient experiences more frequent infections with a narrowing range of therapeutic options. For example, otitis and sinusitis are conditions for which resistant strains have become a major problem. Administering antibiotics for viral infection prophylaxis when not needed also places the patient at increased risk for adverse effects (including allergy, anaphylaxis, and death). Because of recent programs to educate the primary care providers about the dangers of overuse of antibiotics, the inappropriate prescription of antibiotics for viral infections has decreased for many groups in the past few years. Research documents that elderly patients still seem to have a high rate of inappropriate prescription of antibiotics.

Despite pressures from the patient for quick relief, it is good practice to culture first and treat second. Culturing first provides results that direct definitive therapy with an antibiotic to which the organism is susceptible. If the patient is acutely ill, treat empirically until the results of the culture are available. Be sure to check the culture results to see if the organism is susceptible to the drug prescribed. If the site cannot be cultured, treat empirically and cover the likely pathogens. If treating empirically, be sure to check with the patient in 2 to 3 days to see if he or she is improving. Determine the most likely pathogen by assessing the location of the infection and the patient setting such as community, nursing care facility, or recent hospitalization.

Gram Positive versus Gram Negative

Identification of an organism as gram positive or gram negative helps the clinician move to the next critical decision in choosing an antibiotic that will be effective against the specific organism.

The Gram stain is a laboratory test used to divide bacteria into two groups, reflecting basic differences in the cell wall composition. Gram-positive bacteria retain the staining dye and appear deep violet on the microscopic slide. Gram-negative bacteria do not retain the dye and appear red on the slide. Gram-positive cell walls are low in lipids, whereas gram-negative cell walls are high in lipids. Many antibiotics exert their effect by action on cell walls, so the cell wall difference determines whether certain antibiotics will be effective.

Anaerobes are organisms that can grow without oxygen. This characteristic allows them to grow in necrotic tissue and poorly aerated portions of the respiratory tract. Mycobacteria have very tough cell walls and are difficult to kill. Yeasts are gram positive; rickettsiae are gram negative.

Sensitivity Testing

Throat, blood, urine, or other specimens may be sent to commercial laboratories for culture and sensitivity testing. The specimen sample is placed in a special culture medium so that the organism might grow and then be identified. Antibiotic effectiveness against an organism is determined through exposing the organism to various antibiotic disks placed in the culture medium. This is the second piece of critical information needed by the clinician to make an effective treatment decision.

In vitro sensitivity tests are standardized to reflect drug concentrations in plasma. They do not reflect concentrations that can be attained at the site of infection. They also do not take into account local factors that may affect the activity of the drug, for example, the pH.

Resistance to Antibiotics

It is very important for clinicians to pay attention to the organisms that are dominant in the community and to know their local pattern. Patterns of resistance differ from one community to the next, and change rapidly. Clinicians need to search for the patterns in their patient population. For example, children going to the same day care facility are likely to have the same organisms. Keep good patient records and review them. Think about the particular patient, his or her probable exposure, and what the patient's treatment behavior has been. Take every reasonable opportunity to culture and identify organisms. Monitor all culture results and talk to other providers about what type of infections they are seeing. Group practices have an advantage over solo practitioners in this capability.

Mechanisms of Resistance. There are four general mechanisms that are responsible for the development of antibiotic resistance.

1. Mutations occur in the gene encoding the target proteins so it no longer binds the drug. These are random events that confer a selective advantage to the bacteria. This mechanism does not require exposure to the particular drug. It can be either a single-step mutation conferring a high degree of resistance or a several-step mutation, each with a slight alteration in susceptibility. Examples of resistance through mutation include *Mycobacterium tuberculosis, Escherichia coli,* and *Staphylococcus aureus.*
2. Transduction occurs when a virus containing deoxyribonucleic acid (DNA) infects bacteria. The virus that infects the bacteria contains plasmids, bacterial DNA that contains genes for various functions, including one providing drug resistance. Incorporation of this plasmid makes the newly infected bacterial cell resistant and capable of passing on the trait of resistance. One plasmid carries the code for penicillinase. An example is *S. aureus.* Others contain codes for resistance to erythromycin, tetracycline, or chloramphenicol.
3. Transformation involves transferring DNA that is free in the environment into the bacteria. Penicillin resistance in pneumococci and *Neisseria* are examples.
4. Conjugation is transfer of DNA from one organism to another during mating. This occurs predominantly among gram-negative bacilli such as Enterobacteriaceae and *Shigella flexneri.*

DRUG ACTION AND EFFECTS

Antibiotics are classified as either bacteriostatic or bactericidal in action. The bacteriostatic agents inhibit growth; bactericidal agents kill the bacteria. The antibiotics provide these effects through different mechanisms of action. These include:

- Inhibition of cell wall synthesis such as the bactericidal penicillins, cephalosporins, β-lactam antibiotics, vancomycin, antifungal agents, and bacitracin.
- Direct action on the cell membrane to alter permeability and cause leakage of intracellular compounds, for example, bactericidal action of polymyxin and nystatin.
- Affecting function of ribosomal subunits to inhibit protein synthesis; examples are the bacteriostatic action of tetracycline, erythromycin, clindamycin, and chloramphenicol.
- Binding ribosome subunits to alter protein synthesis and cause cell death, for example, the bactericidal action of aminoglycosides.
- Changes in nucleic acid metabolism such as the bactericidal actions of rifampin, quinolones, or metronidazole.

- Blockage of specific essential metabolic steps by antimetabolites, for example, the bactericidal action of sulfonamides and trimethoprim.
- Inhibition of viral enzymes essential for DNA synthesis by nucleic acid analogs producing bacteriostatic activity.

DRUG TREATMENT PRINCIPLES

Cardinal to any discussion of infection is the emphasis on prevention. Knowledge of the pathogenesis of disease, including the microbiology underlying infectious disease, makes it clear that many infections may be prevented by good hygiene and improved sanitation. Health care providers and patients of all ages should practice the basic principles of washing hands after going to the bathroom and before eating or preparing foods, good personal hygiene, avoidance of polluted air and water, and eating balanced meals. Together these good health habits work to increase resistance to disease. Clinicians send a powerful message to patients when they wash their hands before and after performing any physical examination.

Prophylaxis

There are some occasions when prophylaxis is indicated. If a single effective nontoxic drug can be used to prevent an infection by a specific organism or to eradicate the organism immediately after it has been introduced, then prophylaxis may be successful. Prophylaxis is often not successful in preventing colonization or preventing infection by microorganisms present in the environment. An example of a traditionally used prophylaxis is for prevention of bacterial endocarditis by group A streptococci, but this procedure has been challenged in some studies. Treatment for a sexually transmitted disease after exposure is often effective. Attempts are being made to provide prophylaxis for human immunodeficiency virus (HIV) postexposure. Immunization when indicated and treatment after positive skin tests for tuberculosis are other examples of prophylaxis.

Prophylaxis of patients at increased risk of bacterial infection, such as those undergoing organ transplantation, cancer chemotherapy, and HIV treatment, is sometimes attempted. However, prophylactic treatment may kill off normal flora of the host and allow infection to occur with drug-resistant strains, defeating the purpose of the prophylaxis.

Selection of an Antibiotic

Choose the most effective, narrowest spectrum, lowest toxicity, lowest potential for allergy, least expensive single agent to decrease risk of resistance.

The idea for first-line therapy is to begin with a BB gun, not a shotgun or a cannon! Table 58-1 indicates common primary care problems and the antibiotics to which each organism is usually susceptible. Consider both drug characteristics and patient characteristics when choosing an antibiotic.

Drug Characteristics. All antibiotics alter the normal flora of the patient. Normal flora helps prevent overgrowth and infection by pathogenic bacteria. Change in this flora places the patient at risk for superinfection. The wider the spectrum of the antibiotic, the greater is the alteration in normal flora and the greater the risk of a superinfection. Choose the antibiotic with the narrowest spectrum that is effective against the organism causing the infection.

Certain antibiotics are more likely to produce allergic reactions than others. Patients with a history of atopic allergy seem particularly susceptible to the development of allergic reactions to antibiotics. The penicillins and sulfonamides are the most frequent causes of allergic reactions.

Certain viral infections increase the frequency of rash in response to penicillin. This often happens when amoxicillin is given to a patient with mononucleosis. This is not necessarily an allergic reaction. Antibiotics can also cause a drug fever that may be mistakenly blamed on the infection. It is important to differentiate the cause of the fever and discontinue the antibiotic if drug fever is suspected.

Toxic effects from antibiotics vary with the particular antibiotic. Antibiotics differ in frequency and severity of adverse reactions. When possible, choose the least toxic of the available alternatives. See individual drug chapters for the adverse reactions associated with each particular drug.

Consider the volume of distribution of the drug. Some antibiotics penetrate different sites of infection better than others. Antibiotics that are extensively plasma protein bound may not penetrate to infection sites as well. Lipid-soluble antibiotics will cross the blood-brain barrier. For example, for skin infections tetracyclines and fluoroquinolones are effective.

The liver metabolizes some antibiotics. The macrolides clarithromycin, erythromycin, and troleandomycin are inhibitors of the cytochrome P450 3A4 system. Clindamycin and erythromycin are substrates of the 3A4 system. It is important to check for drug interactions before prescribing multiple products. Alterations in dosage are often required if the patient has hepatic dysfunction.

The kidney is involved in elimination of most antibiotics. Monitor renal function and decrease dose if impaired. This is especially important when using aminoglycosides. All clinicians must know how to calculate creatinine clearance and how to reduce dosage in those patients with renal impairment.

Host Factors that Affect Selection of Antibiotic. In primary care it is usually not important whether the antibiotic is bacteriostatic or bactericidal. If the host is immunocompromised, a bactericidal antibiotic may be more effective than a bacteriostatic drug. This is particularly true in patients with AIDS.

Local factors such as pus, hemoglobin, pH, decreased oxygen, and presence of a foreign body (such as prosthetic valve) affect healing. These are variables the clinician must consider in evaluating the therapeutic regimen.

Research suggests that patient compliance decreases as the frequency of dosing increases. The clinician should not fail to make sure the patient is able to take the medication as directed.

Severity of illness is a factor in deciding how aggressively to treat the infection and how long to treat. If patients are unable to take the medication orally or drink enough fluids, they will probably need to be admitted to the hospital.

Concurrent illness is an important factor. Older patients tend to have more chronic illnesses. They are more susceptible to infection and harder to treat, generally requiring longer duration of treatment. Conditions that reduce circulation, such as diabetes or congestive heart failure, may limit delivery of the antibiotic to infected sites.

Location of the infection must also be considered. The antibiotic must reach the site of the infection. If the infection is in the brain, the antibiotic must pass the blood-brain barrier. A lipid-soluble drug may work better. Drugs that are extensively protein-bound may not penetrate tissue as well.

Administer Antibiotic According to Accepted Guidelines

Clinical guidelines have been developed for the treatment of many common infections. Many of these guidelines have been developed from analysis of valid research and scientific studies and issued by federal agencies or professional groups. Evidence-based research will validate and legitimize these guidelines over time. To practice in accordance with legally defensible standards, the clinician will be expected to be knowledgeable about the guidelines and to follow them. For example, when the Centers for Disease Control and Prevention (CDC) issue a guideline that says strep throats must be treated for 10 days, that is the standard of practice to which clinicians must adhere.

The half-life of the drug will determine the frequency of dosing. It is important to follow the appropriate dosing schedule to maintain the serum and tissue concentration of the antibiotic. The medication must be taken at regular intervals. The clinician should write a prescription describing precisely how the patient is to take the medication. For example, an antibiotic to be taken three times a day should be taken every 8 hours, not at each of the patient's three meals, so the clinician must be precise in writing the prescription. Stress the importance of not skipping doses.

Adequate hydration is mandatory, especially in respiratory infections or any febrile infection. Forcing fluids to 3 to 4 quarts of water per day is recommended for almost all patients to thin mucous secretions and prevent dehydration. Adequate nutrition is also important. A short course of high doses of vitamin C (2000 to 3000 mg/day) is helpful in reducing symptoms in some patients. Patients with asthma, COPD, or URIs should be encouraged to stop smoking.

How Long to Treat

Always establish a definite duration of treatment; do not begin an open-ended course. If necessary, a course of therapy can be extended if the patient evaluation indicates the need to continue beyond the originally defined period.

Whether to discontinue a course of antibiotics once started can be a difficult choice. If the culture shows the bacteria are resistant to the agent being used, it is clear the provider must discontinue the drug and substitute one to which the bacteria are susceptible. In general, providers should emphasize to their patients that it is important to complete a course of antibiotics even if the symptoms are gone. This is to completely eradicate the offending organism, not just the ones most susceptible to the antibiotic leaving resistant bacteria alive. On the other hand, the clinician should discontinue an antibiotic that was started based on empiric evidence if the culture is negative. Many providers are reluctant to do so for a variety of reasons.

Skin, eye, and vaginal infections can be treated by local application of medication. Drainage of the site, as in some sinus infections and empyema, is necessary. Abscesses usually need to be drained. Antibiotics do not replace local treatment such as incision and drainage.

Foreign objects often must be removed in order to control an associated infection.

The most important complication of antibiotic treatment is superinfection by an organism resistant to the antibiotic. This can be from bacteria, for example, in colitis caused by *Clostridium difficile*. Fungal infections can also be a problem. Women frequently get vaginal yeast infections when treated with an antibiotic.

Antibiotics are the most commonly prescribed group of medications in primary care. The primary care provider should have a good understanding of the general principles and be familiar with the use of the many classes of antiinfectives. The Chapter 59 discusses the infections most common in primary care. Subsequent chapters will discuss specific antiinfectives.

RESOURCES FOR PATIENTS AND PROVIDERS

Centers for Disease Control and Prevention, www.cdc,gov.
Major reporting and monitoring center for disease.

International Society for Infectious Diseases, www.isid.org.
Internet source for policy, trends, protocols.

National Flu Surveillance Network, www.fluwatch.com.
Federal monitoring system for clinicians to monitor flu prevalence.

National Foundation for Infectious Diseases, www.nfid.org.
National source for policy, trends, protocols.

Sanford JP, Gilbert DN, Moellering RC Jr, et al: *The Sanford Guide to Antimicrobial Therapy 2002*. Available from 800 Towers Crescent Drive, Suite 270, Vienna, VA 22182; (703) 847-4441 or 5910 N. Central Expressway, Suite 1955, Dallas, TX 75206; (214) 750-5783.

BIBLIOGRAPHY

Baddour LM, Groback SL: *Therapy of infectious diseases*, Philadelphia, 2003, Saunders.

Betts RF, Chapman SW, Penn RL: *Practical approach to infectious diseases*, ed 5, Philadelphia, 2002, Lippincott Williams & Wilkins.

Close W: *The Medical Letter: drugs and therapeutics handbook of antimicrobial therapy*, ed 16, New Rochelle, NY, 2002, The Medical Letter.

Conlon C, Pasvol G: *Color atlas and text of infectious diseases*, St Louis, 2000, Mosby.

Cunha BA: *Infectious disease pearls*, St Louis, 1998, Mosby.

Gates RH: *Infectious disease secrets*, St Louis, 1998, Mosby.

Gilbert DN, Moellering RC, Sande MA: The Sanford Guide to antimicrobial therapy, ed 33, Hyde Park, Ver., 2003, Antimicrobial Therapy, Inc.

Gorbach B, Bartlett M, Blacklow M: *Infectious diseases*, ed 2, Philadelphia, 1998, WB Saunders.

Mandel GL, Bennett JE, Dolin R, editors: *Principles and practice of infectious diseases*, ed 5, vols 1 and 2, New York, 2000, Churchill Livingstone.

Manian FA: *Mosby's curbside clinician: infectious diseases*, St Louis, 1998, Mosby.

Tierney LM, McPhee SJ, Papadakis MA: *Current medical diagnosis & treatment 2003*, ed 42, New York, 2002, McGraw-Hill/Appleton & Lange.

CHAPTER 59

Treatment of Specific Infections and Miscellaneous Antibiotics

Drug Names

Class	Subclass	Generic Name	Trade Name
Antibiotics	Lincosamide	(200) clindamycin	Cleocin
	Tricyclic glycopeptide	vancomycin	Vancocin
	Synthetic nitrofurantoin	(200) nitrofurantoin	Macrobid
Miscellaneous		fosfomycin (as tromethamine)	Monurol

(200), Top 200 drug.

General Uses

Because of all the information available about antibiotics, the student or beginning clinician may be overwhelmed by the choices. Table 59-1 serves as a general summary of common offending organisms for different infections. Both the first treatment choice and alternative treatment suggestions are listed, based on a compendium of various authorities.

Disease or site-specific infections are also discussed. These treatment guidelines include recommendations for both children and adults when available. These are general guidelines for simple infections, with no complicating factors. See specific drug information and check dosages before prescribing, especially for children.

Skin and Soft Tissue Infections

Impetigo

- Group A streptococci, *Staphylococcus aureus*, and group A β-hemolytic streptococci

Impetigo is a contagious infection of the skin common in children. The lesions are macules, vesicles, bullae, pustules, and honey-colored crusts, usually on the face and other exposed skin. Systemic antibiotics are usually required. However, mupirocin (Bactroban) can be used for topical treatment of mild impetigo.

Cellulitis

- Cellulitis, erysipelas, extremities: group A strep, occasionally group B, C, G; *S. aureus* (uncommon)
- Necrotizing fasciitis "flesh eating bacteria": group A, C, G strep, polymicrobic
- Diabetic: group A strep, *Staph. aureus*, Enterobacteriaceae, clostridia (rare)

Duration of treatment is usually until 3 days after resolution of inflammation.

Because the more common skin and soft tissue infections are caused by gram-positive streptococci and staphylococci, the appropriate penicillin or cephalosporin should be the first-line therapy. *Staph. aureus* remains a possibility and should be considered if first-line treatment is not successful. Culturing an open wound seldom produces useful information; usually the report comes back with multiorganisms. Site and how infection was acquired will often determine most likely causative organism.

Animal Bites

- Cat: *Pasteurella multocida, Staph. aureus*
- Dog: *P. multocida, S. aureus,* Bacteroides sp., *Fusobacterium*
- Human: *Strep. viridans, Staph. epidermidis, Corynebacterium, S. aureus, Eikenella,* Bacteroides sp., *Peptostreptococcus*

The location and type of the wound are important factors as well as the type of animal in determining treatment of the bite wound. Unprovoked animal bites should raise the suspicion of rabies. Cat bites are more likely to become infected than human or dog bites. Human bites by children are not likely to become infected; whereas bites by adults are more likely. Dog bites are very unlikely to become infected.

Infected Postoperative Wound

- *Staph. aureus,* group A streptococci, Enterobacteriaceae

Superficial infected wounds may be treated by primary care.

If the infection is deeper, the treatment will depend on the type of surgery.

Respiratory Tract Infections

By far, the most common causative agent is a virus, which causes an acute self-limiting disease that should not be treated with an antibiotic. Influenza is caused by a virus and can be treated by drugs listed in Chapter 70.

Otitis Media

- *Strep. pneumoniae, Haemophilus influenzae, Moraxella catarrhalis,* virus; group A strep; *Staph. aureus,* and Enterobacteriaceae (uncommon)

Duration of treatment is generally 10 days.

TABLE 59-1 Empiric Antimicrobial Treatment

Site of Infection	Usual Causes	First-Choice Treatment, Oral	Alternative Treatment
SKIN AND SOFT TISSUE			
Impetigo	*S. aureus* and group A strep	dicloxacillin or cloxacillin	mupirocin topical, azithromycin, clarithromycin, erythromycin, oral cephalosporin second-generation (cephalexin)
Cellulitis, extremities	Group A strep, occasionally group B, C, G	dicloxacillin	erythromycin, AM/CL azithromycin, clarithromycin
Cellulitis: diabetic	Group A strep, *S. aureus*, Enterobacteriaceae	AM/CL	IV
ANIMAL BITES			
Cat	*P. multocida, S. aureus*	AM/CL 875 mg bid or 500 mg tid	cefuroxime 500 mg q12hr, doxycycline 100 bid
Dog	*P. multocida, S. aureus, Bacteroides* sp., *Fusobacterium*	AM/CL 875 mg bid or 500 mg tid	Adults: clindamycin 300 mg qid and fluoroquinolone Children: clindamycin + TMP/SMX
Human	*Streptococcus viridans, Strep. epidermidis, Corynebacterium, Strep. aureus, Eikenella,* bacteroides	AM/CL 875 mg bid × 5 days	clindamycin + either ciprofloxacin or TMP/SMX
Infected postoperative wound	*S. aureus*, group A strep, Enterobacteriaceae	Oral cephalosporin, first-generation or AM/CL	dicloxacillin
RESPIRATORY			
Otitis media			
No antibiotics in past month	*S. pneumoniae, H. influenzae, M. catarrhalis*, group A strep, Enterobacteriaceae	amoxicillin	azithromycin, clarithromycin
Antibiotics in past month		amoxicillin, AM/CL, cefdinir, cefpodoxime, cefprozil, or cefuroxime	
Acute sinusitis			
No antibiotics in past month	*S. pneumoniae, H. influenzae, M. catarrhalis*	amoxicillin, AM/CL, cefdinir, cefpodoxime, cefuroxime × 10 days	clarithromycin, azithromycin, TMP/SMX, doxycycline, or fluoroquinolones
Antibiotics in past month		AM/CL or fluoroquinolones Q (adults) × 10 days	
Treatment failure		Mild to moderate: AM/CL + extra amoxicillin or cefpodoxime, cefuroxime, or cefdinir	Severe: gatifloxacin, levofloxacin, moxifloxacin
Pharyngitis	Group A, C, G strep, *C. diphtheriae, A. haemolyticum, M. pneumoniae*	penicillin V po × 10 days	erythromycin × 10 days, oral cephalosporin second-generation × 4-6 days, clindamycin or azithromycin × 5 days, clarithromycin × 10 days
Acute bacterial exacerbation of COPD	*S. pneumoniae, H. influenzae, M. catarrhalis*	Mild: no antibiotics Moderate: amoxicillin, doxycycline, (TMP/SMX), cephalosporin	Severe: AM/CL, azithromycin, clarithromycin, oral cephalosporin, fluoroquinolones with enhanced activity versus *S. pneumoniae*
PNEUMONIA			
Age 1-3 months	*C. trachomatis*, RSV virus, bordetella	erythromycin IV	
Age 1-24 months	*S. pneumoniae, H. influenzae*, chlamydia, mycoplasma	cefuroxime IV	
Age 3 months-5 years	*S. pneumoniae*, mycoplasma, chlamydia	erythromycin, clarithromycin, azithromycin	

TABLE 59-1 Empiric Antimicrobial Treatment—cont'd

Site of Infection	Usual Causes	First-Choice Treatment, Oral	Alternative Treatment
PNEUMONIA—cont'd			
Age 5-18 years	Mycoplasma, *S. pneumoniae*, *C. pneumoniae*	clarithromycin 500 bid, azithromycin	doxycycline, erythromycin
Age 18 and older	Mycoplasma, chlamydia, *S. pneumoniae*	azithromycin, clarithromycin	fluoroquinolone with enhanced activity versus *S. pneumoniae*, oral cephalosporin second-generation, AM/CL, doxycycline
GI INFECTIONS			
Mouth	Oral microflora infection, polymicrobial	clindamycin 300-450 mg q6hr	AM/CL 875 mg bid or 500 mg tid
Gastroenteritis	Usually viral; amebiasis, *L. monocytogenes*, *V. cholerae*	Culture, treat cause	
Diarrhea, traveler's	*E. coli*, shigella, salmonella, *Campylobacter*, *C. difficile*, amebiasis	Mild: ciprofloxacin 750 mg × 1 dose; severe: fluoroquinolone bid × 3 days	azithromycin usual dose, or 1000 mg × 1 dose
Diarrhea, severe	Shigella, salmonella, *C. jejuni*, *E. coli* 0157 H7, *E. histolytica*	fluoroquinolone (Cipro) 500 mg q12hr × 3-5 days	TMP/SMX bid (resistance common)
	C. difficile	metronidazole 500 mg tid × 10-14 days	Vancomycin 125 mg qid po × 10-14 d
Diverticulitis	Enterobacteriaceae, *P. aeruginosa*, *Bacteroides* sp., enterococci	TMP/SMX bid or ciprofloxacin 500 mg bid + metronidazole 500 mg q6hr × 7-10 days	AM/CL 500 mg tid po × 7-10 days
RENAL/GU			
UTI	*E. coli*, *S. saprophyticus*, enterococci	fluoroquinolone × 3 days	TMP/SMX, oral cephalosporin, doxycycline, AM/CL
Pyelonephritis	*E. coli*, *S. saprophyticus*, enterococci	fluoroquinolone × 7 days	AM/CL, oral cephalosporin, TMP/SMX DS
PROSTATITIS			
Younger than 35 years	*N. gonorrhoeae* or *C. trachomatis*	See STDs; ofloxacin, ceftriaxone then doxycycline	
Older than 35 years	Enterobacteriaceae	fluoroquinolone, TMP/SMX DS	
STDs			
Gonorrhea	*N. gonorrhoeae*	cefixime 400 mg × 1 dose, ceftriaxone 125 mg IM × 1 dose, ciprofloxacin 500 mg × 1 dose ofloxacin 400 mg × 1 dose, levofloxacin 250 mg × 1 dose	spectinomycin 2 g IM × 1 dose, ceftizoxime 500 mg IM, cefoxitin 2 mg IM with probenecid 1 g po, cefotaxime 500 mg IM, gatifloxacin 400 mg, norfloxacin 800 po, lomefloxacin 400 mg × 1 dose
Ophthalmia neonatorum	Prophylaxis for *N. gonorrhoeae*	silver nitrate (1%) aqueous solution × 1 dose, erythromycin (0.5%) ophthalmic ointment × 1 dose, tetracycline ophthalmic ointment (1%) × 1 dose	
Syphilis	*T. pallidum*	benzathine penicillin G 2.4 million units IM × 1 dose	
Chlamydia	*C. trachomatis*	azithromycin 1 g × 1 dose; doxycycline 100 mg bid × 7 days	erythromycin base 500 mg qid × 7 days, ofloxacin 300 mg bid × 7 days, levofloxacin 500 mg qd × 7 days
FEMALE REPRODUCTIVE			
Mastitis	*S. pneumoniae*, *S. pyogenes*, *S. aureus*, *H. influenzae*, *P. aeruginosa*	dicloxacillin 500 mg q6hr	clindamycin 300 mg q6hr

Continued

TABLE 59-1 Empiric Antimicrobial Treatment—cont'd

Site of Infection	Usual Causes	First-Choice Treatment, Oral	Alternative Treatment
SYSTEMIC FEBRILE			
Lyme disease	*B. burgdorferi*	doxycycline 100 mg bid × 10 days; or amoxicillin 500 mg tid, cefuroxime 500 mg bid, × 14-21 days	erythromycin 250 mg qid
Rocky Mountain spotted fever	*R. rickettsii*	doxycycline 100 mg po bid × 7days	chloramphenicol 500 mg qid po or IV × 7days

AM/CL, Augmentin; *S. pneumo*, Streptococcus pneumoniae.
Fluoroquinolones with enhanced activity versus *S. pneumo*: gatifloxacin, levofloxacin, or moxifloxacin.

Signs and symptoms that indicate a need for antibiotic treatment include otalgia, fever, otorrhea, or a bulging yellow or red tympanic membrane. Simple effusion (presence of fluid in the middle ear with no signs or symptoms of acute infection) does not need to be treated with antibiotics. Patients with tympanic membrane perforation, chronic or recurrent infections, or craniofacial abnormalities, or immunocompromised patients should be referred. There are Agency for Health Care Policy and Research (AHCPR) guidelines on treatment of otitis media. How recently the patient has been treated with antibiotics will affect the antibiotic choice.

Sinusitis

- Sinusitis, acute: *Staph. pneumoniae, H. influenzae, M. catarrhalis*
- Sinusitis, chronic: anaerobic bacteria often present (Bacteroides sp., Peptostreptococcus, *Fusobacterium*)

Duration of treatment is usually 10 to 14 days.

Less frequent bacteria include group A strep, anaerobes, *Staph. aureus, Strep.* sp., *Neisseria* sp., and gram-negative rods. This infection has a very similar pattern to that of otitis media with perhaps more unusual bacteria seen. Most sinus infections are viral. The common cold frequently involves the sinuses. Evidence of bacterial infection include prolonged symptoms without improvement for 10 to 14 days or longer, fever higher than 102° F (39° C), unilateral pain, sinus tenderness, or tooth pain. Nasal discharge is not a reliable indicator of bacterial sinusitis. Viral upper respiratory infections (URIs) may have the nasal discharge change from clear to yellow during the first few days of the infection. Suspect a bacterial infection if the discharge changes to green. If the patient starts to improve then worsens, this may indicate a secondary bacterial infection.

Unfortunately younger children may not present with the classic signs or symptoms of sinusitis. Congestion and cough lasting for more than 10 days, high fever, and purulent nasal discharge are the most likely symptoms.

Because the causative organisms are similar to otitis media, treatment will be very similar. Nonantibiotic therapy of sinusitis is not well researched. Decongestants and mucolytics may improve drainage. Nonpharmacologic remedies such as drinking hot fluids, applying moist heat, inhaling steam, and saltwater nasal spray or rinses may decrease congestion.

Pharyngitis

- Pharyngitis: Group A, C, G strep, *C. diphtheria, A. haemolyticum*, and *Mycoplasma pneumoniae*

Duration of therapy is at least 10 days.

Once again, virus (including mononucleosis) causes the majority of cases of pharyngitis. The classic infection to be treated with antibiotics is group A β-hemolytic streptococci. It is impossible to accurately diagnose a bacterial pharyngitis by history and physical alone. A throat culture is necessary. Symptoms such as pharyngeal pain, dysphagia, fever, tonsillar exudate, and lymphadenopathy with absence of cough increase the likelihood of a diagnosis of strep, but still only approximately one half of the patients with these characteristics will have strep throat upon culture.

Because of the diagnostic vagueness, the provider has the option of waiting 2 days for the culture results or treating empirically. Immediate empirical treatment is tempting because of symptom relief and decreased transmission, but will result in substantial overtreatment. To avoid this dilemma, a rapid antigen detection test can be used. If used carefully, these tests can be very accurate. If the rapid test is positive, initiate antibiotic treatment. If it is negative, await culture results before initiating antibiotic treatment.

Bronchitis

- Infants/children (<5): virus
- Adolescents and adults: virus, *M. pneumoniae, Chlamydia pneumoniae, Bordetella pertussis*

Bronchitis is a poorly defined illness, involving a cough. A virus causes almost all cases of bronchitis. Rarely, a child older than 5 years will have bronchitis caused by *M. pneumoniae* or *C. pneumoniae*. If the child does not get better in 10 to 14 days, consider treatment with a macrolide.

Acute Bacterial Exacerbation of COPD

- *Strep. pneumoniae, H. influenzae, M. catarrhalis*
- Mycoplasma or chlamydia (rare)

Many acute exacerbations of COPD are viral. The patient may have any one of a wide variety of bacteria, depending on previous hospitalizations, etc. These patients are likely to be frail, to have a history of smoking, and to have been previously treated with many antibiotics. A sputum culture may be difficult to obtain but will be very useful. Obtaining a sputum sample after a nebulization treatment may be necessary. Try to get the patient to stop smoking.

Community-Acquired Pneumonia (CAP)

- Ages 1 to 3 months: *Chlamydia trachomatis*, respiratory syncytial virus (RSV), virus, *Bordetella*
- Ages 1 to 24 months: RSV, viruses, *Strep. pneumoniae*, *H. influenzae*, chlamydia, mycoplasma, *Staph. aureus* (rare)
- Ages 3 months to 5 years: viruses, *Strep. pneumoniae*, mycoplasma, chlamydia
- Ages 5 to 18 years: Mycoplasma, respiratory viruses, consider S. *pneumoniae*, *C. pneumoniae*
- Age 18 and older
- No comorbidity: Mycoplasma, chlamydia, *S. pneumoniae*, viral
- Smokers: *Strep. pneumoniae, H. influenzae, M. catarrhalis*
- Postviral: *Strep. pneumoniae*, rarely *S. aureus*
- Alcoholic: *Strep. pneumoniae*, anaerobes, coliforms
- Epidemic: Legionnaire' s disease

Duration of treatment is until afebrile for at least 5 days for pneumococcal pneumonia. Pneumonia caused by Enterobacteriaceae, *Pseudomonas*, or *Staphylococcus* is treated 21 to 28 days.

Because so many different bacteria can cause pneumonia, determining empiric treatment can be problematic. Mycoplasma or chlamydial infections are common, and a macrolide is recommended. However, penicillin-resistant pneumococci occur regularly and may be resistant to a macrolide or doxycycline. Frail elderly patients may need to be treated with one of the fluoroquinolones.

Tuberculosis. See Chapter 67.

Cardiovascular Infections

Prophylaxis of Infective Endocarditis

- Endocarditis is most frequently caused by streptococcus viridans, other *Streptococcus* spp., enterococci, staphylococci
- Oral medications are given 1 hour before procedure
- IM or IV medications are given within 30 minutes before procedure

Prophylactic Regimens for Dental, Oral, Respiratory Tract, or Esophageal Procedures

- Standard treatment: amoxicillin: adult, 2 g; child, 50 mg/kg/po
- Unable to take oral medication: ampicillin: adult, 2 g IM or IV; child, 50 mg/kg IM or IV
- Allergy to
  penicillin: clindamycin: adult, 600 mg; child, 20 mg/kg po
  cephalexin or cefadroxil: adult, 2 g; child, 50 mg/kg 1 hour before procedure
  azithromycin or clarithromycin: adult, 500 mg; child, 15 mg/kg po
  penicillin and unable to take oral medication: clindamycin: adult, 600 mg; child, 20 mg/kg

GI Infections

Mouth

- *Strep. mutans*, other *Strep* spp., *Actinomyces* spp.
- Oral microflora, infection often polymicrobial

Duration of treatment is 2 to 3 weeks.

Mouth infections can be caused by a large variety of bacteria. Because uncontaminated cultures are hard to obtain, treatment with a broad-spectrum agent is often necessary.

Gastroenteritis

- Mild: virus, bacterial (see below), parasitic

Most diarrhea is viral in cause, not severe, and self-limiting.

Traveler's Diarrhea

- Traveler's diarrhea
- Acute: *E. coli, Shigella, Salmonella, Campylobacter, C. difficile*, amebiasis
- Chronic: *Cyclospora, Cryptosporidium, Giardia, Isospora*

Duration of treatment is usually 3 days.

If the patient is traveling to an area with endemic infections and may be unable to adequately observe safety precautions (bottled water, etc.), a course of antibiotics may be provided so that the patient is able to initiate treatment immediately upon onset of symptoms. Treatment may also include loperamide and/or Pepto-Bismol.

Severe Diarrhea

- Diarrhea, severe: *Shigella, Salmonella, C. jejuni, E. coli* 0157 H7, *C. difficile, Entamoeba histolytica*, many others.

Duration of treatment is 7 to 14 days.

Symptoms of severe diarrhea include more than six liquid stools per day, temperature greater than 101° F, tenesmus, blood, or fecal leukocytes. These patients always require a culture. Treatment is based on culture results.

C. difficile is often a consequence of treatment with antibiotics, especially the wide-spectrum products. *C. difficile* is usually associated with copious liquid diarrhea. It can be less than acute in onset and moderate in amount of liquid stool produced. Suspect *C. difficile* in any patient who develops diarrhea after taking an antibiotic. Onset of symptoms can be delayed for weeks after treatment with the antibiotic. Treatment of C. *difficile* is either metronidazole or oral vancomycin for 14 days. Vancomycin and metronidazole are discussed in detail at the end of this chapter.

Diverticulitis

- Diverticulitis: Enterobacteriaceae, *P. aeruginosa, Bacteroides* sp., enterococci

Duration of treatment is until patient is afebrile for 3 days.

Diverticulosis is a common problem in the elderly, not requiring antibiotics. Diverticulitis symptoms include acute abdominal pain and fever, lower left abdominal tenderness and mass, and leukocytosis. There is a wide range of severity from mild to severe disease. Treatment requires a broad-spectrum oral antibiotic with anaerobic activity.

Peptic Ulcer Disease. *H. pylori* is implicated in many cases of peptic ulcer disease. See Chapter 32 for treatment regimens.

Renal/Genitourinary Infections

Urinary Tract Infections (UTIs)

- UTI: *E. coli, Staph. saprophyticus*, enterococci, and many others
- Pyelonephritis: same

Duration of treatment of uncomplicated UTI is generally 3 to 10 days. In general, single-dose treatments are less effective.

Duration of treatment of pyelonephritis is at least 14 days.

Most resources state that a urine culture is not necessary for the management of a simple UTI. An acute uncomplicated UTI can be treated empirically. A patient who has been in the hospital or had previous UTIs may have any one of a large number of bacteria, including *P. aeruginosa*.

For many patients, particularly the elderly, treatment is more accurately determined with urine for culture and urinalysis before treatment is initiated. The urinalysis validates culture results or shows if the specimen was contaminated. A dipstick urinalysis will confirm the presence of a UTI, but it does not provide information about susceptibility. The culture confirms the organism and its sensitivity.

If patients have symptoms making them uncomfortable, treat with phenazopyridine (Pyridium) or treat empirically pending culture results. If the patient' s symptoms are not a problem, waiting for culture results allows the clinician to put the patient on a narrow-spectrum yet effective medication.

Prostatitis

- Prostatitis in men younger than 35 years: *Neisseria gonorrhoeae* or *C. trachomatis*.

See treatment of sexually transmitted diseases (STDs) for the treatment of these organisms.

Prostatitis in older men is likely to be caused by Enterobacteriaceae. Other possible organisms are enterococci or *P. aeruginosa*.

Duration of treatment of chronic prostatitis is 1 month.

Sexually Transmitted Diseases (STDs)

Patterns of resistance to STDs are rapidly changing, and treatment recommendations change frequently. Check with the most recent Centers for Disease Control and Prevention (CDC) or state resources before treating. The local health department is a good source of information on local patterns of resistance and effective treatments.

Many patients who present with one STD will have other concomitant STDs. When diagnosed with gonorrhea or urethritis/cervicitis, treat for both *N. gonorrhoeae* and Chlamydia. Concurrent treatment covering syphilis should also be considered.

Gonorrhea

- Gonorrhea: *N. gonorrhoeae*

Men present with urethritis with mucopurulent or purulent discharge. Women present with mucopurulent cervicitis. Newborn infants can get a gonococcal infection in their eyes. Because this can cause blindness, most states require treatment. Laboratory testing is Gram stain of secretions and culture.

Surveillance for antimicrobial resistance is crucial for guiding therapy recommendations. Treatment recommendations change rapidly; make sure you have up-to-date recommendations.

Quinolone-resistant *N. gonorrhoeae* (QRNG) is common in parts of Asia and the Pacific and has spread to the West Coast. Quinolones are no longer recommended for treatment of gonorrhea in Hawaii or of infections acquired in Asia or the Pacific. Use of quinolones for treatment of gonorrhea in California is inadvisable.

For ophthalmia neonatorum, one of the recommended preparations should be instilled into both eyes of every neonate as soon as possible after delivery. It is not known if this prevents chlamydial ophthalmia.

Syphilis

- Syphilis: *Treponema pallidum*

Syphilis is a systemic disease. Primary infection consists of ulcer or chancre at the infection site. Secondary infection includes skin rash, mucocutaneous lesions, and lymphadenopathy. Tertiary infection syphilis consists of cardiac, ophthalmic, and auditory abnormalities and gummatous lesions. Latent syphilis lacks clinical manifestations. Darkfield examinations and direct fluorescent antibody tests of lesion exudate or tissue are the definitive methods for diagnosing early syphilis. Parenteral penicillin remains the preferred drug for treatment of all stages of syphilis.

Chlamydia

- Chlamydial genital infection, lymphogranuloma venereum, ophthalmia neonatorum, infant pneumonia: *C. trachomatis*

Men present with urethritis with mucopurulent or purulent discharge. Women present with mucopurulent cervicitis. Untreated chlamydial infections can result in pelvic inflammatory disease, ectopic pregnancy, and infertility. Because treatment of chlamydia (doxycycline) costs less than the diagnostic testing, many providers treat patients diagnosed with gonorrhea for chlamydia without testing.

Lymphogranuloma venereum is caused by *C. trachomatis* serovars L1, L2, or L3. It occurs rarely in the United States. It causes genital ulcers with unilateral tender inguinal and/or femoral lymphadenopathy.

Other

- Chancroid: *Haemophilus ducreyi*

Criteria for diagnosis are clinical picture of one or more painful genital ulcers with regional inguinal lymphadenopathy, and there must be no evidence of *T. pallidum* or herpes simplex virus (HSV) by standard laboratory tests.

- Granuloma inguinale (donovanosis): *Calymmatobacterium granulomatis*

Rare in the United States, it is common in certain tropical and developing areas. It presents as painless, progressive ulcerative lesions without regional lymphadenopathy. The ulcers bleed easily on contact.

- Virus: HIV, herpes simples, human papillomavirus (HPV), condyloma acuminatum

See Chapter 70 for discussion of treatment of viral disease.

Female Reproductive Infections

Mastitis

- Acute outpatient: *S. aureus, S. pneumoniae, S. pyogenes, H. influenzae, P. aeruginosa*

Mastitis usually begins with 3 months of delivery; it may start with a sore nipple. Symptoms of cellulitis will be obvious. Apply cold compresses.

Vaginitis

- Candidiasis: *Candida albicans*
- Trichomoniasis: *Trichomonas vaginalis*
- Bacterial vaginosis: *Gardnerella, Bacteroides,* others

See Chapter 57 for more information.

Musculoskeletal Infections

Gangrene

- Gas gangrene: *Clostridium perfringens,* Clostridium spp.

This infection generally occurs in tissue that is not adequately perfused. The onset is sudden with pain, decreased blood pressure, tachycardia, and fever. It can be rapidly fatal and should be treated in the hospital with IV antibiotics.

Septic Arthritis

- Children: *S. aureus, S. pyogenes, S. pneumoniae, H. influenzae,* gram-negative bacteria
- Adult, sexually active: *N. gonorrhoeae*
- Adult, not sexually active: *S. aureus,* streptococci, gram-negative bacilli

It is important to aspirate the joint to obtain a culture and sensitivity. The joint often needs local aspiration, sometimes daily. In general these infections should be treated by a specialist.

Osteomyelitis

- Osteomyelitis: *S. aureus*, gram-negative bacilli, group B streptococcus

Patients should be referred to an infectious disease specialist and an orthopedic surgeon if osteomyelitis is suspected. Blood and infected bone should be cultured. Intravenous antibiotics are required, especially for initial treatment. Occasionally chronic osteomyelitis treatment will be completed orally in the outpatient setting. The offending organism is most commonly *S. aureus*.

Infections of the Central Nervous System

Meningitis

- Age less than 1 month: Group B streptococcus, *E. coli, Listeria*, miscellaneous gram negative, miscellaneous gram positive
- Ages 1 month to 50 years: *S. pneumoniae*, meningococci, *H. influenzae* (rare)
- Age older than 50 years: S. *pneumoniae, Listeria*, gram-negative bacilli, no meningococcus

Patients should be hospitalized for treatment.

Systemic Febrile Syndrome

There are many causes of systemic febrile syndrome. Rickettsial diseases include typhus, Rocky Mountain spotted fever (RMSF), ehrlichiosis, and Q fever. Only Lyme disease and Rocky Mountain spotted fever are discussed here.

Lyme Disease. Lyme disease is caused by the spirochete *Borrelia burgdorferi* and transmitted to humans by ticks. The tick must feed for 24 hours or longer in order to transmit the disease. Shortly after the bite the patient may experience erythema migrans and central nervous system and musculoskeletal symptoms. Confirm the diagnosis by serologic testing.

Rocky Mountain Spotted Fever. RMSF is caused by *Rickettsia rickettsii* and is transmitted by the bite of wood and dog ticks. It occurs most commonly in the middle and southern Atlantic states and in the central Mississippi valley. Symptoms include an influenza-like prodrome, followed by fever, chills, headache, myalgias, and restlessness. A red macular rash appears on the wrists and ankles and spreads centrally. It appears between the second and sixth days of the fever. Onset is 2 to 14 days after the tick bite.

PATIENT VARIABLES

Geriatrics

Geriatric patients are at considerably increased risk of infection, and the infections are often more serious. Because of their low body mass, they may need a lower dose. They are particularly susceptible to the toxic effects of aminoglycosides.

Pediatrics

Infants are at increased risk for infection until their immune system is more mature. They are also at greater risk for toxicity until their renal and hepatic function is adequate. Tetracyclines bind to teeth and discolor tooth enamel if given when the teeth are developing and can result in retardation of bone growth. Fluoroquinolones affect growth of cartilage in developing bone.

Use caution to ensure an overweight child does not receive an overdose of antibiotics.

Children younger than 12 usually need more frequent dosing with shorter dosing intervals because of increased metabolism and clearance.

Pregnancy/Lactation

Many antibiotics are contraindicated in pregnancy. Pregnancy will affect the pharmacokinetics of antibiotics. Most antibiotics are passed into the breast milk.

Gender

Certain antibiotics interact with oral contraceptive pills. Use alternative method of contraception.

Women are at risk for vaginal yeast infections when treated with an antibiotic.

HOW TO MONITOR

- Check culture to make sure growth is susceptible to the antibiotic chosen.
- Resolution of infection varies with severity of illness but should start to improve in 2 to 3 days. Continued elevation of temperature of the patient may indicate lack of efficacy or drug fever.
- Consider monitoring the WBC count in a moderately ill patient.

PATIENT EDUCATION

- Take all of the medication even if condition improves.
- Call the provider if there is no improvement within 2 to 3 days.
- Warn of most common side effects of the specific antibiotic. Caution patients about adverse effects such as yeast infection and pseudomembranous enterocolitis (*C. difficile* infection).

- Stop the medication if allergic reaction occurs, and notify provider.
- Most antibiotics should be taken on an empty stomach, with a full glass of water 1 hour before or 2 hours after eating.
- Lemon yogurt, other citrus flavors, or chocolate masks the bitter flavor of many medications. Gum can be used to mask aftertaste.
- Certain antibiotics may interfere with the effectiveness of oral contraceptives. Use alternative contraception method during the month in which antibiotics are taken.
- Be specific about when the patient should take the medication. Evenly spaced dose intake should be emphasized to maintain therapeutic blood levels.
- Prescriptions for antibiotics should never be shared with others or kept and taken for another occasion of illness.
- Daily ingestion of yogurt with active cultures or acidophilus may help prevent some of the diarrheal effects of certain antibiotics and may also decrease overgrowth of yeast infections.
- Report to the provider if they are not getting better within a few days of administration of antibiotic.
- Report any rash, fever, chills, or if any other sensitivity to the drug develops.

Specific Drugs

clindamycin (Cleocin)

Indications. Reserve this drug for serious infections when less toxic antimicrobial agents are inappropriate. Used for serious infections caused by susceptible strains of streptococci, pneumococci, and staphylococci.

In primary care, clindamycin is combined with tretinoin gel formulations and is used in the topical treatment of noninflammatory and inflammatory lesions of acne vulgaris. The addition of clindamycin to tretinoin enhances the comedolytic efficacy of tretinoin in moderate to severe acne of the face, maintaining at the same time its antiinflammatory efficacy, thus accelerating resolution of all types of acne lesions without affecting the safety of response to both components.

Mechanism of Action. Clindamycin binds exclusively to the 50S subunit of bacterial ribosomes and suppresses protein synthesis.

Warnings
- Can cause severe and possibly fatal colitis. Symptoms include severe persistent diarrhea, severe abdominal cramps, and passage of blood and mucus. May be aggravated by antiperistaltic agents.
- Reserve for serious infections where less toxic antimicrobial agents are inappropriate.
- Hypersensitivity reactions: use with caution in patients with a history of asthma or significant allergies.
- Renal/hepatic function impairment: use with caution in patients with severe renal or hepatic disease accompanied by metabolic aberrations. Monitor serum clindamycin levels during high-dose therapy.

Precautions
- Monitor liver/kidney function, blood counts with prolonged therapy
- Use caution with patients with GI disease, particularly colitis
- Superinfection is a risk

Adverse Effects
- Cardiovascular: hypotension
- GI: diarrhea (2% to 20%), pseudomembranous colitis (0.01% to 10%), nausea, vomiting, abdominal pain, esophagitis, glossitis, stomatitis
- Hematologic: neutropenia, leukopenia, agranulocytosis, thrombocytopenic purpura, aplastic anemia
- Hepatic: Increased transaminases
- Renal: dysfunction characterized by azotemia, oliguria, and proteinuria

Dosage and Administration
- May be taken without regard to meals
- Take each dose with a full glass of water

Patient Variables

Geriatrics. Older patients may not tolerate the diarrhea; monitor carefully.

Pediatrics. Use with caution.

Pregnancy. *Category B:* safety has not been established. Appears in breast milk. The American Academy of Pediatrics considers clindamycin to be compatible with breast-feeding.

vancomycin (Vancocin)

Indications. Vancomycin IV is most often used in serious or life-threatening staphylococcal or streptococcal infections. There has been a substantial increase in the colonization of vancomycin-resistant enterococci. Many hospitals are now restricting the use of the drug unless prescribed under strict guidelines and approved by a pharmacist.

The primary care use of vancomycin is for pseudomembranous colitis caused by *C. difficile.* It is given in oral form when treatment by metronidazole is contraindicated or ineffective. Metronidazole is preferred because of the high cost of vancomycin and the increase in the incidence of vancomycin-resistant enterococcal infections. However, vancomycin remains the drug of choice for severe cases of *C. difficile.*

Mechanism of Action. It works by preventing synthesis of the bacterial cell wall by blocking peptidoglycan strand formation.

Warnings
- Ototoxicity has occurred; may be permanent.
- Hypotension, reversible neutropenia, nephrotoxicity, and renal failure are among the warnings. Must be monitored closely.
- The "red man" syndrome may be stimulated by too rapid IV infusion. It is not an allergic reaction. It is characterized by

a sudden and profound fall in blood pressure with or without a maculopapular rash over the face, neck, upper chest, and extremities.

Adverse Effects
- Anaphylaxis, drug fever, nausea

Dosage and Administration
- Give 500 mg to 2 g/day po in three or four divided doses for 7 to 10 days.
- Alternately give 125 mg po three or four times daily for 7 to 10 days.

nitrofurantoin (Macrobid, Macrodontic, generic)

Indications. Used in treating UTIs caused by susceptible strains of *E. coli*, enterococci, *S. aureus*, and some strains of *Klebsiella* and *Enterobacter* spp. Least expensive antibiotic.

Contraindications
- Renal function impairment
- Pregnancy

Warnings/Precautions
- Pulmonary reactions may be seen with acute, sudden onset of dyspnea, chest pain, cough, fever, and chills. More chronic pulmonary reactions may be associated with prolonged therapy.
- Hemolytic anemia may be induced.
- Hepatic reactions, including hepatitis and cholestatic jaundice, occur rarely with fatalities.

Adverse Effects
- Peripheral neuropathy may occur and may be severe or irreversible.
- Superinfection may occur.
- Most common problems are anorexia, nausea, and emesis.

Drug Interactions
- Anticholinergics increase nitrofurantoin bioavailability.
- Magnesium salts decrease absorption of nitrofurantoin.
- Uricosurics such as probenecid increase serum levels of nitrofurantoin.

Patient Education
- May cause GI upset; take with food or milk
- May cause brown discoloration of the urine
- Notify health care provider if patient develops fever, chills, cough, chest pain, difficult breathing, skin rash, or numbness or tingling of the fingers or toes, or if intolerable GI upset occurs

Dosage and Administration
- Adult: 50 to 100 mg qid for 7 to 10 days
- Children: 5 to 7 mg/kg/day in single or two divided doses

Patient Variables

Pediatrics. Contraindicated in infants less than 1 month of age.

Pregnancy. *Category B.*

Lactation. Product is excreted in milk.

fosfomycin (Monurol)

Indications. Used in treatment of UTIs.

Adverse Effects. Main adverse effects are diarrhea, nausea, dyspepsia, vaginitis, headache, dizziness, and asthenia.

Drug Interactions. Serum level may be lowered by drugs that increase GI motility, such as metoclopramide.

Dosage and Administration. Mix 3-g packet with 3 to 4 oz cold water and drink immediately. One dose per episode of UTI.

Patient Variables

Pediatrics. Contraindicated in children.

Pregnancy. *Category B.*

Lactation. Concurrent use not recommended.

RESOURCES FOR PATIENTS AND PROVIDERS

Centers for Disease Control and Prevention (CDC), www.cdc.gov.
Provides multiple types of information such as prevention guidelines online and Morbidity and Mortality Weekly Report.

Mediconsult, www.mediconsult.com.
This site is designed primarily for patients. It offers a variety of options for individuals to choose from. Site devoted to information concerning STDs.

World Health Organization, www.who.int.
Provides information of infectious disease and advice for travelers.

BIBLIOGRAPHY

AHCPR: *Otitis media with effusion, clinical practice guideline* (SN 017-026-00116-6), Springfield, VA, 1997, NTIS.

Centers for Disease Control and Prevention. Sexually transmitted diseases treatment guidelines. *MMWR Morb Mortal Wkly Rep,* 51(No. RR-6), 2002. Available on line through www.guidelines.gov.

Close W: *The Medical Letter: drugs and therapeutics handbook of antimicrobial therapy*, ed 16, New Rochelle, NY, 2002, The Medical Letter.

Conlon C, Pasvol G: *Color atlas and text of infectious diseases,* St Louis, 2000, Mosby.

Gilbert DN et al: The Sanford guide to antimicrobial therapy, ed 33, 2003.

Rennie RP, Jones RN, Mutnick AH: Occurrence and antimicrobial susceptibility patterns of pathogens isolated from skin and soft tissue infections: report from the SENTRY Antimicrobial Surveillance Program (United States and Canada, 2000), *Diagn Microbiol Infect Dis* 45(4):287-293, 2003.

Wormser GP et al: Duration of antibiotic therapy for early Lyme disease, *Ann Intern Med* 138(9):697-704, 2003.

CHAPTER 60

Penicillins

Drug Names

Class	Subclass	Generic Name	Trade Name
Penicillins	Natural penicillins	penicillin G	Crysticillin AS
	(P)(200)	penicillin VK	Veetids, Pen-Vee K
Penicillinase-resistant penicillins		cloxacillin	Tegopen, Cloxapen
		dicloxacillin	Dynapen, Dicloxacil
		nafcillin	Unipen, Nafcil
		oxacillin	Prostaphlin, Bactocill
Aminopenicillins		ampicillin	Omnipen, Ampican, Polycillin
	(200)	amoxicillin	Amoxil, Polymox, Trimox, etc
		bacampicillin	Spectrobid
	(200)	amoxicillin and potassium clavulanate (AM/CL)	Augmentin
		ampicillin/sulbactam	Unasyn
Extended-spectrum penicillins		carbenicillin	Geocillin
		mezlocillin	Mezlin
		piperacillin	Pipracil
		piperacillin sodium and tazobactam sodium	Zosyn
		ticarcillin	Ticar
		ticarcillin/potassium clavulanate	Timentin

(200), Top 200 drug; (P), prototype drug.

General Uses

Indications

See Table 60-1 for specific indications.

- Otitis media
- Streptococcal pharyngitis
- Sinusitis
- Pneumococcal pneumonia
- Animal bite
- Impetigo
- Syphilis
- Gonorrhea
- Bacterial endocarditis prophylaxis

• • •

Penicillins remain an extremely important class of antibiotics. The different penicillins are active against a large number of infectious diseases. They are generally indicated in the treatment of mild to moderately severe infections caused by penicillin-sensitive microorganisms. They are extensively used for empiric therapy as well therapy determined by culture. This chapter focuses on the outpatient use of oral penicillins. The extended-spectrum penicillins are generally given IV in a hospital setting and are not discussed.

Sir Alexander Fleming, a British scientist, discovered penicillin in 1928 and the medicine has been available since the 1940s. The different penicillins have different antimicrobial activity. Microbial resistance to the penicillins is a major limitation to their use. Penicillinase resistance is now common. Methicillin-resistant *Staphylococcus aureus* (MRSA) is now resistant to most antibiotics and is very difficult to treat. Methicillin is no longer marketed in the United States because of resistance and toxicity.

DRUG ACTION AND EFFECTS

Penicillin is a derivative of 6-aminopenicillanic acid. It is composed of a distinct four-membered β-lactam ring fused to a five-membered thiazolidine ring that comprises the chemical structure. Penicillin subclasses have additional chemical constituents that bestow differences in antimicrobial activity, susceptibility to acid, enzyme hydrolysis, and biodisposition. Many biosynthetic types of penicillin have been created through the introduction of diverse acids, amines, or amides in developing penicillin molds in order to render products superior to the natural penicillins.

Penicillins are bactericidal against susceptible organisms. Penicillins disrupt synthesis of the bacterial cell wall and

TABLE 60-1 Penicillin Indications with Dosage and Administration

Drug	Bacteria	Site/Disease	Dosage (mg Oral Except Penicillin G)
penicillin G IM	*Pneumococcus, Staphylococcus*	Moderate to severe URIs, skin, soft tissue	Adult: 600,000-1 million U/day Child (<60 lb): 300,000 U/day
	Group A streptococcus	Tonsil, URI, skin, soft tissue	Adult: 600,000-1 million U/day × 10 days Child (<60 lb): 300,000 U/day
	C. diphtheriae	Diphtheria	300,000-600,000 U/day × 14 days
	T. pallidum	Syphilis	Adult and child >12: 600,000 U/day 8 days
penicillin V	*Streptococcus*	URI, scarlet fever, erysipelas	125-250 mg q6-8 hr × 10 days
	Streptococcus	Pharyngitis in children	Child: 25-50 mg/kg/day divided q6hr × 10 days
	Pneumococcus	URI, otitis media	250-500 mg q6-8 hr until afebrile × 2 days
	Staphylococcus	Skin and soft tissue	250-500 mg q6-8 hr
	Group A streptococcus	Prevention of recurrence following rheumatic fever	125-250 mg bid continuous
dicloxacillin	Penicillinase-resistant *Staphylococcus*	Mild to moderate infection	Adult: 125 mg q6hr Child: 12.5 mg/kg/day in divided doses q6hr
		Severe infection	Adult: 125-250 to 500 mg q6hr Child: 25 mg/kg/day divided doses q6hr
oxacillin	Penicillinase-resistant *Staphylococcus*	Mild infection	Adult: 500 mg q4-6 hr Child: 50 mg/kg/day in divided doses q6hr
		Severe infection (following parenteral therapy)	Adult: 1 g q4-6 hr Child: 100 mg/kg/day in divided doses q4-6 hr
ampicillin	*H. influenzae, Staphylococcus, S. pneumoniae,* and spp.	URI, soft tissue	≤20 kg: 50 mg/kg/day in divided doses q6-8 hr >20 kg: 250 mg q6hr
	Shigella, E. coli, Salmonella, P. mirabilis, enterococci	GI, GU infections	Adult, child >20 kg: 500 mg q6hr Child: ≤20 kg: 100 mg/kg/day q6hr
	N. gonorrhoeae		3.5 g with 1 g probenecid
amoxicillin	ENT: *Streptococcus* α- and β-hemolytic, *S. pneumoniae, Staphylococcus* sp, *H. influenzae*	Mild/moderate Severe	Adult, child >40 kg: 500 mg q12hr or 250 mg q8hr Child >3 mo and <40 kg: 25 mg/kg/day in divided doses q12hr or 20 mg/kg/day in divided doses q8hr
	Skin: *Streptococcus* sp. α- and β-hemolytic, *Staphylococcus* sp., *E. coli*		Adult, child >40 kg: 875 mg q12hr or 500 mg q8hr Child >3 mo and <40 kg: 45 mg/kg/day in divided doses q12hr or 40 mg/kg/day in divided doses q8hr
	GU tract: *E. coli, P. mirabilis, Enterococcus faecalis* *Streptococcus* sp., α- and β-hemolytic, *S. pneumococcus, Staphylococcus* sp., *H. influenzae*	Lower respiratory tract	Adult, child >40 kg: 875 mg q12hr or 500 mg q8hr Child >3 mo and <40 kg: 45 mg/kg/day in divided doses q12hr or 40 mg/kg/day in divided doses q8hr
	N. gonorrhoeae	Gonorrhea	Adult: 3 g as single oral dose Prepubertal children >2 yr: 50 mg/kg with probenecid 25 mg/kg as single dose
amoxicillin and potassium clavulanate	*H. influenzae, M. catarrhalis*	Otitis media, sinusitis	Adult, child >40 kg: 500 mg q12hr or 250 mg q8hr Child <3 mo: 30 mg/kg/day divided q12hr (duration otitis media 10 d)
	H. influenzae, M. catarrhalis	Lower respiratory, severe infection	Adult: 875 q12h or 500 q8h
Augmentin XR	*H. influenzae, M. catarrhalis, H. parainfluenzae, K. pneumoniae* or methicillin-susceptible *S. aureus, S. pneumoniae*	Pneumonia, sinusitis	4000/250/day given as two tabs q12hr × 10 days sinusitis, × 7-10 days for pneumonia

U, units.

compete for and bind to specific enzyme proteins that catalyze transpeptidation and cross-linking. The enzymes to which they bind are called penicillin-binding proteins (PBPs). They consist of transpeptidases, transglycosylases, and D-alanine carboxykinases and are implicated in the final phases of building and reshaping the bacterial cell wall while it is growing and dividing. This action interferes with the biosynthesis of mucopeptides and prevents linkage of structural components of the cell wall. After the penicillin molecules bind and inhibit the transpeptidase enzymes, susceptible bacteria are no longer able to lay protein cross-links across the peptidoglycan backbone of the cell wall. In addition to being structurally weak, this formation is thought to catalyze the activation of autolytic enzymes in the cell wall that cause a progressive bacterial lysis.

Resistance can occur to penicillin, primarily through the formation of β-lactamases (penicillinases). An example of this mechanism is the resistance of *S. aureus* to penicillin G. Other significant factors contributing to penicillin resistance include diminished permeability of the drug through the bacterial outer cell membrane and decreased binding of the drug at its target sites on the inner bacterial membrane. Inhibitors of the β-lactamases, including clavulanic acid, sulbactam, and tazobactam, are often used in combination therapy with certain penicillins to prevent their inactivation.

DRUG TREATMENT PRINCIPLES

Before prescribing any penicillin, check for drug allergy. Oral penicillins are generally indicated for the treatment of mild to moderately severe infections caused by penicillin-sensitive microorganisms. They are broad-spectrum antibiotics used as empiric treatment for many infections, according to the site of infection, while awaiting the results of a culture.

Many penicillins including penicillin G (IM), penicillin V, cloxacillin, dicloxacillin, amoxicillin, amoxicillin, and potassium clavulanate (AM/CL) are indicated as first-choice empiric treatment for many infections including skin infections and animal bites, otitis media, sinusitis, pharyngitis, acute exacerbation of COPD, syphilis, mastitis, and Lyme disease (see Table 60-1). Penicillin V remains the drug of choice for group A β-hemolytic streptococcus. Penicillin G remains the drug of choice for syphilis.

A minimum 10 days of treatment is recommended for any infection caused by group A β-hemolytic streptococci to prevent the occurrence of acute rheumatic fever or acute glomerulonephritis. In severe staphylococcal infections, continue therapy with penicillinase-resistant penicillins for at least 14 days.

The natural penicillins are generally active against non–penicillinase-producing staphylococci and streptococci and most gram-positive organisms. They are active against some gram-negative organisms and active against most anaerobic bacteria. The penicillinase-resistant penicillins are active against penicillinase-producing staphylococci and some streptococci.

The aminopenicillins are active against non–penicillinase-producing staphylococci, some streptococci, and some gram-negative and anaerobic bacteria. The addition of a β-lactam product increases the spectrum to include more gram-positive and gram-negative bacteria and anaerobes. The combination of amoxicillin and clavulanate is very commonly used and increases the spectrum of amoxicillin effectiveness to cover *S. aureus, Moraxella catarrhalis, Haemophilus influenzae, Salmonella,* and *Shigella.* The combination of ampicillin and sulbactam has the widest spectrum of activity of the oral penicillins. The extended-spectrum penicillins have increased penicillin's activity against gram-negative and anaerobic bacteria.

HOW TO MONITOR

- Monitoring is particularly important in newborns, infants, and when high dosages are used.
- Perform bacteriologic studies to determine causative organisms and their susceptibility so that appropriate therapy is administered
- Monitor for resolution of the infection, resistance.
- *Clostridium difficile* infection of the bowel may develop.
- Penicillin G potassium can cause hyperkalemia.
- Penicillin G with procaine: monitor for sensitivity to procaine.
- Penicillinase-resistant penicillins: obtain blood cultures, WBC, and differential cell counts prior to initiation and at least weekly during therapy with penicillinase-resistant penicillins. Measure AST and ALT during therapy to monitor for liver function abnormalities.
- Penicillinase-resistant penicillins: perform periodic urinalysis, BUN, and creatinine determinations during therapy and consider dosage alterations if these values become elevated. If renal impairment is known or suspected, reduce the total dosage and monitor blood levels to avoid possible neurotoxic reactions.
- When administering penicillin parenterally, the practitioner should monitor the patient for at least 30 minutes postadministration to rule out any allergic or anaphylactic reaction to the drug.
- Avoid SC and fat layer injections; pain and induration may occur.
- Inadvertent intravascular administration of IM injections has resulted in severe neurovascular damage. Damage has occurred after injections into the buttock, thigh, and deltoid areas. These reactions occur most frequently in infants and small children.
- Some products contain tartrazine and sulfites.

PATIENT VARIABLES

Geriatrics

Oral penicillins are generally well tolerated. Ask specifically about a penicillin allergy because the patient may have difficulty remembering old allergies. The high sodium content of certain parenteral penicillins such as carbenicillin disodium and ticarcillin disodium may pose a danger for patients with cardiac and renal conditions.

Pediatrics

For infants less than 3 months old, investigate history of penicillin allergy in the mother. Pediatric renal tubular function appears to mature more slowly than the glomerular filtration rate and reaches adult levels at approximately 7½ to 8 months of age. Penicillins are secreted by the renal tubules, and therefore clearance is reduced at birth but appears to increase swiftly during the first year of the child's life.

Safety and efficacy of carbenicillin, piperacillin, and the β-lactamase inhibitor/penicillin combinations have not been established in infants and children less than 12 years old.

Pregnancy

Category B: no adequate studies. Use during pregnancy only if clearly needed. Penicillin crosses the placenta and is excreted in breast milk; it may cause diarrhea, candidiasis, or allergic response in the nursing infant. Ampicillin use by nursing mothers may lead to sensitization of infants.

Gender

Women taking ampicillin, bacampicillin, and penicillin V should be educated to use an alternative method of contraception if they are using estrogen-containing contraceptives because their effectiveness is compromised.

PATIENT EDUCATION

Patient should take medication on an empty stomach 1 hour before or 2 hours after meals, with a full glass of water. Penicillin V may be given with meals, although drug levels may be higher when given on an empty stomach. Amoxicillin, bacampicillin, and AM/CL may be given without regard to meals.

Patients should notify the health care provider if skin rash, itching, hives, severe diarrhea, shortness of breath, urticaria, black tongue, sore throat, nausea, vomiting, fever, swollen joints, or any unusual bleeding or bruising occurs.

Those patients with penicillin allergies or hypersensitivity should be urged to wear some kind of emergency identification informing others of their allergy.

Patients or family should report any type of symptoms of developing allergic reactions. Intradermal skin tests may detect previous drug sensitivity.

Store tablets at 15° to 30° C (59° to 86° F). Reconstituted solutions remain stable for 14 days if refrigerated.

Specific Drugs

Ⓟ Prototype VK

Penicillin VK

All penicillins share the following characteristics, except as noted.

Contraindications

- History of hypersensitivity to penicillins, cephalosporins, or imipenem
- Severe infections with an oral penicillin during the acute stage
- AM/CL: History of AM/CL-associated cholestatic jaundice or hepatic dysfunction

Warnings

Hypersensitivity reactions are often serious and occasionally fatal. The incidence of anaphylactic shock is between 0.015% and 0.04%. Accelerated reactions (urticaria and laryngeal edema) and delayed reactions (serum sickness) may also occur. They are more likely in patients with a history of atopic conditions. Hypersensitivity myocarditis may occur at any time. The initial symptoms include rash, fever, and eosinophilia.

An urticarial rash (nonallergic) occasionally occurs with ampicillin. This is common in patients with mononucleosis.

There is a risk of cross-sensitivity of penicillins with cephalosporins. Estimated incidence is between 3% and 16%. Skin testing and desensitization are available. Desentization is most often used for treatment of syphilis.

Treatment of allergy includes antihistamines and if necessary, corticosteroids. Anaphylaxis requires emergency measures.

The dosage of penicillin G should be reduced in patients with severe renal impairment, with additional modifications when hepatic disease accompanies the renal impairment.

Precautions

- Patients with a history of rheumatic fever or chorea and receiving continuous prophylaxis may harbor increased numbers of penicillin-resistant organisms.
- Probenecid increases serum concentrations of penicillin.
- Cystic fibrosis patients have a higher incidence of side effects.
- With streptococcal infections, therapy must be sufficient to eliminate the organism within 7 to 10 days to prevent sequelae (endocarditis, rheumatic fever).
- Resistance may occur.
- Pseudomembranous colitis may occur.
- Superinfection may result.
- Some products contain tartrazine or sulfites that also may provoke hypersensitivity reactions.
- Other products contain aspartame, which is contraindicated in patients with PKU.

Pharmacokinetics

See Table 60-2. Absorption is variable. Penicillins are widely distributed into the body fluids, into the pleural and pericardial cavities, passing into joints, into bile, to the placenta, and to breast milk. Adequate penicillin levels in the cerebrospinal fluid are attainable when the meninges are inflamed.

Most penicillin products undergo rapid renal elimination, with approximately 85% to 90% being excreted by tubular secretion. The half-life of penicillin in serum varies from approximately 0.4 to 1.3 hours and can last as long as 20 hours in the anuric patient. Nafcillin, oxacillin, cloxacillin, and dicloxacillin levels usually do not increase in anuric patients, due to increased compensation for diminished urinary elimination by hepatic metabolism or biliary excretion. The amount of penicillin excreted by the liver is minimal except for nafcillin and oxacillin.

Adverse Effects

Hypersensitivity occurs in about 10% to 15% of patients receiving penicillins, depending on the type of preparation and the route of administration. The risk of anaphylaxis is approximately 0.05%. The frequency of reaction is least when the penicillin is given orally (po), somewhat higher with IV administration, and distinctly higher when it is combined with procaine and administered IM.

Table 60-3 lists important adverse reactions by body system. Elevated BUN and creatinine occurs very rarely and photosensitivity does not occur with penicillins.

Drug Interactions

The penicillins interact with many other drugs. Table 60-4 lists major drug interactions.

Overdosage

Symptoms are neuromuscular hyperexcitability, convulsions, agitation, and confusion.

TABLE 60-2 Pharmacokinetic Parameters of Penicillin

Drug	Absorption	Onset of Action	Time to Peak	Half-Life	Protein Bound	Metabolism	Excretion
penicillin G	15%-30%	po 0.5-1 hr IM 15-30 min	30-60 15-30	0.5 hr	60%	None	Renal
penicillin V	60%	0.5-1 hr	0.5-1	1 hr	80%	None	Renal
cloxacillin	49%	1-2 hr	1-2	0.4 hr	95%	Liver	Renal
dicloxacillin	50%-85%	0.5-1 hr	0.5-1.5	0.8 hr	98%	Liver	Renal
nafcillin	Low	1-2 hr	1-2	0.5 hr	90%	Liver	Renal/bile
oxacillin	33%	0.5-1 hr	0.5-1	0.4 hr	94%	Liver	Renal/bile
ampicillin	30%-50%	1.5-2 hr	1.5-2	1.0 hr	20%	None	Renal, 60%
amoxicillin	93%	2 hr	1-2	1.7 hr	20%	None	Renal, 86%

TABLE 60-3 Adverse Reactions to Penicillin by Body System

Body System	Common Minor	Serious Adverse Reactions
Skin, appendages	Maculopapular and erythematous rashes, photosensitivity, onycholysis and discoloration of nails	Exfoliative dermatitis, minocycline: blue-gray pigmentation, Stevens-Johnson syndrome
Hypersensitivity		Rash, fever, anaphylaxis, urticaria, laryngeal edema, serum sickness
GI	Anorexia, nausea, vomiting, diarrhea, epigastric distress, bulky loose stools, stomatitis, sore throat, glossitis, hoarseness, black hairy tongue	Dysphagia, enterocolitis, inflammatory lesion in anogenital region
Hematologic		Neutropenia, eosinophilia, thrombocytopenia
Hepatic		↑ LFTs
CNS	Headache	Transient myopathy, confusion

TABLE 60-4 Penicillin Drug Interactions

Penicillin	Drug Acted On	Drug	Penicillin Acted On
Penicillins	↓ Oral contraceptives	β-blockers	May potentiate anaphylactic reactions to penicillin
ampicillin may reduce bioavailability	atenolol	tetracycline	↓ penicillins
		aspirin, sulfonamides, indomethacin, thiazides, furosemide	↑ penicillin G
		probenecid	↑ penicillins renally excreted
		allopurinol	↑ Rate of ampicillin-induced rash

Dosage and Administration

- Dosage and administration recommendations vary according to age of patient. Table 60-1 provides general recommendations. Dosage and administration must be adjusted to the individual conditions.
- Because the absorption of penicillins is affected by food, they should be taken on an empty stomach. However, penicillin V amoxicillin, bacampicillin, and AM/CL can be given without regard to meals.

Other Drugs in Class

Other drugs in this class are similar to the prototype except as follows.

Natural Penicillins

penicillin G (Crysticillin AS)

- This is the only parenteral penicillin in common use in the outpatient setting.

penicillin V (Pen-Vee K, Beepen VK, V-cillin K)

- *Unlabeled uses:* prophylactic treatment of children with sickle cell anemia, anaerobic infections, and Lyme disease

Penicillinase-Resistant Penicillins

cloxacillin (Tegopen), dicloxacillin (Dynapen), nafcillin (Unipen), oxacillin (Prostaphlin)

- Nafcillin is available as IV only and is not discussed further.

Indications

- Treatment of infections caused by penicillinase-producing staphylococci that have demonstrated susceptibility to the drug. May be used to initiate therapy in suspected cases of resistant staphylococcal infections prior to the availability of susceptibility test results. Do not use in infections caused by organisms susceptible to penicillin G.

Aminopenicillins

ampicillin (Omnipen, Ampicen, Polycillin), amoxicillin (Amoxil, Polymox, Trimox)

- Amoxicillin has better absorption and causes less diarrhea than ampicillin.

bacampicillin (Spectrobid)

- Better absorbed than ampicillin or amoxicillin. Spectrobid needs only every-12-hour administration, promoting compliance.

amoxicillin and potassium clavulanate (AM/CL) (Augmentin)

Dosage and Administration. The 12-hour dosing regimen causes less diarrhea. The 200 and 400 mg suspension and chewable tablets contain aspartame. AM/CL comes as 250, 500, and 875 mg amoxicillin and 125 mg clavulanic acid. This means two 250-mg tablets are not equivalent to one 500-mg tablet (has more potassium clavulanate). AM/CL also comes in tablets, chewable tables, and powder for oral suspension in different strengths. Augmentin XR comes as 1000 mg amoxicillin and 62.5 mg potassium clavulanate.

ampicillin/sulbactam (Unasyn)

Indications. Used in skin, intraabdominal, gynecologic infections caused by β-lactamase–producing strains of bacteria. It is a very broad-spectrum product; thus it should be reserved for mixed or complicated infections.

RESOURCES FOR PATIENTS AND PROVIDERS

Centers for Disease Control and Prevention, www.cdc.gov.
Federal data collection and monitoring agency.

BIBLIOGRAPHY

Baker CJ et al: 1997 AAP guidelines for prevention of early-onset group β streptococcal disease, *Pediatrics* 103(3):701, 1999.

Bouza E: Antibiotic resistance and therapeutic options in lower respiratory tract infections, *Int J Antimicrob Agents* 11(suppl 1):S3-6, March, 1999.

Craig TJ et al: Common allergic and allergic-like reactions to medications. When the cure becomes the curse, *Postgrad Med* 105(3):173, 1999.

Curtin-Wirt C et al: Efficacy of penicillin vs amoxicillin in children with group A beta hemolytic streptococcal tonsillopharyngitis, *Clin Pediatr (Phila)* 42(3):219-225, 2003.

DiGrego GJ, Barbieri EJ: *Handbook of commonly prescribed drugs,* West Chester, PA, 1998, Medical Surveillance.

Gilbert DN, Moellering RC, Sande MA: The Sanford Guide to antimicrobial therapy, ed 33, Hyde Park, Ver., 2003, Antimicrobial Therapy, Inc.

Jones RN, Biedenbach DJ, Beach ML: Influence of patient age on the susceptibility patterns of *Streptococcus pneumoniae* isolates in North America (2000-2001): report from the SENTRY Antimicrobial Surveillance Program, *Diagn Microb Infect Dis* 46(1):77-80, 2003.

Todd J: Antimicrobial therapy of pediatric infections. In Hay W et al, editors: *Current pediatric diagnosis and treatment,* ed 12, Norwalk, CT, 1995, Appleton & Lange.

CHAPTER 61

Cephalosporins

Laurie Scudder

Drug Names

Class	Subclass	Generic Name	Trade Name
Cephalosporins	First-generation drugs	(P)(200) cephalexin	Keflex
		cefadroxil	Duricef
	Second-generation drugs	(200) cefuroxime	Ceftin
		(200) cefprozil	Cefzil
		cefaclor	Ceclor
		cefpodoxime	Vantin
		loracarbef	Lorabid
	Third-generation drugs	cefixime	Suprax
		ceftriaxone	Rocephin
		cefdinir	Omnicef
		cefditoren	Spectracef

(200), Top 200 drug; (P), prototype drug.

General Uses

Indications

First-generation drugs
- Skin and soft tissue
- Urinary tract infection (UTI)

Second- and third-generation drugs
- Otitis media
- Gonorrhea
- Acute bronchitis or pneumonia in COPD patients
- Pneumonia, community-acquired
- Pharyngitis
- Sinusitis
- Lyme disease

• • •

Cephalosporins comprise a large category of antimicrobials with a wide spectrum of activity, superior to penicillin (Table 61-1). They are generally very safe and effective, with minimal side effects. This chapter discusses the oral cephalsporins with one exception, ceftriaxone, which can be given intramuscularly (IM) in the primary care setting. There are many cephalosporins used intravenously (IV) for serious infections that are not discussed.

All cephalosporins are active against most gram-positive cocci and many strains of gram-negative bacilli. Cephalosporins are classified by "generation," with each successive generation boasting better efficacy against gram-negative organisms although at the expense of action against gram-positive organisms.

In general, if a patient has had an anaphylactic reaction to penicillin, do not use cephalosporins if other treatments are available.

The common wisdom is that approximately 10% of individuals with penicillin allergy will also be allergic to the cephalosporin antibiotics. A recent study found that the incidence of cephalosporin reactions in penicillin-allergic individuals is only minimally increased, if at all. They also found that penicillin skin tests did not identify those few potential reactors.

DRUG ACTION AND EFFECTS

Cephalosporins are β-lactam antibiotics that have the ability to resist bacterial enzymes, specifically β-lactamase. They have a similar mechanism of action as that of penicillin. They interfere with cell wall synthesis by inhibition of the synthesis of the bacterial peptidoglycan in the cell wall. This makes the cell wall osmotically unstable. Cephalosporins are bactericidal and usually more effective against rapidly growing organisms.

The most common mechanism of resistance to cephalosporins is destruction by hydrolysis of the β-lactam ring by β-lactamase.

TABLE 61-1 Cephalosporin Indications with Dosage and Administration

Drug	Bacteria	Site/Disease	Dosage
FIRST GENERATION			
cephalexin (Keflex)	GABHS, *S. pneumoniae, Staph, H. influenzae, E. coli, Klebsiella, Proteus*	URI, UTI, skin	Adult: 250-500 mg q6hr Child: 25-50 mg/kg/day in divided doses Otitis media: 75-100 mg/kg/day in four divided doses
cefadroxil (Duricef)	GABHS, *S. pneumoniae, Staph, H. influenzae*	Pharyngitis, tonsillitis	Adult: 1 g/day in single or two divided doses × 10 days Child: 300 mg/kg/day in single or two divided doses × 10 days
	E. coli, Klebsiella, Proteus	UTI, skin	Adult: 1 g/day in single or two divided doses Child: 30 mg/kg/day in single or two divided doses
SECOND GENERATION			
cefuroxime (Ceftin)	GABHS, *Staph*	Pharyngitis, tonsillitis	Adult: 250 mg bid × 10 days Child (3 mo-12 yr): 20 mg/kg/day divided bid × 10 days
	GABHS, *S. pneumoniae, H. influenzae, M. catarrhalis*	Otitis media, impetigo	Child: 30 mg/kg/day divided bid × 10 days
	S. pneumoniae, H. influenzae, M. catarrhalis; Strep, Staph	Acute exacerbation of COPD, skin, soft tissue	Adult: 250-500 mg bid × 10 days
	E. coli, Klebsiella, Proteus, Morganella, Citrobacter	UTI	Adult: 125-250 mg bid × 7-10 days
	N. gonorrhoeae	Gonorrhea	Adult: 1000 once, single dose
	B. burgdorferi	Early Lyme disease	Adult: 500 mg bid × 10 days
cefprozil (Cefzil)	GABHS	Pharyngitis, tonsillitis	Adult (>13 yr): 500 mg q24hr × 10days Child (2-12 yr): 7.5 mg/kg q12hr × 10 days
	S. pneumoniae, H. influenzae, M. catarrhalis	Otitis media	Child: 15 mg/kg q12hr × 10 days
	Same	Sinusitis	Adult: 250-500 mg q12hr × 10 days Child: 7.5-13mg/kg q12hr × 10 days
	Same	Exacerbation of COPD	Adult: 500 mg q12hr × 10 days
	Strep, Staph	Skin, soft tissue	Adult: 250-500 mg q12hr × 10 days Child: 20 mg/kg q24hr × 10 days
cefaclor (Ceclor)	Same	Mild to moderate infection	Adult: 250 mg q8hr
		Acute exacerbation of COPD	Adult: 500 mg q12hr × 7 days
		Pharyngitis, tonsillitis	Adult: 375 mg q12hr × 10 days Child: 20 mg-40/kg/day in divided doses q8hr
cefpodoxime (Vantin)	*S. pneumoniae, H. influenzae, M. catarrhalis, S. pyogenes*	Pneumonia, bronchitis	Adult: 200 q12hr × 14 days
		Pharyngitis, tonsillitis	Adult: 100 q12hr × 5-10 days
		Skin	Adult: 400 q12hr × 7-14 days
		Otitis media	Child (5 mo-12 yr): 10 mg/kg/day × 10 days
		Pharyngitis/tonsillitis	Child (5 mo-12 yr): 10 mg/kg/day × 5-10 days

GABHS, Group A β-hemolytic *Streptococcus pyogenes.*

Continued

TABLE 61-1 Cephalosporin Indications with Dosage and Administration—cont'd

Drug	Bacteria	Site/Disease	Dosage
SECOND GENERATION—cont'd			
loracarbef (Lorabid)	*S. pyogenes, S. pneumoniae, H. influenzae, M. catarrhalis*	Pharyngitis/ tonsillitis	Adult: 200 mg q12hr × 10 days
	Same	Sinusitis	Adult: 400 q12hr × 10 days
	Same	Lower respiratory tract	Adult: 400 mg q12hr × 7-14 days
	Strep, Staph	Skin	Adult: 200 mg q12hr
	Same	UTI	
THIRD GENERATION			
cefixime (Suprax)	*H. influenzae, M. catarrhalis, S. pyogenes*	Otitis media, pharyngitis, tonsillitis, acute exacerbations of COPD	Adult: 400 mg/day as single dose or 200 mg bid Child (<50 kg or <12 yr): 8 mg/kg/day suspension as single daily dose or a 4 mg/kg q12hr
ceftriaxone (Rocephin)	*S. pneumoniae, S. aureus, H. influenzae, H. parinfluenzae, K. pneumoniae, S. marcescens, E. coli, E. aerogenes, P. mirabilis, S. pyogenes*	Lower respiratory, skin and skin structure, UTI	Adult: 1-2 g qd × 4-14 days IM Child: 50-75 mg/kg/day in divided doses q12hr IM × 10-14 day
	N. gonorrhoeae	Gonorrhea	Single IM dose of 250 mg
cefdinir (Omnicef)	Same	Pharyngitis tonsillitis, sinusitis	Adult: 300 mg q12hr or 600 q24hr × 10 days Child: 7 mg/kg q12hr or 14 mg/kg q24hr × 10 days
		Acute exacerbation of COPD	Adult: 300 q12hr or 600 q24hr × 10 days
		Pneumonia, skin, soft tissue	Adult: 300 q12hr × 10 days Child: 7 mg/kg q12hr × 10 days
		Otitis media	Child: 7 mg/kg q12hr or 14 mg/kg q24hr × 10 days
cefditoren (Spectracef)	*S. pyogenes, S. aureus*	Pharyngitis, tonsillitis, skin, soft tissue	Adult: 200 mg bid × 10 days
	H. influenzae, H. parainfluenzae, S. pneumoniae, M. catarrhalis	Acute exacerbation of COPD	Adult: 400 mg bid × 10 days

DRUG TREATMENT PRINCIPLES

Cephalosporins have a very wide spectrum of activity. They are useful for empirical treatment of many of the most common infections seen in primary care.

The first-generation agents are the most active against gram-positive cocci, including β-lactamase–producing *Staphylococcus aureus*, group A β-hemolytic streptococci (GABHS), and *Pneumococcus*. However, penicillin remains the drug of choice for treating GABHS pharyngitis. Cephalosporins have moderate activity against gram-negative bacilli, including *Escherichia coli, Klebsiella,* and *Proteus mirabilis*. They are inactive against *Bacteroides fragilis, Citrobacter, Enterobacter, Pseudomonas, Serratia,* and all other *Proteus* spp. First-generation cephalosporins are not effective against *Haemophilus influenzae*. Two first-generation cephalosporins are available as oral products and are commonly used. Cephalexin (Keflex) must be given every 6 hours, whereas cefadroxil (Duricef) may be dosed twice daily.

Second-generation cephalosporins continue to exhibit efficacy against gram-positive organisms with the added advantage of increased gram-negative activity and β-lactamase stability. These drugs are generally active against some strains of *Acinetobacter, Citrobacter, Enterobacter, Klebsiella, Neisseria, Proteus, Providencia,* and *Serratia* spp. In addition, second-generation products have good activity against *E. coli*. They are effective against most strains of *H. influenzae*, including those strains that produce β-lactamase. There are many second-generation cephalosporins. The manufacturers suggest that second-generation cephalosporins may be appropriate for bid dosing. An examination of their half-life suggests that this may not be appropriate (Table 61-2).

Third-generation cephalosporins have the broadest spectrum of activity of all the cephalosporins and are extremely effective against gram-negative organisms. The gram-positive activity is, as a whole, sharply reduced. Their activity against anaerobes varies with the agent. This generation of antibiotics is able to achieve excellent penetration into blood and body fluids, including the cerebrospinal fluid. Due to their lack of toxicity, even at high doses, they are a good alternative to aminoglycosides.

TABLE 61-2 Pharmacokinetics of Common Cephalosporins

Drug	Absorption	Time to Peak Concentration	Half-Life	Protein Bound	Excretion
cephalexin (Keflex)	Well absorbed 90%	1 hr	1 hr	14%	Urine
cefadroxil (Duricef)	Rapid	12 hr	1.5 hr	20%	Urine
cefuroxime (Ceftin)	Give IM, IV, or po; dosage forms not bioequivalent; absorption better after food	2-3 hr	1.3 hr	33%-50%	Urine; give with probenecid to slow clearance
cefprozil (Cefzil)	Well absorbed		1.25 hr	36%	Urine
cefaclor (Ceclor)	With or without food	30-60 min	To 1 hr	25%	Urine
cefpodoxime (Vantin)	Slowed with food; use film-coated tablet	2-3 hr	2-3 hr	21%-29%	Urine
loracarbef (Lorabid)	Well absorbed		1 hr	25%	Urine
cefixime (Suprax)	40%-50% absorbed; reduced with food; oral suspension absorbed better than tablet	2-6 hr	3-4 hr	65%	Urine
ceftriaxone (Rocephin)	Given IM or IV	2-3 hr	6-8 hr	85%-95%	Urine
cefdinir (Omnicef)	With or without food		1.7 hr	60%-70%	Urine
cefditoren (Spectracef)	Absorbed faster with high-fat meal		1.5-3 hr	88%	Urine

The third-generation cephalosporin cefixime (Suprax) is available in oral form. Although ceftriaxone (Rocephin) is available only in IM and IV forms, it is used in primary care as a once-daily IM injection. Ceftriaxone IM is used in outpatient settings as a one-time dose for treatment of sexually transmitted diseases and sometimes as adjunct therapy in Lyme disease.

Clinicians need to be aware of the limitations of cephalosporin effectiveness. Cephalosporins do not have activity against a number of common organisms, including penicillin-resistant *Pneumococcus*, methicillin-resistant *S. aureus* and *S. epidermidis*, *Enterococcus*, *Listeria*, *Mycoplasma*, clostridia, *Campylobacter*, *Chlamydia pneumoniae*, or *C. trachomatis*.

HOW TO MONITOR

These drugs have a wide safety margin and do not require routine monitoring of drug levels.

PATIENT VARIABLES

Geriatrics

Products are generally safe and effective. Dosage adjustments based on decreased renal function may be necessary.

Pediatrics

The products are generally safe and effective. In neonates, accumulation of cephalosporins has occurred. Each cephalosporin has a different age for established safety, ranging usually from 1 to 9 months. Cefaclor extended-release tables and cefonicid, cefmetazole, cefoperazone, cephalexin, and cefotetan are not indicated in children.

Pregnancy

Category B. Moxalactam is Category C. Cephalosporins appear safe for pregnant patients, but relatively few controlled studies exist. Use only when potential benefits outweigh potentia hazards to the fetus.These products cross the placenta and are excreted in breast milk.

PATIENT EDUCATION

- Take these products with food or milk to prevent gastrointestinal (GI) upset.
- Notify provider of any nausea, vomiting, or diarrhea that might develop.
- Notify provider if there is any response that would suggest an allergic reaction.

Specific Drugs

Ⓟ **Prototype Drug**

cephalexin (Keflex)

All cephalosporins share the following characteristics, except as noted.

Contraindications

- Hypersensitivity to any cephalosporin

Warnings

- Some patients may express cross-allergenicity with penicillin.

- Serum sickness–like reactions (erythema multiforme, skin rashes with polyarthritis, arthralgia, fever) have been reported.
- Products have triggered seizures in some patients.
- Coagulation abnormalities have been reported with moxalactam, cefamandole, cefoperazone, ceftriaxone, and cefotetan.
- Pseudomembranous colitis may occur because of *C. difficile*.
- Immune hemolytic anemia has been observed; it is rarely serious.
- Renal function impairment: products may be nephrotoxic; use with caution in patients with renal impairment.
- Hepatic function impairment: cefoperazone is excreted in bile. Half-life is increased in hepatic disease.
- Hypersensitivity reactions range from mild to life threatening.

Precautions

- Inject intramuscular preparations deep IM.
- Superinfection may occur.

Pharmacokinetics

Most cephalosporins are excreted by the kidneys and thus require moderate dosage adjustments in patients with renal insufficiency. There is no need, however, for routine monitoring of renal function. See Table 61-2 for product pharmacokinetic comparisons.

Adverse Effects

See Table 61-3. Most symptoms are GI, including nausea, vomiting, and diarrhea. These are usually mild and only rarely require discontinuation of the drug. Cefixime (Suprax) is the exception to the rule; diarrhea severe enough to require discontinuation of the drug may occur in as many as 10% of patients taking this drug. Cefaclor may cause serum sickness. There are no photosensitivity reactions.

Drug Interactions

See Table 61-4.

TABLE 61-3 Adverse Reactions to Cephalosporins by Body System

Body System	Common Minor Effects	Serious Adverse Reactions
Body, general	Malaise, asthenia, dysgeusia	Fever, chills, pain/tightness in chest
Skin, appendages	Diaphoresis, flushing	Urticaria, cutaneous moniliasis
Hypersensitivity		Fever, maculopapular rash, anaphylaxis, angioedema, Stevens-Johnson syndrome, erythema multiforme, toxic epidermal necrolysis
Respiratory		Asthma, dyspnea, interstitial pneumonitis, bronchospasm, pneumonia, rhinitis (loracarbef)
Cardiovascular	Palpitations, tachycardia	Hypotension, chest pain, vasodilation, syncope
GI	Nausea, vomiting, diarrhea, constipation, dyspepsia, anorexia, thirst, glossitis, abdominal pain, flatulence, stomach cramps	Melena, bleeding peptic ulcer, ileus, gallbladder sludge, colitis, including pseudomembranous colitis
Hemic and lymphatic		Eosinophilia, neutropenia thrombocytopenia, agranulocytosis, hemolytic anemia, decreased platelet function, aplastic anemia
Metabolic and nutritional	Glucosuria	
Musculoskeletal	Muscle cramps, stiffness neck spasms	Myalgia, arthralgia, rhabdomyolysis
Nervous system	Headache, dizziness, vertigo, lethargy, fatigue	Paresthesia, confusion, anxiety, hyperactivity, nervousness, insomnia, hypertonia, somnolence
Hepatic		↑ LFTs, hepatomegaly, hepatitis, jaundice, cholestasis
enitourinary	Dysuria	Transitory elevations in BUN, creatinine, reversible interstitial nephritis, hematuria, toxic nephropathy, acute renal failure (rare), ceftriaxone—casts in urine

TABLE 61-4 Cephalosporins Drug Interactions

Cephalosporin	Action on Other Drugs	Drug	Action on Cephalosporin
cephalosporins	↑ Aminoglycoside nephrotoxicity	probenecid, loop diuretics	↑ cephalosporins
cefazolin, cefmetazole, cefoperazone, cefotetan	↑ Ethanol, anticoagulants	antacids	↓ cefaclor, cefdinir, cefpodoxime
		H_2 antagonists	cefpodoxime, cefuroxime
		Iron supplements	↓ cefdinir

Overdosage

The most common symptom associated with overdosage is development of seizures. Treatment is supportive.

Generalized tonic-clonic seizures, mild hemiparesis, and extreme confusion after large doses in renal failure with cefazolin.

Dosage and Administration

Virtually all cephalosporins can be administered with food without affecting total amount of drug absorption, although a delay in absorption and peak concentration may result.

BIBLIOGRAPHY

Betts RF, Chapman SW, Penn RL: *Practical approach to infectious diseases,* ed 5, Philadelphia, 2002, Lippincott Williams & Wilkins.

Close W: *The Medical Letter: drugs and therapeutics handbook of antimicrobial therapy,* ed 16, New Rochelle, NY, 2002, The Medical Letter.

Conlon C, Pasvol G: *Color atlas and text of infectious diseases,* St Louis, 2000, Mosby.

Gilbert DN, Moellering RC, Sande MA: The Sanford Guide to antimicrobial therapy, ed 33, Hyde Park, Ver., 2003, Antimicrobial Therapy, Inc.

Mandel GL, Bennett JE, Dolin R, editors: *Principles and practice of infectious diseases,* ed 5, vols 1 and 2, New York, 2000, Churchill Livingstone.

McCarty JM et al: A randomized trial of short-course ciprofloxin, ofloxacin, or trimethoprim/sulfa-methoxazole for the treatment of acute urinary tract infection in women, Ciprofloxacin Urinary Tract Infection Group, *Am J Med* 106(3):292, 1999.

Tierney LM, McPhee SJ, Papadakis MA: *Current medical diagnosis & treatment 2003,* ed 42, New York, 2002, McGraw-Hill/Appleton & Lange.

CHAPTER 62

Tetracyclines

Drug Names

Class	Subclass	Generic Name	Trade Name
Tetracyclines		(P)(200) tetracycline	Achromycin, Panmycin, Sumycin, Tetra
		demeclocycline	Declomycin
		(200) doxycycline	Vibramycin, Doxy Caps, Doxycin, Vibra-Tabs
		methacycline	Rondomycin
		(200) minocycline	Minocin
		oxytetracycline	Terramycin, Uri-Tet

(200), Top 200 drug; (P), prototype drug.

General Uses

Indications

See Table 62-1 for specifics.

- Acute exacerbation of COPD
- Sinusitis
- Pneumonia
- Chlamydia
- Rickettsial infections
- UTIs
- Demeclocycline has an unlabeled use to treat syndrome of inappropriate antidiuretic hormone (SIADH)

• • •

Tetracyclines are active against a wide range of aerobic and anaerobic gram-positive and gram-negative bacteria. Their greatest usefulness is against rickettsia, mycoplasma, and chlamydia. Tetracyclines are not active against fungi or viruses.

All of the tetracyclines have similar antimicrobial activity, and cross-resistance is common. Resistance has reduced their usefulness in recent years. Another major restriction to their use is the contraindication for use in children younger than 8 years old or in pregnant women. If used in children or in pregnant women, may permanently stain teeth.

DRUG ACTION AND EFFECTS

The basic tetracycline structure is a hydronaphthacene nucleus that contains four fused six-carbon rings. Each of the tetracyclines differs on the basis of substitutions on the fifth, sixth, or seventh positions of the basic tetracycline structure. These substitutions affect the lipid solubility, serum half-life, and the effect that food has on the bioavailability of the drug.

The tetracyclines are bacteriostatic antibiotics. The mechanism of action is to inhibit protein synthesis in the susceptible organism by binding to the 30S ribosome subunit, impeding the binding of aminoacyl tRNA to the receptor site on the messenger RNA ribosome complex. Tetracyclines also may reversibly bind to 50S ribosomal subunits and possibly alter cytoplasmic membranes of susceptible organisms, resulting in the leakage of cytosolic nucleotides. This action requires active microbial growth, distinguishing the tetracyclines as bacteriostatic and not bactericidal agents.

Resistance to tetracyclines is plasmid mediated and occurs by decreased influx into the cell, decreased access to the ribosome, and enzymatic inactivation.

DRUG TREATMENT PRINCIPLES

There is not much difference in microbial activity between the different tetracyclines. Tetracyclines are wide-spectrum antibiotics useful for empiric therapy. They are one of the drugs of first choice for acute bacterial exacerbation of COPD, chlamydia, rickettsial infections, and are a second-line consideration for many other infections, especially in a patient with allergy to other antibiotics.

The choice between tetracyclines is determined by drug characteristics. Doxycycline and minocycline are the two most commonly used tetracyclines. Most tetracyclines must not be taken with milk or antacids. Doxycycline does not have this complicating factor. It is easier to get the patient to take it correctly. Also doxycycline has a longer half-life than tetracycline. Doxycycline also has less gastrointestinal disturbance than the other tetracyclines. Overall, doxycycline is the most useful tetracycline in primary care.

Tetracyclines are active against many Rickettsieae and STDs. It is commonly used for Lyme disease. Doxycycline has been used to prevent traveler's diarrhea. Gram-negative organisms usually sensitive include *Haemophilus ducreyi*, *Yersinia pestis*, and *Bacteroides*. Most gram-positive bacteria are now resistant to tetracyclines. They are not the drugs of choice for *Streptococcus* or *Staphylococcus*.

HOW TO MONITOR

- Baseline tests for renal and hepatic function and a CBC should be taken and repeated every 3 months for chronic therapy.

TABLE 62-1 Tetracycline Indications with Dosage and Administration Recommendations

Drug	Bacteria/Organism	Site/Disease	Dosage
tetracycline	*S. pneumoniae, M. catarrhalis, H. influenzae, Brucella, Legionella, Mycoplasma*	Mild to moderate	Adult: 1-2 g/day in two or four equal doses Child (>8): 25-50 mg/kg in four equal doses
	N. gonorrhoeae	Gonorrhea; allergic to penicillin	1.5 g initially, then 500 mg q6hr to a total of 9 g
		Severe acne, long term	Initially 1 g/day in divided doses. Maintenance, 125-500 mg/d
doxycycline	Same as tetracycline	Mild to moderate	Adult: first day 100 mg q12hr, then 100 mg qd Child (>8): <45 kg: 4.4 mg/kg divided into two doses on first day, then 2.2 mg/kg qd or in divided doses bid
		More severe	100 mg bid
		Gonorrhea	200 mg immediately, then 100 at bedtime that day, then 100 mg bid × 3 days or single dose 300 then 300 in 1 hr
	B. burgdorferi	Lyme disease	100 mg bid × 14-21 days
methacycline	Same as tetracycline	Mild to moderate	Adult: 200 mg initially, followed by 100 mg q12hr Child (>8): initially 4 mg/kg, follow with 2 mg/kg q12hr
	N. gonorrhoeae	Gonorrhea, urethritis	
minocycline	*Chlamydia trachomatis, Ureaplasma urealyticum*	Urethritis	100 mg bid for at least 7 days
	N. gonorrhoeae	Gonorrhea; sensitive to penicillin	200 initially, then 100 mg q12hr × 4 days
	N. meningitidis	Asymptomatic carriers	100 mg q12hr × 5 days
oxytetracycline	*Actinomycosis*	Actinomycosis	IM: 200 mg
	N. gonorrhoeae	Acute gonococcal problems	
	Chlamydia	Vaginal infections, CAP	

- Loss of appetite, jaundice, or abdominal pain may indicate possible hepatotoxicity.
- Minocycline: A change in mental status could indicate possible intracranial hypertension.

PATIENT VARIABLES

Geriatrics

Tetracyclines are well absorbed in the elderly, even in patients with achlorhydria or low gastric pH. With the exception of doxycycline and minocycline, serum levels of tetracyclines are increased by impaired renal function and dosages should be reduced. Because the primary routes of excretion with doxycycline and minocycline are biliary, and the serum half-life of these is unaffected by renal insufficiency, either doxycycline or minocycline would be a good choice for a tetracycline in the elderly, particularly if there is a concern of deteriorating renal function.

Pediatrics

Tetracyclines should not be given to children younger than 8 years of age. These products will cause permanent damage to teeth and bone.

Pregnancy

Category D: tetracyclines cross the placenta and, because of the chelating effect, bind with calcium, resulting in discoloration of deciduous teeth, enamel hypoplasia, and inhibition of fetal skeletal growth. The period for greatest risk of discoloration of the anterior deciduous teeth is between the middle of the second trimesters and up to 6 months of age in the newborn. Tetracyclines should never be given to pregnant patients.

Lactation

Relatively high concentrations of tetracyclines are excreted in breast milk. Therefore they are contraindicated during lactation.

Gender

Tetracyclines may decrease the pharmacologic effects of oral contraceptives; breakthrough bleeding or pregnancy may occur. Use an alternative form of contraception.

PATIENT EDUCATION

All tetracyclines should be taken with a full glass of water (240 ml) to avoid esophagitis or esophageal ulceration. The patient should not lie down for approximately one-half hour after taking each dose because most of the reported cases of esophageal ulceration involve patients lying down immediately after taking a tetracycline dose.

All tetracyclines, with the exceptions of doxycycline and minocycline, should be taken on an empty stomach (i.e., 1 hour before or 2 hours after meals) to maximize absorption.

With the exceptions of doxycycline and minocycline, use of iron preparations, antacid products, or other products containing aluminum, magnesium, calcium, zinc, and milk products will substantially decrease absorption from oral administration.

Because of the potential for tetracycline-induced photosensitivity, the patient should avoid unnecessary exposure to the sun. If sun exposure is unavoidable, the use of sunscreens with a minimum sun-protection factor (SPF) of 15 should be used.

Patients should report any signs and symptoms of hepatotoxicity (i.e., persistent nausea, vomiting, or anorexia with or without yellow coloring of the skin or eyes, dark urine, or pale stools).

Specific Drugs

Ⓟ Prototype Drug

Tetracycline

All tetracyclines share the following characteristics, except as follows.

Contraindications

- Hypersensitivity

Warnings

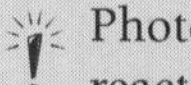
Photosensitivity manifested by exaggerated sunburn reaction.

- Demeclocycline long-term therapy has resulted in diabetes insipidus syndrome (polyuria, polydipsia, and weakness).
- Minocycline has caused light-headedness, dizziness, and vertigo. Patients should use caution during hazardous tasks.
- Except doxycycline and minocycline, tetracyclines will accumulate in patients with renal function impairment. Except doxycycline, tetracyclines may cause increase in BUN levels.
- High doses of tetracyclines can cause liver failure.

Precautions

- Benign intracranial hypertension with severe headaches and blurred vision has occurred.

Unused tetracyclines should be discarded to prevent Fanconi-like renal toxicity on proximal renal tubules from the ingestion of outdated and degraded tetracycline.

- Superinfection may occur.
- Some products contain sulfites that may provoke reactions in sensitive individuals.

Pharmacokinetics

See Table 62-2. Tetracyclines are incompletely absorbed when patients are fasting; absorption is decreased with food except doxycycline and minocycline. Doxycycline is the best absorbed.

TABLE 62-2 Comparison of Tetracycline Pharmacokinetics

Drug	Percent	Oral Absorption	Lipid Solubility	Half-life	Half-life in Anuria	Usual Adult Oral Daily Dosage	Metabolism	Routes of Excretion
tetracycline HCl	75-77	Slowed	Intermediate	6-11 hr	57-108 hr	250-500 mg q6hr	None	Renal/biliary
chlortetracycline HCl	25-30	Slowed				Topical	None	
demeclocycline HCl	66	Slowed	Intermediate	10-17 hr	40-60 hr	150 mg q6hr; increase up to 300 mg q12hr	None	Renal/biliary
doxycycline	90-100	Reduced by 20%, not clinically significant	High	12-22 hr	12-22 hr	50 mg every 12 hr to 100 mg q24hr	None	Biliary/renal
methacycline HCl		Slowed				150 mg every 6 hr; increase up to 300 mg q12hr		None
minocycline HCl	90-100	Not significant	High	11-23 hr	11-23 hr	100 mg q12hr	Possibly hepatic	Biliary/renal/hepatic
oxytetracycline HCl	58	Slowed	Low	6-10 hr	47-66 hr	250-500 mg q6hr	None	Renal/biliary

Doxycycline and minocycline are highly lipid soluble and readily penetrate into the cerebrospinal fluid, brain, eye, and prostate. The other tetracyclines are intermediate in their lipid solubility.

The tetracyclines are concentrated by the liver in the bile and excreted unchanged in the urine and feces. Reduction in dosing and/or interval is required in renal impairment, except for doxycycline and minocycline.

Because tetracycline is excreted unchanged in the urine via glomerular filtration, with a secondary biliary excretion route, reduction in dosing and/or interval is required in renal impairment. See Table 62-2 for comparison of tetracycline pharmacokinetics.

Adverse Effects

Hypersensitivity is rare. Doxycycline is believed to be associated with less nephrotoxicity than the other tetracyclines, even though there have been reports of doxycycline and renal failure.

See Table 62-3.

Drug Interactions

See Table 62-4.

Overdosage

If overdosage had just occurred with oral administration, antacids or milk products could be administered in an attempt to prevent and minimize absorption.

Dosage and Administration

! With the exception of both doxycycline and minocycline, tetracyclines interact with divalent and trivalent cations to form insoluble and nonabsorbable chelate. Therefore it is critical that tetracyclines not be taken at the same time with products containing calcium, magnesium, zinc, or iron (e.g., antacids, milk products, calcium- or iron-containing supplements, iron preparations, etc.).

TABLE 62-3 Adverse Reactions to Tetracyclines by Body System

Body System	Common Minor Effects	Serious Adverse Reactions
Body, general	Deposition in teeth	Superinfections
Skin, appendages	Maculopapular and erythematous rashes, photosensitivity, onycholysis and discoloration of nails	Exfoliative dermatitis, minocycline: blue-gray pigmentation, Stevens-Johnson syndrome
Hypersensitivity	Photosensitivity	Urticaria, angioneurotic edema; anaphylaxis, anaphylactoid purpura, pericarditis, exacerbated systemic lupus erythematosus (SLE), polyarthralgia, serum sickness–like reactions (fever, rash, arthralgia), pulmonary infiltrates with eosinophilia
Gastrointestinal	Anorexia, nausea, vomiting, diarrhea, epigastric distress, bulky loose stools, stomatitis, sore throat, glossitis, hoarseness, black hairy tongue	Esophageal ulcers dysphagia, enterocolitis, inflammatory lesions in anogenital region
Hemic and lymphatic		Hemolytic anemia, thrombocytopenia, thrombocytopenic purpura, neutropenia, eosinophilia
Central nervous system	Headache; minocycline—light-headedness, dizziness, vertigo	Transient myopathy
Hepatic		Fatty liver, hepatotoxicity, hepatitis (rare), ↑ LFTs, hepatic cholestasis (rare, with high levels)
Renal		↑BUN, creatine

TABLE 62-4 Tetracycline Drug Interactions

Tetracycline	Action on Other Drugs	Drug Acting	Action on Tetracycline
Tetracycline	Anticoagulants: ↑ hypoprothrombinemia effects ↑ Serum levels of digoxin ↓ insulin requirements ↓↑ lithium levels ↓ Pharmacologic effects of oral contraceptives ↓ Effect of penicillins	Antacids	↓ Absorption (except doxycycline and minocycline)
		Barbiturates, carbamazepine and hydantoins	↓ Levels of doxycycline
		cimetidine	↓ GI absorption
		iron salts	↓ GI absorption
		sodium bicarbonate	↓ GI absorption

Bismuth subsalicylate, kaolin, and pectin reduce absorption of oral tetracyclines and should be avoided. Food inhibits the absorption of the tetracyclines, again with the exceptions of doxycycline and minocycline. Therefore except for doxycycline and minocycline, the tetracyclines should be taken on an empty stomach, 1 hour before or 2 hours after meals or any other medication that contains divalent or trivalent cations.

Other Drugs in Class

doxycycline (Vibramycin, Doxy Caps, Doxycin, Vibra-Tabs)

Doxycycline is associated with fewer reports of renal failure than the other tetracyclines.

minocycline (Minocin)

Minocycline is almost completely absorbed orally, even when taken with food or milk. Although minocycline does bind to divalent and trivalent cations in the gut, oral absorption is reduced by only 20% when given with milk. With its long half-life, minocycline can be taken twice a day. It has good tissue penetration because of high lipid solubility. Minocycline does not require dosing adjustment in renal impairment.

BIBLIOGRAPHY

Gilbert DN, Moellering RC, Sande MA: The Sanford Guide to antimicrobial therapy, ed 33, Hyde Park, Ver., 2003, Antimicrobial Therapy, Inc.

Goulden V: Guidelines for the management of acne vulgaris in adolescents, *Paediatr Drugs* 5(5):301-313, 2003.

Klein NC, Cunha BA: Tetracyclines, *Med Clin North Am* 79:789, 1995.

Knigge K et al: Eradication of *Helicobacter pylori* infection after ranitidine bismuth citrate, metronidazole and tetracycline for 7 to 10 days, *Aliment Pharmacol Ther* 13(3):323, 1999.

Loewen PS et al: Systematic review of the treatment of early Lyme disease, *Drugs* 57(2):157, 1999.

Marshall E: Lyme disease. Patients scarce in test of long-term therapy, *Science* 5:283(S407):14, 1999.

Reese RE, Betts RF: *A practical approach to infectious diseases,* ed 4, Boston, 1996, Little, Brown.

Wormser GP et al: Duration of antibiotic therapy for early Lyme disease. A randomized double-blind placebo-controlled trial, *Ann Intern Med* 138(9):697-704, 2003.

CHAPTER 63

Macrolides

Drug Names

Class	Subclass	Generic Name	Trade Name
Macrolides	Erythromycins	(P) erythromycin base	E-Mycin, Ery-Tab, Eryc
		erythromycin estolate	Ilosone, Erythrozone
		erythromycin stearate	Eramycin
		erythromycin ethylsuccinate	EryPed, E.E.S.
	Newer macrolides	(200) azithromycin	Zithromax, Z-Pack Oral suspension,
		(200) clarithromycin	Biaxin, Biaxin XL
		dirithromycin	Dynabac
		troleandomycin	Tao

(200), Top 200 drug; (P), prototype drug.

General Uses

Indications

See Table 63-1 for specifics.

- Otitis media
- Acute bronchitis or pneumonia in COPD patient
- Community-acquired pneumonia
- Pharyngitis
- Sinusitis

The macrolides are used primarily for respiratory tract infections. Erythromycin is traditionally used as an alternative in patients allergic to penicillin for a number of infections, including as a prophylaxis for endocarditis. A major limitation to erythromycin use is the frequent problem of GI side effects. However, the newer macrolides (azithromycin, clarithromycin, and dirithromycin) rarely cause problematic GI side effects.

Another limitation is that of drug interactions. Macrolides, with the exception of dirithromycin, affect the cytochrome P450 3A4 system, thereby inhibiting the metabolism of certain drugs. A careful patient history of concurrent medications will prevent potentially adverse drug interactions.

DRUG ACTION AND EFFECTS

Macrolides consist of a large lactone ring to which sugars are attached. The structural modifications in clarithromycin and azithromycin make them more acid stable, improve tissue penetration, and broaden the spectrum.

Macrolides may be bacteriostatic or bactericidal. They inhibit protein synthesis by binding specifically to the 50S ribosomal subunit. This causes the RNA to dissociate from the ribosome and prevents protein synthesis. It inhibits a specific step in the synthesis where the new tRNA moves from the ribosome to the new site.

Resistance usually results from movement of the drug from the bacteria by an active pump, decreased drug binding, or hydrolysis.

DRUG TREATMENT PRINCIPLES

Most practitioners consider the macrolides to be a safe first-line choice for uncomplicated infections. Erythromycin products are usually relatively inexpensive; however the newer macrolides are more expensive. When prescribing a macrolide, caution should be taken with dosing in the presence of severe renal or hepatic impairment.

Erythromycin is a first-choice drug for treatment of pneumonia in children (ages 3 months to 5 years) and in ophthalmia neonatorum. Erythromycin is an alternative treatment for impetigo, cellulitis, otitis media, pharyngitis, chlamydia, and Lyme disease. Erythromycin is an alternative treatment for prevention of bacterial endocarditis in patients allergic to penicillin. Azithromycin is another first-choice drug for treatment of pneumonia in children (ages 3 months to 5 years and older). It is a first-choice drug for treatment of chlamydia in adults. Azithromycin is an alternative treatment for impetigo, cellulitis, sinusitis, pharyngitis, acute exacerbations of COPD, and traveler's diarrhea. Clarithromycin is used for pharyngitis, sinusitis, otitis media, acute exacerbation of COPD, pneumonia, and skin infections in adults.

One major difference between erythromycins and the newer macrolides is GI tolerability. Another is drug regimen. Erythromycins must be taken three or four times a day. Azithromycin offers the advantage of once-daily dosing. Clarithromycin requires twice-daily dosing. The longer drug action can make a critical difference in patient compliance.

The strength of each erythromycin product is expressed as erythromycin base equivalents. As a result of differences in absorption and biotransformation, varying quantities of each

TABLE 63-1 Macrolide Indications with Dosage and Administration Recommendations

Drug	Bacteria	Site/Disease	Dosage
erythromycin	GABHS, *S. pneumoniae*	Upper respiratory infection (URI) mild to moderate, lower respiratory infection	Adult: 250-500 mg qid × 10 days Child: 20-50 mg/kg/day in divided doses × 10 days
	M. pneumoniae	Respiratory tract	Adult: 500 mg q6hr × 5-10 days
	S. pyogenes, S. aureus	Skin and skin structure	Adult: 250-500 mg qid × 10 days Child: 20-50 mg/kg/day in divided doses × 10 days
	B. pertussis	Whooping cough	Adult: 500 mg qid × 10 days Child: 40-50 mg/kg/day in divided doses × 10 days
	C. diphtheria	Diphtheria; eradicate carriers	500 mg q6hr × 10 days
	GABHS	Prevention	250 mg bid
clarithromycin	GABHS	Pharyngitis, tonsillitis	250 mg q12hr × 10 days
	H. influenzae, M. catarrhalis, S. pneumoniae	Acute sinusitis	500 mg q12hr × 14 days
	H. influenzae	Acute exacerbation of COPD	500 mg q12hr × 7-14 days
	S. pneumoniae, M. catarrhalis	CAP (pneumonia)	250 mg q12hr × 7-14 days
	S. pneumoniae, M. pneumoniae, C. pneumoniae	CAP (pneumonia)	250 mg q12hr × 7-14 days
	H. influenzae	CAP (pneumonia)	250 mg q12hr × 7 days
	Streptococcus, Staphylococcus	Skin	250 mg q12hr × 7-14 days
azithromycin	*S. aureus, S. pyogenes, S. pneumoniae, H. influenzae, M. catarrhalis, Legionella*	Acute exacerbation of COPD, CAP, pharyngitis, tonsillitis, skin	Adult: 500 mg × 1 day, then 250 mg × 4 days
		Otitis media	Child: 30 mg/kg × one dose, or 10 mg/kg qd × 3 days, or 10 mg/kg × 1 day, then 5 mg/kg × 4 days
		CAP	Child: 10 mg/kg × 1 day, then 5 mg/kg × 4 days

CAP, Community-acquired pneumonia; *GABHS,* group A β-hemolytic *Streptococcus pyogenes.*

erythromycin salt form are required to produce the same free erythromycin serum levels. Erythromycin base is acid labile and is usually formulated in enteric- or film-coated forms for oral administration. Acid-stable salts and esters (estolate, ethylsuccinate, and stearate) are well absorbed.

The macrolides are active primarily against gram-positive organisms including *Streptococcus pyogenes* (GABHS) and *S. pneumoniae.* The newer macrolides have added effectiveness against gram-negative bacteria and anaerobes. Macrolides are of tremendous value for their unique ability to treat atypical pathogens such as *Mycoplasma pneumoniae* seen in community-acquired pneumonias.

Azithromycin and clarithromycin have significantly increased potency against gram-negative bacteria and anaerobes, and are generally reserved for more complicated infections, that is, community-acquired pneumonia, exacerbation of COPD, and sinusitis.

HOW TO MONITOR

When used long term, monitoring hepatic function is prudent, especially for erythromycin estolate.

PATIENT VARIABLES

Geriatrics

Lower doses of macrolides are generally not necessary in the elderly, providing they do not have severe renal or hepatic impairment.

Pediatrics

Age, weight, and severity of illness are important factors in determining dosage for children in the prescribing of erythromycin, azithromycin, troleandomycin, and clarithromycin. Safety and efficacy in children younger than 12 years of age has not been established for the use of dirithromycin.

Pregnancy

- Erythromycin: *category B.* Erythromycin estolate has been associated with elevated liver function tests in 10% of pregnant women and should be used cautiously in pregnancy.
- Azithromycin: *category B.*
- Clarithromycin, dirithromycin: *category C.* These drugs should not be used in pregnancy except in clinical circumstances when no alternative is available.
- Troleandomycin: safety for use has not been established.

Lactation

Erythromycin is considered compatible with breast-feeding. The drug is, however, transferred via breast milk, and the nursing woman should be aware that the nursing child will be exposed to the drug as well. Azithromycin, clarithromycin, dirithromycin, and troleandomycin may be excreted in breast milk, and caution should be exercised as well when administering these drugs to a nursing woman.

TABLE 63-2 Pharmacokinetics of Macrolides

Drug	Absorption	Drug Availability (After First Pass)	Onset of Action	Time to Peak Concentration	Half-Life	Protein Bound	Metabolism	Excretion
erythromycin	30%-50%	Varies, depending on formulation, food presence, and gastric emptying	Varies depending on formulation	Varies between 1 and 4 hr	1.4	70%-96%	Hepatic; demethylation 1A2 inhibitor 3A4 substrate and inhibitor	Urine, 5%-15%; significant quantity in bile
azithromycin	37%, GI tract	~40%	2 hr	2-3 hr	12-68	12-50	3A4	Primarily hepatic
clarithromycin	50%	~50%	1-3 hr	Tabs: 2 hr Susp: 3 hr	250 mg: 3-4 hr; 500 mg 5-7 hr	65%-70%	Metabolized to active metabolite 3A4	Urine, 20%-30%
dirithromycin			4 hr	4 hr	8 hr	15%-32%	Converted to nonenzymatic hydrolysis to active compound	Hepatic

PATIENT EDUCATION

- Do not chew, cut, or crush the tablets.
- Most of the erythromycin products should be taken with food.
- Clarithromycin may be taken with or without food.
- Azithromycin tablets can be taken without regard to food. The oral suspension should be given on an empty stomach.
- Clarithromycin suspension should not be refrigerated. It should be shaken well before each use.
- Patients using oral contraceptives for birth control should be advised that macrolides can reduce their efficacy and that they should consider using a back-up method of contraception.

Specific Drugs

Ⓟ Prototype Drug

erythromycin

All macrolides share the following characteristics, except as noted.

Contraindications

- Hypersensitivity to any macrolide
- Erythromycin estolate: Preexisting liver disease

Warnings

- Superinfection has occurred.
- Pseudomembranous colitis *(Clostridium difficile)* has occurred.
- Clarithromycin: do not use with ranitidine bismuth citrate in patients with history of acute porphyria.
- Azithromycin: do not use for pneumonia in patients judged as inappropriate for oral therapy of pneumonia.
- Cardiac effects: ventricular arrhythmia, including ventricular tachycardia and torsades de pointes in individuals with prolonged QT intervals, has been reported with macrolide antibiotics; however it has not occurred with azithromycin.
- Hepatotoxicity: erythromycin has been associated with infrequent cholestatic hepatitis, especially with erythromycin estolate. Findings include abnormal hepatic function, peripheral eosinophilia, and leukocytosis.
- Erythromycin may aggravate the weakness of patients with myasthenia gravis.
- Azithromycin: rare serious allergic reactions, including angioedema, anaphylaxis and Stevens-Johnson syndrome, and toxic epidermal necrolysis have occurred rarely.
- Serious allergic reactions including anaphylaxis have occurred with erythromycin
- Renal/hepatic function impairment: clarithromycin is principally excreted via the liver and kidney and may be administered without dosage adjustment to patients with hepatic impairment and normal renal function. However, in severe renal impairment the dosage should be halved or the dosing intervals doubled. Because azithromycin is principally eliminated via the liver, exercise caution when administering to patients with impaired hepatic function. Erythromycin is excreted by the liver. Exercise caution in administering to patients with impaired hepatic function. There have been reports of hepatic dysfunction without jaundice.

Precautions

Superinfection may result.

Pharmacokinetics

See Table 63-2. Food delays the onset of clarithromycin. Azithromycin is absorbed faster when taken with food.

Erythromycin stearate and certain formulations of erythromycin bases must be taken 3 hours before or after a meal. Because the erythromycins can cause GI upset, this can be an issue with compliance.

Macrolides readily distribute into body tissues and fluids. Tissue levels are higher than serum levels, thus they are effective at reaching the site of infection.

Macrolides are one of the many drugs that depend on P450 3A4 as a major route of metabolism, and toxicity may occur when the route is blocked.

Adverse Effects

See Table 63-3. Allergic reactions are rare. Erythromycin has significantly more adverse GI effects than the newer macrolides.

Erythromycin also has a wider range of adverse effects. It is more likely to cause a serious allergic reaction and cardiac arrhythmias. The cardiac effects occur mainly in patients who have a prolonged QT interval.

Of the erythromycin salts, erythromycin estolate is most commonly associated with hepatotoxicity. Clarithromycin, azithromycin, and dirithromycin have not been associated with jaundice; however they are also principally excreted via the liver and kidney, and caution should be taken with regard to dosing of these drugs in the presence of severe renal or hepatic impairment.

Drug Interactions

See Table 63-4. The macrolides are metabolized by the CYP450 3A4 system and interact with drugs also metabolized by that system.

Overdosage

Symptoms include nausea, vomiting, epigastric distress, and diarrhea. Hearing loss may occur with erythromycin, especially in patients with renal insufficiency.

Dosage and Administration

See Table 63-1.

Erythromycin base comes in enteric-coated tablets 250 mg for every 6-hour use, and 333 mg for every 8-hour use. It also comes in delayed-release 250 mg capsules. Erythromycin estolate comes in tablets (500 mg), capsules (250 mg), and suspension, either 125 or 250 mg/5 ml. Erythromycin stearate comes in 250 and 500 mg tablets. Erythromycin ethylsuccinate comes in chewable 200 mg tablets, 400 mg tablets, and suspension 200 and 400 mg/5 ml.

TABLE 63-3 Macrolide Adverse Reactions by Body System

Body System	Common Minor Effects	Serious Adverse Reactions
Body, general		Superinfections
Skin, appendages	erythromycin: rash; azithromycin: photosensitivity	
Hypersensitivity		erythromycin: urticaria; Stevens-Johnson syndrome, anaphylaxis; azithromycin: angioedema
Cardiovascular		↑ QT interval, ventricular arrhythmias, torsades de pointes (not with azithromycin)
GI	Abdominal distress, diarrhea, dyspepsia, nausea, vomiting	
Hemic		Neutropenia, thrombocytopenia
CNS	Erythromycin: insomnia, headache, dizziness, asthenia	erythromycin: seizures
Hepatic		↑ ALT, AST, hepatotoxicity; erythromycin: cholestatic hepatitis
Genitourinary		↑ BUN, creatinine

TABLE 63-4 Macrolide Drug Interactions

Macrolide	Action on Other Drugs	Drug	Action on Macrolide
Macrolides	↑ Oral anticoagulants, benzodiazepines, buspirone, carbamazepine, cyclosporine, digoxin, disopyramide, ergot alkaloids, statins, tacrolimus, theophylline	pimozide	↑ Macrolides
erythromycin	↑ bromocriptine, felodipine, grepafloxacin, sparfloxacin, methylprednisone ↓ lincosamide	rifampin, theophylline	↓ Macrolides
Newer macrolides	↑ omeprazole, clarithromycin	clarithromycin, fluconazole	↑ Newer macrolides

Newer Macrolides

azithromycin (Zithromax, Z-Pack)

It is important to give a loading dose, without which, minimum plasma concentrations take 5 to 7 days to reach steady state.

BIBLIOGRAPHY

Brown RB et al: Impact of initial antibiotic choice on clinical outcomes in community-acquired pneumonia: analysis of a hospital claims-made database, *Chest* 123(5):1503-1511, 2003.

Gilbert DN, Moellering RC, Sande MA: The Sanford Guide to antimicrobial therapy, ed 33, Hyde Park, Ver., 2003, Antimicrobial Therapy, Inc.

McConnell SA et al: Review and comparison of advanced-generation macrolides clarithromycin and dirithromycin, *Pharmacotherapy* 19(4):404, 1999.

Prunier AL et al: High rate of macrolide resistance in *Staphylococcus aureus* strains from patients with cystic fibrosis reveals high proportions of hypermutable strains, *J Infect Dis* 187(11):1709-1716, 2003.

Reese RE, Betts RF: *A practical approach to infectious diseases,* ed 4, Boston, 1996, Little, Brown.

Thadepalli H, Mandal AK: Antibiotic prophylaxis in the surgical patient, *Infect Med* 6(2):71-80, 1998.

Waterer GW: Combination antibiotic therapy with macrolides in community-acquired pneumonia: more smoke but is there any fire? *Chest* 123(5):1328-1329, 2003.

CHAPTER 64

Fluoroquinolones

Drug Names

Class	Subclass	Generic Name	Trade Name
Fluoroquinolones		(P)(200) ciprofloxacin	Cipro
		enoxacin	Penetrex
		norfloxacin	Noroxin
		grepafloxacin	Raxar
		lomefloxacin	Maxaquin
		ofloxacin	Floxin
		sparfloxacin	Zagam
Fluroquinolones with enhanced activity versus *Streptococcus pneumoniae*		(200) levofloxacin	Levaquin
		(200) gatifloxacin	Tequin
		moxifloxacin	Avelox

(200), Top 200 drug; (P), prototype drug.

General Uses

Indications

See Table 64-1 for specifics.

- Lower respiratory infections
- Skin and skin structure infections
- Bone/joint infections
- Infectious diarrhea
- Sexually transmitted diseases
- Complicated urinary tract infections
- Prostatitis

• • •

Fluoroquinolones are very important agents that have a broad range of activity against both gram-positive and gram-negative organisms. Fluoroquinolones have a good safety profile, less tendency for development of resistant strains, and excellent absorption after oral administration. All of the marketed fluoroquinolones also have a piperzyl group at position C7, resulting in greater activity against staphylococci and *Pseudomonas*. CNS adverse reactions may occur with fluoroquinolones, especially with prolonged use. Trovafloxacin is associated with liver failure, which limits its use. It will not be discussed here. The other fluoroquinolones have not demonstrated this effect.

DRUG ACTION AND EFFECTS

Earlier quinolone products were of limited use due to toxicity and rapid development of bacterial resistance. Addition of a fluorine substituent has increased their usefulness.

The mechanism of action of the fluoroquinolones is the inhibition of deoxyribonucleic acid (DNA) gyrase, an enzyme that is essential in the transcription, replication, and repair of DNA in bacteria. The blocking of DNA gyrase that occurs at concentrations of 0.1 to 10 g/ml, promotes superhelical formation of bacteria DNA with resultant destruction of the DNA. The activity of topoisomerase II, an enzyme with similar activity in eukaryotic cells, is also inhibited, but only at much higher concentrations, between 100 and 1000 g/ml.

Resistance does not develop rapidly. It occurs by mutation. No quinolone-modifying abilities have been seen in bacteria.

DRUG TREATMENT PRINCIPLES

The fluorquinolones are a group of potent antibiotics with a wide spectrum of action. They usually should not be considered first choice antibiotics for mild infections; however they are first choice for UTIs because of the frequency of resistant bacteria. In general they should be reserved for moderate infections and for bacteria that are resistant to other antibiotics. Because they have good tissue penetration, they are effective for skin, bone, and genital infections. CNS penetration, however, is not enough to be effective. Fluoroquinolones should always be given orally when possible because oral absorption is excellent.

Fluoroquinolones are considered first-choice drugs for empiric treatment of complicated sinusitis, severe diarrhea, UTIs, pyelonephritis, prostatitis, and gonorrhea. They are an alternative treatment for dog bite, acute sinusitis, severe sinusitis, and chlamydia. Fluoroquinolones with enhanced activity vs. *S. pneumoniae* are alternative therapy for acute exacerbation of COPD and pneumonia in adults.

Fluroquinolones are active against many gram-positive organisms; gram-negative organisms, including *Moraxella catarrhalis, Haemophilus influenzae, Escherichia coli,* chlamydia,

TABLE 64-1 Fluoroquinolone Indications with Dosage and Recommendations

Drug	Bacteria	Site/Disease	Dosage and Administration
ciprofloxacin	*E. coli, Klebsiella, Proteus, Enterobacter*	Uncomplicated UTI	100-250 mg bid × 3 days
		Moderate UTI	250 mg bid × 7-14 days
	M. catarrhalis, H. influenzae, M. pneumoniae, Listeria, Legionella, Staphylococcus	Lower respiratory tract, skin, and skin structure	500 mg bid × 7-14 days
		Sinusitis	500 mg q12hr × 10 days
	Shigella, Serratia, Salmonella	GI	750 mg bid × 10 days
enoxacin	Same as ciprofloxacin	Uncomplicated UTI	200 mg q12hr × 3 days
norfloxacin	Same as ciprofloxacin	Uncomplicated UTI	400 q12hr × 3 days
gatifloxacin	Same plus GABHS	Acute exacerbation of COPD	400 mg qd × 5 days
		Sinusitis	400 mg qd × 10 days
		CAP	400 mg qd × 7-14 days
		Uncomplicated UTI	400 mg qd × 7-10days
		Gonorrhea	400 mg in single dose
grepafloxacin	Same as ciprofloxacin	Exacerbation of COPD, CAP, gonorrhea	
levofloxacin	Same plus GABHS, many gram negative	Acute exacerbation of COPD	500 mg qd × 7 days
		CAP	500 mg qd × 7-14 days
		Sinusitis	500 mg qd × 10-14 days
		Skin, soft tissue	500 mg qd 7-10 days
		Uncomplicated UTI	250 mg qd × 3 days
lomefloxacin	Same as ciprofloxacin	Lower respiratory tract	400 mg qd × 10 days
		Uncomplicated UTI	400 mg qd × 3 days
moxifloxacin	Same as ciprofloxacin	Sinusitis	400 mg qd × 10 days
		Acute exacerbation of COPD	400 mg qd × 5 days
		CAP	400 mg qd × 7-14 days
		Skin and soft tissue	400 mg qd × 7 days
ofloxacin	Same as ciprofloxacin	Lower respiratory tract	400 mg q12hr × 10 days
		Uncomplicated UTI	200 mg q12hr × 3 days
sparfloxacin	Same plus GABHS, many gram negative	CAP, acute bacterial exacerbation of COPD	Two 200 mg tabs as loading dose, then 200 qd × 9 more days

CAP, Community-acquired pneumonia; *GABHS,* group A β-hemolytic *Streptococcus pyogenes.*

Mycoplasma pneumoniae; and many anaerobes. They are not active against *Clostridium difficile.*

HOW TO MONITOR

- Monitor renal, hepatic, and hematopoietic function during prolonged therapy.
- Patients on warfarin anticoagulation should be monitored closely for prothrombin times and INR at baseline, daily for the first week of therapy, and weekly thereafter. The patient should be instructed to immediately report any sign of bleeding.
- Patients on any theophylline product (e.g., theophylline, oxtriphylline, aminophylline) should have serum theophylline levels monitored because theophylline clearance may be decreased with concomitant quinolone use.
- Renal and hepatic function should be evaluated at baseline and every 6 weeks if therapy is to be continued.
- Hematology parameters should be monitored periodically for evidence of leukopenia, hemolytic anemia, and thrombocytopenia.
- Monitor for CNS side effects.

PATIENT VARIABLES

Geriatrics

Elderly patients are more likely to have reduced renal function, which will increase the half-life. Dosages should be adjusted in patients with impaired renal function.

Pediatrics

These agents are not recommended in the pediatric age group (<18 years of age) because of documented permanent articular damage in young, experimental animals (i.e., dogs, rats, and rabbits) and reported transient arthropathies in children. There is a lack of safety and efficacy clinical trial data in the pediatric population.

Pregnancy

Category C: there are no adequate studies. Use during pregnancy only if the potential benefit justifies the potential risk to the fetus.

Fluoroquinolones reach breast milk concentrations equal to serum levels within 2 hours of administration. Due to the association of fluoroquinolones and articular damage, these agents are not recommended in nursing mothers.

Dosage in Renal Impairment

Even though the quinolones are metabolized in the liver, elimination depends on renal function. Fluoroquinolones are primarily excreted renally, and adjustment of the dose is essential in patients with impaired renal function.

PATIENT EDUCATION

- The patient should drink plenty of fluids while taking these products.
- Norfloxacin, enoxacin, and ofloxacin should be taken on an empty stomach.

Ciprofloxacin and lomefloxacin can be taken without regard to meals.

Fluoroquinolones should not be taken with milk, antacids, iron preparations, or any product containing aluminum, magnesium, calcium, iron, or zinc. Sucralfate, an aluminum salt of a sulfated glyceride, should also be avoided. Absorption of the fluoroquinolone can be reduced by as much as 98% by chelation and therefore should be taken at least 2 hours before or 6 hours after divalent- or trivalent-cation–containing products.

- Use caution when driving, operating machinery, or performing any task that requires attentiveness because fluoroquinolones can cause dizziness, drowsiness, or confusion.
- Avoid undue exposure to the sun or use a sunscreen to prevent the occurrence of a photosensitivity reaction.

Specific Drugs

Ⓟ Prototype Drug

ciprofloxacin (Cipro)

Cipro is the most commonly used fluoroquinolone in primary care. All fluoroquinolones share the following characteristics, except as noted.

Contraindications

- Hypersensitivity to any of the fluroquinolones
- Tendinitis or tendon rupture associated with quinolone use
- Patients receiving QT-prolonging drugs or drugs reported to cause torsades de pointes

Warnings

Phototoxicity: moderate to severe phototoxic reactions have occurred in patients exposed to direct or indirect sunlight or to artificial ultraviolet light during or following treatment with lomefloxacin, sparfloxacin, or ofloxacin. These reactions have occurred with light through glass and with the use of sunblocks. Ciprofloxacin and levofloxacin can also cause photosensitivity.

- Moxifloxacin, gatifloxacin, and sparfloxacin have been shown to prolong the QT interval in some patients.
- Convulsions: increased intracranial pressure, convulsions, and toxic psychosis have occurred. CNS stimulation may also occur, which may lead to tremor, restlessness, light-headedness, confusion, dizziness, depression, hallucinations, and rarely, suicidal thoughts or acts. Use with caution in patients with known or suspected CNS disorders or other factors that predispose the patient to seizures or lowers the seizure threshold.
- Tendon rupture/tendinitis: ruptures of the shoulder, hand, and Achilles tendons that required surgical repair or resulted in prolonged disability have been reported. Discontinue therapy if the patient experiences pain, inflammation, or rupture of a tendon.
- Syphilis: ofloxacin, ciprofloxacin, norfloxacin, gatifloxacin, and enoxacin are not effective for syphilis. High doses to treat gonorrhea may mask or delay symptoms of incubating syphilis. Test for syphilis before treating for gonorrhea.
- Pseudomembranous colitis has been reported.
- Hypersensitivity reactions: serious and occasionally fatal reactions have occurred in patients, some following the first dose. Some reactions were accompanied by cardiovascular collapse, loss of consciousness, tingling, pharyngeal or facial edema, dyspnea, urticaria, and itching.
- Renal function impairment: alteration in dosage regimen is necessary.

Precautions

- Crystalluria: needle-shaped crystals were found in the urine of patients on norfloxacin and ciprofloxacin. Ensure proper hydration to reduce chances of renal irritation.
- Hemolytic reactions: rarely, hemolytic reactions have occurred in patients with G6PD activity.
- Myasthenia gravis: fluorquinolones may exacerbate the signs and lead to life-threatening weakness of the respiratory muscles.
- Blood glucose abnormalities have been reported usually in diabetic patients.
- Superinfection may occur.

Pharmacokinetics
Fluoroquinolones are well absorbed after oral administration and are widely distributed to most body tissues and fluids. High tissue concentrations are achieved in the kidneys, gallbladder, liver, lungs, cervix, endometrium, prostate, and phagocytes. High concentrations are achieved in the urine, sputum, and bile. Ciprofloxacin and ofloxacin are also distributed to skin, fat, muscle, bone, and cartilage and have been found to penetrate into the cerebrospinal fluid. See Table 64-2 for a comparison of pharmacokinetics in the quinolones.

Adverse Effects
Fluoroquinolones are generally well tolerated. The most common adverse effects are gastrointestinal (GI) (e.g., nausea, vomiting, diarrhea, abdominal pain), CNS (e.g., headache, dizziness, confusion, restlessness, sleep disorders, seizures), and dermatologic (e.g., rash, pruritus). Hypersensitivity is rare (Table 64-3).

Drug Interactions
See Table 64-4. Antacids, vitamins, enteral formulas, sucralfate, or other medications containing divalent or trivalent cations (e.g., magnesium, calcium, aluminum, zinc) significantly reduce the absorption of fluoroquinolones. They should be given either 2 hours before or 6 hours after administration of such products.

Overdosage
Overdosage may result in confusion, hallucinations, seizures, and renal failure.

TABLE 64-2 Pharmacokinetics of Fluoroquinolones

Medication	Absorption	Time to Peak Concentration	Half-Life	Protein Bound	Metabolism (%)	Excretion
ciprofloxacin	60%-70%	0.5 hr	3-5 hr	20%-40%	20	Renal, 50%; bile 20%-35%
enoxacin	90%		5-7 hr	40%	20	Renal, 90%; bile 18%
norfloxacin	35%		3-4 hr	10%-15%	20	Renal, 30%; bile 30%
lomefloxacin	95%		8 hr	10%	5	Renal, 40%; bile 10%
ofloxacin	98%		9 hr	32%	3	Renal, 90%; bile 5%
levofloxacin	99%	1.5 hr	7 hr	30%		Renal, 75%
gatifloxacin	96%	2 hr	7.5-14 hr	20%		Renal, 83%
moxifloxacin	86%	2 hr	15 hr	40%		Renal, 22%

TABLE 64-3 Fluoroquinolone Adverse Reactions by Body System

Body System	Common Minor Effects	Serious Adverse Reactions
Body, general	Fever, edema	Superinfections
Skin, appendages	Rash, pruritus, phototoxicity	
Hypersensitivity		Anaphylaxis, urticaria, toxic epidermal necrolysis, Stevens-Johnson syndrome, exfoliative dermatitis
Cardiovascular	Palpitations	sparfloxacin, moxifloxacin and gatifloxacin prolong the QT interval
GI	Nausea, abdominal pain, diarrhea, vomiting, dry/painful mouth, dyspepsia, constipation, flatulence	Pseudomembranous colitis
Hemic and lymphatic		Leukopenia, eosinophilia, g6Pd—hemolytic reactions
Metabolic and nutritional		Hypoglycemia
Musculoskeletal		Rupture of shoulder, hand, and Achilles tendons
CNS	Headache, dizziness, fatigue/lethargy/malaise, somnolence/drowsiness, insomnia, paresthesias, light-headedness	Seizure, increased intracranial pressure, toxic psychosis, CNS stimulation, tremor, restlessness, confusion, depression, hallucination
Special senses		Visual disturbances
Hepatic		↑ LFTs
Genitourinary		↑ BUN, creatinine, renal failure, crystalluria (rare)

TABLE 64-4 Fluoroquinolone Drug Interactions

Fluoroquinolone	Action on Other Drugs	Drug	Action on Fluoroquinolone
Fluoroquinolones	↑ theophylline	cimetidine	↑ fluoroquinolones
sparfloxacin, gatifloxacin, moxifloxacin	↓ Antiarrhythmic agents	sucralfate, iron salts,	↓ fluoroquinolone
ciprofloxacin, enoxacin, norfloxacin	↑ caffeine	probenecid	↑ norfloxacin, gatifloxacin, lomefloxacin
enoxacin	↑ digoxin	nitrofurantoin	↓ norfloxacin
sparfloxacin	↑ astemizole, terfenadine, bepridil, erythromycin, phenothiazine, TCAs	bismuth subsalicylate	↓ enoxacin
ofloxacin	↑ procainamide	cisapride	↑ sparfloxacin
ciprofloxacin, norfloxacin	↑ cyclosporine		

Other Drugs in Class

enoxacin (Penetrex), norfloxacin (Noroxin)

Used for UTIs only.

grepafloxacin (Raxar)

Offers no significant advantage over ciprofloxacin.

sparfloxacin (Zagam)

Increased risk of cardiac adverse effects.

levofloxacin (Levaquin)

No increased risk of cardiac adverse effects.
Increased activity against *S. pneumoniae.*

gatifloxacin (Tequin) and moxifloxacin (Avelox)

Increased risk of cardiac adverse effects.
Increased activity against *S. pneumoniae.*
The fluoroquinolones with increased activity against *S. pneumoniae* are useful for moderate to severe respiratory infections. Oral dosing ability can prevent hospitalizations for IV antibiotics.

BIBLIOGRAPHY

Balfour JA et al: Moxifloxacin, *Drugs* 57(3):363, 1999.

Blondeau JM: Expanded activity and utility of the new fluroquinolones: a review, *Clin Ther* 21(1):3, 1999.

Borcherding SM et al: Quinolones: a practical review of clinical uses, dosing considerations, and drug interactions, *J Fam Prac* 42:69, 1996.

Gilbert DN, Moellering RC, Sande MA: The Sanford Guide to antimicrobial therapy, ed 33, Hyde Park, Ver., 2003, Antimicrobial Therapy, Inc.

Jones RN et al: Epidemiologic trends in nosocomial and community-acquired infections due to antibiotic-resistant gram-positive bacteria, *Diagn Microbiol Infect Dis* 33(2):101, 1999.

Longworth DL: Microbial drug resistance and the roles of the new antibiotics, *Clev Clin J Med* 68(6):496-497, 501-502, 504, 2001.

McKinnon PS, Tam VH: New antibiotics for infections caused by resistant organisms, *Support Care Cancer* 9(1):8-10, 2001.

O'Donnell JA, Gelone SP: Fluroquinolones, *Infect Dis Clin North Am* 14(2):489-513, 2000.

Pau AK et al: Antibiotics in primary care: focus on fluroquinolones and other new and investigational antimicrobial agents, *Lippincott's Prim Care Pract* 3(1):39, 1999.

Reese RE, Betts RF: *A practical approach to infectious diseases,* ed 4, Boston, 1996, Little, Brown.

Stratton CW: Avoiding fluoroquinolone resistance. Strategies for primary care practice, *Postgrad Med* 101(3):247-250, 255, 1997.

The choice of antibacterial drugs, *Med Lett* 40(1023):33, March 27, 1998.

CHAPTER 65

Aminoglycosides

Drug Names

Class	Subclass	Generic Name	Trade Name
Aminoglycosides		(P) gentamicin	Garamycin, Jenamicin
		amikacin	Amikin
		kanamycin	Kantrex, Klebcil
		neomycin	Cortisporin, Mycifradin, Neobiotic, Neosporin
		streptomycin	Generic
		tobramycin	Nebcin, TobraDex

(200), Top 200 drug; (P), prototype drug.

General Uses

Indications

Oral

- Suppression of oral bacterial flora

Topical

- Irrigation of infected wounds

Parenteral

- Complicated UTIs
- Complicated respiratory infections
- Skin/bone/soft tissue infections
- CNS infection
- GI infection (peritonitis)

Susceptible organisms

- Enterobacter
- *Escherichia coli*
- Klebsiella
- Proteus
- Pseudomonas
- Serratia
- Penicillin- or methicillin-resistant strains of Staphylococcus

Aminoglycosides are reserved for treatment of gram-negative infections not sensitive to less toxic agents. They are not generally used in primary care, but they are important antibiotics and all providers should be familiar with their use.

Aminoglycosides have a narrow therapeutic window, so careful dosing is required.

They are associated with significant nephrotoxicity and ototoxicity. They are excreted renally, so patients with impaired renal function are at increased risk for toxicities. Their use in treatment of infections is either IV or IM. Oral aminoglycosides are poorly absorbed; their only use is for suppression of intestinal bacteria. Table 65-1 provides a summary of indications for each product. The primary care provider will find topical aminoglycosides also covered in Chapters 14 and 15 for localized treatment of eye, skin, ear, and so forth.

DRUG ACTION AND EFFECTS

The aminoglycosides are bactericidal antibiotics. Aminoglycosides irreversibly bind to the 30S subunit of bacterial ribosomes, blocking the recognition step in protein synthesis and causing misreading of the genetic code. The ribosomes separate from messenger RNA; cell death ensues.

DRUG TREATMENT PRINCIPLES

Oral Use

Aminoglycosides are used for suppression of GI bacterial flora and in treatment of hepatic coma.

Topical Use

Aminoglycosides have a wide variety of topical uses.

Aminoglycosides are quickly and almost totally absorbed when applied topically in association with surgical procedures, except to the urinary bladder.

> ! Irreversible deafness, renal failure, and death due to neuromuscular blockade have occurred following irrigation of both small and large surgical fields with an aminoglycoside preparation.

Consider potential toxicity when ordering aminoglycoside irrigation of a wound.

Parenteral Use

These drugs are reserved for short-term treatment of serious infections caused by susceptible strains of gram-negative bacteria. Bacteriologic studies should be performed to identify causative organisms and their susceptibility to specific aminoglycosides. They may be considered as initial therapy in suspected gram-negative infections, and therapy may be instituted before obtaining the results of susceptibility testing. Clinical trials have demonstrated that some of these products are

TABLE 65-1 Indications for Aminoglycoside Agents

Indications	amikacin	gentamicin	kanamycin	neomycin	streptomycin	tobramycin
Systemic infections*						
Gram-negative bacteremia/sepsis	+	+				
Peritonitis	+	+				+
Meningitis	+	+			+	+
Pneumonia		+			+	+
Urosepsis		+	+		+	+
Tuberculosis			+		+	
Endocarditis		+			+	
MRSA/penicillinase-resistant strains		+				
Infectious diarrhea			+	+		
GI sterilization			+	+		
Pyoderma		+		+		
Superficial *Staphylococcus, Streptococcus, Pseudomonas* infections		+		+		

*Aminoglycosides are not a first-line drug and are used only with life-threatening infection.

ineffective in infections caused by gentamicin- and/or tobramycin-resistant strains of gram-negative organisms. The decision to continue therapy with the drug should be based on results of the susceptibility tests, the severity of the infection, the response of the patient, and the important additional considerations of state of hydration, renal status, and other medications that may be taken concomitantly.

HOW TO MONITOR

- Serum peak (drawn approximately 1 hour after dosing) and trough (drawn immediately before dosing) levels should be monitored after the second or third dose and every 3 to 4 days thereafter for the duration of therapy.
- During treatment, collect urine specimens for examination during therapy.
- Monitor serum calcium, magnesium, and sodium.
- Test eighth cranial nerve function by serial audiometric tests.
- Monitor kidney function using creatinine and BUN.

PATIENT VARIABLES

Geriatrics

Diminished glomerular filtration rate related to aging may prolong the drug's half-life and increase the risk of toxicity.

Pediatrics

Premature infants and neonates have immature renal systems resulting in a prolonged half-life of aminoglycosides.

Pregnancy

Category D: aminoglycosides cross the placenta, but the distribution in breast milk is unknown.

PATIENT EDUCATION

- It is necessary to monitor blood values during therapy to ensure effectiveness and prevent toxicity.
- If any visual, hearing, or urinary problems develop, the health care provider should be contacted immediately.
- When IM injections are given, the injection site may be uncomfortable for a short time. Warm moist heat to the area and mild analgesics may reduce localized pain.

Specific Drugs

Because these drugs are not generally used in primary care, only the more important information is presented. Dosage and administration are not discussed.

(P) Prototype Drug

gentamicin (Garamycin, Jenamicin)

Contraindications

- Hypersensitivity

Warnings

- Aminoglycosides are associated with significant nephrotoxicity and ototoxicity.
- Carefully monitor BUN, creatinine, and creatinine clearance values. Recovery of renal function occurs if the drug is stopped at the first sign of renal impairment.
- Electrolyte imbalance may be seen as decreased serum levels of sodium, potassium, calcium, and magnesium.
- Superinfection (especially by fungi) may occur.
- It is essential to maintain adequate hydration, especially with children and the elderly.
- Hypomagnesemia occurs in more than one third of patients whose oral diet is restricted or who are eating poorly.

TABLE 65-2 Pharmacokinetics of Aminoglycoside Antibiotics

Drug	Absorption	Onset of Action	Time to Peak	Half-Life	Duration of Action	Protein Bound	Metabolism	Excretion	Therapeutic Serum Level
gentamicin	Tissues good; CNS poor	1-2 hr	IV 30 min; IM 1 hr	2-3 hr	8 hr	0%-30%	100% excreted unchanged	Renal	Peak 12 μg/ml; trough 2 μg/ml; serum 4-8 μg/ml
amikacin	Tissues good; CNS poor	1-2 hr	IV 30 min; IM 1 hr	2-3 hr	8 hr	1%-10%	100% excreted unchanged	Renal	Peak 15-30 μg/ml; trough 5-10 μg/ml; serum 16-32 μg/ml
kanamycin	Tissues good; CNS poor	Rapid	30 min-2 hr	2-4 hr		1%-10%	>90%	Renal	Peak 15-30 μg/ml; trough 5-10 μg/ml; serum 15-40 μg/ml
neomycin	Tissues good; CNS and GI poor		2-3 hr			0%-30%	Fecal	97% unchanged; renal, 3%	Not applicable
streptomycin	Tissues good; CNS poor	1-2 hr	1 hr	5-6 hr	24 hr	None	100% excreted unchanged	Renal	Peak 50 μg/ml; serum 20-30 μg/ml
tobramycin	Tissues good; CNS poor	1-2 hr	30 min	2-3 hr	8 hr	None	100% excreted unchanged	Renal	Peak 4-10 μg/ml; trough 1-2 μg/ml; serum 4-8 μg/ml

TABLE 65-3 Aminoglycoside Adverse Reactions by Body System

Body System	Common Minor Effects	Serious Adverse Reactions
Body, general		Drug fever, ↓ calcium, sodium, potassium, magnesium
Skin, Appendages		See hypersensitivity
Hypersensitivity		Rash, urticaria, itching, anaphylaxis/anaphylactoid reaction
Respiratory		Apnea
Cardiovascular		Hypotension
GI	Nausea vomiting, diarrhea	
Hemic and lymphatic		Anemia, eosinophilia, leukopenia, thrombocytopenia, granulocytopenia
Musculoskeletal		Acute muscular paralysis
CNS	Headache	Encephalopathy, confusion, lethargy, disorientation, neuromuscular blockade, paresthesia, seizures, numbness, peripheral neuropathy
Special senses	Dizziness, tinnitus, vertigo, roaring in ears	Hearing loss/deafness, loss of balance, visual disturbances/blurred vision
Hepatic		↑ Liver function tests (LFTs)
Genitourinary		↓ Renal function

- Neuromuscular blockade can occur and may result in respiratory paralysis.

Pharmacokinetics
Table 65-2 compares pharmacokinetics for aminoglycoside products.

Adverse Effects
See Table 65-3. Serious adverse reactions are common. Impaired renal function occurs in 5% to 25% of patients, ototoxicity in 3% to 14%, and vestibular toxicity in 4% to 6%.

Drug Interactions
See Table 65-4.

Overdosage
Drug serum levels or signs and symptoms of toxicity can suggest overdosage.

TABLE 65-4 Aminoglycoside Drug Interactions

Aminoglycoside	Action on Other Drugs	Drugs	Action on Aminoglycoside
Aminoglycosides	↑ Neuromuscular blockers, polypeptide antibiotics	cephalosporins, vancomycin, loop diuretics, penicillins	↑ Aminoglycosides

Other Drugs in Class

Other drugs in this class are similar to the prototype except as follows.

neomycin (Cortisporin, Mycifradin, Neobiotic, Neosporin)

Indications. Oral administration of neomycin decreases intestinal bacteria levels and may be useful in treating bacterial diarrhea or preoperative bowel sterilization. It is used topically (Neosporin, Cortisporin), otically (Cortisporin), and ophthalmologically (Neobiotic, Neosporin) for superficial infections of the skin, ears, and eyes.

Irrigation of the urinary bladder with neomycin is effective in preventing bacteriuria in patients with indwelling urinary catheters. Patients with UTIs should have a urine culture and sensitivity done for appropriate antibiotic therapy.

Warnings/Precautions. Superinfection (especially fungi) may occur. Irrigant is intended for genitourinary use only as irrigation of other wounds or sites increases systemic absorption risk.

Risk of systemic absorption of the irrigating solution is increased when therapy exceeds 10 days.

Adverse Effects. Poor absorption from the GI tract decreases the risk of systemic toxicity with oral administration (see Table 65-3). Likewise, it negates the need for serum peak and trough levels.

Irrigant should not be used if open wounds or mucosal excoriation exists because of an increased risk of systemic absorption.

Drug Interactions. Neomycin and polymyxin antibiotic (Neosporin) combinations have a cumulative toxic effect when absorbed systemically.

BIBLIOGRAPHY

Bates DE: Aminoglycoside ototoxicity, *Drugs Today* 39(4):277-285, 2003.

Gilbert DN, Moellering RC, Sande MA: The Sanford Guide to antimicrobial therapy, ed 33, Hyde Park, Ver., 2003, Antimicrobial Therapy, Inc.

Gonzalez LS, Spencer JP: Aminoglycosides: a practical review, *Am Fam Physician* home.aafp.org/afp.981115ap/gonzalez.html.

Group A streptococcus www.cdc/gov/ncidod/diseases/bacter/strep_a.htm.

Kreiger JA et al: Gentamicin contaminated with endotoxin, *N Engl J Med* 340(14):1122, 1999.

Reese RE, Betts RF: *A practical approach to infectious diseases,* ed 4, Boston, 1996, Little, Brown.

Wise R: A review of the mechanisms of action and resistance of antimicrobial agents, *Can Resp Int* 6(suppl A):20A, 1999.

CHAPTER 66

Sulfonamides

Drug Names

Class	Subclass		Generic Name	Trade Name
Sulfonamides	Short acting		sulfisoxazole	Generic
			sulfamethoxazole	Gantanol
			sulfadiazine	Generic
		(P)(200)	trimethoprim and sulfamethoxazole [TMP/SMX])	Bactrim DS, Septra DS
	Active in gut		sulfasalazine	Azulfidine, discussed in Chapter 32
	Topical		sulfacetamide	Discussed in Chapter 15
			silver sulfadiazine	Silvadene

(200), Top 200 drug; (P), prototype drug.

General Uses

Indications

See Table 66-1 for specifics.

- UTIs
- Acute exacerbation of COPD
- Pneumonia
- Traveler's diarrhea
- Diverticulitis
- Sinusitis

The sulfas have a wide antibacterial spectrum that includes both gram-positive and gram-negative organisms, and are most commonly used for UTIs. Frequent allergic reactions and drug resistance limit their use. Sulfa combined with trimethoprim (TMP/SMX) is the most commonly used sulfa because it has fewer problems with resistance.

Sulfonamides are divided into four classes. Two are systemic antibiotics (short acting and long acting); topical and bowel classes. Short acting are rapidly absorbed and rapidly eliminated. The long acting are rapidly absorbed but excreted slowly. Topicals are sulfonamides that are not absorbed systemically; they are used topically particularly in the eye and ear. The poorly absorbed sulfonamides are use to treat infections of the bowels and prepare individuals for surgery.

DRUG ACTION AND EFFECTS

Sulfonamides exert a bacteriostatic activity. They are competitive antagonists that inhibit the enzyme responsible for the utilization of para-aminobenzoic acid (PABA) for the synthesis of folic acid. This mechanism prevents bacteria that synthesize folic acid from reproducing. Those bacteria that do not require folic acid and those that can use folic acid absorbed from the gastrointestinal (GI) tract, are unaffected by the sulfonamides. Human cells are not affected by this mechanism because they do not synthesize folic acid. Trimethoprim bonds to dihydrofolate reductase, the required enzyme of dihydrofolic acid to produce tetrahydrofolic acid, another enzymatic pathway involving folate production.

Bacterial resistance to sulfonamides is presumed to originate by random mutation; transfer of resistance occurs through plasmids. Transfer resistance is probably due to a lower affinity for sulfonamides by the enzyme that utilizes PABA and by decreased bacterial permeability.

DRUG TREATMENT PRINCIPLES

The increasing frequency of resistant organisms has limited the usefulness of the sulfonamides. Resistance develops quickly to sulfa alone, and cross-resistance is common. The addition of trimethoprim improves sulfa activity somewhat. Sulfa allergy is fairly common and can be serious with severe skin reactions. This also limits its usefulness. One advantage is low cost.

TMP/SMX is a first-line treatment of an acute bacterial exacerbation of COPD and diverticulitis. It is an alternative treatment for dog and human bites, acute sinusitis, diarrhea, urinary tract infections (UTIs), and pyelonephritis.

Sulfonamides are active against some gram-positive and some gram-negative bacteria, but no anaerobes. They may be effective against *Streptococcus pneumoniae, Moraxella catarrhalis, Escherichia coli, Klebsiella* sp., *Enterobacter*, and *Legionella* organisms.

HOW TO MONITOR

- Wide variation in blood levels may result with an identical dose. Blood levels should be measured in patients receiving sulfonamides for serious infections.
- Patients should be observed very carefully for the development of severe adverse effects.
- Symptomatic evaluation should also give an indication of effectiveness.

TABLE 66-1 Indications for Sulfonamides with Dosage and Administration

Drug	Bacteria	Site/Disease	Dosage
sulfisoxazole	*H. influenzae, S. pneumoniae, Pneumocystis carinii*	UTI, otitis media, bronchitis, pneumonia, traveler's diarrhea, diverticulitis, sinusitis, dog bite	Adult: loading dose 2-4 g, maintenance 4-8 g/day in four to six divided doses Child (>2 yr): initial dose 75 mg/kg, then 150 mg/kg/day in four to six divided doses
sulfamethoxazole	Same	Same	Adult: 2 g initially, maintenance dose is 1 g bid Child (>2 yr): initially 50-60 mg/kg, maintenance dosage 25-30 mg/kg bid
sulfadiazine	Same	Same	Adult: loading dose 2-4 g, then 2-4 g/day in three to six divided doses Child (>2 yr): loading 75 mg/kg, maintenance 150 mg/kg/day in four to six divided doses
TMP/SMX	Same plus *Shigella flexneri*	UTI and otitis media shigellosis (× 5 days)	Adult: 160 TMP/ 800 SMX q12hr × 10-14 days Child (0.2 m): 8 mg/kg TMP/40 mg/kg SMX/day in two divided doses × 10 days

PATIENT VARIABLES

Geriatrics

The use of TMP/SMX in the elderly results in an increased risk of severe reactions, especially when used in conjunction with other drugs or in those with impaired renal or liver function.

The most frequently reported severe adverse reactions in the elderly include skin reactions, bone marrow depression, and decreased platelets, with or without purpura. The elderly patient who is also taking certain diuretics, especially thiazides, may have an increased incidence of thrombocytopenia with purpura.

Pediatrics

Limited data exists on the safety of repeated courses of TMP/SMX in children younger than 2 years of age. Sulfonamides are not recommended in children younger than 2 months.

Pregnancy

Category C: do not use at term. Because TMP/SMX may interfere with folic acid metabolism, use during pregnancy only if the potential benefits outweigh the potential hazards to the fetus. Lactation: excreted in breast milk.

PATIENT EDUCATION

- Patients should be instructed to drink one 8-ounce glass of water with each dose and several times a day to prevent crystalluria.
- Take on empty stomach with a full glass of water.
- Patients should avoid prolonged exposure to sunlight because photosensitivity may occur.
- Patients should notify provider if hematuria, rash, tinnitus, dyspnea, fever, sore throat, or chills develop.
- For patients taking the oral suspension: Product should be shaken well and refrigerated after opening.

Specific Drugs

Ⓟ Prototype Drug

trimethoprim and sulfamethoxazole (TMP/SMX) (Bactrim DS, Septra DS)

Contraindications

- Hypersensitivity to SMX or TMP
- Megaloblastic anemia due to folate deficiency
- Pregnancy at term and lactation, or infants younger than 2 months of age

Warnings

- Do not use to treat streptococcal pharyngitis due to greater incidence of resistance than with penicillin.
- Hematologic effects: agranulocytosis, aplastic anemia, and other blood dyscrasias. Both TMP and SMX can interfere with hematopoiesis. In patients with G6PD deficiency, hemolysis may occur.
- Hypersensitivity: although rare, fatalities associated with the sulfonamides have occurred from hypersensitivity of the respiratory tract.
- Stevens-Johnson syndrome, toxic epidermal necrolysis.
- Fulminant hepatic necrosis may occur.

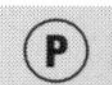

The presentation of a rash, sore throat, fever, arthralgia, cough, shortness of breath, pallor, purpura, or jaundice may be early signs of serious reactions. The drug should be discontinued at the first sign of any adverse reaction.

TMP/SMX should be used with caution in patients with impaired renal or liver function, those with chronic folate deficiency, asthma, or severe allergies.

TABLE 66-2 Pharmacokinetics of Sulfonamides

Drug	Absorption	Time to Peak Concentration	Half Life	Protein Bound	Metabolism	Excretion
sulfisoxazole	96%	1.5-3 hr	5-6 hr	90%	Liver	Kidney, 50%
sulfamethoxazole	100%	4 hr	11 hr	55%	Liver	Kidney, 14%
sulfadiazine	100%	3-6 hr	10 hr	40%	Liver	Kidney
trimethoprim and sulfamethoxazole	70%-100%	2-4 hr	10 hr	55%	Liver, 15%-40%	Kidney

TABLE 66-3 Adverse Reactions to Sulfonamides by Body System

Body System	Common Minor Effects	Serious Adverse Reactions
Body, general		Chills, fever, L.E. phenomenon
Skin, appendages	Photosensitivity	Morbilliform, scarlatinal, erysipeloid, pemphigoid, purpuric, petechia
Hypersensitivity		Stevens-Johnson type erythema multiforme, generalized skin eruptions, epidermal necrolysis, urticaria, periarteritis nodosum, serum sickness, pruritus, exfoliative dermatitis, anaphylactoid reactions, periorbital edema, conjunctival or scleral injection
Respiratory		Allergic decreased pulmonary function
Cardiovascular		Allergic myocarditis
GI	Nausea, vomiting, abdominal pains, diarrhea, anorexia	Pancreatitis, stomatitis, pseudomembranous enterocolitis, glossitis
Hemic and lymphatic		Agranulocytosis, aplastic anemia, thrombocytopenia, leukopenia, hemolytic anemia, purpura, hypoprothrombinemia, neutropenia, eosinophilia, methemoglobinemia
Musculoskeletal		Allergic arthralgia
CNS	Headache, insomnia, apathy, drowsiness,	Peripheral neuropathy, mental depression, convulsions, ataxia, hallucinations, tinnitus, vertigo, polyneuritis, neuritis, optic neuritis, transient myopia
Hepatic		Hepatitis, hepatocellular necrosis
Genitourinary		Crystalluria, elevated creatinine, toxic nephrosis with oliguria and anuria

TABLE 66-4 Sulfonamide Drug Interactions

Sulfa Product	Action on Other Drugs	Drugs	Action on Sulfa Product
sulfonamides	↑ Oral anticoagulants, hydantoins, methotrexate, sulfonylureas, tolbutamide, uricosuric agents	Thiazide diuretics, indomethacin, methenamine, probenecid, salicylates	↑ Sulfonamides
sulfonamides	↓ cyclosporine		
TMP/SMX	↑ Diuretics, zidovudine		

Precautions

Use with caution in patients with possible folate deficiency (elderly, chronic alcoholics, anticonvulsant therapy, malabsorption, malnutrition), severe allergy, or bronchial asthma.

Superinfection may occur.

Pharmacokinetics

The sulfas are readily absorbed from the GI tract. They are distributed throughout the body tissues, entering the cerebrospinal fluid (CSF), pleura, synovial fluids, and the eye. Different patients bind sulfa to plasma proteins to varying degrees, resulting in wide interpatient variation in serum levels. They are not metabolized by the cytochrome P450 enzyme system in the liver, but are metabolized in the liver by conjugation and acetylation. Patients who are slow acetylators have an increased risk of toxicity. Renal excretion is mainly by glomerular filtration. Table 66-2 provides pharmacokinetics.

Adverse Effects

Hypersensitivity reactions are common. Although the blood dyscrasias are relatively rare, they can be fatal.

The incidence of adverse effects to sulfonamides is higher in patients with acquired immunodeficiency syndrome Table 66-3 lists common adverse effects.

Drug Interactions

In elderly patients receiving diuretics, especially the thiazides, there is an increased incidence of thrombocytopenia with purpura.

See Table 66-4.

Overdosage

Symptoms of overdose of TMP/SMX have not been reported. Signs and symptoms of overdose with the sulfonamides include anorexia, colic, nausea, vomiting, dizziness, headache, drowsiness, and unconsciousness.

Dosage and Administration

- The total daily dose should not exceed 350 mg TMP and 1600 mg SMX.
- Decrease dosage in patients who have impaired renal function.
- See Table 66-1.

BIBLIOGRAPHY

Craig TJ et al: Common allergic and allergic-like reactions to medications: when the cure becomes the curse, *Postgrad Med* 105(3):171, 1999.

Gilbert DN, Moellering RC, Sande MA: The Sanford Guide to antimicrobial therapy, ed 33, Hyde Park, Ver., 2003, Antimicrobial Therapy, Inc.

Ibarra C et al: High-dose trimethoprim sulfamethoxazole therapy with corticosteroids in previously intolerant patients with AIDS-associated *Pneumocystis carinii* pneumonia, *Arch Dermatol* 135(3):350, 1999.

Kim DS et al: Antibiotic use at a pediatric age, *Bonsai Med J* 39(6):595, 1998.

Lu KC et al: Is combination antimicrobial therapy required for urinary tract infection in children? *J Microbiol Immunol Infect* 35(1):56-60, 2003.

Nicolle L: Best pharmacological practice: urinary tract infections, *Expert Opin Pharmacother* 4(5):693-704, 2003.

CHAPTER 67

Antitubercular Agents

Drug Names

Class	Subclass	Generic Name	Trade Name
Antibiotic		isoniazid (INH)	Laniazid, generic
		rifampin (RIF)	Rifandin, Rimactane
		pyrazinamide (PZA)	Generic
		ethambutol HCl (EMB)	Myambutol
		streptomycin (SM)	Generic
		cycloserine	Seromycin
		ethionamide	Trecator-SC

General Uses

Indications

- Prevention and treatment of tuberculosis (TB)

This chapter will discuss common antibiotics used in the prevention and treatment of tuberculosis. Their mechanisms of action differ and are discussed in the specific drug sections. There is no prototype drug for this chapter because each antibiotic differs from the others in many aspects.

TB is a highly contagious, reportable disease whose treatment should be initiated by an infectious disease specialist. The primary care provider should be attentive to the possibility that patients may have TB, especially if they come from a high-risk population such as those with HIV/AIDS. These patients should be referred for initial workup and treatment. The primary care provider frequently follows the patient while on therapy. Prophylaxis of TB is an important component of primary care. The use of isoniazid should be a part of every primary care provider's armamentarium.

DISEASE PROCESS

Pathophysiology

TB is caused by *Mycobacterium tuberculosis,* a thick-walled bacterium. The primary route of infection is inhalation of infectious particles. The bacilli are also spread to the lymphatic system and may lodge in bone or other organ systems. A cellular-mediated immune response results in tubercle formation.

The Disease

TB is an infection that has been known for centuries. Its incidence decreased from 1963 to 1985 because of better diagnosis and treatment methods. The current increase in incidence is clearly linked to increases in HIV infection. A normal adult exposed to the disease (reacts positively to a tuberculin skin test) has a 10% chance of developing clinical illness. Patients infected with HIV have an essentially 100% chance of developing the disease. Also, TB in an AIDS patient is extremely difficult to treat.

Clusters of TB patients are considered recently transmitted cases that occur within geographic localities, demographic groups, or individuals sharing certain behaviors and lifestyles. Neighborhoods associated with clustered cases and recent transmission tend to be characterized by low socioeconomic status, inadequate housing, and high rates of drug abuse, poverty, and crime. Unclustered cases are those most likely associated with reactivation of old infection and are usually found in middle-class neighborhoods.

The most common site of TB infection is the pulmonary system. It can also infect the bone, causing bone pain, and the urinary tract, causing urinary tract infection (UTI) symptoms. It then can become disseminated, causing systemic symptoms. Pulmonary TB is seen predominantly in urban areas, whereas rural areas have an increased incidence of urinary and bone TB.

Reactivation disease occurs in a patient who was infected in the past. When the patient becomes old or develops animmunosuppressive illness, the disease may reactivate. This can occur in a patient with chronic obstructive pulmonary disease (COPD) taking prednisone (see Box 67-1 for risk factors for TB).

Assessment

The clinical symptoms of pulmonary TB include cough, pain in chest when breathing or coughing, and cough productive of sputum or blood. The general symptoms of TB, either pulmonary or disseminated, include weight loss, fatigue, malaise, fever, and night sweats.

Testing for Exposure to TB. The Mantoux tuberculin skin test is the preferred test for TB because it is the most accurate. The tine test should no longer be used. With the Mantoux tuberculin skin test, 0.1 ml of purified protein derivative (PPD) tuberculin containing 5 tuberculin units (TU) is injected

BOX 67-1

PATIENTS AT RISK FOR TUBERCULOSIS

Persons with HIV infection.
Close contacts of a person with infectious TB.
Persons with certain medical conditions that decrease resistance to infection, such as diabetes mellitus, lymphoma, certain GI surgeries, 10% below ideal body weight, chronic renal failure, certain cancers, silicosis, immunosuppressive therapy.
Persons who inject drugs.
Foreign-born persons from areas where TB is common.
Medically underserved, low-income populations.
Residents and employees of long-term care facilities such as nursing homes, correctional facilities.
Locally identified high-prevalence groups such as migrant workers, homeless.
Health care workers at risk of exposure to TB in the workplace.

BOX 67-2

CRITERIA FOR A POSITIVE TUBERCULIN SKIN TEST

Greater than 5 mm Induration
Children younger than 1 year of age
X-ray or clinical evidence of TB
Close contact of person with active disease
Evidence of old, healed TB lesions
Persons with HIV infection
Persons with risk factors for HIV
Persons who inject drugs

Greater than 10 mm Induration
Children between 1 and 4 years old
Foreign-born persons from high-prevalence countries
HIV seronegative IV drug users
Persons with medical conditions known to increase risk
Employees and residents of certain long-term and health care facilities

Greater than 15 mm Induration
All others

intradermally to produce a discrete, pale elevation of skin 6 to 10 mm in diameter.

The interpretation of the tuberculin skin test changed in 1997. The new criteria are listed in Box 67-2. The test should be read 48 to 72 hours after the injection. Positive reactions may still be measurable up to 1 week after testing. If the patient returns in more than 3 days and the results appear negative, the test must be repeated. The test site is measured crosswise to the axis of the forearm. Only the induration (hardness) is measured. Erythema is not measured. The result is recorded in millimeters, not positive or negative.

Candidates for testing include all high-risk patients (as indicated in Box 67-1), plus employees or residents in congregate settings, such as hospitals, prisons and jails, homeless shelters, nursing homes, etc., or people from areas of the world with high prevalence of TB. Close contacts of someone with infectious TB who has a negative PPD should be retested 10 weeks after the contact. Previously it was taught to never give a PPD to a patient who had received a bacille Calmette-Guérin (BCG) vaccination. However, previous vaccination with BCG usually should not influence the need for tuberculin skin testing. However, most patients who have received BCG have been told they must never have a PPD because of the risk for serious adverse reaction and will refuse the PPD.

Patients who are immunocompromised should be evaluated for anergy prior to receiving the PPD. Mumps skin test antigen (MSTA) and tetanus toxoid (fluid) may be used. Give 0.1 ml of the antigen intradermally. Read at 48 to 72 hours. Any induration greater than 2 mm is considered positive (reactive), so PPD testing can proceed.

The two-step method should be used in patients who may have diminished skin test reactivity, such as geriatric patients. The procedure is to give a PPD followed by a second PPD in 1 to 3 weeks if the first is negative. Yearly administration of the PPD obviates the need for further two-step testing. If the first test is negative but the second is positive, the patient is considered to have a positive PPD. This reaction is commonly called "boosted." Evaluate elderly patients and high-risk employees by the two-step procedure. It is important to know if a patient has truly converted from negative to positive or if he or she was boosted by a two-step PPD to avoid the false impression of a conversion.

Diagnosis of TB. A chest x-ray (CXR) examination should be obtained on all patients who have a positive PPD. Both posteroanterior and lateral views should be obtained. An apical lordotic view should be obtained if the history is suggestive of TB and the initial films are normal. A person with a normal x-ray is unlikely to have pulmonary TB, making the chest x-ray a very sensitive test.

The goal of x-ray examination is detection of lung abnormalities that indicate active disease. However, the films do not confirm that TB causes any detected abnormalities. A biopsy showing caseation granulomas would confirm the diagnosis. Previously an annual chest x-ray was required for all persons with a positive PPD. Although state policies may vary, most people are considered cleared of TB indefinitely if their chest x-ray is clear, and another chest x-ray is required only if they again develop signs or symptoms of TB.

The culturing of the TB organism takes 6 weeks. Thus for diagnosing TB and determining the severity of a patient's illness, TB control programs worldwide rely on the acid-fast bacilli (AFB) smear. In this test, a sample of sputum is inspected under a light microscope for the presence of tuberculosis bacteria. It is a fast, cheap, and simple method for diagnosing TB. Positive results mean that a patient should immediately be placed in isolation in a hospital because every cough could launch enough bacteria to infect many other people. Negative results have generally been interpreted to mean that the patient is noninfectious and requires no special precautions.

However, theoretic and experimental results have cast doubt on the ability of this test to detect infectious patients. Although as few as five TB bacteria in the lungs can start a new infection, a sample must contain 5000 to 10,000 bacteria per milliliter to reach the test's threshold of detection. Epidemiologic investigations confirm an elevated rate of TB among people exposed to patients who tested negative. Thus there is growing awareness worldwide that persons with negative smears but positive cultures of sputum cause a significant number of infections.

Direct examination of sputum samples will show the presence of acid-fast bacilli. Patients with a positive smear are considered contagious. Culturing sputum, which takes 6 weeks, makes the classic definitive diagnosis. A sputum test, the *Mycobacterium tuberculosis* Direct Test, can give results in 4 to 5 hours. However, this test will miss TB in about 5% of cases, so a culture is still required.

In conclusion, the presumptive diagnosis of active TB is made when the patient has any of the following:

- Recent conversion to positive PPD associated with characteristic signs/symptoms
- Positive sputum smear
- Characteristic chest x-ray
- Biopsy showing caseating granulomas
- Some clinicians add HIV/AIDS to this list because of the high rate of concurrent infection of these patients with TB

The confirmed diagnosis of active TB is made by a positive culture from any body fluid or biopsy specimen.

DRUG ACTION AND EFFECTS

All of the drugs used in the treatment of TB are antibiotics. Each drug is quite different. See specific drug for specific mechanism of action.

DRUG TREATMENT PRINCIPLES

Critical decisions about drug therapy concern whether to provide prophylaxis, choice of drugs for treating active disease, and whether the patient is compliant and responding to prescribed drugs.

Drug resistance to the medications commonly used to treat TB is a major problem. In the past 40 years many inner-city patients have frequently taken inadequate amounts of medication or discontinued therapy prematurely, leading to bacilli that are resistant to many antitubercular drugs in these geographic areas. These resistant organisms then infect other people. The tubercle bacilli may be resistant to several of the standard antituberculous drugs: isoniazid, rifampin, and ethambutol. Some strains are resistant to all known antitubercular drugs. The incidence of resistance is high, and the patterns of resistance are different in different geographic locations. Thus patterns of resistance determine local treatment, which continually changes in response to the development of new resistance.

Prophylaxis

It is important to clarify who should receive preventive treatment. Certainly anyone who fits into the following two categories should be treated:

Recent skin test converters: Persons with a positive tuberculin skin test who have normal chest x-ray results, and no other evidence of active TB.

Close contacts of individuals with infectious, clinically active TB.

Individuals in these two groups should be evaluated to rule out active TB. The health care provider should assess for a history of hepatitis, heavy alcohol ingestion, liver disease, or age older than 35. If the history is positive, LFTs should be obtained to determine whether the patient has any contraindications to therapy. The risk vs. benefits must be weighed for each patient.

Prophylactic treatment includes:

- Isoniazid (INH) 300 mg po daily
- Length of treatment
  Children younger than 18 years old: 9 months
  Adults: 6 months
  Immunocompromised or abnormal chest x-ray findings: 12 months
- Dispense medication 1 month's supply at a time. Monitor patient monthly

If the patient has been exposed to TB known to be resistant to INH, consult the local health department for treatment recommendations.

Treatment of Active Disease

Report all presumptive or confirmed TB cases within 24 hours to your health department. Maintain respiratory isolation.

A patient is assumed to be contagious in any of the following circumstances:

- Cough is present
- Undergoing cough-inducing procedures
- Sputum smear is positive and until there are three negative sputum smears
- Until the patient has been on therapy for at least a week
- Showing poor response to therapy

To prevent the spread of TB in patients being seen in a clinic setting, health care providers should maintain high suspicion of TB, isolate suspected cases immediately, see TB patients when no patients who are at increased risk for TB are in the clinic setting, maintain proper ventilation in the facility, and maintain a TB isolation room in clinics where TB patients are seen frequently.

Inpatient treatment guidelines were established by the CDC. Many states have introduced these treatment guidelines into law in order to protect the public safety.

Multidrug regimens are required for treatment of TB. The initial therapy for TB usually requires four drugs: isoniazid, rifampin, pyrazinamide, and ethambutol or streptomycin. It is essential to never add single drugs to a failing regimen. Generally an infectious disease specialist initiates treatment and follows the patient.

Compliance is the key to successful treatment of tuberculosis. Direct observed therapy (DOT) is now the standard of care in many areas, including Maryland and New York City. In DOT, every dose of antituberculosis medication taken by the patient is observed and supervised by a health care worker. Patients not compliant with medication therapy may be sent to prison to ensure that DOT is carried out. Emerging results from numerous state health departments suggest that DOT programs for TB reduce the prevalence of multidrug-resistant disease, cuts the cost per case of individuals treated, and improves the rate of treatment completion.

Health care providers and institutions that fail to recommend and register TB patients for DOT when resources are available are probably and unnecessarily putting their community at increased risk for TB.

HOW TO MONITOR

isoniazid Prophylaxis

See patients on a monthly basis and ask about signs/symptoms of liver damage or other toxic effects: anorexia, nausea or vomiting, fatigue, weakness, new and persistent paresthesias of the hands and feet, persistent dark urine, icterus, rash, or elevated temperature. Obtain routine liver function tests monthly for patients at high risk of developing INH hepatitis. These include patients more than 35 years old, daily drinkers, those with concomitant medications toxic to liver, or a those with a history of liver disease. Discontinue INH immediately if a patient develops signs or symptoms of toxicity.

Patients with Active TB

Obtain chest x-ray at baseline and at 6 months. Collect sputum smear and culture at baseline, and monthly until negative. Measure levels of hepatic enzymes, bilirubin, serum creatinine, CBC, platelets, and serum uric acid at baseline and monthly.

There are also some potential problems for which patients taking specific drugs should be monitored: For patients taking INH, obtain periodic ophthalmologic examinations; for those taking pyrazinamide, collect blood glucose levels (may be particularly difficult to control glucose levels of patients with diabetes mellitus [DM]); ethambutol, monitor color vision for red-green at baseline and at 2 and 3 months; streptomycin, have audiogram before beginning drug and at 2 and 3 months, as well as monitoring drug serum concentrations of streptomycin; cycloserine, monitor blood level weekly in patients with reduced renal function.

PATIENT VARIABLES

Geriatrics

Patients are at increased risk for toxic effects, especially liver and CNS.

Pediatrics

Treatment of TB in children is difficult, especially with young children unable to report symptoms reliably or cooperate with tests such as visual acuity. Risk vs. benefits must be weighed for the individual patient. Whereas dosages for some of these products may be listed for pediatric patients, safety and dosages may not have been established for many drugs.

INH, rifampin, and pyrazinamide are commonly used with children. Ethambutol is not recommended for use in children younger than 13 years. Streptomycin is not recommended for use in children. Cycloserine and ethionamide have not had safety and dosage established for pediatric use.

Pregnancy

Category C: prescribe only when necessary to the pregnant mother

Category D: aminoglycosides; ethionamide: teratogenic effects demonstrated in animals

Lactation

INH, rifampin, pyrazinamide, ethambutol, and cycloserine all appear in breast milk.

PATIENT EDUCATION

Patients need extensive education about the nature of the disease and the need to follow instructions exactly. The most important points are summarized as follows:

Compliance

- Take medication exactly as directed.
- Keep all appointments for follow-up.
- Adequate testing will be required to determine if TB is being halted.
- Maintain respiratory isolation while contagious.
- Avoid intimate contact with others.
- Cough into tissue, dispose of tissue in closed plastic bags.

For information about the particular medications, see *Patient Education* under the specific drug.

Specific Drugs

isoniazid (INH) (generic, Laniazid)

Mechanism of Action. INH is bacteriostatic for resting organisms and bactericidal for dividing organisms. It interferes with lipid and nucleic acid biosynthesis in growing organisms.

Contraindications

- Known contact with an isoniazid-resistant TB case
- Previous INH-associated adverse effect
- Acute liver disease, severe chronic liver disease

Warnings

- Watch for hypersensitivity reactions
- Monitor patients with renal or hepatic function impairment
- Carcinogenesis: INH induces tumors in mice
- Malnourished patients or those predisposed to peripheral neuropathy should receive pyridoxine
- Periodic ophthalmic examinations are recommended

Pharmacokinetics. Table 67-1 compares pharmacokinetics for all anti-tubercular products. INH is metabolized primarily by acetylation and dehydrazination. The rate of acetylation is genetically determined, with approximately 50% of blacks and whites being "slow acetylators" and the rest rapid acetylators; the majority of Eskimos and Asians are "rapid acetylators."

Adverse Effects. Table 67-2 summarizes major side effects of all anti-TB products according to body system affected.

The most frequent adverse effects to INH involve the nervous system and the liver.

Drug Interactions

- Isoniazid is a P450 1A2 inhibitor and a 2C inhibitor
- Concomitant use of alcohol is associated with higher incidence of hepatitis

TABLE 67-1 Pharmacokinetics of Major Antitubercular Medications

Drug	Absorption	Time to Peak Concentration	Half-Life	Protein Bound	Metabolism	Excretion	Therapeutic Serum Level
isoniazid	Food may interfere with absorption	1-2 hr	Varies widely	24 hr	Diffuses to all body tissues	Hepatic: acetylation; rate of metabolism genetically determined	Renal
rifampin	Readily absorbed	Varies widely	2-3 hr	Distribution to all body tissues; 80% protein bound	Hepatic	Bile, 70%; urine, 30%	4-32 μg/ml
pyrazinamide	Well absorbed	2 hr	9-10 hr	Most tissues	Hepatic	Renal	9-12 μg/ml
ethambutol	75%-80%	2-4 hr	24 hr	Most tissues	Hepatic: oxidation	Renal: 80%; feces: 20%	Requires special assay
streptomycin	PO: poor; IM: rapid	1 hr	5-6 hr	Well distributed	Renal: glomerular filtration		25-50 μg/ml
cycloserine	Well absorbed	4-8 hr	12 hr	Wide		Renal	25-30 μg/ml
ethionamide	80%, rapid	3 hr		Wide	Hepatic	Renal: active drug and metabolites	

- Benzodiazepine activity may be increased
- Disulfiram: acute behavioral and coordination changes
- Phenytoin: increased levels
- Carbamazepine: toxicity or INH hepatotoxicity may result
- Ketoconazole: serum concentration decreased
- Anticoagulants, oral: activity may be enhanced
- Cycloserine: increased CNS side effects, especially dizziness
- Meperidine: hypotension or CNS depression
- Rifampin: high rate of hepatotoxicity
- Aluminum-containing antacids: reduce oral absorption, administer separately
- INH has some monoamine oxidase (MAO) inhibitor activity and may cause interactions with tyramine-containing foods. Diamine oxidase may also be inhibited, causing reactions to foods containing histamine.

Overdosage. Symptoms of nausea, vomiting, dizziness, slurring of speech, blurring of vision, and visual hallucination are early signs. Later symptoms are respiratory distress and CNS depression and can be fatal.

Patient Education
- Take on an empty stomach 1 hour before or 2 hours after a meal.
- Minimize alcohol consumption.
- Avoid foods containing tyramine (see MAO inhibitors) and histamine (tuna, sauerkraut, and yeast extract).
- Notify health care provider if fatigue, weakness, nausea/vomiting, loss of appetite, yellowing of skin or eyes, darkening of urine, or numbness and tingling in hands or feet occur.

Dosage and Administration. Table 67-3 indicates dosage, administration, and available formulations for all antitubercular products.

rifampin (RIF) (Rifadin, Rimactane)

Mechanism of Action. Rifampin inhibits DNA-dependent RNA-polymerase activity, suppressing RNA synthesis. It can be bacteriostatic or bactericidal and is most active against bacteria undergoing cell division.

Contraindications. Hypersensitivity.

Warnings
- Hepatotoxicity with fatalities has developed. Monitor liver function carefully. Adjust dose with impaired liver function.
- Hyperbilirubinemia may occur.
- Porphyria may be exacerbated.
- Meningococci resistance may emerge rapidly.
- Hypersensitivity reactions may occur during intermittent therapy or if therapy is resumed after interruption.
- May be associated with carcinogenesis.
- Monitor CBC and LFTs.
- Urine, feces, saliva, sputum, sweat, and tears may be colored red-orange. Soft contact lenses may be permanently stained.
- Thrombocytopenia has occurred, primarily with high-dose intermittent therapy or after resumption of interrupted treatment. It occurs rarely during well-supervised daily therapy. It is usually reversible, but fatalities have occurred.

Adverse Effects. GI symptoms and rash are common adverse effects. High doses may cause flulike syndrome, hematopoietic reactions, and other serious side effects.

Drug Interactions
- P450: rifampin is a 1A2 substrate, 2C inducer, 2D6 inducer, and a 3A4 inducer and substrate.

TABLE 67-2 Important Adverse Effects of Antituberculosis Agents by Body System

Body System	isoniazid	rifampin	pyrazinamide	ethambutol	streptomycin	cycloserine	ethionamide
Body, general		Stains urine orange-red		Fever, malaise, dizziness, headache			
Skin, appendages				Dermatitis, pruritus		Rash	Rash, alopecia
Hypersensitivity	Fever, rash, vasculitis				Rash, fever		
Cardiovascular						CHF	Postural hypotension
GI	Nausea, vomiting	Distress	Disturbances	Nausea, vomiting, anorexia, abdominal pain			Anorexia, nausea/ vomiting, diarrhea, metallic taste, jaundice
Hematologic and lymphatic	Agranulocytosis, thrombocytopenia	Thrombocytopenia	Thrombocytopenia	Thrombocytopenia			Thrombocytopenia
Metabolic and nutritional			↓ DM control			Anemia: B_{12}, folic megaloblastic	
Musculoskeletal		Gout, myalgias, arthralgias	Gout, joint pain				
Nervous system	Peripheral neuropathy, numbness, tingling of extremities		Mental confusion			Drowsiness, somnolence, dizziness, headache, lethargy, depression, tremor, paresthesia, anxiety, vertigo, memory loss, seizures, possible suicidal tendencies	Depression, drowsiness, asthenia, peripheral neuritis, neuropathy, headache, tremors, psychosis
Special senses				Optic neuritis, loss of acuity, loss of red-green discrimination	Ototoxicity		
Hepatic	Jaundice, abnormal liver function tests (LFTs)	Hepatic toxicity	Hepatic toxicity			Elevated LFTs	
Genitourinary		Hyperbilirubinemia			Nephrotoxicity		

TABLE 67-3 Antituberculosis Drugs: Dosage, Administration, How Supplied

Drug	Dosage	Administration	How Supplied
isoniazid	Route: PO, IM Adult: Daily dose is 5 mg/kg; higher doses may be given. Pediatric dose: 10-20 mg/kg/day (max 300 mg). Give as a single daily dose, may be divided. Give pyridoxine (15-50 mg a day) while patient is on INH.	Take on an empty stomach; 1 hr before or 2 hr after a meal. Minimize alcohol consumption. Avoid foods containing tyramine (see MAO inhibitors) and histamine (tuna, sauerkraut, and yeast extract).	Tablets: 50 mg, 100 mg, 300 mg Syrup: 50 mg/5 ml Injection: 500 mg/ml
rifampin	Oral and IV Adult: 600 mg once daily. Pediatric: 10-20 mg/kg/day (max 600 mg).	Take on an empty stomach, 1 hr before or 2 hr after meals. Avoid missing doses. May cause a red-orange discoloration of body fluids.	Capsules: 150 mg, 300 mg Powder for injection: 600 mg
pyrazinamide	Oral Usual dose: 15-30 mg/kg/day (max 3 g/day). Pediatric: 15-30 mg/kg/day (max 2 g/day); divide dose. Alternative dose: 50-70 mg/kg; twice a week.	Stress importance of not missing any doses. Store medication at 59°-86° F.	Tablets: 500 mg
ethambutol	Initial treatment: 15 mg/kg/day (single dose). Pediatric dose (≥6 yr): Same as above. Retreatment: 25 mg/kg/day; after 60 days of therapy decrease dose to 15 mg/kg/day.	May cause GI upset; take with food. Aluminum-containing antacids may interfere with absorption; separate administration by several hours.	Tablets: 100 mg, 400 mg
streptomycin	IM route only Usual dose: 15 mg/kg/day in divided doses given every 12 hours. Do not exceed 2 g day. Adjust dosage according to renal function. Pediatric dose: 20-30 mg/kg/day.	Watch for symptoms of ototoxicity and nephrotoxicity.	Injection: 400 mg/ml
cycloserine	Initial: 250 mg twice daily for first 2 wk; 500 mg to 1 g daily in divided doses; (maximum daily dose 1 g). Pediatric dose: 10-20 mg/kg/day; 500 mg/day.	Avoid alcohol consumption. Monitor blood levels.	Capsules: 250 mg
ethionamide	Oral: 500 mg to 1 gm daily in divided doses. Concomitant administration of pyridoxine is recommended. Pediatric dose: 15-20 mg/kg/day; take in two divided doses.	May cause stomach upset, metallic taste, or loss of appetite. Take with food to minimize GI upset. Notify practitioner if GI effects persist. Keep in tightly closed containers.	Tablets: 250 mg

- Rifampin may decrease the therapeutic effects of the following drugs: acetaminophen, oral anticoagulants, barbiturates, benzodiazepines, β-blockers, oral contraceptives, corticosteroids, cyclosporine, disopyramide, estrogens, phenytoin, methadone, quinidine, sulfonylureas, theophyllines, and verapamil.
- Digoxin serum concentrations may be decreased by rifampin.
- Rifampin inhibits assays for folate and vitamin B_{12}.

Overdosage
- Symptoms: nausea, vomiting, and lethargy. Liver toxicity may occur; patient must be hospitalized.

Patient Education
- Take on empty stomach 1 hour before or 2 hours after meals.
- Avoid missing doses.
- May cause a red-orange discoloration of body fluids.
- Notify practitioner if "flulike" symptoms, yellow discoloration of skin or eyes, skin rash, or itching occurs.

Dosage and Administration. See Table 67-3.

pyrazinamide (PZA)

Mechanism of Action. The mechanism of action is unknown. It may be bacteriostatic or bactericidal against *M. tuberculosis*, depending on the concentration.

Contraindications
- Hypersensitivity, liver damage, or acute gout

Warnings/Precautions
- Inhibits renal excretion of urates and may cause hyperuricemia and gout.

- Use with caution in patients with renal function impairment. Reduction in dosage is not usually necessary.
- Monitor patients with hepatic function impairment closely.
- In patients with DM, control may be more difficult.

Adverse Effects. Mild arthralgia and myalgia are frequent. The most common serious adverse reactions are gout and hepatic toxicity.

Drug Interactions. No P450 interactions are known.

Overdosage. Experience is limited. Liver toxicity may develop.

Patient Education. Patient reports fever, loss of appetite, malaise, nausea and vomiting, darkened urine, yellowish discoloration of skin or eyes, pain or swelling of joints.

Dosage and Administration. See Table 67-3.

ethambutol HCl (EMB) (Myambutol)

Mechanism of Action. Ethambutol impairs cellular metabolism, causing cell multiplication to stop and cell death. It is bactericidal and active only against mycobacteria.

Contraindications. Hypersensitivity or known optic neuritis

Warnings/Precautions

> ! Visual testing should be conducted before initiating ethambutol therapy and periodically while on therapy. Vision testing should be done on each eye individually and on both eyes together. It should include visual acuity, ophthalmoscopy, peripheral fields, and color discrimination.

Renal impairment requires dose adjustment.

Adverse Effects. See Table 67-2.

Drug Interactions. Aluminum salts may delay and reduce the absorption of ethambutol; administer separately.

Patient Information
- May cause GI upset; take with food.
- Aluminum-containing antacids may interfere with absorption; separate administration by several hours.
- Notify practitioner if changes in vision occur blurring, red-green color blindness or skin rash occurs.

Dosage and Administration. See Table 67-3.

streptomycin (SM)

See aminoglycosides, Chapter 65 for complete information.

Mechanism of Action. Streptomycin is a bactericidal antibiotic. It acts by interfering with normal protein synthesis.

Adverse Effects. Ototoxicity and nephrotoxicity are serious adverse effects.

Dosage and Administration. See Table 67-3. Drug is given by IM injection.

cycloserine (Seromycin)

Mechanism of Action. Cycloserine inhibits cell wall synthesis and can be either bacteriostatic or bactericidal.

Warnings/Precautions
- CNS toxicity, dysarthria, or allergic dermatitis warrants discontinuation or reduction in dosage.
- Toxicity is related to high blood levels; the therapeutic index is narrow.
- In renal function impairment, cycloserine will accumulate and toxicity will develop.
- Anticonvulsant drugs or sedatives may be effective in controlling symptoms. Pyridoxine may also help.
- Has been associated with B_{12}, folic acid deficiency, megaloblastic anemia, and sideroblastic anemia.

Adverse Effects. CNS symptoms such as convulsions, psychosis, somnolence, depression, confusion, hyperreflexia, headache, tremor, vertigo, and paresis are the most problematic.

Drug Interactions
- Isoniazid (increase in dizziness)
- Alcohol (increases risk and possibility of epileptic episodes)

Overdosage
- Symptom: CNS depression

Patient Information
- Notify practitioner if signs of dizziness, mental confusion, skin rash, or tremor occur.
- Avoid alcohol consumption.
- May cause drowsiness; use caution when operating dangerous machinery.

Dosage and Administration. See Table 67-3.

ethionamide (Trecator-SC)

Indications
- Treatment of tuberculosis when first-line therapy (INH, rifampin) has failed

Mechanism of Action. Ethionamide probably inhibits peptide synthesis and is bacteriostatic or bactericidal, depending on concentration attained and susceptibility of the organism. It is highly specific against *Mycobacterium*.

Contraindications
- Hepatic damage or hypersensitivity

Warnings/Precautions
- Hepatitis occurs more frequently; monitor LFTs.
- Management of diabetes may be more difficult.

Drug Interactions. Temporarily raises serum concentrations of INH. It may potentiate the adverse effects of other antitubercular drugs if administered concomitantly, especially with cycloserine. Avoid excessive ethanol ingestion because it may produce psychotic reaction.

Patient Information

- May cause stomach upset, metallic taste, or loss of appetite.
- Take with food to minimize GI upset.
- Notify practitioner if these effects persist.

Dosage and Administration. See Table 67-3.

RESOURCES FOR PATIENTS AND PROVIDERS

Internet

Antimicrobial Use Guidelines, www.medsch.wisc.edu/clinsci/amcg/amcg.html.

Interdisciplinary guide to antimicrobials from the University of Wisconsin.

CDC, www.cdcna.org.

CDC guidelines for prevention of TB.

BIBLIOGRAPHY

AAP Committee on Infectious Diseases: update on tuberculosis skin testing of children, *Pediatrics* 97:282, 1996.

AAP 2003 Red Book, Report of the Committee on Infectious Diseases, Washington, DC, 2003, American Academy of Pediatrics.

Agrawal S et al: Bioequivalence assessment of rifampicin, isoniazid and pyrazinamide in a fixed dose combination of rifampicin, isoniazid, pyrazinamide and ethambutol vs separate formulations, *Int J Clin Pharmaco Ther* 40(10):474-481, 2002.

Gilbert DN, Moellering RC, Sande MA: The Sanford Guide to antimicrobial therapy, ed 33, Hyde Park, Ver., 2003, Antimicrobial Therapy, Inc.

Iseman MD: Tuberculosis therapy: past, present and future, *Eur Respir J Suppl* 36:87s-94s, 2002.

Pablos-Mendez A, Gowda D, Frieden TR: Controlling multidrug resistant tuberculosis and access to expensive drugs: a rational framework, *Bull World Health Org* 80(6):489-495; discussion 495-500, 2002.

Zhu M et al: Population pharmacokinetics of ethionamide in patients with tuberculosis. *Tuberculosis* 82(2-3):91-96, 2002.

Zwolska Z, Augustynowicz-Kopec E, Niemirowska-Mikulska H: The pharmacokinetic factors and bioavailability of rifampicin, isoniazid and pyrazinamide fixed in one dose capsule, *Acta Pol Pharm* 59(6):448-452, 2002.

CHAPTER 68

Antifungals

Drug Names

Class	Subclass	Generic Name	Trade Name
Azoles	Imidazoles	ketoconazole	Nizoral
	Triazoles	(200) fluconazole	Diflucan
		itraconazole	Sporanox
Allylamine		terbinafine	Lamisil
Griseofulvin		griseofulvin	Grisactin, Fulvicin, Gris-PEG

(200), Top 200 drug.

General Uses

Indications

- Onychomycosis
- Tinea
- Candida
- Histoplasmosis
- Blastomycosis
- Pneumocystosis
- Cryptococcosis
- Aspergillosis

This chapter discusses the use of oral antifungals in the treatment of two types of fungal infections: systemic fungal infections and superficial fungal infections not responsive to topical therapy. Treatment of superficial fungal infections with topical antifungal agents is discussed in Chapter 14. All of these drugs except fluconazole have black box warnings regarding either hepatic toxicity or drug interactions.

The azoles are synthetic compounds with broad antifungal activity effective against most yeast and filamentous fungi. Ketoconazole, the only imidazole on the market, is effective in systemic fungal infections but has a warning about hepatic toxicity, including some fatalities. The triazole fluconazole is fairly safe given orally. Itraconazole has a warning regarding chronic heart failure (CHF) and may not be used in patients with evidence of cardiac dysfunction. It also has many serious drug interactions involving the 3A4 system.

Terbinafine also has a warning regarding hepatic failure, some situations leading to death. Griseofulvin is fairly safe but has a limited spectrum of action. Caspofungin and the triazole, voriconazole, are new antifungals for the treatment of invasive aspergillosis and other serious fungal infections refractive to other therapy, and are not discussed in this chapter. Amphotericin B is an older drug that is not discussed because it is only used by specialists for progressive and potentially fatal fungal infections.

DISEASE PROCESS

Anatomy and Physiology

Fungi can be divided into two broad categories based on morphology: yeasts and molds. Yeasts are unicellular fungi that are typically round or oval and reproduce by budding. When buds do not separate, they form long chains of yeast cells known as pseudohyphae. Molds are multicellular colonies composed of tubular structures called hyphae that grow by branching and longitudinal extension. Some fungi are dimorphic and can grow as either yeast or molds, depending on environmental conditions.

Fungal and mammalian cells are eukaryocytes. Unlike bacteria, which are prokaryocytes, eukaryocytes have a distinct nucleus, specialized organelles, and a protective cell membrane. A key difference between fungal and mammalian cells is the sterol used in the synthesis of their respective cell membranes ergosterol in fungi, cholesterol in mammals.

Pathophysiology

Mycosis is the presence of parasitic fungi in or on the body. Most fungi that are pathogenic in humans grow as yeast, are nonmotile, and with rare exceptions are not transmissible. Fungal infections can be superficial (confined to the keratinous layers), subcutaneous, or deeply invasive.

The Disease

Fungal infections have increased dramatically over the past 20 years. This increase is associated with the widespread use of broad-spectrum antibiotics, a rise in the number of invasive procedures, immunosuppression associated with organ transplants and chemotherapy, the treatment of autoimmune disorders, and AIDS. The AIDS epidemic has radically altered the spectrum and frequency of fungal infections. Fungal infections in transplant and AIDS patients tend to be severe and usually require indefinite treatment.

Fungal infections of the nails remain prevalent, and demand for treatment has increased as safer drugs have been developed. A factor limiting this treatment is the refusal of many health insurance companies to reimburse for these medications, which are expensive and must be used for an extended period. However, infections of the nails are generally impervious to superficial treatment. Ciclopirox (Penlac) is a new topical medication effective for skin and nail infections; however, it too is expensive (see Chapter 14).

Some tinea infections require systemic treatment. Tinea capitis (most commonly caused by *Trichophyton tonsurans*) usually requires systemic treatment. Tinea corporis (usually caused by *T. rubrum*) usually responds to topical therapy, but may require systemic treatment. Tinea versicolor (caused by *Malassezia furfur* or *Pityrosporum orbiculare*) frequently requires systemic treatment.

Candida albicans is part of the normal flora of the mouth, vagina, and feces of most people. Overgrowth of candida organisms causes mucosal candidiasis, which may include the mouth, esophagus, and vulvovagina. It is also frequently found on the skin, especially in skinfolds. Vulvovaginal candida is discussed in Chapter 57. Topical candida is discussed in Chapter 14. Risk factors for invasive candidiasis (fungemia and endocarditis) include neutropenia, recent surgery, broad-spectrum antibiotic therapy, indwelling catheters (intravenous [IV] or bladder), and immunodeficiency. HIV infection should be suspected if patient has invasive candidiasis.

The primary care provider should be aware of endemic fungal infections in rural and regional populations and maintain a high index of suspicion. Skin tests are available to aid in the diagnoses of some of these. Most of these fungi cause few infections in immune competent persons. Patients at risk are immunocompromised, especially those with HIV. There are a great many of these fungi and only a few of the most common are mentioned.

Histoplasmosis is caused by *Histoplasma capsulatum*. *H. capsulatum* can be found in bird droppings and bat exposure along river valleys, especially the Ohio and Mississippi river valleys. Symptoms are those of respiratory system. Most cases, in healthy people, are asymptomatic or mild and unrecognized. More severe infections present as atypical pneumonia. It also can be acute and severe or progressive disseminated and fatal. Severe symptoms are marked prostration, fever, dyspnea, and loss of weight.

Coccidioidomycosis is caused by *Coccidioides immitis*, a mold that grows in soil in arid regions of the southwestern United States, Mexico, and Central and South America. Few immunocompetent people get these infections, but among those who do, the mortality is high. Symptoms are respiratory tract symptoms with fever, chills, and arthralgia.

Blastomycosis is caused by *Blastomyces dermatititidis*. It occurs primarily in healthy men, infected during outdoor activities in the south-central and midwestern United States and Canada. Symptoms are of a pulmonary infection. Dissemination may occur with lesions on the skin, in bones, and in the urogenital system.

Pneumocystosis is caused by *Pneumocystis carinii*. It is a fungus found in the lungs of many domesticated and wild mammals and is distributed worldwide in humans. It seldom causes illness in immunocompetent people. It causes an acute pneumonia in premature or debilitated infants in hospitals in underdeveloped countries and older children and adults who have weakened cellular immune systems, most commonly by HIV. It is an important cause of death in AIDS patients.

Cryptococcosis is caused by *Cryptococcus neoformans*, a yeast that is found worldwide in soil and in dried pigeon dung. It is acquired by inhalation. Immunocompetent people rarely develop clinically apparent pneumonia. Progressive lung disease and dissemination occur in patients with immunodeficiency, including HIV.

Aspergillosis is caused by *Aspergillus fumigatus*. This fungus often colonizes in burn eschar and detritus in the external ear canal. Clinical symptoms are bronchospasm and pulmonary infiltrates. It can become invasive, again most commonly in patients who are immunocompromised, such as HIV.

DRUG ACTION AND EFFECTS

The azoles are primarily fungistatic rather than fungicidal. They are classified as either imidazoles or triazoles, depending on whether the azole has two or three nitrogens in the five-membered azole ring.

The azoles' primary antifungal effect is the inhibition of ergosterol synthesis. This is accomplished by disrupting C-14 α-demethylase, an enzyme dependent on cytochrome P450. Without ergosterol, fungal cell membranes become more permeable and leak cell contents. Cell growth and replication are thereby inhibited.

Terbinafine blocks the biosynthesis of ergosterol, an essential component of fungal cell membranes.

Griseofulvin is derived from a species of *Penicillium*. It is deposited in the keratin of diseased tissue, making it resistant to fungal infection. The diseased tissue is gradually exfoliated and replaced by noninfected tissue.

DRUG TREATMENT PRINCIPLES

Cultures should be obtained whenever possible to confirm a diagnosis of fungal infection. If infections are unresponsive to empiric therapy, cultures must be obtained to confirm the diagnosis and rule out resistant organisms. Table 68-1 summarizes the drugs of choice for treatment of fungal infections, depending upon the identified organism. Use the least toxic drug possible for the particular infection. It is clear that these drugs have the potential for serious adverse reactions and drug interactions are a problem.

The optimal duration of treatment with antifungal therapy is not clear. Depending on the infection, they are continued for weeks, months, or, as is frequently the case with AIDS patients, indefinitely.

Fluconazole has been approved for single-dose treatment of vulvovaginal candidiasis, although the CDC still recommend topical therapy with an imidazole-derivative antifungal as preferable due to the appearance of fluconazole-resistant candidiasis in both HIV and non-HIV patients.

Terbinafine is not effective against *Epidermophyton floccosum*, *C. albicans*, and *Scopulariopsis brevicollis*.

Griseofulvin is used for tinea infections of the skin, hair, and nails not responsive to topical therapy, caused by *Trichophyton*, *Microsporum*, and *Epidermophyton* fungi. It is

TABLE 68-1 Indications for Antifungals with Dosage and Administration

Drug	Site/Disease	Dosage and Administration
ketoconazole	Candidiasis, blastomycosis, histoplasmosis, severe tinea, onychomycosis	Adult: 200-400 mg qd Child (>2 yr): 3.3-6.6 mg/kg/day as single daily dose Candida × 2 wk; systemic 6 mo
fluconazole	Candidiasis	Adult vaginal: 150 mg as single oral dose Adult oral: 200 mg × 1 d, then 100 mg qd × 2 wk Adult esophageal: 200 mg × 1 day, then 100 mg qd × 3 wk
	Cryptococcal meningitis	
itraconazole	Tinea	Corporis/cruris: 100 mg qd × 14 d Pedis: 100 qd × 28 day Versicolor: 200 mg qd × 7 days
	Onychomycosis	200 mg bid × 7 days, 3 wk; drug free then repeat × 2 for fingernail or × 3 for toenail
	Candidiasis	Oral 100-200 mg qd × 2-4 wk
	Blastomycosis/histoplasmosis	200-400 mg qd × 3 mo or more
	Aspergillosis	200 mg qd-bid × 3-4 mo
terbinafine	Onychomycosis	Fingernail: 250 mg/day × 6 wk Toenail: 250 mg/day × 12 wk
griseofulvin	Tinea corporis, tinea cruris, tinea capitis	Adult: single or divided daily dose of 500 microsize (330-375 mg ultramicrosize)
	Tinea pedis, tinea unguium	Adult: 0.75-1 g microsize (660-750 ultramicrosize)/day in divided doses

ineffective against other organisms, such as candidiasis, blastomycosis, coccidioidomycosis, and histoplasmosis. Griseofulvin used for tinea requires lengthy treatment, and recurrences are common. Topical treatment of tinea capitis is usually ineffective because the fungus invades the hair shaft. Once-daily dose of griseofulvin for 4 to 6 weeks is usually effective.

HOW TO MONITOR

All Antifungals

Perform initial cultures. Assess response to therapy by repeat cultures as necessary.

Assess for signs or symptoms of hepatitis such as fatigue, anorexia, nausea, vomiting, jaundice, dark urine, or pale stools.

Perform LFTs before initiating therapy and periodically thereafter (e.g., baseline studies, then biweekly for 2 months and every 1 to 2 months thereafter).

Azoles

Assess for inhibition of steroidogenesis with high-dose ketoconazole. Patients receiving itraconazole 600 mg/day may experience adrenal suppression. High doses and/or prolonged therapy with itraconazole have been associated with hypokalemia and secondary ventricular fibrillation.

terbinafine

Immunodeficiency: consider monitoring CBC in patients receiving treatment for more than 6 weeks.

griseofulvin

Check baseline and periodic renal, liver, and hematopoietic function.

PATIENT VARIABLES

Geriatrics

- Elderly patients tend to be more susceptible to hepatotoxicity and are likely to be on other medications that may interact with these drugs. These products require lower dosages in patients with reduced renal function.
- Itraconazole oral solution should be used with caution.

Pediatrics

- Ketoconazole, griseofulvin: the safety for use in children younger than 2 years has not been established.
- Fluconazole: has been used in immunocompromised children 6 months and older.
- Itraconazole: has been used in children with serious system infections 3 months to 12 years. Safety and efficacy have not been established.
- Terbinafine: safety and efficacy have not been established.
- Griseofulvin may produce estrogen-like effects in children, including enlarged breasts and hyperpigmentation of areolae, nipples, and external genitalia.

Pregnancy

- *Category B:* terbinafine, not recommended, present in breast milk.
- *Category C:* ketoconazole, fluconazole, itraconazole, griseofulvin: teratogenic effects have been seen in animals.
- Women taking itraconazole or griseofulvin should use contraception during and for 1 month after therapy.

Lactation

- Excreted in breast milk. Do not prescribe to nursing women.

PATIENT EDUCATION

All Antifungals

- Take as prescribed. Inadequate treatment periods may result in a poor response or early recurrence of symptoms.
- Immediately report any signs or symptoms of hepatitis such as fatigue, anorexia, nausea, vomiting, jaundice, dark urine, or pale stools.
- Griseofulvin and ketoconazole many cause photosensitivity.

Azoles

- Do not take ketoconazole or itraconazole within 2 hours of taking antacids.
- Fluconazole may be taken without regard to food or gastric acidity.
- Women of childbearing age should use contraception or abstain from sexual intercourse while on azole therapy.

griseofulvin

- Bioavailability improves when given with food.
- Headaches, if they occur, usually disappear with continued therapy or when griseofulvin is taken with food.
- Notify provider if skin rash or sore throat appears.
- May potentiate effects of alcohol.

Specific Drugs

AZOLES

The azoles have enough differences between them that they will be discussed separately.

Imidazoles

ketoconazole (Nizoral)

Contraindications

- Hypersensitivity
- Fungal meningitis due to poor penetration into the cerebrospinal fluid (CSF)
- Concomitant use with oral triazolam

Warnings. Hepatic toxicity: asymptomatic elevations of plasma aminotransferase occur in less than 10% of patients on azole therapy.

Ketoconazole, and rarely the triazoles, can cause clinically significant and even fatal hepatitis. Therapy must be stopped immediately if signs or symptoms of hepatitis develop, or with laboratory evidence of persistent or progressive hepatic dysfunction.

- In one series, the median time for development of symptomatic hepatitis associated with ketoconazole therapy was 28 days but occurred in as few as 3 days. Toxicity is usually hepatocellular, but a cholestatic or mixed pattern of injury may occur and is associated with an elevated alkaline phosphatase. Hepatic injury is usually reversible with recovery in several weeks to months after discontinuation of the drug.
- Prostatic cancer has been associated with ketoconazole but the causal relationship is not known.
- Hypersensitivity reactions: anaphylaxis occurs rarely after the first dose. Other hypersensitivity reactions, including urticaria, have been reported.

Precautions. Steroidogenesis: ketoconazole can directly inhibit adrenal cortisol and testosterone synthesis. Testosterone levels (and therefore estradiol) are lowered with ketoconazole doses greater than 400 mg/day and eliminated altogether with 1600 mg/day. A variety of hormonal disturbances are seen, including low sperm counts, decreased libido, impotence, gynecomastia, and menstrual irregularities. High doses may also inhibit adrenal cortisol production and, in rare cases, cause adrenal insufficiency. These effects have been exploited therapeutically in the treatment of prostate cancer and Cushing syndrome (hypercortisolism).

The products require gastric acidity for dissolution and absorption. They should not be taken with antacids, anticholinergics, or H_2 blockers.

Pharmacokinetics. See Table 68-2.

Adverse Effects. See Table 68-3. Ketoconazole is associated with the least favorable toxicity profile among the azoles.

Drug Interactions. See Table 68-4.

Dosage and Administration. See Table 68-5. Ketoconazole: bioavailability depends on an acidic pH for absorption. Administration with food may decrease absorption.

Triazoles

fluconazole (Diflucan)

Contraindications

- Hypersensitivity. Use with caution in patients with hypersensitivity to other azoles.

Warnings

- Hepatotoxicity: see ketoconazole; incidence and severity is less with fluconazole.
- Allergic/dermatologic reaction: anaphylaxis and exfoliative skin disorders have occurred rarely in patients with serious underlying conditions such as AIDS or malignancy while on fluconazole. These reactions have, in some cases, resulted in death.
- Carcinogenesis: hepatocellular adenomas have been observed in rats.
- Fertility impairment has occurred in rats. The hormone change has not been observed in women treated with fluconazole.

Precautions

- Dose reduction is recommended for patients with renal dysfunction.
- Care should be exercised when prescribing fluconazole to elderly patients.

TABLE 68-2 Pharmacokinetics of Antifungals

Drug	Absorption	Drug Availability (After First Pass)	Time to Peak Concentration	Half-Life	Protein Bound	Metabolism	Excretion
ketoconazole	Variable	NI	1-2 hr	2 hr then 8 hr	99%	Liver, 3A4 potent 1A2, 2C	Bile
fluconazole	90%		1-2 hr	30 hr	10%	2C and 3A4 inhibitor	Renal, 80%
itraconazole			2-5 hr	30-40	99.8%	Liver 3A4	Renal; inactive metabolites
terbinafine	70%	40%	2 hr	36 hr	99%	Liver 2D6	Renal; inactive metabolites
griseofulvin	Variable		4 hr	NI	NI	No P450	

NI, No information.

TABLE 68-3 Adverse Reactions to Antifungals by Body System

Body System	ketoconazole	fluconazole	itraconazole	terbinafine	griseofulvin
Body, general	Fever, chills		Edema, fatigue, fever, hypokalemia		Fatigue
Skin, appendages	Photophobia, pruritus	Exfoliative dermatitis, Stevens-Johnson syndrome, alopecia	Rash, alopecia	Rash, pruritus, exfoliative, dermatitis, Stevens-Johnson syndrome	Photosensitivity
Hypersensitivity	Urticaria, anaphylaxis	Angioedema, anaphylaxis		Urticaria	Rash, urticaria, angioneurotic edema, erythema multiforme
Respiratory			Bronchitis/ bronchospasm, cough, dyspnea		
Cardiovascular			Arrhythmias, CHF, pulmonary edema		
GI	Nausea, vomiting (5%), abdominal pain, diarrhea	Nausea, abdominal pain, diarrhea, dyspepsia, vomiting	Nausea, diarrhea, vomiting abdominal pain, dyspepsia	Diarrhea, dyspepsia, abdominal pain	Oral thrush, nausea, vomiting, epigastric distress, diarrhea
Hemic and lymphatic	Thrombocytopenia, leukopenia, hemolytic anemia	Leukopenia		Neutropenia	Leukopenia
Metabolic	Lower serum testosterone				
CNS	Headache, dizziness, somnolence	Headache, dizziness, seizures	Headache, dizziness, neuropathy	Headache	Headache, dizziness, insomnia, mental confusion, impairment of performance
Special senses		Taste perversion	Taste perversion	Ophthalmic changes, taste disturbance	
Hepatic	Hepatic toxicity	Hepatic toxicity (less than other antifungals)	Hepatic toxicity	Hepatic toxicity	Hepatic toxicity
Genitourinary	Impotence				Proteinuria, nephrosis
Other	Suicidal tendencies, severe depression, gynecomastia, bulging fontanels				

TABLE 68-4 Drug Interactions with Antifungal Agents

Antifungal	Action on Other Drugs
ketoconazole	↑ benzodiazepines, buspirone, carbamazepine, corticosteroids, cyclosporine, donepezil, nisoldipine, protease inhibitors, quinidine, sulfonylureas, tacrolimus, TCAs, warfarin, zolpidem
ketoconazole	↓↑ Oral contraceptives
ketoconazole	↓ theophylline
fluconazole	↑ alfentanil, zolpidem, benzodiazepines, buspirone, corticosteroids, cyclosporine, losartan, nisoldipine, phenytoin, sulfonylureas, tacrolimus, theophylline, TCAs, warfarin, zidovudine?
fluconazole	↓↑ Oral contraceptives
itraconazole	↑ Alfentanil, benzodiazepines, buspirone, calcium channel blockers, carbamazepine, cisapride, corticosteroids, cyclosporine, digoxin, haloperidol, HMG-CoA reductase inhibitors, hydantoins, oral hypoglycemic agents, pimozide, protease inhibitors, quinidine, rifampin, tacrolimus, tolterodine, warfarin, zolpidem
terbinafine	↑ caffeine, dextromethorphan ↓ cyclosporine
griseofulvin	↓ Anticoagulants, oral contraceptives, cyclosporine, salicylates

Drugs	Act on Antifungals
Antacids, didanosine, sucralfate, proton pump inhibitors H_2 antagonists, isoniazid, rifampin	↑ ketoconazole ↓ ketoconazole
hydrochlorothiazide	↑ fluconazole
cimetidine, rifampin	↓ fluconazole
Hydantoins, antacids, proton pump inhibitors H_2 antagonists	↓ itraconazole
cimetidine	↑ terbinafine
rifampin	↓ terbinafine
Barbiturates	↓ griseofulvin

TABLE 68-5 Oral Treatment of Selected Fungal Infections

Disease	First-Line Treatment	Alternative
Onychomycosis, fingernail	terbinafine 250 mg qd × 6 wk	itraconazole 200 mg po qd × 3 mo fluconazole 150-300 mg po qwk × 3-6 mo
Onychomycosis toenail,	terbinafine 250 mg po qd × 12 wk	itraconazole 200 mg po qd × 3 mo *OR* 200 mg bid × 1 wk/mo × 3-4 mo; fluconazole 150-300 mg po qwk × 6-12 mo
Tinea capitis	terbinafine 250 mg po qd × 4-8 wk Child: 125 mg po qd	itraconazole 3-5 mg/kg/day for 30 days fluconazole 8 mg/kg qwk × 8-12 wk griseofulvin: adult: 500 mg po qd × 4-6 wk; child: 10-20 mg/kg × 6-8 wk
Tinea corporis, cruris, or pedis	Topical terbinafine 250 mg po qd × 2 wk	ketoconazole 200 mg po qd × 4 wk fluconazole 150 mg q wk × 2-4 wk griseofulvin: adult: 500 mg po qd × 4-6 wk; child: 10-20 mg/kg/d × 2-4 wk for corporis, 4-8 wk for pedis
Tinea versicolor	ketoconazole 400 mg × single dose *OR* 200 mg qd × 7 day *OR* topical	fluconazole 400 mg po single dose *OR* itraconazole 400 mg po qd × 3-7 days
Histoplasmosis	itraconazole 200 mg/day sol po × 9 mo	
Coccidioidomycosis, primary pulmonary	Treatment not indicated	
Blastomycosis	itraconazole oral solution 200-400 mg/day po × 6 mo	fluconazole 400-800 mg/day × 6 mo
Cryptococcosis	IV treatment	
Aspergillosis	Corticosteroids, many different antifungal regimens	
Candida, chronic mucocutaneous	ketoconazole 400 mg/day × 3-9 mo	Child: fluconazole 3-6 mg/kg/day
Candida, oral thrush	fluconazole 200 mg × 1 dose or 100 mg/day × 5-14 days	itraconazole oral solution 200 mg (20 ml) qd × 7 days
Candida, vaginitis	fluconazole 150 mg po × 1 or topical	itraconazole 200 mg po bid × 1 day

- Single-dose use: carries a higher incidence of adverse reactions (26%) than intravaginal agents (16%).

Pharmacokinetics
- Food or gastric pH does not affect fluconazole.
- Fluconazole is excreted renally with therapeutic concentrations achieved in the urine.
- Fluconazole is unique among the azoles in that it crosses the blood-brain barrier and has good penetration into the CSF.

Adverse Effects. See Table 68-3. Systemic side effects (26%) are common as compared with local symptoms associated with intravaginal imidazole or triazole (17%). Gastrointestinal side effects are the most common (15%) and may include transient nausea, vomiting, diarrhea, and abdominal pain. Headache and anaphylaxis (rare) have been reported with a single dose of fluconazole.

Dosage and Administration. See Table 68-5. Administration of a loading dose on day one of twice the usual daily dose results in steady state concentration in 1 or 2 days instead of 5 to 10 days.

itraconazole (Sporanox)

Contraindications
- CHD: patients with evidence of ventricular dysfunction such as CHF or a history of CHF
- Coadministration of pimozide, quinidine, cisapride, triazolam, or oral midazolam, HMG-CoA reductase inhibitors metabolized by the CYP 3A4 system (lovastatin, simvastatin)
- Pregnant women or in women contemplating pregnancy
- Hypersensitivity to azoles

Warnings

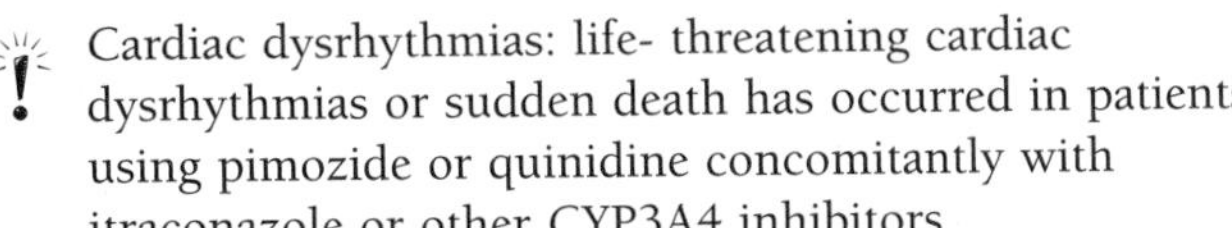
Cardiac dysrhythmias: life- threatening cardiac dysrhythmias or sudden death has occurred in patients using pimozide or quinidine concomitantly with itraconazole or other CYP3A4 inhibitors.

- CHF: itraconazole has a negative inotropic effect. Risk factors for CHF should be taken into consideration, including ischemic and valvular disease, COPD, and renal failure.
- Hepatotoxicity: hepatitis, including liver failure and death, has been reported. Monitor hepatic enzymes.
- Hepatic function impairment: itraconazole is predominantly metabolized in the liver. The half-life is prolonged in patients with liver failure.
- Bioequivalency: do not use itraconazole capsules and oral solution interchangeably. Drug exposure is greater with the oral solution.
- HIV patients may have decreased absorption of drug.
- Renal function impairment: use with caution; monitor serum potassium.
- Absorption is decreased with decreased gastric acidity. Do not take at the same time as drugs that decrease acidity.
- Carcinogenesis: rats had a slightly increased incidence of soft tissue sarcoma. It has not been found in humans.

Pharmacokinetics. See Table 68-3. Reduced absorption when administered with drugs that decrease gastric acidity. Therapeutic concentrations may persist in fingernails and toenails for up to 6 months after discontinuation of the drug.

terbinafine (Lamisil)

Contraindications
- Hypersensitivity

Warnings
- Hepatic failure: rare cases of liver failure, some leading to death have occurred. The severity of hepatic events may be worse in patients with liver disease.
- Ophthalmic: changes in the ocular lens and retina have been reported. The clinical significance of these changes is unknown.
- Neutropenia: isolated cases of severe neutropenia have been reported but were reversible with discontinuation.
- Dermatologic: isolated reports of Stevens-Johnson syndrome, toxic epidermal necrolysis.
- Renal function impairment: do not use with significant renal impairment.
- Hepatic function impairment: not recommended for patients with chronic or active liver disease. Assess liver function before prescribing.

griseofulvin (Grisactin, Fulvicin, Gris-PEG)

Contraindications
- Hypersensitivity (5% to 7%)
- Hepatocellular failure, porphyria

Warnings
- Hypersensitivity has been reported in 5% to 7% of patients. It may include skin rashes, urticaria, and angioneurotic edema and necessitates withdrawal of therapy.
- Prophylaxis: the safety and efficacy of griseofulvin prophylaxis for fungal infections have not been established.
- Carcinogenesis: liver tumors in mice, but not in other species.
- Fertility impairment: men should wait 6 months after completing therapy before attempting to father a child; women should avoid risk of pregnancy while receiving therapy.

Precautions
- Prolonged therapy: renal, hepatic, and hematopoietic functions must be monitored periodically.

Penicillin cross-sensitivity. Because griseofulvin is derived from a species of penicillin, cross-sensitivity is possible; however, patients with known sensitivity to penicillin have been treated without adverse effects.

- Lupus erythematosus: exacerbation of lupus erythematosus and lupuslike syndromes have occurred in patients receiving griseofulvin.

- Photosensitivity: patients on griseofulvin should take protective measures against the sun (i.e., sunblocks or protective clothing).

Dosage and Administration

- Absorbed better when taken with meals high in fat content. The ultramicrosized griseofulvin is better absorbed than conventional microsized griseofulvin.

RESOURCES FOR PATIENTS AND PROVIDERS

Antimicrobial Drug Use, www.medsch.wisc.edu/clinsci/amcg/amcg.html.
University of Wisconsin Hospital.

Journal of the International Association of Physicians in AIDS Care, www.iapac.org.
Information and current news on antiretroviral therapies, opportunistic diseases, conferences, and report summaries.

National AETC HIV/AIDS, itsa.ucsf.edu/warmline and (800) 933-3413 phone line.
Telephone Consultation Service. Useful for providers where HIV expertise is not readily available.

BIBLIOGRAPHY

Albougy HA, Naidoo S: A systematic review of the management of oral candidiasis associated with HIV/AIDS, *SADJ* 57(11):457-466, 2002.

Bennett JE: Mycoses. In Mandell GL, Bennet JE, editors: *Principles and practice of infectious diseases,* ed 5, New York, 2000, Churchill Livingstone.

Gupta AK: Factors that may affect the response of onychomycosis to oral antifungal therapy, *Australas J Dermatol* 39(4):222, 1998.

Hulisz D: Systemic antifungal therapy for onychomycoses, *US Pharm* p. 29, December 1995.

Klepser ME et al: Therapy of candida infections: susceptibility testing, resistance, and therapeutic options, *Ann Pharmacother* 32(12):1353, 1998.

Richardson MD et al: Diagnosis and prevention of fungal infection in the immunocompromised patient, *Blood Rev* 12(4):241, 1998.

Systemic antifungal drugs, *Medical Rec* 96-100, 1998.

CHAPTER 69

Antiretrovirals

Victoria L. Anderson and Susan Orsega

Drug Names

Class	Subclass	Generic Name	Trade Name
Antiretrovirals	Nucleoside reverse transcriptase inhibitors (NRTIs)	(P) zidovudine (ZDV, AZT)	Retrovir
		lamivudine (3TC)	Epivir
		abacavir (ABC)	Ziagen
		didanosine (ddl)	Videx, Videx EC
		stavudine (d4T)	Zerit
		tenofovir disoproxil fumarate (TDF)	Viread
		zalcitabine (ddC)	Hivid
		zidovudine/lamivudine	Combivir
		zidovudine/lamivudine/abacavir	Trizivir
		emtricitabine (FTC)	Emtriva
	Nonnucleoside reverse transcriptase inhibitors (NNRTIs)	(P) delavirdine (DLV)	Rescriptor
		efavirenz (EFV)	Sustiva
		nevirapine (NVP)	Viramune
	Protease inhibitors (PIs)	(P) ritonavir (RTV)	Norvir
		amprenavir (APV)	Agenerase
		indinavir (IDV)	Crixivan
		nelfinavir (NFV)	Viracept
		saquinavir (SQV)	Invirase, Fortovase
		lopinavir/ritonavir (LPV/RTV)	Kaletra
		atazanavir	Reyataz
		fosamprenavir (f-APV)	Lexiva
	Fusion inhibitor	(P) enfuvirtide	Fuzeon, T-20

(P), Prototype drug.

General Uses

Indications

Nucleoside Analogue Reverse Transcriptase Inhibitors (NRTIs)

- Alone or in combination therapies for the treatment of patients with HIV infection
- Zidovudine: reduces neonatal transmission of HIV and as postexposure prophylaxis
- Lamivudine: treatment of chronic hepatitis B
- Tenofovir: In combination therapy, newly treated HIV-infected patients and in those who have failed other antiretroviral regimens; also hepatitis B

Nonnucleoside Reverse Transcriptase Inhibitors (NNRTIs)

- Used alone or in combination therapies are for the treatment of patients with HIV infection

Protease Inhibitors (PIs)

- Alone or in combination therapies are for the treatment of patients with HIV infection

Entry (Fusion) Inhibitors

- Enfuvirtide can be used as part of a medication regimen in patients with limited treatment options. Enfuvirtide should be used only in patients who have previously used other anti-HIV drugs and have ongoing evidence of viral replication.

The recommended use of antiretroviral agents in clinical practice will continue to evolve as new information from clinical trials and research becomes available. Infectious disease specialists generally provide treatment of patients with symptomatic HIV infection because of the difficulty in keeping current with the latest treatment protocols. Primary care providers generally are concerned with prevention of the transmission of the virus. Yet having knowledge of the current drug therapies and the side effects is necessary because HIV-infected patients will rely on their primary care provider to help them evaluate their complaints as well as provide the treatment to some of them even on a limited degree.

DISEASE PROCESS

The Virus

HIV is a retrovirus. Retroviruses are viruses that replicate through the use of the reverse transcriptase enzyme. This key enzyme transcripts the RNA into the double-stranded DNA, which then continues integration into the genome. There are three primary categories of human retroviruses: the T cell leukemia retroviruses, endogenous viruses, and the human immunodeficiency viruses (HIV-1 and HIV-2). This chapter discusses in detail only HIV-1.

Pathophysiology

The HIV virus attaches to the CD4 protein with the help of coreceptors (CXCR4 or CCR5) found on T-helper lymphocytes and other cells such as macrophages and dendritic cells. The HIV then fuses its membrane with that of the host cell and inserts its genetic material into the cytoplasm. The viral genetic material is then transcribed into double-stranded DNA called proviral DNA (see Figure 69-1). The HIV enzyme, reverse transcriptase, is responsible for creating the double-stranded DNA from the viral RNA. Once produced, this DNA often becomes integrated into the chromosomal DNA of the host cell. The HIV DNA is expressed using the host cell's genetic machinery. Expression of HIV DNA creates new HIV RNA genetic material and messenger RNA. The messenger RNA codes for the development of HIV polyproteins that must be cleaved, or separated, into individual proteins by the HIV enzyme protease in order for infectious virions to be produced. Once this occurs, new virions are assembled and bud from the host cell's membrane, able to infect new cells.

The Disease

The defining stages of HIV infection through progression to AIDS have changed over the years as drug treatments have become extremely effective in preventing the opportunistic infections that once led to severe debilitation and death. The natural history of the disease follows this course: primary infection then early, middle, and advanced or late-stage HIV infection or AIDS (see Figure 69-2).

The disease seems to be divided into a primary phase that includes initial acute infection that almost always presents with a mild to moderate viral syndrome. This stage includes the development of antibody production and stabilization of viral load levels. The early and middle stages of HIV infection can be fairly asymptomatic and represent the time when the virus entrenches itself in the architecture of the host's immune system. The virus during this time destroys normal lymphoid architecture and creates reservoirs difficult to eradicate despite the best drug treatment. CD4 and CD8 cells too undergo immunologic changes that render them useless in effectively killing and or controlling HIV infection, leading to rapid HIV replication and mutation. It is during this stage that CD4 counts decrease dangerously to 200 to 300 cells/mm^3.

The advanced or late stages of HIV infection show continued falling of CD4 counts, with drops to 50 cells/mm^3. The patient develops neurologic changes heralded by dementia, peripheral neuropathy, and myelopathy. Further immune system collapse occurs with the onset of recurrent opportunistic infections such as *Pneumocystis carinii* (PCP), cryptosporidium diarrhea, mycobacterium avium complex, and multiple viral primary or reactivated infections such as herpes simplex, or varicella zoster. Chronic illness produces constitutional disease with muscle wasting, weight loss, fevers, and severe fatigue. Malignancy with Kaposi's sarcoma is also seen. The compilation of AIDS and the sequelae of opportunistic infections result finally in death.

Assessment. The following baseline information should be obtained before starting a patient on antiretrovirals:

- Documentation of all medications and dosages.
- Past history and current medical problems including hepatitis, pancreatitis, alcohol use.
- Helper T-lymphocyte count (CD4) and plasma HIV RNA measurement. These studies help to assess a patient's immunologic status and severity of infection. They also provide a means of measuring the efficacy of therapy.
- CBC, including a WBC with differential. Also evaluation of folate, vitamin B_{12}, ferritin, iron, and percentage of iron saturation.
- LFTs and hepatitis B, C, and A serologies.
- Rapid plasma reagin or VDRL test for syphilis.
- Amylase. Triglyceride and lipase levels may also be warranted in cases in which antiretrovirals that may cause pancreatitis are being used (Table 69-1). An isoamylase fractionates the amylase into pancreatic and salivary amylase. This should be determined in patients with elevated amylase levels to differentiate salivary from pancreatic because some patients with an elevated amylase are found to have an elevated salivary amylase with a normal pancreatic amylase. An elevated salivary amylase is not an indication of pancreatitis and is therefore not an indicator for stopping medication.
- Triglyceride levels. Hypertriglyceridemia is often seen in HIV infection. There are reports of elevated triglyceride levels in some patients before the development of pancreatic symptoms.
- Pregnancy testing. This will determine specific antiretroviral treatment choices.
- Peripheral neuropathy. A vitamin B_{12} level should be checked because vitamin B_{12} deficiency is common in HIV-infected patients. Use a 128-cycle/second tuning fork to obtain a timed vibratory sensation at the metatarsal joint of both great toes. A normal timed vibratory sensation is the ability to feel the vibration for greater than 10 seconds. Documenting a patient's timed vibratory sensation before starting an antiretroviral agent allows the practitioner to evaluate whether any changes in vibratory sensation may be due to antiretroviral agents that cause peripheral neuropathy.

DRUG ACTION AND EFFECTS

Antiretroviral agents act to stop the production of new retroviruses by interfering with the ability of the retrovirus to replicate (Figure 69-1). NRTIs disrupt replication of the virus at the point in which the virion is replicating its RNA to make DNA via the reverse transcriptase, the enzyme that copies viral RNA into DNA. NNRTIs resemble false nucleotides by binding in a mechanism to inhibit the reverse transcriptase enzyme activity. PI's prevent the protease enzyme from cleaving essential proteins into the HIV virion (Figure 69-2). Fusion inhibitors prevent the HIV from entering into target cells.

Reverse Transcriptase Inhibitors

Reverse transcriptase inhibitors prevent the HIV enzyme reverse transcriptase from creating HIV proviral DNA from the viral RNA. This in turn prevents new viruses from being produced. There are two primary categories of reverse transcriptase inhibitors: nucleoside analog reverse transcriptase inhibitors and nonnucleoside reverse transcriptase inhibitors.

TABLE 69-1 Baseline and Screening Laboratory Studies for HIV/AIDS

Laboratory Test	Frequency, Indication
CD4 count	At diagnosis, every 3-6 months, monitor response to antiretroviral.
HIV viral load	At diagnosis, before treatment, 2-8 weeks after start of new treatment.
Complete blood count with differential	Every 3-6 months, more frequently for low values and bone marrow toxicities (AZT).
Vitamin B_{12}	As needed for evaluation of B_{12} deficiency neuropathy versus HAART therapy induced neuropathy.
Serum chemistries	Every 3-6 months, glucose monitoring every 3-4 months. More frequently for abnormal values and those that cause hyperglycemia (all PIs, NRTIs, and NNRTIs). Lipodystrophy syndrome may be associated with increased lactate and alanine aminotransferase and lower levels of albumin, cholesterol, triglycerides, glucose, and insulin.
Liver function tests (LFTs)	Every 3-6 months, more frequently for abnormal values and elevated LFTs (D4T, delavirdine, nevirapine, PIs). Increased bilirubin (indinavir). LFTs should be closely monitored with nevirapine at baseline, 2 weeks × 1 month, then monthly × 12 weeks, and then every 1-3 months thereafter.
Amylase/lipase	Every 3-6 months, monitor closely for pancreatitis.
Lipid profile	Every 3-4 months, monitor for patients taking PI's or NNRTIs. If increased at baseline, monitor within 1-2 months of HAART initiation.
Serum lactate	No current recommendations because of significant technical blood drawing difficulties. If patient symptomatic of lactic acidosis seen in NNRTIs, experts suggest evaluation will reveal hypercalcemia, increased anion gap, elevated aminotransferase, CPK, LDH, amylase, and lipase.
Urinalysis	As indicated for indinavir, monitor for nephrolithiasis and UA may show crystalluria, increased urine pH, proteinuria, hematuria, and pyuria.

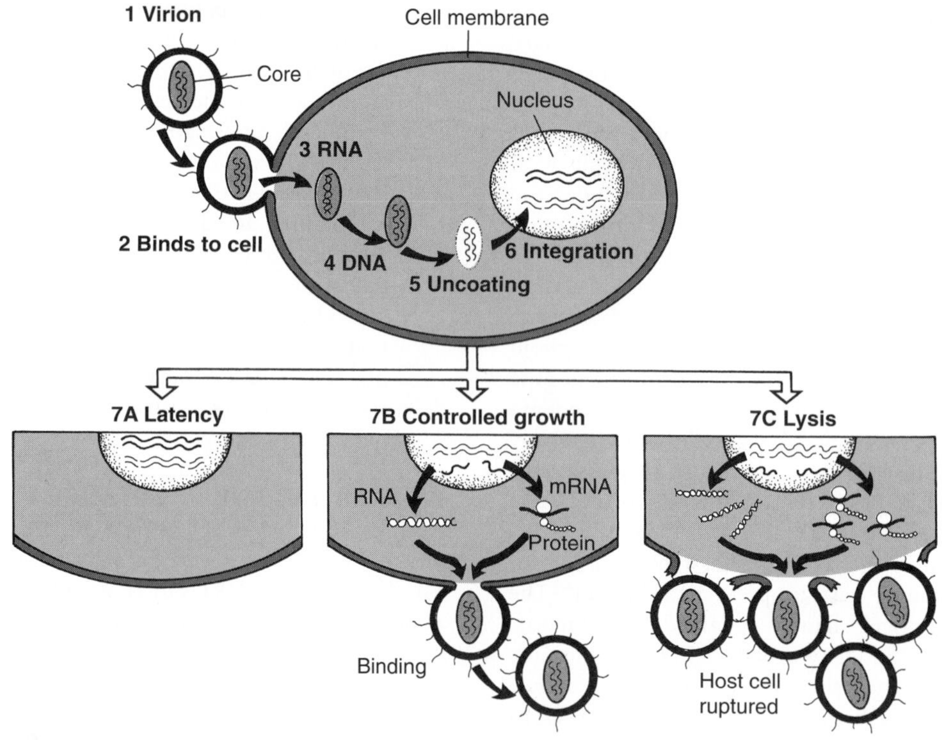

FIGURE 69-1

Infection and cellular outcomes of HIV. HIV infection begins (1) when a virion, or virus particle, (2) binds to the outside of a susceptible cell and fuses with it, (3) injecting the core proteins and two strands of viral RNA. Uncoating occurs, during which the core proteins are removed and the viral RNA is released into the infected cell's cytoplasm. (4) The double-stranded DNA (provirus) migrates to the nucleus, (5) uncoats itself, and (6) is integrated into the cell's own DNA. The provirus then can do a couple of things: (7A) remain latent or (7B) activate cellular mechanisms to copy its genes into RNA, some of which is translated into viral proteins or ribosomes. The proteins and additional RNA then are assembled into new virions that bud from the cell. The process can take place slowly, sparing the host cell (7B), or so rapidly that the cell is lysed or ruptured (7C). (From McCance KL, Huether SE: *Pathophysiology,* ed 2, St Louis, 1994, Mosby.)

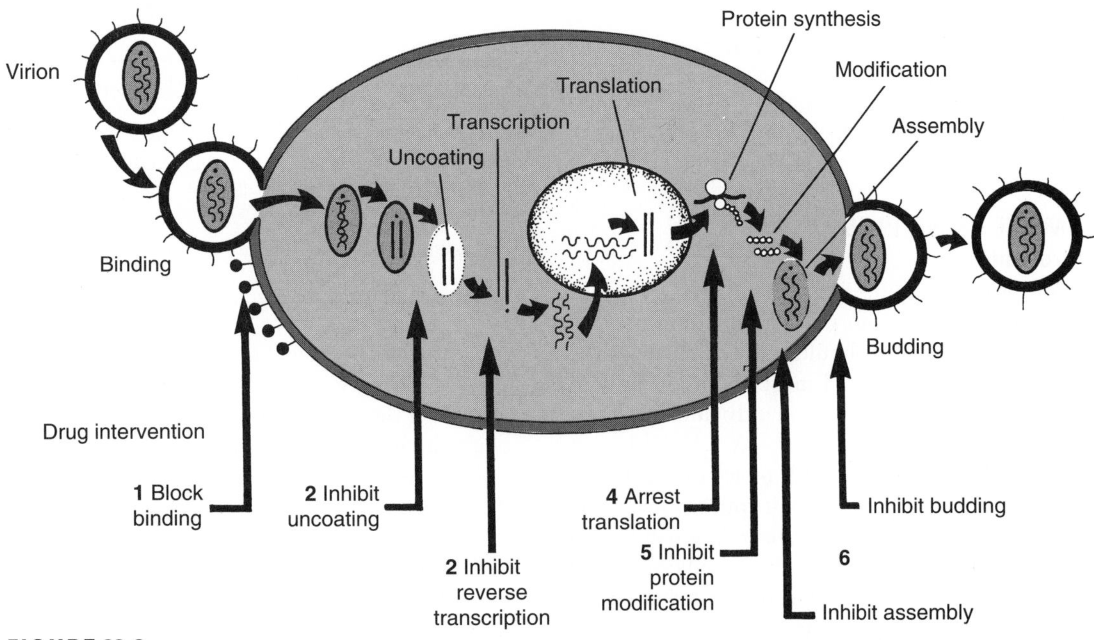

FIGURE 69-2

HIV is subject to attack by drugs at several stages. Certain agents could block the binding of the HIV to CD4 receptors on the surface of helper T cells (1). Other agents might keep viral RNA and reverse transcriptase from leaving their protein coat (2). Drugs such as AZT and other dideoxynucleosides prevent the reverse transcription of viral RNA into viral DNA (3). Later, antisense oligonucleotides could block the translation of mRNA into viral proteins (4). Certain compounds could interfere with viral assembly by modifying such processes (5), and finally, antiviral agents such as interferon could keep the virus from assembling itself and budding out of the cell (6). (Modified from Yarchoan R, Mitsuya H, Broder S: AIDS therapies. In *The science of AIDS: readings from Scientific American*, New York, 1989, WH Freeman.)

The nucleoside analog reverse transcriptase inhibitors must be phosphorylated in the target cells to their active triphosphate form. It is important to note that there is a nucleotide analog reverse transcriptase inhibitor, tenofovir, that is under the same category as a nucleoside subclass. However, the structural difference between nucleotides and nucleosides is that the nucleotides already have a phosphate group, so it only requires two steps of phosphorylation instead of three steps. Once these medications are in the active triphosphate form they work by at least two mechanisms: chain termination and competitive inhibition.

Chain termination occurs when reverse transcriptase adds the reverse transcriptase inhibitor into the growing chain of HIV proviral DNA. Antiretroviral nucleoside analogs all have a modification in their sugar ring that prevents further nucleotides (the building blocks of DNA) from being added. This stops the production of HIV proviral DNA, therefore preventing new HIV viruses from being formed.

Competitive inhibition of the endogenous nucleoside-5′-triphosphates is a process in which the phosphorylated reverse transcriptase inhibitor competes with and replaces the endogenous nucleoside-5′-triphosphates. The endogenous nucleoside-5′-triphosphates are necessary for the production of HIV proviral DNA. By competing with and replacing the nucleoside-5′-triphosphates, HIV proviral DNA is not produced, and therefore new HIV viruses are not produced.

NNRTIs do not require phosphorylation or intracellular processing to be activated. They are noncompetitive, binding to reverse transcriptase and inhibiting the function of this enzyme by binding at sites distinct from the nucleoside binding sites.

Protease Inhibitors

One of the final stages of the HIV life cycle is the production of HIV polyproteins coded for by the viral messenger RNA. These polyproteins must be cleaved or separated into individual proteins by the HIV enzyme known as protease in order for infectious virions to be produced. Protease inhibitors block the HIV enzyme protease and therefore prevent certain HIV polyproteins from being cleaved or separated into the individual proteins necessary for the production of new infectious virions. This causes noninfectious HIV virions to be produced.

Fusion Inhibitors

Entry fusion inhibitors work by attaching themselves to proteins on the surface of T cells or proteins on the surface of HIV. In order for HIV to bind to T cells, the proteins on HIV's outer coat must bind to the surface receptors on T cells. Fusion inhibitors prevent this from happening. Some fusion inhibitors target the gp120 or gp41 or target the CD4 protein or the CCR5 or CXCR4 receptors. If entry inhibitors are successful, HIV is unable to bind to the surface of T cells and gain entry into the cells. Enfuvirtide, the only FDA approved fusion inhibitor, binds to glycoprotein 41 molecule which is involved in viral entry and prevent the folding mechanism or fusion required for entry into the cell.

DRUG TREATMENT PRINCIPLES

Prophylaxis/Prevention

As a primary care provider, counseling regarding the risk for HIV and AIDS should include information regarding prevention and prophylaxis. The patient should be made aware of the disease, its route of transmission, and most important how to prevent infection. Regimens change frequently and the latest information should be followed.

Prevention of HIV infection, according to the CDC, is accomplished best by abstaining from sexual intercourse or by being in a long-term, mutually monogamous relationship with a partner who has been tested and who is confirmed uninfected (CDC HIV/AIDS prevention fact sheet). Otherwise the *correct* and *consistent* use of a male latex condom is the only other way to reduce the risk of transmission. Eliciting information on sexual habits and counseling male and female patients on how to use a condom is an effective way to promote safe sexual behavior.

Antiretrovirals are used as prophylaxis to prevent HIV seroconversion in health care workers who have been recently exposed to HIV (≤72 hours). A multicenter study sponsored by the CDC revealed that the use of postexposure prophylaxis (PEP) with zidovudine was associated with a 79% decrease in the risk of HIV seroconversion. PEP should be initiated within 1 to 2 hours after exposure. Currently the PEP guidelines recommend the use of zidovudine in addition to lamivudine and a protease inhibitor. These recommendations vary according to the type of exposure and the patient population.

Use in a non–health care worker exposure is still controversial because assessing of risk exposure is difficult. There are no current data to suggest that PEP in this setting is safe, or effective. The decision should be made carefully and be based on the circumstances of the exposure, and the patient should be well informed of the regimen's risk and benefits.

Treatment

Once infection has been identified, the patient should be referred to an infectious disease specialist or a center that provides care to HIV-infected individuals. Consideration regarding insurance is unfortunate, but a realistic concern because the care and the treatments are costly. The patient should be reassured that the infectious disease experts are partners to primary care providers and that your relationship will continue. Patients should be counseled on what tests they can expect and what kinds of treatments may be recommended. Patients should be counseled about the risks of transmission of their infection and that all past and present partners should be notified of the infection. Reporting of the infection should occur following state guidelines.

TABLE 69-2 Department of Health and Human Services Guidelines for Initiation of Antiretroviral Therapy

Category	CD4/μl	Recommendations
Symptomatic	Any	Treat
Asymptomatic	<200	Treat
Asymptomatic	200-349	Treat; some defer especially if viral loads <20,0000 copies/ml
Asymptomatic	>350	Defer; some treat if viral load is >55,000 copies/ml

The primary care provider will be seeing the patient and assessing the complications of any antiretroviral therapy along with the infectious disease team.

The decision to start antiretrovirals in a patient who is not being treated in a "prophylactic" manner is controversial. However, almost all experts agree that starting therapy is necessary in those patients with symptomatic disease; those with a decreasing CD4+ T-cell counts and a high viral load, and those experiencing acute primary HIV infection. Treatment for patients who do not fall into this category remains controversial and is based on open discussion between the patient and his or her health care providers.

Guidelines have been developed for clinical management of HIV-infected adults and adolescents that discuss details of treatment strategies and adverse effects, initiation of therapy, and other treatment principles. The current treatment methodology is based on the use of multiple antiretrovirals with the goal of suppressing HIV replication for months or perhaps even years. This concept is the driving force for today's management of a patient with HIV infection who is in need of antiretroviral treatment (Table 69-2).

Highly Active Antiretroviral Treatment (HAART)

HAART therapy is used to describe the combination of multiple antiretrovirals to achieve the maximum effect in viral load suppression to a goal of undetectable viral load levels. In using HAART treatment, the following management strategy is recommended when changing therapy:

1. Base changes on drug regimen on:
   CD4 decline measured on two occasions
   Virologic failure demonstrated by increases in HIV RNA viral load
   Toxicity
   Patient tolerance
   Inability to comply with the regimen
2. Obtain genotypic or phenotypic resistance testing while the patient is still on the old regimen and use the results to help choose new regimen.
3. Always change at least two of the antiretrovirals in the regimen.
4. Avoid choosing agents with overlapping resistance patterns with those the patient has failed.
5. Avoid choosing agents with similar side effects as those to which the patient is intolerant.
6. Try to make the next regimen simpler if at all possible.

Genotypic or phenotypic testing is available as an in vitro tool to understand resistance of HIV to antiretroviral agents. Genotypic assays detect drug resistance mutations that are present in reverse transcriptase and protease genes. Phenotypic assays measure the ability of the virus to grow in concentrations of the antiretrovirals. These aid in selection of antiretroviral agents when changing drug regimens. It is best to consult with an expert to assist interpretation of these results. The Department of Health and Human Services (DHHS) antiretroviral guidelines are a comprehensive reference for changing medications.

HOW TO MONITOR

Baseline laboratory studies and screening testing should be performed as described in the initial evaluation section. It is important to note that this table is a general reference. If patients are symptomatic or have other comorbidities, then more scrupulous testing may be indicated. After the initiation of antiretroviral therapy. Monitor response through laboratory tests outlined in Table 69-1.

PATIENT VARIABLES

Special Populations

Renal and hepatic insufficiency patients can pose a therapeutic challenge to the practitioner caring for HIV-infected patients. Renal-impaired patients may require dose modifications due to decreased drug clearance in most antiretrovirals. See reputable product information for guidance.

Patients with severely impaired liver function may be at greater risk of toxicity and should be monitored closely.

Geriatrics

Except for geriatric patients, the life expectancy of HIV-infected persons receiving HAART is now extended, most likely due to the immune reconstitution resulting from potent antiretroviral therapy. The limited data available about combined antiretroviral therapy in the elderly seem to show a similar virologic success rate but a slower immune recovery compared with younger patients. When selecting an antiretroviral, the practitioner should be should be cautious when dosing for an elderly patient because of the greater risk for decreased hepatic, renal, or cardiac function, and of concomitant disease or other medication therapy. As an increasing number of HIV-infected individuals become older than 50 years of age, more studies should begin to explore their tolerance to antiretroviral, pharmacokinetics, drug-to-drug interactions, and toxicities.

Pediatrics

As of March 2004, there were 20 antiretroviral agents approved for use in HIV-infected adults and adolescents in the United States; 12 of these have an approved pediatric treatment indication. Of the available, the following are approved for pediatric use: NRTIs (zidovudine, didanosine, stavudine, lamivudine, and abacavir), NNRTIs (nevirapine and efavirenz), and PI's (ritonavir, nelfinavir, amprenavir, and lopinavir/ritonavir). No current treatment guidelines exist for NRTIs (zalcitabine and tenofovir), NNRTIs (delavirdine), or PI's (saquinavir hard and soft gel capsules, and indinavir). Fusion inhibitor (enfuvirtide) safety profile has not been established for patients younger than 6 years of age and doses are based upon weight for patients between 6 and 16 years of age.

Pregnancy and Lactation

Clinicians who care for HIV-infected women should provide family planning services and counseling to optimize the medications and health prior to a pregnancy. Before treating any HIV-positive pregnant women with any antiretroviral, it is highly encouraged for the practitioner to enroll the patient in the Antiretroviral Pregnancy Registry by calling (800) 258-4263. This registry was established to monitor the maternal-fetal outcome of pregnant women who receive antiretrovirals. Fatal lactic acidosis occurred in pregnant women treated with a combination of stavudine and didanosine.

All HIV-positive women should be warned of the high risk of HIV transmission in breast milk. The CDC advise all HIV-infected women not to breast-feed.

Category B: nelfinavir, ritonavir, didanosine, enfuvirtide, saquinavir, tenofovir

Category C: abacavir, amprenavir, delavirdine, efavirenz, indinavir, lamivudine, lopinavir, nevirapine, stavudine, tenofovir, zalcitabine, zidovudine

Category D: hydroxyurea

PATIENT EDUCATION

Adherence is essential. Patients need to be instructed to take their medications as prescribed. Some strategies such as providing a written schedule, use of pill boxes, alarm clocks, pagers, and other mechanical devices aid adherence. Underdosing, partial adherence, or nonadherence may result in the development of a resistant strain(s) of HIV that will not be susceptible to treatment. Taking less than the prescribed dose can be more harmful than not taking the drug at all. Patients should be informed that antiretrovirals do not cure HIV infection and the use of these medications does not preclude the ongoing need to prevent transmission through safe sex practices and universal precautions.

Specific Drugs

REVERSE TRANSCRIPTASE INHIBITORS

Zidovudine and lamivudine are used in prophylaxis and are discussed in detail.

(P) Prototype Drug

zidovudine (ZDV, AZT) (Retrovir)

Reduces neonatal transmission of HIV and as postexposure prophylaxis.

Contraindications

- Life-threatening allergic reactions
- Concomitant use of ribavirin

Warnings

- Hypersensitivity: rare reports, including anaphylaxis, have occurred. If rash develops, careful evaluation is warranted.

- Zidovudine should be used with particular caution in patients who have an absolute granulocyte count of less than 1000 cells/mm^3 or a hemoglobin level less than 9.5 g/dl because of worries about bone marrow suppression.
- Myalgias and inflammatory frank myositis may occur with long-term zidovudine therapy.
- Rare occurrence of lactic acidosis/severe hepatomegaly with steatosis. Close monitoring is required, especially in obese women with risk factors for liver disease.
- Zidovudine is eliminated by renal excretion after the liver metabolizes it. In patients with renal impairment dose reduction is recommended (see Dosage and Administration). Patients with very severely impaired liver function may be at greater risk of toxicity.

Precautions
Be particularly cautious of other medications that cause myelosuppression such as ganciclovir and interferon-α. Be aware of other underlying causes of bone marrow suppression in AIDS. Patients taking zidovudine generally have an elevated mean corpuscular volume (MCV).

Adverse Effects
See Table 69-3.

Drug Interactions
Probenecid may increase zidovudine levels. Trimethoprim increases serum levels of zidovudine; however, dosage adjustment is not indicated. Phenytoin levels may be

TABLE 69-3 Adverse Reactions to Antiretroviral Agents

Drug	Important Adverse Reactions
NRTIs	Lactic acidosis/hepatic steatosis/failure, hypersensitivity
zidovudine (ZDV, AZT)	Myelosuppression (macrocytic anemia or granulocytopenia, myalgias, and malaise), headache, nausea, myopathy/myositis, hepatic steatosis, lactic acidosis/hepatic steatosis, elevated creatine phosphokinase, excessive eyelash growth, and nail hyperpigmentation.
lamivudine (3TC)	Neutropenia, amylasemia, headache, nausea, malaise, fatigue, peripheral neuropathy, insomnia, pancreatitis in children
abacavir	Systemic hypersensitivity reaction, nausea, vomiting, transaminitis, anemia, neutropenia
didanosine (ddl)	Pancreatitis, peripheral neuropathy, retinal depigmentation, diarrhea, headache, dry mouth, insomnia, nervousness, amylasemia, transaminitis, hyperuricemia, lactic acidosis/hepatic steatosis, hepatic dysfunction, retinal changes, and optic neuritis
stavudine (d4T)	Lactic acidosis/hepatic steatosis/failure, peripheral neuropathy, diarrhea, nausea, vomiting transaminitis, hypersensitivity, pancreatitis, headache, fat redistribution
tenofovir (TDF)	Lactic acidosis/hepatic steatosis/failure GI symptoms (nausea, diarrhea, flatulence, vomiting, abdominal pain, anorexia), headache
zalcitabine (ddC)	Lactic acidosis/ hepatic steatosis/failure, pancreatitis, peripheral neuropathy, rash, esophageal ulceration, pancreatitis (rare) amylasemia, transaminitis, lactic acidosis/hepatic steatosis. GI symptoms (nausea, diarrhea, flatulence, stomatitis, and aphthous esophageal ulcers), maculopapular rash, cardiomyopathy, fevers.
emtricitabine (FTC)	Lactic acidosis, hepatic stenosis
NNRTIs	Hepatotoxicity
delavirdine (DLV)	Transaminitis, rash, pruritus, headache, bilirubinemia, myalgia, arthralgia, headache, nausea, diarrhea, and fatigue, neutropenia, anemia
efavirenz (EFV)	Transaminitis, rash, CNS and psychiatric disturbances
nevirapine (NVP)	Transaminitis hepatotoxicity, rash (Stevens-Johnson), hypersensitivity, fever, nausea, headache
PIs	Hepatotoxicity, insulin resistance/hyperglycemia, hyperlipidemia and bleeding episodes in hemophiliac patients
ritonavir	Nausea, diarrhea, taste perversion, circumoral paresthesias, transaminitis, elevated triglycerides, thrombocytopenia, granulocytopenia
amprenavir	Rash, nausea, perioral paresthesias, diarrhea, transaminitis, elevated triglycerides
indinavir	Nephrolithiasis, nausea, abdominal pain, fat redistribution. Crix belly,* indirect bilirubinemia, hematuria, sterile pyuria, crystalluria
nelfinavir	Diarrhea, nausea, neutropenia, increased creatine phosphokinase, vomiting
saquinavir	Diarrhea, nausea, abdominal pain, ataxia, neutropenia, hemolytic anemia, transaminitis
lopinavir/ritonavir	Pancreatitis, nausea, diarrhea, elevated triglycerides
fosamprenavir (f-APV)	Skin rash, diarrhea, nausea, headache, transaminase elevation, hyperglycemia, fat maldistribution, lipid abnormalities, bleeding episodes in hemophiliacs
atazanavir	Indirect hyperbilirubinemia, prolonged PR interval, fat maldistribution, hyperglycemia, increased bleeding episodes in hemophiliacs
ENTRY INHIBITOR	
enfuvirtide	Hypersensitivity, local site reaction, diarrhea, nausea, fatigue

*Crix belly is characterized by elevated levels of triglycerides, cholesterol, and plasma glucose with a weight gain of 40 pounds or greater. Fat accumulates in the lower abdomen and flanks and tissue is often lost in the arms and legs. Named after Crixivan; however, it may be associated with other protease inhibitors.

altered with concomitant use of zidovudine. Zidovudine and acyclovir in combination may cause drowsiness and lethargy in some patients. Methadone increases the area under the curve (AUC) of zidovudine by approximately 43%, increasing the possibility of zidovudine-related toxicities.

Dosage and Administration

Zidovudine should not be taken with meals if possible, but it's not absolutely necessary. Zidovudine (AZT) monotherapy is *not* recommended. Because these dosing recommendations are constantly being revised by infectious disease specialists, consult the latest product information. evolve For a summary of general dosing information, see the supplemental tables on the Evolve Learning Resources website.

If a patient's hemoglobin is less than 7.5 g/dl or decreases more than 25% from baseline and/or the granulocyte count is less than 750/mm^3 or decreases by more than 50% from baseline, interruption of zidovudine may be necessary until there is an indication of bone marrow recovery. If less severe anemia or granulocytopenia occurs, reducing the dose may be adequate. Many practitioners chose to place their patients on cytokines such as epoetin alfa (Epogen) and G-CSF to treat the anemia and/or granulocytopenia.

The nausea associated with zidovudine use may improve if taken on a full stomach or with the syrup formulation. Patients with poor tolerance can start at a low dose and gradually be escalated by 100 mg every few days until full dosage is achieved (600 mg daily).

The results of the ACTG 076 clinical trial demonstrated that treating women with zidovudine during pregnancy significantly decreased perinatal transmission from 25% to approximately 8%. Due to these important data, the USPHS guidelines currently recommend specific zidovudine dosing for this population. Practitioners should call the Antiretroviral Pregnancy Registry at (800) 258-4263.

Other Drugs in Class

Other drugs in this class are similar to the prototype except as follows.

lamivudine (3TC) (Epivir)

Used also in treatment of chronic hepatitis.

Contraindications

- Hypersensitivity
- Concomitant use of lamivudine

Warnings. Lactic acidosis and severe hepatomegaly with steatosis have been reported with the use of nucleoside analogs alone or in combination, including lamivudine and other antiretrovirals. There have been rare cases of pancreatitis.

Important Differences Among lamivudine-Containing Products. Epivir tablets and oral solution contain a higher dose of the same active ingredient (lamivudine) than in Epivir-HBV that is used for patients with chronic hepatitis B. The formulation and dosage of Epivir-HBV are not appropriate for patients dually infected with HIV and HBV. If a decision is made to administer lamivudine to these patients, Epivir or Combivir (lamivudine/zidovudine) tablets should be used.

Precautions. Reduction in dosage is recommended in patients with renal impairment.

Adverse Effects. See Table 69-3. Lamivudine has limited toxicities compared with the other antiretrovirals.

Drug Interactions. There are few drug interactions with lamivudine. Trimethoprim/sulfamethoxazole significantly increases the area under the curve (AUC) of lamivudine by 43%, and it decreases the renal clearance by 35%.

Dosage and Administration

- Epivir comes in 150 mg tablets and oral solution 10 mg/ml and is administered with or without food
- Adults and children older than 12 years of age: dosage is based on weight in kilograms (kg): 50 kg or greater: 150 mg twice daily; less than 50 kg: 2 mg/kg twice daily
- Pediatric dosage is 4 mg /kg every 12 hours up to 300 mg once daily
- Combination therapy: AZT 300 mg/3TC 150 mg, 150 mg twice daily
- Renal impairment: these patients should have dose modifications due decreased drug clearance. Consult package insert

abacavir (Ziagen)

Adverse Effects. Hypersensitivity syndrome. Fever is a key feature; it occurs 1 to 3 days following exposure to the drug.

Dosage and Administration

- Patients should carry a wallet medication card to notify emergency personnel of the use of abacavir in case of a hypersensitivity reaction.
- Patients should be warned that interruption in abacavir therapy for reasons other than hypersensitivity could result in a hypersensitivity reaction once the drug is restarted.
- All patients should be registered. Registry: 1-800-270-0425.

didanosine (ddI) (Videx)

Dosage and Administration

- To be taken on an empty stomach (>½ hour before or >2 hours after meals).
- Space apart from all protease inhibitors (except for Videx EC, which can be taken with indinavir).
- To be taken with water or apple juice.
- Can be taken with light meal if taken with tenofovir. Still must be spaced apart from protease inhibitors.

tenofovir disoproxil fumarate (Viread)

Drug Interactions

- Acyclovir, cidofovir, ganciclovir, valacyclovir, valganciclovir may increase the serum concentrations of tenofovir.
- Tenofovir may increase levels of ddI.

Nonnucleoside Reverse Transcriptase Inhibitors (NNRTIs)

Ⓟ Prototype Drug

delavirdine mesylate (DLV) (Rescriptor)

Contraindications
- Hypersensitivity

Precautions
Diffuse, maculopapular, pruritic skin rash. When a severe rash occurs, or a rash with other symptoms such as fever, blistering, oral lesions, conjunctivitis, swelling, myalgias, or arthralgias, delavirdine must be discontinued immediately.

Drug Interactions

Administration of delavirdine with certain medications may result in potentially serious and/or life-threatening events. See latest manufacturer information.

Delavirdine inhibits cytochrome P450 enzymes; therefore it is not recommended for concurrent use with astemizole, alprazolam, terfenadine, midazolam, cisapride, rifabutin, rifampin, triazolam, ergot derivatives, amphetamines, calcium channel blockers (nifedipine), and anticonvulsants (phenytoin, carbamazepine, phenobarbital).

Delavirdine increases levels of dapsone, clarithromycin, quinidine, warfarin, indinavir, and saquinavir. A reduction of indinavir to 600 mg three times a day should be considered when combined with delavirdine. H_2-receptor antagonists may reduce the absorption of delavirdine.

Other Drugs in Class

Other drugs in this class are similar to the prototype except as follows.

efavirenz (Sustiva)

Must not be used as a single agent to treat HIV.

Drug Interactions. Because of cytochrome P450 induction, this medication may affect levels of indinavir, aprenavir, lopinavir, or saquinavir. Dose adjustment may be necessary and use with caution with these antiretroviral medications.

nevirapine (Viramune)

Adverse Effects
- Hepatotoxicity occurs in >10% of patients with or without clinical hepatitis. Increasing reports of serious, even life-threatening hepatic necrosis. Two thirds occur in the first 12 weeks of therapy. Liver function testing includes baseline, 2 weeks prior to dose escalation, 2 weeks post dose escalation, and monthly during first 12 weeks or beyond.
- Severe life-threatening skin rash, Stevens-Johnson syndrome, has been reported—more commonly in females. When a severe rash occurs, or a rash with other symptoms such as fever, blistering, oral lesions, conjunctivitis, swelling, myalgias, or arthralgias, nevirapine must be discontinued immediately.

Protease Inhibitors

A protease inhibitor may be used in prophylaxis of HIV.

Ⓟ Prototype Drug

ritonavir (Norvir)

Contraindications
- Hypersensitivity

Warnings
Because ritonavir is primarily metabolized by the liver, it should be used with extreme caution in patients with hepatic impairment.

Precautions
- Tobacco decreases the AUC of ritonavir

Drug Interactions
Concurrent use with amiodarone, astemizole, bepridil, cisapride, dihydroergotamine, ergonovine, ergotamine, flecainide, lovastatin, methylergonovine, midazolam, pimozide, propafenone, quinidine, simvastatin, St John's wort, terfenadine, or triazolam is contraindicated. Ritonavir may also cause large increases in the levels of hypnotic and sedative drugs. These drugs include alprazolam, clorazepate, diazepam, estazolam, flurazepam, triazolam, and zolpidem. Because these drugs compete for the CYP3A, there is a potential for life-threatening reactions.

Ritonavir contains alcohol in its formulation; therefore coadministration of disulfiram (Antabuse) or metronidazole can cause Antabuse-type reactions.

There are many drug interactions with ritonavir and it is highly recommended to review pharmaceutical information prior to initiation of any new medication. Ritonavir decreases levels of ethinyl estradiol, theophylline, sulfamethoxazole, and zidovudine. Ritonavir decreases the levels of rifabutin to one quarter of standard dose; ritonavir increases levels of clarithromycin and also, desipramine. Those patients with ritonavir and clarithromycin with renal impairment should have further dose reduction and reference to a pharmaceutical source is warranted.

Dosage and Administration
- Administer 600 mg twice daily by mouth. It should be taken with meals if possible. Oral solution may be mixed in chocolate milk or nutritional supplements such as Ensure or Advera within 1 hour of dosing for improved taste.
- Adult dosage is 600 mg twice a day when used as a single PI or 100 to 400mg twice a day when used with another PI.
- Dose escalation regimen to improve GI tolerance: 300 mg every 12 hours for 1 day, 400 mg twice a day for 2 days, 500 mg twice a day for 1 day, and then 600 mg twice a day.
- Pediatric dosage is 400 mg/m^2 twice daily by mouth and should not exceed 600 mg twice daily. Dose escalation as follows: start at 250 mg/m^2 twice daily on day 1, then increased at 2- or 3-day intervals by 50 mg/m^2 twice daily until 400 mg/m^2 twice daily dosing is achieved.
- Renal impairment: dose reduction is not necessary. In pediatric patients ritonavir should be used with as

combination therapy with other antiretrovirals. For patients who are also taking other antiretroviral medications, refer to product information for specifics on antiretroviral dosage adjustments. Ritonavir may be better tolerated when used in combination with another antiretroviral by initiating ritonavir alone before adding subsequently adding the second agent.

Other Drugs in Class

There are now multiple drugs in this class. Refer to recent dosing information as food affects absorption of some drugs in this class.

Fusion Inhibitor

Ⓟ Prototype Drug

enfuvirtide (Fuzeon, T-20)

Contraindications

- Hypersensitivity

Warnings

- Local injection site reaction is the most common adverse effect and symptoms may include pain, induration, erythema, nodules, cysts, pruritus, and ecchymosis.
- An increased rate of bacterial pneumonia was observed in trials. It is unclear if there is a relationship, but patients on this medication should be carefully monitored for signs and symptoms of pneumonia.
- Hypersensitivity reactions have occurred and may occur on rechallenge. Patients developing symptoms suggestive of a systemic hypersensitivity reaction should discontinue enfuvirtide.

RESOURCES FOR PATIENTS AND PROVIDERS

With the increasing number of antiretrovirals and continuous HIV research, the greatest challenge is keeping up with treatment information. These are some of useful resources for basic clinical information, patient information, and clinical trials. They have been found to be useful, accurate, and updated regularly.

The Eighth Annual HIV Drug Guide: *Positively Aware,* Jan/Feb:36-30, 2004.
Journal published annually for the lay public with detailed information about AIDS drugs.

HRSA-AETC National HIV Telephone Consultation Service (for health care providers only): (800) 933-3413 (7:30 AM-5:00 PM Pacific Time, Monday-Friday) or www.ucsf.edu/hivcntr/services.html#warmline.
The telephone number or consultation hotline for medical professionals, staffed by physicians and pharmacists, is made available to provide updated HIV treatment information. In addition, the same website provides a national telephone hotline for clinicians needing information on postexposure prophylaxis (PEP) at (888) HIV-4911.

Panel on Clinical Practices for Treatment of HIV Infection, *Guidelines for the Use of Antiretroviral Agents in HIV-Infected Adults and Adolescents,* March 2004. Available from the Centers for Disease Control and Prevention (CDC) National AIDS Clearinghouse at (800) 458-5231 and from the HIV/AIDS Treatment Information Service (ATIS) at (800) 448-0440 or www.hivatis.org.
In November 1997 the Panel on Clinical Practices for Treatment of HIV Infection, convened by the Department of Health and Human Services (DHHS) and the Henry J. Kaiser Family Foundation, developed these guidelines. The guidelines continue to be updated by an expert panel on a regular basis, with the most recent update in March 2004. It is important to note that these guidelines stress that the treatment of HIV-infected patients should be directed by a clinician with extensive experience in the care of HIV-infected patients.
Updated information about HIV PEP is also available on the ATIS website.

Other Internet Sites

Johns Hopkins AIDS Service, http://hopkins-aids.edu.
Information on AIDS service publications, treatments, consultations, resources, education, prevention. It also has HIV guidelines, outcomes research, with special section on women and the reference to the text. The Medical Management of HIV Infection, by John Bartlett and Joel Gallant.

AIDS Education Global Information System (AEGIS), www.aegis.com.
A nonprofit site that has exceptional resource for HIV/AIDS information for both the patient and the provider.

Anti-HIV Compound list, www.niaid.nih.gov/daids/dtpdb.
This National Institutes of Health/National Institutes of Allergy and Infectious Diseases database contains list of all anti-HIV compounds with references and links to other sites.

Association of Nurses in AIDS Care (ANAC), www.anacnet.org.
Nursing specialty group.

HIV Insite, http://hivinsite.ucsf.edu/.
HIV insite is a product from University of California at San Francisco and provides news, textbook, and links to other sites. Also good site for patients.

Journal of the International Association of Physicians in AIDS Care, www.iapac.org.
Information and current news on antiretroviral therapies, opportunistic diseases, conferences, and report summaries.

National Institutes of Health (NIH) Clinical trials, http://clinicaltrials.gov.
NIH site lists all NIH-sponsored trials.

The body, www.thebody.com.
Widely acclaimed as a top site for basic information, latest news, advice from HIV experts for both the patient and the provider.

BIBLIOGRAPHY

Bartlett JG, Gallant JE: 2001-2002 Medical management of human immunodeficiency virus infection, Baltimore, 2001, Johns Hopkins University.

Dybull M et al: Guidelines for using antiretroviral agents among HIV-infected adults and adolescents. The Panel on Clinical Practices for the Treatment of HIV, Ann Intern Med 137:381, 2002.

Department of Health and Human Services: *Guidelines for the use of antiretroviral agents in HIV-infected adults and adolescents,* Washington, DC, 2002, Department of Health and Human Services.

Dolin R, Mazur H, Saga M: *Aids therapy,* ed 2, New York, 2003, Churchill Livingstone.

Drugs for HIV infection: *Med Lett* 39(1015):111, 1997.

Grasala T et al: Analysis of potential risk factors associated with the development of pancreatitis in phase I parents with AIDS or AIDS-related complex receiving didanosine, *J Infect Dis* 169:1250, 1994.

Guidelines for antiretroviral agents in pediatric HIV infection, *MMWR Morb Mortal Wkly Rep* 1998; 47(RR-4);1-43. (August 2001 update available at http: //www.hiatus.org).

Hanna GH, Hirsch MS: Antiretroviral therapy for human immunodeficiency virus infection. In Mandell,GL, Bennett, J and Dolin,R, editors: *Mandells, Douglas, and Bennett's principles and practice of infectious diseases,* ed 5, Philadelphia, 2000, Churchill Livingstone.

Kopp JB et al: Crystalluria and urinary tract abnormalities with indinavir, *Ann Intern Med* 127:119, 1997.

Manfredi R: HIV disease and advanced age: an increasing therapeutic challenge, *Drugs Aging,* 19(9):647-69, 2002.

Masur H, Kaplan JE, Holmes KK: Guidelines for preventing opportunistic infections among HIV-infected persons—2002. Recommendations of the U.S. Public Health Service and the Infectious Diseases Society of America, *Ann Intern Med* 137 (5 Pt 2):435-478, 2002.

Serchuck LK, Welles L, Yarchoan R: Antiretroviral treatment for human immunodeficiency virus infection. In Merigan TC Jr, Bartlett JG, Bolognesi D, editors: *The textbook of AIDS medicine,* ed 2, Baltimore, 1998, Williams & Wilkins.

Stenzel MS, Carpenter CC: The management of the clinical complications of antiretroviral therapy, *Infect Dis Clin N Am* 14(4): 51-878, 2000.

Watts DH: Management of human immunodeficiency virus in pregnancy, *N Engl J Med* 346(24):1879-1891, 2002.

CHAPTER 70

Antivirals and Antiprotozoal Agents

Drug Names

Class	Subclass	Generic Name	Trade Name
Antivirals	Antiherpes	(200) acyclovir	Zovirax
		famciclovir	Famvir
		(200) valacyclovir	Valtrex
		penciclovir	Denavir
	Antiinfluenza	amantadine	Symmetrel
		rimantadine	Flumadine
		zanamivir	Relenza
		oseltamivir	Tamiflu
Antiprotozoal		metronidazole	Flagyl
		chloroquine	Plaquenil

(200), Top 200 drug.

General Uses

Indications

acyclovir, famciclovir, valacyclovir, and penciclovir

- Herpes simplex (types 1 and 2): treatment of acute infection and chronic suppression
- Varicella-zoster viruses (chickenpox and shingles)
- Epstein-Barr virus (mononucleosis)

amantadine and rimantadine

- Influenza A

zanamivir, oseltamivir

- Influenza A and B

metronidazole

- Many protozoa

chloroquine

- Malaria

This group includes the antiviral drugs, and the two common antiprotozoal medications that are used in primary care. Acyclovir, famciclovir, and valacyclovir are closely related. They are used in the treatment of initial and frequently recurrent (more than 6 outbreaks per year) mucosal and cutaneous herpes simplex types 1 and 2 in immunocompromised and nonimmunocompromised patients and for treatment of acute herpes simplex virus (HSV) infections. Acyclovir has the greatest antiviral activity in vitro against herpes simplex virus type 1 followed, in decreasing order of potency, by HSV type 2 (HSV-2), varicella-zoster virus, Epstein-Barr virus, and cytomegalovirus. Penciclovir is structurally similar but is only used topically. See Chapter 14.

Amantadine, rimantadine, zanamivir, and oseltamivir are used for prevention and treatment of influenza virus infections. Amantadine is also used in Parkinson's disease. See Chapter 47.

Metronidazole has several uses in addition to treatment of protozoa, including bacterial and amebic infections. Chloroquine is used for malaria; however, many strains of malaria are now resistant to chloroquine. There are many antiparasitic and antiprotozoal medications that are important in international travel but only rarely encountered in primary care. These are not discussed.

DISEASE PROCESS

Anatomy and Physiology

Virus. A virus is a single- or double-stranded DNA or RNA molecule enclosed in a protein coat. Some may also have a lipoprotein envelope. They may contain proteins that can cause antigenic reactions or enzymes that can initiate viral replication. They lack metabolic functions and must rely on the host cell for metabolism. According to the definition of life, viruses are not alive. They do not eat or produce waste. They do not reproduce independently.

DNA viruses include herpesviruses (chickenpox, shingles, herpes), adenoviruses (conjunctivitis, pharyngitis), hepadnaviruses (hepatitis B), and papillomaviruses (warts). RNA viruses include rubella (German measles), rhabdoviruses (rabies), and picornaviruses (poliomyelitis, meningitis, colds), arboviruses (yellow fever), orthomyxoviruses (influenza), and paramyxoviruses (measles and mumps). The retroviruses are a subgroup of RNA viruses that are discussed in Chapter 69.

Protozoa. The word *parasite* is used to discuss protozoa, helminths, and arthropods. Parasites are metabolically dependent on a host. This chapter discusses only a few of the many protozoa that are most commonly seen in the United States. Malaria is included because it is such an important disease worldwide.

Protozoa are small and unicellular. They are the simplest organisms in the animal kingdom. They are divided into categories based on their type of locomotion. Important protozoal diseases include amebiasis, caused by *Entamoeba histolytica*; giardiasis, caused by *Giardia lamblia*; and trichomoniasis, caused by *Trichomonas vaginalis*.

Protozoa also cause malaria. *Plasmodium falciparum, P. vivax, P. malariae*, and *P. ovale* all cause malaria.

The Disease

Herpes Simplex. Herpes simplex virus type 1 (HSV-1) causes infections of the mouth and face (herpes labialis), and of the skin, esophagus, and brain. Vesicles form moist ulcers after several days and epithelialize over 2 to 3 weeks. In some geographic locations, HSV-1 infections are a common cause of first episodes of genital herpes. They may occur in stable, monogamous relationships and are less likely to recur than genital infections caused by HSV-2.

HSV-2 causes infection of the genitals, rectum, skin, hands, and meninges. Asymptomatic shedding of the virus is commonly the mechanism of transmission. Thus the disease can be transmitted sexually. Recent serologic surveys, employing type-specific antibody assays, show a rising prevalence of previous HSV-2 infections in postadolescent populations in developed countries; many of these infections have been asymptomatic.

Herpes simplex can be a primary infection (which can be asymptomatic) or activation of a latent infection. It is unknown what triggers activation. Type 2 is latent in the presacral ganglia. Both type 1 and type 2 can also cause keratitis, encephalitis, recurrent meningitis, disseminated infection, and Bell's palsy.

The varicella-zoster virus (VZV) is the herpesvirus 3. The virus causes the disease chickenpox in children, which is highly contagious, being spread by inhalation of infective droplets or contact with lesions. In older adults or immunocompromised patients, the virus can cause shingles. Shingles is caused by reactivation of the virus that is latent in the nerve ganglion. It causes a vesicular rash on an erythematous base in a dermatome pattern, accompanied by pain and systemic symptoms.

Influenza. Influenzavirus causes epidemics of acute illness that are transmitted by the respiratory route. Influenza is diagnosed by association with an epidemic that is confirmed by viral cultures. The standard trivalent influenzavirus vaccine provides partial immunity to certain strains of influenza A and B that vary from year to year.

Protozoal Diseases: Giardia and Malaria. Giardia is the most common cause of waterborne diarrheal disease in the United States. It is transmitted by fecal-oral spread of cysts via contaminated food or water. It is resistant to chlorination levels found in water supplies and can survive freezing for several days. Symptoms include diarrhea, fatigue, malaise, abdominal cramps, and weight loss. A diagnostic test is available to detect antigens in the stool.

Malaria is the most significant protozoal disease in the world, causing 1.5 to 2.7 million deaths annually. Symptoms of malaria include periodic attacks of chills, fever and sweating, headache, myalgia, splenomegaly, anemia, and leukopenia. Increasing drug resistance has caused treatment of malaria to be problematic. An additional complication is the fact that plasmodia go through distinct stages that affect its susceptibility to different agents. For example, chloroquine is active against asexual blood stages but not sexual blood stages or asexual liver stages. Prophylaxis of malaria in travelers depends on risk factors, including area to be visited and the type of malaria active in that area. Chloroquine and primaquine are used in nonchloroquine-resistant areas.

DRUG ACTION AND EFFECTS

Antivirals

In order to be effective an antiviral drug must enter the infected cells and act at the site of infection. Effective agents have a narrow spectrum of activity, inhibiting replication but not killing the virus. They target a specific viral protein, usually an enzyme involved in viral nucleic acid synthesis. Resistance may develop quickly. The difference between in vitro sensitivity testing and in vivo effectiveness is not clear. The human must still have a good immune system to recover from infection.

Acyclovir is a synthetic purine nucleoside analog. Valacyclovir and famciclovir are pro-drugs of acyclovir, with chemical structures similar to acyclovir. They work by inhibiting viral DNA synthesis. The drugs are activated by the enzyme thymidine kinase, which is found only in cells that are infected with the virus. Consequently they are relatively nontoxic to cells that are not infected with the virus. They are selectively and preferentially taken up by the infected cells; the drug incorporates itself into the DNA chain and interferes with DNA replication, stopping viral production. In chemical terms, activation of the antiviral first occurs in the infected cells, followed by phosphorylation by the enzyme thymidine kinase. Finally, acyclovir triphosphate (the active derivative obtained from monophosphate by host cell enzymes) inhibits viral DNA polymerase, thereby blocking viral replication.

Amantadine and rimantadine are structurally similar tricyclic amines. They both inhibit an early step in viral replication, and they also have an effect in the viral assembly. The locus of action is the influenza A virus M2 protein, which is an integral membrane protein.

Zanamivir and oseltamivir are thought to inhibit the virus neuraminidase; this alters virus particle aggregation and release.

Antiprotozoals

metronidazole. Metronidazole is considered a cytotoxic agent, but its exact mechanism of action is not well understood. Metronidazole damages DNA synthesis, resulting in cell death. Most probably, metronidazole initially enters cells by passive diffusion and is then activated by an enzymatic system present only in certain cells, such as anaerobic cells and protozoa. A reaction occurs; a nitrogen group is reduced. The metabolites are toxic substances that bind to DNA and RNA and interrupt synthesis.

chloroquine. The exact mechanism of action is unknown. Chloroquine raises the internal pH of parasites. It may also influence hemoglobin digestion or interfere with parasite/ nucleoprotein synthesis.

DRUG TREATMENT PRINCIPLES

acyclovir, famciclovir, and valacyclovir

Herpes Simplex Treatment. All of these agents are useful in the treatment of herpes viruses. They are used as a treatment of acute infections as well as an agent for chronic suppressive therapy. Systemic therapy for initial episodes does not prevent either the establishment of latency or the development of future recurrences even when used in high or prolonged dosage. Oral acyclovir is the most useful and effective form of the drug for treatment of herpes simplex viruses and varicella infections. In patients with frequent recurrences, oral acyclovir has prevented or reduced the frequency or severity of recurrences in more than 95% of patients. Topical acyclovir is significantly less effective, but will shorten healing time and the duration of viral shedding and pain in patients with an initial outbreak of herpes. No clinical benefit was found using the topical form in recurrent episodes of genital herpes.

When prescribing these drugs, the practitioner should understand two important principles. First, the peak of viral activity and reproduction occurs prior to the appearance of any symptoms. Therefore therapy is prescribed late in the disease process. Second, viral agents work by inhibiting reproduction but not eradicating latent viruses. Elimination of the virus is not complete, but they can assist in reducing and suppressing symptoms. The effectiveness of the drug depends on how early treatment is initiated.

Almost all persons with initially symptomatic HSV-2 infection have symptomatic recurrences. More than 35% of such patients have frequent recurrences. Recurrence rates are especially high in persons with an extended first episode of infection, regardless of whether they receive antiviral chemotherapy with acyclovir or not. Men with genital HSV-2 infection have about 20% more recurrences than do women, a factor that may contribute to the higher rate of HSV-2 transmission from men to women than from women to men and to the continuing epidemic of genital herpes in the United States.

These antiviral drugs are indicated for treating genital herpes in the following circumstances: initial episode of genital herpes, frequently recurring episodes (more than six per year), immunocompromised patients (treatment or chronic suppression), and severe genital herpes. Antivirals should not be used in mildly affected patients because resistance to the medication can occur. Although resistance is rare, it is more likely to occur with prolonged or repeated therapy in severely immunocompromised patients. Use of acyclovir, valacyclovir, and famciclovir in the nonpregnant and pregnant woman can significantly alter the disease and influence transmission rates along with decreasing the morbidity and mortality associated with HSV infections.

Herpes Zoster Treatment. Antiviral drugs have been shown to enhance healing of lesions and decrease or stop the pain frequently associated with the zoster lesions (paresthesia, dysesthesia, hyperesthesia), particularly in the generally more severe cases of shingles found in patients 50 years of age or older. Treatment has been more successful when started within the first 48 hours following the onset of the rash.

Antiinfluenza Drugs

These drugs are used as short-term prophylaxis during the course of an influenza outbreak. These drugs are used to prevent influenza in exposed, unvaccinated individuals. They should be started immediately and continued for 10 days.

They may be used as an adjunct to late immunization of high-risk individuals. (Response to vaccine takes about 2 weeks.) They also may be used to supplement vaccination protection in those patients with impaired immune responses, and they may be used as chemoprophylaxis for patients at high risk for whom influenza vaccine is contraindicated.

Antiprotozoal Drugs

metronidazole. Metronidazole has both antibiotic and antiprotozoal actions. It is useful for a wide variety of infections. Metronidazole has excellent activity against most gram-negative and gram-positive anaerobes and is indicated for use in many serious infections. Because metronidazole reaches high concentrations in most body tissues, it is very successful in the treatment of intraabdominal, intrapelvic, and cerebral infections as well as endocarditis, bone and joint infections, and head and neck infections caused by susceptible anaerobes. Metronidazole also reaches high concentrations in abscesses (e.g., cerebral, hepatic, abdominal abscesses) and is often indicated in their treatment. Metronidazole does not cover gram-positive cocci or aerobic organisms; hence it is usually used in combination with another drug in treating complicated infections.

In primary care settings, metronidazole is the drug of choice in treating *T. vaginalis*. Because trichomonas is a sexually transmitted disease, both partners need to be treated in order to obtain a cure (i.e., to prevent reinfection of the other partner). The practitioner has the option of prescribing a 1- or 7-day course of treatment. A single oral dose (2 g) is usually as effective as the 7-day course. Although some evidence has shown that the 7-day treatment may have a slightly higher cure rate, the 1-day treatment may be justified if patient compliance is in question. Metronidazole is also indicated in treating bacterial or nonspecific vaginitis.

Metronidazole is the current treatment of choice for symptomatic intestinal infections caused by *G. lamblia* and *E. histolytica*. Both parasites are found worldwide and are usually contracted by ingesting contaminated water or food. Sporadic outbreaks of *Giardia* occur throughout the United States and are occasionally seen in the primary care setting.

The high cost of vancomycin and the increase in the incidence of vancomycin-resistant enterococcal infections have now made metronidazole the recommended initial treatment of *Clostridium difficile*. Studies have shown that metronidazole is effective in the majority of cases of *C. difficile*. However, vancomycin remains the drug of choice for severe cases of *C. difficile*.

Much attention has been focused on the use of metronidazole in treating *Helicobacter pylori*, an organism involved in the etiology of gastritis and peptic ulcer disease. Metronidazole, in conjunction with bismuth (and sometimes omeprazole or a histamine blocker), appears to be effective in treating *H. pylori*.

The addition of tetracycline may increase the length of remission (see Chapter 28).

chloroquine. Chloroquine is used for chemoprophylaxis of malaria. It is effective against *P. falciparum* and *P. malariae* infections that are not resistant. Chloroquine is given weekly starting 1 week before travel, during travel, and continuing for 4 weeks after leaving. Chloroquine is also used for treatment of malaria.

HOW TO MONITOR

Antivirals

- Monitor closely for toxicity and adverse effects, especially in patients with renal impairment.

Antiprotozoals

- Metronidazole: Perform total and differential leukocyte counts before and after therapy.
- Chloroquine: Perform baseline and periodic ophthalmologic examinations.
- Monitor for muscular weakness, question and examine patient, and test knee and ankle reflexes.
- Monitor CBC periodically.

PATIENT VARIABLES

Geriatrics

- Medications are generally very effective and well tolerated.
- Antiherpes agents: reduce dosage in elderly and those with decreased in renal failure. Elderly are more likely to have renal or CNS adverse events.
- Amantadine and rimantadine: reduce dosage in patients older than 65 years.
- Zanamivir and oseltamivir: no dosage adjustment is necessary.
- Metronidazole: dosage adjustment may be necessary.

Pediatrics

- Famciclovir and valacyclovir: safety and efficacy in children younger than 18 years old have not been established.
- Acyclovir: safety and efficacy in children younger than 2 years have not been established.
- Amantadine, rimantadine: safety and efficacy in children younger than 1 year old have not been established.
- Zanamivir: safety and efficacy have not been established in patients younger than 7 years old.
- Metronidazole: safety and efficacy have not been established, except for the treatment of amebiasis.
- Chloroquine: children are especially sensitive to these drugs. Fatalities following accidental ingestion of relatively small doses and sudden deaths from parenteral chloroquine have been recorded. Do not exceed a single dose of 5 mg base/kg of chloroquine HCl in infants or children.

Pregnancy

- *Category B:* famciclovir, valacyclovir, and metronidazole. Do not use metronidazole during first trimester
- *Category C:* acyclovir, amantadine, rimantadine, zanamivir
- Chloroquine: no category; use only when clearly needed and when potential benefits outweigh potential hazards to the fetus

Lactation

- Acyclovir, amantadine, rimantadine, metronidazole, chloroquine: appear in breast milk. Use is not recommended.
- Famciclovir and valacyclovir, zanamivir: safety and use in lactation are unknown.

PATIENT EDUCATION

Antivirals

Antiherpes Agents

- Avoid sexual intercourse when visible herpes lesions are present.

amantadine, rimantadine

- Blurred vision or impaired mental acuity may occur. Use caution in performing tasks that require acute vision or physical coordination.
- Avoid excessive alcohol use, as it will exacerbate CNS effects.

zanamivir

- Instruct patients in use of the delivery system.
- The use of zanamivir for treatment of influenza has not been shown to reduce the risk of transmission of influenza to others.
- Stop use of drug if the patient experiences bronchospasm.

Antiprotozoals

metronidazole

- May cause GI upset; take with food
- May cause darkening of the urine or metallic taste

> ! Avoid alcoholic beverages or any products containing alcohol because together they may cause severe nausea, vomiting, flushing, and/or heart palpitations, a disulfiram-like reaction.

chloroquine

- May cause GI upset; take with food.
- Report visual disturbances or difficulty in hearing or ringing in ears, diarrhea, vomiting, muscle weakness, or rash.
- Keep out of reach of children; overdosage is especially dangerous in children.
- Medication may cause diarrhea, loss of appetite, nausea, stomach pain or vomiting. Notify provider if pronounced or bothersome.

Specific Drugs

ANTIVIRALS

Antiherpes Agents

acyclovir (Zovirax), famciclovir (Famvir), valacyclovir (Valtrex)

Contraindications

- Hypersensitivity or intolerance to the drug or any of its components

Warnings

- Acyclovir and famciclovir: testicular toxicity has occurred in rats.
- Famciclovir: carcinogenesis—increase in incidence of mammary adenocarcinoma was seen in rats.
- Famciclovir caused chromosomal aberrations in mice.
- Valacyclovir does not appear to be mutagenic.
- Valacyclovir: thrombotic thrombocytopenic purpura/hemolytic-uremic syndrome has occurred in patients with advanced HIV.

Precautions

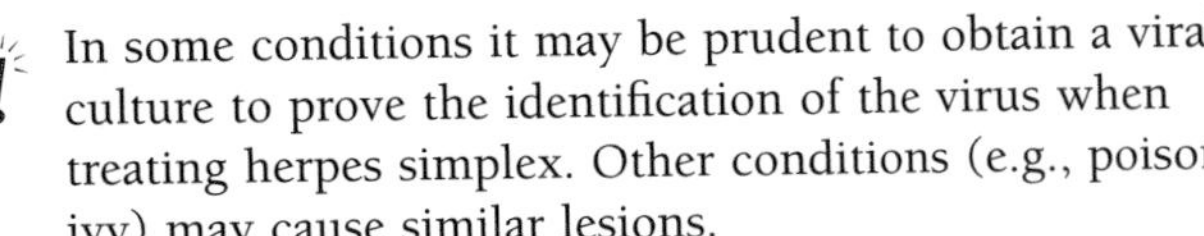

In some conditions it may be prudent to obtain a viral culture to prove the identification of the virus when treating herpes simplex. Other conditions (e.g., poison ivy) may cause similar lesions.

- Renal function impairment: reduce dosage according to the guidelines given in the package insert. Drugs are excreted mainly through the kidneys. Use caution in patients with decreased renal function (creatinine clearance less than 60 ml/min). Use with caution in patients who are poorly hydrated or are on other nephrotoxic medications because these predispose the patient to acute renal failure.
- Ensure adequate hydration.
- Use cautiously in patients who have underlying neurologic disorders or who have had prior neurologic reactions to drugs. A small percentage (1%) of patients receiving parental acyclovir have had major neurologic symptoms such as lethargy, obtundation, tremors, confusion, hallucinations, agitation, seizures, or coma.
- Use can result in emergence of resistant viruses. HSV and varicella-zoster virus strains resistant to one drug have generally been cross-resistant to other drugs in this class.

Pharmacokinetics. See Table 70-1. The drug is widely distributed in body tissues and fluids, including brain, kidney, lung, liver, muscles, spleen, uterus, vaginal mucosa and secretions, cerebral spinal fluid, and herpetic vesicular fluid.

Adverse Effects. See Table 70-2. Common side effects experienced with oral acyclovir include GI symptoms such as nausea, vomiting, and diarrhea. In general, more side effects have been noted with long-term or chronic use of the drug.

Drug Interactions. See Table 70-3.

Dosage and Administration. Table 70-4 provides common primary care usage. Parenteral dosages for acute or severe infections are not included. Medication may be taken without regard to meals. Begin as soon as a diagnosis is made. These drugs are most effective if given within 24 to 48 hours of onset of signs and symptoms. Give reduced dose with any indication of renal impairment.

Antiinfluenza Agents

amantadine (Symmetrel), rimantadine (Flumadine)

Amantadine and rimantadine are similar and are discussed together.

Contraindications

- Hypersensitivity to either drug

Warnings

- Deaths have been reported from overdose with amantadine. Suicide attempts have been seen, some of which have been fatal in some patients without history of psychiatric illness.

Amantadine can exacerbate emotional problems in patients with a history of psychiatric disorders or substance abuse.

TABLE 70-1 Pharmacokinetics of Antivirals and Antiprotozoals

Drug	Absorption	Time to Peak Concentration	Half-Life	Protein Bound	Metabolism	Excretion
acyclovir	15%-30%	1.5-2 hr	2.5 hr	9%-33%	Liver	14.4%
famciclovir	77%	1 hr	2.3 hr		Liver	82%
valacyclovir	54%		2.5-3.3 hr	15%	Liver	45%
amantadine	Well	3.3 hr	17 hr			Renal
rimantadine		6 hr	25 hr		Liver	Renal, 25%
zanamivir	Inhaled, 4%-17% systemically absorbed	1-2 hr	2.5-5 hr			Renal
oseltamivir	Well			3%	Liver	Renal
metronidazole	Well	1-2 hr	8 hr		Liver	Renal

TABLE 70-2 Adverse Reactions to Antivirals and Antiprotozoals by Body System

Body System	acyclovir	famciclovir	valacyclovir	amantadine	rimantadine	zanamivir	oseltamivir	metronidazole	chloroquine
Body, general	Malaise	Fatigue, pain, fever		Fatigue	Fatigue	Malaise, fatigue, fever	Fatigue	Bacterial infection, influenza-like symptoms, moniliasis	
Skin, appendages	rash	Pruritus		Photosensitivity, rash	Rash	Urticaria			Hair loss, pruritus, rash, pigment changes
Hypersensitivity				Anaphylaxis					
Respiratory		Pharyngitis, sinusitis		Respiratory failure	Dyspnea	Nasal symptoms, bronchitis, sinusitis	Cough	Rhinitis, sinusitis, pharyngitis	
Cardiovascular				Orthostatic hypotension, congestive heart failure (CHF), hyper-tension, arrhythmias	Hypertension, CHF, heart block				Hypotension, electrocardiogram (ECG) changes, cardiomyopathy
GI	Nausea, vomiting, diarrhea, constipation	Nausea, vomiting, diarrhea, abd pain, dyspepsia, constipation, anorexia	Nausea, vomiting, abd pain	Nausea, anorexia, dry mouth, con-stipation, diarrhea, vomiting	Nausea, vomiting, anorexia, dry mouth, abd pain	Diarrhea, nausea, vomiting, abd pain	Nausea, vomiting, diarrhea abd pain	Nausea, abd pain, diarrhea, dry mouth	Anorexia, nausea, vomiting, diarrhea, abd cramps
Genitourinary								Vaginitis, genital pruritus, dysmenorrhea	
Hemic and lymphatic			Leukopenia, thrombocytopenia	Leukocytosis					Agranulocytosis, blood dyscrasias
Musculoskeletal		Back pain, arthralgia	arthralgia			Myalgia, arthralgia			Neuromyopathy
CNS	Headache	Headache, dizziness, insomnia, somnolence, paresthesia	Headache, dizziness	Dizziness, insomnia, depression, anxiety, restlessness, irritability, hallucinations, ataxia, headache psychosis	Insomnia, dizziness, headache, asthenia, nervousness, ataxia, somnolence, agitation, ataxia, hallucination, confusion, seizure	Headache, dizziness, peripheral neuropathy	Headache, dizziness, insomnia, vertigo	Headache, dizziness	
Special senses				Visual disturbance	Tinnitus, eye pain			Metallic taste, disulfiram-like reaction	Irreversible retinal damage, blurred vision, scotoma

abd, Abdominal.

TABLE 70-3 Drug Interactions with Antivirals and Antiprotozoals

Antiviral/Antiprotozoal	Action on Other Drugs	Other Drugs	Action on Antivirals/Antiprotozoals
famciclovir	↑ digoxin	probenecid, zidovudine	↑ acyclovir
amantadine	↑ CNS stimulants	cimetidine, probenecid, theophylline	↑ famciclovir
metronidazole	↑ hydantoins, lithium	cimetidine, probenecid	↑ valacyclovir
chloroquine	↓ kaolin or magnesium trisilicate	Anticholinergic agents, quinidine, quinine, triamterene, thiazide diuretics, trimethoprim/sulfamethoxazole	↑ amantadine
		cimetidine	↑ rimantadine
		acetaminophen, aspirin	↓ rimantadine
		cimetidine	↑ chloroquine

TABLE 70-4 Dosage and Administration Recommendations for Antivirals and Protozoals

Drug	Disease	Stage	Dosage and Administration	Max Dose
acyclovir	Herpes simplex, genital	Initial	200 mg q4hr, 5 ×/day × 10 days	
		Chronic suppressive therapy	400 mg bid × 12 mo	
	Herpes zoster	Acute	800 mg q4hr, 5 ×/day × 7-10 days	
		Chickenpox	20 mg/kg qid × 5 days	800 mg
famciclovir	Herpes simplex, genital	Recurrent episodes	125 mg bid × 5 days	
	Herpes zoster	Acute	500 mg q8hr × 7 days	
valacyclovir	Herpes simplex, genital	Initial	1 g bid × 10 days	
		Recurrent	500 mg bid × 3 days	
		Suppressive	1 g qd × 1 yr	
	Herpes simplex, labialis	Treatment	2 g bid × 1 day	
	Herpes zoster	Acute	1 g tid × 7 days	
amantadine	Influenza A	Prophylaxis, treatment	1-9 yr: 4.4-8.8 mg/kg/day qd or divided bid 9-12 yr: 100 mg bid 13-64 yr: 200 mg qd or 100 bid 65+: 100 mg qd	150 mg/d
rimantadine	Influenza A	Prophylaxis	Adult: 100 mg bid Child (<10 yr): 5 mg/kg/day qd	150 mg/d
		Treatment	Adult: 100 mg bid	
zanamivir	Influenza A and B	Treatment	Age >7 yr: 2 inh bid × 5 days	
oseltamivir	Influenza A and B	Prophylaxis, exposure	Age >13 yr: 75 mg qd × 7 days	
		Prophylaxis, epidemic	Age >13 yr: 75 qd × 6 wk max	
		Treatment	Age >13 yr: 75 mg bid × 5 days Child <13 yr: see PI	
metronidazole	Bacterial vaginosis	Treatment	7.5 mg/kg q6hr × 7-10 days 500 mg bid or 750 ER qd × 7 days	
	C. difficile		500 mg tid	

- Seizures and other CNS effects: observe patient with a seizure history carefully for increased seizure activity. Reduced dosage may be required. Caution patients who note CNS effects or blurring of vision against performing tasks that require alertness and motor coordination.
- Use with caution in patients with history of recurrent eczematoid rash; or psychosis or severe psychoneurosis not controlled by chemotherapeutic agents.
- Chronic heart failure may occur. Use caution in patients with cardiac history.
- Use amantadine with caution in patients with liver disease.
- Renal function impairment may require reduced dose because amantadine accumulates in plasma.
- Rimantadine safety and pharmacokinetics in renal and hepatic insufficiency have only been evaluated after single-dose administration. In renal failure, the half-life was

increased. In hepatic failure, apparent clearance was decreased.

Precautions

- Do not discontinue abruptly in patients with Parkinson's disease because it may precipitate a parkinsonian crisis.
- Sporadic cases of possible neuroleptic malignant syndrome have been reported with dose reduction or withdrawal. Observe carefully when dosage is reduced or discontinued.
- Notify primary care provider if patient develops mood or mental changes, swelling of the extremities, difficult urination, or shortness of breath.

Overdosage

- Symptoms include cardiac, respiratory, renal, and CNS toxicity. Death has occurred from overdose with amantadine; the lowest reported acute lethal dose was 1 g. Acute toxicity may be attributable to the anticholinergic effects of amantadine.

zanamivir (Relenza), oseltamivir (Tamiflu)

Contraindications

- Hypersensitivity

Warnings. See *Patient Variables.*

Precautions

- Zanamivir: allergic reactions, including oropharyngeal edema and serious skin rashes, have been reported.
- Bacterial infections may begin with influenza-like symptoms, may coexist, or may be a complication of influenza. These agents do not prevent such complications
- Underlying respiratory disease: safety and efficacy have not been demonstrated in patients with underlying COPD. Some patients with underlying respiratory disease have experienced bronchospasm or decline in lung function with zanamivir. Zanamivir is not generally recommended for treatment of patients with underlying airway disease such as asthma or COPD.
- Zanamivir has not been shown to prevent influenza and should not replace annual influenza immunizations.
- Safety and efficacy have not been demonstrated in patients with high-risk underlying medical conditions.

Dosage and Administration

- Prophylaxis: therapy should begin within 2 days of exposure. The duration of protection lasts for as long as dosing is continued.
- Treatment: begin within 2 days of onset of symptoms.
- May be taken without regard to food, although tolerability may be enhanced with food.

ANTIPROTOZOALS

metronidazole (Flagyl)

Contraindications

- History of hypersensitivity to metronidazole or other nitroimidazole derivatives.
- Pregnancy

This medication should not be given to patients who will ingest any type of alcohol. This includes alcoholic drinks, alcohol-based cough syrups, flavorings, or other products. Although the extent of risk is unknown, in sensitive individuals the product will cause a severe and immediate disulfiram (Antabuse)-like reaction if the patient has drunk alcohol while taking the medication.

Warnings

- Neurologic effects: seizures and peripheral neuropathy have been reported in patients treated with metronidazole. Administer metronidazole with caution to patients with CNS disease.
- Patients with severe hepatic disease may experience an accumulation of metronidazole and its metabolites; therefore the dose prescribed for these patients may need to be adjusted. A 50% dose reduction has been recommended in cases of severe liver failure.
- Carcinogenesis has been found in rodents with chronic oral administration.

Precautions

- Crohn's disease patients are known to have an increased incidence of GI and extraintestinal cancers. It is not known if metronidazole increases the risk.
- Known or previously unrecognized candidiasis may present more prominent symptoms during therapy and requires treatment with a candicidal agent.
- Use with caution in patients with evidence or history of blood dyscrasia. Mild leukopenia has been seen during administration; however no persistent hematologic abnormalities attributable to the drug have been observed. Perform total and differential leukocyte counts before and after therapy with metronidazole.

Pharmacokinetics. Metronidazole is well absorbed orally with peak serum levels occurring 1 to 2 hours after administration. Food does not alter the oral bioavailability of the drug but can delay peak serum levels by 1 to 2 hours. Plasma concentrations are proportional to the administered dose for both oral and intravenous use. For instance, oral administration of 250 mg and 500 mg tablets produces peak serum levels of 6 μg/ml and 12 μg/ml. The half-life of metronidazole is approximately 8 hours.

Metronidazole has a large volume of distribution. Less than 20% of the drug is bound to plasma proteins. It is well absorbed and concentrated in all body tissues and fluids, including bone, pelvic tissue, cerebral spinal fluid, meninges, bile, saliva, seminal fluid, breast milk, placenta, abscesses (including brain and hepatic), empyema fluid, and middle ear fluid.

Metabolism of metronidazole occurs in the liver. The metabolites of the drug have very strong bactericidal activity against most strains of anaerobic bacteria and *Trichomonas*. Plasma clearance of metronidazole is decreased in patients with decreased liver function; consequently such patients may require altered doses. A 50% dose reduction has been recommended in patients with severe liver failure.

The major route of elimination of metronidazole and its metabolites is through the urine. Although some of the drug's metabolites may accumulate in patients with renal failure, it is unlikely to cause toxicity. Therefore a dose reduction is not usually required in patients with decreased renal function. However, the literature does suggest a reduced dose in patients with severe renal failure.

Drug Interactions. The most severe reaction may occur with concurrent ingestion of alcohol, producing a disulfiram-like reaction. In sensitive individuals, this is a violent reaction causing immediate nausea, vomiting, diarrhea, and cardiovascular effects. Table 70-3 lists other common drug interactions.

Overdosage. Single oral doses of up to 15 g have been reported with symptoms including nausea, vomiting, and ataxia. Neurologic symptoms (including seizures and peripheral neuropathy) have been reported after 5 to 7 days of doses of 6 to 10.4 g every other day.

Dosage and Administration. See Table 70-4. The pharmacokinetics of metronidazole may be altered in elderly patients or patients with hepatic failure. Therefore monitoring of serum levels in certain cases may be necessary in adjusting the dosage properly. Take metronidazole (Flagyl ER) tablet while fasting. Reduce dosage in patients with hepatic disease. Dosage reduction is not needed in renal insufficiency.

chloroquine (Plaquenil)

Contraindications
- Hypersensitivity
- Retinal or visual field changes
- Long-term therapy in children (hydroxychloroquine)

Warnings
- Resistance easily develops to this product. Certain strains of *P. falciparum* are resistant. Treat with other therapy if resistance develops.
- May cause irreversible retinal damage. Monitor vision frequently during treatment.
- Use with caution in patients with G6PD deficiency.
- Muscular weakness may occur; discontinue if symptoms develop.
- May exacerbate psoriasis or porphyria.
- Use with caution in hepatic disease or alcoholism or with other hepatotoxic drugs.

Precautions
- Monitor CBC; see *How to Monitor.*

Adverse Effects. See Table 70-2. Cardiovascular, ophthalmic retinal damage, and agranulocytosis are some of the more important severe adverse effects.

Overdosage. Headache, drowsiness, visual disturbances, cardiovascular collapse, convulsions, and death can occur. Treatment is symptomatic.

Dosage and Administration. See Centers for Disease Control and Prevention (CDC) recommendations for use of chloroquine.

BIBLIOGRAPHY

Baker DA: Antiviral therapy for genital herpes in nonpregnant and pregnant women, *Int J Fertil Womens Med* 43(5):243, 1998.

Carr PL et al: Evaluation and management of vaginitis, *J Gen Intern Med* 13(5):353, 1998.

Gutierrez K, Arvin AM: Long term antiviral suppression after treatment for neonatal herpes infection, *Pediatr Infect Dis J* 22(4):371-372, 2003.

Johnson RW, Dworkin RH: Treatment of herpes zoster and postherpetic neuraligia, *BMJ* 5:327(7392):748-750, 2003.

Majeroni BA: Bacterial vaginosis: an update, *Am Fam Physician* 57(6):1285, 1998.

Mandell GL, Douglas RG, Bennett JE: *Principles and practice of infectious diseases,* ed 5, Philadelphia, 2000, Churchill Livingstone.

Miller KE, Ruiz DE, Graves JC: Udpate on the prevention and treatment of sexually transmitted diseases, *Am Fam Physician* 67(9):1915, 1922, 2003.

Reis AJ: Treatment of vaginal infections; candidiasis, bacterial vaginosis, and trichomoniasis, *J Am Pharm Assoc (Wash)* NS37(5):563, 1997.

Roberts CM: Genital herpes: evolving epidemiology and current management, *JAAPA* 16(2):36-40, 2003.

What you need to know about...herpes zoster (shingles), *Nurs Times* 99(11):28, 2003.

UNIT 15

Health Promotion

Unit 15 offers a description of those drugs commonly seen in outpatient primary care settings. As society is increasingly turning its attention to health promotion and disease prevention, the ways in which drug products may help individuals maintain or regain health is increasingly important.

The common factor in most of the drugs in these final chapters is that patients are required to get involved in the selection and continuation of more of these drug products than is typical of drug treatment for disease entities. These products are all prescribed in relatively healthy patients. Thus, the success of drug utilization will be intimately related to the client-provider relationship.

- **Chapter 71** describes the latest guidelines for immunization, including a growing focus on those immunizations that adults should maintain.
- **Chapter 72** features the latest NIH guidelines on managing obesity and the medications available to help patients lose weight safely.
- **Chapter 73** evaluates the theory and practice of smoking cessation and identifies how and why different nicotine replacement therapies may be helpful.
- **Chapter 74** updates the latest research information about vitamin and mineral use.
- **Chapter 75** is an expanded chapter identifying what scientists really know about complimentary and alternative products. The scientific knowledge and scholarly rigor of research about these products; so it is difficult, sometimes impossible, to know whether a product may be used safely. However, patients are taking these herbal products. Thus, clinicians need to learn as much as possible about how to help patients reduce risks and adverse effects, especially when patients are taking prescription drugs and herbal supplements simultaneously.

CHAPTER 71

Immunizations and Biologicals

Laurie Scudder

Common Immunization and Biologic Agents Used in Primary Care

Disease	Active Immunity	Passive Immunity	Testing
Hepatitis B	Hepatitis B vaccine	Hepatitis B immune globulin	
Diphtheria	DPaT	Diphtheria antitoxin	
Tetanus/pertussis	DPT-HIB vaccine, DTaP, Td, tetanus toxoid	Tetanus immune globulin	
Haemophilus pneumonia	*Haemophilus influenzae* B vaccine		
Polio	Poliovirus vaccine, inactivated		
Rubeola (measles)	MMR, measles (rubeola) vaccine	Immune globulin, IM	Rubella titer
Mumps	Mumps vaccine, rubella and mumps vaccine, MMR		
Rubella (measles)	MMR (rubella vaccine)		
Varicella zoster	Varicella virus vaccine	Varicella zoster immune globulin	
Influenza	Influenza virus vaccine		
Pneumococcal pneumonia	Pneumococcal polysaccharide vaccine, polyvalent and pneumococcal conjugate vaccine		
Meningitis	Meningococcal polysaccharide vaccine		
Hepatitis A	Hepatitis A vaccine, inactivated	Immune globulin, IM	Antibody levels
Rabies	Rabies vaccine (HDCV)	Rabies immune globulin, human	
Tuberculosis	BCG vaccine		Tuberculin tests
Yellow fever	Yellow fever vaccine		
Typhoid	Typhoid vaccine		

General Uses

Indications

The individual immunizations mentioned in the above table are not discussed in equal detail. The routine immunizations that almost everyone receives are discussed in detail. Maintaining the patient's vaccination status is a major component of primary care. Nurse practitioners should keep up to date with the latest recommendations from CDC's Advisory Committee on Immunization Practices (ACIP) and keep their patients' immunizations up to date.

Vaccines and biologicals for testing that are not in common use are mentioned. The skin tests for coccidioidomycosis and histoplasmosis are used to help with the diagnosis of these diseases; these organisms are most commonly found in rural areas. The *Candidiasis* skin test is primarily used to test for anergy, because everyone has been exposed to yeast.

DISEASE PROCESS

The goal of immunization is the eradication of disease. Numerous infectious diseases, many of which are potentially fatal, have been sharply curtailed worldwide through vigilant adherence to immunization strategies and public health control measures. In the United States, diphtheria, measles, polio, and tetanus are almost unknown. Children who are not vaccinated for religious, cultural, or other reasons are at risk for disease and increase societal risk by contributing to the pool of unvaccinated individuals who are capable of transmitting infection to susceptible and high-risk individuals. However, it is estimated that 5% to 20% (National Committee for Quality Assurance: see http://www.ncqa.org/somc2001/CHILD_IMM/SOMC_2001_CIS.html) of all 2-year-olds in the United States have not received the recommended four doses of the diphtheria-tetanus-pertussis (DTP) vaccine, three doses of the polio vaccine, and the single dose of the measles-mumps-rubella

(MMR) vaccine that should be completed by that time. State and national statistics suggest the need to improve public education on the importance of immunization. The immunization goals set forward in *Healthy People 2000* are not yet met.

ANATOMY AND PHYSIOLOGY: THE IMMUNE SYSTEM

Organs of the immune system consist of primary and secondary organs. Primary organs are responsible for the development and storage of lymphocytes. The bone marrow and the thymus gland are the primary organs of the immune system. Secondary organs are the lymph nodes, spleen, and Peyer's patches. These secondary organs of the immune system entrap foreign substances, produce antibodies, and stimulate T-cell production, all with the main objective of destroying the antigen.

The immune system is the third line of defense against the invasion of antigens. The first line of defense is the skin, mucous membranes, body hair, and body secretions. The second line of defense is the inflammatory response.

The main function of the immune system is to protect the body from damage caused by the introduction of a foreign substance. These foreign substances (antigens), such as viruses, bacteria, and protozoa, invade organs and tissues and can multiply and destroy or impede organ and cellular functions. The immune system acts to rid the body of these foreign bodies/antigens before they can impede or retard body function.

White Blood Cells

The immune system is composed of three categories of WBCs: (1) polymorphonuclear (PMN) leukocytes (neutrophils, eosinophils, basophils, and mast cells), (2) monocytes/macrophages, and (3) lymphocytes (B and T cells) (Figure 71-1). All WBCs originate from a stem cell in the bone marrow. The stem cells first differentiate into myeloid and lymphoid cells. The myeloid cells differentiate into PMN leukocytes and into monocyte/macrophages. The lymphoid cells differential into the B and T lymphocytes

The immune system is responsible for the development of immunity. Immunity to disease occurs when the body, in response to exposure to a foreign substance (antigen), is able to produce antibodies to combat these antigens. The antibody reaction is very specific. This means that antibodies will only fight that antigen for which they were formed. Protective antibodies or immunoglobulin stimulate the body to react to foreign substances (antigens) through phagocytic action. Neutralization of foreign substances is another way the body's immune system fights invaders. Chemotaxic factors are released through the activation of PMNs into the area of invasion, where they dilute the toxin's effect and decrease tissue damage caused through contact with chemotaxic factors.

Specific Immune System Functions

1. *PMN leukocytes* or *granulocytes* are composed of neutrophils, eosinophils, basophils, and mast cells. They are the most active cells and the largest number of immune cells in the body. They arrive first at a site of injury, infection, or inflammation and function in several ways. They phagocytize foreign substances, release chemotaxic substances that encircle the area of invasion, killing and preventing contamination by foreign substance into other areas, and

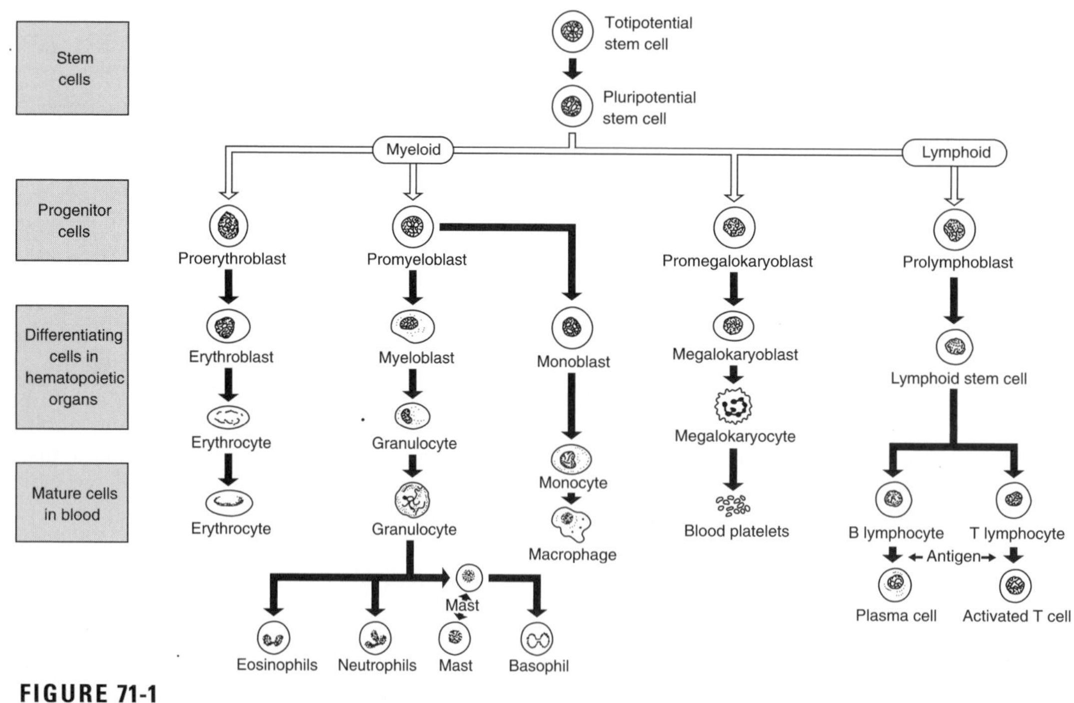

FIGURE 71-1

Bone marrow and stem cell systems. Probable pathways of differentiation, from the totipotential cell to mature blood cells. (*PMN*, Granulocytes.) (From McCance KL, Heuther SE: *Pathophysiology*, ed 3, St Louis, 1998, Mosby.)

stimulate the release of antimicrobial substances that aid in the destruction of the foreign material.

a. *Neutrophils* contain large granules. These granules degranulate when they come in contact with antigens and release enzymes that destroy foreign substances and can injure surrounding tissue. Debris from this destructive action produces an exudate/pus. The enzymes that are secreted from these granules are known as chemotaxic factors: leukotrienes, vasoactive kinins, and toxic metabolites.
b. *Eosinophils* are very similar to neutrophils. They contain granules and engage in the phagocytosis process. They seem to congregate in the respiratory and gastrointestinal tracts. They are especially prominent during allergic reactions and parasitic infections, and they carry certain enzymes that neutralize chemicals responsible for allergic responses. They release potent chemotaxic factors that cause inflammation, bronchospasm, and tissue damage.
c. *Basophils* also contain granules that produce histamine and heparin, which play a role in the immune response. The basophil is not a strong structure and is easily damaged, which causes the granules to release histamine and heparin. Vasospasm, increased vascular permeability, and increased inflammation are the major effects seen when this occurs. This reaction increases the severity of allergic responses.
d. *Mast cells* are the guards of the immune system and are found in cutaneous and mucosal tissue. They can immediately recognize entering non-self foreign antigens without the aid of macrophages or lymphocytes. They are the effectors of immediate hypersensitivity reactions. They contain most of the body's IgE. When this IgE and an antigen meet, there is immediate degranulation and release of histamine, prostaglandin, and leukotrienes, and arachidonic acid metabolism, which potentiate the hypersensitivity response.

2. *Monocytes/macrophages.* When the monocytes are released into the bloodstream, they migrate to various tissue sites where they differentiate (mature) and become macrophages. Macrophages serve three functions in the immune response. The first is to secrete biologically active compounds/molecules such as prostaglandins, interleukins, interferons, tumor necrosis factors, growth factors, proteins, and enzymes, which serve to provide host defense from specific antigens. The second is to remove excess dead or damaged antigens. The third is to engulf and present antigens to lymphoid cells for elimination. Macrophages are found in connective tissue (histocyte), the liver (Kupffer's cells), alveolar tissue in the lung, and microglial cells in the nervous system. They are also found in the spleen, lymph nodes, and other organs.
3. *Lymphocytes are B and T cells.* These cells have the ability to react with antigens to produce reactions that will create a specific response that will destroy the antigen. The B lymphocytes are those cells that produce antibodies. They undergo a specific differentiation when exposed to an antigen and become plasma cells that are the major secretor of antibodies (Figure 71-2). These antibodies' major function is to destroy a specific antigen and remove it from the body. In a response to a specific antigen, a single antibody is produced (each antigen has a specific antibody). The antibodies are grouped into five different classes known as immunoglobulins. These classes contain formed chains of immunoglobulins expressed on the cell surface and labeled IgG, IgA, IgM, IgE, and IgD. Table 71-1 describes the features of these antibodies. B lymphocytes provide humoral immunity through the secretion of these immunoglobulins.
4. *T-cell lymphocytes* make up 65% to 80% of all lymphocytes in the blood. There are three different types of T cells: helper, suppressor, and cytotoxic. *Helper cells* aid in the initiation of the immune response by helping B cells synthesize antibodies for action. *Suppressor cells* help keep the B-cell antibody production in check. They hold back the immune response or restrict antibody production because, if left unchecked, these B cells can do more harm that good. *Cytotoxic cells,* or *killer cells,* circulate to kill cells not recognized as self cells (such as tumor cells). Activation of these cells occurs through interaction of antigen with macrophages. Through the secretion of the special products produced by the macrophages, T-cell proliferation occurs. These activated T cells release substances known as lymphokines that influence the growth of other cells necessary for body defense, thus amplifying the immune reaction (Figure 71-3).

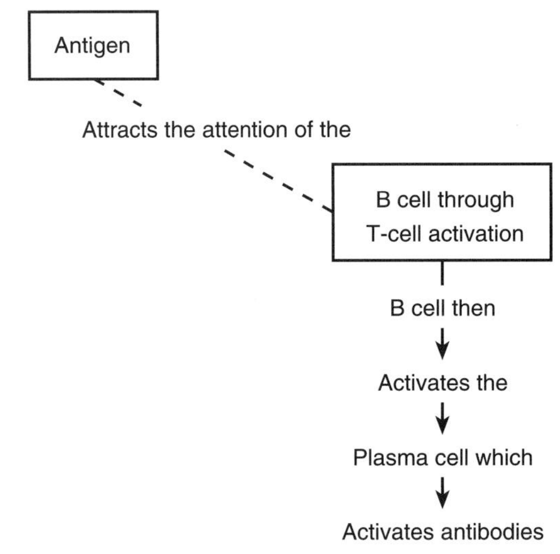

FIGURE 71-2

Immune response—humoral.

The Immune Response

The immune response is activated through generation of humoral or cellular immunity. *B lymphocytes* are the cells involved in antibody-mediated or humoral immunity. *T lymphocytes* are the effectors for cell-mediated immunity. This response can be summarized as follows:

- A foreign substance (the antigen) invades.
- Macrophage engulfs it and presents it on its cell surface.
- The expressed antigen stimulates T-cell activity.

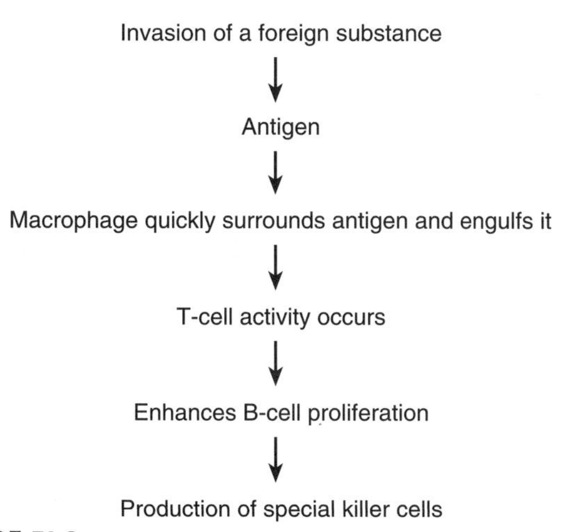

FIGURE 71-3

Immune response—cell-mediated.

- T helper cells are activated to enhance B-cell differentiation into plasma cells and the production of antibodies/immunoglobulin (IgG, IgM, IgA, IgE, IgD).
- Proliferation of B and T cells produces clones with a memory that enables them to recognize a returning invader. This memory produces a more potent and rapid immune response should the invader return.

DRUG ACTION AND EFFECTS

Immunizations act to confer immunity to a particular disease. There are two types of immunity: active and passive.

Active Immunity

Active immunization involves the administration of all or a part of a microorganism to evoke a response. Antigens are taken from living or dead organisms, and small amounts are given intradermally or subcutaneously. This process stimulates the body's immune response, and antibodies are stimulated to protect the immunized person from greater exposure to this particular disease-producing antigen. This immunity is retained for a prolonged period, thereby protecting the person from the disease whenever he or she may be exposed to that antigen. This immunity can be "boosted" at specific intervals.

Active immunization is accomplished with three different types of agents:

1. *Inactivated vaccines (killed agents)*. Most bacterial vaccines, and some viral, involve the use of inactivated agents. These agents are not capable of replicating within the host and thus present little risk to the recipient. Maintenance of lifelong immunity requires the administration of multiple doses. Mucosal protection after the use of killed vaccines is less than with the use of live vaccines. Thus, local infection or colonization with the agent can occur, with potential for transmission, although systemic disease is prevented.
2. *Live vaccines (attenuated)*. Most viral vaccines involve the use of live virus that has been chemically changed to decrease its virulence. Active infection, with replication of the virus, occurs in the host following administration of the product, although few adverse effects occur. This route generally produces a superior response, including mucosal immunity, and does not require the use of multiple doses.
3. *Active immunization*. This may be accomplished with use of a modified product of an organism, such as a toxoid, which are modified bacterial toxins and retain the ability to stimulate antibody formation but are nontoxic. This is the route of immunization used against diphtheria and tetanus. The maintenance of protective titers of antitoxin requires periodic administration of booster doses of toxoid.

Passive Immunity

Passive immunity occurs when antibodies acquired from a human or an animal (who already has acquired immunity to a specific organism) are given to people who do not have immunity to the organism. Newborn infants can achieve this naturally from their mothers through the placenta and through breastfeeding. It can also be achieved through injections of gamma globulins (for hepatitis protection) or antiserums or antitoxins. This process temporarily provides the same protection as that of a person who achieved active acquired immunity because the antibodies naturally break down and are eliminated from the body. (See Table 71-1 for a summary of characteristics and function of immunoglobulins.)

TABLE 71-1 Characteristics and Functions of Immunoglobulins

Immunoglobulins	Amount in Serum	Location of Concentration	Stimulated By	Functions
IgG	Most abundant in the blood 75%	Intravascular Extravascular	Allergic response Second immunoglobulin	Provides immunity against bloodborne infection (i.e., bacteria, viruses, some fungi)
IgA	15%	Intravascular Secretions	Presence of antigens Antiviral antibody	Most common antibody in secretions, where it protects mucous membranes Bacteriocidal with lysosome
IgM	10%	Intravascular	Allergic response	First immunoglobulin produced during an immune response Activates complement
IgD	1%	On the surface of B cell	Presence of antigens	Antigen-specific receptor on B cells

Antisera, which are antibodies of animal origin used to counteract the effects of a toxin, and human plasma are used after exposure. Very specific indications and guidelines govern the use of these products; they will not be discussed in detail in this chapter. Contact your local health department or the CDC for guidelines concerning use of antisera.

Incompetent immune systems do not develop active immunity in response to vaccines and toxoid. These patients need protection from infection, and this protection can be accomplished through passive immunity, identification of the deficient immune mediators and replacement of those mediators, or by giving these patients antiinfective drugs. Agents that are classified as immune mediators are agents such as interferon, interleukins, and immunoglobulin.

All immunizations contain several different components, such as the following:

- *Immunizing agent.* This is the active component of the product and may be a killed or attenuated vaccine or a toxoid.
- *Suspending fluid.* This may be either sterile water or saline or a complex tissue-culture fluid. It may contain proteins derived from the medium in which the vaccine was produced, such as egg antigen in measles and influenza vaccines. Individuals who experience anaphylactic reactions to egg may be allergic to these vaccines.
- *Preservatives.* Trace amounts of preservatives, stabilizers, or antibiotics are often added to prevent bacterial overgrowth in multiuse vials of vaccines. Individuals may have allergic reactions to products such as neomycin that may be present in minute amounts. Thimerosal, a mercury-containing organic compound widely used as a preservative, was removed from or reduced to trace amounts in all vaccines in 2001 secondary to concerns about the potential of neurodevelopmental pathology in infants who may receive multiple vaccines containing thimerosal and be unable to adequately clear this product due to hepatic immaturity (see http://www.fda.gov/cber/vaccine/thimerosal.htm).
- *Adjuvants.* This is often an aluminum-based compound that is added to enhance the immunogenicity of an agent and prolong the stimulatory effect. This is necessary for some inactivated vaccines and for toxoids.

Comparable vaccines made by different manufacturers may be used interchangeably, if used according to recommended guidelines. Available data suggest that adequate response occurs even when products from different manufacturers are used during the same series. Table 71-1 contains a summary of the immunizations generally used in primary care.

DRUG TREATMENT PRINCIPLES

Guidelines concerning the use of immunizations are one of the most carefully studied areas of pharmacology. Guidelines have been revised frequently in the last decade as new products have been introduced and recommendations for use of older products change; these guidelines determine the standard of care that all primary care providers are expected to provide. With the increase in the immunocompromised population, and the increasing numbers of immigrants living in the United States who require catch-up vaccination, the greatest challenge for primary care providers is in mastering the exceptions to the recommended schedule. Table 71-2 provides the recommendations for adult and pediatric immunizations from the CDC Advisory Committee on Immunization Practices and the American Academy of Pediatrics. The latest updates are available at http://www.cdc.gov/nip/recs/child-schedule.pdf. It is important to stress that these are general guidelines. The specific requirements of each patient must be individualized.

Critical decisions to be made in immunization include what products to give and when to give them. Before using any biological, the health care provider should take all precautions known for the detection or prevention of allergic or any other adverse reaction. This should include a review of the patient's history regarding possible sensitivity, the ready availability of epinephrine 1:1000 and other appropriate agents used for control of immediate allergic reactions, and a knowledge of the recent literature pertaining to use of the biological to be used, including the nature of side effects and adverse effects that may follow its use.

Individuals with impaired immune responsiveness, whether the result of the use of immunosuppressive therapy, a genetic defect, HIV/AIDS, or other causes, may have a reduced antibody response to active immunization procedures. Deferral of the administration of vaccine may be considered in individuals receiving immunosuppressive therapy. Other groups should receive vaccines according to the usual recommended schedule.

Schedule for Immunization of Children

Both the CDC, ACIP, and the American Academy of Pediatrics Committee on Infectious Disease issue immunization guidelines for children that are revised annually and published each January. Recommendations from these two bodies may vary slightly, and these variances are noted in a joint Recommended Vaccine Schedule last issued in January 2004.

Immunization of Adult and Elderly Persons

Although significant emphasis has been placed on the subject of childhood immunizations, recommendations for adult immunization have been lacking. However, in recognition of the fact that almost 50,000 adults a year die in the United States as a result of vaccine-preventable disease (http://www.medscape.com/viewarticle/449845), the CDC issued the first schedule for adult immunizations in October 2002. This schedule may be found at http://www.cdc.gov/nip/recs/adult-schedule.pdf.

At-Risk and Postexposure Patients

Certain populations are considered to be at risk and require modification of the routine vaccination schedule. Details for these exceptions may be found at http://www.cdc.gov/nip/ACIP/default.htm.

A summary of important exceptions is as follows:

1. In compliance with recommendations for all individuals, it is particularly important that all health care workers be immunized against hepatitis B. In addition, health care workers in emergency department settings and on emergency response teams, such as emergency medical technicians and paramedics, may elect to be

Text continued on p. 740

TABLE 71-2 Combined Immunization Schedule for Children and Adults

Recommended Childhood and Adolescent Immunization Schedule (United States, January-June 2004)

Vaccine	Age: Birth	1 mo	2 mo	4 mo	6 mo	12 mo	15 mo	18 mo	24 mo	4-6 yr	11-12 yr	13-18 yr
Hepatitis B[1]	HepB #1		HepB #2			HepB #3					HepB Series	
Diphtheria, tetanus, pertussis[2]			DTaP	DTaP	DTaP			DTaP		DTaP	Td	Td
Haemophilus influena type b[3]			Hib	Hib	Hib[3]	Hib						
Inactivated poliovirus			IPV	IPV		IPV				IPV		
Measles, mumps, rubella[4]						MMR #1				MMR #2	MMR #2	
Varicella[5]							Varicella				Varicella	
Pneumococcal[6]			PCV	PCV	PCV	PCV			PCV		PPV	
Vaccines below line are for selected populations												
Hepatitis A[7]											Hepatitis A Series	
Influenza[8]								Influenza (Yearly)				

This schedule indicates the recommended ages for routine administration of currently licensed childhood vaccines, as of December 1, 2003, for children through age 18 years. Any dose not given at the recommended age should be given at any subsequent visit when indicated and feasible. ■ Indicates age groups that warrant special effort to administer those vaccines not previously given. Additional vaccines may be licensed and recommended during the year. Licensed combination vaccines may be used whenever any components of the combination are indicated and the vaccine's other components are not contraindicated. Providers should consult the manufacturers' package inserts for detailed recommendations. Clinically significant adverse events that follow immunization should be reported to the Vaccine Adverse Event Reporting System (VAERS). Guidance about how to obtain and complete a VAERS form can be found on the Internet: *www.vaers.org* or by calling 800-822-7967.

Range of recommended ages | Only if mother HBs | Preadolescent assessment | Catch-up vaccination

1. **Hepatitis B (HepB) vaccine.** All infants should receive the first dose of hepatitis B vaccine soon after birth and before hospital discharge; the first dose may also be given by age 2 months if the infant's mother is hepatitis B surface antigen (HBsAg) negative. Only monovalent HepB can be used for the birth dose. Monovalent or combination vaccine containing HepB may be used to complete the series. Four doses of vaccine may be administered when a birth dose is given. The second dose should be given at least 4 weeks after the first dose, except for combination vaccines which cannot be administered before age 6 weeks. The third dose should be given at least 16 weeks after the first dose and at least 8 weeks after the second dose. The last dose in the vaccination series (third or fourth dose) should not be administered before age 24 weeks.

   Infants born to HBsAg-positive mothers should receive HepB and 0.5 mL of Hepatitis B Immune Globulin (HBIG) within 12 hours of birth at separate sites. The second dose is recommended at age 1 to 2 months. The last dose in the immunization series should not be administered before age 24 weeks. These infants should be tested for HBsAg and antibody to HBsAg (anti-HBs) at age 9 to 15 months.

   Infants born to mothers whose HBsAg status is unknown should receive the first dose of the HepB series within 12 hours of birth. Maternal blood should be drawn as soon as possible to determine the mother's HBsAg status; if the HBsAg test is positive, the infant should receive HBIG as soon as possible (no later than age 1 week). The second dose is recommended at age 1 to 2 months. The last dose in the immunization series should not be administered before age 24 weeks.
2. **Diphtheria and tetanus toxoids and acellular pertussis (DTaP) vaccine.** The fourth dose of DTaP may be administered as early as age 12 months, provided 6 months have elapsed since the third dose and the child is unlikely to return at age 15 to 18 months. The final dose in the series should be given at age ≥4 years. **Tetanus and diphtheria toxoids (Td)** is recommended at age 11 to 12 years if at least 5 years have elapsed since the last dose of tetanus and diphtheria toxoid–containing vaccine. Subsequent routine Td boosters are recommended every 10 years.
3. ***Haemophilus influenzae* type b (Hib) conjugate vaccine.** Three Hib conjugate vaccines are licensed for infant use. If PRP-OMP (PedvaxHIB or ComVax [Merck]) is administered at ages 2 and 4 months, a dose at age 6 months is not required. DTaP/Hib combination products should not be used for primary immunization in infants at ages 2, 4, or 6 months but can be used as boosters following any Hib vaccine. The final dose in the series should be given at age ≥12 months.
4. **Measles, mumps, and rubella vaccine (MMR).** The second dose of MMR is recommended routinely at age 4 to 6 years but may be administered during any visit, provided at least 4 weeks have elapsed since the first dose and both doses are administered beginning at or after age 12 months. Those who have not previously received the second dose should complete the schedule by the 11- to 12-year-old visit.
5. **Varicella vaccine.** Varicella vaccine is recommended at any visit at or after age 12 months for susceptible children (i.e., those who lack a reliable history of chickenpox). Susceptible persons age ≥13 years should receive 2 doses, given at least 4 weeks apart.
6. **Pneumococcal vaccine.** The heptavalent **pneumococcal conjugate vaccine (PCV)** is recommended for all children age 2 to 23 months. It is also recommended for certain children age 24 to 59 months. The final dose in the series should be given at age ≥12 months. **Pneumococcal polysaccharide vaccine (PPV)** is recommended in addition to PCV for certain high-risk groups. See *MMWR* 2000; 49(RR-9):1-38.
7. **Hepatitis A vaccine.** Hepatitis A vaccine is recommended for children and adolescents in selected states and regions and for certain high-risk groups; consult your local public health authority. Children and adolescents in these states, regions, and high-risk groups who have not been immunized against hepatitis A can begin the hepatitis A immunization series during any visit. The two doses in the series should be administered at least 6 months apart. See *MMWR* 1999; 48(RR-12):1-37.
8. **Influenza vaccine.** Influenza vaccine is recommended annually for children age ≥6 months with certain risk factors (including but not limited to children with asthma, cardiac disease, sickle cell disease, human immunodeficiency virus infection, and diabetes; and household members of persons in high-risk groups [see *MMWR* 2003; 52(RR-8):1-36]) and can be administered to all others wishing to obtain immunity. In addition, healthy children age 6 to 23 months are encouraged to receive influenza vaccine if feasible, because children in this age group are at substantially increased risk of influenza-related hospitalizations. For healthy persons age 5 to 49 years, the intranasally administered live-attenuated influenza vaccine (LAIV) is an acceptable alternative to the intramuscular trivalent inactivated influenza vaccine (TIV). See *MMWR* 2003; 52(RR-13): 1-8. Children receiving TIV should be administered a dosage appropriate for their age (0.25 mL if age 6 to 35 months or 0.5 mL if age ≥3 years). Children age ≤8 years who are receiving influenza vaccine for the first time should receive 2 doses (separated by at least 4 weeks for TIV and at least 6 weeks for LAIV).

Continued

Recommended Adult Immunization Schedule by Age Group by Medical Conditions (United States, 2003-2004)

Vaccine	Age Group: 19-49 yr	50-64 yr	65 yr and Older
Tetanus, diphtheria (Td)*	1 dose booster every 10 years[2]		
Influenza	1 dose annually[2]	1 dose annually[2]	
Pneumococcal (polysaccharide)	1 dose[3,4]		1 dose[3,4]
Hepatitis B*	3 doses (0, 1-2, 4-6 months)[5]		
Hepatitis A	2 doses (0, 6-12 months)[6]		
Measles, mumps, rubella (MMR)*	1 dose if measles, mumps, or rubella vaccination history is unreliable; 2 doses for persons with occupational or other indications[7]		
Varicella*	2 doses (0, 4-8 weeks) for persons who are susceptible[8]		
Meningococcal (polysaccharide)	1 dose[9]		

- For all persons in this group
- Catch-up on childhood vaccinations
- For persons with medical/exposure indications

*Covered by the Vaccine Injury Compensation Program. For information on how to file a claim call 800-338-2382. Please also visit www.hrsa.gov/osp/vicp To file a claim for vaccine injury contact: US Court of Federal Claims, 717 Madison Place, NW, Washington DC, 20005, 202-219-9657.

This schedule indicates the recommended age groups for routine administration of currently licensed vaccines for persons 19 years of age and older. Licensed combination vaccines may be used whenever any components of the combination are indicated and the vaccine's other components are not contraindicated. Providers should consult the manufacturers' package inserts for detailed recommendations.

Report all clinically significant post-vaccination reactions to the Vaccine Adverse Event Reporting System (VAERS). Reporting forms and instructions on filing a VAERS report are available by calling 800-822-7967 or from the VAERS website at www.vaers.org.

For additional information about the vaccines listed above and contraindications for immunization, visit the National Immunization Program Website at www.cdc.gov/nip/ or call the National Immunization Hotline at 800-232-2522 (English) or 800-232-0233 (Spanish).

Approved by the Advisory Committee on Immunization Practices (ACIP), and accepted by the American College of Obstetricians and Gynecologists (ACOG) and the American Academy of Family Physicians (AAFP)

Medical Conditions	Tetanus-diphtheria (Td)*,[1]	Influenza[2]	Pneumococcal (polysaccharide)[3,4]	Hepatitis B*,[5]	Hepatitis A[6]	Measles, Mumps, Rubella (MMR)*,[7]	Varicella*,[8]
Pregnancy		A					
Diabetes, heart disease, chronic pulmonary disease, chronic liver disease, including chronic alcoholism		B	C		D		
Congenital immunodeficiency, leukemia, lymphoma, generalized malignancy, therapy with alkylating agents, antimetabolites, radiation or large amounts of corticosteroids			E			F	
Renal failure/end stage renal disease, recipients of hemodialysis or clotting factor concentrates			E	G			
Asplenia including elective splenectomy and terminal complement component deficiencies		H	E, I, J				
HIV infection			E, K			L	

- For all persons in this group
- Catch-up on childhood vaccinations
- For persons with medical/exposure indications
- Contraindicated

Special Notes for Medical Conditions

A. For women without chronic diseases/conditions, vaccinate if pregnancy will be at second or third trimester during influenza season. For women with chronic diseases/conditions, vaccinate at any time during the pregnancy.
B. Although chronic liver disease and alcoholism are not indicator conditions for influenza vaccination, give one dose annually if the patient is age 50 years or older, has other indications for influenza vaccine, or if the patient requests vaccination.
C. Asthma is an indicator condition for influenza but not for pneumococcal vaccination.
D. For all persons with chronic liver disease.
E. For persons <65 years, revaccinate once after 5 years or more have elapsed since initial vaccination.
F. Persons with impaired humoral immunity but intact cellular immunity may be vaccinated. *MMWR* 1999; 48 (RR-06): 1-5.
G. Hemodialysis patients: Use special formulation of vaccine (40 μg/ml) or two 1.0 ml 20 μg doses given at one site. Vaccinate early in the course of renal disease. Assess antibody titers to hep B surface antigen (anti-HBs) levels annually. Administer additional doses if anti-HBs levels decline to <10 milliinternational units (mIU)/ml.
H. There are no data specifically on risk of severe or complicated influenza infections among persons with asplenia. However, influenza is a risk factor for secondary bacterial infections that may cause severe disease in asplenic individuals.
I. Administer meningococcal vaccine and consider Hib vaccine.
J. Elective splenectomy: vaccinate at least 2 weeks before surgery.
K. Vaccinate as close to diagnosis as possible when CD4 cell counts are highest.
L. Withhold MMR or other measles containing vaccines from HIV-infected persons with evidence of severe immunosuppression. *MMWR* 1998; 47 (RR-8): 21-22; *MMWR* 2002; 51 (RR-02): 22-24.

1. **Tetanus and diphtheria (Td) toxoids?** Adults, including pregnant women with uncertain histories of a complete primary vaccination series should, receive a primary series of Td. A primary series for adults is 3 doses: the first 2 doses given at least 4 weeks apart and the 3rd dose, 6-12 months after the second. Administer 1 dose if the person had received the primary series and the last vaccination was 10 years ago or longer. Consult *MMWR* 1991; 40 (RR-10): 1-21 for administering Td as prophylaxis in wound management. The ACP Task Force on Adult Immunization supports a second option for Td use in adults: a single Td booster at age 50 years for persons who have completed the full pediatric series, including the teenage/young adult booster. *Guide for Adult Immunization.* 3rd ed. ACP 1994: 20.
2. **Influenza vaccination?** Medical indications: chronic disorders of the cardiovascular or pulmonary systems including asthma; chronic metabolic diseases including diabetes mellitus, renal dysfunction, hemoglobinopathies, or immunosuppression (including immunosuppression caused by medications or by human immunodeficiency virus [HIV]), requiring regular medical follow-up or hospitalization during the preceding year; women who will be in the second or third trimester of pregnancy during the influenza season. Occupational indications: health-care workers. Other indications: residents of nursing homes and other long-term care facilities; persons likely to transmit influenza to persons at high-risk (in-home care givers to persons with medical indications, household contacts and out-of-home caregivers of children birth to 23 months of age, or children with asthma or other indicator conditions for influenza vaccination, household members and care givers of elderly and adults with high-risk conditions); and anyone who wishes to be vaccinated. For healthy persons aged 5-49 years without high-risk conditions, either the inactivated vaccine or the intranasally administered influenza vaccine (Flumist) may be given. *MMWR* 2003; 52 (RR-8): 1-36; *MMWR* 2003; 53 (RR-13): 1-8.
3. **Pneumococcal polysaccharide vaccination?** Medical indications: chronic disorders of the pulmonary system (excluding asthma), cardiovascular diseases, diabetes mellitus, chronic liver diseases including liver disease as a result of alcohol abuse (e.g., cirrhosis), chronic renal failure or nephrotic syndrome, functional or anatomic asplenia (e.g., sickle cell disease or splenectomy), immunosuppressive conditions (e.g., congenital immunodeficiency, HIV infection, leukemia, lymphoma, multiple myeloma, Hodgkins disease, generalized malignancy, organ or bone marrow transplantation), chemotherapy with alkylating agents, anti-metabolites, or long-term systemic corticosteroids. Geographic/other indications: Alaskan Natives and certain American Indian populations. Other indications: residents of nursing homes and other long-term care facilities. *MMWR* 1997; 46 (RR-8): 1-24.
4. **Revaccination with pneumococcal polysaccharide vaccine?** One-time revaccination after 5 years for persons with chronic renal failure or nephrotic syndrome, functional or anatomic asplenia (e.g., sickle cell disease or splenectomy), immunosuppressive conditions (e.g., congenital immunodeficiency, HIV infection, leukemia, lymphoma, multiple myeloma, Hodgkins disease, generalized malignancy, organ or bone marrow transplantation), chemotherapy with alkylating agents, anti-metabolites, or long-term systemic corticosteroids. For persons 65 and older, one-time revaccination if they were vaccinated 5 or more years previously and were age less than 65 years at the time of primary vaccination. *MMWR* 1997; 46 (RR-8): 1-24.
5. **Hepatitis B vaccination?** Medical indications: hemodialysis patients, patients who receive clotting-factor concentrates. Occupational indications: health-care workers and public-safety workers who have exposure to blood in the workplace, persons in training in schools of medicine, dentistry, nursing, laboratory technology, and other allied health professions. Behavioral indications: injecting drug users, persons with more than one sex partner in the previous 6 months, persons with a recently acquired sexually-transmitted disease (STD), all clients in STD clinics, men who have sex with men. Other indications: household contacts and sex partners of persons with chronic HBV infection, clients and staff of institutions for the developmentally disabled, international travelers who will stay more than 6 months in countries with high or intermediate prevalence of chronic HBV infection, inmates of correctional facilities. *MMWR* 1991; 40 (RR-13): 1-19. (www.cdc.gov/travel/diseases/hbv.htm)
6. **Hepatitis A vaccination?** For the combined HepA-HepB vaccine use 3 doses at 0, 1, 6 months. Medical indications: persons with clotting-factor disorders or chronic liver disease. Behavioral indications: men who have sex with men, users of injecting and noninjecting illegal drugs. Occupational indications: persons working with HAV-infected primates or with HAV in a research laboratory setting. Other indications: persons traveling to or working in countries that have high or intermediate endemicity of hepatitis A. *MMWR* 1999; 48 (RR-12): 1-37. (www.cdc.gov/travel/diseases/hav.htm)
7. **Measles, mumps, rubella vaccination (MMR)?** Measles component: adults born before 1957 may be considered immune to measles. Adults born in or after 1957 should receive at least 1 dose of MMR unless they have a medical contraindication, documentation of at least 1 dose, or other acceptable evidence of immunity. A second dose of MMR is recommended for adults who:
   - Are recently exposed to measles or in an outbreak setting
   - Were previously vaccinated with killed measles vaccine
   - Were vaccinated with an unknown vaccine between 1963 and 1967
   - Are students in post-secondary educational institutions
   - Work in health care facilities
   - Plan to travel internationally

   Mumps component: 1 dose of MMR should be adequate for protection. Rubella component: give 1 dose of MMR to women whose rubella vaccination history is unreliable and counsel women to avoid becoming pregnant for 4 weeks after vaccination. For women of child-bearing age, regardless of birth year, routinely determine rubella immunity and counsel women regarding congenital rubella syndrome. Do not vaccinate pregnant women or those planning to become pregnant in the next 4 weeks. If pregnant and susceptible, vaccinate as early in postpartum period as possible. *MMWR* 1998; 47 (RR-8): 1-57; *MMWR* 2001; 50: 1117.
8. **Varicella vaccination?** Recommended for all persons who do not have reliable clinical history of varicella infection, or serological evidence of varicella zoster virus (VZV) infection who may be at high risk for exposure or transmission. This includes health-care workers and family contacts of immunocompromised persons, those who live or work in environments where transmission is likely (e.g., teachers of young children, day care employees, and residents and staff members in institutional settings), persons who live or work in environments where VZV transmission can occur (e.g., college students, inmates and staff members of correctional institutions, and military personnel), adolescents and adults living in households with children, women who are not pregnant but who may become pregnant in the future, international travelers who are not immune to infection. Note: more than 95% of U.S.-born adults are immune to VZV. Do not vaccinate pregnant women or those planning to become pregnant in the next 4 weeks. If pregnant and susceptible, vaccinate as early in postpartum period as possible. *MMWR* 1996; 45 (RR-11): 1-36; *MMWR* 1999; 48 (RR-6): 1-5.
9. **Meningococcal vaccination (quadrivalent polysaccharide vaccine for serogroups A, C, Y, and W-135)?** Consider vaccination for persons with medical indications: adults with terminal complement component deficiencies, with anatomic or functional asplenia. Other indications: travelers to countries in which disease is hyperendemic or epidemic ("meningitis belt" of sub-Saharan Africa, Mecca, Saudi Arabia for Hajj). Revaccination at 3-5 years may be indicated for persons at high risk for infection (e.g., persons residing in areas in which disease is epidemic). Counsel college freshmen, especially those who live in dormitories, regarding meningococcal disease and the vaccine so that they can make an educated decision about receiving the vaccination. *MMWR* 2000; 49 (RR-7): 1-20.
   Note: the AAFP recommends that colleges should take the lead in providing education on meningococcal infection and vaccination and offer it to those who are interested. Physicians need not initiate discussion of the meningococcal quadrivalent polysaccharide vaccine as part of routine medical care.

Pediatric data from www.cdc.gov/nip/recs/child-schedule.htm; adult data from www.cdc.gov/nip/recs/adult-schedule.pdf.

vaccinated against smallpox. Specific recommendations for the use of smallpox vaccine are discussed later in this chapter.

2. Food handlers should receive hepatitis A and typhoid immunizations. State requirements differ. Contact your local health department for details.
3. Travelers to many underdeveloped nations may require specific immunizations depending on where they are traveling. The CDC publishes information on vaccine recommendations for travel. These can be found by calling (800) CDC-SHOT or online at www.cdc.gov.

Principles of Administration of Vaccines

Numerous myths exist about contraindications to administration of vaccines. For all currently available products, the following principles apply:

- Minor upper respiratory infection or gastroenteritis, with or without fever, is not an appropriate indication for withholding a scheduled vaccine dose.
- Concurrent administration of an antibiotic is not a contraindication to immunization.
- In most cases, preterm infants should be immunized at the usual recommended chronologic age.
- Pregnancy in a mother or other household member is not an indication for the withholding of immunizations, including live virus vaccines such as oral polio or measles-mumps-rubella (MMR).
- Women who are breastfeeding may be immunized with all products with the exception of small pox vaccine. There is no evidence that trace amounts of a vaccine present in breast milk are harmful to infants.
- A lapse in the recommended immunization schedule does not require that the entire series be restarted. Needed doses should be given at the first opportunity as though the usual interval had occurred.
- Half doses of vaccine in individuals who had a significant reaction to a previous dose are *never* indicated. In addition, reduced or divided doses are not recommended for preterm or low birth weight infants.
- Family history of an adverse event with an immunizing agent, family history of seizures, or a family history of sudden infant death are not appropriate indications for withholding of recommended immunizations.

All immunizing agents do have specific contraindications that will be discussed separately.

Notification of Risks and Benefits of the Vaccine

The National Childhood Vaccine Injury Act of 1986 mandates the notification of patients and parents of the risks and benefits of individual vaccines. This legislation requires the distribution of standardized information to these individuals. A simplified version of information pamphlets was approved by federal legislation in 1993 and is available from vaccine manufacturers, the CDC, and most state health departments.

The legislation requires health care providers who administer vaccines to keep permanent records of all immunizations given along with specific information about the manufacturer of the product and lot number of all doses. In addition, the provider is required to report occurrences of events suspected to be the result of vaccine through a mechanism entitled the Vaccine Adverse Event Reporting System (VAERS). Reports may be made online at: http://www.vaers.org. The specifics of reportable events for each agent are discussed separately. In addition, this act established a Vaccine Injury Compensation Table that determined the injuries, disabilities, and conditions for which compensation may be made.

Information about the legislation as well as the injury compensation program may be obtained from state health departments or by writing to the program directly:

National Vaccine Injury Compensation Program
Health Resources and Services Administration
Parklawn Building, Room 8-05
5600 Fishers Lane
Rockville, MD 20857
Telephone: (800) 338-2382 or (301) 443-6593
www.hrsa.dhhs.gov/bhpr/vicp/new.htm

HOW TO MONITOR

Vaccines that are administered as recommended induce protective immunity in over 95% of recipients. It is not recommended or necessary to obtain serum titers to document immunity.

PATIENT VARIABLES

Geriatrics

The immune systems of the elderly are less active.

Pediatrics

Immunizations are an integral part of the primary health care of children.

Pregnancy

Live vaccines are usually contraindicated in pregnancy (see individual drugs).

Lactation

It is usually safe to give vaccines while the mother is breastfeeding.

PATIENT EDUCATION

For most vaccines, the arm in which the vaccine is given may become sore; this can be treated with a warm compress. Some patients develop generalized flu-type symptoms. For any feeling of malaise or flu, the patient is often instructed to take acetaminophen. Most symptoms are mild and self-limited. Anything more severe should be reported.

Notify the patients and parents of the risks and benefits of each individual vaccine, and distribute the standardized information pamphlets.

Specific Vaccines

IMMUNIZATIONS

Hepatitis B Vaccine

Currently available vaccine is produced through recombinant DNA technology using genetically modified baker's yeast to synthesize hepatitis B surface (HBs) antigen (Ag). Three intramuscular doses induce protective antibody in 90% to 95% of adults and children. Long-term studies indicate that protection appears to be long lasting even in the face of low or undetectable anti-HBs concentrations.

Contraindications, Warnings, Precautions. Because of the long incubation period for hepatitis B, it is possible for unrecognized infection to be present at the time the vaccine is given. The vaccine may not prevent hepatitis B in such patients.

Epinephrine should be available for immediate use should a rare anaphylactoid reaction occur. Any serious active infection is reason for delaying use of the vaccine except when, in the opinion of the health care provider, withholding the vaccine entails a greater risk.

Caution should be exercised in administering the vaccine to those who have a severely compromised cardiopulmonary status or to others in whom a febrile or systemic reaction could pose a significant risk.

Pregnancy category C: The vaccine should be given to pregnant women only if clearly needed. It is not known if it is excreted in human milk. It is well tolerated and highly immunogenic in infants and children of all ages.

Adverse Effects. Pain and low-grade fever are the most frequently reported side effects, with an incidence between 1% and 6%. Allergic reactions are infrequent; anaphylaxis is exceedingly rare and has been reported only in adults.

Dosage and Administration

Children. Hepatitis B vaccination is recommended for all infants, regardless of their mothers' hepatitis status. Three doses of vaccine, administered intramuscularly in the thigh or deltoid, should be given before the age of 18 months. In populations with a high incidence of hepatitis, such as Alaskan Natives and immigrants from countries in which hepatitis B virus (HBV) is endemic, special effort should be made to complete the series by 6 months. The recommended three-dose schedule should be begun by 2 months of age; the second dose is given 1 to 2 months later and the final 6 to 18 months after the first. The first dose should be given in the newborn period to infants born to HBsAg-positive mothers; infants born to HBsAg-negative mothers may delay the first dose until 2 months of age.

Preterm infants should be immunized after they reach a weight of 2 kg or by 2 months of age. For most children in the United States, the risk of infection is low until adolescence. The exception is children from high-risk populations; these children should be vaccinated in the first 5 years of life. All adolescents should also be vaccinated. The American Academy of Pediatrics recommends that children complete this series of immunization by the age of 11 or 12 years old; this has the advantage of lower cost and potentially better compliance.

Adults. Routine immunization of adults is not currently recommended. However, those who are members of a high-risk group should receive immunization. These groups include the following:

- Health care and public safety workers, including those in training, and others with occupational exposure to blood and blood-contaminated body fluids
- Residents and staff of institutions for the developmentally disabled, long-term correctional facilities
- Hemodialysis patients
- Patients with bleeding disorders who receive blood products
- Household contacts and sexual partners of HBV carriers
- Immigrants, adoptees, and family members from countries where HBV is endemic
- International travelers who will be visiting countries with moderate or high rates of HBV infection (a list of these countries can be found at www.cdc.gov/travel/diseases/hbv.htm)
- Individuals with more than one sex partner in the previous 6 months, persons with a recent sexually transmitted infection, clients in sexually transmitted disease (STD) clinics, and men who have sex with men
- Injecting drug users

Pregnancy. Routine screening for HBV is recommended for all women early in pregnancy; it should be repeated late in pregnancy for negative women who are at high risk for infection. No adverse effects on the developing fetus have been noted when vaccine is administered during pregnancy. Pregnancy and lactation are not a contraindication to HBV vaccination.

How Supplied. There are two commercially available recombinant preparations in the United States containing between 10 and 40 µg/ml of HBsAg protein. The immune response of the two is interchangeable, and therefore an individual who begins a series with one brand may safely complete with the second. In addition, a *Haemophilus* B conjugate–hepatitis B combination is available (Comvax; Merck & Co.). Only monovalent vaccine should be used if the first dose is given in the newborn period; four doses of hepatitis B may be given if the schedule is completed with combination vaccine at 2, 4, and 12 months.

Diphtheria-Tetanus-Pertussis Vaccine (DTP, DP, DT, DTaP)

The incidence of these three diseases has decreased by 99% in the United States since the introduction of this vaccine. Diphtheria and tetanus preparations are both toxoids that are made by treating toxins with formaldehyde. The pertussis component is available as an acellular preparation containing detoxified pertussis toxin and pertussis proteins. The five commercially available pertussis preparations available in the United States vary in formulation of pertussis antigen; immunogenicity is similar.

Contraindications, Warnings, Precautions. When pertussis component is contraindicated, primary series should be completed with DT. In addition, unstable, changing neurologic disorders (e.g., uncontrolled epilepsy, infantile spasms, and progressive encephalopathy) are reasons to delay immunization until the condition is clarified. Stable neurologic disorders (e.g., well-controlled epilepsy, cerebral palsy, developmental delay) are not a contraindication.

See the following *Adverse Effects* section for a list of effects that contraindicate another dose being given.

Adverse Effects. Localized redness, induration, and tenderness at injection site are common, especially as the doses in a series increase. Temperature of more than 38°C (100.4°F), drowsiness, fretfulness, and anorexia are common; they occur significantly more often after DTaP than after DT and are self-limited; their likelihood decreases as the number of doses increases. The pertussis component of the vaccine is responsible for the majority of these reactions. None of these reactions result in sequelae and are not contraindications to subsequent doses.

Moderate-to-severe systemic reactions are infrequent. The *2004 Red Book* suggests these may include the following:

- Fever (temperature >40.5°C or >105°F) occurring in less than 0.3% of recipients
- Persistent, inconsolable crying that lasts more than 3 hours was reported to occur in 1:100 doses of older whole-cell preparations of DTP; incidence following acellular pertussis preparations is significantly less.
- Seizures were reported to occur in 1:1750 doses of older whole cell preparations. The incidence with DTaP is substantially less.
- Hypotonic-hyporesponsive episodes were known to occur with older preparations. The incidence with DTaP is unknown, but is significantly less.
- Acute encephalopathy and permanent neurologic deficit had been reported to rarely occur following whole cell DTP. However, numerous studies have not supported a causal relationship between DTP vaccine and neurologic injury. It is unknown if there is a temporal association between these events and DTaP.

Side effects can often be managed with acetaminophen or ibuprofen. In addition, warm tub baths and ice packs may relieve local side effects.

Absolute contraindications to administration of pertussis-containing preparations are the following effects noted after previous doses of DTP or DTaP:

- Allergic hypersensitivity reactions. Anaphylaxis, if it occurs at all, is extremely rare. Urticaria may follow pertussis vaccine. If the appearance is delayed, it is unlikely to represent an IgE-mediated process and is not a contraindication to subsequent doses.
- Encephalopathy within 7 days

The following conditions were previously considered to be contraindications but have not been demonstrated to cause permanent sequelae and are now listed as precautions to further administration of DTaP:

- Temperature above 105°F within 48 hours
- Collapse or shocklike state within 48 hours
- Persistent, inconsolable crying that lasts longer than 3 hours
- Unusual, high-pitched crying within 48 hours
- Seizures with or without fever

Vaccination with pertussis should be delayed in children with progressive neurologic disorders, conditions known to be associated with neurologic deficit such as tuberous sclerosis, or a history of recent onset of seizures of unknown etiology. A decision to vaccinate these children should be made on a case-by-case basis and will need to be reevaluated with changes in their condition.

Dosage and Administration. Give 0.5 ml intramuscularly according to primary immunization schedule.

Children. Children should receive a first dose of (DTP or) DTaP between 6 and 8 weeks of life, with subsequent doses at 4 and 6 months. There should be at least 6 weeks between doses. A fourth dose should be given after the age of 15 months; there should be at least 6 months between the third and fourth dose. A fifth dose is indicated after the age of 48 months.

Subsequent booster doses of Td, a preparation containing a lower dose of diphtheria toxoid, should be given every 10 years.

Adults. Currently, pertussis vaccination is not indicated in individuals over the age of 7 years, although it is recognized that adults with asymptomatic infection are a significant reservoir of disease. Td, that is, adult-type tetanus and diphtheria toxoids, should be given every 10 years as routine prophylaxis.

Pregnancy. To prevent neonatal tetanus, previously unimmunized women should receive two doses of Td administered at least 4 weeks apart with the second dose given at least 2 weeks before delivery. Pregnancy is not a contraindication for the administration of routine booster doses.

How Supplied

DTaP: Diphtheria, tetanus toxoids combined with acellular pertussis vaccine.

DT: For infants and children over 7 years in whom pertussis is contraindicated.

Td: Tetanus and diphtheria toxoids for persons over 7 years old. The diphtheria component is reduced in concentration because adverse effects are age and dose related.

DTaP-Hib (Tri HIBit): DTaP combined with *Haemophilus influenzae* type b vaccine

DTaP-IPV-Hepatitis B (Pediarix): Approved by the Food and Drug Administration in 2003, the vaccine combines DTaP, injectable polio vaccine, and hepatitis B vaccine and may be given at 2, 4, and 6 months of life.

Haemophilus *B Conjugate Vaccine (Hib)*

This product is a polysaccharide conjugated with a carrier protein coat to increase immunogenicity. This protein is more antigenic because of its ability to invoke a T-cell response. T cells allow a "memory" response with successively increased antibody production occurring after each exposure. The carrier protein alone invokes this T-cell response. Carrier proteins include diphtheria toxoid, a nontoxic mutant diphtheria toxin, an outer membrane protein complex of *Neisseria meningitidis*, or tetanus toxoid. It is used for the immunization of children against *Haemophilus* type b.

Contraindications, Warnings, Precautions. Children with impaired immune systems, such as those infected with HIV, may not mount sufficient immunity with the recommended vaccine schedule and may require an additional dose.

Adverse Effects. Very few side effects occur with any of the conjugate preparations. Localized swelling, tenderness, and redness occur in less than 25% of recipients. Systemic effects such as fever are very uncommon. There are no known serious side effects.

Dosage and Administration. The product is a suspension and must be shaken vigorously to obtain a uniform suspension before withdrawing each dose from a multidose vial.

Children. Immunize all children beginning at 2 months with subsequent doses (boosters) at 4, 6, and 12 to 15 months. Children aged 12 to 14 months require at least two doses; infants over 2 months but under 12 months should receive two doses with a booster at 12 to 15 months. Children who were not immunized as infants who are now over the age of 15 months need only one dose.

Children who have had invasive Hib disease younger than 24 months of age may, despite this illness, have low antibody concentrations and are at risk for a subsequent episode. Any vaccine given before this disease should be ignored, and conjugate vaccine should be re-administered beginning within 1 month using the recommended schedule for non-immunized children of the same age. Children who are over 24 months at the time of disease do not require immunization irrespective of previous status.

Adults. Vaccine is not indicated in those over 60 months of age.

How Supplied. There are four commercial preparations available in the United States, and recommendations for each vary. All contain an Hib capsular polysaccharide covalently linked to a carrier protein. HbOC Hib (oligosaccharides conjugated to diphtheria CRM197 toxin protein, HibTITER; Lederle) and PRP-T Hib (polyribosylribitol phosphate polysaccharide conjugated to tetanus toxoid, ActHIB; Pasteur Merieux) require three doses in the primary series with a booster at 12 to 15 months. PRP-OMP, a purified capsular polysaccharide (PRP) conjugated to the outer membrane protein (OMP) of *Neisseria meningitidis* serotype B (Pedvax; Merck), requires only three doses at 2, 4, and 12 to 15 months. Vaccines may be used interchangeably. In such causes, the recommended number of doses to complete the series is determined by the HbOC or PRP-T product, not by the PRP-OMP vaccine. PRP-D (ProHIBit; Connaught) is not indicated for use in children under the age of 12 months. All other preparations are recommended for infants. PRP-OMPHib is also available combined with hepatitis B vaccine (Comvax; Merck). PRP-T is available combined with DTP (OmniHIB; Pasteur Merieux) and may be used for the primary series.

Polio Vaccine (IPV, OPV)

The poliovirus is an *Enterovirus* classified as types 1, 2, and 3. Thus vaccines are trivalent; that is, they provide protection against all three subtypes. Inactivated, or killed, polio vaccine is administered parenterally. Oral vaccines, which use attenuated, live viruses, because they are absorbed through the intestinal tract, provide systemic immunity, as well as mucosal, IgA-mediated immunity; oral preparations are no longer recommended for use in the United States because of concerns about the rare incidence of vaccine-acquired paralytic polio (VAPP).

Contraindications, Warnings, Precautions. Oral poliovirus vaccine (OPV) is no longer recommended for routine use in the United States and availability is limited; it is contraindicated in persons with immunodeficiency disorders resulting from underlying disease, chemotherapy, or radiation. It may be used in the unlikely event of a mass vaccination campaign in response to an outbreak of polio, for unimmunized children who are traveling to countries where polio is endemic who do not have sufficient time to receive two doses of IPV, or for the third or fourth dose in children who refuse injectable vaccine. If OPV should be given to a close contact of an immunodeficient patient (i.e., chemotherapy, transplant, HIV, long-term steroid use defined as more than 2 weeks of systemic, not topical, use), close contact should be avoided for 1 month.

IPV contains trace amounts of streptomycin, neomycin, and polymyxin B; thus allergic reactions to one of these three antibiotics may rarely occur.

Adverse Effects. VAPP is the most serious risk and does not occur with IPV. Paralytic polio occurs in 1 : 560,000 first doses of OPV and in 1 : 10 million subsequent doses. Risk is highest in close contacts of vaccine recipients, adults, and those with immunodeficiency conditions.

Dosage and Administration

Children. Children should be vaccinated with four doses, beginning at 2 months of life; subsequent doses are administered at 4 months, 6 to 18 months, and 4 to 6 years. When accelerated protection is indicated, the first dose may be administered as early as 6 weeks, with a second dose a minimum of 4 weeks later. Giving the third dose at 6 months may lead to increased compliance.

Adults. IPV is recommended for use in individuals over the age of 7 years who have never been immunized. Adults who previously completed primary series with OPV may be given a booster dose of IPV. Unimmunized adults should receive two doses at intervals of 4 to 8 weeks, with a booster dose 6 to 12 months later.

Pregnancy. Do not vaccinate during pregnancy unless necessary for epidemic control.

How Supplied. Preparations are available in two formulations.

1. *Inactivated polio virus (IPV).* This killed virus preparation is administered parenterally, either subcutaneously or intramuscularly. This preparation provides excellent systemic immunity; current IPV preparations are of enhanced potency and produce seroconversion rates equal to or better than OPV.
2. *Attenuated polio virus (APV).* This live virus is administered orally. Systemic immunity is equal to that achieved by IPV with the addition of excellent mucosal immunity.

Measles-Mumps-Rubella Vaccine

MMR vaccine is a live, attenuated vaccine that is prepared in chick embryo cell culture. After the administration of a single dose of live virus vaccine, 95% of individuals develop adequate serum antibody.

Contraindications, Warnings, Precautions. MMR vaccination is contraindicated in the following situations:

- Pregnancy
- Egg anaphylaxis
- Significantly immunocompromised individuals or those receiving immunotherapy, with the exception of those with HIV infection, should not be given live-virus vaccines.
- Individuals who have received immunoglobulin antibody–containing blood products within the preceding 3 months should not be vaccinated until at least 3 months after receipt. If these products are given less than 14 days after MMR, the vaccine should be repeated in 3 months.
- Tuberculin skin test may be performed at time of immunization; otherwise, it should be postponed until 4 to 6 weeks after because immunization can temporarily suppress tuberculin reaction.

Adverse Effects. There are many reported side effects to these preparations; the majority are not serious. They include the following:

- From 5% to 15% of vaccinated patients experience temperature of at least 103° F, which begins 7 to 12 days after vaccination and commonly lasts 1 to 2 days; fever has been reported to last up to 5 days. The majority of these individuals are otherwise asymptomatic.
- Five percent of recipients may experience transient rashes on days 7 to 12.
- Frank arthritis rarely occurs in children, although 10% to 15% of adult women may experience significant joint pain, particularly in peripheral small joints. There have been no reports of permanent joint destruction.
- Transient thrombocytopenia has been reported, although the incidence is unknown.
- Side effects are markedly less common with second doses, presumably because most individuals are already immune.
- No side effects have been reported in immune persons who were inadvertently vaccinated.
- Seizure risk is slightly elevated following measles vaccination, although a known seizure disorder is not a contraindication to vaccine administration.
- Measles vaccine is not causally linked to a risk of developing autism spectrum disorders

Rarely, side effects that are more serious may occur. Allergic reactions occur rarely and are usually attributable to trace amounts of neomycin; children with known anaphylaxis to topical or systemic neomycin should receive vaccine in settings where such a reaction can be treated. A history of contact dermatitis to neomycin is not a contraindication. The measles component of the vaccine is produced in chick embryo cell culture but does not contain significant amount of egg protein. Children with egg allergy are at low risk for anaphylactic reactions to measles-containing vaccine. The incidence of subacute sclerosing panencephalitis (SSPE) after vaccine is significantly lower than the risk of acquiring this condition from measles infection.

Dosage and Administration

Children. The first dose is recommended at 12 to 15 months of age with a booster dose at elementary school entry. Children who have had physician-diagnosed measles or who have laboratory evidence of immunity do not require vaccinations.

Adults. Persons born before 1957 have probably been naturally infected and do not require vaccination. All individuals born after 1957 who do not have laboratory evidence of immunity or evidence of appropriate vaccination should receive two doses of MMR at least 1 month apart.

Pregnancy. Live virus vaccines should not be administered during pregnancy. In addition, women of childbearing age who receive a rubella-containing preparation should be counseled to defer pregnancy for 3 months. If vaccination should occur during the first trimester, the pregnant woman should be counseled on possible risks to the fetus. It is currently suggested that inadvertent rubella vaccination during pregnancy is not sufficient reason to recommend termination of the pregnancy. MMR preparations may be given to children with pregnant mothers.

How Supplied. Monovalent preparations of measles, mumps, and rubella are available. In epidemic areas, it may be indicated to immunize infants under the age of 12 months with one of these preparations. For routine use, however, a trivalent preparation should be used. This is true in both children and adult populations where protection against all three diseases is desirable.

Varicella Vaccine

Varicella vaccine was licensed for general use in March 1995. Preparations contain cell-free live attenuated varicella zoster virus; trace amounts of neomycin are also found. In well children over the age of 12 months, a single dose results in a seroconversion rate of greater than 95%. There is an age-related decrease in the ability of the immune system to mount and maintain a primary response after the age of 12 years. In adolescents over the age of 12 and adults, seroconversion rates after one dose range from 79% to 82%; two doses result in a seroconversion rate of 94%. The rate of disease after immunization appears to be about 1% to 3% per year. Even more importantly, there appears to be a very high rate of protection from severe varicella disease. In those individuals who do contract the virus after vaccination, disease is reported to be much milder.

Contraindications, Warnings, Precautions. Varicella vaccine may be given simultaneously with MMR; however, if not given simultaneously, the interval between administration should be at least 1 month. Varicella vaccine does not appear to have any effect on the administration of any other vaccine.

Varicella vaccine should not be given routinely to immunocompromised individuals. This includes those with malignancies, HIV disease where CD4 T-lymphocyte counts are less than 25%, or congenital immunodeficiencies or those who are receiving immunosuppressive therapy or long-term systemic steroids. Children with acute lymphocytic leukemia who have been in remission for at least 1 year may be immunized if they have documented adequate lymphocyte and platelet counts.

Varicella virus should not be given to those individuals receiving high-dose systemic corticosteroids (>2 mg/kg/day of prednisone); after discontinuation of steroids, vaccination should be delayed for 3 months. In children who are on lower doses (1 to 2 mg/kg/day of prednisone), the risk of vaccination with an attenuated live virus must be weighed against the risk of infection with wild virus. Some experts recommend vaccination of these children if steroid use is discontinued for a period of 1 or more weeks both before and after administration. Decisions to vaccinate these children must be made after consultation with appropriate physicians. Inhaled steroid use is not a contraindication to use of the vaccine.

As with other live virus vaccines, administration should be withheld if an individual has received immune globulin in the preceding 5 months.

The association between wild virus varicella, salicylate use, and the development of Reye's syndrome is well known. No such association has been found with use of varicella vaccine; however, the manufacturer recommends that salicylates not be given for 6 weeks after administration of the vaccine.

Vaccine should not be given to individuals who have an anaphylactic reaction to neomycin. As with other vaccines, moderate-to-severe illness is reason to withhold vaccination.

Adverse Effects. Adverse effects are minimal. Less than 25% of children and adults report mild pain and erythema at the injection site. Approximately 7% to 8% of vaccinees develop a mild maculopapular or morbilliform rash within 1 month of receiving vaccine. Rarely, varicella virus has been recovered from these skin lesions. There has been no disease reported in susceptible individuals who have contact with vaccinees with a rash.

Dosage and Administration

Children. Children should be routinely vaccinated at 12 months. Unimmunized children between the age of 12 months and 13 years should be vaccinated with a single dose; over 13 years, two doses administered at least 4 weeks apart are recommended.

Adults. Adults who lack a reliable history of varicella vaccine should be vaccinated at the earliest opportunity; two doses spaced 4 to 8 weeks apart are necessary. Serologic testing before administration of the vaccine is optional. No adverse sequelae have been noted in immune individuals who receive vaccine.

Pregnancy. As with all live viruses, pregnancy is a contraindication to administration of the vaccine. Pregnancy should be avoided for 1 month following vaccination. A pregnant household member is not a contraindication to the administration of vaccine to susceptible individuals.

How Supplied. There is only one licensed product available in the United States.

Influenza Vaccine (Various Strains)

Although *Healthy People 2000* set a goal of 60% vaccination rates in older and other high-risk individuals, success in meeting this goal has been mixed, with minority populations and adults over 65 not residing in nursing homes less likely to be immunized. Despite rising vaccination rates, continuing epidemics of influenza occur during the winter months and are responsible for an average of approximately 20,000 deaths per year in the United States. Rates of infection are highest among children, but rates of serious illness and death are highest among persons older than 65 years and persons of any age who have medical conditions that place them at increased risk for complications from influenza.

Current influenza vaccines are produced in embryonated eggs. The vaccines are multivalent and contain three different viral subtypes; the composition is changed annually in anticipation of expected prevalent influenza strains. Efficacy of vaccines is difficult to document because of both yearly variations in circulating strains and the difficulty of distinguishing clinically between true influenza disease and that caused by other viruses. Thus influenza vaccine is not effective against all possible strains of influenza virus, and protection is afforded only against those strains of virus from which the vaccine is prepared or against closely related strains. The impact of immunization is most noticeable in adult populations, probably because of the lower frequency of colds and other viral disease. Protection against disease is probably in the range of 70% to 80%, with duration of efficacy of less than 1 year.

Contraindications, Warnings, Precautions. Influenza vaccine should be withheld in the following conditions:

- Individuals receiving chemotherapy should not receive vaccine until at least 4 weeks after discontinuation of therapy.
- The effect of steroid therapy on influenza vaccine immunogenicity is unknown. Steroid therapy should not necessarily delay the administration of vaccine, particularly in those individuals in whom influenza can be expected to be particularly severe.
- The American Academy of Pediatrics recommends that influenza virus vaccine should not be administered within 3 days of immunization with a pertussis-containing vaccine because both vaccines may cause febrile reactions in young children.

Adverse Effects. Because influenza vaccine contains only noninfectious viruses, it cannot cause influenza. Occasional cases of respiratory disease following vaccination represent coincidental illnesses unrelated to influenza vaccination.

Febrile reactions in children younger than 13 are uncommon; adults and children over the age of 13 infrequently experience fever; malaise and local soreness and erythema occur in approximately 10% of cases.

There is a slightly increased risk of developing Guillain-Barré syndrome, or other temporary neurologic disorders, after vaccination.

Individuals with severe, anaphylactic reaction to eggs or chickens or gentamicin sulfate may, on rare occasions, experience similar reactions after influenza vaccine. In view of the need for yearly administration and the availability of chemoprophylaxis against influenza A, it is recommended that these individuals not receive vaccine. Individuals who would benefit from the vaccine should be given a skin test or other allergy-evaluating test, using the influenza virus vaccine as the antigen.

Immunocompromised individuals may have a reduced antibody response to active immunization procedures.

Influenza vaccine often contains one or more antigens used in previous years. However, immunity declines during the year after immunization. Therefore revaccination on a yearly basis is necessary to provide optimal protection for the current season.

Dosage and Administration. Providers should begin vaccination efforts in October in persons at high risk and health care workers. Vaccination of children under the age of 9 who are receiving vaccine for the first time should also begin in October as these children require a booster dose 1 month after the initial dose. Vaccination of all other groups should begin in November, including household members of persons at high risk, healthy persons aged 50 to 64 years, and any other individuals who wish to receive vaccine. Vaccine should continue to be offered in December and throughout the influenza season as long as vaccine supplies are available.

Children. Efficacy has not been evaluated in children under the age of 6 months. Yearly immunization is recommended for all children between the ages of 6 and 24 months and siblings of children under the age of 2 years with particular emphasis for those siblings of children under 6 months of age who, due to their young age, may not be vaccinated.

Children over the age of 24 months in the following high-risk categories should also be vaccinated:

- Children with chronic pulmonary, renal, metabolic, or cardiovascular disorders, including asthma and diabetes mellitus
- Hemodynamically significant cardiac disease
- Hemoglobinopathies, including sickle cell disease
- Any disease that requires the use of immunosuppressive therapy
- HIV infection
- Receiving long-term aspirin therapy

Vaccination should also be considered for children in living situations where rapid transmission of disease is likely. This includes residents of group homes or college dormitories or those who are members of athletic teams that live and travel together. In addition, children who live in close contact with an at-risk child should be considered for immunization to decrease the potential for spread to others.

Two doses spaced at least 1 month apart are recommended for those individuals receiving vaccine for the first time. If strains have not changed significantly, immunization in subsequent years may be achieved with the administration of only one dose.

Adults. Adults in the following categories should be considered for routine administration:

- Persons older than 50 years
- Residents of nursing homes and other long-term care facilities
- Adults with chronic pulmonary, cardiovascular, metabolic, or renal disorders
- Adults with hemoglobinopathies, or immunosuppression (including immunosuppression caused by medications or by HIV)
- Health care workers, employees of long-term care facilities, child care workers, and household members of individuals in high-risk categories

Two doses spaced 1 month apart are recommended for those individuals receiving the vaccine for the first time. If strains have not changed significantly, immunization in subsequent years may be achieved with the administration of only one dose.

Pregnancy. Women who will be in their second or third trimester during influenza season should be vaccinated. Women who are breastfeeding may safely be vaccinated.

How Supplied. There are several different preparations currently in use:

- Inactivated whole-virus vaccines prepared from purified virus particles
- Subvirion vaccines, which are prepared by another step of disrupting the lipid-containing outer membrane of the virus
- Purified surface antigen vaccines

These last two preparations are termed "split-virus vaccines"; they are the only products licensed for use in children under the age of 13. All are equally safe and immunogenic.

A limited amount of thimerosal free vaccine began to be available during the 2002 influenza season; these products currently are only licensed for use in children over the age of 4 years.

A nasal spray flu vaccine (FluMist; Aviron), a cold-adapted, live-attenuated, trivalent influenza virus vaccine, is now available for use in individuals between the ages of 5 and 49.

Pneumococcal Vaccine

Two types of pneumococcal vaccine are available. The first, PS23, is a polyvalent product that is a mixture of highly purified capsular polysaccharides from the 23 most prevalent or invasive pneumococcal type. It is recommended for use in adults and children over 2 years of age. A pneumococcal conjugate vaccine, PCV7, was also approved in 2000 (Prevnar; Wyeth). This product conjugates the capsular polysaccharides from the seven most invasive types of pneumococci with diphtheria protein; it is approved for use in children between the ages of 2 months and 10 years.

Contraindications, Warnings, Precautions. In patients who require penicillin (or other antibiotic) prophylaxis against pneumococcal infection, such prophylaxis should not be discontinued after vaccination with this vaccine.

The polysaccharide vaccine is a pregnancy category C product and should be given to a pregnant woman only if clearly needed.

Adverse Effects. With both the polysaccharide and conjugate vaccines, local reactions are the most common side effect and include local injection site soreness, erythema, and swelling, usually lasting no more than 2 days; local induration occurs less frequently. Rash, urticaria, arthritis, arthralgia, adenitis, and serum sickness have occasionally been reported. Malaise, myalgia, headache, and asthenia have also been seen. Fever is more common following administration of conjugate vaccine, occurring in about one-fourth of all children; older children are less likely to experience fever.

Dosage and Administration. Infants should be vaccinated using the pneumococcal conjugate product at 2, 4, 6, and 12 to 15 months. Children receiving their first pneumococcal vaccination between 2 and 6 months of age should receive three doses, 6 to 8 weeks apart, with a booster at 15 to 18 months. Children who do not receive their first dose until 7 and 1 months of age should be given two doses, 6 to 8 weeks apart, with a booster at the recommended age. Children receiving their first dose at 12 and 23 months of age, should be administered two doses, 6 to 8 weeks apart and will not require a booster dose. High-risk children between 24 and 59 months of age should receive one dose; high-risk categories include the following:

- Children with anatomic asplenia or who have splenic dysfunction from sickle cell disease or other causes
- Children with chronic illnesses in which there is an increased risk of pneumococcal disease, such as those with functional impairment of cardiorespiratory, hepatic, and renal systems
- Children with immunosuppression including HIV infection

Children in high-risk groups who are over the age of 59 months should be vaccinated with polysaccharide vaccine. In addition, adults in the following categories should be considered for vaccination:

- Persons 50 years of age or older
- Patients with other chronic illnesses who may be at greater risk of developing pneumococcal infection or having more severe illness as a result of alcohol abuse or coexisting diseases
- Patients with Hodgkin's disease if immunization can be given at least 10 days before treatment

Vaccine should also be considered for adults residing in closed-group communities such as residential schools and nursing homes, groups epidemiologically at risk in the community, and patients at high risk of influenza complications.

The polysaccharide vaccine should be administered as a single 0.5-ml dose subcutaneously or intramuscularly, preferably in the deltoid muscle or lateral midthigh.

How Supplied. Polysaccharide product comes in multidose vials of either 14-valent or 23-valent vaccines.

Respiratory Syncytial Virus Prophylaxis

Although this is not a vaccine but rather an antibody that is given to high-risk infants under the age of 24 months, it is included because it is now part of the routine recommendations for these infants.

Respiratory syncytial virus (RSV) is recognized to be the most significant etiologic agent in acute respiratory tract illness in infants and young children, causing significant morbidity in high-risk infants, including preterm babies. The American Academy of Pediatrics recommends that infants and children under the age of 2 who are at risk for complications from RSV, including infants born at less than 35 weeks' gestation and those with chronic lung disease, receive prophylaxis for RSV within 6 months of the anticipated RSV season, which typically is from winter to early spring in temperate climates. A monoclonal antibody product, palivizumab (Synagis; Medimmune), for use in high-risk children under the age of 24 months was approved by the Food and Drug Administration in 1998. In addition, RSV prophylaxis may be accomplished with administration of RSV intravenous immunoglobulin (RSV-IGIV). Although RSV-IGIV and palivizumab are both approved as prophylactic agents, palivizumab is preferred due to its easier administration, safety profile, and equivalent efficacy. Most infants will only require RSV prophylaxis for their first RSV season, but children with significant lung disease may benefit from therapy for two seasons.

Contraindications, Warnings, Precautions. Palivizumab is the preferred agent for most infants, but RSV-IGIV has been shown to reduce the numbers of non-RSV respiratory infections in high-risk infants. Therefore it may be preferable to provide IGIV rather than palivizumab for infants younger than 6 months who cannot receive influenza vaccination due to their age. It also should be considered for infants and children with severe pulmonary disease in whom respiratory infections other than those caused by RSV may be serious.

Adverse Effects. The administration of palivizumab does not require alteration in the routine vaccination schedule and does not interfere with immunologic response to these agents. However, children receiving RSV-IGIV should not receive MMR and Varivax until at least 9 months after their last dose of immunoglobulin. The product does not interfere with response to inactivated polio vaccine or hepatitis B vaccine.

The incidence of adverse effects after the administration of palivizumab is similar to that of placebo.

Dosage and Administration. RSV prophylaxis should be begun at the start of RSV season, between October and December in most parts of the United States, and be terminated at the end of the season, typically March to May.

RSV-IGIV should be given at a dose of 750 mg/kg at the outset of RSV season and monthly during the season. Palivizumab is administered intramuscularly, at a dose of 15 mg/kg, monthly during RSV season.

Prophylaxis should be considered in the following instances:

1. Infants and children younger than 2 years of age with chronic lung disease who require medical therapy during the 6 months before RSV season.
2. Infants born at less than 32 weeks' gestation without chronic lung disease also may benefit from RSV prophylaxis. Infants born at less than 28 weeks' gestation should be considered for prophylaxis up to 12 months of age.

Infants born between 29 and 32 weeks' gestation should be considered for prophylaxis until 6 months of age.

3. Infants born between 32 and 35 weeks who have additional risk factors, such as immunosuppression or non-cyanotic heart disease, should be considered for prophylaxis. RSV-IGIV is contraindicated in children with cyanotic heart disease.

How Supplied. Palivizumab is supplied in 50-mg and 100-mg single-dose vials.

Meningococcal Vaccine

Neisseria meningitides is the second most common cause of bacterial meningitis in the United States and has a case-fatality rate of approximately 10% to 20% despite therapy with antimicrobial agents to which all strains remain highly sensitive. For uncertain reasons, there has been a significant increase in outbreaks of infection in the past 10 years; over one-third of these outbreaks have occurred in the college dormitory setting. Meningococcal vaccine is a quadrivalent vaccine containing 50 μg of each of four purified bacterial capsular polysaccharides from serogroups A, C, Y, and W-135 antigens from *N. meningitidis*. The vaccine is highly effective, but it does not provide protection against all forms of meningococcal meningitis. Historically, most disease outbreaks were the result serogroup C; however, recently outbreaks resulting from serogroups Y and B have occurred. Disease in infants under the age of 1 year is most likely to be the result of infection with serogroup B, for which there is no vaccine. Antibodies against the serogroup A and C polysaccharides decline markedly over the first 3 years after a single dose of vaccine, with the decline being most pronounced in the youngest children. It is recommended for use in persons 2 years of age and above in epidemic or endemic areas; individuals who are high risk, such as those with asplenia; and travelers to countries recognized as having hyperendemic or epidemic disease. In addition, U.S. military recruits are routinely vaccinated on entrance. Vaccinations should also be considered for household or institutional contacts of persons with meningococcal disease. In 1997, the American College Health Association recommended that college health centers proactively inform entering college students who would be residing in dormitories and their parents about the risk of disease and that vaccine be offered. In 2000, both the American Academy of Pediatrics and the ACIP issued their own recommendation that these students be offered vaccine; in addition, the American Academy of Pediatrics and the ACIP stated that although the risk of meningococcal disease was not elevated in students not residing in dormitories, there was no contraindication to vaccinating these students and they should be given vaccine if desired. Protective antibodies are usually seen within 7 to 10 days after vaccination.

Contraindications, Warnings, Precautions. Pregnancy is not a contraindication to vaccination.

Adverse Effects. Adverse effects are mild and infrequent, consisting of localized erythema lasting 1 to 2 days. Young children may have transient mild fever.

Dosage and Administration. The immunizing dose is a single injection of 0.5 mg given subcutaneously. The vaccine may be given at the same time as other immunizations.

Although it is recognized that antibody levels decrease very rapidly, usually within 3 to 5 years, after vaccination, there is no recommendation that high- risk individuals routinely be revaccinated. In some select individuals, including children who were first immunized under 4 years of age, revaccination may be warranted, but those decisions should be made on an individual basis.

How Supplied. The vaccine is available in 1-, 10-, and 50-dose vials.

Hepatitis A Vaccine

Hepatitis A is highly contagious, with the predominant mode of transmission being person-to-person via the fecal-oral route. Infection has been shown to be spread by contaminated water or food, infected food handlers, after breakdown in usual sanitary conditions or after floods or natural disasters, by ingestion of raw or undercooked shellfish from contaminated waters, during travel to areas of the world with poor hygienic conditions, among institutionalized children and adults, in day care centers where children have not been toilet trained, by parenteral transmission, and by either blood transfusions or sharing needles with infected people. The incubation period for hepatitis A averages 28 days, with an extremely variable course. Although many children may have asymptomatic infection, most older children and adults are symptomatic, with a self-limiting course characterized by fever, malaise, nausea, and jaundice. Recovery is usually complete and followed by protection against hepatitis A virus (HAV) infection.

Hepatitis A vaccine, inactivated (Havrix; GlaxoSmithKline, and Vaqta; Merck), is a whole-cell, purified sterile suspension of inactivated viral proteins.

Contraindications, Warnings, Precautions. Because hepatitis A has a relatively long incubation period (15 to 50 days), this vaccine may not prevent hepatitis A infection in individuals who have an unrecognized hepatitis A infection at the time of vaccination.

The vaccine may be given at the same time as other immunizations.

Safety data in pregnancy are limited, but there appears to be little risk from administration of this inactivated product.

Adverse Effects. Generally, the vaccine is associated with only mild and short-term effects: 1% to 10% of patients may have local reactions at injection site with induration, redness, and swelling. They may also experience fatigue, mild fever, malaise, anorexia, or nausea. Serious side effects have not been reported.

Dosage and Administration. Routine vaccination is not recommended for children or adults residing in the United States, with the exception of individuals living in an area that experiences a significant increase in infection rates.

Individuals traveling to developing countries with high rates of infection, including Mexico, should be considered for vaccination. In addition, men who have sex with men, individuals using intravenous drugs, or those who work in high-risk settings such as research settings where hepatitis A is present or with infected animals, should be considered for vaccination. Finally, individuals at high risk for fulminant liver disease, such as those with chronic liver disorders or recipients of clotting factors, should be considered for immunization.

The vaccine is not approved for use in children under the age of 2 years. Dosing varies according to age of recipient and product; check the manufacturer's recommendations. Both products require a two-dose schedule, with the initial dose followed by a booster 6 to 18 months later. While preferable to complete the series with the same product, they may be used interchangeably.

How Supplied. Single-use vials are available; concentrations vary by manufacturer.

Rabies Vaccine and Rabies Immune Globulin (RVA, RIG)

Rabies vaccine is given prophylactically to individuals at high risk of exposure to rabid animals: veterinarians, animal handlers, and certain laboratory workers. It should be given as a series and started immediately after any bite from a suspicious animal. Rabies immunoglobulin gives passive protection when started immediately after exposure to rabies virus. It takes approximately 1 week for antibodies to develop.

Rabies vaccine is available as a human diploid-cell vaccine (HDCV), an adsorbed vaccine (RVA), and a purified chick embryo cell (PCEC) (RabAvert; Chiron Behring GmbH and Company).

Contraindications, Warnings, Precautions. There are no known contraindications to administration of rabies IG or vaccine. Pregnancy is not a contraindication. The product does not pose a risk for nursing infants of children.

Adverse Effects. Although adverse reactions are less common with currently available products, 15% to 25% of adults may experience local reactions, such as pain and swelling, and systemic reactions including headache, muscle pain, nausea, and dizziness. Reactions are much less frequent in children. Severe reactions, including several cases of a Guillain-Barré–like syndrome, do not appear to be causally linked to vaccine.

Dosage and Administration. Postexposure prophylaxis should begin as soon as possible, preferably within 24 hours, and requires administration of both RIG and vaccine. Vaccine dosing varies for children and adults.

For both adults and children, RIG at a dose of 20 IU/kg should be given as soon as possible, with as much of the dose as possible used to infiltrate the wound; RIG may be diluted with saline to increase volume and allow penetration of the entire wound. The remaining volume should be given intramuscularly at a distant site. Vaccine should be given at the same time; dose is 1.0 ml, intramuscularly, of the three available vaccines on days 0, 3, 7, 14, and 28. The same product should be used for all doses. Adults should receive an intramuscular injection in the deltoid; the anterolateral thigh may be used in young children. In individuals who have been previously vaccinated, RIG is not given. Two doses of vaccine should be given, with the first on the day of exposure followed by a second dose 3 days later.

Both adults and children should be administered a three-dose regimen consisting of a 1.0-ml dose of any available product on day 0, 7, and 21 or 28. Booster doses at 2-year intervals may be necessary, as determined by serum antibody levels.

How Supplied. All preparations are available in single-dose vials.

Yellow Fever Vaccine

This vaccine is a live attenuated virus preparation that provides immunity in 7 to 10 days with continued efficacy for about 10 years. Indicated for travelers to areas where yellow fever is endemic. Updated information on endemic area can be found at Travelers' Health, Division of Global Migration and Quarantine, National Center for Infectious Diseases, CDC, at http://www.cdc.gov/travel/index.htm, or from the Division of Vector-Borne Infectious Diseases, National Center for Infectious Diseases, CDC, at http://www.cdc.gov/ncidod/dvbid/yellowfever/index.htm.

Contraindications, Warnings, Precautions. Children under the age of 9 months should not be vaccinated, although in special, high-risk cases, vaccination may be considered for children aged 6 to 9 months. Vaccination should never be given to children under the age of 6 months. The safety of yellow fever vaccination during pregnancy has not been established, and vaccination should only be considered when travel to endemic regions, with an associated high risk of exposure, is unavoidable. The seroconversion rate after vaccination in pregnant women is uncertain, and serologic testing to determine immunity should be considered. Although there have been no cases reported of transmission through breast milk, vaccination of nursing women should be avoided unless there is a high risk of exposure. Vaccinated patients should continue to take precautions to avoid mosquito bites.

Adverse Effects. Fever or malaise usually appears 7 to 14 days after administration. Myalgia and headache may also develop. Anaphylaxis or encephalitis may rarely occur; the majority of yellow fever vaccine associated cases of encephalitis have occurred in children under the age of 6 months.

Dosage and Administration. *Adults and children:* Administer a single immunizing dose of 0.5 ml subcutaneously. Booster doses are not currently recommended.

Limited available data suggest that vaccine may be safely administered at the same time as other commercially available vaccines.

How Supplied. Vaccine is available as single-dose, 5-dose, and 20-dose vials.

Typhoid Vaccine

Vaccine is estimated to be about 70% effective in preventing typhoid fever, partly depending on the degree of exposure. Vaccine is available as a live attenuated oral product (Ty21a), a polysaccharide preparation that is delivered by intramuscular injection (ViCPS) and a killed whole cell vaccine that may be given subcutaneously. Researchers at the National Institute of Child Health and Human Development have recently developed an oral product that reportedly has 91% efficacy and may be given to children as young as 2 years.

Of the 400 cases of typhoid fever occur in the United States each year, 70% are reported to be acquired outside of the United States. Indicated for those traveling to areas where typhoid fever is endemic, when contact with infected individuals is expected, and in laboratory workers handling organisms.

Contraindications, Warnings, Precautions. Do not give the oral formulation to immunocompromised individuals because it contains live virus.

Administration of the live oral product should be delayed until 24 hours before or after a dose of mefloquine, an antimalarial drug. Similarly, administration should be delayed until 24 hours after use of any antimicrobial drugs.

Adverse Effects. Oral and polysaccharide preparations cause minimal systemic adverse reactions; local reactions are infrequently reported from the polysaccharide. More significant local pain and swelling, in up to 35% of individuals, are reported with use of the killed product that is delivered subcutaneously. In addition, systemic reactions such as fever and headache are more common.

Dosage and Administration. *Oral:* Vaccine may be given to individuals over the age of 6 years. Take one enteric-coated capsule on alternate days (days 1, 3, 5, and 7) for four doses. Swallow capsule whole 1 hour before a meal with cold or lukewarm water. Complete at least 1 week before travel or contact. Current recommendations are to repeat the entire four-dose course every 5 years for booster protection as indicated.

Polysaccharide: Vaccine may be given to individuals over the age of 2 years. Give a single 0.5-ml dose intramuscularly, with a booster dose every 2 years if the risk of exposure remains high.

Killed whole cell preparation: This is the only product approved for use in children under the age of 2 years who are at high risk for infection, although many experts avoid use in these children because of the high rate of side effects. Give two 0.25-ml doses subcutaneously a minimum of 4 weeks apart. Booster doses should be given every 3 years if indicated with one of the other commercially available products.

How Supplied. *Oral:* Single foil blister containing four doses in a single package

Parenteral: Vials of 5, 10, 20, and 50 ml, depending on the suspension

Smallpox Vaccine

Routine administration of smallpox vaccine was discontinued in the United States in 1972 when the virus was declared to be eradicated in the wild. Current concerns about its use as a weapon of mass destruction have led to reinstitution of immunization in selected at-risk populations. The smallpox vaccine currently available in the United States (Dryvax; Wyeth) is a live virus preparation of infectious vaccinia virus. Smallpox vaccine does not contain smallpox (variola) virus.

Contraindications, Warnings, Precautions. Due to the incidence of potentially severe reactions, routine immunization is not recommended. Vaccine is contraindicated in the following situations:

1. Individuals who have ever been diagnosed with eczema or atopic dermatitis should not be vaccinated, even if their skin condition is well controlled. These individuals are at high risk of developing eczema vaccinatum, a potentially severe and sometimes fatal complication. Persons living with these individuals should similarly not be vaccinated. Individuals with other acute, chronic, or exfoliative skin conditions, and their household contacts, should not be vaccinated until resolution.
2. Individuals with diseases or conditions that cause immunodeficiency or immunosuppression, including HIV/AIDS, organ transplant, and malignancy, should not be vaccinated because of the higher risk of developing progressive vaccinia, a condition that results in dangerous replication of the vaccine virus.
3. Individuals receiving treatments which cause immunodeficiency or immunosuppression such as radiation, chemotherapy, high-dose corticosteroids. Household contacts of individuals undergoing such treatment should not receive smallpox vaccine until they or their household contact have been off immunosuppressive treatment for 3 months.
4. Live virus vaccines should not be given during pregnancy. Pregnant women who receive the smallpox vaccine are at risk of fetal vaccinia, a very rare condition that results in stillbirth or death of the infant shortly after delivery. Women who are pregnant or intend to become pregnant in the next month, and their household contacts, should not be vaccinated.
5. Previous allergic reaction to smallpox vaccine or any of the vaccine's components
6. Moderate or severe acute illness should prompt a delay until the illness is resolved.
7. Smallpox vaccine is contraindicated for children under 12 months of age and should not be administered in nonemergency settings in persons younger than 18 years of age.
8. Breastfeeding mothers should not receive the smallpox vaccine as it is not known whether vaccine virus or antibodies are excreted in human milk.
9. Following reports of cardiac events after vaccination, it is currently recommended that individuals with known cardiac disease such as previous myocardial infarction,

angina, chronic heart failure, or cardiomyopathy not be vaccinated. It is unknown if these events are causally linked to vaccination, and this recommendation is being studied.

During a smallpox emergency, such as a weapons of mass destruction attack, all contraindications to vaccination would be reconsidered in the light of the risk of smallpox exposure.

Adverse Effects. Smallpox vaccination, although generally safe, has been associated with a significant incidence of adverse reactions. Most are benign, but they may be alarming in appearance and occasionally serious and life threatening. Severe adverse reactions are more common in persons receiving primary vaccination compared with those being revaccinated.

Local reactions, such as local edema, satellite lesions, pain, and swelling of regional lymph nodes, may occur 3 to 10 days after vaccination and may persist for up to 4 weeks. The resultant viral cellulitis may be confused with bacterial cellulitis. In up to a third of recipients, these reactions may be severe enough to prompt the individual to seek treatment.

Systemic reactions include fever in 17% of primary vaccinees, malaise, myalgia, and erythematous or urticarial rashes. As with local reactions, up to a third of these recipients are ill enough to miss work.

The lesion produced at the vaccination site contains high vaccinia virus titers and is frequently pruritic. The itching that results may result in transfer of virus to face, eyes, genital, and rectum with secondary lesions, which usually heal without treatment. Successful vaccination produces a lesion at the vaccination site. Beginning about 4 days after vaccination, the florid site contains high titers of vaccinia virus. This surface is easily transferred to the hands and to fomites, especially because itching is a common part of the local reaction. The most severe manifestation is vaccinia keratitis, which may result in lesions of the cornea and, if untreated, corneal scarring with resultant visual impairment.

Generalized vaccinia results in vesicles or pustules on normal skin distant from the vaccination site; this generally resolves without specialized treatment and without residual. Progressive vaccinia, also known as vaccinia necrosum, is a severe, potentially fatal illness characterized by progressive necrosis in the area of vaccination, often with distant lesions. Prompt hospitalization and aggressive use of massive doses of VIG are required.

Eczema vaccinatum results in localized and systemic spread of vaccinia virus, producing extensive lesions. This may occur even in those individuals who do not have active dermatitis at the time of vaccination. Treatment includes hospitalization and vaccinia immunoglobulin.

The Food and Drug Administration has recommended that vaccinees be deferred from donating blood for 21 days or until the scab has separated.

Dosage and Administration. Vaccination is achieved with a single-use bifurcated needle using a technique called multiple puncture vaccination. Three insertions are necessary for primary vaccination, and 15 insertions are necessary for revaccination. A trace of blood should appear at the site of vaccination within 15 to 20 seconds. During primary vaccination, if no trace of blood is visible after three insertions, an additional three insertions should be made using the same bifurcated needle without reinserting the needle into the vaccine vial.

How Supplied. Licensed Dryvax vaccine for civilian is only available through the CDC.

RESOURCES FOR PATIENTS AND PROVIDERS

Internet

American Academy of Pediatrics. Available at www.aap.org/family/parents/immunize.htm.
Immunization schedule updates and information.

Centers for Disease Control and Prevention National Immunization Program. Available at www.cdc.gov/nip.

Centers for Disease Control and Prevention Travel Information. Available at www.cdc.gov/travel/.

National Library of Medicine. Available at www.nlm.nih.gov/.

FDA/CDC Vaccine Adverse Event Reporting System. Available at www.fda.gov/cber/vaers.html.

Brochure

Division of Vaccine Injury Compensation: *Commonly asked questions about the National Vaccine Injury Compensation Program,* Washington, DC, July 1998, US Department of Health and Human Services, Public Health Service.

BIBLIOGRAPHY

American Academy of Pediatrics Committee on Infectious Disease: *2004 Red book: report of the Committee on Infectious Diseases,* ed 26, Elk Grove Village, IL, 2004, The Academy.

American Academy of Pediatrics Committee on Infectious Disease: Policy statement: recommendations for the prevention of pneumococcal infections, including the use of pneumococcal conjugate vaccine (Prevnar), pneumococcal polysaccharide vaccine, and antibiotic prophylaxis, *Pediatrics* 106:362-366, 2000.

Atkinson WL et al: General recommendations on immunization: recommendations of the Advisory Committee on Immunization Practices (ACIP) and the American Academy of Family Physicians (AAFP), *Morb Mortal Wkly Rep* 51(RR02):1-36, 2002.

CHAPTER 72

Weight Management

Drug Names

Class	Subclass	Generic Name	Trade Name
Anorexiants	Mixed neurotransmitter reuptake inhibitor	sibutramine	Meridia
	Sympathomimetic	phentermine	Adipex-P, Ionamin
Lipase inhibitors		orlistat	Xenical

General Uses

Indications

Major advances have recently been made in medications for weight loss. In the past, dexfenfluramine and fenfluramine received great attention, but their association with primary pulmonary hypertension and heart valve problems led to their removal from the market. Because of this negative experience, all weight loss products should be used with caution. Sibutramine and orlistat currently are the dominant products used in helping patients lose weight. Phentermine can be used in the short term only.

This chapter incorporates the new obesity guidelines issued in 2003 from the National Heart, Lung, and Blood Institute at NIH.

DISEASE PROCESS

Pathophysiology

Obesity involves both genetic and environmental factors. There is a segment of the population that is genetically predisposed to obesity. Another segment of the population succumbs to adverse environmental conditions: fast food, sedentary jobs, and few opportunities to exercise. These individuals phenotypically express obesity.

Taking in more calories than are expended causes obesity. Overweight individuals tend to eat too many grams of fat, as well as consuming too many calories. Although decreasing fat intake is important in reducing cardiovascular risk factors and lowering cholesterol, it is calories that really count with weight gain.

An individual's energy expenditure must be closely examined. This is divided into three categories. First, resting energy expenditure is what the body consumes just resting and that is about 60% of energy used in a day. This depends on the amount of lean body mass and age. Resting energy goes down with age and up with lean body mass. A person who has more muscle will have higher resting energy expenditure. It is very difficult to change this level to any significant degree. However, it does determine most of the energy that a person burns.

The second category of energy expenditure is the exercise or activity energy expenditure. This is about 30% of the energy burned and is highly variable. People who fidget burn about 600 more calories a day than the sedentary bradykinetic individual. Thus it is clear that patients who wish to lose weight should be more physically active.

The third category of energy expenditure comes from the thermic effect of food and is responsible for about 10% of the energy expenditure. There are small decreases in obese individuals in their thermic-effect-of-food rates, but this does not explain the obese state.

Adipose tissue in the body is used primarily to store energy in the form of triglyceride. During a famine, or during periods of time when food is not eaten, the adipose tissue becomes a reservoir to store what is needed to help the individual survive. The store of triglycerides remains available to be broken down into fatty acids to use as energy. There is a lot of interest in trying to understand if obese individuals are more efficient at storing triglycerides than lean people. It has been observed that an obese person who takes in 100 g fat might be more likely to deposit that as adipose tissue, whereas a lean person might oxidize it and burn it off as heat.

In discussing obesity at the cellular level two factors must be considered: (1) how many fat cells does the individual have and (2) to what extent are these fat cells filled with fat. To answer these questions, it is important to understand that there are two compartments for fat storage: the fat cells and the stromal vascular or supporting connecting tissue. Fat cells start out as preadipocytes. These are fibroblast-like cells that do not respond to insulin, and they do not store fat. They are small, spindle-like cells that are within the fat cell that divide and can turn into fat cells with the excess stimulation of nutrients. These fat cells can also enlarge and make huge fat cells. There is a limit to how stretched these fat storage cells can become. After fat cells reach a certain level, they recruit more preadipocytes to make more fat cells.

In determining how many fat cells an individual has, there are two critical times in life when many preadipocytes are made and thus the person will develop a larger pool of fat cells for the body to use. One time is age 2, and the second is at puberty. An individual who becomes obese at 2 or at puberty has a bigger supply of precursor cells and thus may be more resistant to long-term weight loss. It is not correct to say that at puberty people have all the fat cells they will ever have and will die with that number. People can accumulate fat cells throughout life if they give in to the environmental stimulus, that is, overeating. Some metabolic diseases also contribute to the development of more fat cells.

The reason why it is very difficult to lose weight, once an individual has formed extra fat cells, is that fat cells do not divide once they are differentiated, but they also do not die. There is a process called *programmed cell death,* or *apoptosis,* that cells go through to get rid of excess cells. But adipocytes, as a rule, do not go through apoptosis and die; they are around for life. Obesity needs to be prevented because once the individual has fat, it is very difficult to lose. Even if fat cells contain no fat, they remain prepared and waiting to take up more triglycerides.

Obesity and adipose tissue mass are tightly regulated. Patients complain, "I just get so hungry, I start eating again, and then I gain weight back." If individuals have a certain mass of adipose tissue, the body does whatever possible to defend that mass. As soon as patients start reducing adipose tissue in the form of diet and exercise, the body thinks it is starving, so it makes these individuals hungry. Many physiologic mechanisms kick in. Neuropeptides in the brain and enzymes in the lining of the stomach help accomplish this. They stimulate the body to say it is hungry and to eat. All of these factor interactions in brain, environment, and adipose tissue try to work to restore fat mass to its previous level.

Hazards of Obesity

Obesity, or being overweight, is associated with increased morbidity and mortality. Obesity is an independent risk factor for coronary heart disease. Hypertension and diabetes mellitus are more difficult to control in the obese patient. The patient is at increased risk for CAD, CHF, stroke, gallbladder disease, osteoarthritis, and sleep apnea or other respiratory problems. Levels of triglycerides, total serum cholesterol, and low-density lipoprotein (LDL) are elevated and levels of high-density lipoprotein (HDL) are decreased. Obesity is associated with increased risk of certain cancers such as endometrial, breast, colon, and prostate. Obesity is associated with gynecologic problems such as complications of pregnancy, menstrual irregularities, hirsutism, and stress incontinence. In addition, patients who are obese are at increased risk for depression and are higher surgical risks.

THE DISEASE

Obesity is an excess of body fat relative to lean body mass. *Overweight* is defined as body mass index (BMI) of 25 to 29.9 kg/m^2. *Obesity* is defined as a BMI of 30 kg/m^2 or more according to the *Clinical Guidelines on the Identification, Evaluation, and Treatment of Overweight and Obesity in Adults* published by the National Heart, Lung, and Blood Institute (NHLBI) in June 1998. These guidelines provide the basic information underlying the diagnosis and management of obesity and should be consulted by all clinicians. (See list of resources at the end of the chapter to obtain copies using the Internet.)

Obesity is increasing in prevalence, both in this country and throughout the world in all segments of the population. The prevalence of obesity increases with age. In the United States, obesity is more prevalent in some minority groups and in patients with lower incomes and less education.

The economic costs associated with people who are overweight or obese are tremendous. The total cost attributable to obesity was over $99 billion in 1995. One half of these costs were direct medical costs from diseases attributed to obesity. The indirect costs represent the lost productivity due to obesity and are similar to those of smoking. Because obesity is associated with the development of other chronic diseases such as diabetes, coronary heart disease, and arthritis, additional indirect costs associated with obesity increase dramatically. Thus costs are both individual and societal.

Assessment

The most useful estimate of body fat is the BMI. The BMI is a powerful indicator of health risk that should be included in the comprehensive evaluation of any patient.

When considering patients for a weight reduction program, assess their BMI, weight, waist circumference, and overall risk status and their motivation to lose weight.

The BMI is a number measured by dividing the weight in kilograms by the height in meters squared. The easiest way for most individuals to do the calculation is to multiply 704.5 by the patient's weight in pounds. Divide that number by the patient's height in inches multiplied by itself. There are conversion charts easily available.

$$\text{BMI} = 704.5 \times \text{Weight in pounds}/(\text{Height in inches})^2$$

The normal BMI is considered to be 19 to 24.9 kg/m^2. By way of reference, the average fashion model has a BMI of about 16.5. Tiger Woods has a BMI of 21.

Persons with a BMI of 20 to 25 have the lowest mortality. For the most part, increasing BMI is associated with increasing mortality. If the BMI is less than 25, the health risk is minimal. Patients with BMI above 27 are in the moderate range; above 40 it is more likely that they will develop diabetes or some other obesity-related condition. Obese geriatric patients have less upper and lower body function. The incidence of obesity does not change, but the functional status changes in the geriatric population.

In individuals who are overweight, where the fat is located is also an important consideration. Waist circumference is an independent predictor of risk factors and morbidity and is correlated to abdominal fat content. Men at high risk have a waist greater than 102 cm (40 in). Women at high risk have a waist greater than 88 cm (35 in). The Nurses' Health Study has documented that women whose waist measurement is 38 inches or more have 3 times the risk of heart disease as do women whose waists measure 28 inches or less. Women who are apple-shaped, with a high waist-to-hip ratio, have a greater risk of heart disease than do pear-shaped women, whose weight is concentrated in their hips and thighs. A large waist correlates with the metabolic syndrome.

The metabolic syndrome, formerly known as syndrome X, has been recognized as an important factor in obese patients as a risk factor for diabetes and cardiovascular disease. Fat cells release substances such as free fatty acids, complement D and cytokines (which promote inflammation), prothrombic agents, and angiotensinogen. Free fatty acids increase insulin resistance. This raises insulin levels. Increased insulin leads to increased sodium reabsorption leading to increased blood pressure. Insulin resistance leads to increased blood sugar and diabetes mellitus. Free fatty acids lead to increased lipids with raises the risk of CAD.

Metabolic syndrome must have three or more of the following:

Abdominal fat (waist circumference)	35 inches (men, 40)
Insulin resistance (fasting sugar)	≥110 mg/dL
Triglycerides	≥150 mg/dL
HDL cholesterol	<50 (men, 40)
High blood pressure	≥135/85 mm Hg

Evaluation for overall risk status looks at other conditions that put the patient at increased risk from obesity or overweight. These include cardiovascular risk factors, CAD, atherosclerosis, diabetes mellitus (DM), sleep apnea, osteoarthritis, gallstones, physical inactivity, and high levels of serum triglycerides. Their presence increases the importance of weight reduction for that patient.

Patient motivation is essential to weight loss success. The clinician must evaluate the patient's reasons and motivation for weight loss, previous weight loss attempts, the patient's understanding of the problem, physical activity, diet, and financial constraints.

DRUG ACTION AND EFFECTS

Anorexiants are indirect-acting sympathomimetic amines. They are thought to provide a direct stimulant effect on the satiety center in the hypothalamus. The different anorexiants act through different pathways.

Sibutramine is from a new class of reuptake inhibitors that increases levels of serotonin and norepinephrine in the brain (SNRI). Sibutramine inhibits the reuptake of norepinephrine, serotonin, and dopamine. Serotonin works in the hypothalamus, the center that regulates food intake. Sibutramine increases serotonins, reduces appetite, and increases satiety. Patients are less hungry, and they get full faster. Lower levels of serotonin are also associated with depression, which may explain why people eat to improve their mood. A desirable side effect of sibutramine is reduced depression.

Phentermine acts by modulating central norepinephrine and dopamine receptors through the promotion of catecholamine release.

Orlistat works by a completely different mechanism. Orlistat blocks about 30% of fat absorption in the GI tract. It acts locally and is minimally absorbed. The GI tract enzyme, lipase, together with a colipase, breaks down fat molecules before they can be absorbed. Orlistat interferes with lipase. It works in the jejunum to inhibit pancreatic lipase.

DRUG TREATMENT PRINCIPLES

The treatment goals in working with the overweight or obese individual are to (1) prevent further weight gain, (2) reduce body weight, and (3) maintain a lower body weight over the long term. An initial goal is to reduce body weight by about 10% from baseline. A reasonable time frame for this loss is 6 months. A treatment algorithm from the NHLBI addresses the management of patients who are obese or overweight. A stepped-care model has also been devised by Shape Up America, C. Everett Koop's group, and a new group called the American Obesity Association.

Nonpharmacologic Treatment

Helping patients to lose weight begins with an assessment of the patient's motivation to lose weight. Even with patients who are very motivated, the clinician must spend time to understand their concerns and tailor a program to fit their situation. Individuals who have always been 100 lbs or more overweight may never be able to get to their ideal body weight. They will also not lose weight at the rate at which they would desire. Helping them develop realistic expectations is foundational to success.

How do you determine what is an appropriate weight for an individual? The answer to this question has changed over the years. The normal weight chart developed from actuarial data of the Metropolitan Life Insurance Company was the standard used for years. These charts have been modified over time to reflect heavier weights due to better nutrition and changing views of what a "normal" person weighs. National guidelines stipulate that the BMI is a better indication of obesity than weight; therefore, many clinicians now use the weight needed for a normal BMI as the goal.

It is important to set specific goals. An overall target goal and a time period in which to accomplish the goal are helpful. More meaningful for both monitoring and motivational purposes are monthly goals of a 2- to 4-lb weight loss. A successful strategy included in many weight loss programs is a system of built-in rewards the patients give themselves when they reach the goal: for example, new haircuts, cosmetic makeovers. Some patients may do better meeting their goals through an organized program such as Weight Watchers; others do better alone.

The foundation of any successful weight loss regimen includes reduction of caloric intake and increase in physical exercise. Without both of these, weight loss is generally transient. Medications may be helpful in both foundational areas through suppressing appetite and also helping keep energy levels high so that the patient feels like exercising.

Diet. Lowering calorie intake every day will result in a reasonable, slow, steady weight loss. There are several valid methods for arriving at the proper dietary prescription for an individual.

The total daily allotment of calories is based on the requirements of the patient and depends on his or her nutritional status when the diet is instituted and on the estimate of daily activity. During their peak growth period, active adolescent boys need 3100 to 3600 cal/day and adolescent girls 2400 to 2700 cal/day. Children generally require 1000 cal/day plus an additional 100 calories for every year of age. Accordingly, a 10-year-old child should receive approximately 2000 calories daily.

A general rule of thumb is that it takes approximately 10 calories to support each pound of weight. For example a 150-lb woman is probably eating 1500 calories. To lose weight the patient must decrease their intake below the level needed to maintain their weight. The patient must decrease their daily intake by 500 calories for each pound they wish to lose weekly. Weight loss of about 1 to 2 lb/week commonly will occur for up to 6 months. After 6 months, the rate of weight loss will plateau. This is because the patient has a lower energy expenditure at the lower weight. Once a patient has plateaued, evaluate if he or she needs to lose more weight. If so, reevaluation of diet and exercise is required. The patient must further decrease calories and/or increase physical activity.

Rapid weight loss is not advisable. Studies have shown that regaining weight almost always follows rapid weight reduction. There is also increased risk for gallstones and electrolyte abnormalities when weight loss is excessive.

Once the patient has reached a weight loss goal, the goal changes to weight maintenance at the lower weight. It is important to continue to monitor these patients to assist them in staying at the lower weight.

Exercise. An increase in physical activity is the second essential component of weight reduction. Exercise leads to increased expenditure of energy, inhibits food intake, and reduces overall CAD risk. Efforts to lose weight by exercise alone without calorie reduction usually produces a 2% to 3% weight decrease. Exercise may be useful in decreasing abdominal fat in addition to weight. A regular exercise program such as walking is something almost every patient can tolerate, and patients can integrate more activity into their lives by walking up stairs, parking at the far end of the lot, and so on.

Behavior. To achieve long-term weight loss, the patient must change basic eating and activity patterns. Specific strategies include keeping a food diary, stress management, stimulus control (avoid situations that precipitate overeating), problem solving (self-correcting problems), contingency management, cognitive restructuring (setting realistic goals), and social support.

These three components of weight reduction (i.e., treatment diet, exercise, and behavior therapy) work best when used together under the supervision of a health care provider.

Pharmacologic Treatment

Critical decisions to be made concern whether it is appropriate to use pharmacologic therapy and, if so, whether the patient has any conditions that would be contraindications to these products. Drugs seem to help the patient lose 5 to 20 lbs, or up to 10% of excess weight, although a few patients will lose larger amounts. Weight-loss drugs should be used only for patients who are at increased medical risk because of their weight and should not be used for "cosmetic" weight loss. The NHLBI guidelines state that these drugs may be useful for a patient with a BMI of 30 or more with no concomitant obesity-related risk factors or diseases or for a patient with a BMI of 27 or more with concomitant obesity-related risk factors or diseases.

Medications work by helping the patient stay on a diet and exercise plan. The drug will not cause weight loss if the patient continues to eat at the same level. Most of the weight loss will occur in the first 6 months of treatment with the drug. If the patient does not respond within the first month of therapy, the likelihood of response is very low.

Sibutramine is the only anorexiant currently available for long-term use. It is generally used for no more than 6 months. It should be stopped after 1 month if it is not effective. Safety and efficacy have not been determined beyond 2 years at this time. It can help with modest weight loss and help keep weight off. Sibutramine can cause increases in blood pressure and pulse. People with a history of high blood pressure, CAD, CHF, arrhythmias, or stroke should not take this medication, and blood pressure should be monitored regularly.

Phentermine is used as a short-term adjunct in weight reduction. It should not be used for longer than a few weeks. It may be tried if sibutramine is not effective. However, there are significant serious risks in its use.

Orlistat (Xenical) acts to increase fecal fat excretion. The extent of drug activity may be determined by measuring the amount of fat in the stool. The maximum amount of fat excretion is around 25% to 30%. (If 100 g of fat is consumed in a day, 30 g will end up in the stool.) Once the medication is stopped, fecal fat excretion goes back down to normal.

The overall effectiveness of orlistat shows that it is about as effective, or perhaps a little less effective, as the sympathomimetics. In a short-term study, there was about a 10% reduction in initial weight. In long-term studies, most of the weight loss occurred in the first months and was maintained for up to 2 years.

Orlistat is associated with irritating GI side effects: soft liquid stools and oil in the stool. Some people had oily spotting, necessitating the use of minipads. These symptoms appear to be dose dependent. Long-term use might also be associated with development of vitamin deficits. Levels of vitamin D and beta carotene both decreased 20% to 24%, but they remained within the normal range. Fat-soluble vitamin supplementation may be required (taken at a different time than orlistat).

There are also many herbal and OTC products advertised to help with weight loss that the patient may ask about. The lay literature is filled with information about fat substitutes such as Olestrin (currently limited to snack foods). Patients might also ask about medications derived from the exoskeletons of shrimp and lobsters. These products absorb fat and have been used for the cleanup of oil spills. These fat absorbers are available in some health food stores. There are no data in the professional literature on these products. OTC products used for weight loss has often contained ephedrine, which was available in herbal form. Ephedrine can be very dangerous, causing stokes, headache, tachycardia, hypertension, and catecholamine-like symptoms: restlessness, dry mouth, insomnia, fatigue, and other central nervous system effects. Ephedrine use should be discouraged. Adverse effects from ephedrine have caused the FDA to remove this product from most preparations.

Surgery

Surgery is having an increasingly larger place in the treatment of extremely obese individuals with comorbid problems. There are two surgical procedures that are not associated with higher morbidity and mortality as were the operations of earlier years. The first is the vertical banded gastroplasty, which makes a smaller stomach by use of a ring or band that the food has to pass through. This restrictive procedure leads to about a 50% reduction in excess weight. A 350-pound person could lose 50% of excess weight and maintain it over time with this procedure. Mortality is about 1% to 1.5%. The second procedure is the Ruin-Wey gastroplasty, which reconnects the small bowel to the stomach. Patients requiring surgical intervention should find a specialist interested in obesity.

For patients who have gastric surgery, the clinician may need to deal with surgically created malabsorption or physical restriction. Regurgitation is a significant problem with restriction. People have high intolerance to food; they will need to make major changes in diet. Malabsorption syndromes may lead to micronutrient or macronutrient deficiency, anemias, protein malnutrition, dumping syndrome, etc. Gastric leaking may also be a problem at anastomosis or banding, which leads to peritonitis. These patients need medical and psychologic monitoring.

Evaluating Patients Who Have Taken dexfenfluramine or fenfluramine

Dexfenfluramine (Redux) and fenfluramine (Pondimin) were effective anorexiants that acted centrally to suppress appetite. They were the first drugs successfully associated with weight loss, and the public demand for them was enormous. Clinicians and patients began using fenfluramine in association with phentermine, the "phen-fen" regimen. The combination was very effective in depressing appetite; however, the medications were not intended to be used together.

Phen-fen was voluntarily taken off the market because of growing complaints of pulmonary hypertension and valvular heart disease in patients who had used the products. Approximately 5% to 25% of the patients using the combination developed valvular heart disease.

Patients with pulmonary hypertension or valvular disease exhibit the following signs and symptoms: dyspnea, shortness of breath (SOB), decrease in exercise tolerance, angina, syncope, and lower extremity edema. If the patient has symptoms, the patient should be referred to a cardiologist. It is a wise precaution to have all patients who took these drugs to have an echocardiogram, perhaps repeating the study in asymptomatic people within 6 months to 1 year after the first echocardiogram.

HOW TO MONITOR

- Monitor the patient's progress at least monthly. Initially the patient may benefit from weekly assessments. Weight should be measured monthly.
- *sibutramine:* Monitor blood pressure periodically

PATIENT VARIABLES

Geriatrics

- *sibutramine, phentermine:* Use with caution in the elderly because of the possibility of reduced hepatic or cardiac function.
- *orlistat:* Monitor nutritional status.

Pediatrics

- *Do not use sibutramine* (under age 16), *phentermine, or orlistat;* safety and efficacy have not been established.

Pregnancy

- *Category B:* orlistat, not recommended
- *Category C:* sibutramine
- *Category X:* phentermine
- Sibutramine has caused fertility impairment in rats at high doses.

Lactation

- sibutramine, phentermine, orlistat not recommended.

PATIENT EDUCATION

sibutramine

- Patient must keep regular monthly follow-up visits.
- Notify the primary care provider if a rash or hives develops.
- Avoid taking any OTC cold preparations that may contain decongestants.
- Blood pressure must be monitored closely.

phentermine

- The drug may cause insomnia; avoid taking the medication late in the day.
- Avoid alcohol or other CNS active drugs and anorectic agents.
- Notify primary care provider if the patient experiences palpitations, nervousness, or dizziness.
- The drug may cause dry mouth and constipation.
- It also may produce dizziness or blurred vision, which may interfere with driving or performing other tasks requiring alertness.
- Take on an empty stomach.

orlistat

- Take with a meal.
- Take multiple vitamins at a different time from taking orlistat.
- May cause leakage of stool.

Specific Drugs

ANOREXIANTS

sibutramine (Meridia)

Contraindications

- MAOIs
- Hypersensitivity
- Anorexia nervosa
- Other centrally acting appetite suppressant drugs

Warnings

- Sibutramine substantially increased blood pressure in some patients. Regular monitoring of blood pressure is required when prescribing this product.
- Use caution with prescribing sibutramine with other agents that may raise blood pressure or heart rate, including decongestants, cough, cold, and allergy medication that contain agents such as ephedrine or pseudoephedrine.

- Serotonin syndrome is rare but serious constellation of symptoms. It may occur especially if the patient is taking sibutramine along with an SSRI or triptans for migraine, certain opioids, or tryptophan. Symptoms include excitement, hypomania, restlessness, loss of consciousness, confusion, myoclonus, tremor, ataxia, and dysarthria. This requires emergency medical attention.
- Treatment with sibutramine has been associated with increases in heart rate or blood pressure. Do not use in patients with a history of CAD, CHF, arrhythmias, or stroke.
- *Glaucoma:* because sibutramine can cause mydriasis, use with caution in patients with narrow-angle glaucoma.
- Exclude organic causes of obesity before prescribing sibutramine.
- *Renal/hepatic function impairment:* do not use in patients with severe renal impairment or severe hepatic dysfunction.

Precautions

- *Abuse/physical and psychologic dependence:* evaluate patient for history of drug abuse and follow closely for signs of misuse or abuse (development of tolerance, incremental increase of doses, drug-seeking behavior).
- *Primary pulmonary hypertension (PPH):* certain centrally acting weight loss agents that cause release of serotonin have been associated with PPH, a rare but lethal disease. No cases of PPH have been reported with sibutramine. However, it is not known whether or not sibutramine may cause this disease.
- *Seizures* were reported in less than 0.1% of patients. Use with caution in patients with a history of seizures.
- *Gallstones:* weight loss can precipitate or exacerbate gallstone formation.
- *Interference with cognitive and motor performance:* although sibutramine did not affect psychomotor or cognitive performance, any CNS active drug has the potential to impair judgment, thinking, or motor skills.

Pharmacokinetics. See Table 72-1.

Adverse Effects. See Table 72-2.

Drug Interactions. See Table 72-3. The product is extensively metabolized by the cytochrome P450 3A4 system.

Dosage and Administration

- Take once a day without regard to meals.
- Initial dose is 10 mg po qd; may be increased to 15 mg po qd.

phentermine (Fastin, Ionamin)

Contraindications

- Advanced arteriosclerosis, symptomatic cardiovascular disease, moderate-to-severe hypertension, hyperthyroidism, known hypersensitivity to the sympathomimetic amines, or glaucoma, highly nervous or agitated states, history of drug abuse, during or within 14 days following MAOIs, and coadministration with other CNS stimulants.

Warnings

- Indicated for short-term use only. Tolerance to the anorexic effect usually develops within a few weeks. When this occurs, the recommended dose should not be exceeded in an attempt to increase the effect; rather, the drug should be discontinued.

PPH is a rare, frequently fatal disease of the lungs that has been reported in chemically related anorexiants. Monitor closely for development of symptoms.

- Valvular heart disease has also been reported in chemically related anorexiants. Monitor closely for development of symptoms

Precautions

- Psychologic disturbances have occurred in patients who received an anorectic agent together with a restrictive diet.
- *Cardiovascular disease:* exercise caution in patients with even mild hypertension.
- The least amount feasible should be prescribed or dispensed at one time to minimize the possibility of overdosage.
- Insulin requirements in DM may be altered.
- These drugs are chemically and pharmacologically related to the amphetamines and have abuse potential. Intense psychological dependence and severe social dysfunction may occur. If this occurs, gradually reduce the dosage to avoid withdrawal symptoms (extreme fatigue, sleep EEG changes, mental depression). Chronic intoxication is manifested by severe dermatoses, marked insomnia, irritability, hyperactivity, and personality changes and psychosis.
- The drug may impair the ability of the patient to engage in potentially hazardous activities such as operating machinery or driving a motor vehicle.

Adverse Effects. The adverse effects can be serious (see Table 72-2).

TABLE 72-1 Pharmacokinetics

Drug	Absorption	Drug Availability (after first pass)	Time to Peak Concentration	Half-Life	Protein Bound	Metabolism	Excretion
sibutramine	Rapid, 77%	Metabolized to active form	3-4 hr	14-16 hr	95%	Liver 3A4	Renal, 85%
phentermine							Renal
orlistat	Minimal		8 hr		99%	In GI wall	Feces

TABLE 72-2 Adverse Reactions by Body System: Weight Loss Agents

Body System	sibutramine	phentermine	orlistat
Skin, appendages	Rash, sweating	Hair loss, excessive sweating, ecchymosis, flushing	
Hypersensitivity		Urticaria, rash, erythema	
Respiratory	Rhinitis, pharyngitis	Dyspnea	
Cardiovascular	Tachycardia, vasodilation, migraine, hypertension, palpitation	Palpitations, tachycardia, arrhythmias, including ventricular, precordial pain, PPH, valvular disease, ↑ BP	
GI	Anorexia, constipation, increased appetite, nausea, dyspepsia, dry mouth	Dry mouth, nausea, vomiting, abdominal discomfort, diarrhea, GI disturbances, constipation, stomach pain	Oily spotting, flatus with discharge, fecal urgency, fatty/oily stool, oily evacuation, increased defecation, fecal incontinence, abd pain, gingival disorder, nausea, rectal discomfort
Hemic and lymphatic		Bone marrow depression, agranulocytosis, leukopenia	
Musculoskeletal	Arthralgia, myalgia	Muscle pain	
Nervous system	Headache, insomnia, dizziness, nervousness, anxiety, depression, paresthesia, somnolence, CNS stimulation, emotion lability	Malaise, overstimulation, CVA, nervousness, restlessness, dizziness, insomnia, anxiety, euphoria, drowsiness, depression, agitation, dysphoria, dyskinesia, tremor, headache, psychosis, agitation, jitteriness, depression following withdrawal	
Special senses	Taste perversion	Unpleasant taste, mydriasis, blurred vision	
Genitourinary	Dysmenorrhea	Dysuria, polyuria, urinary frequency, impotence, menstrual upset, gynecomastia, changes in libido	Menstrual irregularity

BP, Blood pressure; *CNS*, central nervous system; *CVA*, cerebrovascular accident; *GI*, gastrointestinal; *PPH*, primary pulmonary hypertension.

TABLE 72-3 Drug Interactions: Weight Loss Agents

Medications	Acts on Other Drugs	Other Drugs	Act on Weight Loss Agents
sibutramine	↑ Other agents that ↑ BP, MAOIs, SSRIs, ergot, lithium, opioids, triptans, tryptophan	alcohol	↑ sibutramine
		cimetidine, erythromycin, ketoconazole	↓↑ sibutramine
phentermine	↓ guanethidine ↑ TCAs	MAOIs	↑ phentermine
orlistat	↑ pravastatin ↓ Fat-soluble vitamins ↑↓ cyclosporine, warfarin		

BP, Blood pressure; *MAOIs*, monoamine oxidase inhibitors; *SSRIs*, selective serotonin-reuptake inhibitors; *TCAs*, tricyclic antidepressants.

Dosage and Administration

- A dose of 30 mg daily has been found to be adequate in appetite suppression for 12 to 14 hours.
- Take 8 mg three times daily, one-half hour before meals, or 16 to 37.5 mg as a single dose before breakfast or 10 to 14 hours before retiring.

LIPASE INHIBITORS

orlistat (Xenical)

Contraindications

- Chronic malabsorption syndrome
- Cholestasis
- Hypersensitivity

Warnings. Organic causes of obesity should be excluded before prescribing orlistat.

Precautions

- *Diet:* Advise patients to adhere to dietary guidelines.
- GI adverse reactions may increase when orlistat is taken with a diet high in fat.
- Patients should take a multiple vitamin to ensure adequate nutrition because orlistat reduces the absorption of some fat-soluble vitamins and beta-carotene. Do not take at the same time as orlistat.
- Some patients may develop increased levels of urinary oxalate with treatment.
- Diabetic patients with weight loss may improve metabolic control, which might require a reduction in oral hypoglycemic medication.
- As with any weight loss agent, the potential exists for misuse of orlistat, especially with anorexia nervosa or bulimia.

Overdosage. Single doses of 800 mg and multiple doses of up to 400 mg tid for 15 days have caused no significant adverse reactions.

Dosage and Administration. Take 1 tablet po tid with meals.

RESOURCES FOR PATIENTS AND PROVIDERS

American Dietetic Association, www.eatright.org.

American Obesity Association, www.obesity.org.

NIDDK (National Institute of Diabetes and Digestive and Kidney Diseases, www.niddk.gov.

NHLBI (National Heart Lung and Blood Institute) Obesity Guidelines (NIH), www.nhlbi.nih.gov/guidelines/obesity.

Shape that Body, www.shapethatbody.com

Excellent material for weight reduction.

BIBLIOGRAPHY

Apfelbaum M: Maintenance of weight loss after a very low calorie diet: a randomized blinded trail of the efficacy and tolerability of sibutramine, *Am J Med* 106:179-184, 1999.

Davidson MH et al: Weight control and risk factor reduction in obese subjects treated for 2 years with orlistat, *JAMA* 281:235-242, 1999.

Early JL et al: Treatment strategies for weight management in primary care, *Cardiol Rev* 17:suppl, 2000.

Ludwig DS: The glycemic index: physiological mechanisms relating to obesity, diabetes, and cardiovascular disease, *JAMA* 287:21414-2423, 2002.

Nawaz H, Katz DL: American College of Preventive Medicine Practice Policy statement. Weight management counseling of overweight adults, *Am J Prev Med* 21:73-78, 2001.

Sachiko T et al: Dietary protein and weight reduction. A statement for healthcare professionals from the Nutrition Committee of the Council on Nutrition, Physical Activity, and Metabolism of the American Heart Association, *Circulation* 104:1869-1874, 2001.

CHAPTER 73

Smoking Cessation

Drug Names

Class	Generic Name	Trade Name	Formulation
Nicotine replacement therapy	nicotine polacrilex	Nicorette	Gum
	nicotine	Nicoderm CQ	Transdermal
		Habitrol	Transdermal
		Nicotrol	Transdermal
		Prostep	Transdermal
		Nicotrol NS	Nasal spray
		Nicotrol inhaler	Oral inhaler
		Commit	Lozenge
Antidepressant	bupropion	Zyban, Wellbutrin	Tablet

General Uses

Many chemicals have been developed to help people stop smoking. In current use are the nicotine replacement therapy (NRT) products and bupropion (Zyban, Wellbutrin). This chapter discusses methods for assisting the patient to stop smoking. The only drugs that are discussed in detail in this chapter are the NRT products because bupropion is discussed in Chapter 49. Many NRTs are now available over-the-counter (OTC), but the patient still benefits from professional guidance on how to use these products.

DISEASE PROCESS

Tobacco use is the single most preventable cause of death and disease in the United States. Smoking is strongly correlated to age. An estimated 27.9% of those aged 18 to 24 smoke, followed by 27.3% of those aged 25 to 44, 23.3% of those aged 45 to 64, and only 10.5% of people who are 65 or older. (The relatively low number of older smokers may be due to the fact that many smokers die prematurely as a result of their smoking.) There is an inverse relationship with increased years of education.

Smoking has been associated with greater than 420,000 deaths annually, causing risk for cancer of the lung, larynx, and esophagus and others. Cigarette smoking is associated with coronary artery disease/myocardial infarction, chronic obstructive pulmonary disease (COPD), peripheral artery disease, and cerebral vascular disease. Cancer and respiratory diseases have also been associated with passive (environmental) smoking. Nicotine and other tobacco-related components (tar and aromatic hydrocarbons) are probable causative factors for both the psychologic and pathologic sequelae of smoking. Individuals, especially children, subjected to passive smoke have a higher risk for developing asthma. Current research suggests that children already in danger of developing heart disease because of high cholesterol blood levels face a triple jeopardy if they live in smoke-filled homes, because the passive smoke lowers by about 10% the level of the child's high-density lipoprotein (HDL), or the good cholesterol that protects against heart attacks.

Primary care is an ideal setting in which to institute smoking cessation measures. Most smokers see a primary care provider each year. The provider should screen all patients for smoking behaviors as the "fifth vital sign" and recommend that all patients stop smoking. Research suggests that many health care providers fail to take advantage of opportunities to recommend that the patient stop smoking. Primary care clinicians should especially be knowledgeable about the components of successful smoking cessation programs.

DRUG ACTION AND EFFECTS

Nicotine is rapidly absorbed across the pulmonary capillary membrane and delivered to the brain in high concentration within seconds of inhalation. The typical smoker delivers 200 to 300 boluses of the addictive drug nicotine to the brain each day.

Nicotine increases heart rate, elevates blood pressure, and causes peripheral vasoconstriction. It enhances platelet aggregateability and fibrinogen levels. It decreases nitric oxide and blunts its vasodilatory effects. It increases carbon monoxide levels, which reduces oxygen delivery to the myocardium. Nicotine activates the sympathetic nervous system and can induce coronary vasospasm. It has been shown that smokers may lose their cognitive abilities, such as remembering, thinking, or perceiving, more rapidly than elderly nonsmokers.

Cigarette smoking has been found to be particularly hazardous to those who already have some pathologic condition. The risk of vasospasm following subarachnoid hemorrhage is increased in smokers. Cigarette smoking exaggerates risk factors for cardiovascular disease by significantly increasing a protein known as thromboglobulin that increases the activity and clotting functions of platelets in hypertensive smoking patients. Smoking also increases epinephrine, stimulating the heart and blood pressure in the hypertensive smoking patient.

Even patients who suffer the results of smoking continue to engage in the behavior. For smokers who undergo angioplasty or coronary artery bypass surgery, almost three in five smokers continue to smoke after their procedure.

Nicotine, the chief alkaloid in tobacco products, binds stereoselectively to acetylcholine receptors at the autonomic ganglia, in the adrenal medulla, at neuromuscular junctions, and in the brain. Two types of CNS effects are believed to be the basis of nicotine's positively reinforcing properties: a simulating effect (exerted mainly in the cortex via the locus ceruleus), which produces increased alertness and cognitive performance; and a reward effect via the "pleasure system" in the brain in the limbic system. At low doses, the stimulant effects predominate, whereas at high doses, the reward effects predominate.

Regular nicotine consumption through smoking is associated with neuroadaptation of nicotinic receptors, resulting in increasing numbers of receptors and the development of tolerance and drug dependence. Symptoms from abrupt withdrawal include irritability, restlessness, anxiety, difficulty concentrating, lethargy, depression, increased appetite, weight gain, and minor somatic complaints (headache, myalgia, constipation, fatigue). These symptoms may be reduced by using nicotine-containing smoking deterrents, which produce lower nicotine plasma concentrations (approximately 3 to 17 ng/ml) than those achieved through smoking (approximately 20 to 50 ng/ml).

DRUG TREATMENT PRINCIPLES

Nicotine replacement products are effective as an aid in smoking cessation and for the relief of nicotine withdrawal symptoms and may be used as part of a comprehensive behavioral smoking-cessation program.

Table 73-1 lists actions and strategies for the primary care clinician from the Agency for Health Care Policy and Research (AHCPR) guidelines. Current research from the National Ambulatory Medical Care Surveys of 1991 through 1995 has documented that physicians reported counseling patients about smoking or prescribing nicotine replacement far less than called for by current practice guidelines, thus missing many opportunities to help their patients quit smoking.

Prevention and Early Intervention

With each visit to a health care provider, it is critical to ask patients if they smoke. If patients do not smoke, praise them for their wisdom and encourage them not to start. This is very important in children and adolescents. Emphasize the immediate effects of tobacco, such as bad breath, stains on the fingers and teeth, reduced exercise performance, and dry skin and hair. Patients are not fully addicted for 3 years after starting to smoke, so this is the time to encourage them to stop.

NRTs reduce the physical effects from nicotine withdrawal but do not address the psychologic aspects of smoking cessation. Therefore smoking deterrents are usually efficacious only when used in conjunction with a comprehensive behavioral modification program.

Components of Smoking Cessation

With all patients who do smoke, the provider should assess their willingness to attempt to quit (Figure 73-1). If they are unwilling or unready to quit, the provider should focus on motivational issues. The negative consequences of smoking should also be emphasized. Patients are often not influenced by remote events such as COPD or lung cancer but may be motivated by immediate effects such as fewer and milder respiratory infections or asthma. They may particularly respond to suggestions they are hurting their family, particularly small or unborn children. Positive consequences of stopping smoking should also be discussed, such as saving money, better tasting food, and feeling better physically.

Once the patient is ready to try to quit, the provider should help the patient plan to quit and monitor his or her progress. The patient should be offered specific help on how to quit successfully. Brief interventions are often still successful.

Most patients have tried unsuccessfully to quit. They should be encouraged to try again by reminding patients that most people who succeed in stopping smoking make several attempts before their final successful attempt. Each attempt should not be seen as a failure but as a trial for the next attempt. They should try to find out what went wrong the last time they tried and how they can plan to avoid the problem situation.

Nonpharmacologic therapy is the mainstay of therapy. How to encourage the patient to explore these strategies is the first critical treatment decision. Patients should have a realistic idea about the difficulty of smoking cessation. They will probably experience withdrawal symptoms such as craving, irritability, restlessness, and increased appetite. With a clear understanding of the difficulties, the patient should set a realistic quit date.

Find out why the patient uses nicotine. Is it for stimulation, handling, pleasure, stress reduction, craving, or habit? The patient should then develop specific strategies to cope with their reasons for smoking. Patients for whom it is a habit should plan to alter their patterns of behavior to avoid common cues to light a cigarette. Those who like to handle cigarettes need to find something to keep their hands busy to replace handling cigarettes. Patients who use cigarettes for stimulation should replace cigarettes with another stimulating exercise, such as walking, and avoid fatigue. Develop other methods for stress reduction such as deep breathing or other relaxation exercises.

All patients should make plans for how to handle difficult situations. Exercise such as walking can promote the feeling of well-being. They should set up a reward system for staying nicotine free, such as using the money saved to buy something they have been wanting.

Many patients are concerned about weight gain if they stop smoking. They should be warned that they may gain weight but watching their diet and increasing their exercise can minimize this. They should be prepared by having healthful, low-calorie meals and snacks available.

Specific nonpharmacologic approaches include aversive conditioning, hypnosis, acupuncture, behavior modification,

Text continued on p. 766

TABLE 73-1 Actions and Strategies for the Primary Care Clinician to Use in Smoking Cessation

Action	Strategies for Implementation
STEP 1. ASK: SYSTEMATICALLY IDENTIFY ALL TOBACCO USERS AT EVERY VISIT	
Implement an office-wide system that ensures that for *every* patient at *every* clinic visit, tobacco-use status is queried and documented.*	Expand the vital signs to include tobacco use: Data should be collected by the health care team. The action should be implemented using preprinted progress note paper that includes the expanded vital signs, a vital signs stamp, or, for computerized records, an item assessing tobacco-use status. Alternatives to the vital signs stamp are to place tobacco-use status stickers on all patients' charts or to indicate smoking status using computerized reminder systems.
STEP 2. ADVISE: STRONGLY URGE ALL SMOKERS TO QUIT	
In a *clear, strong,* and *personalized* manner, urge every smoker to quit.	Advice should be *Clear:* "I think it is important for you to quit smoking now, and I will help you." "Cutting down while you are ill is not enough." *Strong:* "As your clinician, I need you to know that quitting smoking is the most important thing you can do to protect your current and future health." *Personalized:* tie smoking to current health or illness and/or the social and economic costs of tobacco use, motivational level/readiness to quit, and the impact of smoking on children and others in household. Encourage clinic staff to reinforce the cessation message and support the patient's attempt to quit.
STEP 3. IDENTIFY SMOKERS WILLING TO ATTEMPT TO QUIT	
Ask every smoker if he or she is willing to make an attempt to quit at this time.	If the patient is willing to attempt to quit at this time, provide assistance (see Step 4). If the patient prefers a more intensive treatment or the clinician believes more intensive treatment is appropriate, refer the patient to interventions administered by a smoking cessation specialist and follow up with the patient regarding quitting (see Step 5). If the patient clearly states unwillingness to attempt to quit at this time, provide a motivational intervention.

STEP 4. ASSIST: AID THE PATIENT IN QUITTING

Help the patient with a plan for quitting.

Set a quit date: ideally, the quit date should be within 2 weeks, taking patient preference into account.

Help the patient prepare for quitting: the patient must

- *Inform* family, friends, and coworkers of quitting and request understanding and support.
- *Prepare* the environment by removing cigarettes from it. Prior to quitting, the patient should avoid smoking in places where he or she spends a lot of time (e.g., home, car).
- *Review* previous attempts at quitting. What helped? What led to the relapse?
- *Anticipate* challenges to the planned quit attempt, particularly during the critical first few weeks.

Encourage nicotine replacement therapy except in special circumstances.

Encourage the use of the nicotine patch or nicotine gum therapy for smoking cessation.

Give key advice on successful quitting.

Abstinence: total abstinence is essential. "Not even a single puff after the quit date."

- Alcohol: drinking alcohol is highly associated with relapse. Those who stop smoking should review their alcohol use and consider limiting or abstaining from alcohol use during the quit process.
- Other smokers in the household: the presence of other smokers in the household, particularly a spouse, is associated with lower success rates. Patients should consider quitting with their significant others and/or developing specific plans to maintain abstinence in a household where others still smoke.

Provide supplementary materials.

Source: federal agencies, including the National Cancer Institute and the Agency for Health Care Policy and Research; nonprofit agencies (American Cancer Society, American Lung Association, American Heart Association); or local or state health departments.

Selection concerns: the material must be culturally, racially, educationally, and age appropriate for the patient.

Location: readily available in every clinic office.

STEP 5. ARRANGE: SCHEDULE FOLLOW-UP CONTACT

Schedule follow-up contact, either in person or via telephone.

Timing: follow-up contact should occur soon after the quit date, preferably during the first week. A second follow-up contact is recommended within the first month. Schedule further follow-up contacts as indicated.

Actions during follow-up: congratulate success. If smoking occurred, review the circumstances and elicit recommitment to total abstinence. Remind the patient that a lapse can be used as a learning experience and is not a sign of failure. Identify the problems already encountered and anticipate challenges in the immediate future. Assess nicotine replacement therapy use and problems. Consider referral to a more intense or specialized program.

From The Smoking Cessation Clinical Practice Guideline Panel and Staff: the agency for Health Care Policy and Research smoking cessation clinical practice guideline, *JAMA* 275:1270, 1996.

*Repeated assessment is not necessary in the case of the adult who has never smoked or not smoked for many years, and for whom this information is clearly documented in the medical record.

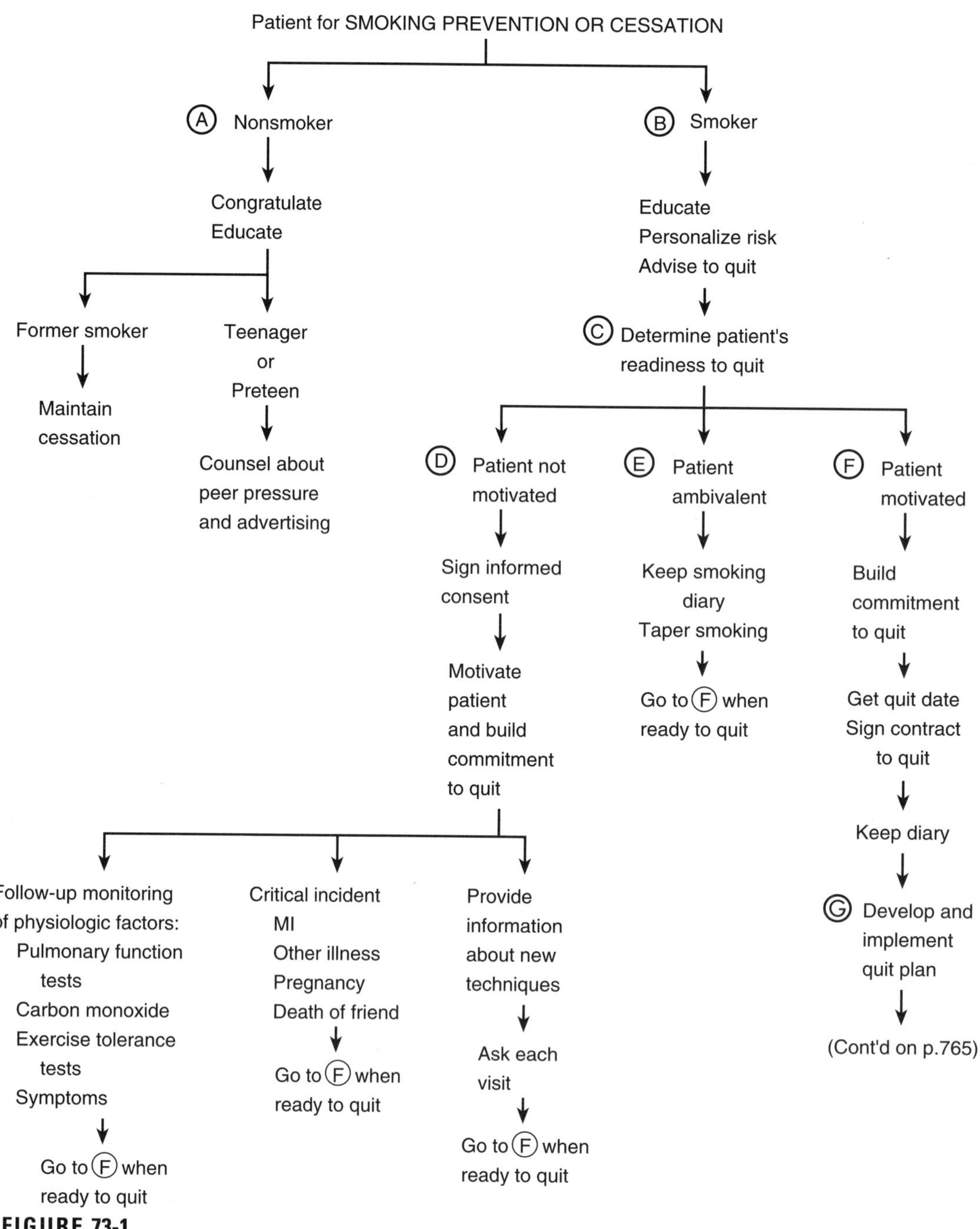

FIGURE 73-1

Smoking cessation algorithm. (Modified from Green HL et al, editors: *Decision-making in medicine,* ed 2, St Louis, 1998, Mosby.)

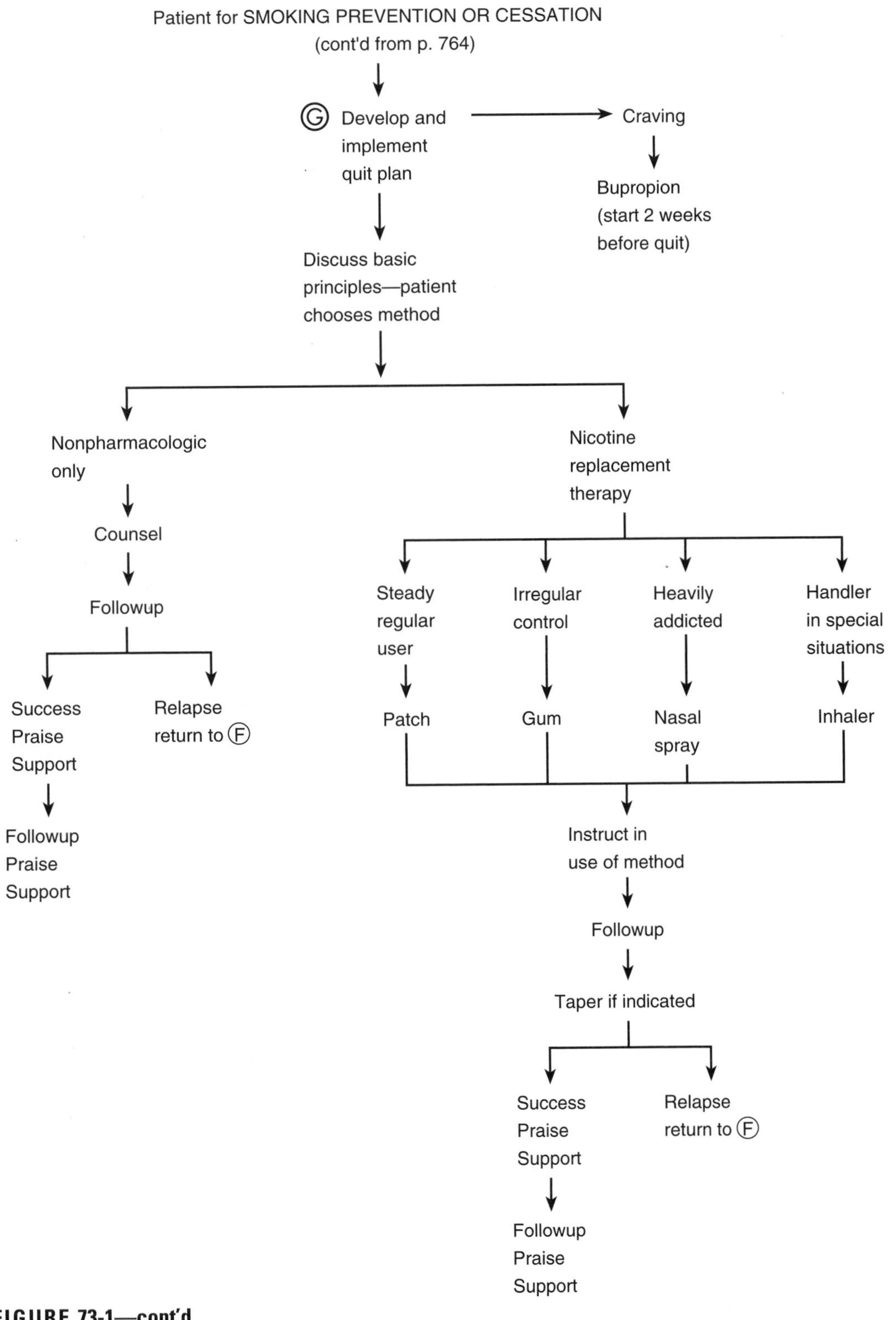

FIGURE 73-1—cont'd

Smoking cessation algorithm.

and multicomponent programs. Intensive treatment programs are often necessary for patients who have great difficulty stopping and have failed several times.

Pharmacologic Therapy

Unless contraindicated, every patient should be offered NRT. Make sure the patient receives an adequate dose; one of the main reasons for failure of nicotine treatment is underdosing. Another cause of failure is incorrect use of product.

First help the patient choose the dosage form that will work best for the patient. The patch is usually best for patients who smoke at regular intervals. The gum may work better for patients who smoke at irregular intervals. The patch is a more convenient, once-a-day application. The gum offers more direct control of the amount of nicotine the patient receives. The gum can be used when the patient has a craving. The nasal spray is useful to respond quickly to a craving. The nasal spray is especially beneficial to highly dependent smokers. The inhaler mimics the act of smoking and will be useful for patients who enjoy handling the cigarettes. The inhaler is also useful when gum will not work because of concomitant consumption of acidic foods or beverages, alcohol, or coffee. Social occasions involving alcohol are often an especially difficult time, and the inhaler might be the most acceptable in this situation. Gum might be more acceptable at work. Patients who have a stomach ulcer or diabetes should not use gum or lozenges but may use patches. However, patients who have an allergy to adhesive tape or preexisting skin problems should not choose NicoDerm CQ or Nicotrol. All replacement products are meant for those who smoke more than 10 cigarettes a day. Nicorette 2 mg is for those who smoke fewer than 25 cigarettes daily, while Nicorette 4 mg is for those who smoke 25 or more daily. Commit Lozenges use a different index for the initial choice. Those who smoke their first cigarette more than 30 minutes after waking should begin with the 2 mg lozenge, and those who smoke their first cigarette within 30 minutes of waking up should begin by using the 4 mg lozenge.

Although many of these NRT products are now available over-the-counter, there are certain patient populations that should seek the advice of a health professional before starting therapy, particularly with the patch. Those include people under age 18, people with heart disease or an irregular heartbeat or who have had a recent heart attack, people with high blood pressure not controlled with medication, people taking prescription medicine for depression or asthma, or people with skin problems or who are allergic to adhesive tape. Pregnant or nursing women should first try to stop smoking without the nicotine patch and seek advice of a health professional before using a nicotine patch.

Using the Patch

The nicotine transdermal system is a multilayered unit containing nicotine as the active agent that provides systematic delivery of nicotine for 16 to 24 hours. Determine the duration of action of patch to use. Some patients find that wearing the patches for only 16 hours prevents bizarre dreams. If patients crave a cigarette when they wake up, they should wear a 24-hour patch. Do not underdose by wearing the same patch for more than the 24-hour period. It is also necessary to use the patch for 8 to 12 weeks and not stop the therapy prematurely.

The patient should start with the highest-dose patch unless he or she is a light smoker (10 or less a day), weighs less than 100 lbs, or has cardiac disease. Use the highest-dose patch for 6 to 12 weeks. Then use the second-strength patch for 2 weeks and the lowest-dose patch for another 2 weeks. If the patient should use a lower dose, start with the second-strength patch for 6 weeks, then the lowest-dose patch for 2 to 4 weeks. Table 73-2 provides the dosing schedule for different brands.

Using Nicorette Gum

Nicotine polacrilex contains nicotine bound to an ion exchange resin in a chewing gum base. The gum comes in two strengths: 2 mg for patients who should use a lower dose and 4 mg for healthy patients who smoke 25 or more cigarettes a day. The patients chew a piece of gum every 1 to 2 hours for 6 weeks. They then taper the dose for the next 6 weeks. Duration of treatment is about 12 weeks. Usually at least 9 pieces of gum per day is necessary. They should not exceed 24 pieces a day. Gradually they should reduce the number of pieces of gum per day and length of time gum is chewed after 6 weeks. Many patients do not use enough gum, hoping to economize. They must be taught the importance of adequately suppressing their nicotine craving.

Using the Nicorette Lozenge Commit

The most recent addition to the NR market, Commit, is a nicotine polacrilex lozenge. Like the gum, Commit lozenges are not tapered in regard to the strength used (e.g., 2 mg versus 4 mg). Rather, the patient tapers the number of pieces used daily, in a schedule identical to that used for Nicorette Gum. Lozenges, although containing nicotine, are free from the carcinogens that are found in chewing tobacco and snuff.

Using the Nasal Spray/Oral Inhaler

The nasal spray and oral inhaler can be used alone or in combination with the gum or patch. The nasal spray is useful for a patient with severe cravings who desires immediate relief. The inhaler might be used for a patient who finds handling the cigarettes particularly difficult to give up. Other individuals can substitute lollipops, chewing on straws, pencils, or other actions that simulate smoking to compensate for cigarettes.

Many people are concerned about the safety of using NRT. The risk of using NRT must be compared to the risk of having the patient continue smoking as well as the risk of the patient using the patch while smoking. The fact is the effects of cigarette smoking promote myocardial ischemia. A patient with coronary artery disease can develop ischemic changes on electrocardiogram (ECG) just by smoking a cigarette. Patients with coronary artery disease (CAD) may be especially vulnerable to the ischemic effects of nicotine. Studies have shown that CAD patients who use NRT to stop smoking do not have an increased incidence of adverse cardiac effects; in fact, the opposite is true. It is especially important that CAD patients stop smoking for their health, and NRT has been shown safe and effective in this population. However, it is mandatory that patients with CAD do not continue to smoke while using NRT, as then the risk of adverse cardiac events does increase.

TABLE 73-2 Comparison of Smoking Cessation Products

Product	Dosage Form	Dosing and Treatment Information	Approximate Cost	Nicotine Release Mechanism	Patient Information Provided	Common Side Effects	Advantages	Disadvantages
Nicoderm CQ	Transdermal patch 16 or 24 hr (OTC)	>10 cig/day: 21 mg × 6 wk; 14 mg × 2 wk; 7 mg × 2 wk <10 cig/day: 14 mg × 6 wk; 7 mg × 2 wk May wear patch for 16 or 24 hr	7 mg (7), $28.00 14 mg (7), $50 21 mg (7), $50 21 mg (14), $50	Rate and diffusion controlling membrane	*Committed Quitters Program* booklet, audiotape, tips for quitting, toll-free support	Local cutaneous reaction (erythema, pruritus, edema); dizziness; cutaneous itching or hypersensitivity; headache; sleep disturbances and abnormal dreams (with 24-hr use).	Convenient, few compliance problems; no special skills for use; concealable; provides 24-hr steady concentration, which may reduce morning cravings.	Allergic reactions to adhesive may occur.
Nicotrol	Transdermal system 16 hr (OTC)	Steps 1, 2, and 3 deliver 15, 10, and 5 mg of nicotine respectively The patches are used once daily in a tapering manner: Step 1: weeks 1-6 Step 2: weeks 7-8 Step 3: weeks 9-10 Step 1 for >10 cig/day smokers Remove patch before sleep (only releases 16 hr) No tapering of dose	Patch $60	Adhesive containing rate-controlling membrane and concentration gradient	*Pathways to Change Program* booklet, audiotape, tips for quitting, toll-free support number	Local cutaneous reactions: erythema, pruritus, edema, hypersensitivity, headache.	One-step process. Few compliance problems. No oral side effects. Easily concealed.	No nicotine through night may reduce occurrence of bizarre dreams but lead to morning cravings. Doses cannot be titrated by patient. Allergic reactions to adhesive may occur.

Continued

TABLE 73-2 Comparison of Smoking Cessation Products—cont'd

Product	Dosage Form	Dosing and Treatment Information	Approximate Cost	Nicotine Release Mechanism	Patient Information Provided	Common Side Effects	Advantages	Disadvantages
Habitrol	Transdermal 24-hr system (Rx)	>100 lb, >10 cigs/day and NO cardiovascular disease: 21 mg × 6 wk; 14 mg × 2-4 wk 7 mg × 2-4 wk <100 lb, <10 cig/day or cardiovascular disease: 14 mg × 6 wk; 7 mg × 2-4 wk	7 mg (30), $110.00 14 mg (30), $116.00 21 mg (30), $122.00	Rate-limiting membrane and a concentration gradient	*Patient Support Kit* cassette, information booklet, guide for family/ friends, prescription refill stickers	Sleep disturbances and abnormal dreams; headache Local cutaneous reactions: erythema, pruritus, edema, hypersensitivity.	Provides 24-hr steady concentration that may reduce morning cravings. Easily concealable. Few compliance problems.	Allergic reactions to adhesive may occur.
Nicorette and generic	Gum (OTC) in regular and mint flavor	2 mg: <25 cig/day 4 mg: >25 cig/day 6 wk: one piece q1-2 hr 3 wk: one piece q2-4 hr 3 wk: one piece q4-8 hr Do not exceed 24 pieces/day STOP ALL SMOKING No acidic foods/ beverages before and during use Chew, park gum between cheek and gum 1-5 min; repeat Use one piece no longer than 30 min	2-mg starter (48), $32; refill (100), $57 4-mg starter (48), $32; refill (110), $50	Ion exchange resin, releases when being chewed only, not when swallowed	*Committed Quitters Program* booklet, CD with tips for quitting, toll-free support number	Nausea/vomiting, jaw soreness, hiccups. From incorrect chewing: headache, mouth/throat soreness, bad taste, indigestion.	Use when prompted by cravings. May satisfy oral craving. Dose easily titrated. Gum chewing part of life style for some people. May delay weight gain.	Must use proper chewing technique to lessen adverse effects and get benefits. Difficult to use with dentures. Gum may be socially inappropriate at times.
Commit nicotine polacrilex lozenge	2-mg, 4-mg lozenges	Patient should suck one lozenge q1-2 hr for weeks 1-6; one q2-4 hr for weeks 7-9; one q4-8 hr for weeks 10-12 Tapering is accomplished by the number of lozenges per day	$43 for 72 lozenges (2 mg and 4 mg)	Ion exchange resin	Go to Quit.com	Nausea, vomiting, bad taste, indigestion	For those who smoke more than 30 min after waking.	May chew and not get even dosing.

Nicotrol inhaler	Oral inhaler (Rx)	6-16 cartridges/day Best effects with continuous puffing for 20 minutes Individualize dosing An open cartridge is good only for 1 day Must use minimum of six cartridges/day for at least 3-6 wk, then continue for 3 months, taper for next 6-12 wk Do not exceed 6 months of use	More expensive	Nicotine release mechanism	*Pathways to Change* materials, booklet, audiotape, tips for quitting, toll-free support number	Local irritation of throat and mouth; headache; dyspepsia; hiccups; coughing; rhinitis; bad taste in mouth.	Mimics act of smoking. Used to reduce cravings. Dose easily titrated by patient.	Cartridges should be stored between 59° and 86°F. May take up to 1 wk to get used to side effects. Dependence to product may develop.
Nicotrol NS	Nasal spray (Rx)	One to two 0.5-mg sprays in each nostril/hr Gradually reduce rate over 6-8 wk Do not exceed five sprays/hr or 40 sprays/day	10 ml, $36.00	Information not applicable	*Pathways to Change* materials, booklet, audiotape, tips for quitting, tool-free support number	Peppery/hot sensation in nose/throat; sneezing; coughing; runny nose; watery eyes.	Used to suppress cravings. Dose easily titrated by patient. Immediate effect.	Often found uncomfortable to use. May take 2 wk to get used to delivery method. Dependence or product may develop. Must avoid contact with skin. Wait 5 minutes before driving.
Bupropion SR (Zyban)	Oral sustained-release 150-mg tablet (Rx)	150 mg qd for 3 days, then increase to 150 mg bid Set quit date at 1-2 wk after beginning Zyban therapy, continue for 7-12 wk Not to exceed 200 mg/day Treatment >3 months generally NOT necessary Dose tapering NOT recommended Can be used with nicotine replacement products	60 150-mg tablets, $77.00	Not applicable	*Advantage Plan* booklet, tips for quitting, toll-free support number	Risk of seizures increases to 1/1000. Nervousness; difficulty concentrating; rash; dry mouth; insomnia; constipation.	No risk of nicotine toxicity if patient continues to smoke. Ease of use may be more beneficial in patients with subclinical depression. Safer to use in pregnancy. Can be used in combination with nicotine replacement.	Seizure risk. Increases cost of smoking cessation program.

Cig, Cigarettes.

bupropion

Bupropion seems to reduce craving for cigarettes or the urge to smoke. Side effects are more serious than with nicotine, most notably the risk of seizures. Bupropion should be started 1 to 2 weeks before the quit date, using 150 mg/day orally for 3 days and then increased to 150 mg orally twice a day. Continue this dosage for 7 to 12 weeks. The patient should not exceed 300 mg/day. Treatment for more than 3 months is usually not necessary, and dose tapering is not needed. Bupropion can be used in addition to nicotine replacement products and may be especially useful for patients who are somewhat depressed.

Whatever method is chosen, the patient should only use one particular product. Patches cannot be combined with gum or lozenges. While using any product, the patient must not use nicotine in any form (e.g., cigars, cigarettes, dip, snuff, pipes). Additional use of any of these products may cause serious nicotine toxicity.

Nicotine replacement products are meant to help patients stop smoking. They are not meant to help get a patient through a long plane flight or an all-day meeting in a nonsmoking building. Additionally, when the time period labeled for use is over, the patient should stop using them (e.g., 10 to 12 weeks, or whatever the course is listed for that product). Any patient who experiences symptoms of nicotine overdose (nausea, vomiting, dizziness, weakness, rapid heartbeat, diarrhea) should stop using the product immediately and see a health care provider to make sure he or she is not toxic or seriously ill.

Products must be kept away from children and pets. If children or pets accidentally swallow either new or used patches, gum, or lozenges, immediately call a poison control center.

HOW TO MONITOR

- The first 2 weeks are critical. Monitor patients closely by telephone. Call to see how they are doing within the first week. Tell them to call the clinician if they are experiencing difficulty.
- Because most relapses occur within the first 3 months of cessation, the patient should be seen frequently to try to problem solve and prevent relapse.
- Because many patients relapse, check on smoking at each visit and encourage patients to try again if they have relapsed.
- In older patients, monitor for cardiovascular effects, monitor blood pressure, and ask about angina.

PATIENT VARIABLES

Hospitalized Patients

The hospital is an ideal place to have the patient stop smoking. Patients with cardiovascular disease should be given a decreased dose of the transdermal systems, to minimize the potential for adverse effects (asthenia, body aches, and dizziness) and cardiovascular complications (arrhythmias and MI).

Geriatrics

Transdermal systems have been found to be just as effective in geriatric patients.

Pediatrics

The safety and effectiveness of transdermal systems have not been tested in the pediatric population. Therefore use in children and adolescents is not recommended.

Pregnancy

- *Category D:* patch.
- *Category X:* gum.
- Risks to the fetus include spontaneous abortion, low birth weight, anencephaly, cleft palate, and congenital heart disease, as does smoking. Pregnant women should be encouraged to stop smoking because of the potential damage of smoking to their children. NRT should be used only if benefits outweigh the risk. Nicotine passes freely into breast milk.

Race/Gender

The increase in smoking by women since 1950 is now showing up in a higher rate of women dying from lung disease. Cigarettes cause more damage to black women than other populations. Black women show less recovery after quitting smoking.

PATIENT EDUCATION

Patients need extensive education. All drug companies that supply NRT medications have patient information and support materials for patients trying to quit. See also patient education material in the reference section of this chapter.

All Forms of NRT

- No smoking while on NRT.
- Dispose of used NRT properly. Patches are particularly hazardous to children.
- Keep out of reach of children and pets.

Patch

- Place a new patch at the start of each day, wear for 16 or 24 hours/day.
- Wear 24 hours if patients crave cigarettes the minute they wake up.
- Wear 16 hours if the patient has vivid dreams or sleep disruptions.
- Place on a new location that is relatively hairless between the neck and the waist.
- Dispose of used patch carefully: fold sticky sides together; insert in disposal tray.
- Wash hands after handling patches.
- Notify provider if the patient has skin reactions.

Gum

- Patients should use one piece at a time.
- They should begin chewing slowly and avoid swallowing saliva immediately.
- They should chew until they experience a peppery taste or a tingle. This usually takes about 15 chews.

- Then they should stop chewing, park the gum between the cheek and gum and leave it there.
- When the taste or tingle fades, usually a minute or so, start to chew slowly again until taste or tingle returns.
- Stop chewing again. Park in a different place.
- Continue this until taste or tingle does not return, usually about 30 minutes.
- Use gum at regular intervals.
- Do not consume acidic foods or beverages, alcohol, fruit, coffee, soft drinks, etc., for 15 minutes before and during use.

Lozenge

Patient must allow the lozenge to dissolve slowly over 20 to 30 minutes, swallowing as little as possible. Lozenge should not be chewed or swallowed. Patient should occasionally move the lozenge from one side of the mouth to the other. A warm feeling or tingling sensation may result.

Specific Drugs

Nicotine Replacement Therapy

All NRT formulations share the following characteristics, except as noted.

Contraindications. Not to be used in patients with hypersensitivity to nicotine or any component. It should also not be used in patients during the immediate postmyocardial infarction period or in patients with life-threatening arrhythmias or severe or worsening angina pectoris. Gum is contraindicated in active temporomandibular joint disease.

Warning/Precautions. Use with caution in patients with cardiovascular disease. Screen for CAD, arrhythmias, or vasospastic diseases. Use in hypertensive patients only when benefit outweighs risk. Monitor BP closely.

Use cautiously in patients with hepatic or severe renal impairment, hyperthyroidism, pheochromocytoma, type 1 diabetes mellitus, active peptic ulcer disease, hypertension, and peripheral vascular and cardiovascular diseases.

Patient MUST stop smoking completely when initiating therapy. Many clinicians require patients to sign a form indicating that they have been told of the risks of continuing to smoke and using NRT.

Transference of addiction from cigarette to patch or gum may occur. They should use NRT no longer than 3 months.

- *Patch:* use with caution in certain dermatologic (atopic dermatitis and eczematous) conditions. Monitor all patients for contact allergy.
- *Gum:* dental problems may be exacerbated.
- *Nasal spray:* use not recommended for patients with known chronic nasal disorders such as allergy, rhinitis, nasal polyps and sinusitis; or asthma, bronchospasm, or reactive airway disease.

Pharmacokinetics. Transdermal systems deliver nicotine systemically through percutaneous absorption. After application to the skin, nicotine plasma concentrations usually peak and plateau within 2 to 4 hours. Nicoderm CQ onset is rapid, and it peaks between 2 and 4 hours; Habitrol onset is 1 to 2 hours and peaks between 6 and 12 hours, and slowly declines over the remaining period of patch application. The nicotine in gum is absorbed bucally. The onset and peak levels are dependent on the vigor, rapidity, and duration of chewing. The nasal inhaler has onset of action of about 4 minutes and half-life of 1 to 2 hours.

Nicotine has a large volume of distribution and is metabolized extensively in the liver as well as in the kidney and lung. It has over 20 metabolites. The main metabolite cotinine has a half-life of 15 to 20 hours. Ten percent is excreted unchanged in the urine.

Adverse Effects

- Systemic effects of NRT include edema, flushing, hypertension, palpitations, tachyarrhythmias, tachycardia, dizziness, confusion, convulsions, depression, euphoria, numbness, paresthesia, syncope, tinnitus, weakness, headache, insomnia, dry mouth, nonspecific GI distress, nausea, vomiting, altered LFTs, constipation, diarrhea, difficulty breathing, cough, hoarseness, sneezing, and wheezing.
- Adverse effects of the patch are primarily skin reactions and rash.
- Patch or gum may provide toxic levels of nicotine for young children who accidentally handle or chew product.
- Effects associated with the gum are the mechanical effects of gum chewing: traumatic injury to oral mucosa, jaw ache, and eructation secondary to air swallowing. Oral mucosal changes include stomatitis, glossitis, gingivitis, pharyngitis, aphthous ulcers, and changes in taste perception.
- Nasal spray is irritating to nasal mucosa.

Drug Interactions

- Nicotine increases general metabolism and lowers blood levels of the following drugs through enzyme induction: acetaminophen, caffeine, imipramine, oxazepam, pentazocine, propranolol, and theophylline.
- Nicotine increases circulating cortisol and cate-cholamines. Adjust doses of adrenergic agonists or blockers accordingly.
- Nicotine may reduce diuretic effects of furosemide, decrease subcutaneous insulin absorption, and decrease first-pass metabolism of propoxyphene.
- Gum interacts with food or drink in the mouth.

Overdosage

- *Symptoms:* nausea and vomiting are early symptoms. Other symptoms are salivation, abdominal pain, headache, dizziness, confusion, weakness, hypotension, difficulty breathing, and tachycardia. Death may result from paralysis of respiratory muscles. Minimum oral lethal dose in adults is 40 to 60 mg. The lethal dose is much lower in children.
- *Treatment of overdosage of gum:* empty stomach.
- *Overdosage for patch:* remove patch and flush skin with water; do not use soap.
- *Ingestion:* refer to health care facility, administer activated charcoal, and provide supportive measures.

Dosage and Administration

See Table 73-2.

RESOURCES FOR PATIENTS AND PROVIDERS

Organizations and symposiums

Action on Smoking and Health, 2013 H St. NW Washington, DC 20006 (202) 659-4310.

National nonprofit charitable organization that serves as the legal action arm of the nonsmoking community.

Doctors Ought to Care (DOC), 5615 Kirby Drive, Suite 440 Houston, TX 77005 (713) 528-1487.

Coalition of health professionals concerned about educating the public about preventable causes of death.

Effective Strategies for Smoking Cessation in Primary Care Practice.

Highlights from a closed symposium, sponsored by SmithKline Beecham Consumer Healthcare.

Medical Information Service: *Smoking: The New Vital Sign.*

A video-plus-print program available from Marion Merrell Dow, Inc. and SmithKline Beecham Consumer Healthcare for health care professionals.

Office on Smoking and Health (OSH), Centers for Disease Control National Center for Chronic Disease Prevention and Health Promotion, Mail Stop K-50 4770 Buford Highway NE Atlanta, GA 30341 (800) CDC-1311, (770) 488-5705.

Office with a wide variety of information on smoking and health; also has an up-to-date fax directory of tobacco, smoking, and health information.

Stop Teenage Addiction to Tobacco (STAT), 311 E Columbus Ave. Springfield, MA 01105 (413) 732-7828.

Nonprofit tax-exempt educational organization dedicated to reducing tobacco addiction among young people.

U.S. Department of Health and Human Services Public Health Service National Institutes of Health, National Cancer Institute, and Cancer Information Service (800) 4-CANCER.

Booklets and charts

Commit to Quit, from SmithKline Beecham

Helping Smokers Quit: A Guide for Advanced Practice Nurses, from the American Nurses Foundation.

How to Stay Quit Over the Holidays, from American Cancer Society.

Wall charts on Nicotrol prescribing information provided by McNeil Consumer Products Company.

Internet

Nursing Center for Tobacco Intervention, www.con.ohio-state.edu/tobacco.

BIBLIOGRAPHY

Fagerstrom K: The epidemiology of smoking, *Drugs* 62(suppl 2):1-9, 2002.

Hughes JR et al: Recent advances in the pharmacotherapy of smoking, *JAMA* 281:72, 1999.

Karnath B: Smoking cessation, *Am J Med* 112:399-405, 2002.

Merrill E: Preventing tobacco use in young people: strategies for the nurse practitioner, *Nurse Pract Forum* 6:343, 1995.

Murray RP et al: Safety of nicotine polacrilex gum used for 3094 participants in the lung health study, *Chest* 109:438, 1996.

Nonprescription options for smoking cessation, *US Pharmacist* 28, 2003 (posted 3/13/03), www.uspharmacist.com.

Sachs DPL: Effectiveness of the 4 mg dose of nicotine polacrilex for the initial treatment of high-dependent smokers, *Arch Intern Med* 155:1973, 1995.

Sargent JD et al: Predictors of smoking cessation in adolescents, *Arch Pediatr Adolesc Med* 152:388, 1998.

Shiffman S et al: Efficacy of a nicotine lozenge for smoking cessation. *Arch Intern Med* 162:1267-1276, 2002.

The Smoking Cessation Clinical Practice Guideline Panel and Staff: the Agency for Health Care Policy and Research smoking cessation clinical practice guideline, *JAMA* 275:1270, 1996.

Transdermal Nicotine Study Group: Transdermal nicotine for smoking cessation six-month results from two multicenter controlled clinical trials, *JAMA* 266:3133, 1991.

CHAPTER 74

Vitamins and Minerals

Drug Names

Class	Subclass	Generic Name	Trade Name
Multivitamins	General multivitamins		Various OTC
			Berocca Tablets
			Nephrocaps
			Nephro-Vite (Rx) Tablets
			Pro-Hepatone Capsules
			Renal Multivitamin formula (Rx)
	Multivitamins with minerals		Various OTC
			Bacmin Tablets
			Berocca Plus Tablets
			Cezin-s Capsules
			Vicon Forte Capsules
			Vitamist Intra-Oral Spray Dietary Supplements
	Multivitamins with fluoride		Poly-Vi-Flor with Iron
			Vi-Daylin/F Chewable Multivitamin Tablets
			Vi-Daylin/F Multivitamin + Iron Chewable Tablets
	Parenteral multivitamins		Aquason A Parenteral
			Neurodep Injection
			Vicam Injection
	Prenatal vitamins (OTC)		Materna Tablets
			Mynatal Capsules
			Natalins Tablets
			Nestabs FA Tablets
			Niferex-PN Tablets
	Prenatal Rx Tablets		Stuartnatal Plus Tablets
Other multivitamin formulations and products	Anti-folic acid antagonists		Leucovorin Calcium for Injection (Rx)
			Leucovorin Calcium Tablets
	Antioxidant combinations		Various OTC
	Geriatric vitamin formulations		Various OTC
	Pediatric vitamin formulations		Various OTC
	Pediatric vitamins with fluoride		Various OTC
	Iron combinations		Multiple OTC
			Berocca Plus
			Fumatinic Capsules
			Iberet-Folic-500
			InFed Injection (Rx)
			Hemocyte-F Tablets
			Nefplex Rx Tablets
			Nephro-Fer (Rx) Tablets
			Nephro-Vite (Rx) + Fe Tablets
			Nephron-A
			Niferex-150 Forte Capsules
			Niferex-PN Tablets
			Theragran Hematinic Tablets
			Vitafol Capsules
	Iron with vitamin B_{12} and intrinsic factor		Chromagen Capsules
			Chromagen Tablets
			Fero-Grad-500 Filmtab

Continued

Drug Names—cont'd

Class	Subclass	Generic Name	Trade Name
Other multivitamin formulations and products—cont'd			Fero-Gradumet Filmtab Iberet Iberet-500 Filmtab Iberet-500 Liquid Iberet-Folic-500 Ironspan Capsules Pronemia Hematinic Capsules
Individual vitamins and minerals	Vitamin A		Aquasol A Drops, Capsules, Injection
	Vitamin B_1 (thiamin)		Thiamine HCl Injection
	Vitamin B_3 (niacin)		Niacon Tablets Nicolar Tablets
	Vitamin B_6 (pyridoxine)		Pyridoxine Injection
	Vitamin B_{12}		Hydrocobalamin Injection
	Vitamin C (ascorbic acid)		Ascorbic Acid Injection Cenolate
	Vitamin D (calcitrol)		Calcijex Injection Rocaltrol Capsules
	Vitamin K		AquaMEPHYTON Injection (Rx) Mephyton Tablets
	Calcium		Calphron Phoslo
	Fluoride		Luride Drops Luride Lozi-Tabs Tablets Pediaflor Drops
	Folic acid		Folvite Injection Folic Acid Tablets
	Niacin		Nicobid Nicolar
	Phosphorus		K-Phos Neutral Tablets Neutra-Phos Tablets Neutra-Phos K Powder Uro-KP Neutral Tablets
	Zinc		Zincate

General Uses

The integrity and the health of the body are maintained through nutrients. Most commonly, these nutrients come from natural sources. With a poor diet or during times of stress or illness, supplementation may be required. Vitamins and minerals may then become important components of the therapeutic regimen. Additionally, new research findings confirm the role that some of these formulations play in improving or preventing some chronic diseases. Listed in this chapter are some of the prescription and OTC formulations of multivitamins currently available. Also included are prescription vitamins and minerals currently being marketed as individual therapies. Many nonprescription vitamin preparations and many other individual vitamins and minerals are sold over-the-counter and are not covered. Prescriptions are often required in order to be covered by insurance.

Vitamins and minerals are by definition essential for human life, and their role in basic metabolism is well researched (Table 74-1). However, much new research documents their role in health promotion and disease prevention. This is a rapidly developing field, and it is necessary for the provider to keep current with the latest research.

In 2003 the American Medical Association made a recommendation for the first time that all Americans should take a general multivitamin daily. This reflects the failure of so many Americans to get all nutrients required daily in their diet, especially if on weight-loss diets.

Nutrients contained in the diet affect a number of cellular metabolic mechanisms that are common in the pathogenesis of chronic disease. Unified dietary guidelines issued jointly by six national organizations (American Heart Association, American Cancer Society, American Dietetic Association, American Academy of Pediatrics, National Institutes of Health, and American Society for Clinical Nutrition) have been proposed to help reduce the risk of cancer, atherosclerosis, obesity, and diabetes. These unified guidelines indicate that the simplest way of achieving a healthy diet would be to include less than 10% saturated fat and no more than 30% total fat, as measured in calories; 55% of total calories should come in the form of carbohydrates; no more than 300 mg of cholesterol should

Text continued on p. 782

TABLE 74-1 Summary of Important Information about Vitamins and Minerals

Nutrient	Major Function	Sources	RDA
FAT-SOLUBLE VITAMINS			
Vitamin A	Essential for vision: especially in the dark Maintains epithelial tissue: needed for proper functioning of the cornea, mucous membranes, GI tract, lungs, vagina, urinary tract, bladder, and skin By maintaining healthy epithelium, prevents infection and possibly cancer	Fat soluble: stored for long periods of time in the liver Retinol sources: liver, butter, fish oils, egg yolk, and fortified dairy products Beta-carotene sources: yellow and dark-green vegetables, orange fruits, watermelon, and cherries; the more intense the color, the more vitamin A it contains	Dependent on body weight Infant 0-6 mo: 2100 IU Infant 6 mo-3 yr: 2000 IU Child 4-6 yr: 2500 IU Child 7-10 yr: 3300 IU Male 11+ yr: 5000 IU Female 11+ yr: 4000 IU Pregnancy: +1000 IU Lactation: +2000 IU
Vitamin D	Main function is calcium management, vitamin D makes sure enough calcium is readily available for retrieval Promotes calcium absorption in the gut, pulls calcium out of bones, deposits calcium into bone, and monitors calcium excretion by the kidney	Sunlight is the best source of vitamin D Most people get their vitamin D through the fortified milk they drink Other sources include seafood: fish oils, and oily fish (salmon, herring, sardines, mackerel)	Vitamin D RDAs are very stable early in life, while bones are growing, but requirements decrease gradually with age Infant and child to 18 yr: 400 IU Male and female to 22 yr: 300 IU Male and female 22+ yr: 200 IU Pregnancy and lactation: +200 IU
Vitamin E	Potent antioxidant (prevents fats in cell membranes from oxidation or spoiling Considered a possible cancer preventative because it protects cell walls from damage that can lead to tumor formation	Vegetable oils (corn, cottonseed, peanut) are the best sources; nuts (almonds, hazelnuts, safflower, sunflower, walnuts) wheat germ, and whole-wheat flour are good sources Vegetables (spinach, lettuce, onions) and fruits (blackberries, apples, pears) also contain vitamin E	Vitamin E requirements are based on body size and fat intake; with increased polyunsaturated fat intake, vitamin E requirements increase (more fats to protect) Elderly people and alcoholics may require supplementation The upper limit amount of vitamin E is 1000 IU; side effects from megadoses include an increased risk of hemorrhage damage due to its anticoagulant properties Infant to 12 mo: 9-12 IU Child 1-7 yr: 15-21 IU Child 11-18 yr: 24 IU Male 18+ yr: 22 IU of natural source vitamin E or 33 IU synthetic form Female 18+ yr: 22 IU of natural source vitamin E or 33 IU synthetic form Pregnancy: +6 IU Lactation: +9 IU
Vitamin K	Plays an essential role in blood clot formation	Two sources of vitamin K: K_1 is plant derived and K_2 produced by bacteria in the human intestine; 50% of each contributes to our daily supply Synthetic vitamin K: K_3 has twice the potency K_1 found in dark-green leafy vegetables (brussels sprouts, spinach, cabbage, cauliflower); also found in oats, soybeans, egg yolks, and green tea	There is a recommended "adequate and safe" range for this vitamin, rather than an official RDA Infant to 6 mo: 12 μg Infant 6-12 mo: 10-20 μg Child 1-3 yr: 15-30 μg Child 4-6 yr: 20-40 μg Child 7-10 yr: 30-60 μg Child 11-17 yr: 50-100 μg Adult: 70-140 μg Pregnancy: consult physician—no recommendations for safe vitamin K supplementation

Continued

TABLE 74-1 Summary of Important Information about Vitamins and Minerals—cont'd

Nutrient	Major Function	Sources	RDA
WATER-SOLUBLE VITAMINS			
Vitamin B_1	B_1 (thiamin), like most B complex vitamins, acts as a coenzyme or catalyst in the production of energy	Most foods (if they contain thiamin at all) contain very small amounts of this vitamin Animal products that are relatively "rich" in thiamin are pork, beef, organ meats, and salmon Some plant sources are relatively rich: rye and whole-wheat flours, rice bran, enriched cereals, nuts, and legumes (peas and beans in particular Brewer's yeast also contains significant amounts of thiamin	Infant to 6 mo: 0.3 mg Infant 6-12 mo: 0.5 mg Child 1-3 yr: 0.7 mg Child 4-6 yr: 0.9 mg Child 7-10 yr: 1.2 mg Male 11-18 yr: 1.4 mg Male 19-50 yr: 1.5 mg Male 51+ yr: 1.2 mg Female 11-22 yr: 1.1 mg Female 23+ yr: 1.0 mg Pregnancy: +0.4 mg Lactation: +0.5 mg Remember the thiamin deficiency associated with alcoholism and supplement accordingly
Vitamin B_2	B_2 (riboflavin) is essential for the formation of two coenzymes, both of which play an important role in energy production; cellular growth cannot occur without B_2	B_2 is present in both plant and animal products, but "excellent" sources are from animals: milk and milk products are probably the best, with liver being second Other good sources are dairy products, chicken, leafy green vegetables, cereal, bread, wheat germ, brewer's yeast, and almonds	Riboflavin is not stored in large amounts, so must be taken in daily Infant to 6 mo: 0.4 mg Infant 6-12 mo: 0.6 mg Child 1-3 yr: 0.8 mg Child 4-6 yr: 1.0 mg Child 7-10 yr: 1.4 mg Male 11-14 yr: 1.6 mg Male 15-22 yr: 1.7 mg Male 23-50 yr: 1.6 mg Male 51+ yr: 1.4 mg Female 11-22 yr: 1.3 mg Female 23+ yr: 1.2 mg Pregnancy: +0.3 mg Lactation: +0.5 mg Athletes (especially women) probably should consider supplementation
Vitamin B_3	B_3 (niacin) is one of the most stable B vitamins and performs tasks similar to riboflavin—taking part in multiple metabolic reactions related to energy production	Best niacin sources are proteins: meats, fish, poultry, nuts, legumes, milk, and eggs Moderate sources include whole-grain cereals and breads; highly processed grains have been stripped of much of their nutrient value, and unless they have been "fortified" are poor sources of niacin (and many other nutrients)	A water-soluble vitamin, B_3 needs to be constantly replenished Infant to 6 months: 6 mg Infant 6-12 months: 8 mg Child 1-3 yr: 9 mg Child 4-6 yr: 11 mg Child 7-10 yr: 16 mg Male 11-18 yr: 18 mg Male 19-22 yr: 19 mg Male 23-50 yr: 18 mg Male 50+ yr: 16 mg Female 11-14 yr: 15 mg Female 15-22 yr: 14 mg Female 23+ yr: 13 mg Pregnancy: +2 mg Lactation: +4 mg
Vitamin B_6	B_6 (pyridoxine) also assists in coenzyme reactions, helping the body process protein, fat, and carbohydrates Stored in muscle tissue, it is readily available when energy is needed	Vitamin B_6 is widely available from dietary sources Animal products high in B_6 include both meats and fish (salmon, shrimp, tuna)	Because excess vitamin B_6 can have toxic effects, limiting supplements to less than 200 mg/day is recommended Infant to 6 mo: 0.3 mg

TABLE 74-1 Summary of Important Information about Vitamins and Minerals—cont'd

Nutrient	Major Function	Sources	RDA
WATER-SOLUBLE VITAMINS—cont'd			
Vitamin B_6—cont'd		Plant products include whole grains (bran, whole-wheat flour, wheat germ, rice), fruits and vegetables (bananas, avocados, carrots), and nuts (hazelnuts, soy, sunflower) Beer seems to be correlated with raised serum levels of vitamin B_6	Infant 6-12 mo: 0.6 mg Child 1-3 yr: 0.9 mg Child 4-6 yr: 1.3 mg Child 7-10 yr: 1.8 mg Male 11+ yr: 2.2 mg Female 11+ yr: 2.0 mg Pregnant: +0.6 mg Lactating: +0.5 mg
Vitamin B_{12}	The most chemically complex of the B vitamins, B_{12} (cobalamin) plays a major role in energy production and growth, as well as nervous system function and blood cell production	B_{12} is found primarily in animal protein (making strict vegetarians at risk for this deficiency) Good sources include fish (many types), dairy products, meats, and eggs	Infant to 6 mo: 0.5 μg Infant 6-12 mo: 1.5 μg Child 1-3 yr: 2 μg Child 4-6 yr: 2.5 μg Child 7-10 yr: 3 μg Adult 11+ yr: 3 μg Pregnancy and lactation: +1 μg
Folic acid	Critical for formation and activity of both DNA and RNA, therefore regulating growth and development; also plays a major role in red blood cell production Dietary folate has been found to reduce stroke risk by 20% Folic acid deficiency has been related to an increase in congenital anomalies (neural tube defects), and supplementation is strongly recommended in reproductive-age women, especially oral contraceptive users (more rapid depletion of this nutrient in these women)	Folic acid is found in plant products almost exclusively; best sources include green leafy vegetables (broccoli, spinach, romaine), fruit (oranges), nuts, and grains (wheat germ, rice, barley), legumes (beans, peas, lentils, soybeans) Due to problems with bioavailability, folic acid supplements and fortified cereals have been found to be more effective than a diet rich in naturally occurring folates in reducing levels of total homocysteine levels It is important to note that cooking these plant products will significantly reduce the amount of available folic acid (heat fragile)	Infant to 6 mo: 30 μg Infant 6-12 mo: 45 μg Child 1-3 yr: 100 μg Child 4-6 yr: 200 μg Child 7-10 yr: 300 μg Adult 11+ yr: 400 μg Pregnancy: +400 μg Lactation: +100 μg
Biotin	Another B vitamin, biotin is often called "vitamin H" Involved in enzymatic reactions related to protein, fat, and carbohydrate metabolism and energy production; also necessary to convert folic acid to its biologically active state	Biotin is produced largely by bacteria in the human intestine Both animal and plant products are rich in biotin with the best sources being liver and organ meats, molasses, and milk Other sources include nuts (cashews, peanuts, walnuts, sunflower seeds), legumes (peas, lentils, soybeans), and whole grains (brown rice, bulgur, wheat, oats)	No official RDA has been established, but estimated adequate intake is: Infant to 6 mo: 35 μg Infant 6-12 mo: 50 μg Child 1-3 yr: 65 μg Child 4-6 yr: 85 μg Child 7-10 yr: 120 μg Adult: 100-200 μg
Pantothenic acid	Pantothenic acid (another B vitamin) is converted to its biologic form—coenzyme A, which, like most B vitamins, is essential for energy production and protein, fat, and carbohydrate metabolism; it also plays roles in red blood cell formation and acetylcholine production	The word *pantos* means everywhere—and that's where this B vitamin can be found—very widely in dietary sources Perhaps the best sources are meat products (liver), but it's widely available in plant products (nuts, cereals, beans)	An RDA has not been established for pantothenic acid; recommended adequate intakes are: Infant to 6 months: 2 mg Child to 3 yr: 3 mg Child 4-6 yr: 3-4 mg Child 7-10 yr: 4-5 mg Adult 10+ yr: 4-7 mg Pregnancy and lactation: not established

Continued

TABLE 74-1 Summary of Important Information about Vitamins and Minerals—cont'd

Nutrient	Major Function	Sources	RDA
WATER-SOLUBLE VITAMINS—cont'd			
Vitamin C	Major role is in collagen formation and stabilization Vitamin C helps repair damaged tissue and has antioxidant properties Vitamin C also supports other nutrients—helping the body activate folic acid and utilize iron	Not present in animal products, vitamin C is available in a wide variety of fruits and vegetables Sources include fruits (oranges and orange juice, lemons, grapefruit, tangerines, strawberries, tomatoes) and vegetables (broccoli, brussels sprouts, cabbage, green peppers, potatoes, spinach, hot peppers)	The upper intake level is 2000 mg/day for adults; high levels could cause adverse effects, including diarrhea Infant to 12 mo: 35 mg Child 1-10 yr: 45 mg Child 11-14 yr: 50 mg Women and men: 90 mg Pregnancy: +20 mg Lactation: +40 mg Adult over age 55 or smoker may need vitamin C supplements
MINERALS			
Calcium	Main function is to grow, support, and maintain bone and tooth structures Only 1% is free in serum, but that small amount is critical in nerve transmission, muscle contraction, and blood clotting	Calcium is present in many foods, but not in large enough quantities to make the "average" diet adequate in calcium; many people require calcium supplementation to meet daily requirements of this mineral Best food source is dairy products; bony fish (salmon, sardines) also have calcium, as do some green leafy vegetables, some nuts (Brazil, almonds), molasses, soybeans, and tofu	Dietary requirements steadily increase through childhood, while bony matrix is being laid down, but even higher calcium intakes should be considered with advancing age—especially postmenopausal women at risk for osteoporosis Infant to 6 mo: 400 mg Infant 6-12 mo: 600 mg Child 1-10 yr: 800 mg Youth 11-24 yr: 1200 mg Adult 18+ yr: 800 mg Pregnancy and lactation: +400 Premenopausal female: 1000 mg Postmenopausal female: 1500 mg
Chromium	Chromium is insulin enhancing and may facilitate the binding of insulin to cell walls, it is therefore necessary for normal carbohydrate metabolism Adult-onset diabetics with normal chromium levels may require less exogenous insulin Pregnant women with (or at risk for) gestational diabetes should	Like most minerals, water and soil content plays a role in dietary sources; in areas where chromium is present in drinking water, up to 70% of the average daily intake comes from this source Other dietary sources include meats (beef, chicken, liver), shellfish (oysters), dairy products, eggs, fruits, and whole grains	No RDA has been established for chromium, but estimated "safe and adequate" intake is: Infant to 6 mo: 1-40 μg Infant 6-12 mo: 20-60 μg Child 1-3 yr: 20-80 μg Child 4-6 yr: 30-120 μg Child 7-10 yr: 50-200 μg Adult: 50-200 μg Pregnancy and lactation: not recommended
Copper	Copper enhances the body's ability to store and use iron as well as being a building block for various enzymes important in collagen formation, myelin sheath maintenance, and energy production	Copper is present mostly in plant products—the only nonplant products are shellfish (mussels, oysters) and bony fish (salmon) Plant sources particularly rich in copper include nuts (Brazil, cashew, hazel, peanuts, and walnuts), grains (barley, wheat germ, oats) natural sweeteners (honey, molasses), lentils, and mushrooms	No RDA established for copper; "safe and adequate" dietary allowances: Infant to 6 mo: 0.5-0.7 mg Infant 6-12 mo: 0.7-1 mg Child 1-3 yr: 1-1.5 mg Child 4-6 yr: 1.5-2 mg Child 7-10 yr; 2-2.5 mg Child 11+ yr: 2-3 mg Adult: 2-3 mg Pregnancy and lactation: not recommended
Cobalt	Cobalt works with B_{12}—enhancing and supporting its function, and without cobalt, B_{12} would be inactive; B_{12} functions include energy production, growth, nervous system functioning, and red blood cell production	Cobalt is present in both animal and plant sources: figs, shellfish (oysters, clams), milk, and buckwheat Other, weak sources include cabbage, spinach, beet greens, lettuce, and watercress; strict vegetarians can become cobalt deficient	No RDAs have been established for cobalt, but the average American diet contains about 5-8 μg of cobalt per day

TABLE 74-1 Summary of Important Information about Vitamins and Minerals—cont'd

Nutrient	Major Function	Sources	RDA
MINERALS—cont'd			
Fluoride	Fluoride works with calcium to make bone and tooth matrixes harder and more resistant to decay, and may help prevent osteoporosis	Fluoridated water is the most common source of dietary fluoride Fluoride occurs naturally in drinking water and soil in many parts of the country, but in other areas, fluoride is deliberately added to public drinking water Food sources generally rich in fluoride (depending on soil and water concentrations of fluoride) include fish, tea, milk, and eggs	No RDA established for fluoride; "safe and adequate" daily intake: Infant to 6 mo: 0.1-0.5 mg Infant 6-12 mo: 0.2-1 mg Child 1-3 yr: 0.5-1.5 mg Child 4-6 yr: 1-2.5 mg Child 7-10 yr: 1.5-2.5 mg Child 11+ yr: 1.5-4 mg Adult: 1.5-4 mg Pregnancy and lactation: controversial—talk with health care provider before supplementing
Iodine	Iodine functions as a building block of thyroid hormone and is therefore involved in cellular metabolism	Ocean water contains iodine (people living near the oceans grew crops and ate foods with naturally high iodine levels and rarely suffered iodine deficiency; the farther away from the ocean people moved, the more problems they experienced with iodine deficiency) The most available source of iodine to Americans is fortified table salt Other foods rich in iodine include seafoods of all kinds (salmon is particularly high in iodine), sea salt, sunflower seeds, and seaweed	Infant to 6 mo: 40 μg Infant 6-12 mo: 50 μg Child 1-3 yr: 70 μg Child 4-6 yr: 90 μg Child 7-10 yr: 120 μg Child 11+ yr: 150 μg Adult: 150 μg Pregnancy: +25 μg Lactation: +50 μg Both inadequate and excessive iodine during pregnancy and lactation can be harmful to developing fetuses and infants
Iron	Iron is an essential part of hemoglobin and is critical for oxygen transport	There are many sources of iron, both animal and plant; this abundance is vital, because humans have trouble absorbing iron—being able to utilize only about 10% of the iron available in the diet The best iron sources are animal—liver and other organ meats Other good sources include dried fruits, beans, dark-green leafy vegetables, shellfish, enriched bread, grains (wheat germ, whole grains), nuts and seeds (cashews, pistachios, walnuts, pumpkin), and natural sweeteners (molasses)	Infant to 6 mo: 10 mg Child 6 mo to 3 yr: 15 mg Child 4-10 yr: 10 mg Male 11-18 yr: 18 mg Male 19+ yr: 10 mg Female 11-50 yr: 18 mg Female 51+ yr: 10 mg Pregnancy and lactation: +30-60 mg
Magnesium	Magnesium plays multiple roles: (1) promoting absorption of other minerals, (2) removing excess amounts of other minerals, (3) assisting in nervous conduction, (4) enhancing protein metabolism, and (5) binding calcium to tooth enamel	Magnesium is important in photosynthesis, so vegetables high in chlorophyll are good sources Animal products contain very small amounts of magnesium (varies depending on the animal's diet), although fish contains relatively high levels Good sources include green leafy vegetables, seafood (many fish and shellfish), fruits and fruit juice, nuts and seeds (almonds, sunflower seeds), molasses, soybeans, and wheat germ	Infant to 6 mo: 50 mg Infant 6-12 mo: 70 mg Child 1-3 yr: 150 mg Child 4-6 yr: 200 mg Child 7-10 yr: 250 mg Male 11-14 yr: 350 mg Male 15-18 yr: 400 mg Male 18+ yr: 350 mg Female 11+ yr: 300 mg Pregnancy and lactation: +150 mg (should come from dietary sources, supplementation during pregnancy and lactation is not recommended)

Continued

TABLE 74-1 Summary of Important Information about Vitamins and Minerals—cont'd

Nutrient	Major Function	Sources	RDA
MINERALS—cont'd			
Manganese	Manganese is a "helper" nutrient—important in some biochemical reactions, but other minerals can perform these roles, so the presence of manganese is not critical The main functions include energy production, glucose management, assisting in vitamin utilization, and helping form proper bone and collagen	Manganese is available from both plan and animal sources Good sources include organ meats, muscle meats, leafy green vegetables (spinach, tea, lettuce), nuts and beans, and whole-grain cereals and breads	Tolerable upper limit in adults is 11 mg/day; neurologic adverse effects, similar to symptoms caused by Parkinson's disease, have been observed in individuals who have consumed high amounts of manganese, and iron absorption by the body may be inhibited Some glucosamine and chondroitin products have excessively high levels of managese Infants to 6 mo: 0.5-0.7 mg Infants 6-12 mo: 0.7-1 mg Children 1-3 yr: 1-1.5 mg Children 4-6 yr: 1.5-2 mg Children 7-10 yr: 2-3 mg Children 11+ yr: 2.5-5 mg Adults: 2.5-5 mg Pregnancy and lactation: supplementation not recommended
Molybdenum	Plays two major roles: (1) assists in maintaining body iron reserves, (2) helps to utilize fat stores for energy Minor role: is an ingredient in tooth enamel—deficiency has been implicated in dental decay	Like other minerals, concentrations in plant and animal foods depend on soil and water concentrations of this mineral; water alone (if rich in molybdenum) can provide more than 40% of the RDA Good sources include dark-green leafy vegetables, organ meats, beans, and grains	No RDA established for molybdenum; estimated "safe and adequate" daily intake: Infant to 6 mo: 30-60 μg Infant 6-12 mo: 40-80 μg Child 1-3 yr: 50-100 μg Child 4-6 yr: 60-150 μg Child 7-10 yr: 100-300 μg Child 11+ yr: 150-500 μg Adult: 150-500 μg Pregnancy and lactation: no recommendations
Phosphorus	Phosphorus plays a major role in bone and tooth structure—it is also present in every cell in the body (appearing as a part of cellular DNA) and is fundamental to body tissue growth, maintenance, and repair	Because it is an essential part of cellular structure, meat is an excellent source of phosphorus Good sources: all types of meat, seafood, milk and milk products, eggs Plant sources rich in phosphorus include nuts and seeds (almonds, peanuts, pumpkin, sunflower), legumes (beans, peas, and soybeans), and whole grains	Infant to 6 mo: 240 mg Infant 6-12 mo: 360 mg Child 1-10 yr: 800 mg Child 11-17 yr: 1200 mg Adult: 800 mg Pregnancy and lactation: +400 mg
Potassium	Almost 100% of the body's potassium stores are intracellular, creating a large concentration gradient across the cell membrane; this sets the stage for depolarization and nerve transmission Potassium also: • Helps maintain water balance • Governs acid/base balance • Helps with muscle contraction • Assists with protein and carbohydrate metabolism • Helps form glycogen and catabolize glucose	Potassium is found in a wide assortment of foods, both animal and plant Some of the best sources are plant: fruits (avocado, banana, citrus, raisins, dried peaches, tomatoes), vegetables (spinach, parsnips, potatoes), nuts (almonds, Brazil, cashews, peanuts, pecans, walnuts), dairy products, whole-grain cereals, legumes, and molasses Animal sources include lean meats and some seafood (sardines)	No RDA for potassium exists; dietary salt intake affects the body's levels of potassium inversely—increased sodium intake = decreased potassium Some experts suggest minimum daily requirements should be 2000-2500 mg; the "average" American diet provides between 2000-6000 mg daily, so potassium deficiency is not common unless disease states or medications interfere with body stores

TABLE 74-1 Summary of Important Information about Vitamins and Minerals—cont'd

Nutrient	Major Function	Sources	RDA
Selenium	Selenium works together with vitamin E; it is a very potent antioxidant and is found in high concentrations in the kidney, heart, spleen, and liver Both selenium and vitamin E must be present in the body—selenium cannot take over vitamin E's role, nor can vitamin E perform in selenium's place	Again, food concentrations of selenium vary depending on the soil and water selenium content Good sources include animal products: liver, kidney, meats, eggs, milk, and seafood Plant products vary more widely, depending on the soil: vegetables (broccoli, cabbage, celery, cucumbers, garlic, mushrooms, onions), whole grains (bran, wheat germ)	The upper intake level is 400 μg/day; side effects from higher doses could induce selenosis, a toxic reaction marked by hair loss and nail sloughing Daily intake: Infant to 6 mo: 10-40 μg Infant 6-12 mo: 20-60 μg Child 1-3 yr: 20-80 μg Child 4-6 yr: 30-120 μg Child 7+: 50-200 μg Adult (women and men): 55 μg Pregnancy and lactation: no supplement advised
Sodium	Like potassium, sodium's major functions are nervous system conduction and acid/base regulation Sodium is the major extracellular ion, creating another large concentration gradient for the nerve cell, promoting nervous conduction Other functions include: • Carbon dioxide transport • Assistance with muscle contraction • Amino acid transport • Prevention of excess water loss	Table salt is the major dietary source of sodium in American diets, but sodium is present in many foods—more in animal than in plant sources; many processed foods contain very high sodium content Good sources include meat (bacon, beef, ham), seafood (clams, sardines), and dairy products Other sources are grains, vegetables (green beans), and fruits (tomatoes)	Unlike other vitamins and minerals, sodium excess is more problematic for most people; staying below the RDA can be a challenge Infant to 6 mo: 0.11-0.35 g Infant 6-12 mo: 0.25-0.75 g Child 1-3 yr: 0.32-1 g Child 4-6 yr: 0.45-1.35 g Child 7-10 yr: 0.6-1.8 g Child 11-17 yr: 0.9-2.3 g Adult: 1.1-3.3 g Pregnant and lactating: no restriction advised
Sulfur	Sulfur has two primary functions: (1) building block of keratin (helps to maintain clear skin, healthy nails, and glossy hair), and (2) assists in bile production, which aids in the digestion of fats	Protein-containing foods are the best sources of sulfur, with eggs being richest in this mineral Other sources include meat, fish, milk, and a few plant sources (dried beans, cabbage, wheat germ)	No RDAs for sulfur exist; deficiency has not been reported
Zinc	Zinc is a very important mineral, even though it is present in only tiny amounts Zinc's two major functions: (1) plays an active role in over 20 different enzymatic reactions, and (2) assists in the stabilization of RNA in protein synthesis Zinc also affects: • Insulin activity • Wound healing • Immune system response • Bone structure • Normal oil gland function • Normal fetal growth and development • Preserves senses of taste and smell Zinc has been found to prevent capsid protein formation in several viruses, including rhinoviruses, the most common cause of colds; zinc lozenges may help reduce the duration of symptoms of the common cold Antioxidant/zinc combinations have been found to be the best treatment to slow the progression of age-related macular degeneration	Animal products contain the best sources of zinc; particularly good sources are meats, seafoods (oysters, herring), milk, and egg yolks Vegetarians can get adequate zinc intakes from whole grains (wheat bran, wheat germ), natural sweeteners (maple syrup, molasses), seeds (sesame and sunflower) and soybeans Most fruits and vegetables are poor sources of zinc	Infant to 6 mo: 3 mg Infant 6-12 mo: 5 mg Child 1-10 yr: 10 mg Child 11+ yr: 15 mg Adult: 15 mg Pregnant: +5 mg Lactating: +10 mg (breast milk contains a zinc-binding protein, improving absorption in the gut; infant formula is not as well absorbed

be consumed each day; and daily salt intake should be limited to less than 6 g. Twenty-five grams of dietary fiber should also be maintained, which is not only cardioprotective but also helps curb the tendency to eat more than is necessary by providing a feeling of fullness. The theory underlying the unified diet also suggests that total calories should be adjusted to achieve and maintain desirable weight. The simplest way to use the guidelines would be to have all people older than 2 years:

- Eat a variety of foods
- Choose most foods from plant sources
- Eat at least 5 servings of fruit and vegetables every day (increases fiber)
- Eat at least 6 servings of whole grain foods each day (increases fiber and provides vitamins and minerals)
- Minimize the consumption of high-fat foods, especially those from animals
- Limit the amount of simple sugars in the diet

There is also special concern for the diet of certain groups of people. Problems exist with the increasing prevalence of obesity in children and women; undernourishment among the elderly; osteoporosis, iron deficiency, and folic acid intake in women; and the special needs of various minority populations.

Eating a well-balanced diet, implementing an exercise program, replacing saturated fats with fish and nuts, and limiting salt and alcohol intake are other key components of a healthy lifestyle. Avoid extreme diets.

VITAMINS

Vitamins are organic materials, essential for human survival, that must be ingested on a regular basis because they are not synthesized by the body. Some are available in their active form, some are ingested as a "precursor" or "provitamin" that is then converted, and two vitamins, vitamin K and biotin, are not ingested at all but are synthesized by bacteria inside the intestinal tract.

Thirteen essential vitamins have been identified to date, and more information about essential nutrients is being discovered every year. Only tiny amounts of vitamins are required on a daily basis, but chronic deprivation of even one vitamin will cause disease, and death can occur. The inverse is also true; some vitamins ingested in large quantities will also result in illness and death. An "adequate" diet is one that includes an appropriate amount of each vitamin on a daily basis but does not include excessive amounts of any of them.

Vitamins primarily serve regulatory functions and assist in the production of energy. They are not used in the body for structural purposes and cannot be used as an energy source. There are two types of vitamins: fat soluble (will dissolve in oil) and water soluble (will dissolve in water). Both are essential but differ markedly in their absorption and potential for toxicity.

Fat-Soluble Vitamins

Fat-soluble vitamins include vitamins A, D, E, and K ("DEAK" for short) and are primarily found in a variety of plant and animal oils or fats. Because these vitamins are stored in our body fat, daily ingestion is not required, but adequate body levels must be maintained in the long term. When ingested, these vitamins are transported through the body by the bloodstream. To remain dissolved in the blood, unique carrier proteins are required for each vitamin. Some people with particular metabolic and genetic diseases are unable to synthesize carrier proteins and can have extreme vitamin deficiency states, despite adequate vitamin intake.

Fat-soluble vitamins have common properties—their ability to be stored, their mode of transport, and the severity of deficiency syndromes in young children—but each vitamin is unique in its function and the physiologic effects of deficiency and toxicities. Development of fat-soluble vitamin deficiencies can be gradual, and the symptoms subtle, but toxicities can present suddenly and be devastating in their effects. Overdosage is more of a problem with fat-soluble vitamins than with water-soluble vitamins because of their ability to be stored and accumulated.

Water-Soluble Vitamins

Water-soluble vitamins include all the B vitamins (B_1, B_2, B_3, B_6, B_{12}, folacin, biotin, and pantothenic acid) and vitamin C. With the exception of B_{12}, these vitamins are rapidly excreted from the body because the body has no way to store them. These vitamins must be ingested on a regular basis or deficiency symptoms will quickly appear. They are not particularly toxic, however, since high levels rarely develop. These products are readily available but are destroyed by heat. Because they are water soluble, the vitamins may leach out into water used for cooking and be discarded if the consumer is not aware of how to properly store and cook them. Overdosage may occur when large quantities are taken chronically and exceed the body's ability to excrete them.

MINERALS

Minerals are inorganic substances present in the body that work in combination with enzymes, hormones, and vitamins. The majority of human minerals are found in the skeleton and make up about 4% of total body weight. Calcium and phosphorus are by far the most predominant minerals in the body.

Minerals, like vitamins, are essential for body functions but are present in much smaller amounts. Both acute and chronic mineral deficiencies, as well as toxicities, can occur, because even though the daily intake may vary enormously, the average adult male will consistently excrete several grams of minerals every day.

Minerals are classified as major or trace. Major minerals must comprise at least 0.01% of body weight (calcium, phosphorus, magnesium, potassium, sodium, and chloride). Trace minerals fall below 0.01% but are still measurable and have metabolic impact (arsenic, chromium, cobalt, copper, fluoride, iodine, iron, manganese, molybdenum, nickel, selenium, silicon, tin, vanadium, and zinc), although the exact biologic significance of some of these trace minerals is still a mystery. The label applied to a particular mineral ("major" or "trace") does not imply significance; excess or deficiency of any of the minerals can be devastating.

Minerals are found in a variety of states as free ions or bound to many different substances (such as iron to hemoglobin or cobalt to vitamin B_{12}). This variety allows minerals to perform many different biologic roles within the body.

PATIENT VARIABLES

Daily requirements of vitamins and minerals vary from person to person and with age, sex, physiologic state (e.g., pregnancy), and physical activity. The development of a completely comprehensive list is impossible, so the Food and Nutrition Board of the National Academy of Sciences, National Research Council, developed a list of recommended dietary allowances (RDAs), first published in 1943. This list is not intended to be comprehensive but attempts to define what amounts of each vitamin and mineral would be appropriate to meet the needs of normal, healthy people. In fact, the RDAs are deliberately set higher than the requirements of an "average" person, to compensate for dietary deficiencies or to offer us a "safety zone."

A healthy individual conscientiously adhering to the RDA will be taking in adequate amounts of essential vitamins and minerals. However, adhering to the RDA may be either excessive or inadequate for a person in poor health or someone who has metabolic or genetic disorders.

Geriatrics

Elderly people may have very different nutritional needs depending on their state of health. Metabolic changes slowed digestive rate, increased fat-to-muscle ratio, and decreased liver and renal functions all have an impact on digestion, absorption, and excretion of vitamins and minerals. Medication use can also have a significant impact on absorption and utilization of nutrients.

Dietary deficiencies in the elderly can occur for many reasons: because they do not eat sufficient food, do not eat the correct foods, or do not eat an adequate variety of foods. There is a risk for vitamin B_{12} deficiency because of decreased acidity of the stomach. The signs of vitamin deficiency may be subtle but should always be considered; for example, thiamine deficiency (associated with alcohol abuse) can cause Wernicke's encephalopathy or organic amnestic syndrome, folic acid deficiency is associated with dementia, and vitamin B_{12} deficiency can result in psychologic changes and peripheral neuropathy.

The benefit of multivitamin/mineral supplementation is not known. The risk of advising routine supplementation to a geriatric population is probably not great, but the risks and benefits to individual patients should always be considered.

Pediatrics

Pediatric RDAs for the various vitamins and minerals vary widely age and body weight are significant factors, and careful attention should be paid to children's diets throughout the growing years. Nutrient deficiency states are always more quickly seen and very often more devastating in children than in adults. Some deficiencies can have lifelong effects as well; for example, vitamin D deficiency causes abnormalities in bone ossification, causing bones to become soft and bend a disease called rickets. Vitamin D therapy will stop further damage but will not correct many of the existing bone deformities.

As children grow, their need for supplementation changes. Breastfed infants get almost all the nutrients they need from their mother. The only supplement these babies may need are fluoride (which is present in only small amounts in breast milk) and an iron supplement after 4 to 6 months of age. Bottle-fed infants receiving infant formula are receiving the RDA through the formula. Consider the use of iron-fortified formula after age 4 months.

As they start to eat solid foods, however, many children develop strong food preferences, and maintaining a balanced diet can be a struggle for parents. Balance *over time* is the important point to remember. Not every meal needs to include every nutrient; ensuring a balance for the day is sufficient. Caution parents to avoid food conflicts by offering small portions of foods from many sources frequently. Vitamin supplementation is not necessary for a child who is willing to eat from many food groups but may be helpful in the child who eats only a small variety of foods.

Pregnancy

In general, almost all vitamin and mineral RDAs increase in pregnancy to support the increase in metabolic rate and the demands of a growing fetus. These nutritional needs can be met dietarily by most women, with the exception of iron. Iron requirements in pregnancy are nearly impossible to reach by diet alone. Folic acid supplementation is being recognized more and more as an essential pregnancy nutrient as well, and many physicians are advising both iron and folic acid supplements to all pregnant women. All women should begin supplementing with a daily multivitamin-mineral supplement. In 1992 the Institute of Medicine recommended that this supplement contain 30 mg iron, 15 mg zinc, 2 mg copper, 250 mg calcium, 2 mg vitamin B_6, 300 μg folic acid, 50 mg vitamin C, and 5 μg vitamin D.

One potential problem in pregnancy is vitamin and/or mineral toxicity. The nutrients that are particularly harmful to a developing fetus if provided in excess (10 times the RDA or more), include iron, zinc, selenium, and vitamins A, B_6, C, and D. Although some vitamins taken in excess just pass through the system and are excreted in the urine, other vitamins may be stored in tissues, and toxicity may develop. In other cases, the body seems to develop a dependency on higher doses of some vitamins, and the patient does not feel good if they are not consuming large quantities of vitamins.

Gender

Men's nutritional needs remain relatively stable from late adolescence into old age. With aging, illness, and injury, dietary needs need to be reassessed, and supplementation might be considered. Elderly men (>80 years) are at risk for osteoporosis. Adequate calcium intake is essential in elderly men as well as women.

Women's needs vary widely throughout their lifetime. Until adolescence, all children's needs are essentially the same, and a gradual increase in the RDAs is seen for most nutrients. During adolescence, however, women's dietary needs undergo striking changes.

With the onset of menses, dietary iron needs increase. Many women do not take in adequate amounts of dietary iron to compensate for monthly blood loss.

It is certainly possible for a woman's diet to provide sufficient iron, but because many women diet to keep their weight down and are taught poor food habits (or learn them in adolescence), most American women's diets are inadequate and iron supplementation should be considered.

Folic acid supplementation (400 μg) should be taken by all reproductive age women. A deficiency in this B vitamin has been shown to be related to an increase in neural tube defects in developing fetuses.

Appropriate calcium intake is a significant problem for American women. Chronic calcium deficiency often starts in young women and worsens with age. As adolescence begins, many women stop drinking milk. Many women become deficient in calcium just when they need it most for pregnancy, lactation, and menopause. Bone loss accelerates in the first 5 to 10 years after menopause and if not stopped can lead to devastating consequences. It is estimated that 25% of white women over age 70 and 50% over age 80 will show evidence of vertebral fractures. By the age of 90, 33% of all white women will have sustained a hip fracture, and many of these women will die as a direct result of complications related to the fracture. Calcium supplementation beginning by age 35 has been proposed by many physicians and should continue through menopause and added as an adjunct to hormone replacement therapy (HRT) when used. Even when the new bone-building medications are used (alendronate), calcium is a critical supplement. See Chapter 40.

Vitamin D is another critical bone-building nutrient of which many women are deficient when they need it most as they age. Vitamin D promotes calcium absorption, and one without the other is useless. Taking a calcium supplement without paying attention to vitamin D does not help bones. Many women become deficient in vitamin D because they stop drinking fortified milk and do not spend sufficient time outside to absorb ultraviolet (UV) radiation to make vitamin D. Many women, worried about the risks of skin cancer, cover all exposed skin if they do go outside, again, blocking vitamin D absorption.

HOW TO MONITOR

Blood studies to determine nutrient levels are generally not indicated. If a patient presents with a particular set of physical symptoms that seem to be related to nutrient deficiencies or toxicities, blood and hair studies may provide the answer. Vitamins are usually evaluated using serum markers. Minerals are also measured using serum markers but are more concentrated in hair, often 10 times or more than will be present in blood and urine, so hair analysis should be considered, especially if the clinician is worried about mineral toxicities. Some studies have shown that for many elements, hair more closely reflects body mineral stores, especially in toxic metal accumulation.

PATIENT EDUCATION

All patients should be counseled on their nutritional needs. Parents should be aware of growing children's needs and how they should be managing children's diets. Young teenagers should be told about the importance of balance in the diet. This is particularly important for youth engaged in vigorous sports, such as wrestling, when forced weight loss may be an issue. Older adolescents should be aware of typical "pitfalls": decreased calcium intake, increased alcohol consumption, fad and weight reduction diets. They should also be informed about the hazards of vitamin and mineral toxicities. Pregnant and lactating women, as well as young mothers, require frequent nutritional "updates" as they progress through the childbearing years. Older women need to be encouraged to supplement with calcium and vitamin D to prevent osteoporosis. Older people of both genders should receive periodic reminders about the importance of balance in the diet, and together with their care provider should consider appropriate nutritional supplementation when illness or injury occurs.

Controversy Over Antioxidants

The hypothesis that antioxidant vitamins might reduce the risk of many degenerative diseases is based on a large body of both basic and human epidemiologic research. One of the most consistent findings in dietary research is that those who consume higher amounts of fruits and vegetables have lower rates of heart disease and stroke, as well as cancer. Recent attention has focused on the antioxidant content of fruits and vegetables as a possible explanation for the apparent protective effects.

There is increasing evidence that free radical reactions are involved in the early stages, or sometimes later, in the development of human diseases, and it is therefore of particular interest to inquire whether vitamin E and other antioxidants that are found in the human diet may be capable of lowering the incidence of these diseases. Low levels of antioxidants, which increase free radical activity, are clearly associated with an increased risk of these diseases. Put simply, the proposition is that by improving human diets by increasing the quantity of antioxidants in them, it might be possible to reduce the incidence of a number of degenerative diseases.

Antioxidant vitamins, which include beta carotene (provitamin A), vitamin E, and vitamin C, are hypothesized to decrease cancer risk by preventing tissue damage by trapping organic free radicals and/or deactivating excited oxygen molecules, a byproduct of many metabolic functions. These micronutrients may be lowered by smoking and passive smoking.

A large number of descriptive, case-control, and cohort studies provide data suggesting that consumption of antioxidant vitamins is associated with reduced risks of cardiovascular disease, and a plausible mechanism has been developed to explain why antioxidants might reduce the risk of atherosclerosis. These data raise the question of a possible role of antioxidants, such as vitamins C and E and beta-carotene, in the primary prevention of cardiovascular disease but do not provide a definite answer. Results from several large-scale randomized trials of antioxidant supplement are now available; however, results are not entirely consistent. The results of the major trials do not prove or disprove the value of antioxidant vitamins, nor do they incriminate them as harmful. They do, however, raise the possibility that some of the benefits from observational epidemiology may have been overestimated and that there may be some adverse effects.

In a multitude of noncomparable studies, the observations are compatible with the following very general conclusions:

- Some dietary antioxidants may protect against cognitive impairment in older people.
- A high dietary intake or high blood concentration of antioxidant vitamins is associated with a reduced risk of cardiovascular diseases and cancer at several common sites.
- A low risk of pathologic conditions may be related to multiple nutrients consumed at nutritional doses and in combination.

- Optimal effects may be expected with a combination of nutrients at levels similar to those found in a healthy diet.
- In a number of studies where dietary and supplementary vitamin E were clearly differentiated, a reduced risk of certain cancers or cardiovascular disease from supplemental vitamin E but not from dietary vitamin E was demonstrated. This provides strong presumptive evidence that high intakes of vitamin E per se provide a health benefit.
- Only a few intervention studies with specific nutrients are available, and results are inconsistent.
- A single antioxidant beta carotene vitamin given at high doses in subjects with high risk of pathologic conditions (smokers, asbestos-exposed subjects) may not have substantial benefits and could even have negative consequences.
- There are inconclusive and insufficient epidemiologic and clinical trial data with regard to the role of vitamin C in cardiovascular protection.

To evaluate the cause-effect relationship of the antioxidant nutrients, prospective population-based studies of large, randomized, double-blind intervention have been started in several European countries, particularly France. The prime objective of these studies is evaluating the effectiveness of a combination of antioxidant minerals and vitamins at nutritional dosages on the morbidity and mortality caused by cancer and ischemic heart disease in a cohort of volunteers of both sexes.

Specific Drugs

FAT-SOLUBLE VITAMINS

Vitamin A (Retinol and Carotenes)

As indicated by its name, vitamin A was the first of the vitamins to be discovered. It was identified in the early 1900s and appears in two forms. Carotenes are converted in the body to vitamin A by the intestines, and although they require some effort by the body to activate, they are more readily absorbed because they are not fat soluble. Because retinol is fat soluble and stored in the liver, daily intake is not essential. Retinol is transported through the blood by retinol-binding protein.

Deficiency. In developing countries, vitamin A deficiency is second only to protein/calorie malnutrition, and in the United States, subclinical vitamin A deficiency syndromes are common in some populations. Vitamin A deficiency is the most common cause of blindness in children around the world. Vitamin A deficiency causes a decrease in visual acuity (especially night vision), and without vitamin As support, the corneal epithelium becomes dry, inflamed, and eventually keratinized, causing permanent scarring.

Epithelial tissue throughout the body is affected by a deficiency in vitamin A and is manifested by keratin deposits. Early in the syndrome, the deposition occurs around hair follicles, and hardened, pigmented "goose bumps" appear on the extremities. As the deficiency progresses, more of the body becomes involved, and skin peeling and scaling occur. Internal effects are also seen: GI tract disturbances, oral and vaginal dryness, and keratinization.

Research is ongoing regarding the relationship between vitamin A and cancer. Vitamin A supplementation has not been shown to be helpful in curing existing cancers, but normal amounts of vitamin A in the diet may help prevent the development of certain forms of cancer.

Toxicity. Vitamin A (especially retinol) taken in excess can be hazardous and even life threatening. Signs of vitamin A toxicity include epithelial lining problems involving the GI tract (nausea, vomiting, and pain, leading to weight loss and anorexia), mouth problems (cracking, drying, scaling, and bleeding lips and mouth corners), and scalp conditions (hair loss and itching). Other effects can include amenorrhea, spleen and liver enlargement, transient hydrocephalus, and bone problems (joint pain, stunting of growth). Effects on the developing fetus are known in animals, and congenital malformations have been clearly documented. In humans, doses in excess of 31,000 to 36,000 IU have been related to an increase in birth defects.

Recommended Daily Allowances. The RDA requirements are based on retinol "equivalents" (RE). (1 RE = 1 μg retinol or 6 μg beta-carotene. This is converted to international units of 1 RE = 5 IU.)

Vitamin D (Vitamin D_2, Ergocalciferol; D_3, Cholecalciferol)

Vitamin D acts as both a vitamin and a hormone. As a vitamin, it is present in food, and when ingested, it is immediately available for use. As a hormone, it is formed in one organ and has effects on another.

Vitamin D_3 is a steroid derivative. After irradiation by UV light, an inactive sterol converts to cholecalciferol. This is converted again in the liver, travels to the kidney, and is converted into the active vitamin D_3. D_3 travels to the bone and to the gut, where it exerts its effects, which are modified by positive and negative feedback loops.

Deficiency. Vitamin D deficiency was extremely common before the early 1900s and resulted in rickets (a childhood disease) and osteomalacia (the adult form of the disease). In both cases, the problem was inadequate bone ossification, causing soft, pliable bones. Clinical symptoms included bowed legs, knock knees, contracted pelvis, skull malformations, and dental eruption delay. Adults experienced problems with bone fractures and, if the deficiency became severe enough, tetany resulted. During the early 1900s, lack of sunlight as the cause for rickets was discovered. Some countries in the Arctic Circle today regularly expose children to UV lamps to promote vitamin D absorption. While many health care providers suggest limiting the exposure of the skin to the sun to prevent skin cancer, vitamin D supplementation may be necessary to provide adequate vitamin D. Some research suggests that women who take vitamin D supplements have a 31% lower risk of death from heart disease compared with women who do not take supplements, regardless of whether it was taken with calcium. In addition to its influence on bones, Vitamin D is involved in blood pressure regulation and acts as a tumor suppressant in some types of cancer. Some researchers urge higher doses for the entire population to prevent osteoporotic fractures.

Toxicity. Vitamin D is highly toxic in large doses, because it is stored in fat cells and is not readily eliminated. After a large dose, it can be found circulating for months. Toxicity is more likely to occur in young children, and the consequences are more serious for them as well. Excess vitamin D causes calcium to deposit in many body tissues, and symptoms include serious GI tract disturbances, permanent kidney damage, aortic stenosis, and mental retardation.

Vitamin E (Alpha-Tocopherol)

Some experts consider vitamin E to be the most important antioxidant because it protects cell membranes and prevents damage to enzymes associated with them. Natural sources of vitamin E include vegetable oils such as sunflower oil, grains, oats, nuts, and dairy products. The values of vitamin E supplements are controversial. There have been suggestions that vitamin E might be neuroprotective, with potential use in helping prevent Alzheimer's disease in selected patients. Vitamin E may also shut down a critical enzymatic pathway to make platelets less sticky, thereby helping prevent narrowing of the arteries.

Deficiency. Vitamin E deficiency is difficult to diagnose because it can be subtle, manifesting itself in many body systems or in only one. Vitamin E deficiency has been well documented in animals but has not been seen in healthy people eating a varied diet. Again, children are more vulnerable to this deficiency, and most present with hematologic symptoms such as severe anemia and hemorrhage.

Because vitamin E absorption is dependent on pancreatic secretions and bile, biliary obstruction or pancreatic insufficiency can result in vitamin E deficiency.

Toxicity. Vitamin E overdose is better tolerated than many of the other fat-soluble vitamins, and toxicity is rarely seen. In animals given very high doses, growth retardation, poor bone calcification, and anemia are seen. Because of these effects in animals, large doses of vitamin E are not recommended in humans.

Vitamin K (K_1, Phylloquinone; K_2, Menaquinone; Synthetic Vitamin K_3, Menadione)

Deficiency. Vitamin K deficiency is rare because vitamin K is so widely available from both dietary and internal sources. Deficiency can be a problem in newborn infants with sterile intestinal tracts, so synthetic vitamin K is given shortly after birth, helping to prevent hemorrhage during the first several days of life.

Several medications can interfere with vitamin K absorption and use. Coumarin, warfarin, heparin, and salicylates all decrease vitamin K effectiveness, usually by competing for biologically active receptor sites.

Toxicity. Toxicity has rarely been seen with vitamin K, despite its fat-soluble nature. Hemolytic anemia has been seen in newborns (especially in the premature infant) and causes an increase in the breakdown of red blood cells. Allergic reactions to vitamin K_3 have also been reported.

WATER-SOLUBLE VITAMINS

Vitamin B_1 (Thiamin)

Deficiency. Vitamin B_1 deficiency was a very common problem in the late nineteenth century, resulting in the disease beriberi. This disease is not commonly seen today except in special populations. Physical symptoms of thiamin deficiency include fatigue, GI problems, muscle weakness and atrophy, bradycardia, and heart enlargement. Multiple peripheral nervous system problems (numbness, tingling, loss of reflexes, etc.) can be present, and more subtle central nervous system changes appear as the disease progresses: memory loss, decreased attention span, irritability, confusion, and depression. Prolonged thiamin deficiency can result in permanent damage to the nervous system.

Alcohol abusers are particularly prone to this disease for several reasons. Their diet is often inadequate, alcohol decreases intestinal absorption of thiamin, and thiamin is required to metabolize alcohol.

Wernicke's encephalopathy, a thiamin-deficiency disease, is seen in both alcoholics and in people with pernicious vomiting. Symptoms can range from mild confusion to coma and death. If the patient survives, permanent damage to the cerebral cortex may result in psychosis. Many of the symptoms of Wernicke's encephalopathy can be reversed with thiamin therapy.

Toxicity. Vitamin B_1 toxicity is rare, and the side effects are mild because thiamin is water soluble and is excreted readily from the body. People ingesting megadoses of thiamin may become drowsy, but hazardous effects have not been reported. Anaphylaxis after multiple thiamin injections has been reported and should be considered when administering this vitamin in an injectable form.

Vitamin B_2 (Riboflavin)

Riboflavin was discovered in the early 1900s as researchers were looking for growth factors in food. Each food identified seemed to have one common characteristic it was yellow. Biochemists working at the same time kept running into a yellow enzyme that seemed to be strongly related to increases in metabolism. The yellow substance was riboflavin.

Deficiency. Vitamin B_2 deficiency does not appear to occur in isolation; it occurs along with multiple nutrient deficiencies. However, symptoms have been isolated resulting from inadequate B_2 intake. These symptoms include cheilosis (cracks at the corner of the mouth) and inflammation of oral mucosa accompanied by a purple-tinged glossitis, eye irritation, dermatitis (unusual in that the symptoms include both dryness and greasy scaling), mood changes, depression and/or hysteria, growth retardation and malformations.

Toxicity. No toxicity symptoms for riboflavin have been reported.

Vitamin B_3 (Niacin, Nicotinic Acid, Nicotinamide)

Deficiency. Niacin deficiency causes a destabilization in cells, causing damage and destruction to cells throughout the body, if not corrected. This disease is called pellagra. Symptoms are seen most clearly in the body systems where cells divide rapidly, such as the skin, GI tract, and nervous system. Initially, patients will complain of weakness, fatigue, anorexia, and indigestion. As the deficiency progresses, symptoms develop. The classic symptoms are dermatitis, diarrhea, and dementia the "three Ds." If uncorrected, the fourth D stands for "death."

Niacin deficiency rarely occurs by itself and is often seen in multiple-nutrient deficiency states. Treatment of pellagra with niacin supplementation alone is usually not sufficient or completely effective without consideration of other possible B-complex deficiencies.

Toxicity. Nicotinic acid overdose will cause skin irritation and flushing as well as GI irritation, possible liver damage, and multiple enzyme changes. All the symptoms are reversible if niacin doses are decreased. Nicotinamide does not seem to cause any toxicity symptoms.

Vitamin B_6 (Pyridoxine)

Deficiency. Because B_6 is involved in so many enzymatic reactions, deficiency presents in a wide array of symptoms. No particular disease is associated with pyridoxine deficiency, but symptoms similar to riboflavin and niacin deficiency are seen.

Toxicity. High doses of vitamin B_6 have not been shown to be particularly harmful, although some reports of nervous system effects (numbness, clumsiness of the hands) have been seen. A water-soluble vitamin, B_6, is rapidly excreted in the urine.

Vitamin B_{12} (Cobalamin)

Deficiency. Vitamin B_{12} deficiency can be caused either by inadequate B_{12} intake or by lack of "intrinsic factor" in the gut that helps absorb vitamin B_{12} from foods. Any disruption of GI architecture (by surgery or disease) will inhibit absorption, as does the development of antibodies to intrinsic factor or inheriting a disease affecting intrinsic factor formation or function.

The "classic" symptom of B_{12} deficiency is pernicious (or megaloblastic) anemia. Other deficiency problems include peripheral nervous system changes (numbness, tingling, ataxia), central nervous system changes (moodiness, confusion, agitation, delusions, hallucinations, and eventually psychosis), and GI problems (loss of appetite, nausea, vomiting).

This deficiency is often found in geriatric populations and is frequently related to a loss of intrinsic factor. The need for supplementation is increased by an increase in metabolic rate (hyperthyroidism), by GI tract diseases, and by pregnancy. Because B_{12} is found in animal fat, vegetarians become deficient unless they supplement their diets. If B_{12} deficiency is caused by lack of intrinsic factor, it must be replaced by injection.

Toxicity. Although B_{12} is stored in the liver in significant quantities, excretion of excess vitamin B_{12} is rapid, and toxicity symptoms are not seen. Synthetic B_{12} (with its cyanide component) can be toxic and should be administered judiciously.

Folacin (Folic Acid)

Deficiency. Folic acid deficiency is one of the most common deficiencies in humans, and the symptoms are very similar to B_{12} deficiency.

Always rule out a B_{12} deficiency before treating a patient for folate deficiency.

Megaloblastic anemia is a worrisome complication. This deficiency is one of the most frequently seen complications in pregnancy and often occurs in the third trimester. If megaloblastic anemia is present before conception, it can result in fetal neural tube defects. Inadequate folic acid intake will be evident in serum in as little as 1 month, and red blood cell and liver stores will be depleted in less than 3 months.

Deficiencies can result from inadequate intake, defective absorption, or abnormal metabolism.

Toxicity. Even though folic acid is water soluble, toxicity symptoms have occurred, the most concerning being permanent nerve damage. Folic acid concentrations are restricted in over-the-counter preparations to guard against inadvertent toxicity.

Biotin

Deficiency. Biotin deficiency is very uncommon but can be induced by consuming large quantities of raw egg white. Avidin, a compound in the white, binds with biotin and inhibits absorption. Symptoms include nonpruritic dermatitis, hypercholesterolemia, ECG changes, anemia, anorexia, nausea, fatigue, and muscle pain. Simply cooking the egg white destroys avidin.

Young infants can develop a biotin deficiency from poor absorption and develop similar symptoms. Treatment with biotin provides prompt resolution of symptoms.

Toxicity. Large doses of biotin have not produced any toxicity symptoms. The water-soluble nature of this nutrient makes it easily excreted when taken in excess.

Pantothenic Acid (B_5, Pantetheine)

This B vitamin can be produced synthetically and is available in an injectable form.

Deficiency. Deficiency of pantothenic acid has not been seen in humans because it is so readily available in food sources.

Toxicity. Megadoses may cause GI upset (diarrhea), but no other toxicities have been reported. Because it is water soluble, it is readily excreted when ingested in excessive amounts.

Vitamin C (Ascorbic Acid)

Vitamin C is a fragile vitamin, being readily destroyed by heat or exposure to air or to alkalis. It is the most common antioxidant found in the skin. It is also found in vegetables and citrus fruits. It is considered important in repairing damage caused by free radicals and preventing them from be coming cancerous or accelerating the aging process.

Deficiency. Vitamin C deficiency is called scurvy. Symptoms are related to a breakdown or lack of repair of collagenous tissue, causing muscle weakness, bleeding/swollen gums, tooth loss, rough skin, delayed wound healing, anemia, fatigue, and depression. This condition is not widespread in the United States, but is still seen in some populations and should be considered when a patient presents with these symptoms.

Children are at higher risk for permanent damage when vitamin C deficiency persists. Damage to the epiphyseal junctions, thinning of the jawbone (causing loose teeth, spongy gums, and resorption of dentine) are among the most disturbing problems seen in children.

Some diseases and illnesses affecting collagen should be treated with vitamin C to facilitate healing. These include infections, burns, trauma, surgery, congestive heart failure, renal and hepatic disease, GI tract problems (gastroenteritis, diarrhea), and malignancies.

Low levels of vitamin C in the blood seem to be correlated with a higher incidence of clinical gallbladder disease. Individuals with higher levels of vitamin C have significantly reduced risk of stroke.

Toxicity. Because vitamin C is water soluble, it is easily excreted, up to a point. Once this renal "saturation point" has been reached, mild toxicity symptoms have been seen. GI tract disturbances (diarrhea, nausea, vomiting, stomach cramps), facial flushing, headaches, dizziness, and faintness have all been seen.

MINERALS

Calcium

Calcium is the most abundant mineral in the human body and is found in the bone. Only 1% of the body's calcium supply is outside the bony skeleton, but this 1% is critical for nerve transmission, muscle contraction, and blood clotting, to name only a few other roles. Other minerals such as magnesium, sodium, phosphorus, strontium, carbonate, and citrate combine with calcium to form the complete bone matrix.

Deficiency. Calcium deficiency can occur at any time in life, although in the United States today it is usually a disease of aging. Recent studies suggest that the amount of calcium an individual consumes may have an impact on the development of such diseases as hypertension and colon cancer. Decreased calcium levels definitely contribute to development of osteoporosis. Yet the health benefits of taking calcium depend on each individual's ability to absorb it—which may vary greatly. Independent predictors of calcium absorption include dietary fat, fiber, alcohol intake, and serum concentrations of vitamin D. In particular, the amount of dietary fat consumed in relation to dietary fiber appears to have an important role in determining the differences in calcium absorption. Fat may increase calcium absorption by slowing its transit time through the intestines and allowing longer contact with the absorptive surface.

Calcium supplements have been demonstrated to help maintain bone density. However, bone loss associated with aging climbs to pretherapy levels if calcium supplementation is discontinued. The calcium supplement formulation calcium citrate is 2.5 times more bioavailable than calcium carbonate, challenging the misperception that all calcium supplements are equal.

If children have inadequate calcium intake, soft bones and weak teeth result. Adults deficient in calcium have condition termed osteoporosis. It has been seen in young adults who have certain diseases or are on certain medications (systemic steroids), but the most common osteoporosis sufferer is the postmenopausal woman and the elderly male. Bone density increases in childhood and young adulthood, peaking in the mid-20s. Very little new bone is laid down in the 30s and 40s, and with the onset of menopause and loss of estrogen from circulation, women's bone densities plummet for 5 to 10 years before assuming a more gradual downward slope. If the postmenopausal woman had inadequate calcium intake, excessive calcium use (with multiple pregnancies), or had a concomitant disease requiring systemic steroids during the bone-building years, bones could become dangerously fragile within the first few years after menopause.

Vitamin D is essential for calcium utilization. Even in the presence of adequate calcium intake, osteoporosis can result from vitamin D deficiency.

Calcium absorption is affected by need. If the body requirements are low, calcium absorption from the gut will drop. During periods of increased calcium requirements (growth, pregnancy, or lactation) absorption from the intestinal tract increases markedly. Excretion of calcium, both from the gut and the kidney, however, remains nearly constant, so a net negative calcium effect can be seen. A daily calcium intake of up to 700 mg may significantly reduce the risk of developing distal colon cancer; 600 mg calcium in women from food or supplements lowered the risk of stroke by one third, probably by reducing cholesterol and possibly inhibiting clot formation.

Calcium interacts with phosphorus in attempting to maintain a phosphorus/calcium ratio of 1 : 1 or 1 : 1.5. The average American diet, however, provides 2 parts phosphorus/1 part calcium daily, and the body compensates by excreting excess phosphorus. Unfortunately, calcium is always attached to the phosphorus, further decreasing body calcium levels. The body responds by pulling more calcium from storage, which demineralizes the bones further. High phosphorus foods include soda (regular and diet), processed foods, eggs, meat, and peanuts.

Toxicity. Normally, calcium toxicity does not occur despite very high oral intake of calcium. In the presence of other mineral imbalances, however, such as magnesium deficiency, soft-tissue calcification can occur. Some disease states cause hypercalcemia and renal stones, but these seem to be related to internal management of calcium sources and not to excess intake.

Chromium

Chromium is a trace mineral, with serum containing only 20 parts per billion.

Deficiency. Chromium deficiency causes diabetes-like symptoms that are reversible when chromium is provided either dietarily or in supplements.

Toxicity. Chromium toxicity can occur. Excess amounts can reverse the beneficial effects and actually cause a decrease in insulin activity.

Cobalt

Deficiency. This deficiency is identical to vitamin B_{12} deficiency.

Toxicity. If excessive amounts of cobalt are ingested, polycythemia will develop because of cobalt's stimulating effect on erythropoietin. This can lead to congestive heart failure in some people. Pericardial effusion, thyroid hyperplasia, and neurologic disorders have also been reported.

Copper

Copper is another trace mineral that is found in almost all body tissues, although it is concentrated in the brain and liver.

Deficiency. Clinical deficiency is rare but does occur in some disease states (kwashiorkor, chronic diarrhea), whereas subclinical deficiencies are much more common and usually result from inadequate intake. Symptoms include anemia, collagen disorders, and nervous system conduction problems.

Toxicity. Copper is toxic in large doses. Wilson's disease (genetically inherited) is a disease of excess tissue copper and inadequate serum copper. Irreversible liver, kidney, and brain damage will result in addition to nervous system damage and blindness unless copper levels are lowered. Mild copper toxicity by ingestion usually results in GI symptoms, headache, dizziness, weakness, and a copper taste in the mouth, whereas extreme toxicity can result in tachycardia, hypertension, jaundice, coma, and death.

Fluoride

Deficiency. Deficiency was common until water began to be fluoridated, but the only symptom appeared to be weak dental structures and a marked increase in cavities.

Toxicity. Fluoride toxicity can be significant but usually requires very high doses over prolonged periods of time to become evident. A one-time dose 2500 times the RDA can be fatal but is rarely seen.

Iodine

Iodine, a trace mineral, is found in most parts of the body, with 50% in muscles, 7% in bones, 20% in the thyroid gland, 10% in the skin, and 13% in endocrine glands.

Deficiency. Goiter is the classic symptom of iodine deficiency and can appear after several months of inadequate iodine intake. This is particularly seen in areas of the United States or the world where the diet is iodine deficient. The pituitary gland in the brain responds to a decrease in thyroid hormone and sends a signal to the thyroid gland, thyroid-stimulating hormone (TSH), to produce more. If no iodine is available to make thyroid hormone, the gland is unable to secrete adequate amounts. The pituitary gland signals the thyroid with ever-increasing amounts of TSH and over time, the thyroid grows larger, forming a goiter.

Iodine deficiency in pregnancy can be very dangerous to a forming fetus. A condition called cretinism can result with serious effects, including poorly formed bones, weak muscles, and severe mental retardation. The widespread use of iodized salt has substantially reduced the incidence of goiter.

Toxicity. Iodine toxicity is usually not a problem for someone with a normal thyroid gland.

Iron (in Hemoglobin, Transferrin, and Ferritin)

Iron is available as a "recycled" mineral or is taken in diet. Once taken in, iron is stored in the liver, spleen, and bone marrow close to the sources of hemoglobin production. During pregnancy or as a result of chronic blood loss (menstruation, slow GI bleed) iron stores can be depleted at a rate of 10 to 40 mg/day. Iron supplementation has been found to provide relief from patients with angiotensin-converting enzyme inhibitor–induced dry cough, according to some research.

Deficiency. Iron deficiency causes the most common form of anemia. Symptoms of anemia demonstrate the importance of oxygen to all living cells. Anemia causes dizziness, headache, drowsiness, fatigue, irritability, heart enlargement, and spoon-shaped nails.

Although anyone can be iron deficient, populations at highest risk for iron deficiency anemia include women of reproductive age, pregnant women, young children, elderly, low-income populations, and minorities.

Toxicity. The body has no effective way to get rid of excess iron. Because the physiologic system is designed to recycle this mineral, iron toxicity is potentially fatal. Populations at risk include young children poisoning themselves with either iron-fortified children's vitamins or their mother's iron-fortified vitamins (usually prescribed for pregnancy), people with genetic conditions that result in no excretion of iron, and alcoholics with chronic liver disease or pancreatitis (who have abnormally high iron absorption), and the elderly taking iron-fortified vitamins needlessly.

Magnesium

Considered a major mineral, magnesium still accounts for only 1.75 oz in a 130-pound person. Bones contain 60% of the body's magnesium, with 27% found in muscle, and serum containing only 3%. Only about 30% of dietary magnesium is absorbed, and that absorption is dependent on several intestinal factors, as well as the presence or absence of dietary fat and other compounds that bind magnesium. Magnesium is a common ingredient in laxatives and antacids. It may be given intravenously for suppression of ventricular ectopy, and in asthma or chronic lung disease when conventional treatment has failed. It may also have a role in the prevention and treatment of vascular headaches.

Deficiency. Because magnesium is so important in cellular metabolism (moving sodium and potassium across the membrane), magnesium deficiency is most visible in the cardiovascular, neuromuscular, and renal systems. Symptoms of mild magnesium deficiency include mental status changes (confusion, personality changes, lack of coordination), GI tract problems (nausea, anorexia, vomiting), and musculoskeletal problems (weakness, muscle tremor). As deficiency worsens, more symptoms appear, such as tetany, bizarre muscle movements, dermatologic problems (alopecia, skin lesions), and cardiovascular changes (myocardial necrosis and lesions of the small arteries).

Toxicity. Magnesium toxicity is rare because the kidneys are efficient at excreting excess amounts of the mineral. Toxicity may occur in geriatric patients with renal insufficiency who use large quantities of milk of magnesia. When toxicity is acute, the symptoms can be dramatic and require immediate treatment. Symptoms include severe nausea and vomiting, extreme muscle weakness, occasionally progressing to paralysis and difficulty breathing that may eventually lead to coma and death.

Manganese

Manganese is another mineral present in only trace amounts and concentrated in specific organs. It is found in measurable amounts only in the pituitary gland, liver, pancreas, kidney, intestinal mucosa, and bones. Very little manganese is stored in the body. Total manganese in the body is usually not more than 20 mg at any one time, and this mineral is excreted primarily through the bowel (via feces and bile). Very little manganese is renally cleared.

Deficiency. Deficiency has not been reported in humans, primarily because other minerals will take over the biochemical roles that manganese usually plays. This could theoretically cause other types of nutrient deficiencies, or more likely, make other deficiencies worse.

Toxicity. Manganese toxicity is possible because this mineral is not quickly excreted. Toxicity symptoms include iron deficiency anemia (manganese interferes with iron absorption), depression, insomnia, impotence, leg cramps, headaches, and speech impairments. In significant toxicity states, symptoms can resemble Parkinson's disease or viral encephalitis with flat facial expressions, muscle rigidity and spasms, and delusions or hallucinations.

Molybdenum

Another trace mineral, molybdenum is found primarily in the liver and kidney, with small amounts occurring in other body tissues (muscle, bone, brain, lung, and spleen).

Deficiency. Molybdenum deficiency is both rare and very mild. The effects of deficiency are seen in the blood (anemia) and in teeth (decay). No other physiologic symptoms are seen.

Toxicity. Toxicity is possible with molybdenum because, like most minerals, excretion is slow and body requirements are very low. Symptoms of excess molybdenum intake include gout symptoms (painful, swollen joints), growth retardation and weight loss (especially in children), and copper deficiencies (because molybdenum and copper compete for the same receptor sites in the intestine).

Phosphorus (Calcium Phosphate and Phosphoric Acid)

Phosphorus is a major mineral, second only to calcium in body requirements. Phosphorus and calcium are linked; that is, decreases in one mineral will cause a concomitant decrease in the other, as the kidney attempts to maintain a stable calcium/phosphorus ratio.

Deficiency. Phosphorus deficiency is not common because of the abundance of phosphorus in the American diet. Phosphorus intake is almost universally higher than calcium intake, making the calcium/phosphorus ratio difficult to maintain and possibly contributing to calcium deficiency syndromes and diseases (like osteoporosis).

Toxicity. Because the kidneys closely regulate phosphorus and calcium serum levels, phosphorus toxicity is uncommon, and direct symptoms are unlikely. The single largest problem with excess phosphorus intake is an imbalance in the calcium/phosphorus ratio.

Potassium

Potassium is a major mineral with very important biochemical roles to play. Almost all of the body stores of this mineral are intracellular, creating a large concentration gradient across cell membranes.

Deficiency. It is relatively easy to develop a potassium deficiency. Common causes include diuretic therapy, trauma (burns in particular), starvation (pay attention to young women with anorexia and bulimia), gastroenteritis (diarrhea, vomiting), and diabetic acidosis.

Symptoms of deficiency range from mild muscle weakness, impaired growth, bone fragility, and mental status changes, to severe paralysis, decreased heart rate, and death.

Toxicity. Potassium toxicity can also be deadly, with symptoms ranging from confusion, fatigue, and intestinal tract changes to irregular or rapid heart rate, dropping blood pressure, and paralysis of arms and legs. Convulsions, coma, and cardiac arrest often occur before death.

Toxicity can be caused by excess potassium supplement intake or by sudden increases in dietary potassium (as in switching to a salt substitute such as potassium chloride, and using it excessively). Other medical conditions can cause potassium excesses: acute or chronic renal failure, adrenal insufficiency, severe acidosis (respiratory or metabolic), or systemic infection.

Selenium

Selenium is a trace mineral that is closely related to sulfur in its behavior. It is found in higher concentrations in the kidney, heart, spleen, and liver but is present in all body tissue except fat. This mineral helps protect the body from cancers, including skin cancer caused by sun exposure. It also preserves tissue elasticity and slows down the hardening of tissues associated with oxidation. Dietary sources of the mineral include whole grain cereals, seafood, garlic, and eggs.

Deficiency. Selenium and vitamin E deficiencies often look very much alike, but selective selenium deficiencies have been seen, and the results can be devastating. In areas of the world that have poor selenium levels in soil, cardiomyopathy with resultant heart-related deaths have been seen along with an increased risk of cancer deaths.

Toxicity. Both the kidney and lung excrete selenium, but toxicities have occurred. People exposed to very high selenium levels who are working in industrial settings have a higher incidence of liver disease and cardiomyopathy. People exposed more gradually (from foods grown in selenium-rich soil) experience milder symptoms, such as dental decay, hair loss, fatigue, and occasionally paralysis.

Sodium

Sodium is one of the major minerals, composing 0.15% of body weight, and is found in every cell in the body. Unlike potassium, sodium is primarily concentrated in extracellular fluid, again creating a concentration gradient.

Deficiency. Sodium deficiency is rare, and when it occurs it is very strongly associated with abnormalities in water management. Both dehydration and excess water intake will cause a sodium imbalance. (Dehydration causes direct sodium loss, and water intoxication dilutes the normal serum sodium content.) Sodium deficiency is seen with diuretic use, starvation, GI tract problems (vomiting, diarrhea), profuse sweating, and excess water intake.

Symptoms of sodium deficiency include muscle weakness, mental status changes, acidosis, and tissue atrophy.

Toxicity. Sodium toxicity results in excess water retention. If too much water is retained, edema and adverse cardiovascular effects are seen: hypertension, dizziness, stupor, and possibly coma.

Sulfur

Sulfur is a major mineral in the body, composing almost 0.25% of total body weight.

Deficiency. Deficiency symptoms are unknown, although it is theoretically possible for deficiencies to develop.

Toxicity. Sulfur toxicity has not been reported, and ingestion of excess amounts has not been shown to be dangerous.

Zinc

Zinc is a trace mineral and is present in only tiny amounts (2 to 3 g total). Zinc supplements are frequently ordered to aid in wound healing.

Deficiency. Because of the many roles zinc plays in the body, deficiency can be devastating. Symptoms include skin and hair changes, growth retardation, anemia, poor wound healing, lethargy, and sterility.

Causes of zinc deficiency include poor dietary intake (especially protein/calorie malnutrition), acute or chronic infection (lots of zinc being used up), alcoholism and liver cirrhosis, renal disease, and malignancy. Populations at risk for zinc deficiency include children, pregnant women, hospitalized patients, low-income persons, elderly persons, athletes (increased loss through sweat), and strict vegetarians.

Zinc is critical in pregnancy for normal fetal growth and development. Inadequate zinc levels during pregnancy can cause congenital malformations (including changes in skeletal, brain, heart, GI tract, eye, and lung tissues) and growth retardation.

Toxicity. Zinc toxicity is rare, and high zinc doses are required to produce toxic symptoms. These symptoms can include GI tract problems (nausea and vomiting), mental status changes (drowsiness, sluggishness, light-headedness, and restlessness), and muscle coordination problems (difficulty writing or walking).

RESOURCES FOR PATIENTS AND PROVIDERS

Dr. Koop, www.drkoop.com.
Comprehensive health information.

New York Online Access to Health, www.noah-health.org.
Includes information in Spanish.

BIBLIOGRAPHY

Antoniades C et al: Effects of antioxidant vitamins C and E on endothelial function and thrombosis/fibrinolysis system in smokers, *Thromb Haemost* 89:990-005, 2003.

By the way, doctor: does selenium interfere with other vitamins? *Harv Health Lett* 28:8, 2003.

Cooper L et al: Vitamin D supplementation and bone mineral density in early postmenopausal women, *Am J Clin Nutr* 77:1324-1329, 2003.

Doyle W: Role of vitamins in healthy eating, *Community Nurse* 6:21-24, 2000.

Feskanich D et al: Dietary intakes of vitamins A, C, and E and risk of melanoma in two cohorts of women, *Br J Cancer* 88:1381-1387, 2003.

Gaziano JM: Antioxidants in cardiovascular disease: randomized trials, *Nutrition* 12:583, 1996.

Hennekens CH: Antioxidant vitamins and cancer, *Am J Med* 26:97, 1994.

Hercberg S et al: The potential role of antioxidant vitamins in preventing cardiovascular diseases and cancers, *Nutrition* 14:513, 1998.

Huggins K: *The nursing mother's companion,* ed 2, Boston, 1990, Harvard Common Press.

Kmietowicz Z. Food watchdog warns against high doses of vitamins and minerals, *BMJ* 326:1001, 2003.

MRC/BHF Heart Protection Study of antioxidant vitamin supplementation in 20,536 high-risk individuals: a randomised placebo-controlled trial, *Lancet* 360(9326):23-33, 2002.

Prestwood KM, Raisz LG: Prevention and treatment of osteoporosis, *Clin Cornerstone* 4:31-41, 2002.

Salonen RM, Nyyssonen K, Kaikkonen J, et al. Six-year effect of combined vitamin C and E supplementation on atherosclerotic progression: the Antioxidant Supplementation in Atherosclerosis Prevention (ASAP) Study, *Circulation* 107(7):947-953, 2003.

Satia J et al: Reliability and validity of self-report of vitamin and mineral supplement use in the Vitamins and Lifestyle Study, *Am J Epidemiol* 157:944-954, 2003.

Schmidt R et al: Plasma antioxidants and cognitive performance in middle-aged and older adults: results of the Austrian Stroke Prevention Study, *J Am Geriatr Soc* 46:1407, 1998.

Vazquez MC et al: The SUVIMAX (France) study: the role of antioxidants in the prevention of cancer and cardiovascular disorders, *Rev Esp Salud Publica* 72:173, 1998.

Yusef S, Dagenais G, Pogne J, et al. Vitamin E supplementation and cardiovascular events in high-risk patients. The Heart Outcomes Prevention Evaluation Study Investigators, *N Eng J Med* 342(3):154-160, 2000.

CHAPTER 75

Complementary and Alternative Medicine

Bonnie R. Bock

In 1993, Dr. David Eisenberg of the Harvard Medical School released a landmark study in *The New England Journal of Medicine,* showing that one third of Americans were using unconventional medicine such as aroma therapy, acupuncture, and therapeutic touch. More recent studies have found that 40% to 50% of Americans are using alternative therapies, and even more are taking herbs and supplements on their own. In 1997, approximately 42% of people in the United States reported using at least one form of alternative medicine in the previous year, and an estimated 70% of people had used at least one complementary or alternative modality over their lifetime (Dobs, 2002). Approximately 20% to 30% of general pediatric patients have used one or more alternative therapies, with a 50% to 70% use among adolescents (Kemper, 2001). The use of alternative therapies rose from 33% in 1990, to 47% in 1997, at a cost of $27 billion.

Based on these statistics, this chapter is included in *Pharmacology for the Primary Care Provider,* second edition, although the information is often excluded from standard pharmacology texts. Although a high level of scientific study and knowledge is not available, and the information in this chapter must of necessity be somewhat brief, it is clear that clinicians must have some exposure to the products because patients are taking them. In general, not enough is known about complementary products to either support or discredit their use. Although Europe has done a great deal of research on some of these products, definitive conclusions cannot be drawn regarding the use of most of them.

A 2002 study by the National Institutes of Health suggests complementary treatment, especially botanical, cannot be recommended without many qualifications by conventional providers because they have not been proven either safe or effective.

DEFINING COMPLEMENTARY AND ALTERNATIVE THERAPIES

Complementary, alternative, untraditional, unconventional, or *"eastern" medicine* are terms used interchangeably to describe diverse medical and health care practices that are considered outside the realm of conventional or allopathic medical therapies and have yet to be validated by scientific methods (Straus, 2002). The term *complementary* describes therapy that is used to supplement more traditional medical care, and the term *alternative* suggests that the therapy has taken the place of usual medical therapy. *Integrative medicine* is a term used to describe the appropriate use of conventional and alternative methods to facilitate the body's innate healing response. Integrative medicine shifts the orientation of medicine to one of healing rather than disease and uses an approach that engages the body, mind, spirit, and community. Complementary or alternative medicine (CAM) are the terms most frequently seen in the lay literature.

HEALTH CARE PROVIDERS AND COMPLEMENTARY AND ALTERNATIVE THERAPIES

Patient interest has far outpaced the resources of the traditional health care system, as providers discover that standard texts and reference books do not cover herbs, supplements, and homeopathic remedies. Patients often believe that they know more than their health care providers and that their providers are not listening to them or respecting their choices. Responsible providers, for their part, desire reliable information about the choices that their patients are making so that they can provide better advice and treatment.

It is crucial that health care providers have up-to-date, balanced, and scientifically founded reference material to assist them in understanding nonconventional therapy, to learn about strengths, weaknesses, clinical indications, proper dosages, toxicities, and interactions of different therapies. It is important for health care providers to be familiar with the many products that do not require prescriptions that are available to patients today. Many of these products contain ingredients that are useful in treating common ailments. If providers are familiar with these products and their ingredients, they can help patients choose the safest product for their ailment in the context of their present state of health or illness. It should be noted, however, that some of the active ingredients in these products may interact with prescribed medications or may even complicate existing medical conditions.

The first rule regarding patient-initiated and controlled therapy is to obtain a thorough medication history. Because many patient-initiated remedies are purchased over the counter, patients often neglect to tell their providers about them. More than 70% of patients who used complementary therapies did not tell their primary care providers of the use. Many Americans consider herbal or over-the-counter products to be safe because they are so readily available. That may not be so for all patients. General knowledge about patient-initiated products will enable providers to evaluate specific regimens their patients report taking and thus decrease the potential for negative outcomes from products that may be harmful (Micozzi, 1998).

Even providers who take a drug history from patients may focus on prescription drug use and fail to adequately document other product use. Questions regarding alternative treatments should be a routine part of the patient's medication history. Some specific questions to ask may include the following:

- Are you using any over-the-counter vitamins, herbs, or supplements?
- Why are you taking the product?
- What dosage are you taking?

- Is it helping?
- Have you experienced any side effects?
- Are you being treated by an alternative therapist—herbalist, acupuncturist, naturopathic practitioner, or chiropractor?

It is also important to have patients bring in any remedies they are using so that an accurate record may be obtained. Seeing products in their original containers will provide additional information that might be required to evaluate the safety of products with which the provider might not be familiar. This research may be important to prevent dangerous drug interactions or complications.

When obtaining a history about complementary health measures, health care providers should try to remain as nonjudgmental or neutral about alternate health care remedies as possible. This approach is essential in earning patients' trust so they will answer completely or honestly. Providers should understand that patients who use alternative therapies or complementary treatments do so for many reasons:

- They seek products that will maintain health, prevent disease, or provide treatment for existing health problems.
- They have tried conventional therapeutic options without success.
- Conventional therapies had undesirable side effects.
- No known therapy will relieve their problem.
- Other respected family or community members may have recommended the product.
- Conventional approaches have disregarded their religious or spiritual beliefs.
- Dissatisfaction with the fragmentation of care by multiple medical specialties.
- Media reports and advertising promote alternative and complementary therapies as being more "natural" and therefore safe.
- Using complementary and alternative modalities give the patient empowerment over their treatment.
- Many complementary/alternative modalities focus on emotional and spiritual well being.
- Complementary and alternative therapists generally provide three elements often not provided by conventional medicine: touch, talk, and time.

COMPLEMENTARY THERAPIES AND HERBAL MEDICINE

Complementary and alternative therapies, in general, have been somewhat mysterious, and the scientific basis for their therapeutic action is uncertain. Over the last several years, as research and interest has increased in this area, more universities and medical schools are incorporating the use and teaching of complementary/alternative modalities, and many are conducting research in this area. In 2000, 64% of medical schools were offering courses that address complementary and alternative therapies.

Because of widespread use of complementary therapies, there has been growing interest in scientifically studying the action of various products. In 1991, the Office of Alternative Medicine (OAM) was established within the National Institutes of Health (NIH), with an Alternative Medicine Advisory Council established in 1993. In November, 1995, the National Institutes of Health established the Office of Dietary Supplements to promote the scientific study of dietary supplements. In October 1998, congress mandated the establishment of the OAM to an NIH center—the National Center for Complementary and Alternative Medicine (NCCAM). In February 1999, a charter creating NCCAM was signed, making it the 25th independent component of the National Institutes of Health. In October 1999, NCCAM and the NIH Office of Dietary Supplements established the first Dietary Supplements Research Center with an emphasis on botanical medicine. Since its inception, NCCAM has funded multiple studies. Several Phase III clinical trials were conducted in 2002, including the following:

- A study of St. John's wort and depression*
- Shark cartilage as adjunctive therapy for lung cancer.
- Ginkgo biloba to prevent dementia.
- Acupuncture for osteoarthritis pain.
- Glucosamine/chondroitin to treat osteoarthritis.
- Vitamin E/selenium to treat prostate cancer.
- EDTA chelation therapy to treat coronary artery disease.
- Saw palmetto/*P. africanum* to prevent progression of benign prostatic hypertrophy

Funding appropriated by Congress for NCCAM rose from $50 million in 1999 to $113 million in 2003.

Common Complementary and Alternative Practices

NCCAM has classified complementary and alternative modalities into five domains: alternate medical systems, mind–body interventions, manipulative and body-based methods, energy therapies, and biologic-based therapies.

Alternate Medical Systems. Alternative medical systems are complete systems of theory and practice. Non-Western systems, such as traditional Chinese medicine and Ayurveda, are ancient systems that have been used for thousands of years, whereas systems developed in Western cultures such as naturopathic medicine, homeopathic, and osteopathic systems have evolved apart from conventional allopathic medical practices used in the United States.

Mind–Body Interventions. Mind–body modalities use various techniques that help to enhance the mind's capacity to affect body functions and symptoms. Examples include meditation, prayer, hypnosis, yoga, biofeedback, and creative therapies such as music therapy, art therapy, and dance. Modalities such as patient support groups and cognitive-behavioral therapy were once considered complementary/alternative medicine (CAM) modalities but are now considered mainstream techniques.

Manipulative and Body-Based Methods. Body-based and manipulative methods are based on the manipulation and/or movement of one or more parts of the body. Modalities such as chiropractic manipulate the spine while osteopathic treatments involve manipulation of the muscles and joints to treat illness. Massage, reflexology, and postural therapies are other modalities that use the hands to treat the patient.

*Study completed; findings revealed that both St. John's wort and prescription setraline were no better than placebo in treating major depression (Davidson et al, 2002).

Energy Therapies. Energy therapies involve the use of the following two types of energy fields:

1. Biofield therapies affect energy fields that purportedly surround and penetrate the human body. The existence of such fields has not yet been scientifically proven. Some forms of energy therapy, such as therapeutic touch, Reiki, and qi gong, manipulate biofields by applying pressure and/or manipulating the body by placing the hands in, or through, these fields.
2. Bioelectromagnetic-based therapies involve the unconventional use of electromagnetic fields, such as magnetic fields, pulsed fields, or alternating current or direct current fields.

Biologic-Based Therapies. Biologically based therapies use substances that are found in nature to treat various conditions or to maintain health. Examples include botanical or herbal therapy, dietary supplements, orthomolecular medicine, and the use of other "natural" therapies, which have yet to be scientifically proved (i.e., shark cartilage to treat lung cancer). Nonherbal biologicals are discussed in Table 75-1.

The five domains are not mutually exclusive. Modalities may overlap domains. For example, acupuncture and acupressure are considered modalities used in traditional Chinese medicine, but they may also be considered forms of energy therapy.

Also, naturopathic medicine uses biologic-based therapies, such as vitamins, herbs, and other natural remedies, to treat illness.

Botanical therapies are discussed in this chapter. For more information on vitamins and nutritional supplements, see Chapter 74.

Botanical Therapy

Use of herbal medicine (drugs from plant sources) has been part of most cultures since the beginning of time. In the United States, medicinal plants were the primary form of medication in nineteenth century medicine. Today, herbal supplements are often used or prescribed like pharmaceuticals for a particular symptom or complaint. Many complementary and alternative modalities incorporate the use of herbal remedies. Traditional Chinese medicine, Ayurveda, naturopathy, and homeopathy make use of botanical therapies. Aromatherapy, often used in massage therapy, uses essential oils extracted from the petals, leaves, bark, resins, rinds, roots, stalks, seeds, and stems of aromatic plants to promote health and well-being. It is also believed that these oils have medicinal properties that fight bacteria, viruses, bacterial toxins, and fungi. It is believed that the scents work by triggering the production of hormones that govern bodily functions.

Some questions have been raised about the government's lack of regulation of complementary medicine practices, particularly those involving herbal products. Legislatively, there are few regulations that oversee complementary therapies or herbal medicines. The Hatch-Richardson Bill of 1992 defines a dietary supplement as different from a food additive or a drug. Under this law, the manufacturer may make health claims without receiving approval from the government if there is adequate data to support the claim. In 1994, the Dietary Supplement Health and Education Act (DSHEA) defined a dietary supplement as a food and not a drug or related item. Vitamins, minerals, amino acids, herbs, and enzymes are all used as dietary supplements and thus can be marketed under this law. The FDA considers a food to be a drug only when it makes a medical claim for curing a certain disease. In only those cases must the product meet rigorous standards of safety and efficacy.

Although the FDA does not regulate herbal medicines, they took action on April 24, 1998, to protect consumers from misleading health claims by the booming herbal remedy industry.

TABLE 75-1 Natural Remedies (Not Herbs or Vitamins)

Name	Source	Uses	Safety and Efficacy/Dosage
Chondroitin	Cattle cartilage	Eases aches and pains, protects and rebuilds cartilage	Safe and effective; 400 mg
Coenzyme Q_{10}	Produced in body and formulated in soybean oil	CHF, cardiovascular disorders	Safe; 100 mg/day bid-tid Angina: 50 mg tid Isolated systolic hypertension: 60 mg bid
Creatine	Muscle tissue or synthetic	Improving exercise performance and increasing muscle mass	Possibly unsafe in high doses 20 g/day for 5 days followed by a maintenance dose of 2 g or more per day
Glucosamine	Crab shells	Eases aches and pains, protects and rebuilds cartilage	Safe and effective if shells are not from polluted water 500 mg qd
DHEA	Androgen hormone synthesized from wild yams	Alleviates cancer, heart disease, and autoimmune disease; antiaging remedy	Felt to be safe, but all side effects not known Toxic to liver in sufficient quantities Efficacy not proven
Melatonin	Hormone If from natural sources, it comes from the pineal glands of cattle	Cure for jet lag, helps the body's clock, sleep aid Antiaging	May inhibit sex drive in men 1-3 mg at HS

Data from McPherson ML: *Over-the-counter medications: syllabus,* 1997 National Nurse Practitioner Conference, Washington, DC, November, 1997, Nurse Practitioner Education Associates; Tyler VE: Herb/drug interactions, *Prevention,* 93-97, Sept 1998; and Natural Medicine Comprehensive Database website; available at http://www.naturaldatabase.com; accessed November 1, 2002.

The goal of the FDA was to clarify for manufacturers what types of claims can and cannot be made on dietary supplement labels so that consumers can make more informed and wise choices.

The FDA actions were a result of the agency's attempt to conform with the Dietary Supplement Health and Education Act passed by Congress in 1994, which distinguished health and disease claims from structure/function claims. The Act says that labels cannot make claims that a product cures a disease or has a special benefit or health effect without special FDA approval. The Act allows general statements about the product's function in the body. The new rules bar makers of vitamins and herbal remedies from claiming to cure, prevent, or alleviate cancer, acquired immunodeficiency syndrome, and other specific diseases. Companies will be limited to making general claims about the product's enhancing the immune system. However, critics claim that most disease treatments can be described in terms of their effects on a structure or function of the body, so it will be difficult to distinguish between allowable structure/function claims and prohibited disease claims.

Advantages and Disadvantages of Herbal Therapy for Primary Care Practice. Herbal preparations are generally thought to have three major advantages: lower cost, fewer side effects, and medicinal effects that tend to normalize physiologic function. When used effectively, the herb's mechanism of action will often correct the underlying cause of a disorder or symptom. A synthetic pharmaceutical is often developed to alleviate a symptom without addressing the underlying cause. Some research has suggested that the whole plant or crude extract of many plants is often much more effective than an isolated compound.

Herbal therapies have historical and cultural traditions that have created the impression that they are safe and natural. These impressions create a false sense of safety and efficacy for the consumer. Just because something is natural does not mean it is safe or effective. Herbal preparations are not regulated anywhere in the world. Chinese medicine has used herbal products for centuries as a standard part of medical practice. These products are just beginning to be scientifically evaluated. The German Commission E, a panel that reviews the safety and efficacy of herbs, has done the most in terms of scientific research into the safety and efficacy of herbs. Although some of these studies have been small and do not begin to meet the scientific standard demanded by the FDA for prescription drugs, the German Commission E Monographs have been considered the gold standard in the field of herbal medicine for many years. There is a growing consensus that if herbs are effective, they should be used under the supervision of a trained health care professional.

Safety, purity, and effectiveness are the major issues in evaluating herbal products. Important questions to consider are the following:

- How much of the relevant herb does this product actually contain?
- What part of the plant was used to make the extract?
- What other chemicals does it contain?
- What are the active ingredients?
- What reliable information exists that this herb is useful, and for what conditions?
- Are there potential herb–drug interactions?

Consumers are using herbal remedies in record numbers, believing that these products are drugs and will prevent disease, treat illness, and improve health. Most of the publications concerning herbal therapies are written to sell products. As expensive new prescription drugs enter the market, cheaper nonprescription products reported to perform the same function also appear. For example, herbal preparations that purportedly have the same actions as Viagra are being heavily marketed. Antiobesity products containing ephedra were sold as herbal alternatives to fenfluramine and dexfenfluramine until ephedra was linked to serious adverse effects, including death, and removed from the market. Recently, herbs used and natural products used to treat menopausal symptoms have increased in popularity significantly since the safety of hormone replacement therapy has been questioned. But black cohosh, one of these menopausal drugs, has been linked to liver toxicity.

In July 2002, the FDA advised consumers of the potential risk of severe liver injury from the use of dietary supplements containing kava (also know as kava kava or *Piper methysticum*). A high-profile death of a baseball player caused restrictions to be placed on drugs containing ephedra. Because of these dangers, the FDA took action to remove some products from the market and post information about high-risk products on their MedWatch homepage at www.fda.gov/medwatch/.

Herbs can be used medicinally in many forms. Many herbs can be consumed raw or in food as a garnish, spice or main ingredient; used in teas made either by infusion or decoction; as a tincture or extract in an alcohol or vinegar base; or for topical use in poultices and compresses. Herbal products are made by grinding up parts of the plant and converting the result into pills, capsules, or liquid. Almost any part of a plant may be used, from the stems to the bark, leaf, flower, root, or seeds.

One of the major criticisms of herbal products is that there is much variability in concentration or dosage because plants make different amounts of chemicals, depending upon the environmental conditions. The weight of a leaf may be the same but the amount of biologically active chemical varies according to the amount of sunlight, the nutrition in the soil, and the extent of dilution. Some herbalists recommend using only herbs that have been standardized. Standardization, unlike the raw, pulverized plant or simple extract, ensures a certain quantity of the plant as well as a certain quantity of one or more of the plant's phytochemicals, making them easier to use in randomized studies. This provides consistent, measurable levels of one or more active ingredients. Standardization of herbs is also more practical. In many cases, huge amounts of unrefined herbs would need to be consumed to get the equivalent beneficial effect of a standardized supplement. A consortium of industry groups led by the Council for Responsible Nutrition has developed voluntary guidelines that some companies are using. Patients need to look for products that have been standardized by the manufacturer through measuring the amount of the key ingredient.

There are no definitive standards or regulations by which to judge the quality of herbal supplements; however, several resources have been developed. In 2000, the United States

Pharmacopoeia (USP) created the Dietary Supplement Verification Program (DSVP) to help inform and safeguard the growing number of consumers who use dietary supplements. The program responds to the need to assure the public that dietary supplement products contain the ingredients stated on the product label. The USP is also developing the USP-NF Botanical Monographs.

The National Nutritional Foods Association (NNFA) also has established a Good Manufacturing Practices (GMPs) Certification Program for its members. This program requires third party inspections of the manufacturing facilities to determine whether NNFA standards are being met. Manufacturers meeting the NNFA's GMPs will be allowed to use a seal to be placed on all product labels, ensuring consumers of a quality product.

Another resource, Consumerlab.com, is a privately held company that independently tests vitamins, herbs, supplements, and nutritional products. Test results are published online (www.consumerlab.com), including a listing of products that have passed testing. These resources for health care professionals and consumers provide helpful information to guide in the selection of the numerous health, wellness, and nutrition products.

In 2003, the FDA took steps to help consumers get uncontaminated and better-labeled products. The agency proposed a rule, which would take effect in 2004 if approved, requiring good manufacturing practices and labels that list the amount and strength of ingredients. Many consumers believe that the rule does not go far enough because it does not require that the products be safe and effective, as is required with over-the-counter drugs.

DRUG–HERB INTERACTIONS

Herbs have been used as medicine for over 2000 years, and until the development of pharmaceuticals there was little knowledge or concern of drug interactions. However, today, with the predominant use of synthetic medications, there are many factors to consider. Interactions between natural products and drugs are based on the same pharmacokinetic and pharmacodynamic principles as drug–drug interactions. Certain herbs may oppose or heighten the effect of synthetic medications; others may mimic effects. Some may reduce the bioavailability or alter cofactors; others act in an additive or complementary manner. Some herbs may actually be beneficial, have no effect on other medications, or cause it to appear that a synthetic drug did not work by virtue that the herb itself is exacerbating the disease. For example, echinacea, an immunostimulant, if taken by a patient with lupus, may increase symptoms of lupus even if the patient is taking immunosuppressants. Table 75-2 lists commonly used herbs and potential drug interactions.

Despite the concern over drug–herb interactions, it is important to put these interactions in perspective and note that drug–herb interactions are generally less severe that drug–drug interactions. Canadian researchers, studying serious and fatal adverse drug reactions (ADRs) in hospitalized patients in the United States, found that even when drugs are properly prescribed and administered, large numbers of ADRs exist. In general, herbals are less toxic than pharmaceuticals, and drug–drug interactions are much more common and severe than drug–herb interactions.

Recent research suggests that few databases or texts on drug–herbal interactions are complete. This requires clinicians to rely on pharmacies with extensive resources to confirm or rule out drug interactions as the source of patient symptoms.

Beneficial Interactions

Many botanical therapies can be used in conjunction with pharmaceuticals to enhance healing by strengthening the body's immune system to protect against infection and disease. An example of an enhanced combination is a blend of herbals with prescription antibiotics. Echinacea, a very popular herbal supplement, can be used as an adjuvant therapy for relapsing infections of the respiratory and urinary tract. All species of echinacea have been found to increase macrophage activity as well as increase levels of tumor necrosis factor and interleukin-2, enhancing replication and phagocytosis of cytokine production by WBCs. Individual components of echinacea also have antibacterial, antiviral, and antimycotic activities. Cranberry, also used as a preventative or adjunct treatment for urinary tract infections, has been shown to be effective by preventing the adhesion of bacteria to the bladder wall.

Botanical remedies can also be used beneficially to protect from side effects of pharmaceuticals. Milk thistle has been shown to protect the liver after exposure to hepatotoxins such as acetaminophen, ethanol, and halothane and to restore liver function in hepatitis and cirrhosis. Silymarin, one of the medicinal compounds in the herb, has been shown to strengthen the outer surface of the liver and encourages an enzymatic action that leads to cellular regeneration, allowing the liver to detoxify the bloodstream more efficiently.

Adverse Interactions

Detrimental Effects. All medicines, natural or synthetic, have side effects or the potential to interact with other substances. As with pharmaceuticals, herbs may have both desirable and detrimental effects. Any substance that interferes with the absorption or excretion of a prescription medication can reduce bioavailability and have a deleterious effect on their intended action. Laxative and fiber-rich herbs (senna, aloe, marshmallow, slippery elm, psyllium) can decrease intestinal transit time and reduce drug absorption.

Herbs that are high in tannin precipitate alkaloids of medications such as atropine, ephedrine, codeine, and theophylline. Other herbs may have antagonistic activities with medications or may compromise a drug's essential metabolism, especially if metabolized in the liver. Natural products, like drugs, can affect CYP isozymes. The best-investigated metabolic interactions are those involving St. John's wort. Claimed be effective for the treatment of mild to moderate depression, St. John's wort appears to be a potent inducer of isozyme CYP 3A4. Table 75-3 lists herbs that are generally considered unsafe.

Additive Effects. Some herbs combined with pharmaceuticals that have similar or comparable actions may have an additive effect. Additive effects may be beneficial or detrimental. In some cases, dosage of the herb or medication can be adjusted

Text continued on p. 804

TABLE 75-2 Actions, Uses, and Drug Interactions of Commonly Used Herbs (Safety and Efficacy Not Confirmed)

Herb	Action	Common Clinical Uses	Drug Interactions
Astragalus *(Astragalus membranaceus; Astragalus mongholicus)*	Antioxidant	Common cold, upper respiratory infections; strengthen immune system; increase production of blood cells in chronic disease	Cyclophosphamide Immunosuppressants
Bilberry *(Vaccinium myrtillus)*	Increases the synthesis of glycosaminoglycans, decrease vascular permeability, reduce basement membrane thickness, and aid in the redistribution of microvascular blood flow and the formation of interstitial fluid; antiulcer, gastroprotective effects, antiinflammatory and antiedema, lowers blood glucose	Cataracts, glaucoma, macular degeneration, poor night vision, retinopathy Topically used for mild inflammation of the mouth, throat, and mucous membranes	Antidiabetes agents
Black cohosh *(Cimicifuga racemosa, Actaea racemosa, Actaea macrotys)*	Menopausal symptoms, PMS	Action unknown	None known
Celery seed *(Apium graveolens)*	Sedative, diuretic, antispasmodic, antiarthritic, antiplatelet	Arthritis and inflammation, gout, flatulence, arrhythmias, angina, hypertension	Anticoagulants, antiplatelet drugs, sedatives, drugs used in PUVA therapy: methoxsalen (8-methoxypsoralen, 8-MOP, Oxsoralen) and trioxsalen (Trisoralen)
Chasteberry *(Vitex agnus-castus)*	Antiandrogenergic, dopaminergic, indirect effects on various hormones	Menstrual irregularities, menopausal symptoms, PMS symptoms, mastalgia	Dopamine antagonists (antipsychotics, metoclopramide), oral contraceptives, hormone replacement therapy
Cranberry *(Vaccinium macrocarpon)*	Interferes with bacterial adherence to the urinary tract epithelial cells, antibacterial	Prevention and treatment of UTIs	Proton pump inhibitors—ansoprazole (Prevacid), omperazole (Prilosec), and rabeprazole (Aciphex)—might increase absorption of dietary vitamin B_{12}
Don quai *(Angelica sinensis)*	Vasodilator, antispasmodic, estrogenic effects	Menstrual problems, menopausal symptoms, hypertension, rheumatism, ulcers, anemia, constipation, allergies, skin depigmentation, psoriasis	Anticoagulants, antiplatelet drugs—warfarin (Coumadin)

Data from Natural Medicine Comprehensive Database web site; available at http://www.naturaldatabase.com; accessed November 1, 2002.

Continued

TABLE 75-2 Actions, Uses, and Drug Interactions of Commonly Used Herbs (Safety and Efficacy Not Confirmed)—cont'd

Herb	Action	Common Clinical Uses	Drug Interactions
Echinacea *(Echinacea angustifolia, Echinacea pallida, Echinacea purpurea)*	Antiviral, immune system stimulatory effects, antibacterial, antifungal, antiinflammatory, promotes tissue granulation, protects collagen from free radical damage	Common cold and upper respiratory infections, UTIs, vaginal candidiasis (yeast infections), genital herpes (HSV type 1 and 2) Topically: skin wounds, ulcers, eczema, psoriasis, UV radiation skin damage, herpes simplex, bee stings, hemorrhoids	Immunosuppressants Cautious use with drugs metabolized by CYP 450, 3A4: lovastatin (Mevacor), ketoconazole (Nizoral), itraconazole (Sporanox), fexofenadine (Allegra), triazolam (Halcion)
Evening primrose oil *(Oenothera biennis, other Oenothera species)*	Antiinflammatory, may lower elevated plasma lipids and inhibit platelet aggregation	PMS, mastalgia, endometriosis, menopausal symptoms, atopic eczema, psoriasis, acne, rheumatoid arthritis, osteoporosis, Raynaud syndrome, multiple sclerosis, Sjogren syndrome	Anesthetics, anticoagulants, antiplatelet drugs, phenothiazines
Fenugreek *(Trigonella foenum graecum)*	Hypoglycemic, improves plasma glucose and insulin response in noninsulin-dependent diabetes	Diabetes, decreased appetite Topical uses: poultice for local inflammation, myalgia, lymphadenitis, gout, wounds, leg ulcers, eczema Food: ingredient in spice blends	Anticoagulants, antiplatelet drugs, corticosteroids, hormone therapy, antidiabetes agents, insulin, MAOIs, warfarin (Coumadin)
Feverfew *(Tanacetum parthenium)*	Antiinflammatory effects	Migraine prophylaxis, arthritis, allergies, asthma, tinnitus	Anticoagulants, antiplatelet drugs, NSAIDs
Garlic *(Allium sativum)*	Antihyperlipidemic, antihypertensive, antifungal effects; antibacterial, anthelminthic, antiviral, antispasmodic, diaphoretic, expectorant, immunostimulant, antithrombotic effects	Hypertension, hyperlipidemia, atherosclerosis, prevention and treatment of bacterial and fungal infections Topically: garlic oil is used for tinea pedis, tinea corporis, tinea cruris, and onychomycosis Intravaginally: used alone or in combination with yogurt for vaginitis	Anticoagulants, antiplatelet drugs, antidiabetes drugs, insulin, cyclosporine (Neoral, Sandimmune), NNRTIs, oral contraceptives, saquinavir (Fortovase, Invirase) Use cautiously with drugs affected by CYP 450, 3A4: lovastatin (Mevacor), ketoconazole (Nizoral), itraconazole (Sporanox), fexofenadine (Allegra), triazolam (Halcion)
German chamomile *(Matricaria recutita)*	Antiallergic, antiflatulent, antispasmodic, mild sedative, antiinflammatory, antiseptic	Restlessness and insomnia, GI disorders, menstrual cramps Topically: hemorrhoids; mastitis; leg ulcers; bacterial skin diseases, including those of the mouth and gums; treating or preventing chemotherapy- or radiation-induced oral mucositis	Anticoagulants, antiplatelet drugs, benzodiazepines, sedatives

Ginger *(Zingiber officinale)*	Antiemetic, antiinflammatory, analgesic, antitussive, cardiac inotropic, sedative, antibiotic, weak antifungal, antipyretic	Motion sickness, morning sickness, colic, dyspepsia, flatulence, chemotherapy-induced nausea, rheumatoid arthritis, osteoarthritis, loss of appetite, postoperative nausea and vomiting, migraine headache, upper respiratory tract infections, cough, bronchitis	Acid-inhibiting drugs, anticoagulants, antiplatelet drugs, barbiturates, antihypertensives, vasopressors, antidiabetes drugs
Gingko *(Ginkgo biloba)*	Antioxidant, antiinflammatory, improves circulation by both decreasing blood viscosity and affecting vascular smooth muscle, increase cerebral and peripheral blood flow microcirculation	Dementia, Alzheimer's disease, cerebral vascular insufficiency, including memory loss, headache, tinnitus, vertigo, dizziness, difficulty concentrating, mood disturbances, hearing disorders, sexual dysfunction caused by SSRI antidepressants, PMS, improvement of cognitive function, intermittent claudication	Anticoagulants, antiplatelet drugs, buspirone (Buspar), fluoxetine (Prozac), insulin, MAOIs, seizure medications, thiazide diuretics, trazodone (Desyrel), warfarin (Coumadin) Can affect CYP 450 enzymes, including 1A2, 2D6, and 3A4
Ginseng, American *(Panax quinquefolius)*	Antihypertensive, antihemolytic, antipyretic, antipsychotic, CNS depressant, ulcer protective activity, increases GI motility, decreases islet insulin concentrations	Stress reduction, stimulant diuresis, digestive aid, anemia, diabetes, insomnia, neurasthenia, gastritis, impotence, fever, hangover symptoms, stimulating immune function, ADHD, and for eradicating *Pseudomonas* infection in cystic fibrosis	Antidiabetic agents, antipsychotics, hormones, MAOIs, stimulants, warfarin (Coumadin)
Ginseng, Panax *(Panax ginseng)*	Interferes with platelet aggregation and coagulation, analgesic, antiinflammatory, potential antiasthmatic, works against stress by affecting the hypothalamic-pituitary-adrenal (HPA) axis, affects immune function, may have anticancer effects	General tonic for improving well-being, stimulating immune function, improving physical and athletic stamina, and improving cognitive function, concentration, memory, depression, anxiety, *Pseudomonas* infection in cystic fibrosis, irritated or inflamed tissues, diuretic	Anticoagulants, antiplatelet drugs, antidiabetes drugs, antipsychotic drugs, caffeine, furosemide, immunosuppressants, insulin, MAOIs, stimulants, warfarin (Coumadin) Can inhibit CYP 450 2D6 enzyme by approximately 6%

Continued

TABLE 75-2 Actions, Uses, and Drug Interactions of Commonly Used Herbs (Safety and Efficacy Not Confirmed)—cont'd

Herb	Action	Common Clinical Uses	Drug Interactions
Ginseng, Siberian *(Eleutherococcus senticosus)*	Antioxidant and possible anticancer effects, hypoglycemic, antiinflammatory, antiviral, sedative, diuretic, gonadotropic, estrogenic activity, protein-anabolic activity, and stimulate the pituitary-adrenocortical system (recent studies suggest it is not effective)	Herpes simplex virus, stress reduction, normalizing high or low blood pressure, atherosclerosis, pyelonephritis, craniocerebral trauma, rheumatic heart disease, neuroses, insomnia, and increasing work capacity, Alzheimer's disease, ADHD, chronic fatigue syndrome, diabetes, fibromyalgia, rheumatoid arthritis, influenza, chronic bronchitis, tuberculosis, improving athletic performance, reducing toxicity of chemotherapy	Alcohol, anticoagulants, antiplatelet drugs, antidiabetic agents, barbiturates, digoxin, kanamycin (Kantrex), sedatives May inhibit the CYP 450 1A2 and 3A4 enzymes
Goldenseal *(Hydrastis canadensis)*	Antibacterial, antifungal, antimycobacterial, antiprotozoal	Common cold and upper respiratory tract infections, nasal congestion, GI disorders, vaginitis, UTIs, to mask urine tests for illicit drugs Topically: used as a mouthwash for sore gums and mouth, skin rashes, ulcers, wound infections, itching, eczema, acne, dandruff, ringworm, herpes blisters, herpes labialis, eyewash for eye inflammation and conjunctivitis Otologically: tinnitus, earache, and catarrhal deafness	Acid-inhibiting drugs, antihypertensives, barbiturates, heparin, sedatives
Gotu kola *(Centella asiatica)*	Antiinflammatory, stimulates collagen synthesis, antiulcer, antibacterial, antiviral against herpes simplex type 2	Reducing fatigue, improving memory and intelligence, chronic venous insufficiency, varicose veins, wound healing Topically: used for skin conditions, including scabies, ulcers, psoriasis, and fungal infections, varicose veins, striae gravidarum, cellulitis, keloids and hypertrophic scarring	Cholesterol-reducing drugs, diabetes drugs, sedatives

Hawthorn *(Crataegus laevigata)*	Acts on the myocardium by increasing force of contraction, lengthening the refractory period, reducing peripheral vascular resistance, vasodilation, increased coronary blood flow, decrease uterine tone and motility, reduces lipid levels, antibacterials, spasmolytic, analgesic	Angina, arrhythmias, atherosclerosis, cardiovascular insufficiency, dyspnea, edema, hypertension, hyperlipidemia, ADHD Topically: used as a poultice for boils, sores, and ulcers	Cardiovascular drugs, CNS depressants, coronary vasodilators, digoxin
Horse chestnut *(Aesulus hippocastanum)*	Antithrombin, decreases the permeability of venous capillaries, constricts veins and reduces the capillary permeability	Varicose veins, hemorrhoids, and phlebitis	Anticoagulants, diabetes therapy, protein-binding drugs
Kava kava *(Piper methysticum)*	Anxiolytic, sedative, anticonvulsant, local anesthetic, spasmolytic, antiinflammatory, and analgesic activities	Anxiety disorders, stress, insomnia, and restlessness, depression	Alprazolam, CNS depressants, hepatotoxic drugs, levodopa (Larodopa, Dopar)
Lemon balm *(Melissa officinalis)*	Sedative, antiflatulent, spasmolytic, antibacterial, antiviral	Promoting digestion, mild tranquilizer, appetite stimulation, antispasmodic, Graves' disease, functional GI disorders with distention and gas Topically used for cold sores	Barbiturates, sedatives, thyroid hormone
Milk thistle *(Silybum marianum)*	Inhibits tumor necrosis factor (TNF), antioxidant, inhibits lipid peroxidation, antiinflammatory	Cirrhosis, hepatitis, liver damage caused by chemicals, medications, or poisonous mushrooms	Estrogen, glucuronidated drugs: lorazepam (Ativan), lamotrignine (Lamictal), entacapone (Comtan) May inhibit the CYP 450 2C9 and 3A4 enzymes
Passion flower *(Passiflora incarnata)*	Sedative, hypnotic, antispasmodic, analgesic	Insomnia, GI upset related to anxiety or nervousness, generalized anxiety disorder (GAD), symptoms of opiate withdrawal	Barbiturates, MAOIs, sedatives, tranquilizers
Sage *(Salvia officinalis, Salvia lavandulaefolia)*	Antiflatulent, antispasmodic, astringent, antibacterial, fungistatic, virustatic, antiperspirant, hypoglycemic	Anorexia, diaphoresis, dysmenorrhea, diarrhea, gastritis, galactorrhea, reduction of saliva secretion, GI disorders including flatulence, bloating, and dyspepsia Gargle for laryngitis, pharyngitis, stomatitis, gingivitis, glossitis, minor oral injuries, and inflammation of the nasal mucosa	Anticonvulsants, sedatives, hypoglycemic drugs

Continued

TABLE 75-2 Actions, Uses, and Drug Interactions of Commonly Used Herbs (Safety and Efficacy Not Confirmed)—cont'd

Herb	Action	Common Clinical Uses	Drug Interactions
Saw palmetto *(Serenoa repens)*	Antiandrogenic, antiproliferative, and antiinflammatory properties	Benign prostatic hyperplasia (BPH)	Anticoagulants, antiplatelet drugs, oral contraceptives, hormone therapy
St. John's wort *(Hypericum perforatum)*	Antidepressant, antiviral, antibiotic	Mild to moderate depression, dysthymia, anxiety, neuropathy, HIV/AIDS	5-HT1 agonists (triptans), amitriptyline (Elavil), antidepressants, barbiturates, carbamapine (Tegretol), cyclosporine (Neoral, Sandimmune), digoxin (Lanoxin), fenfluramine (Pondimin), irinotecan (Camptosar), MAOIs, narcotics, nefazodone (Serzone) NNRTIs, nortriptyline (Pamelor, Aventyl), oral contraceptives, paroxetine (Paxil), photosensitizing drugs, protease inhibitors (PIs), reserpine, sertraline (Zoloft), tacrolimus (Prograf, Protopic), theophylline, warfarin (Coumadin), drugs metabolized by CYP 450 3A4, 2C9, and 2D6 enzymes
Stinging nettle *(Urtica dioica, Urtica urens)*	Analgesic, antiinflammatory, local anesthetic, hemostatic, antibacterial, antiviral, hyperglycemic	Allergies, allergic rhinitis, osteoarthritis	Anticoagulants, antidiabetes agents, antihypertensives, CNS depressants
Valerian *(Valeriana edulis, Valeriana jatamansii)*	Sedative-hypnotic, anxiolytic, antidepressant, anticonvulsant, antispasmodic	Insomnia, restlessness, and sleeping disorders associated with anxiety, improving mood and concentration	Alcohol, barbiturates, benzodiazepines, sedatives
Yohimbe *(Pausinystalia yohimbe)*	Increases penile blood flow, increases central sympathetic excitatory impulses to the genital tissue May not be superior to placebo	Impotence, sexual dysfunction in mean and women, sexual dysfunction caused by SSRIs, as and adjunct to conventional antidepressants for refractory depression	

TABLE 75-3 Herbs Considered Unsafe

Common Name	Use for Which It Is Promoted	Safety/Efficacy/Dosage
Angelica, herb, seed	Diuretic, diaphoretic	Contain furocoumarins, which are photosensitizers and photocarcinogenic
Black cohosh	Menopausal symptoms, PMS	Liver failure
Blue cohosh	Labor induction, reduction of menopausal symptoms	Birth defects in animals, liver toxicity
Borage seed oil	Antidiarrheal, diuretic	Contains pyrrolizine alkaloids that are potentially carcinogenic and toxic to the liver
Broom (broom-tops, Irish broom)	Miscellaneous	Toxic
Calamus	Antipyretic, digestive aid	Contains a known carcinogen associated with kidney damage, tremors, and convulsions
Chaparral	Natural antioxidant, to purify blood, anticancer, acne	Sever liver damage, two cases known where liver transplants were required
Coltsfoot	Antitussive, demulcent	Contains carcinogenic alkaloids
Comfrey	Wound healing	Obstruction of blood flow from liver, has caused cirrhosis and death
Ephedra	Anorectic, bronchodilator	Ineffective as a anorectic, effective for bronchodilation, unsafe for those with HTN, diabetes, or thyroid disease, unsafe with caffeine, may cause serious toxic reactions when taken concurrently with MAOIs; taken off market recently
Germander	Anorectic	Hepatotoxicity
Jin bu huan	Stomachache, insomnia, antitussive	Hepatitis, respiratory depression with bradycardia
Kava kava	Antianxiety	Hepatotoxicity, liver failure
Licorice	Expectorant, antiulcer	Effective, but only safe in small doses for short periods of time; may cause sodium retention and potassium loss
Life root	Diabetes, hypertension	Liver toxicity and possible carcinogenicity and mutagenicity
Lobelia	Bronchodilator	High doses can decrease respiration, raise heart rate, and lower blood pressure
Mistletoe	Smooth muscle stimulant	Contains phoratoxins
Pennyroyal	Abortion agent	Severe hepatotoxicity, interference with clotting
Pokeweed	Emetic	Extremely toxic
Royal jelly	Insomnia, liver ailments	Serious-to-fatal allergic reactions
Rue	Menstrual disorders	Fresh rue can cause severe kidney and liver damage
Sassafras	General tonic	Contains carcinogen safrole
Stephania magnolia	Weight loss	Renal toxicity
Tansy ragwort	Cleansing and purification	Hepatotoxic
Yohimbe	Aphrodisiac, impotence	Toxic in excessive doses

Data modified from McPherson ML: *Over-the-counter medications: syllabus,* 1997 National Nurse Practitioner Conference, Washington, DC, November, 1997, Nurse Practitioner Education Associates; Tyler VE: Herb/drug interactions, *Prevention,* 93-97, Sept 1998; and Natural Medicine Comprehensive Database website; available at http://www.naturaldatabase.com; accessed November 1, 2002.

or reduced. In other cases, accentuated effects could result in overmedication and adverse effects. Many herbal weight-loss and "herbal speed" products rely on the pharmacodynamic interaction between ephedra and caffeine or caffeine-containing herbs, such as cola nut *(Cola acuminata)*, green tea *(Camellia sinesis)*, guarana, and maté *(Ilex paraguariensis)*. The two primary alkaloids contained in ephedra, ephedrine and pseudoephedrine, have additive cardiovascular effects with caffeine. At higher doses, the ephedra–caffeine interaction has been cited as a cause of death. Another example of additive effects includes botanicals such as ginkgo, garlic, ginseng, and ginger, which contain natural coumarins that can increase the effects of synthetic anticoagulants coumarin, wafarin, and even aspirin.

PATIENT VARIABLES

When considering the patient who uses herbal therapies, health care providers must also consider other factors that may be present that could affect the efficacy and safety of herbal use. There are no published studies on the effectiveness of herbal remedies in children. Like prescribed medications, herbal doses may need to be adjusted in the pediatric population based on weight or age. Until safety and efficacy in pediatric populations are studied, caution should be exercised when using any herbal therapy in children. Two pediatric studies currently being funded by NCCAM include "A Randomized Controlled Trial of the Use of Craniosacral Osteopathic Manipulative Treatment and of Botanical Treatment in Recurrent Otitis Media in Children" and "Treatment of Functional Abdominal Pain in Children: Evaluation of Relaxation/Guided Imagery and Chamomile Tea as Therapeutic Modalities."

Similarly, extensive studies in the geriatric population have not been done. Geriatric patients often have multiple medical problems and may be taking one or more prescribed medications that could interact with herbal therapies. Caution and careful assessment of both medical and medication history are necessary in this population.

Herbs, like most medications, are not recommended to be taken during pregnancy. Several herbs can increase the risk of miscarriage. Herbs that should be avoided during pregnancy include balsam pear, barberry root bark, cascara sagrada, chervil, Chinese angelica, feverfew, hernandia, hyptis, juniper berries, mayapple, mountain mint, mugwort, pennyroyal, pokeroot, rue, senna, southernwood, tansy, thuja, and wormwood. Ginger, which has been shown to be helpful with nausea in morning sickness, has not yet been proved safe for use in pregnancy.

SUMMARY

Complementary and alternative modalities, along with botanical therapy, are becoming increasing popular in what is becoming a more integrative health care system. As scientific research tries to keep up with consumer use and demand, it is important that health care providers become familiar with the most commonly used products and have access to information on more unconventional modalities and products. As the results from research studies become more conclusive, it will continue to be the responsibility of health care providers to communicate to patients about the safety, effectiveness, and dangers inherent in these widely available therapies.

RESOURCES FOR PATIENTS AND PROVIDERS

Books

Blumenthal M et al: *Herbal medicine, expanded Commission E monographs*, Newton, MA, 2000, Integrative Medicine Communications.

Duke JA: *Dr. Duke's essential herbs*, Emmaus, PA, 1999, Rodale.

Duke JA: *The green pharmacy*, Emmaus, PA, 1997, Rodale.

Jellin JM et al: *Pharmacist's letter/prescriber's letter natural medicines comprehensive database*, ed 4, Stockton, CA, 2002, Therapeutic Research Faculty.

Novey D: *Clinician's complete reference to complementary & alternative medicine*, St. Louis, 2000, Mosby.

Pizzorno J, Murray M, editors: *Textbook of natural medicine*, New York, 1999, Churchill Livingstone.

Tyler V: *The honest herbal: a sensible guide to the use of herbs and related remedies*, Binghamton, NY, 1993, Hawthorn Press.

Weil A: *Natural health, natural medicine*, New York, 1998, Houghton Mifflin.

Evidence-based resources

CAMLINE. Available at www.camline.org.

Cochrane Library. Available at www.cochranelibrary.com.

Cochrane Complementary Medicine Field Registry. Available at www.compmed.umm.edu.

CAM on PubMed. Available at www.nlm.nih.gov/nccam/camonpubmed.html.

HerbMed. Available at www.herbmed.org.

Databases

Dr. Duke's Phytochemical and Ethnobotanical Databases. Available at www.ars-grin.gov/duke/index.

Natural Medicines Comprehensive Database. Available at www.naturaldatabase.com.

Poisonous Plant Database. Available at http://vm.cfsan.fda.gov/~djw/readme.html.

Other Internet Resources

American Botanical Council. Available at www.herbalgram.org.

American Holistic Health Association. Available at www.ahha.org.

Ask Dr. Weil. Available at www.drweil.com.

Sensitive, well-balanced, research-based discussion of alternative health care.

Consumerlab.com. Available at www.consumerlab.com.

Independently tests vitamins, herbs, supplements, and nutritional products.

Food and Drug Administration. Available at www.fda.gov.

FDA MedWatch. Available at www.fda.gov/medwatch/.

Includes information about herbal products.

Healthnotes. Available at www.healthnotes.com.

Develops and distributes fully referenced, scientific, and balanced information on complementary and alternative medicine.

Health Gate. Available at www.healthgate.com/.

Offers access to information from more than 50 sources for patients. It offers consumers resources such as Healthy Living, The Wellness Center, and the Web version of Our Bodies, Ourselves. Also has extensive pharmacology provider information.

Herb Research Foundation. Available at www.herbs.org.

Offers access to reliable herb information by a nonprofit research and educational foundation. Has useful clinical and research-based information for the practitioner as well as offering the public information about popular herbal remedies.

National Center for Complementary and Alternative Medicine. Available at www.nccam.nih.gov/.

Information about current research on different complementary medicine treatments.

United States Pharmacopeia. Available at www.usp.org/.
Established standards for vitamins, minerals, and botanicals.

Dietary supplements information monographs and botanical monographs

University of Maryland Complementary Medicine Program. Available at www.compmed.ummc.umaryland.edu/ProfessionalResources.pdf.
An extensive list of CAM resources for health professionals and researchers.

WebMD/Medscape. Available at www.medscape.com.
Includes extensive content on alternative and complementary resources for patients. Requires registration.

Organizations

Center for Science in the Public Interest (CSPI). Available at www.cspinet.org.

Cochrane Collaboration Complementary Medicine Field. Available at www.compmed.umm.edu/Compmed/Cochrane/Cochrane.htm.

Cochrane Collaboration Consumer Network. Available at www.cochraneconsumer.com/.

The Alternative Medicine Foundation. Available at www.amfoundation.org.

Periodicals

Alternative Therapies in Health and Medicine, P.O. Box 627, Homes, PA 19043 (800) 345-8112.

Herbal Gram (quarterly publication of the American Botanical Council and the Herb Research Foundation), P.O. Box 201660, Austin, TX, (512) 331-8868.

The Integrative Medicine Consult. Seventeen annual newsletters on integrating complementary therapies into standard medical practice, (617) 720-6002. Available at www.onemedicine.com.

Natural Products Monthly Monographs from Facts and Comparisons, 111 West Port Plaza, Suite 300, St. Louis, MO 63146-9811.

REFERENCES

Astin JA: Why patients use complementary medicine: results of a national study, *JAMA* 279:1548-1553, 1998.

Barnes P, Powell-Griner E, McFann K, Nahin R: Complementary and alternative medicine use among adults: United States, 2002. In CDC Advance Data Report #343, Atlanta, 2004, Centers for Disease Control and Prevention.

Davidson RT et al. Hypericum Depression Trial Study Group. Effect of *Hypericum perforatum* (St. John's wort) in major depressive disorder: a randomized, controlled trial, *JAMA* 287:1807-1814, 2002.

Dobs A, Bimal A: Complementary and Alternative medicine, *WebMD Scientific American Medicine*, 2002. Available at www.medscape.com/viewarticle/439463.

Duke JA: *The green pharmacy*, Emmaus, PA, 1997, Rodale.

Duke JA: *Dr. Duke's essential herbs*, Emmaus, PA, 1999, Rodale.

Eisenberg DM et al: Unconventional medicine in the United States: prevalence, costs, and patterns of use, *N Engl J Med* 328:246-252, 1993.

Green JA: Integrating conventional medicine and alternative therapies, *Altern Ther Health Med* 2:77-81, 1996.

Jellin JM et al: *Pharmacist's letter/prescriber's letter natural medicines comprehensive database,* 4th ed, Stockton, CA, 2002, Therapeutic Research Faculty.

Kemper K: Complementary and alternative medicine for children: does it work? *West J Med* 174:272-276, 2001.

Lazarou J, Paomeranz BH, Corey PN: Incidence of adverse drug reactions in hospitalized patients. A meta-analysis of prospective studies, *JAMA* 279:1200-1205, 1998.

McDermott JH, Motyka TM: *Expert column: assessing the quality of botanical preparations. Medscape pharmacology, 2000.* Available at www.primarycare.medscape.com.

MacLennan AH, Wilson DH, Taylor AW: Prevalence and cost of complementary medicine in Australia, *Lancet* 347:569-573, 1996.

Micozzi MS: Complementary care: when is it appropriate? who will provide it? *Ann Intern Med* 129:65-66, 1998.

Miller LG: Herbal medicinals: selected clinical considerations focusing on known or potential drug-herbal interactions. *Arch Intern Med* 158:2200-2211, 1998.

Neher JO, Borkan JM: A clinical approach to complementary medicine, *Arch Fam Med* 3:859-861, 1994.

Oldendick R et al: Population-based survey of complementary and alternative medicine usage, patient satisfaction, and physician involvement, *South Med J* 93:375-381, 2000.

Pizzorno J, Murray M, editors: *Textbook of natural medicine,* New York, 1999, Churchill Livingstone.

Pennachio D: Drug-herb interactions: how vigilant should you be? *Patient Care Nurse Pract* October 2000. Available at www.patientcareonline.com.

Perkin MR, Pearcy RM, Fraser JS: A comparison of the attitudes shown by general practitioners, hospital doctors, and medical students towards complementary medicine, *J R Soc Med* 87:523-525, 1994.

Piscitelli SC et al: The effect of garlic supplements on the pharmacokinetics of saquinavir, *Clin Infect Dis*, electronic edition, December 3, 2001. Available at www.nih.gov.news/pr/dec2001/niaid-05.htm.

Scott GN, Elmer G: Update on natural product-drug interactions, *Am J Health Syst Pharm* 59:339-347, 2002. Available at www.medscape.com/viewarticle/429776.

Straus S: Exploring the Scientific Basis of Complementary and Alternative Medicine, *NIH Director's Wednesday Afternoon Lecture Series (Webcast)*, March 11, 2002. Available at http://nccam.nih.gov/news/lectures/past.htm.

Tyler V: *The honest herbal: a sensible guide to the use of herbs and related remedies,* Binghamton, NY, 1993, Hawthorn Press.

Bibliography

GENERAL BIBLIOGRAPHY

American Society of Health-System Pharmacists: *Medication teaching manual,* ed 8, Bethesda, Md, 2004, American Society of Health-System Pharmacists.
(301) 657-3000.

Aronoff GR, Berns JS, Brier ME, et al: *Drug prescribing in renal failure: dosing guidelines for adults,* ed 4, Philadelphia, 1999, American College of Physicians.

Atkinson A Jr, Daniels C, Dedrick R, et al: *Principles of clinical pharmacology,* London, 2001, Academic Press.

Ball J: *Mosby's handbook of patient teaching,* St Louis, 1998, Mosby.

Bennett PN, Brown MJ: *Clinical pharmacology,* ed 10, St Louis, 2004, Mosby.

Deck M: *Instant teaching tools for health care educators,* St Louis, 1995, Mosby.

Deck M: *More instant teaching tools for health care educators,* St Louis, 1998, Mosby.

DiPiro JT, et al: *Pharmacotherapy: a pathophysiologic approach,* ed 5, Norwalk, Conn, 2002, McGraw Hill/Appleton & Lange.

Dison N: *Simplified drugs and solutions for nurses,* ed 11, St Louis, 1997, Mosby.

Ferri FF: *Ferri's patient teaching guides,* St Louis, 1999, Mosby.

Greene HL II, Johnston WP, Lemcke D: *Decision making in medicine: an algorithmic approach,* ed 2, St Louis, 1999, Mosby.

Griffith HW, Griffith JA, Moore SW: *Griffith's instructions for patients,* ed 6, Philadelphia, 1998, WB Saunders.

Hardman J, Limbird I, editors: *Goodman & Gilman's: the pharmacological basis of therapeutics,* ed 10, New York, 2001, McGraw-Hill.

Janney C, Timpke J: *Calculation of drug dosages,* ed 6, Penn Valley, Va, 2000, TJ Designs.

Julien RM: *A primer of drug action: a concise, nontechnical guide to the actions, uses and side effects of psychoactive drugs,* ed 9, New York, 2001, Worth Publications.

Kastrup EK, et al, editors: *Drug facts and comparisons,* St Louis, 2004, Facts and Comparisons.

Katzung BG: *Basic and clinical pharmacology,* ed 8, Norwalk, Conn, 2000, Appleton & Lange.

McEvoy GK: *The American hospital formulary service,* Bethesda, Md, 1997, American Society of Hospital Pharmacists.

McCormack R, Ruedy J, Levine M, et al: *Drug therapy decision-making guide,* ed 2, Philadelphia, 2004, WB Saunders.

Mosby's patient teaching guides and *Mosby's patient teaching guides update I and update II,* St Louis, 1996, Mosby.
Available on disk or as a looseleaf notebook for photocopying for patients.

Mowrey D: *Scientific validation of herbal medication,* Norwalk, Conn, 1998, McGraw Hill.

National Health Information Clearing House, Office of Disease Prevention and Health Promotion, U.S. Department of Health and Human Services, PO Box 1133, Washington, DC, 20012-1133, (800) 336-4797.

Olson J: *Clinical pharmacology made ridiculously simple,* ed 2, New York, 2001, MedMaster.

Pharmaceutical Manufacturing Association, 1100 15th Street NW, Washington, DC 20005, (202) 835-3463.
Has guide booklet to 438 health education materials.

Physicians' Desk Reference, ed 53, Montvale, NJ, 2004, Thompson Healthcare.

Radcliff RK, Ogden SJ: *Calculation of drug dosages,* ed 7, St Louis, 2003, Mosby.

Rang HP et al: *Pharmacology,* ed 5, New York, 2003, Churchill Livingstone.

Rice J, Skelley EG: *Medications and mathematics for the nurse,* ed 9, Albany, NY, 2001, Delmar.

Ragland G: *Instant teaching treasures,* St Louis, 1997, Mosby.
Offers creative ideas and exercises for a more effective learning experience.

Rudd R, Moeykens B, Colton T: Health and literacy: a review of medical and public health literature, San Francisco, Calif, 2002, Jossey-Bass.
Annual review of adult learning and literacy.

Schmitt B: *Instructions for pediatric patients,* ed 2, Philadelphia, 1997, WB Saunders.
Also available in Spanish.

Shitzel RE, Craig CR, Stitzel RC: *Modern pharmacology with clinical applications,* ed 6, Lippincott/Williams & Wilkins, 2003, Philadelphia.

Sodeman P: *Instructions for geriatric patients,* Philadelphia, 1995, WB Saunders.

Teaching patients with acute conditions, Springhouse, Pa, 1992, Springhouse.

Teaching patients with chronic conditions, Springhouse, Pa, 1992, Springhouse.

Tierney LM, McPhee SJ, Papadakis MA: *Current medical diagnosis & treatment 2004,* ed 43, New York, 2004, McGraw-Hill/Appleton & Lange.

United States Pharmacopeial Convention: *USP DI Advice for the patient,* vol II, Rockville, Md, 2003, USP.
(800) 227-8772. Yearly, with monthly updates.

United States Pharmacopeial Convention: *USP DI Patient education leaflets,* Rockville, Md, 2003, USP.
(800) 227-8772. Yearly, with monthly updates or as USP leaflet diskette or a software product.

United States Pharmacopeia Dispensing Information: *Drug information for the health care provider,* vol 1; *Advice for the patient,* vol 2; ed 19, Rockville, Md, 1999, United States Pharmacopeial Convention.

Wells BG, DePiro JT, Schwinghammer T: *Pharmacology handbook,* ed 5, New York, 2002, McGraw Hill/Appleton & Lange.

RESOURCES

Important Government Websites

http://chid.nih.gov.
The Combined Health Information Database is a bibliographic database produced by health-related agencies of the Federal Government providing titles, abstracts, and availability information for health information and health education resources.

http://dietary-supplements.info.nih.gov.
The NIH Office of Dietary Supplements.

www.ahcpr.gov.
Agency for Health Care Research and Quality; clinical information on evidence based practice, outcomes and effectiveness, technology assessment, preventive services.

www.cdc.gov.
The Centers for Disease Control and Prevention; includes the MMWR (Morbidity and Mortality Weekly Report).

www.cms.hhs.gov.
Centers for Medicare and Medicaid Services; The CMS Quarterly Provider Update, source of National Medicare Provider Information.

www.fda.gov.
U.S. Food and Drug Administration Center for Food Safety and Applied Nutrition.

www.gpoaccess.gov/index.html.

The U.S. Government Printing Office disseminates official information from all three branches of the federal government.

www.guidelines.gov.

A public resource for evidence-based clinical practice guidelines, sponsored by the Agency for Healthcare Research and Quality, U.S. Department of Health and Human Services. (Note that the web page states the url is wwwlguideline.gov, but really is www.guidelines.gov).

www.health.gov.

A portal to the Web sites of a number of multi-agency health initiatives and activities of the U.S. Department of Heath and Human Services and other federal departments and agencies.

www.healthfinder.gov.

Web site for consumers a resource for finding government and nonprofit heath and human services information, with links to over 1700 sites.

www.medlineplus.gov.

NIH National Library of Medicine with many resources including searching MedlinePlus.

www.nal.usda.gov/fnic/index.html.

U.S. Department of Agriculture (USDA) Food and Nutrition Information Center.

www.nal.usda.gov/fnic/foodcomp/index.html

The USDA National Nutrient Database.

www.ncbi.nlm.nih.gov/PubMed.

Entrez is the text-based search and retrieval system used at NCBI (National Center for Biotechnology Information) for the major databases, including PubMed, Nucleotide and Protein Sequences, Protein Structures, Complete Genomes, Taxonomy, and others.

www.nccam.nih.gov.

National Center for Complementary and Alternative Medicine at the NIH with health information and clinical trials.

www.nci.nih.gov.

The National Cancer Institute at the NIH, with cancer information.

www.niddk.nih.gov.

The NIH National Institute of Diabetes and Digestive and Kidney Disease.

www.nih.gov.

The National Institutes of Health home page with health information and access to the institutes, centers and offices of the NIH.

www.partbnews.com.

Newsletter reporting on the changes in Medicare Part B coverage, coding, billing, and reimbursement rules for physician services.

www.surgeongeneral.gov.

Office of the Surgeon General has publications and information on health topics.

Major Health Organization Websites

www.aafp.org, American Association of Family Physicians.
www.acc.org, American College of Cardiology.
www.acg.gi.org, American College of Gastroenterology.
www.acponline.org, American College of Physicians.
www.alz.org, Alzheimer's and Related Disorders Association.
www.ama-assn.org, American Medical Association.
www.amhrt.org, American Heart Association.
www.arthritis.org, Arthritis Foundation.
www.cancer.org, American Cancer Society.
www.diabetes.org, American Diabetes Association.
www.kidney.org, National Kidney Foundation.
www.liverfoundation.org, American Liver Foundation.
www.lungusa.org, American Lung Association.
www.mayoclinic.com, Mayo Clinic general info for patients.
www.nof.org, National Osteoporosis Foundation.
www.obesity.org, American Obesity Association.

Index

A

Page numbers followed by *f* denote figures, *t* denote tables, and *b* denote boxes.

B

D

E

H

I

J

K

L

M

O

S

U

V